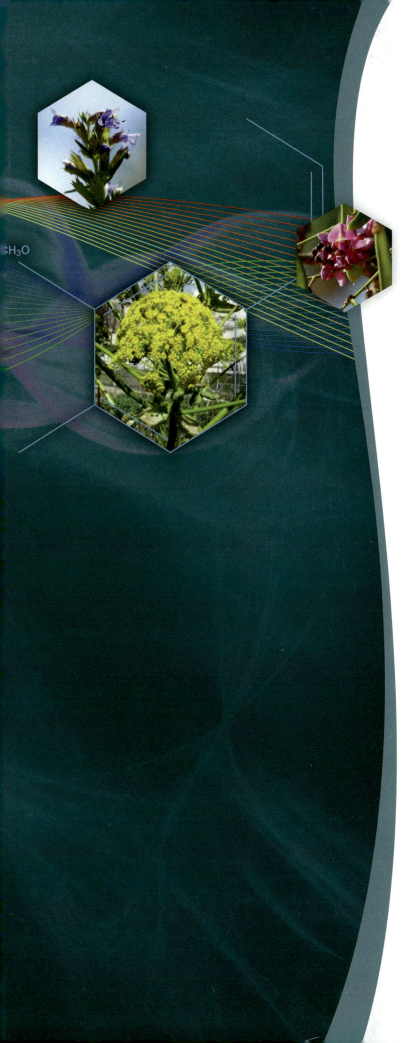

Section Guide

Section 1
Introduction

Section 2
Products

Section 3
Application

Section 4
Special Issues

Section 5
Personal Usage

Section 6
Appendix

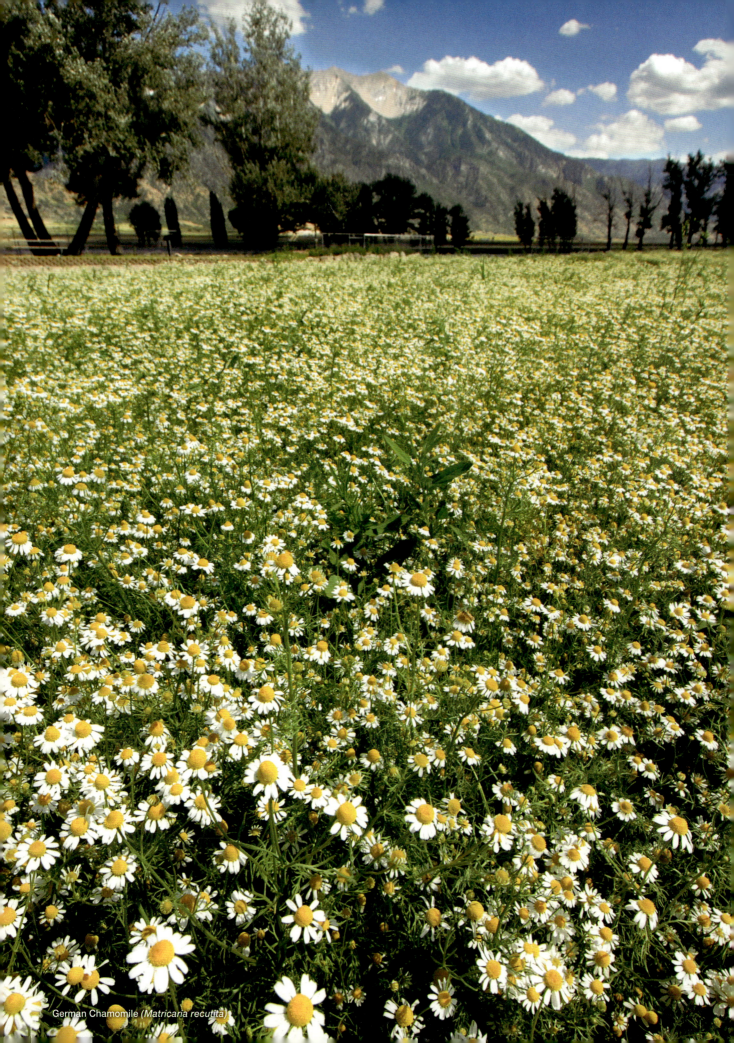

German Chamomile (*Matricaria recutita*)

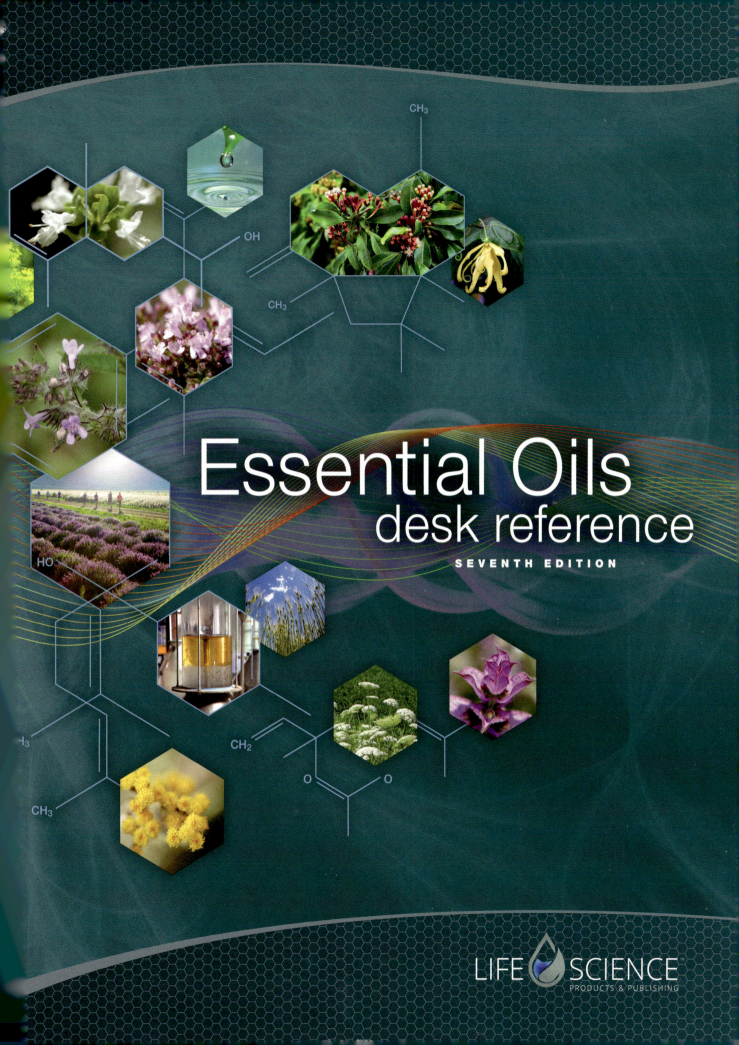

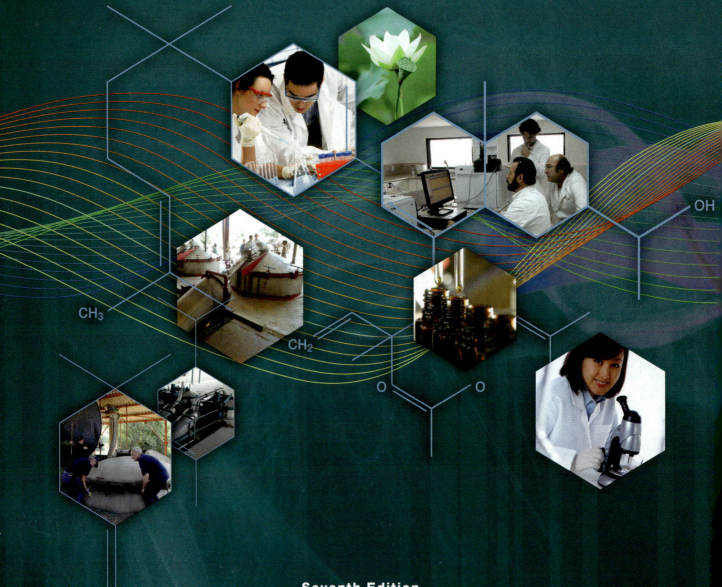

**Seventh Edition**

Copyright © November 2016 • Life Science Publishing
1-800-336-6308 • www.Discoverlsp.com

ISBN 978-0-9966364-9-0

Printed in the United States of America

Printed in the United States of America © Copyright 2016.
All rights reserved. No part of this reference guide may be reproduced or transmitted in any form or by any means, electronic or mechanical, including photocopying, recording, or by any information storage and retrieval system, without permission in writing from the publisher.

Life Science Publishing is the publisher of this reference guide and is not responsible for its content. The information contained herein is for educational purposes only and as a guideline for your personal use. It should not be used as a substitute for medical counseling with a health care professional. Neither the author nor publisher accepts responsibility for such use.

# Table of Contents

Preface . . . . . . . . . . . . . . . . . . . . . . . . . . . . . . . . . . . . . . . . . . . . . . . . . . . v
Acknowledgments . . . . . . . . . . . . . . . . . . . . . . . . . . . . . . . . . . . . . . . . . . vii

## Section 1
### Introduction

**CHAPTER 1 Yesterday's Wisdom, Tomorrow's Destiny** . . . . . . . . . **3**
Essential Oils—The Missing Link in Modern Medicine . . . . . . . . . . . . . . 3
Early History of Essential Oil Extraction . . . . . . . . . . . . . . . . . . . . . . 7
The Rediscovery . . . . . . . . . . . . . . . . . . . . . . . . . . . . . . . . . . . . . . . 9
Biblical References . . . . . . . . . . . . . . . . . . . . . . . . . . . . . . . . . . . . . 12

**CHAPTER 2 How Essential Oils Work** . . . . . . . . . . . . . . . . . . . . . **17**
Understanding Essential Oil Chemistry . . . . . . . . . . . . . . . . . . . . . . . 17
Different Essential Oil Species . . . . . . . . . . . . . . . . . . . . . . . . . . . . . 21
Standards and Testing . . . . . . . . . . . . . . . . . . . . . . . . . . . . . . . . . . 23
Powerful Influence of Aromas . . . . . . . . . . . . . . . . . . . . . . . . . . . . . 26

**CHAPTER 3 Scientific Research and Documentation** . . . . . . . . . . . **29**
Essential Oil Science . . . . . . . . . . . . . . . . . . . . . . . . . . . . . . . . . . . 29
Worldwide Research . . . . . . . . . . . . . . . . . . . . . . . . . . . . . . . . . . . . 31

**CHAPTER 4 Producing Therapeutic-Grade Essential Oils** . . . . . . **35**
Therapeutic-Grade Essential Oils . . . . . . . . . . . . . . . . . . . . . . . . . . . 35
Seed to Seal . . . . . . . . . . . . . . . . . . . . . . . . . . . . . . . . . . . . . . . . . 36
The Distillation Process . . . . . . . . . . . . . . . . . . . . . . . . . . . . . . . . . 42
Plant Parts Used to Distill Essential Oils . . . . . . . . . . . . . . . . . . . . . . 43

**CHAPTER 5 How to Safely Use Essential Oils** . . . . . . . . . . . . . . . **49**
Basic Guidelines for Safe Use . . . . . . . . . . . . . . . . . . . . . . . . . . . . . 49
Essential Oils Certified as GRAS . . . . . . . . . . . . . . . . . . . . . . . . . . . 50
Before You Start . . . . . . . . . . . . . . . . . . . . . . . . . . . . . . . . . . . . . . 52
Topical Application . . . . . . . . . . . . . . . . . . . . . . . . . . . . . . . . . . . . . 53
Diffusing . . . . . . . . . . . . . . . . . . . . . . . . . . . . . . . . . . . . . . . . . . . . 56
Other Uses . . . . . . . . . . . . . . . . . . . . . . . . . . . . . . . . . . . . . . . . . . 58

Seventh Edition | **Essential Oils Desk Reference** | i

**Essential Oils Desk Reference** | Seventh Edition

# Section 2
## Products

**Product Directory** . . . . . . . . . . . . . . . . . . . . . . . . . . . . . **60**

**CHAPTER 6** **Single Oils.** . . . . . . . . . . . . . . . . . . . . . . . . . **65**
Quality Assurance . . . . . . . . . . . . . . . . . . . . . . . . . . . . . 65
Single Essential Oil Application Codes . . . . . . . . . . . . . . . . 67
Single Oils . . . . . . . . . . . . . . . . . . . . . . . . . . . . . . . . . . 68

**CHAPTER 7** **Essential Oil Blends.** . . . . . . . . . . . . . . . . . . **143**
Formulating Essential Oil Blends . . . . . . . . . . . . . . . . . . . . 143
Essential Oil Blends . . . . . . . . . . . . . . . . . . . . . . . . . . . . 143
Essential Oil Blends Application Codes . . . . . . . . . . . . . . . . 144

**CHAPTER 8** **Nutritional Support** . . . . . . . . . . . . . . . . . . . **167**
Nutrition Today . . . . . . . . . . . . . . . . . . . . . . . . . . . . . . . 167
Enzyme Quick Reference Guide . . . . . . . . . . . . . . . . . . . . 168
Nutritional Supplements . . . . . . . . . . . . . . . . . . . . . . . . . 169

**CHAPTER 9** **Ningxia Wolfberry** . . . . . . . . . . . . . . . . . . . . **193**
Chinese Wolfberry Comes to the Modern World . . . . . . . . . . 193
Nutritional Products with Ningxia Wolfberries . . . . . . . . . . . 201
NingXia Red Recipes . . . . . . . . . . . . . . . . . . . . . . . . . . . 202
Personal Care Products with Ningxia Wolfberries . . . . . . . . . 204

**CHAPTER 10** **Hormones and Vibrant Health** . . . . . . . . . . . . **207**
Understanding Hormone Health . . . . . . . . . . . . . . . . . . . . 207
Dangers of Synthetic Hormones . . . . . . . . . . . . . . . . . . . . 211
Products for Hormone Support . . . . . . . . . . . . . . . . . . . . . 212

**CHAPTER 11** **Personal Care** . . . . . . . . . . . . . . . . . . . . . . **217**
Safe, Natural Products . . . . . . . . . . . . . . . . . . . . . . . . . . 217
Bath & Shower Gels . . . . . . . . . . . . . . . . . . . . . . . . . . . 217
Body Lotions . . . . . . . . . . . . . . . . . . . . . . . . . . . . . . . . 218
Deodorants . . . . . . . . . . . . . . . . . . . . . . . . . . . . . . . . . 219
Hair Care . . . . . . . . . . . . . . . . . . . . . . . . . . . . . . . . . . 221
Hand Purifier . . . . . . . . . . . . . . . . . . . . . . . . . . . . . . . . 222
Hormone Balancing . . . . . . . . . . . . . . . . . . . . . . . . . . . . 223
Lip Balms . . . . . . . . . . . . . . . . . . . . . . . . . . . . . . . . . . 224
Lip Gloss/Essential Oil Duos . . . . . . . . . . . . . . . . . . . . . . 224
Oral Health Care . . . . . . . . . . . . . . . . . . . . . . . . . . . . . . 226
Pain Relief . . . . . . . . . . . . . . . . . . . . . . . . . . . . . . . . . . 235
Shaving . . . . . . . . . . . . . . . . . . . . . . . . . . . . . . . . . . . 235
Skin Care . . . . . . . . . . . . . . . . . . . . . . . . . . . . . . . . . . 236
Soaps, All Natural . . . . . . . . . . . . . . . . . . . . . . . . . . . . . 241

**CHAPTER 12** **Healthy Choices for Children** . . . . . . . . . . . . **247**
KidScents Body Care for Children . . . . . . . . . . . . . . . . . . . 247
KidScents Nutritional Support for Children . . . . . . . . . . . . . 248
KidScents Oil Collection . . . . . . . . . . . . . . . . . . . . . . . . . 250

ii | Table of Contents

**Table of Contents**

## Section 2
*(continued)*

### CHAPTER 13 Fortifying Your Home with Essential Oils . . . . . . . 251
Protecting Your Home . . . . . . . . . . . . . . . . . . . . . . . . . . . . . . . . . . . . 251
Thieves Products. . . . . . . . . . . . . . . . . . . . . . . . . . . . . . . . . . . . . . . . 251
Personal Uses for Essential Oils . . . . . . . . . . . . . . . . . . . . . . . . . . . . 254

### CHAPTER 14 Animal Care . . . . . . . . . . . . . . . . . . . . . . . . . . . . . . . . . 257
Veterinary Medicine . . . . . . . . . . . . . . . . . . . . . . . . . . . . . . . . . . . . . 257
Techniques for Different Animal Species . . . . . . . . . . . . . . . . . . . . . 259
Animal Scents Products . . . . . . . . . . . . . . . . . . . . . . . . . . . . . . . . . . . 265
Animal Scents Essential Oil Blends. . . . . . . . . . . . . . . . . . . . . . . . . . . 266
Animal Treatment . . . . . . . . . . . . . . . . . . . . . . . . . . . . . . . . . . . . . . . 267
Specific Care for Horses. . . . . . . . . . . . . . . . . . . . . . . . . . . . . . . . . . . 269
Gary's Equine Essentials . . . . . . . . . . . . . . . . . . . . . . . . . . . . . . . . . . 270
Raindrop Technique for Horses . . . . . . . . . . . . . . . . . . . . . . . . . . . . . 273
Essential Oil Testimonials About Animals. . . . . . . . . . . . . . . . . . . . . . 275

## Section 3
**Application**

### CHAPTER 15 Techniques for Essential Oil Application . . . . . . . 281
The Use of Different Techniques. . . . . . . . . . . . . . . . . . . . . . . . . . . . . 281
Neuro Auricular Technique . . . . . . . . . . . . . . . . . . . . . . . . . . . . . . . . . 282
Lymphatic Pump . . . . . . . . . . . . . . . . . . . . . . . . . . . . . . . . . . . . . . . . . 284
Vita Flex Technique. . . . . . . . . . . . . . . . . . . . . . . . . . . . . . . . . . . . . . . 285
Raindrop Technique . . . . . . . . . . . . . . . . . . . . . . . . . . . . . . . . . . . . . . 290
  Preparation . . . . . . . . . . . . . . . . . . . . . . . . . . . . . . . . . . . . . . . . . . 295
  Overview of Application and Explanation of Terms . . . . . . . . . . . 296

## Section 4
**Special Issues**

### CHAPTER 16 Essential Oils: Spiritual, Mental, and Emotional . 307
Support with Essential Oils. . . . . . . . . . . . . . . . . . . . . . . . . . . . . . . . . 307
"Letting Go" with Essential Oils . . . . . . . . . . . . . . . . . . . . . . . . . . . . . 310
Oils for Specific Emotional Challenges. . . . . . . . . . . . . . . . . . . . . . . . 312

### CHAPTER 17 Cleansing and Diet . . . . . . . . . . . . . . . . . . . . . . . . . . 317
The Importance of Cleansing. . . . . . . . . . . . . . . . . . . . . . . . . . . . . . . 317
Liver Health . . . . . . . . . . . . . . . . . . . . . . . . . . . . . . . . . . . . . . . . . . . . 318
Signs of an Overloaded and/or Toxic Liver . . . . . . . . . . . . . . . . . . . . 320
Alkalinity. . . . . . . . . . . . . . . . . . . . . . . . . . . . . . . . . . . . . . . . . . . . . . . 321
Cleansing Programs . . . . . . . . . . . . . . . . . . . . . . . . . . . . . . . . . . . . . . 323
Establishing and Maintaining Good Health. . . . . . . . . . . . . . . . . . . . . 332
Daily Maintenance. . . . . . . . . . . . . . . . . . . . . . . . . . . . . . . . . . . . . . . 334
Environmental Protection Kits . . . . . . . . . . . . . . . . . . . . . . . . . . . . . . 337
Recipes—Delicious and Nutritious. . . . . . . . . . . . . . . . . . . . . . . . . . . 338

### CHAPTER 18 Building Blocks of Health. . . . . . . . . . . . . . . . . . . . . 343
Enzymes: The Key to Digestion . . . . . . . . . . . . . . . . . . . . . . . . . . . . . 343
Enzyme Quick Reference Guide . . . . . . . . . . . . . . . . . . . . . . . . . . . . . 344
Minerals: We Can't Live Without Them . . . . . . . . . . . . . . . . . . . . . . . . 353
Water: The Purity of Life . . . . . . . . . . . . . . . . . . . . . . . . . . . . . . . . . . . 355

Seventh Edition | **Essential Oils Desk Reference** | iii

**Essential Oils Desk Reference** | Seventh Edition

# Section 4
*(continued)*

**CHAPTER 19 Longevity and Vitality—Special Features** ....... 361

Living Longer with Essential Oils ............................... 361
Aging: The Power of Essential Oils ........................... 361
Brain Function: Essential Oils to the Rescue ................... 363
Clove Oil: A Powerful Antioxidant ........................... 364
Fluoride: Now Classified as a Neurotoxin ................... 365
Frankincense: A Gift to the World ........................... 368
Frequency: Our Electrical Energy ........................... 372
Microbes: How Essential Oils Fight Them ................... 377
Microwave Cooking: The Scientific Facts..................... 377
MSM—Sulfur: An Important Mineral ....................... 382
Radiation: Protecting Our Environment ..................... 383
Environmental Protection Kits ............................... 385
Secrets of Longevity: Living to 100 ......................... 389
Sweeteners: Making the Right Choice ...................... 391

# Section 5
## Personal Usage

**Personal Usage Directory** .............................. 400

**CHAPTER 20 Personal Usage** .......................... 405

Taking Charge of Your Health ............................... 405
Addressing Your Overall Health.............................. 406
Getting Started ........................................... 407
Developing Your Program .................................. 409
Personal Usage Recommendations .......................... 409
Application Guidelines ..................................... 410
Quick Usage Guide......................................... 412
Personal Usage ........................................... 415

# Section 6
## Appendix and Index

**APPENDIX A: Common and Botanical Plant Names** .......... 571

**APPENDIX B: Single Oil Data** ............................ 575

**APPENDIX C: Essential Oil Blends Data** ................... 591

**APPENDIX D: Flash Points for Essential Oils** .............. 597

**APPENDIX E: Product Usage for Body Systems** ............ 601

**INDEX** ................................................ 613

# Preface

The aromatherapy industry has really stepped into the limelight in the last decade. Aromatherapy started as an introduction of the therapeutic usage of essential oils but has since evolved into the synthetic world of misinformation and adulteration of God's oils for financial gain. It is hard to find an aromatherapy-labeled product that does not contain adulterated oils. This is what makes Young Living pure, authentic, therapeutic-grade essential oils so important. Pure essential oils are some of nature's most powerful therapeutic substances available, if only we could get that message to the millions of people who are looking for therapeutic benefits.

Most people today are unaware of the extensive documentation of the use of essential oils and their ancient history of healing and anointing. Many references about essential oils can be found in Judeo-Christian religious texts, and records show that at one time they were used to treat virtually every ailment known to man. Frankincense, myrrh, lotus, cedarwood, and sandalwood oils are some of the oils that were widely used in ancient Egyptian purification and embalming rituals. Oils like cinnamon, clove, and lemon were highly valued as antiseptics hundreds of years before the development of today's laboratory-developed medicines.

With the advancement of over-the-counter and prescription drugs during the last century, the knowledge of natural therapeutic substances, especially essential oils, was lost to the general public. Only about three decades ago in the United States did essential oils begin to gain a place on the shelves in the health food stores and perfume shops.

Many researchers and health care professionals have come to discover that there is a fascinating broad spectrum of therapeutic action in their healing potential. As we have opened the pages of history, we have discovered that in their pure state, essential oils are some of the most concentrated natural extracts known, exhibiting significant and immediate antiviral, anti-inflammatory, antidepressive, antibacterial, and hormone-balancing effects, as well as having calming, sedating, uplifting, and positive emotion-stimulating properties.

In clinical practice, essential oils have been shown to have a profound influence on the central nervous system, helping to reduce or eliminate pain and release muscle tension. The benefits of essential oils are numerous, and years of study are required to learn about the complexity of essential oil chemical constituents.

Even when pure essential oils were available, little was known about their therapeutic effects. The perfume industry was the greatest purchaser of pure oils and, unfortunately, adulterated them for the perfection and consistency of the aroma. It quickly became evident that chemical components were easier and cheaper to produce in the laboratory, which made it possible to increase the volume, putting millions of more dollars into the coffers of the manufacturers.

Today we find synthetic essential oil ingredients in soaps, cleaning agents, cosmetics, skin care, food, and flavorings, as well as, sadly, in the industry of health and wellness. When

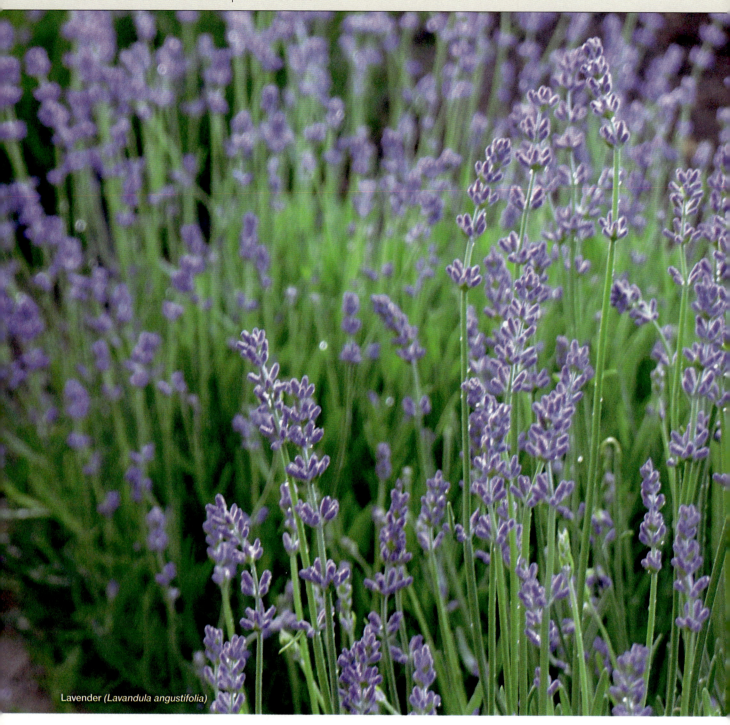

Lavender (*Lavandula angustifolia*)

the oils are extended and adulterated for commercial use, their therapeutic biochemical structure is destroyed, making them useful only as perfume for scenting all types of products and as flavoring compounds.

On the other hand, the chemical structure of a pure essential oil can rapidly penetrate cell membranes, travel throughout the body, and enhance cellular function. For health professionals who have used pure, authentic, therapeutic-grade essential oils on patients, it is very clear that there is a powerful life force inherent in these substances, which gives them an unmatched ability to interact with cells in the human body.

Many people believe that essential oils are God's medicine for mankind and that they will provide critical medical solutions in the future.

Essential oils could very well be the missing link of modern health care, bringing allopathic and holistic practices together for optimal health in the 21st century.

# Acknowledgments

When D. Gary Young brought back 13 essential oils from Europe in 1985, virtually no written information was available about their usage and application. The essential oils that were sold in a few health food and novelty stores were perfume grade with no suggested therapeutic usage.

This opened the door and led the way to a new, exciting frontier that propelled Gary into the research of an ancient knowledge that had been lost to the synthetic production of perfumes and food flavorings. His work began a resurgence of healing modalities from out of the dust of history. He was ridiculed and laughed at for his ideas about therapeutic usage, even though the medical world was beginning to awaken in Europe.

He has spent decades conducting clinical research on the ability of essential oils to combat disease and improve health. He has also developed new methods of application from which thousands of people have benefited, especially his integration of therapeutic-grade essential oils with dietary supplements and personal care products. In our research, we have found no evidence of anyone formulating these types of quality products with essential oils in North America prior to those formulated by D. Gary Young.

Gary grew up learning to love and work the land as a farmer and rancher in Idaho, which made it easy for him to see the vision of developing his own farms. That vision soon became reality as he purchased his first farm in 1992. His passion for extracting God's healing oils from Mother Nature's bounty has made him the world's leading grower of aromatic herbs and plants for the distillation of essential oils.

With eight privately owned farms and distillation operations in Utah, Idaho, Canada, France, Oman, and Ecuador; over 6,000 acres of purchased land under cultivation; and numerous partnerships and contract growers stretching to the far corners of the world, Gary has set new standards for excellence for the production of pure, authentic, therapeutic-grade essential oils in today's modern world.

Gary's long experience as a grower, distiller, researcher, and alternative-care practitioner not only gives him unsurpassed insight into essential oils but also makes him an ideal lecturer and educator on the therapeutic properties of essential oils and their applications. He is sought after by thousands of people to share his knowledge on the powerful potential of essential oils and on how to produce the highest quality therapeutic-grade essential oils.

The dedication to his belief, his *knowing*, brought about the research and discovery that we have compiled into this publication. His tremendous contribution to this new frontier of medicine is immeasurable. The material contained in this book is compiled from his research, lectures, seminars, workshops, and scientific publications, as well as from the work of other practitioners and physicians who are at the forefront of understanding the therapeutic and clinical potential of essential oils to maintain physical and emotional wellness, as well as aid in alleviating physical, emotional, and spiritual dysfunction.

To these researchers, the publisher is deeply indebted to be able to bring this information to all those in search of natural healing modalities found in the world of essential oils.

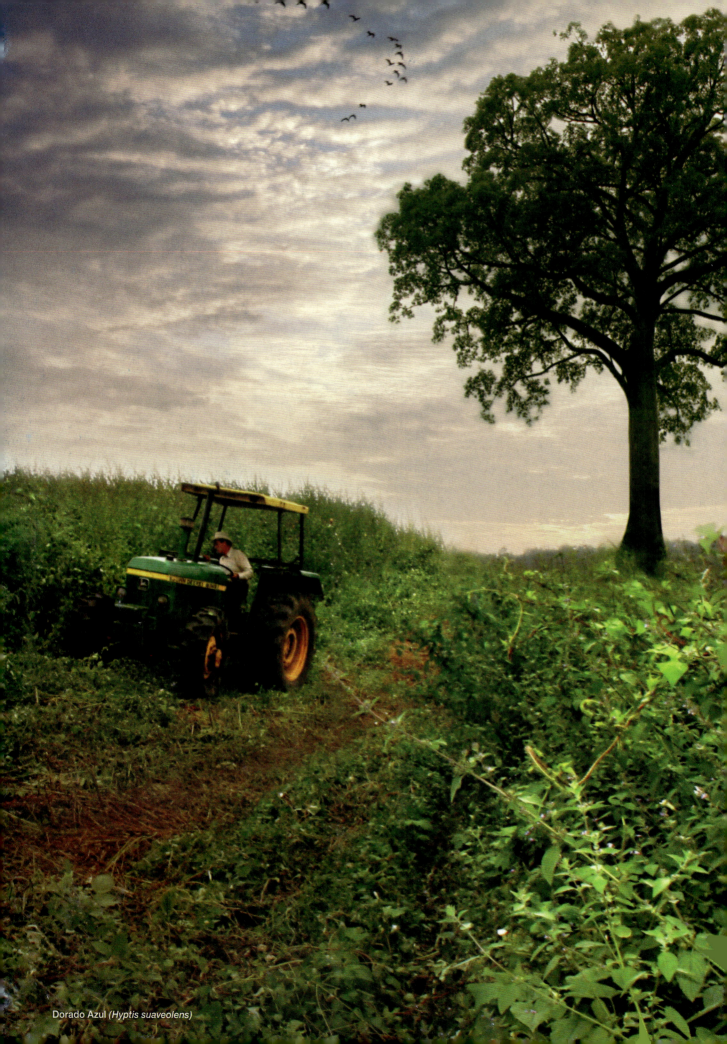

Dorado Azul *(Hyptis suaveolens)*

# Section 1
## Introduction

**CHAPTER 1** Yesterday's Wisdom, Tomorrow's Destiny . . . . . . . . . . . 3

**CHAPTER 2** How Essential Oils Work . . . . . . . . . . . . . . . . . . . . . . . . 17

**CHAPTER 3** Scientific Research and Documentation . . . . . . . . . . . . . 29

**CHAPTER 4** Producing Therapeutic-Grade™ Essential Oils . . . . . . . 35

**CHAPTER 5** How to Safely Use Essential Oils . . . . . . . . . . . . . . . . . . 49

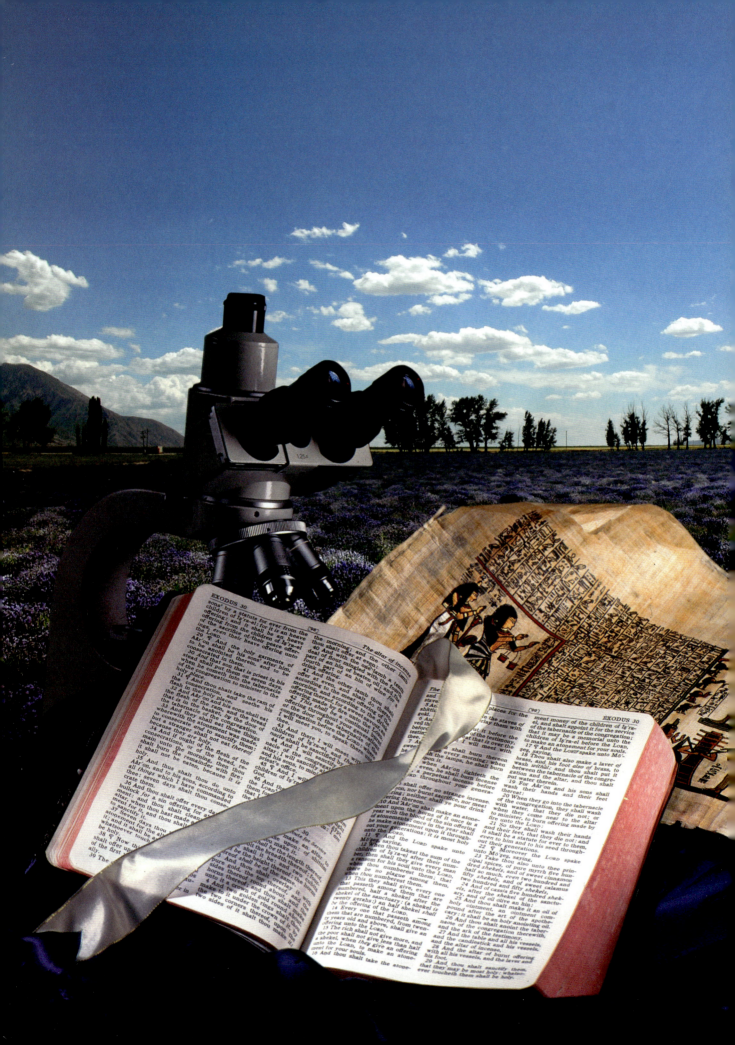

# Chapter 1
## Yesterday's Wisdom, Tomorrow's Destiny

## Essential Oils—The Missing Link in Modern Medicine

Plants not only play a vital role in the ecological balance of our planet, but they have also been intimately linked to the physical, emotional, and spiritual well-being of mankind since the beginning of time.

The plant kingdom continues to be the subject of an enormous amount of research and discovery. Most often prescription drugs are based on naturally occurring compounds from plants. Each year millions of dollars are allocated to private laboratories and universities that are searching for new therapeutic compounds that lie undiscovered in the bark, roots, flowers, seeds, and foliage of jungle canopies, river bottoms, forests, hillsides, and vast wilderness regions throughout the world.

Essential oils and plant extracts have been woven into history since the beginning of time and are considered by many to be the missing link in modern medicine. They have been used medicinally to kill bacteria, fungi, and viruses and to combat insect, bug, and snake bites in addition to treating all kinds of mysterious maladies. Oils and extracts stimulate tissue and nerve regeneration.

Essential oils also provide exquisite fragrances to balance mood, lift spirits, dispel negative emotions, and create a romantic atmosphere.

### Definition of an Essential Oil

An essential oil is that aromatic, volatile liquid that is within many shrubs, flowers, trees, roots, bushes, and seeds and that is usually extracted through steam distillation.

The chemistry of an essential oil is very complex and may consist of hundreds of different and unique chemical compounds. Moreover, essential oils are highly concentrated and far more potent than dried herbs because of the distillation process that makes them so concentrated. It requires a large volume of plant material to produce small amounts of a distilled essential oil. For example, it takes 5,000 pounds of rose petals to produce 1 kilo of rose oil.

Essential oils are also different from vegetable oils such as corn oil, peanut oil, and olive oil. Vegetable oils are greasy and may clog the pores. They also oxidize and become rancid over time and have no antibacterial properties. Most essential oils, on the other hand, do not go rancid and are powerful antimicrobials. Essential oils that are high in plant waxes, such as patchouli, vetiver, and sandalwood, if not distilled properly, could go rancid after time, particularly if exposed to heat for extended periods of time.

Essential oils are substances that definitely deserve the respect of proper education. Users should have a basic knowledge about the safety of the oils, and having a basic understanding of the chemistry of essential oils is very helpful. However, it is difficult to find this knowledge taught in universities or private seminars. Chemistry books are difficult to understand for most people, and they don't usually address the specific chemistry of essential oils. There is very little institutional information, knowledge, and training on essential oils and the scientific approach to their use.

The European communities have tight controls and standards concerning botanical extracts and who may administer them. Only practitioners with proper training and certification can practice in the discipline called "aromatherapy."

In the United States, regulatory agencies have not recognized these disciplines or mandated the type and degree of training required to distribute and use essential oils. This means that in the United States, individuals can call themselves "aromatherapists" after attending brief classes in essential oils and can apply oils to anyone—even though the so-called "aromatherapists" may not have the experience or training to properly understand and use essential oils. This may not only undermine and damage the credibility of the entire discipline of aromatherapy, but it is also dangerous to the patient.

Essential oils are not simple substances. Each oil is a complex structure of hundreds of different chemicals. A single essential oil may contain anywhere from 80 to 300 or more different chemical constituents. An essential oil like lavender is very complex, with many of its constituents occurring in minute quantities—but all contributing to the oil's therapeutic effects to some degree. To understand these constituents and their functions requires years of study.

Even though an essential oil may be labeled as "basil" and have the botanical name *Ocimum basilicum*, it can have widely different therapeutic actions, depending on its chemistry. For example, basil high in linalool or fenchol is primarily used for its antiseptic properties. However, basil high in methyl chavicol is more anti-inflammatory than antiseptic. A third type of basil high in eugenol has both anti-inflammatory and antiseptic effects.

Additionally, essential oils can be distilled or extracted in different ways that will have dramatic effects on their chemistry and medicinal action. Oils derived from a second or third distillation of the same plant material are usually not as potent as oils extracted during the first distillation. Yet with certain oils, there may be additional chemical constituents that are released only in the second or third distillation.

Oils subjected to high heat and high pressure have a noticeable simpler and inferior profile of chemical constituents, since excessive heat and temperature fracture can break down many of the delicate aromatic compounds within the oil—some of which are responsible for its therapeutic action. In addition, oils that are steam distilled are far different from those that are extracted with solvents.

Of greatest concern is the fact that some oils are adulterated, engineered, or "extended" with the use of synthetic-made compounds that are added to the oil. For example, pure frankincense is often extended with colorless, odorless solvents such as diethylphthalate or dipropylene glycol. The only way to distinguish the "authentic" from the "adulterated" is through analytical testing using gas chromatography, mass spectroscopy, and an optical refractometer. So-called "nature identical" lab-created constituents can be detected only by using GC/IRMS (Gas Chromatography, Isotope Ratio, and Mass Spectrometry) technology.

Unfortunately, a large percentage of essential oils marketed in the United States fall in this adulterated category. When you understand the world of synthetic oils as well as low-grade oils cut with synthetic chemicals, you realize why the vast majority of consumers never know the difference. However, if you do know the smell of the pure oil or the technique for recognizing adulteration through scent, it may be possible to perceive a difference.

## Different Schools of Application

Therapeutic treatment using essential oils follows three different models: the English, French, and German.

The English model puts a small amount of an essential oil in a large amount of vegetable oil to massage the body for the purpose of relaxation and relieving stress.

The French model prescribes neat (undiluted) topical application of therapeutic-grade essential oils and/or the ingestion of pure essential oils. Typically, a few drops of an essential oil are added to agave nectar, honey, a small amount of vegetable oil, or put on a piece of bread. Many French practitioners have found that taking the oils internally yields excellent benefits.

The German model focuses on inhalation of essential oils—the true aromatherapy. Research has shown that the effect of fragrance on the sense of smell can exert strong effects on the brain—especially on the hypothalamus (the hormone command center of the body) and limbic system (the seat of emotions). Some essential oils high in sesquiterpenes, such as myrrh, sandalwood, cedarwood, vetiver, and melissa can dramatically increase oxygenation and activity in the brain, which may directly improve the function of many systems of the body.

Together, these three models show the versatility and power of essential oils. By integrating all three models with various methods of application such as Vita Flex, auricular technique, lymphatic massage, and Raindrop Technique, the best possible results may be obtained.

In some cases, inhalation of essential oils might be preferred over topical application, if the goal is to increase growth hormone secretion, promote weight loss, or balance mood and emotions. Sandalwood, peppermint, vetiver, lavender, and eucalyptus oils are effective for inhalation.

In other cases, however, topical application of essential oils would produce better results, particularly in the case of back or muscle injuries or defects. Topically applied, marjoram is excellent for muscles, lemongrass for ligaments, and wintergreen for bones. For indigestion, a drop or two of peppermint oil taken orally or put in a glass of water may be very effective. However, this does not mean that peppermint cannot produce the same results when massaged on the stomach. In some cases, all three methods of application (topical, inhalation, and ingestion) are interchangeable and may produce similar benefits.

The ability of essential oils to act on both the mind and the body is what makes them truly unique among natural therapeutic substances. The fragrance of some essential oils can be very stimulating—both psychologically and physically. The fragrance of other essential oils may be calming and sedating, helping to overcome anxiety or hyperactivity. On a physiological level, essential oils may stimulate immune function and regenerate damaged tissue. Essential oils may also combat infectious disease by killing viruses, bacteria, and other pathogens.

Probably the two most common methods of essential oil application are cold-air diffusing and neat (undiluted) topical application. Other modes of application include incorporating essential oils into the disciplines of reflexology, Vita Flex, and acupressure. Combining these disciplines with essential oils enhances the healing response and often produces amazing results that cannot be achieved by acupuncture or reflexology alone. Just 1–3 drops of an essential oil applied to an acupuncture meridian or Vita Flex point on the hand or foot can produce results within a minute or two.

Several years ago, a professor well known in the field of aromatherapy ridiculed the use of essential oils against disease. However, many people are living proof that essential oils dramatically aided in the recovery of serious illness. Essential oils have been pivotal in helping many people live pain free after years of intense pain. Patients have also witnessed firsthand how essential oils have helped with scoliosis and even restored partial hearing in those who were born deaf and complete hearing with someone who had had some loss of hearing.

For example, a woman from Palisades Park, California, developed scoliosis after surviving polio as a teenager, which was further complicated by a serious fall that dislocated her shoulder. Suffering pain and immobility for 22 years, she had traveled extensively in a fruitless search to locate a practitioner who could permanently reset her shoulder. Upon learning about essential oils, she topically applied the oils of helichrysum and wintergreen, among others, to the shoulder. Within a short time, her pain began to diminish and eventually was completely gone, and she was able to raise her arm over her head for the first time in 22 years.

When one sees such dramatic results, it is difficult to discredit the value and the power of essential oils and the potential they hold. One would certainly think that it would be well worth investigating further. It is so sad that many turn away because of lack of knowledge.

## Man's First Medicine

From ancient writings and traditions, it seems that aromatics were used for religious rituals, the treatment of illness, and other physical and spiritual needs. Records dating back to 4500 BC describe the use of balsamic substances with aromatic properties for religious rituals and medical applications. Ancient writings tell of scented barks, resins, spices, and aromatic vinegars, wines, and beers that were used in rituals, temples, astrology, embalming, and medicine. The evidence certainly suggests that the people of ancient times had a greater understanding of essential oils than we have today.

Science and technology historian E. J. Holmyard wrote that the process of distillation "is of very great antiquity; a primitive form of distillation-apparatus dating from about 3500 BC has been unearthed at Tepe Gawra in north-east Mesopotamia [today's Iraq] and described by Martin Levey of Pennsylvania State University."[1]

The Egyptians were masters in using essential oils and other aromatics in the embalming process. Historical records describe how one of the founders of "pharaonic" medicine was the architect Imhotep, who was the Grand Vizier of King Djoser (2780 - 2720 BC). Imhotep is often given credit for ushering in the use of oils, herbs, and aromatic plants for medicinal purposes. In addition, the Egyptians may have been the first to discover the potential of fragrance. They created various aromatic blends for both personal use and religious ceremonies.

Many hieroglyphics on the walls of Egyptian temples depict the blending of oils and describe numerous oil recipes. An example of this is the Temple of Edfu, located on the west bank of the Nile River. Over the centuries it was buried beneath sand drifts, which preserved the temple nearly intact. The smaller of two hypostyle halls leads to a small room called a laboratory, where perfumes and ointments were compounded. On the walls are hieroglyphics listing recipes for these aromatic perfumes, including two recipes for kyphi, a blend of incense that contained frankincense, myrrh, honey, raisins soaked in wine, sweet flag, pine resin, and juniper. Another recipe was for "Hekenu," with wood pitch, fresh frankincense, dry white frankincense, and acacia flowers, used to anoint "divine limbs" of the gods in the temple. Similar medicinal formulas and perfume recipes were used by alchemists and high priests to blend aromatic substances for rituals.

Well before the time of Christ, the ancient Egyptians collected essential oils and placed them in alabaster vessels. These vessels were specially carved and shaped for housing scented oils. In 1922, when King Tutankhamen's tomb was opened, some 50 alabaster jars designed to hold 350 liters of oils were discovered. Tomb robbers had stolen nearly all of the precious oils, leaving the heavy jars behind that still contained traces of oil. The robbers literally chose oils over a king's wealth in gold, showing how valuable the essential oils were to them.

**Essential Oils Desk Reference** | Seventh Edition

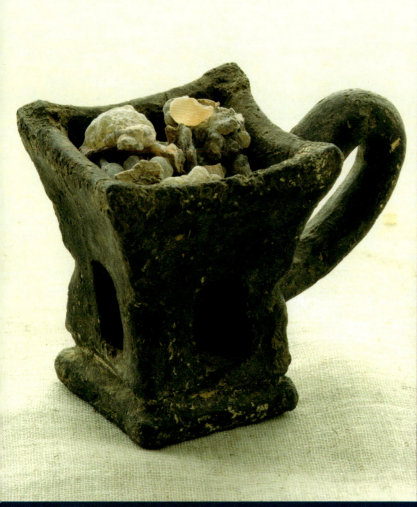

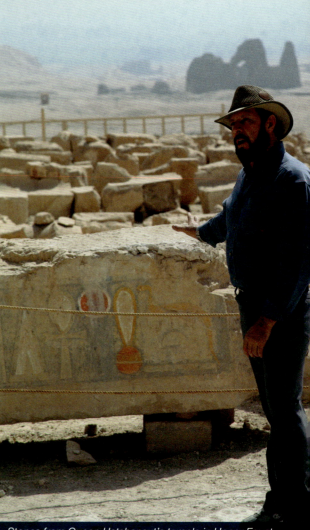

3,500-year-old stone incense burner dug out of the ground in Shabwah, Yemen, in 2009 by D. Gary Young.

Stones from Queen Hatshepsut's temple in Upper Egypt, with reliefs depicting healing with plants and the lotus oil.

In 1817 the Ebers Papyrus, a medical scroll over 870 feet long, was discovered that dated back to 1500 BC. The scroll included over 800 different herbal prescriptions and remedies. Other scrolls described a high success rate in treating 81 different diseases. Many of the remedies contained myrrh and honey. Myrrh is still recognized for its ability to help with infections of the skin and throat and to regenerate skin tissue. Because of its effectiveness in preventing bacterial growth, myrrh was also used for embalming.

The physicians of Ionia, Attia, and Crete, ancient civilizations based on islands of the Mediterranean Sea, came to the cities of the Nile to increase their knowledge. At this time, the school of Cos was founded and was attended by Hippocrates (460-377 BC), whom the Greeks, with perhaps some exaggeration, named the "Father of Medicine."

The Romans purified their temples and political buildings by diffusing essential oils and also used aromatics in their steam baths to invigorate themselves and ward off disease.

6 | Chapter 1 | Yesterday's Wisdom, Tomorrow's Destiny

Yesterday's Wisdom, Tomorrow's Destiny | **Chapter 1**

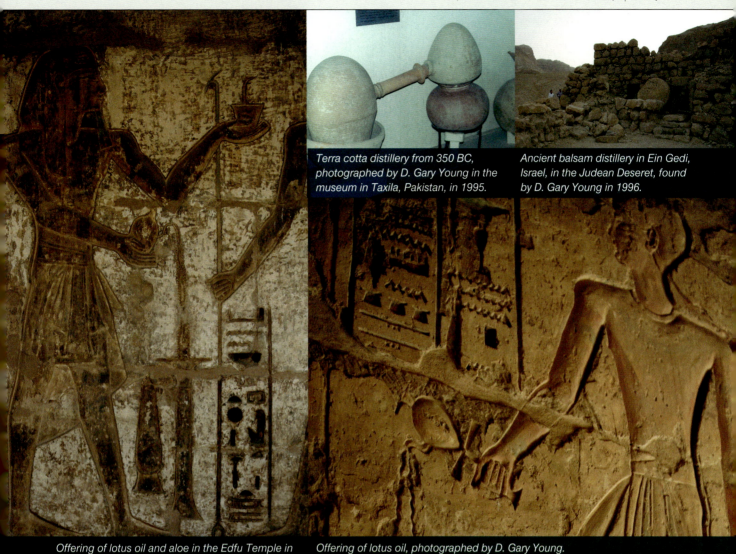

*Terra cotta distillery from 350 BC, photographed by D. Gary Young in the museum in Taxila, Pakistan, in 1995.*

*Ancient balsam distillery in Ein Gedi, Israel, in the Judean Deseret, found by D. Gary Young in 1996.*

*Offering of lotus oil and aloe in the Edfu Temple in Upper Egypt, photographed by D. Gary Young.*

*Offering of lotus oil, photographed by D. Gary Young.*

# Early History of Essential Oil Extraction

Ancient cultures found that aromatic essences or oils could be extracted from the plant by a variety of methods. One of the oldest and crudest forms of extraction was known as enfleurage. Raw plant material such as stems, foliage, bark, or roots was crushed and mixed with olive oil, animal fat, and some vegetable oils. Cedar bark was stripped from the trunk and branches, ground into a powder, soaked with olive oil, and placed in a wool cloth. The cloth was then heated. The heat pulled the essential oil out of the bark particles into the olive oil, and the wool was pressed to extract the essential oil. Sandalwood oil was also extracted in this fashion.

Enfleurage was also used to extract essential oils from flower petals. In fact, the French word enfleurage means literally "to saturate with the perfume of flowers." For example, petals from roses or jasmine were placed in goose or goat fat. The essential oil droplets were pulled from the petals into the fat and then separated from the fat. This ancient technique was one of the most primitive forms of essential oil extraction.

Other extraction techniques were also used such as:

- Soaking plant parts in boiling water
- Cold-pressing
- Soaking in alcohol
- Steam distillation, meaning that as the steam travels upward, it saturates the plant material, causing the plant membranes containing the oil to break open

and release the oil, which then becomes a vapor that travels with the steam into the condenser, where it returns to its liquid form and is then separated from the water.

Many ancient cosmetic formulas were created from a base of goat and goose fat and camel milk. Ancient Egyptians made eyeliners, eye shadows, and other cosmetics this way. They also stained their hair and nails with a variety of ointments and perfumes. Fragrance "cones" made of wax and essential oils were worn by women of royalty, who enjoyed the rich scent of the oils as the cones melted with the heat of the day.

In the temples oils were commonly poured into evaporation dishes so that the aroma could fill the chambers associated with sacred rituals and religious rites throughout the day.

Ancient Arabians also developed and refined the process of distillation. They perfected the extraction of rose oil and rose water, which were popular in the Middle East during the Byzantine Empire (330 AD-1400 AD).

## Biblical History of Essential Oils

The Bible contains over 200 references to aromatics, incense, and ointments. Aromatics such as frankincense, myrrh, galbanum, cinnamon, cassia, rosemary, hyssop, and spikenard were used for anointing and healing the sick. In Exodus, the Lord gave the following recipe to Moses for a holy anointing oil:

| | |
|---|---|
| *Myrrh* | *"five hundred shekels" (about 1 gallon)* |
| *Cinnamon* | *"two hundred and fifty shekels"* |
| *Calamus* | *"two hundred and fifty shekels"* |
| *Cassia* | *"five hundred shekels"* |
| *Olive Oil* | *"an hin" (about 1 1/3 gallons)* |

Psalms 133:2 speaks of the sweetness of brethren dwelling together in unity: "It is like the precious ointment upon the head, that ran down the beard, even Aaron's beard: that went down to the skirts of his garments." Another scripture that refers to anointing and the overflowing abundance of precious oils is Ecclesiastes 9:8: "Let thy garments be always white; and let thy head lack no ointment."

The Bible also lists an incident where an incense offering by Aaron stopped a plague. Numbers 16:46-50 records that Moses instructed Aaron to take a censer, add burning coals and incense, and "go quickly into the congregation to make an atonement for them: for there is a wrath gone out from the Lord; the plague is begun." The Bible records that Aaron stood between the dead and the living, and the plague was stayed. It is significant that according to the biblical and Talmudic recipes for incense,

three varieties of cinnamon were involved. Cinnamon is known to be highly antimicrobial, anti-infectious, and antibacterial. The incense ingredient listed as "stacte" is believed to be a sweet, myrrh-related spice, which would make it anti-infectious and antiviral as well.

The New Testament records that wise men presented the Christ child with frankincense and myrrh. There is another precious aromatic, spikenard, described in the anointing of Jesus in Mark 14:3:

> And being in Bethany in the house of Simon the leper, as he sat at meat, there came a woman having an alabaster box of ointment of spikenard very precious; and she brake the box, and poured it on his head.

The anointing of Jesus is also referred to in John 12:3:

> Then took Mary a pound of ointment of spikenard, very costly, and anointed the feet of Jesus, and wiped his feet with her hair: and the house was filled with the odour of the ointment.

See additional biblical references at the end of this chapter.

## Other Historical References

Throughout world history, fragrant oils and spices have played a prominent role in everyday life.

Herodotus, the Greek historian who lived from 484 BC to 425 BC, recorded that during the yearly feast of Bel, 1,000 talents' weight of frankincense was offered on the great altar of Bel in Babylon.

The Roman historian Pliny the Elder (23-79 AD) complained that "by our lowest reckoning India, China and the Arabian peninsula take from our empire 100 million sesterces every year, for aromatics."

Diodorus of Sicily lived in the 1st century BC and wrote of the abundance of frankincense in Arabia and how it "suffices for the service and worship of gods all the world over."

Napoleon is reported to have enjoyed cologne water made of neroli and other ingredients so much that he ordered 162 bottles of it.

After conquering Jerusalem, one of the things the Crusaders brought back to Europe was solidified essence of roses.

The 12th-century herbalist Hildegard of Bingen used herbs and oils extensively in healing. This Benedictine nun founded her own convent and was the author of numerous works. Her book, *Physica,* has more than 200 chapters on plants and their uses for healing.

Yesterday's Wisdom, Tomorrow's Destiny | Chapter 1

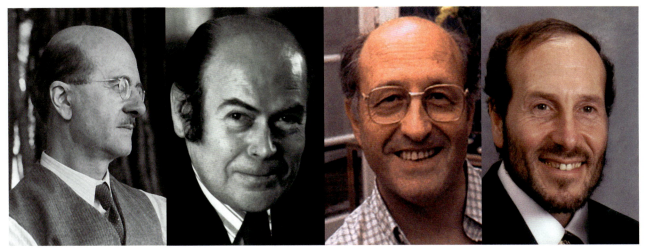

René-Maurice Gattefossé, PhD    Jean Valnet, MD    Jean-Claude Lapraz, MD    Daniel Pénoël, MD

## The Rediscovery

The reintroduction of essential oils into modern medicine first began during the late 19th and early 20th centuries.

During World War I, the use of aromatic essences in civilian and military hospitals became widespread. One physician in France, Dr. Moncière, used essential oils extensively for their antibacterial and wound-healing properties and developed several kinds of aromatic ointments.

René-Maurice Gattefossé, PhD, a French cosmetic chemist, is widely regarded as the father of aromatherapy. He and a group of scientists began studying essential oils in 1907.

In his 1937 book, *Aromatherapy*, Dr. Gattefossé told the real story of his now-famous use of lavender essential oil that was used to heal a serious burn. The tale has assumed mythic proportions in essential oil literature. His own words about this accident are even more powerful than what has been told over the years.

Dr. Gattefossé was literally aflame—covered in burning substances—following a laboratory explosion in July 1910. After he extinguished the flames by rolling on a grassy lawn, he wrote that "both my hands were covered with rapidly developing gas gangrene." He further reported that "just one rinse with lavender essence stopped the gasification of the tissue. This treatment was followed by profuse sweating and healing which began the next day."

Robert B. Tisserand, editor of *The International Journal of Aromatherapy*, searched for Dr. Gattefossé's book for 20 years. A copy was located and Tisserand edited the 1995 reprint. Tisserand noted that Dr. Gattefossé's burns "must have been severe to lead to gas gangrene, a very serious infection."

Dr. Gattefossé shared his studies with his colleague and friend Jean Valnet, a medical doctor practicing in Paris. Exhausting his supply of antibiotics as a physician in Tonkin, China, during World War II, Dr. Valnet began using essential oils on patients suffering battlefield injuries. To his surprise, the essential oils showed a powerful effect in fighting infection. He was able to save the lives of many soldiers who might otherwise have died.

Two of Dr. Valnet's students, Dr. Paul Belaiche and Dr. Jean-Claude Lapraz, expanded his work. They clinically investigated the antiviral, antibacterial, antifungal, and antiseptic properties in essential oils.

In 1990, Dr. Daniel Pénoël, a French medical doctor, and Pierre Franchomme, a French biochemist, collaborated together to co-author the first reference book that cataloged the various medical properties of over 270 essential oils and how to use them in a clinical environment. Their work was based on Franchomme's laboratory experience and Pénoël's clinical experience of administering the oils to his patients. The book, published in French, was titled *l'aromathérapie exactement* and became the primary resource for dozens of authors worldwide in writing about the medical benefits of essential oils.

D. Gary Young sought out the best and brightest experts in clinical use, distillation, and chromatographic analysis as he began his essential oil company. He first studied essential oils with Dr. Jean-Claude Lapraz in

**Essential Oils Desk Reference** | Seventh Edition

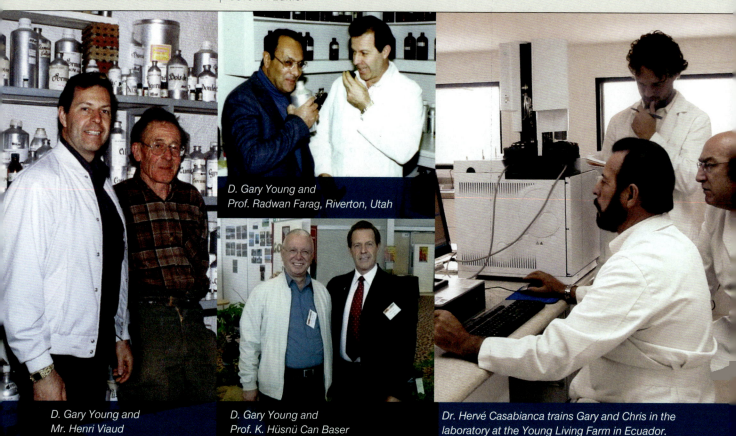

D. Gary Young and Mr. Henri Viaud

D. Gary Young and Prof. Radwan Farag, Riverton, Utah

D. Gary Young and Prof. K. Hüsnü Can Baser

Dr. Hervé Casabianca trains Gary and Chris in the laboratory at the Young Living Farm in Ecuador.

1985 in Geneva, Switzerland. Then he went to Paris to study with one of Jean Valnet's students, Paul Belaiche, MD. Gary also studied with Daniel Pénoël, co-author of *l'aromathérapie exactement*. In the early '90s, he studied with Professor Radwan Farag, PhD, at Cairo University and Professor K. Hüsnü Can Baser at the Andalou University in Eskisehir, Turkey.

Gary Young's training in the art of distillation and essential oil testing began with his lavender partnership with Jean-Noël Landel in Provence, France. Jean-Noël introduced Gary to Marcel Espieu, the president of the Lavender Growers Association in Southern France, and Henri Viaud, a chemist and distiller of essential oils and author of the 1983 book on quality considerations for essential oils (*Huiles Essentielles—Hydrolats*). Mr. Viaud had his own laboratory and small distiller, and Gary was his only student to whom he taught the finer points of distilling.

After studying at the Albert Vieille Laboratory in Grasse, France, in 1994, Gary traveled to Lyon, France, where he studied with the world's foremost authority in chromatography, Hervé Casabianca, PhD. Dr. Casabianca traveled to Young Living laboratories in the U.S. and Ecuador to train staff scientists in gas chromatography/mass spectrometry.

From D. Gary Young to Jean-Claude Lapraz to Jean Valnet to René-Maurice Gattefossé—D. Gary Young is a pioneer in the world of essential oils, just as they were.

From 1994 to 2016, knowledge and use of essential oils has spread throughout the world (see map), making Young Living Essential Oils a billion-dollar company and the World Leader in Essential Oils.®

Health-minded people the world over have learned the value of using high quality natural herbs. Interestingly, most therapeutic herbs can be distilled into an essential oil. The key difference is that of concentration. The essential oil can be from 100 to 10,000 times more concentrated—and therefore more potent—than the herb itself. Even though they are many times more potent than natural herbs, essential oils, unlike prescription drugs, very rarely generate any negative side effects, which carries profound implications for those wanting to maintain or regain their health naturally.

Sometimes the effects of administering essential oils are so dramatic that the patients themselves call it "miraculous"; and while no one fully understands yet "why" or "how" essential oils provide such significant benefits, the fact is that they do. With pure essential oils, millions of people can find relief from disease, infections, pain, and even

Yesterday's Wisdom, Tomorrow's Destiny | Chapter 1

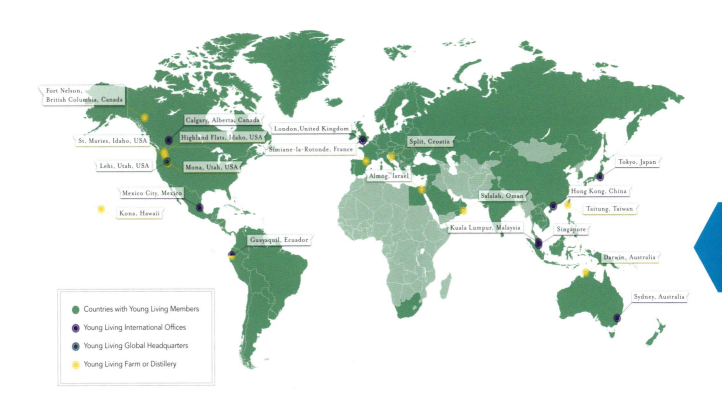

mental difficulties. Their therapeutic potential is enormous and is only just beginning to be tapped.

Because of the research being conducted by many scientists and doctors, the healing power of essential oils is again gaining prominence. Today, it has become evident that we have not yet found permanent solutions for dreaded diseases such as Zika and Ebola viruses, hanta virus, AIDS, HIV, and new strains of tuberculosis and influenza like bird and swine flu.

Essential oils may assume an increasingly important role in combating new mutations of bacteria, viruses, and fungi. More and more researchers are undertaking serious clinical studies on the use of essential oils to combat these types of diseases.

Research conducted at Weber State University in cooperation with D. Gary Young, as well as other documented research, indicates that most viruses, fungi, and bacteria cannot live in the presence of most essential oils, especially those high in phenols, carvacrol, thymol, and terpenes. It may also help us understand why a notorious group of thieves, reputed to be spice traders and perfumers, was protected from the Black Plague as they robbed the bodies of the dead and dying during the 15th century.

A vast body of anecdotal evidence (testimonials) suggests that those who use essential oils are less likely to contract infectious diseases. Moreover, oil users who do contract an infectious illness tend to recover faster than those using antibiotics.

Our modern world has only begun the discovery of the power of God's healing oils—something that the ancient world knew well. Their time was one without laboratories, manufacturing facilities, high technology and equipment, or chemicals. The earth and its healing gifts were the ancient world's medicine—something our modern world should take note of and embrace. Modern medicine is certainly not without its miracles. Millions of lives have been saved in crisis and malfunctions of the body. But the way to live with strength and vitality without pain and disease lies in what God has created, not in what man has altered.

Essential oils are no longer the missing link in modern medicine. Millions of people are applauding their power, and millions more are being introduced and educated to their potential each year. As more and more health practitioners, doctors, scientists, and users of all ages venture into the world of this ancient knowledge, the methods of medicine will take on new dimensions, and exciting discoveries will be made that will benefit mankind today and tomorrow.

# Biblical References

## Cedarwood

Leviticus 14:51—"And he shall take the cedar wood, and the hyssop, and the scarlet, and the living bird, and dip them in the blood of the slain bird, and in the running water, and sprinkle the house seven times:"

Leviticus 14:52—"And he shall cleanse the house with the blood of the bird, and with the running water, and with the living bird, and with the cedar wood, and with the hyssop, and with the scarlet."

Numbers 19:6—"And the priest shall take cedar wood, and hyssop, and scarlet, and cast *it* into the midst of the burning of the heifer."

Numbers 24:6—"As the valleys are they spread forth, as gardens by the river's side, as the trees of lign aloes which the Lord hath planted, *and* as cedar trees beside the waters."

2 Samuel 5:11—"And Hiram king of Tyre sent messengers to David, and cedar trees, and carpenters, and masons: and they built David an house."

2 Samuel 7:2—"That the king said unto Nathan the prophet, See now, I dwell in an house of cedar, but the ark of God dwelleth within curtains."

2 Samuel 7:7—"In all *the places* wherein I have walked with all the children of Israel spake I a word with any of the tribes of Israel, whom I commanded to feed my people Israel, saying, Why build ye not me an house of cedar?"

1 Kings 4:33—"And he spake of trees, from the cedar tree that *is* in Lebanon even unto the hyssop that springeth out of the wall: he spake also of beasts, and of fowl, and of creeping things, and of fishes."

1 Kings 5:6—"Now therefore command thou that they hew me cedar trees out of Lebanon; and my servants shall be with thy servants: and unto thee will I give hire for thy servants according to all that thou shalt appoint: for thou knowest that *there is* not among us any that can skill to hew timber like unto the Sidonians."

1 Kings 5:8—"And Hiram sent to Solomon, saying, I have considered the things which thou sentest to me for: *and* I will do all thy desire concerning timber of cedar, and concerning timber of fir."

1 Kings 5:10—"So Hiram gave Solomon cedar trees and fir trees *according to* all his desire."

1 Kings 6:9—"So he built the house, and finished it; and covered the house with beams and boards of cedar."

1 Kings 9:11—"(*Now* Hiram the king of Tyre had furnished Solomon with cedar trees and fir trees, and with gold, according to all his desire,) that then king Solomon gave Hiram twenty cities in the land of Galilee."

2 Kings 19:23—"By thy messengers thou hast reproached the Lord, and hast said, With the multitude of my chariots I am come up to the height of the mountains, to the sides of Lebanon, and will cut down the tall cedar trees thereof, *and* the choice fir trees thereof: and I will enter into the lodgings of his borders, *and into* the forest of his Carmel."

1 Chronicles 22:4—"Also cedar trees in abundance: for the Zidonians and they of Tyre brought much cedar wood to David."

2 Chronicles 1:15—"And the king made silver and gold at Jerusalem *as plenteous* as stones, and cedar trees made he as the sycomore trees that *are* in the vale for abundance."

2 Chronicles 2:8—"Send me also cedar trees, fir trees, and algum trees, out of Lebanon: for I know that thy servants can skill to cut timber in Lebanon; and behold, my servants *shall be* with thy servants,"

2 Chronicles 9:27—"And the king made silver in Jerusalem as stones, and cedar trees made he as the sycomore trees that *are* in the low plains in abundance."

Ezra 3:7—"They gave money also unto the masons, and to the carpenters; and meat, and drink, and oil, unto them of Zidon, and to them of Tyre, to bring cedar trees from Lebanon to the sea of Joppa, according to the grant that they had of Cyrus king of Persia."

Isaiah 41:19—"I will plant in the wilderness the cedar, the shittah tree, and the myrtle, and the oil tree; I will set in the desert the fir tree, *and* the pine, and the box tree together:"

Ezekiel 17:3—"And say, Thus saith the Lord God; A great eagle with great wings, longwinged, full of feathers, which had divers colours, came unto Lebanon, and took the highest branch of the cedar:"

Ezekiel 17:22—"Thus saith the Lord God; I will also take of the highest branch of the high cedar, and will set *it*; I will crop off from the top of his young twigs a tender one, and will plant *it* upon an high mountain and eminent:"

Ezekiel 17:23—"In the mountain of the height of Israel will I plant it: and it shall bring forth boughs, and bear fruit, and be a goodly cedar: and under it shall dwell all fowl of every wing; in the shadow of the branches thereof shall they dwell."

Zechariah 11:2—"Howl, fir tree; for the cedar is fallen; because the mighty are spoiled: howl, O ye oaks of Bashan; for the forest of the vintage is come down."

## Cinnamon

Proverbs 7:17—"I have perfumed my bed with myrrh, aloes, and cinnamon."

The Song of Solomon 4:14—"Spikenard and saffron; calamus and cinnamon, with all trees of frankincense; myrrh and aloes, with all the chief spices:"

Revelation 18:13—"And cinnamon, and odours, and ointments, and frankincense, and wine, and oil, and fine flour, and wheat, and beasts, and sheep, and horses, and chariots, and slaves, and souls of men."

## Fir

1 Kings 6:15—"And he built the walls of the house within with boards of cedar, both the floor of the house, and the walls of the ceiling: *and* he covered *them* on the inside with wood, and covered the floor of the house with planks of fir."

1 Kings 6:34—"And the two doors *were of* fir tree: the two leaves of the one door *were* folding, and the two leaves of the other door *were* folding."

1 Kings 9:11—"(*Now* Hiram the king of Tyre had furnished Solomon with cedar trees and fir trees, and with gold, according to all his desire,) that then king Solomon gave Hiram twenty cities in the land of Galilee."

2 Kings 19:23—"By thy messengers thou hast reproached the Lord, and hast said, With the multitude of my chariots I am come up to the height of the mountains, to the sides of Lebanon, and will cut down the tall cedar trees thereof, *and* the choice fir trees thereof: and I will enter into the lodgings of his borders, *and into* the forest of his Carmel."

2 Chronicles 2:8—"Send me also cedar trees, fir trees, and algum trees, out of Lebanon: for I know that thy servants can skill to cut timber in Lebanon; and, behold, my servants *shall be* with thy servants."

2 Chronicles 3:5—"And the greater house he cieled with fir tree, which he overlaid with fine gold, and set thereon palm trees and chains."

Psalms 104:17—"Where the birds make their nests: *as for* the stork, the fir trees *are* her house."

The Song of Solomon 1:17—"The beams of our house *are* cedar, *and* our rafters of fir."

Isaiah 14:8—"Yea, the fir trees rejoice at thee, *and* the cedars of Lebanon, *saying*, Since thou art laid down, no feller is come up against us."

Isaiah 37:24—"By thy servants hast thou reproached the Lord, and hast said, By the multitude of my chariots am I come up to the height of the mountains, to the sides of Lebanon; and I will cut down the tall cedars thereof, *and* the choice fir trees thereof: and I will enter into the height of his border, *and* the forest of his Carmel."

Isaiah 41:19—"I will plant in the wilderness the cedar, the shittah tree, and the myrtle, and the oil tree; I will set in the desert the fir tree, *and* the pine, and the box tree together:"

Isaiah 55:13—"Instead of the thorn shall come up the fir tree, and instead of the brier shall come up the myrtle tree: and it shall be to the Lord for a name, for an everlasting sign [that] shall not be cut off."

Isaiah 60:13—"The glory of Lebanon shall come unto thee, the fir tree, the pine tree, and the box together, to beautify the place of my sanctuary; and I will make the place of my feet glorious."

Ezekiel 27:5—"They have made all thy *ship* boards of fir trees of Senir: they have taken cedars from Lebanon to make masts for thee."

Ezekiel 31:8—"The cedars in the garden of God could not hide him: the fir trees were not like his boughs, and the chestnut trees were not like his branches; nor any tree in the garden of God was like unto him in his beauty."

Hosea 14:8—"Ephraim *shall say*, What have I to do any more with idols? I have heard *him*, and observed him: I *am* like a green fir tree. From me is thy fruit found."

Nahum 2:3—"The shield of his mighty men is made red, the valiant men *are* in scarlet: the chariots *shall be* with flaming torches in the day of his preparation, and the fir trees shall be terribly shaken."

Zechariah 11:2—"Howl, fir tree; for the cedar is fallen; because the mighty are spoiled: howl, O ye oaks of Bashan; for the forest of the vintage is come down."

## Frankincense

Leviticus 2:15—"And thou shalt put oil upon it, and lay frankincense thereon: it *is* a meat offering."

Leviticus 2:16—"And the priest shall burn the memorial of it, *part* of the beaten corn thereof, and *part* of the oil thereof, with all the frankincense thereof: *it is* an offering made by fire unto the Lord."

Leviticus 5:11—"But if he be not able to bring two turtledoves, or two young pigeons, then he that sinned shall bring for his offering the tenth part of an ephah of fine flour for a sin offering; he shall put no oil upon it, neither shall he put *any* frankincense thereon: for it *is* a sin offering."

Leviticus 6:15—"And he shall take of it his handful, of the flour of the meat offering, and of the oil thereof, and all the frankincense which *is* upon the meat offering, and shall burn *it* upon the altar *for* a sweet savour, *even* the memorial of it, unto the Lord."

Leviticus 24:7—"And thou shalt put pure frankincense upon *each* row, that it may be on the bread for a memorial, *even* an offering made by fire unto the Lord."

Numbers 5:15—"Then shall the man bring his wife unto the priest, and he shall bring her offering for her, the tenth *part* of an ephah of barley meal; he shall pour no oil upon it, nor put frankincense thereon; for it *is* an offering of jealousy, an offering of memorial, bringing iniquity to remembrance."

1 Chronicles 9:29—"*Some* of them also *were* appointed to oversee the vessels, and all the instruments of the sanctuary, and the fine flour, and the wine, and the oil, and the frankincense, and the spices."

Nehemiah 13:5—"And he had prepared for him a great chamber, where aforetime they laid the meat offerings, the frankincense, and the vessels, and the tithes of the corn, the new wine, and the oil, which was commanded *to be given* to the Levites, and the singers, and the porters; and the offerings of the priests."

Nehemiah 13:9—"Then I commanded, and they cleansed the chambers: and thither brought I again the vessels of the house of God, with the meat offering and the frankincense."

The Song of Solomon 3:6—"Who *is* this that cometh out of the wilderness like pillars of smoke, perfumed with myrrh and frankincense, with all powders of the merchant?"

The Song of Solomon 4:6—"Until the day break, and the shadows flee away, I will get me to the mountain of myrrh, and to the hill of frankincense."

The Song of Solomon 4:14—"Spikenard and saffron; calamus and cinnamon, with all trees of frankincense; myrrh and aloes, with all the chief spices:"

Matthew 2:11—"And when they were come into the house, they saw the young child with Mary his mother, and fell down, and worshiped him: and when they had opened their treasures, they presented unto him gifts; gold, and frankincense, and myrrh."

Revelation 18:13—"And cinnamon, and odours, and ointments, and frankincense, and wine, and oil, and fine flour, and wheat, and beasts, and sheep, and horses, and chariots, and slaves, and souls of men."

## Hyssop

Leviticus 14:49—"And he shall take to cleanse the house two birds, and cedar wood, and scarlet, and hyssop:"

Leviticus 14:51—"And he shall take the cedar wood, and the hyssop, and the scarlet, and the living bird, and dip them in the blood of the slain bird, and in the running water, and sprinkle the house seven times:"

Leviticus 14:52—"And he shall cleanse the house with the blood of the bird, and with the running water, and with the living bird, and with the cedar wood, and with the hyssop, and with the scarlet:"

Numbers 19:6—"And the priest shall take cedar wood, and hyssop, and scarlet, and cast *it* into the midst of the burning of the heifer."

Numbers 19:18—"And a clean person shall take hyssop, and dip *it* in the water, and sprinkle *it* upon the tent, and upon all the vessels, and upon the persons that were there, and upon him that touched a bone, or one slain, or one dead, or a grave:"

1 Kings 4:33—"And he spake of trees, from the cedar tree that *is* in Lebanon even unto the hyssop that springeth out of the wall: he spake also of beasts, and of fowl, and of creeping things, and of fishes."

Psalms 51:7—"Purge me with hyssop, and I shall be clean: wash me, and I shall be whiter than snow."

John 19:29—"Now there was set a vessel full of vinegar: and they filled a spunge with vinegar, and put *it* upon hyssop, and put *it* to his mouth."

Hebrews 9:19—"For when Moses had spoken every precept to all the people according to the law, he took the blood of calves and of goats, with water, and scarlet wool, and hyssop, and sprinkled both the book, and all the people."

## Myrrh

Esther 2:12—"Now when every maid's turn was come to go in to king Ahasuerus, after that she had been twelve months, according to the manner of the women, (for so were the days of their purifications accomplished, *to wit*, six months with oil of myrrh, and six months with sweet odours, and with *other* things for the purifying of the women;)"

Psalms 45:8—"All thy garments *smell* of myrrh, and aloes, *and* cassia, out of the ivory palaces, whereby they have made thee glad."

Proverbs 7:17—"I have perfumed my bed with myrrh, aloes, and cinnamon."

The Song of Solomon 1:13—"A bundle of myrrh *is* my well-beloved unto me; he shall lie all night betwixt my breasts."

The Song of Solomon 3:6—"Who *is* this that cometh out of the wilderness like pillars of smoke, perfumed with myrrh and frankincense, with all powders of the merchant?"

The Song of Solomon 4:6—"Until the day break, and the shadows flee away, I will get me to the mountain of myrrh, and to the hill of frankincense."

The Song of Solomon 4:14—"Spikenard and saffron; calamus and cinnamon, with all trees of frankincense; myrrh and aloes, with all the chief spices:"

The Song of Solomon 5:1—"I am come into my garden, my sister, [my] spouse: I have gathered my myrrh with my spice; I have eaten my honeycomb with my honey; I have drunk my wine with my milk: eat, O friends; drink, yea, drink abundantly, O beloved."

The Song of Solomon 5:5—"I rose up to open to my beloved; and my hands dropped *with* myrrh, and my fingers *with* sweet smelling myrrh, upon the handles of the lock."

The Song of Solomon 5:13—"His cheeks *are* as a bed of spices, *as* sweet flowers: his lips *like* lilies, dropping sweet smelling myrrh."

Matthew 2:11—"And when they were come into the house, they saw the young child with Mary his mother, and fell down, and worshiped him: and when they had opened their treasures, they presented unto him gifts; gold, and frankincense, and myrrh."

Mark 15:23—"And they gave him to drink wine mingled with myrrh: but he received *it* not."

John 19:39—"And there came also Nicodemus, which at the first came to Jesus by night, and brought a mixture of myrrh and aloes, about an hundred pound *weight*."

## Myrtle

Zechariah 1:8—"I saw by night, and behold a man riding upon a red horse, and he stood among the myrtle trees that *were* in the bottom; and behind him *were there* red horses, speckled, and white."

Zechariah 1:10—"And the man that stood among the myrtle trees answered and said, These *are they* whom the Lord hath sent to walk to and fro through the earth."

Zechariah 1:11—"And they answered the angel of the Lord that stood among the myrtle trees, and said, We have walked to and fro through the earth, and, behold, all the earth sitteth still, and is at rest."

## Spikenard

The Song of Solomon 4:14—"Spikenard and saffron; calamus and cinnamon, with all trees of frankincense, myrrh and aloes, with all chief spices."

Mark 14:3—"And being in Bethany in the house of Simon the leper, as he sat at meat, there came a woman having an alabaster box of ointment of spikenard very precious; and she brake the box, and poured *it* on his head."

John 12:3—"Then took Mary a pound of ointment of spikenard, very costly, and anointed the feet of Jesus, and wiped his feet with her hair: and the house was filled with the odour of the ointment."

---

ENDNOTES

1. Holmyard, EJ. *Alchemy*, Dover Publications, 1990, page 44.

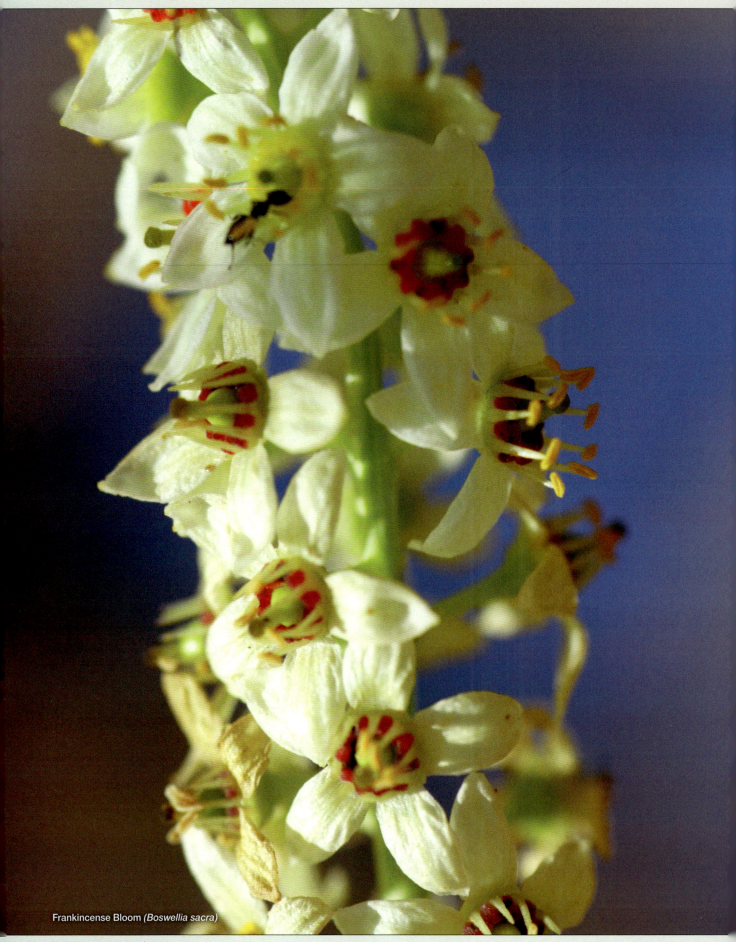

Frankincense Bloom *(Boswellia sacra)*

# Chapter 2
## How Essential Oils Work

# Understanding Essential Oil Chemistry

Essential oils are nature's volatile aromatic compounds generated within shrubs, flowers, trees, roots, bushes, and seeds. They are usually extracted through steam distillation, hydrodistillation, or cold-pressed extraction.

The power of an essential oil lies in its constituents and their synergy. Essential oils are composed of 200-500 different bioconstituents, which makes them very diverse in their effects. No two oils are alike.

Lavender oil, for example, contains approximately 200 different constituents, of which linalyl acetate, linalool, cis-beta-ocimene, trans-beta-ocimene, and terpinene-4-ol are the major components. Lavender oil has been used for burns, insect bites, headaches, PMS, insomnia, stress, and hair growth. Because essential oils are composites of hundreds of different constituents, each oil can exert many different effects on the body.

Essential oils have a unique ability to penetrate cell membranes and travel throughout the blood and tissues. The unique lipid-soluble structure of essential oils is very similar to the makeup of our cell membranes, and the molecules of essential oils are also relatively small, which enhances their ability to penetrate into the cells. When topically applied to the feet or soft tissue, essential oils can travel throughout the body in a matter of minutes.

## Basic Structure of Essential Oil Constituents

The aromatic constituents of essential oils (i.e., terpenes, monoterpenes, phenols, aldehydes, etc.) are constructed from long chains of carbon and hydrogen atoms, which have a predominantly ring-like structure. Links of carbon atoms form the backbone of these chains, with oxygen, hydrogen, nitrogen, sulfur, and other carbon atoms attached at various points of the chain.

Essential oils have different chemistry than fatty oils (also known as fatty acids). In contrast to the simple linear carbon-hydrogen structure of fatty oils, essential oils have a far more complex ring structure and contain sulfur and nitrogen atoms that fatty oils do not have.

The terpenoids found in all essential oils are actually constructed out of the same basic building block—a five-carbon molecule known as isoprene. When two isoprene units link together, they create a monoterpene; when three join, they create a sesquiterpene; and so on.

## Essential Oil Constituent Categories

There are 14 categories of essential oil constituents. We will list each category with examples of oils containing such constituents. The information below has been adapted from *The Chemistry of Essential Oils* by David Stewart, PhD,[1] which is highly recommended, and from *l'aromathérapie exactement*[2] by Pierre Franchomme and Daniel Pénoël.

1. **Alkanes:** Few essential oils contain alkanes, and those that do usually contain less than 1 percent. The alkanes undecane, dodecane, and hexadecane are found in ginger oil. Alkane alcohols are found in lemon oil and ginger oil. Rose oil stands alone as an essential oil that contains 11 to 19 percent alkanes, which may be why this exquisite oil exhibits so many unique characteristics.

2. **Phenols:** Common phenols found in essential oils are thymol (thyme and mountain savory) and eugenol (clove, cinnamon, basil, and bay laurel). Phenol is found in very minute quantities (<1 percent) in cassia, cinnamon, and ylang ylang. Phenols are believed to be antiseptic, antimicrobial, and may boost the immune system in various ways. Some phenols are strong and may cause skin irritation.

Seventh Edition | **Essential Oils Desk Reference** | 17

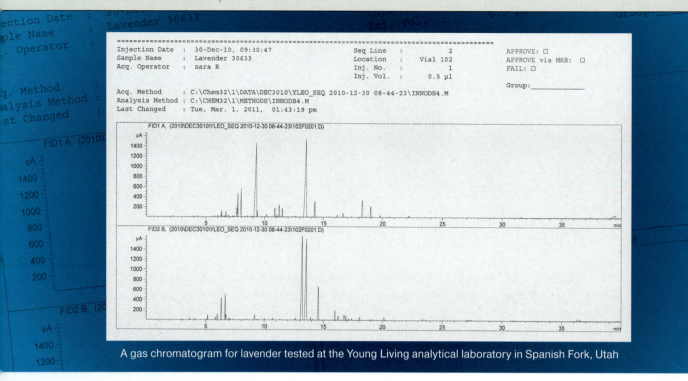

A gas chromatogram for lavender tested at the Young Living analytical laboratory in Spanish Fork, Utah

3. **Monoterpenes:** This class of constituents is the most common and is found in every essential oil. It is estimated that there are 1,000 different monoterpenes found in essential oils. Monoterpenes contain 10 carbons and are characteristically similar to alkanes. Many oils are composed of mostly monoterpenes, including grapefruit and frankincense. They have light fragrances, are supportive, and enhance the therapeutic talents of other constituents. They are commonly the first aroma detected when smelling an essential oil. The monoterpenes α-pinene, d-limonene, l-limonene, sabinene, myrcene, β-phellandrene, camphene, and ocimene are abundant in pine, orange, balsam fir, juniper, frankincense, ginger, spruce, and basil, respectively.

4. **Sesquiterpenes:** As many as 3,000 different sesquiterpenes are found in essential oils. This class of constituents contains 15 carbons and is characteristically similar to alkanes and monoterpenes. The sesquiterpenes beta-caryophyllene, bisabolen, and guaiene are found in black pepper, myrrh, and patchouli, respectively. Oils with high sesquiterpene content include cedarwood, patchouli, sandalwood, ginger, vetiver, blue cypress, and myrrh. Many sesquiterpenes are specific to one oil only, and most have light aromas, but not all. Caryophyllene, for example, is one exception, that has a strong, woody, spicy aroma and is found in a variety of oils. Sesquiterpenes are soothing to inflamed tissue and can also produce profound effects on emotions and hormonal balance.

**Other terpenes:**

Diterpenes (20 carbons) are the heaviest molecules found in distilled essential oils. Jasmine essential oil contains about 14 percent diterpenes. Therapeutically, diterpenes have some of the same properties as sesquiterpenes and are considered to be expectorants and purgatives.

Triterpenes (30 carbons) and tetraterpenes (40 carbons) are larger molecules than diterpenes and are found mostly in the cold-pressed citrus oils of orange, tangerine, lemon, grapefruit, and lime and also in absolutes like jasmine.

It was once believed that diterpene and triterpene molecules were too large to make it through distillation, but diterpenes like incensole have been documented in essential oils through GC-MS analyses, and triterpenic acids (such as boswellic acids) are detectable in frankincense essential oil through High Performance Liquid Chromatography (HPLC) testing.

5. **Alcohols:** The names of these constituents end in –ol. Borneol is found in lavandin; citronellol is in rose; linalool is in rosewood; α-terpineol and terpinen-4-ol are in melaleuca; and lavandulol is in lavender. Alcohols are also found in eucalyptus and fennel oils, as well as many more. Alcohols are energizing, cleansing, antiseptic, antiviral, and have a sweet floral aroma.

How Essential Oils Work | **Chapter 2**

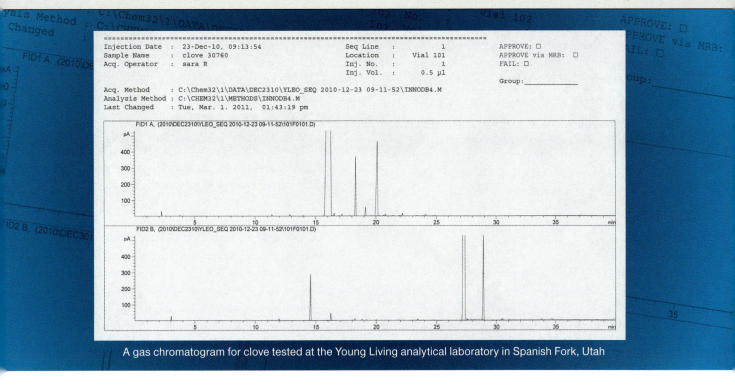

A gas chromatogram for clove tested at the Young Living analytical laboratory in Spanish Fork, Utah

6. **Ethers:** This constituent form is not as common in essential oils as others like terpenes, alcohols, or ketones. The names of these constituents end in "-ole," "-cin," or "-ether." Examples of ethers are anethole, in fennel and anise; estragole, in tarragon; elemicin, in elemi; myristicin, in nutmeg; and eugenol methyl ester found in some melaleuca species. Ethers are balancing and calming, help release emotions, and have an antidepressant effect.

7. **Aldehydes:** The names of these constituents end in "-al" or "-aldehyde." Benzoic aldehyde is found in onycha; cinnamaldehyde, in cassia; citral, in lemongrass; cuminal, in cumin; neral, in melissa; and phellandral, in eucalyptus dives. The aldehyde octanal is in rose, lavender, and citrus oils. Decanal is found in coriander, lemongrass, and mandarin oils. Aldehydes are antimicrobial, anti-inflammatory, cooling, and have strong aromas. They can also be calming to the nervous system, emotional stress relievers, and blood pressure reducers.

8. **Ketones:** A strong, distinctive odor characterizes ketones. Ketones usually end in "-one." Camphor is found in rosemary; fenchone, in fennel; jasmone, in jasmine; pentanone, in myrrh; piperitone, in peppermint; β-thujone, in Idaho tansy; and α-vetivone, in vetiver. Ketones are thought to be calming, with decongesting and analgesic benefits; promote healing (cell regeneration); and cleanse receptor sites.

9. **Carboxylic acids:** These constituents are only minor parts of an essential oil, rarely comprising more than 1-2 percent. They are easy to recognize because they always have the word "acid" in their name. Examples are cinnamic acid, in cinnamon; geranic acid, in geranium; and valerinic acid, in valerian. Carboxylic acids are stimulating and cleansing and are very reactive with other components.

10. **Esters:** Oils composed mainly of esters include birch and wintergreen. The names of esters end in "-ate." Esters usually have a strong, sweet aroma. Linalyl acetate is found in bergamot; neryl acetate, in helichrysum; isobutyl angelate, in Roman chamomile; citronellyl formate, in geranium; menthyl acetate, in peppermint; and bornyl acetate, the main constituent in pine, spruce, juniper, and fir. To make an ester, a carboxylic acid and an alcohol are combined. Esters are soothing, balancing, antifungal, and stress and emotional releasing.

11. **Oxides:** These are oxygenated hydrocarbons and are usually derived from terpenes, alcohols, or ketones that have been oxidized. Examples are bisabolol oxide found in German chamomile; piperitone oxide, in peppermint; linalool oxide, in hyssop; rose oxide, in rose; sclareol oxide, in clary sage; and humulene oxide, in clove. These oxides are in very small quantities, but most oils produce the oxide 1,8-cineole, also known as eucalyptol, in varying amounts. This is more

Seventh Edition | **Essential Oils Desk Reference** | 19

abundantly found in eucalyptus (*E. globulus*), rosemary, and thyme. Oils with 1,8-cineole are known for respiratory-decongesting and sinus-clearing benefits.

12. **Lactones:** This constituent group is characterized by tongue-twisting names. Bergaptene is found in fennel essential oil; furanogermacrene, in myrrh; and umbelliferone, in anise. Celery seed is an oil with higher amounts of lactones. Lactones, like ketones, are generally decongesting and expectorant. They generally have mild aromas. They seem to have antiseptic, antiparasitic, and anti-inflammatory properties, according to Dr. Daniel Pénoël.

13. **Coumarins:** Dr. Stewart notes that coumarins are a subgroup of lactones and are found widely in nature. Because there is a similarity to the name of the blood-thinning drug Coumadin®, he explained that coumarins and Coumadin are *not* similar. One is natural, one synthetic, and they have very different chemical formulas. Coumarins have the fragrance of freshly cut hay or grass. In fact, when you mow your lawn, you are releasing coumarins into the air. They are found in fleabane, bitter orange, lavandin (in very minute quantities), and cassia essential oils. Coumarins are powerful and can have strong therapeutic effects, even in small quantities. Coumarins have antispasmodic, antiviral, antibacterial, and antifungal properties.

14. **Furanoids:** Furanoids or furans are lactones or coumarins with names starting with "furano-" or "furo-" or ending with "furan." Most of the essential oils that contain furans are certain expressed citrus oils. Some essential oils with furanoids are photosensitive (they amplify the effects of the sun) like angelica, bergamot, bitter orange, grapefruit, lemon, lime, petitgrain, and ruta (*R. graveolens*). Other oils containing furanoids, like myrrh, mandarin, sweet orange, and tangerine are not photosensitive. Myrrh is interesting in that it contains more furanoid components than any other essential oil (up to 27 percent), yet it is not photosensitive. Furanoids can have the benefits of lactones or coumarins.

With this brief explanation of constituent chemistry, lavender's components are categorized as esters (linalyl acetate), alcohols (linalool and terpinen-4-ol), and monoterpenes (cis-β-ocimene and trans-β-ocimene).

*Boswellia sacra* essential oil constituents tell us that it is composed of monoterpenes (α-pinene, limonene, sabinene, myrcene, α-thujene, p-cymene), the sesquiterpene β-caryophyllene, and many more components.

Lemon's constituents can be categorized as monoterpenes (limonene, gamma-terpinene, β-pinene, α-pinene, and sabinene).

The constituents of peppermint are categorized as alcohols (menthol), ketones (menthone), furanoids (menthofuran), monoterpenes (1,8-cineole and pulegone), and esters (menthyl acetate).

These constituents listed are only a small percentage of the total number of constituents present in each essential oil.

## Plant Chemotypes and Constituent Variability

A single species of plant can have several different chemotypes (biomolecularly unique variants within one species) based on molecular composition. This means that basil (*Ocimum basilicum*) grown in one area might produce an essential oil with different chemistry than a basil grown in another location. The plant's growing environment, such as soil pH and mineral content, can dramatically affect the plant's ultimate chemistry as well. Different chemotypes of basil are listed below:

- *Ocimum basilicum* CT linalool fenchol (Germany)—antiseptic

- *Ocimum basilicum* CT methyl chavicol (Reunion, Comoro, or Egypt)—anti-inflammatory

- *Ocimum basilicum* CT eugenol (Madagascar)—anti-inflammatory, pain-relieving

Another plant species that occurs in a variety of different chemotypes is rosemary (*Rosmarinus officinalis*).

- *Rosmarinus officinalis* CT camphor is high in camphor, which serves best as a general stimulant and works synergistically with other oils, such as black pepper (*Piper nigrum*), and can be a powerful energy stimulant.

- *Rosmarinus officinalis* CT cineole is rich in 1,8-cineole, which is used in other countries for pulmonary congestion and to help with the elimination of toxins from the liver and kidneys. Young Living offers this chemotype of rosemary because of its great value.

- *Rosmarinus officinalis* CT verbenone is high in verbenone and is the most gentle of the rosemary chemotypes. It offers powerful regenerative properties and has outstanding benefits for skin care.

How Essential Oils Work | **Chapter 2**

# Different Essential Oil Species

**Chamomile (Roman)**
1. *Anthemis nobilis*)
   (Syn. *Chamaemelum nobile*)

**Chamomile (German)**
2. *Chamomilla recutita*
   (Syn. *Matricaria recutita*)

**Chamomile (Morrocan)**
3. *Ormenis mixta* (Syn.
   *Chamaemelum nobile*)
   (not a true chamomile but
   sold as such because it
   contains chamazulene)

**Cinnamon**
1. *Cinnamomum verum*
   (cinnamon bark)
2. *Cinnamomum zeylanicum*
   (synonym for *C. verum*)
3. *Cinnamomum aromaticum*

**Eucalyptus**
1. *Eucalyptus citriodora*
2. *Eucalyptus dives*
3. *Eucalyptus globulus*
4. *Eucalyptus polybractea*
5. *Eucalyptus radiata*

**Frankincense**
1. *Boswellia ameero*
2. *Boswellia bullata*
3. *Boswellia carterii*
4. *Boswellia dalzielii*
5. *Boswellia dioscorides*
6. *Boswellia elongata*
7. *Boswellia frereana*
8. *Boswellia nana*
9. *Boswellia neglecta*
10. *Boswellia ogadensis*
11. *Boswellia papyrifera*
12. *Boswellia pirottae*
13. *Boswellia popoviana*
14. *Boswellia rivae*
15. *Boswellia sacra*
16. *Boswellia serrata*
17. *Boswellia socotrana*

**Juniper**
1. *Juniperus communis*
2. *Juniperus osteosperma*
3. *Juniperus communis ssp alpine*

**Lavandin**
1. *Lavandula x hybrida abrialis*
2. *Lavandula intermedia
   var. Grosso*
3. *Lavandula hybrida reydovan*
4. *Lavandula x intermedia Super*
   (has a higher linalyl acetate
   and ester content)

**Lavender**
1. *Lavandula angustifolia*
   (also known as *L. officinalis*)
2. *Lavandula latifolia*
   1,8-cineole
3. *Lavandula vera*
   (thought once to be the
   original species now
   grown in Bulgaria)
4. *Lavandula stoechas* (also
   known as Spanish lavender)
5. Spike lavender (*Lavandula
   latifolia*) (known for its
   strong cineole/camphor
   content)

**Lemon**
1. *Citrus limon*
2. Verbena (*Lippia citriodora*)
   (lemon-scented verbena)

**Lemongrass**
1. *Cymbopogon flexuosus*
2. *Cymbopogon citratus*

**Marjoram**
1. *Origanum majorana*
   (terpinen-4-ol, sweet)
2. *Thymus mastichina* cineole
   (wild-growing Spanish)

**Melaleuca**
1. *M. alternifolia* (terpinen-4-ol)
2. *M. cajuputii* monoterpenes
3. *M. leucadendron*
4. *M. linariifolia* cineolifera
5. *M. quinquenervia* cineolifera
6. *M. quinquenervia*
   nerolidolifera–sesquiterpenes
7. *M. uncinata* monoterpenes

**Myrrh**
1. *Commiphora myrrha*
2. *Commiphora molmol*
3. *Commiphora erythraea*
4. *Commiphora ornifolia*
5. *Commiphora parvifolia*
6. *Commiphora socotrana*

**Orange**
1. *Citrus aurantium* (bitter)
2. *Citrus sinensis* (sweet)

**Sage**
1. *Salvia officinalis*
2. *Sage lavandulifolia*
   (Spanish sage)
3. *Salvia sclarea* (clary sage)
4. *Salvia apiana*

Seventh Edition | **Essential Oils Desk Reference** | 21

Common thyme (*Thymus vulgaris*) produces several different chemotypes, depending on the conditions of its growth, climate, and altitude. The following are just two chemotypes out of many more.

- *Thymus vulgaris* CT thymol is germicidal and anti-inflammatory.

- *Thymus vulgaris* CT linalool is anti-infectious.

One chemotype of thyme will yield an essential oil with high levels of thymol, depending on the time of year it is distilled. The later it is distilled in the growing season (e.g., mid-summer or fall), the more thymol the oil will contain.

Another example of this variability in chemotype is shown in a Turkish study on *Origanum onites*.[3] Researchers found that the altitude at which the plants grew affected the morphology of the plant and amount of volatile oil the plant produced. The plant produced more volatile oil the higher the altitude in which it grew. Even on the same mountainside, wildcrafted plants produced varying levels of oil.

Proper cultivation assures that more variable-specific chemotypes, like *Thymus vulgaris* and *Origanum compactum*, will maintain more consistent levels of constituents and oil produced.

## Purity and Potency of Essential Oils

One of the factors that determines the purity of an oil is its constituents. These constituents can be affected by a vast number of variables, including the part(s) of the plant from which the oil was produced, soil condition, fertilizer (organic or chemical), geographical region, climate, altitude, harvesting methods, and distillation processes.

The key to producing a therapeutic-grade essential oil is to preserve as many of the delicate aromatic components within the essential oil as possible. Fragile aromatic components are easily destroyed by high temperature and pressure, as well as by contact with reactive metals such as copper or aluminum. This is why all therapeutic-grade essential oils should be distilled in stainless steel cooking chambers at low pressure and low temperature.

The plant material should also be free of herbicides and other agrichemicals. These can react with the essential oil during distillation to produce toxic compounds. Because many pesticides are oil-soluble, they can also mix into the essential oil.

Although chemists have successfully recreated the main constituents and fragrances of some essential oils in the laboratory, these synthetic oils lack therapeutic benefits and may even carry risks. Pure essential oils contain hundreds of different bioconstituents, which lend important therapeutic properties to the oil when combined. Also, many essential oils contain molecules and isomers that are impossible to manufacture in the laboratory.

Today approximately 300 essential oils are distilled or extracted worldwide. Several thousand constituents and aromatic molecules are identified and registered in these 300 essential oils. Ninety-eight percent of essential oil volume produced today is used in the perfume and cosmetic industry. Only about 2 percent of the production volume is for therapeutic and medicinal applications.

Young Living requires all distillers who want to sell to Young Living to submit samples to be analyzed to ensure that all the constituents are present at the right percentage to be therapeutic. You can have pure oils, but if the plants are distilled at the wrong time of day or with incorrect distillation procedures, the constituents that make the oils therapeutic will not be there, and you will not have a therapeutic-grade profile.

In addition, Young Living requires that the farms and the essential oil distillation facilities be subject to site inspection. Of oil samples submitted between May 2007 and October 2011 by distillers wanting to partner with Young Living, over 34 percent did not meet Young Living standards and were rejected.

Because Young Living interacts with the end-users who purchase essential oils, the company is able to monitor human response to and determine the actual therapeutic benefits of various oils, thereby comparing the constituents of different oils to determine their maximum, health-giving potential. Quality and efficacy are moving, evolving targets. No one understands this more than Young Living.

How Essential Oils Work | **Chapter 2**

# Standards and Testing

## Young Living Standards

Over the years, Young Living has bought and compiled an essential oil retention index and mass spectral reference library that contains over 400,000 components. Using this research reference library, Young Living developed its own standards to guarantee the highest possible therapeutic potency for its essential oils.

Young Living's research and quality control laboratories in Utah have four gas chromatograph (GC) instruments, two of which also have a mass spectrometer (GC-MS). The Young Living Ecuador laboratory has a GC-MS. These instruments are the only ones in the world that are matched and calibrated for therapeutic essential oil analysis to the instruments used at the National Center for Scientific Research in France (CNRS: *Centre National de la Recherche Scientifique*) by Dr. Hervé Casabianca.

As a general rule, if one or more marker components in an essential oil fall outside the prescribed percentages, the oil does not meet Young Living's pure, therapeutic-grade essential oil standards.

A lavender essential oil produced in one region of France might have a slightly different chemistry than that grown in another region and as a result may not meet the standard. It may have excessive camphor levels (1.0 instead of 0.5), a condition that might be caused by distilling lavender that was too green, or the levels of lavandulol may be too low due to certain weather conditions at the time of harvest.

By comparing the gas chromatograph chemistry profile of a lavender essential oil with the Young Living pure, therapeutic-grade standard, one may also distinguish true lavender from various species of lavandin (hybrid lavender). Usually lavandin has high camphor levels, almost no lavandulol, and is easily identified. However, Tasmania produces a lavandin that yields an essential oil with naturally low camphor levels that mimics the composition of true lavender. Only by analyzing the essential oil composition of this Tasmanian lavandin using high resolution gas chromatography and comparing it with the Young Living pure, therapeutic-grade standard for genuine lavender can this hybrid lavender be identified.

## Testing Instruments

In the United States, few companies use the proper analytical instruments and methods to properly analyze essential oils. Most labs use equipment best suited for synthetic chemicals—not for natural essential oil analysis.

Young Living Essential Oils uses the proper instruments and has made great effort to calibrate Young Living's GC-MS instruments to the column-wall thickness set by Dr. Casabianca, laboratory director of Natural Product Research, at CNRS labs in France. This ensures identification of more components that otherwise might be missed. In addition to operating its analytical instruments with the same calibration as the CNRS laboratories, Young Living is continually expanding its analytical component library in order to perform a more thorough compositional analysis.

## Gas Chromatography and Mass Spectrometry

Properly analyzing an essential oil by gas chromatography (GC) is a complex undertaking. The injection mixture, capillary column diameter, column length, and oven temperature must fall within certain parameters. GC is the analytical instrumentation used to separate the many natural components biogenerated by the aromatic plant that make up the essential oil. The key components of a GC are the injector, capillary GC column, detector, and oven. A small sample of essential oil is injected into the capillary GC column with a syringe. The capillary GC column is slowly heated within the oven to separate the essential oil components. Finally, the separated components exit the GC column, and the percentage of each component is determined by a Flame Ionization Detector (FID).

Using a longer capillary GC column length increases the separation of each of the components in a complex essential oil. We have found that a 50- or 60-meter-long capillary GC column provides the best separation for essential oil components. Shorter 25- or 30-meter columns provide adequate separation of many components, but they are too short to properly analyze the complex mosaic of natural bioconstituents found in an essential oil. A more detailed analysis of an essential oil can be obtained using a 100-meter-long capillary GC column.

Every capillary GC column has an internal polymer coating (stationary phase) that helps separate the essential oil components. The most common stationary phase for essential oil separations is the polydimethylsiloxane phase that generates a separation based on the boiling points of

Seventh Edition | **Essential Oils Desk Reference** | 23

each essential oil component. In addition, using a "wax-based" stationary phase composed of polyethylene oxide, the GC operator can obtain a separation based on both the boiling points and the polarity of each essential oil component. We use both of these phases simultaneously in one GC to provide two separations from a single injection of essential oil. This process allows us to make more certain identification of essential oil components.

Another common analytical instrument for the separation and identification of essential oil components is the GC-MS (gas chromatograph-mass spectrometer). The MS is a special detector attached to the instrument that can identify by name each essential oil component from a library of known essential oil components. The MS identifies the components based on the arrangement of their individual carbon, hydrogen, and oxygen atoms. The GC-MS is used in the first stages of research in order to separate and identify each component of a new essential oil. After the initial research, the GC (with an FID detector) is used for routine quality control to determine percentages of each component in the essential oil.

## Chiral GC-MS

While GC-MS is an excellent tool to analyze essential oils, it does have limitations. Sometimes it can be difficult to distinguish between natural and synthetic bioconstituents using GC-MS analysis alone. If synthetic linalyl acetate is added to pure lavender, a GC-MS analysis cannot confidently determine whether that constituent is synthetic or natural, only that it is linalyl acetate. Adding a chiral (pronounced "ky-ral") capillary GC column in the GC-MS can help in distinguishing between synthetic and natural components.

Research scientists can use chiral GC-MS to identify whether an essential oil is composed of its natural proportions of chiral components. Some components have what is called chiral polarity. This means they have "left" or "right" versions of the component, called enantiomers.

To see the perfect example of "chirality," bring your hands up, palms facing you. They are mirror images but exact opposites. They are different in that you could not put a right-handed glove on your left hand. The term used to identify rotating to the right is *dextrorotary,* or "d," and rotating to the left, *levorotary,* or "l." Not all essential oil molecules have chirality, but many do.

A trained scientist can check for adulteration by looking at the ratio between the two chiral enantiomers. Nature tends to favor one over the other. For instance, in a 2012 study[4] on chiral differences in the frankincense constituent α-pinene, *Boswellia sacra* is +8.24 while *Boswellia carterii*

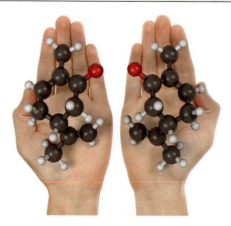

Two chiral forms of the constituent carvone. The left enantiomer is found in dill and caraway essential oils, while the form on the right is found in spearmint essential oil.

is -0.68. When adding an unspecified synthetic, you get equal amounts of both enantiomers. It is possible to purify a synthetic mixture down to the individual enantiomers, but this is not seen much because of the expense.

IRMS (Isotope Ratio Mass Spectrometry) takes it to another extreme. This is needed because sometimes people get really clever and adulterate oils where we can't determine naturalness by chirality alone. IRMS measures the isotopic ratios of the individual atoms in oil. By comparing these ratios to both a natural standard and a synthetic one, we can determine adulteration at the atomic level.

Young Living researchers use a polarimeter to identify the optical rotation of molecules. If the "d" or "l" form deviates from what is listed in a chiral library of left and right enantiomers, the sample will be further analyzed with IRMS testing. Adulterated or synthetic-based oil would then be rejected.

This complexity is why oils must be analyzed by an analytical chemist specially trained on the interpretation of gas chromatography and mass spectroscopy. The chemist examines the entire essential oil composition to determine its purity, measuring how various components in the oil occur in relation to each other. If some components occur in higher quantities than others, these provide important clues to determine if the oil is adulterated or pure.

Adulteration is such a major concern that each essential oil Young Living offers is tested initially by GC-MS, and every subsequent batch of essential oil is tested using GC-FID by Young Living's trained research and quality control scientists. Batches that do not meet established standards are rejected and returned to the sender.

Adulteration of essential oils will become more and more common as the supply of top-quality essential oils dwindles, and demand continues to increase. Adulteration may occur by diluting the essential oil with fatty lipid oils. This is a common practice by some essential oil companies

How Essential Oils Work | **Chapter 2**

to increase supply and reduce cost. Other methods include adulterating with synthetic components or using a cheaper essential oil to increase volume and maximize profits. These adulterated essential oils will jeopardize the integrity of aromatherapy and essential oil use.

## Adulterated Oils and Their Dangers

Today much of the lavender oil sold in America is a hybrid called lavandin, grown and distilled throughout the world. Lavandin is often heated to evaporate the camphor, mixed with synthetic linalyl acetate to improve the fragrance, and then sold as lavender oil. Most consumers don't know the difference and are happy to buy it for $7 to $10 per half ounce in various stores and on the Internet. This is one of the reasons why it is important to know about the integrity of the essential oil company or vendor.

Adulterated and mislabeled essential oils may present dangers for consumers. One woman who had heard of the ability of lavender oil to heal burns used "lavender oil" purchased from a local health food store when she spilled boiling water on her arm. But the pain intensified and the burn worsened, so she later complained that lavender oil was worthless for healing burns. When her "lavender" oil was analyzed, it was found to be lavandin, a hybrid of lavender that is biologically different from pure *Lavandula angustifolia*. Lavandin contains higher levels of camphor (7-18 percent), which may burn the skin. In contrast, true lavender contains almost no camphor and has burn-healing agents not found in lavandin.

Jean Valnet, MD, wrote about a similar instance in his book, *The Practice of Aromatherapy*:

> A man was being treated for a fistula [an abnormal channel or opening in the skin] of the anus by instillation of pure and natural drops of lavender essence. The patient had begun to recover when he went on a journey, and, discovering he had left his essence at home, bought a fresh supply at a chemist's [drugstore]. Unfortunately this essence was neither natural nor pure: one single installation was followed by a painful inflammation of such severity that the unfortunate person was unable to sit down for more than a fortnight.[5]

In France production of true lavender oil (*Lavandula angustifolia*) dropped from 87 tons in 1967 to only 12 tons in 1998. During this same period, the worldwide demand for lavender oil grew over 100 percent. So where did essential oil marketers obtain enough lavender to meet the demand? They probably used a combination of synthetic and adulterated oils. There are huge chemical companies on the east coast of the U.S. that specialize in creating synthetic chemicals that can mimic every common essential oil. For every kilogram of pure essential oil that is produced, an estimated 10 to 100 kilograms of synthetic oil are created.

Adulterated oils that are mixed with synthetic extenders can be very detrimental, causing rashes, burns, and skin irritations. Common additives such as propylene glycol, DEP, or DOP (solvents that have no smell and increase the volume) can cause allergic reactions, besides being devoid of any therapeutic effects.

Some people assume that because an essential oil is "100 percent pure," it will not burn their skin. This is not true. Some pure essential oils may cause skin irritation if applied undiluted. If straight oregano oil is applied to the skin of some people, it may cause severe reddening. Citrus and spice oils like orange and cinnamon may also produce rashes. Even the terpenes in conifer oils like pine may cause skin irritation on sensitive people.

Many tourists in Egypt are eager to buy local essential oils, especially lotus oil. Vendors convince the tourists that the oils are 100 percent pure by touching a lighted match to the neck of the oil container to show that the oil is not diluted with alcohol or other petrochemical solvents. However, this test provides no reliable indicator of purity. Many synthetic compounds that are not flammable can be added to an essential oil, including propylene glycol. Furthermore, some natural essential oils high in terpenes can be flammable.

Some researchers feel that because of their complexity, essential oils do not disturb the body's natural balance or homeostasis: if one constituent exerts too strong an effect, another constituent may block or counteract it. However, synthetic chemicals, like pharmaceuticals, usually have only one action and may disrupt the body's homeostasis and cause various adverse side effects.

Seventh Edition | **Essential Oils Desk Reference** | 25

**Essential Oils Desk Reference** | Seventh Edition

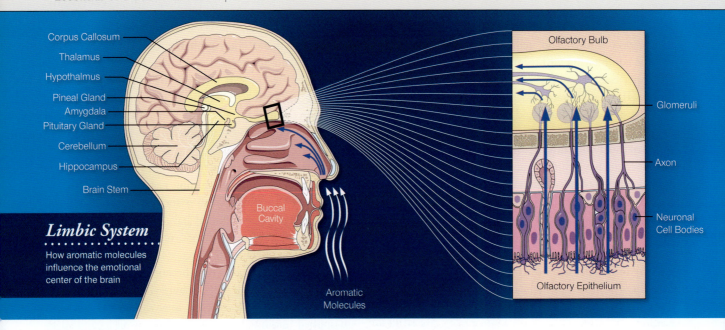

## Powerful Influence of Aromas

The fragrance of an essential oil can directly affect everything from your emotional state to your lifespan. The specific mechanics of the sense of smell are still being explored by scientists but have been described as working like a lock and key or an odor molecule fitting a specific receptor site.

When a fragrance is inhaled, the airborne odor molecules travel up the nostrils to the olfactory epithelium or the center of olfactory sensation. At the olfactory epithelium, which is only about 1 square inch of the nasal cavity, olfactory receptor cells are triggered and send an impulse to the olfactory bulb. Each olfactory receptor type sends an impulse to a particular microregion, or glomerulus, of the olfactory bulb. There are around 2,000 glomeruli in the olfactory bulb, which receive the impulses from the olfactory receptors and allow us to perceive many smells. The olfactory bulb then transmits the impulses to other parts of the brain, including the gustatory center (where the sensation of taste is perceived), the amygdala (where emotional memories are stored), and other parts of the limbic system.

Because the limbic system is directly connected to those parts of the brain that control heart rate, blood pressure, breathing, memory, stress levels, and hormone balance, essential oils can have profound physiological and psychological effects.

An article in *Scientific American* December 15, 2006, raised an interesting question regarding the lock and key theory: "the shape theory doesn't explain why some nearly identically shaped molecules smell vastly different, such as ethanol, which smells like vodka, and ethane thiol (rotten eggs)."[6]

Another theory of smell, called the vibration theory, is proposed by an Italian scientist named Luca Turin in a paper published in 1996. He theorizes that rather than the "lock and key" theory of olfaction, it is the vibrational properties of molecules that enable us to distinguish smells. He suggests that the olfactory receptors sense the quantum vibration of each odorants' atoms, which would allow humans to perceive almost limitless numbers of odors, as olfactory receptors are tuned to different frequencies.

While the vibrational theory is still somewhat controversial, Jennifer Brookes, a University College London researcher based at MIT, was lead author on a study that discusses models of receptor selectivity, including those based on shape and other factors like vibrational frequencies.[7] Speaking of Turin's theory, she told the BBC in March 2011, "It's a very interesting idea; there's all sorts of interesting biological physics that implement quantum processes that's cropping up. I believe it's time for the idea to develop and for us to get on with testing it." A colleague of Brookes, A. P. Horsfield, of Imperial College London, was also interviewed by the BBC about the vibrational theory and said, "There's still lots to understand, but the idea that it cannot possibly be right is no longer tenable really. The theory has to at least be considered respectable at this point."[8]

In February of 2015 writer Christina Agapakis discussed the reasoning of the original proponent of the vibration theory, chemist Malcom Dyson, who proposed the theory in 1928.

> For Dyson, the idea that molecular vibrations might underlie our sense of smell suggested a tantalizing symmetry with our other senses. The rods and cones in our retinas respond to the vibrating wavelengths of light; the hair cells in our ear activate in response to the frequencies of sound waves vibrating in the air. Is smell also a vibrational sense?[9]

Whatever the mechanism, the sense of smell is the only one of the five senses directly linked to the limbic lobe of the brain, the emotional control center. Anxiety, depression, fear, anger, and joy all emanate from this region. The scent of a special fragrance can evoke memories and emotions before we are even consciously aware of it. When smells are concerned, we react first and think later. All other senses (touch, taste, hearing, and sight) are routed through the thalamus, which acts as the switchboard for the brain, passing stimuli onto the cerebral cortex (the conscious thought center) and other parts of the brain.

The limbic lobe (a group of brain structures that includes the hippocampus and amygdala located below the cerebral cortex) can also directly activate the hypothalamus, which is one of the most important parts of the brain. It controls body temperature, hunger, thirst, fatigue, sleep, and circadian cycles. It acts as our hormonal control center and releases hormones that can affect many functions of the body. The production of growth hormones, sex hormones, thyroid hormones, and neurotransmitters such as serotonin are all governed by the hypothalamus.

Essential oils—through their fragrance and unique molecular structure—can directly stimulate the limbic lobe and the hypothalamus, which is responsive to olfactory stimuli. Not only can the inhalation of essential oils be used to combat stress and emotional trauma, but it can also stimulate the production of hormones from the hypothalamus. This results in increased thyroid hormones (our energy hormone) and growth hormones (our youth and longevity hormone).

Essential oils may also be used to reduce appetite and increase satiety through their ability to stimulate the hypothalamus, which governs our feeling of satiety or fullness following meals. In a large clinical study, Alan Hirsch, MD, used fragrances, including peppermint, to trigger weight loss in a large group of patients (over 3,000 individuals) who had previously been unsuccessful in any type of weight-management program.[10] The amount of weight loss among the subjects directly correlated with the frequency of their use of their aroma inhalers. One group in the study lost an average of 4.7 pounds per month over the course of the six months. Hirsch suggests that by inhaling certain aromas, individuals with good olfaction may have induced and sustained weight loss over a 6-month period.

Another double-blind, randomized study by Hirsch documents the ability of aroma to enhance libido and sexual arousal.[11] When 31 male volunteers were subjected to the aromas of 30 different essential oils, each one exhibited a marked increase in arousal, based on measurements of brachial penile index and the measurement of both penile and brachial blood pressures. Among the scents that produced the highest increase in penile blood flow was a combination of lavender and pumpkin fragrances. This study shows that fragrances can enhance sexual arousal by stimulating the limbic system, the emotional center of the brain.

People who have undergone nose surgery or suffer olfactory impairment may find it difficult or impossible to completely detect an odor. These people may not derive the full physiological and emotional benefits of essential oils and their fragrances.

Proper stimulation of the olfactory nerves may offer a powerful and entirely new form of therapy that could be used as an adjunct against many forms of illness. Essential oils, through inhalation, may occupy a key position in this relatively unexplored frontier in medicine.

No one need ever dismiss essential oils as simple perfumes. Now you can understand the complexity and value of each essential oil with its hundreds of different components.

## ENDNOTES

1. Stewart D. *The Chemistry of Essential Oils Made Simple: God's Love Manifest in Molecules.* Care Publications, Marble Hill, MO: 2006.

2. Franchomme P, Pénoël D. *L'aromathérapie exactement.* Roger Jollois, ed., France 31 Août 2003.

3. Gönüz A, Özörgüzü B. An investigation on the morphology, anatomy and ecology of *Origanum onites* L. Tr. *J. of Botany* 1999 23:19-32.

4. Woolley CL, Young DG, et al. Chemical differentiation of *Boswellia sacra* and *Boswellia carterii* essential oils by gas chromatography and chiral gas chromatography-mass spectrometry. *J Chromatog A.* 2012 Oct 26;1261:158-63.

5. Valnet J. *The Practice of Aromatherapy.* Healing Arts Press, Rochester, VT, 1982, p. 27.

6. Minkel JR. Is Sense of Smell Powered by Quantum Vibrations? *Scientific American,* December 15, 2006.

7. Brookes JC, Horsfield AP, Stoneham AM. Odour character differences for enantiomers correlate with molecular flexibility, *J.R. Soc. Interface* (2009) 6, 75-86.

8. Palmer J. Quantum physics explanation for smell gains traction, BBC, March 24, 2011.

9. Agapakis C, Osmic Frequencies, *The New Inquiry,* February 13, 2015.

10. Hirsch AR, Gomez R. Weight reduction through inhalation of odorants. *J. Neurol. Orthop. Med. Surg.* 1995 16:28-31.

11. Hirsch AR, Gruss JJ. Human male sexual response to olfactory stimuli. *J. Neurol. Orthop. Med. Surg.* 1999 19(1):14-19.

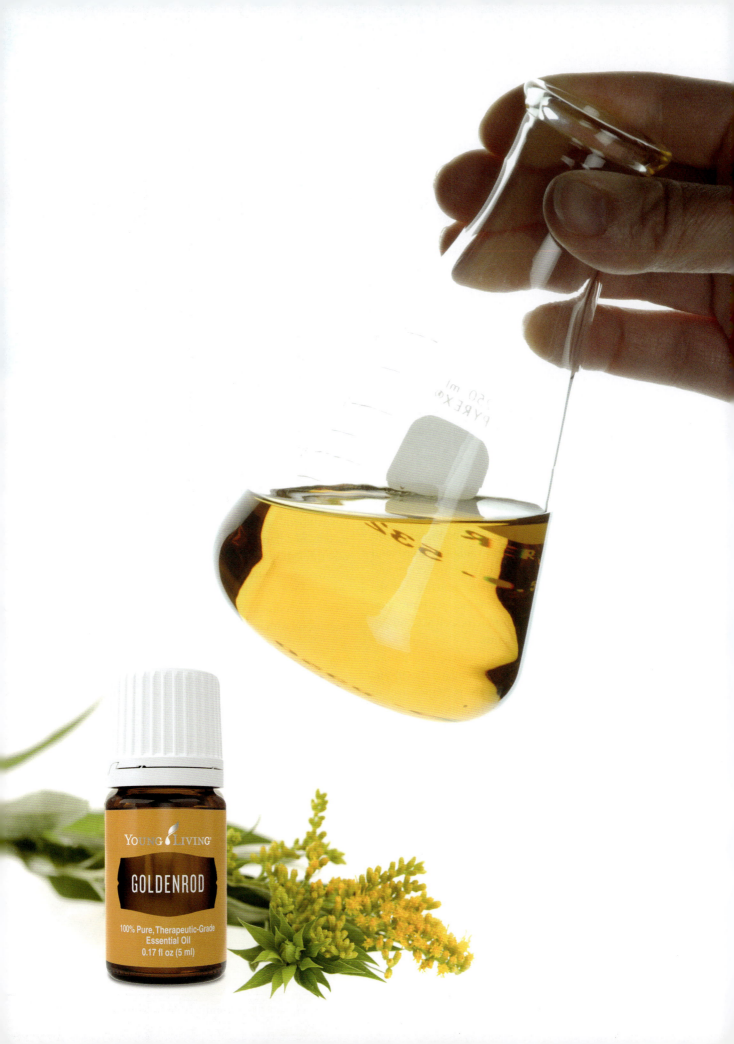

# Chapter 3
## Scientific Research and Documentation

## Essential Oil Science

In 1937 the man who coined the term "aromatherapy," Dr. René Maurice Gattefossé, published the first modern book on the discipline of using essential oils therapeutically. In the foreword to his groundbreaking work, Dr. Gattefossé wrote, "Besides their antiseptic and bactericidal properties widely used today (in part thanks to our work), essential oils possess anti-toxic and antiviral properties, have a powerful vitalizing action, an undeniable healing power and extensive therapeutic properties, as we have demonstrated and this work documents."[1]

"From time immemorial," he wrote, "in every country, aromatic plants have always been considered the most effective treatment for the diseases afflicting mankind. In many cases, the essential oil is used, which is evidence that the volatile part is the most effective."

At the time his book was published, Dr. Gattefossé observed, "The numerous papers, theses and observations made on this subject by the large number of scientists interested since 1907 when our work on the subject commenced, and published in journals and special bulletins, are hard and sometimes impossible to find."[2]

From this humble, modern-day beginning, researchers and scientists from around the world have continued Gattefossé's work. Surely Dr. Gattefossé would be gratified to know that his beloved essential oils remain on the cutting edge of science in solving problems he never could have imagined.

### An Agricultural Practice Births Killer Microbes

The 1940s brought the glory days of antibiotics. Dr. Gattefossé would not have believed just six decades later resistant bacteria would hurtle medicine back to the pre-antibiotic era.

How deadly are the antibiotic-resistant bacteria? The U.S. Centers for Disease Control and Prevention (CDC) reports that every year in the U.S. at least 2 million people are infected with antibiotic-resistant bacteria, and at least 23,000 people die each year as a direct result of these infections.

These statistics are no longer the worst of the bacterial bad news. From a study[3] published in November 2015, the worst news is that the last-resort antibiotic has now been conquered by a bacterial enemy: *Escherichia coli*, popularly known as E. coli.

The bacterial onslaught of antibiotic resistance started with Methicillin-Resistant *Staphylococcus aureus* (MRSA), then progressed to bacteria that were *Multidrug*-Resistant, quickly expanding to *Extensively* Drug Resistant, and now, alas, we have *Pan-Drug*-Resistant. That's "*pan*" meaning "*all*" (as in pandemic). We now have pan-drug resistant bacteria that are resistant to *all known antibiotics*. As of this writing, no research has been conducted on essential oils against the pan-drug resistant E. coli bacteria.

A leading cause of antibiotic resistance? Concentrated Animal Feeding Operations (CAFO). Animals raised for food are given *sub-inhibitory* amounts of antibiotics to increase growth. The sub-inhibitory amounts kill weaker bacteria but allow the stronger bacteria to become resistant. (This is why doctors always tell you to finish an antibiotic because if don't take it all, you are teaching the bacteria how to defeat the antibiotic.) The numbers are shocking: *80 percent* of antibiotics used in the United States are used for livestock farming. The last-resort antibiotic, colistin, no longer effective against E. coli (this pan-resistant E. coli strain is now found in China and has spread to Europe in Denmark), is given to food animals in China in horrific numbers. "China alone uses 12,000 tons of colistin in animal farming each year. The US uses 800 tons annually, and another 400 tons is used in Europe."[4] Until this practice is stopped, antibiotic resistance will continue to grow.

Antibacterial soaps containing the chemical triclosan have become a popular answer to antibacterial resistance.

Seventh Edition | **Essential Oils Desk Reference** | 29

Thankfully, on September 2, 2016, the FDA issued a final ruling that triclosan (for liquid soaps) and triclocarban (bar soaps) cannot be marketed because manufacturers failed to prove the ingredients "are both safe for long-term daily use and more effective than plain soap and water in preventing illness and the spread of certain infections."[5]

It is not surprising that many virulent strains of bacteria became resistant to triclosan. *E. coli, Salmonella enterica, Staphylococcus aureus,* and *Mycobacterium tuberculosis* are able to fight triclosan with a cellular mechanism called a bacterial efflux pump that discharges the antibacterial agent and any other antimicrobial or antibiotic away from the cell. Chicago hospitals and nursing homes reported an increase of a drug-resistant bacteria *Klebsiella pneumoniae Carbapenemase* (KPC) that kills 40 percent of its victims. The superbug *Clostridium difficile* (C-diff, for short) sickens about 500,000 Americans a year, causing 15,000 to 20,000 deaths. It is now considered a rival to MRSA (methicillin-resistant *Staphylococcus aureus*).

## The New, But Ancient, Weapon Against Drug-resistant Bacteria

As the number of antibiotics known to fight these virulent killers dwindles, the amazing natural power of essential oils has captured researchers' attention. A 2008 study by D. Gary Young, ND; Sue Chao; Craig Oberg, PhD; and Karen Nakaoka, PhD, published in the *Flavour and Fragrance Journal,* reported that 78 out of 91 essential oils tested inhibited MRSA.[6] Lemongrass, Lemon Myrtle, Mountain Savory, Cinnamon, and Melissa essential oils had the highest rates of inhibition against MRSA. The oil blends R.C., Motivation, and Longevity had the strongest inhibition of oil blends tested.

Cinnamon essential oil was tested and found to enhance the antimicrobial drug clindamycin against C. difficile.[7] The chemical constituents of *Eucalyptus globulus,* aromadendrene, 1,8-cineole, and globulol, were also effective against multidrug-resistant bacteria. The 2010 study reported, "The oil exerted a marked inhibition against multidrug-resistant bacteria such as methicillin-resistant *Staphylococcus aureus* (MRSA) and vancomycin-resistant enterococci (VRE) *Enterococcus faecalis.*"[8] The individual constituents worked in "a synergistic effect."

A British study tested geranium and lemongrass essential oil vapors against antibiotic-sensitive and -resistant bacteria, including MRSA, vancomycin-resistant *enterococci* (VRE), *Acinetobacter baumanii,* and *Clostridium difficile.* The combined oil vapor effected an 89 percent reduction of airborne bacteria.[9]

## *Pneumonia Superbug Strikes California*

On March 23, 2011, it was reported that medical facilities in Los Angeles County, California, had been hit with 356 cases of a multiresistant pneumonia with a high mortality rate. Most cases were in long-term care facilities, but some cases have been found in hospitals.

The bacterium is called Carbapenem-resistant *Klebsiella pneumoniae,* or CRKB. It causes pneumonia-like symptoms and has a prominent polysaccharide capsule surrounding the cell that defends against the super-antibiotics called carbapenem.

*The Mercury News* quoted infectious disease expert Dr. Brad Spellberg, a physician at County Harbor–UCLA Medical Center, who said, "This is scary stuff. It cannot be treated with any antibiotic that we know of. . . . We're at the point with some of this [resistant bacteria] that we're just mixing a bunch of crap together, throwing it at the patient and crossing our fingers."[10]

A December 2015 study reported that the essential oils of a variety of eucalyptus showed synergy with three conventional antibiotics: ciprofloxacin, gentamicin, and polymyxin B (a pharmaceutical cousin to colistin) against multidrug-resistant *Acinetobacter baumannii,* leading to hopes for new treatment strategies against multidrug-resistant strains.[11]

## Essential Oil Complexity: A Weapon Against Bacterial Resistance

An infectious disease specialist at Louis Stokes Cleveland V.A. Medical Center and Case Western Reserve University, Dr. Louis B. Rice, warned, "There are strains out there, and they are becoming more and more common, that are resistant to virtually every antibiotic we have."[12] Antibiotics may crumble before these "germs on steroids," but essential oils do not.

The multitude of chemical constituents that make up a single essential oil present bacteria with a puzzle that cannot be solved. The mosaic of hundreds of chemical constituents simply do not allow for bacterial resistance.

Beginning in the mid-'90s, scientists began to notice the unexpected gift of essential oils against resistant bacteria. The earliest study is a 1995 Australian study that found 68 isolates of MRSA were susceptible to tea tree oil.[13] In a study on an essential oil-containing dentifrice on dental plaque microbial composition, researchers observed, "Additionally, there was no evidence of the development of bacterial resistance to the antimicrobial activity of the essential oils or the emergence of opportunistic pathogens."[14]

Scientific Research and Documentation | **Chapter 3**

A study of lemon verbena and lemongrass essential oil against the bacteria that causes ulcers caused the scientists to marvel about the power of lemongrass: "Resistance to lemongrass did not develop even after 10 sequential passages, whereas resistance to clarithromycin developed under the same conditions."[15]

Two antiseptic mouthwashes were compared for their control of plaque and gingivitis. While the chemically based mouthwash can cause brown spots on the teeth and tongue, the essential oil mouthwash was effective with no adverse effects and "no evidence of antimicrobial resistance."[16]

In 2009 essential oils were tested against several common and hospital-acquired bacterial and yeast isolates (6 Staphylococcus strains, including MRSA, 4 Streptococ-cus strains, and 3 Candida strains, including *Candida krusei*). The oils tested were eucalyptus, tea tree, white thyme, lavender, lemon, lemongrass, cinnamon, grapefruit, clove bud, sandalwood, peppermint, Kunzea, and sage.

The strongest inhibition was observed with white thyme, lemon, lemongrass, and cinnamon oils, while the other oils showed "considerable efficacy." The control group produced no efficacy. The conclusion: ". . . essential oils represent a cheap and effective antiseptic topical treatment option even for antibiotic-resistant strains [such] as MRSA and antimycotic-resistant Candida species."[17] Keep an eye on the website of the National Library of Medicine, PubMed, for upcoming research on essential oils against pandrug-resistant bacteria.

## Worldwide Research

The U.S. National Library of Medicine (pubmed.gov) is the largest medical library in the world. This online library contains more than 25 million citations for biomedical literature from MEDLINE, life science journals, and online books. Essential oils are represented in 17,483 peer-reviewed medical studies, as of August 29, 2016.

The most recent research on essential oils includes a wide array of topics. Italian researchers studied the neuroprotective effects of bergamot. In Iceland, researchers tested basil against otitis media (ear infection). Texas Southern University researchers looked at the antioxidant and free radical scavenging power of essential oils. In Germany, a study observed the effects of myrtol (from myrtle), eucalyptus, and orange oil for patients with chronic obstructive pulmonary disease. In Iran, researchers found lavender oil inhalation lowered plasma cortisol levels in patients awaiting open-heart surgery.

We now know it is feasible to wash away *Salmonella enterica* contamination on grape tomatoes with thyme oil, thymol, and carvacrol instead of a chlorine-based washing solution. This 2010 study at the University of Delaware concluded that thymol was the most effective without affecting color or taste of the tomatoes.

Brazilian scientists studied the gastroprotective activity of clove oil, while Iranian researchers discovered the healing advantages of lavender essential oil in healing episiotomies following childbirth. The immune-modifying and antimicrobial effects of eucalyptus oil were studied, and frankincense oil was found to induce tumor cell specific toxicity at the University of Oklahoma by HK Lin, PhD.

Clinical research during the last several decades indicates that essential oils have enormous potential to treat conditions ranging from acne to obesity. The following are just a few examples of the on-going research in the world of natural solutions for dysfunction and disease.

Peppermint (*Mentha piperita*) has been reviewed for its ability to block pain, relieve headaches,[18] combat indigestion,[19] boost mental alertness,[20] induce weight loss,[21] kill lice,[22] and inhibit tumor growth.[23]

Tea Tree (*M. alternifolia*) has been used to treat acne,[24] kill fungi,[25] and inhibit bacteria growth.[26,27] Lavender (*Lavandula angustifolia*) fights travel sickness,[28] reduces atherosclerosis,[29] acts as a local anaesthetic,[30] has anticonvulsant properties, and initiates human immune response to *Staphylococcus aureus,* responsible for the most important nosocomial (hospital acquired) infection.[31]

Clove (*Syzygium aromaticum*) has been researched for its action against tooth decay[32] as well as its antifungal[33] and anticonvulsant activities.[34]

Rosemary (*Rosmarinus officinalis*) has been shown to enhance alertness,[35] combat fungi such as Candida albicans,[36] and act as an antioxidant.[37]

Orange (*Citrus sinensis*) halts fungus infection[38,39] and inhibits tumor formation.[40] Limonene, an important component of orange and lemon oil, has demonstrated similar tumor-suppressing effects in studies at Indiana University.[41]

Basil (*Ocimum basilicum*) has been shown to have anticancer properties.[42]

Eucalyptus (*E. radiata*) contains 1,8-cineole (eucalyptol), which has been studied for reducing inflammation,[43]

Seventh Edition | **Essential Oils Desk Reference** | 31

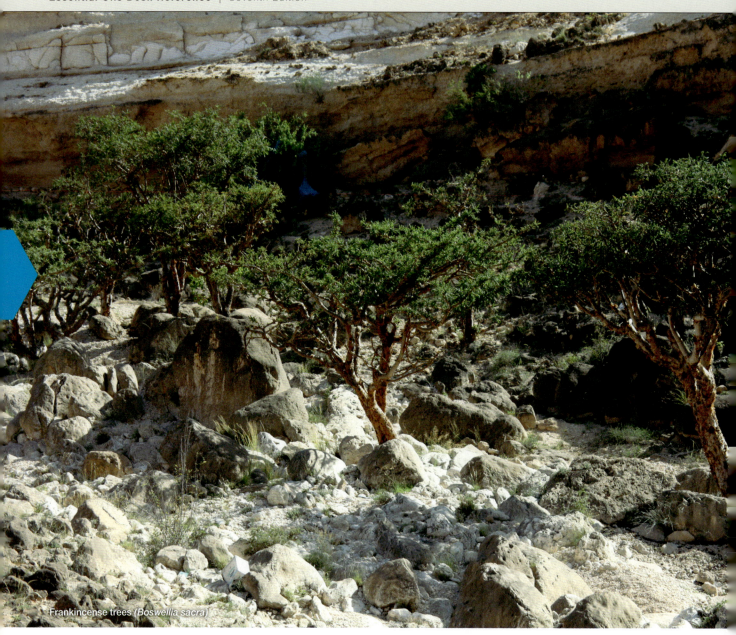

Frankincense trees (*Boswellia sacra*)

improving cerebral blood flow,[44] inhibiting Candida growth,[45] and treating bronchitis.[46]

Many other documented benefits of aromatics have been recorded in recent medical literature.[47-50]

Research conducted at two universities was published in 2002 showing that 58 percent of 60 essential oils and 5 essential oil blends showed general cancer inhibition of 50 percent or better.[51] Researchers continue to open new frontiers of study on the health-supporting effects of essential oils.

Whether the topic is mood enhancement, memory, hypertension, Alzheimer's disease, anxiety in a dental office, cancer, or anti-inflammatory action, current medical research on essential oils can be found by searching the PubMed website.

### Recent Research by D. Gary Young

From 2011-2013 D. Gary Young, ND, published four studies on *Boswellia sacra*, known as Sacred Frankincense, in collaboration with Cole Woolley, PhD; Mahmoud Suhail, MD; and HK Lin, PhD.[52-55] In 2014 Gary co-authored a study[56] on *Boswellia carterii*, and in 2015 he published a review study[57] in the *Journal of Environmental Analytical Chemistry* on detecting essential oil adulteration.

## ENDNOTES

1. Réne-Maurice Gattefossé, *Gattefossé's Aromatherapy*, 1993, CW Daniel Co. LTD, page *xii*.

2. Ibid, page *xi*.

3. Liu YY, et al. Emergence of plasmid-mediated colistin resistance mechanism MCR-1 in animals and human beings in China: a microbiological and molecular biological study. *Lancet Infect Dis.* 2015 Nov 18. [Epub ahead of print]

4. Mercola J. http://articles.mercola.com/sites/articles/archive/2015/12/02/antibiotic-resistance-apocalypse.aspx.

5. http://www.fda.gov/NewsEvents/Newsroom/PressAnnouncements/ucm517478.htm.

6. Chao SC, et al. Inhibition of methicillin-resistant *Staphylococcus aureus* (MRSA) by essential oils, *Flavour Frag. J. 2008* Nov;23:444-449.

7. Shahverdi AR, et al. Trans-cinnamaldehyde from Cinnamomum zeylanicum bark essential oil reduces the clindamycin resistance of Clostridium difficile in vitro. *J Food Sci.* 2007 Jan;72(1):S055-8.

8. Mulyaningsih S, et al. Synergistic properties of the terpenoids aromadendrene and 1,8 cineole from the essential oil of *Eucalyptus globulus* against antibiotic-susceptible and antibiotic-resistant pathogens, *Phytomedicine.* 2010 Nov;17(13):1061-1066.

9. Doran AL, et al. Vapour-phase activities of essential oils against antibiotic sensitive and resistant bacteria including MRSA, *Lett Appl Microbiol.* 2009 Apr;48(4):387-392.

10. Evans M. 356 'superbug' cases found in county medical facilities, *The Mercury News,* March 24, 2011.

11. Knezevic P, et al. Antimicrobial activity of *Eucalyptus camaldulensis* essential oils and their interactions with conventional antimicrobial agents against multi-drug resistant *Acinetobacter baumannii. J Ethnopharmacol.* 2015 Dec 6. [Epub ahead of print]

12. https://cwrumedicine.wordpress.com/2010/02/28/ny-times-id-expert-dr-louis-rice-discusses-rising-threat-of-infections-unfazed-by-antibiotics/.

13. Carson CF, et al. Susceptibility of methicillin-resistant *Staphylococcus aureus* to the essential oil of *Melaleuca alternifolia. J Antimrob Chemother,* 1995 Mar;35(3):421-4.

14. Charles CH, et al. Effect of an essential-oil containing dentifrice on dental plaque microbial composition, *Am J Dent.* 2000 Sep;13(Spec No):26C-30C.

15. Ohno T, et al. Antimicrobial activity of essential oils against *Helicobacter pylori. Helicobacter.* 2003 Jun;8(3):207-215.

16. Santos A. Evidence-based control of plaque and gingivitis, *J Clin Periodontol.* 2003 30(Suppl 5):13-16.

17. Warnke PH, et al. The battle against multi-resistant strains: Renaissance of antimicrobial essential oils as a promising force to fight hospital-acquired infections. *J Craniomaxillofac Surg.* 2009 Oct;37(7):392-397.

18. Gobel H, et al. Effect of peppermint and eucalyptus oil preparations on neurophysiological and experimental algesimetric headache parameters. *Cephalalgia.* 1994 Jun;14(3):228-234.

19. Dalvi SS, et al. Effect of peppermint oil on gastric emptying in man: a preliminary study using a radiolabelled solid test meal. *Indian J Physiol Pharmacol.* 1991 Jul;35(3):212-4.

20. Dember WN, et al. Olfactory Stimulation and Sustained Attention. *Compendium of Olfactory Research 1982-1994, Kendall/Hunt Publishing Company* 1995; 39-46.

21. Hirsch A. A Scentsational Guide to Weight Loss. Rockport, MA: Element, 1997.

22. Veal L. The potential effectiveness of essential oils as a treatment for headlice, Pediculus humanus capitis. *Complement Ther Nurs Midwifery* 1996 Aug;2(4):97-101.

23. Russin WA, et al. Inhibition of rat mammary carcinogenesis by monoterpenoids. *Carcinogenesis* 1989 Nov;10(11):2161-2164.

24. Bassett IB, et al. A comparative study of tea-tree oil versus benzoylperoxide in the treatment of acne. *Med J Aust* 1990 Oct;153(8):455-458.

25. Nenoff P, et al. Antifungal activity of the essential oil of Melaleuca alternifolia (tea tree oil) against pathogenic fungi in vitro. *Skin Pharmacol* 1996;9(6):388-394.

26. Cox SD, et al. The mode of antimicrobial action of the essential oil of Melaleuca alternifolia (tea tree oil). J Appl Microbiol 2000 Jan;88(1):170-175.

27. Carson CF, Riley TV. Antimicrobial activity of the major components of the essential oil of *Melaleuca alternifolia. J Appl Bacteriol* 1995 Mar;78(3):264-269.

28. Bradshaw RH, et al. Effects of lavender straw on stress and travel sickness in pigs. *J Altern Complement Med* 1998;4(3):271-275.

29. Nikolaevskii VV, et al. Effect of essential oils on the course of experimental atherosclerosis. *Patol Fiziol Eksp Ter* 1990 Sep-Oct;5:52-53.

30. Ghelardini C, et al. Local anaesthetic activity of the essential oil of *Lavandula angustifolia. Planta Med* 1999 Dec;65(8):700-703.

31. Giovannini D, et al. *Lavendula angustifolia* Mill. Essential Oil Exerts Antimicrobial and Anti-Inflammatory Effect in Macrophage Mediated Immune Response to *Staphylococcus aureus.* Immunol Invest. 2016 Jan;45(1):11-28.

32. Cai L, Wu CD. Compounds from Syzygium aromaticum possessing growth inhibitory activity against oral pathogens. *J Nat Prod* 1996 Oct;59(10):987-990.

33. Fu Y, et al. Antimicrobial activity of clove and rosemary essential oils alone and in combination. *Phytother Res* 2007;21(10):989-994.

34. Pourgholami MH, et al. Evaluation of the anticonvulsant activity of the essential oil of *Eugenia caryophyllata* in male mice. *J Ethmopharmacol* 1999 Feb;64(2):167-171.

35. Diego MA, et al. Aromatherapy positively affects mood, EEG patterns of alertness and math computations. *Int J Neurosci.* 1998 Dec;96(3-4):217-224.

36. Fu Y, et al. Antimicrobial activity of clove and rosemary essential oils alone and in combination. *Phytother Res* 2007;21(10):989-994.

37. Lopez-Bote CJ, et al. Effect of dietary administration of oil extracts from rosemary and sage on lipid oxidation in broiler meat. *Br Poult Sci* 1998 May;39(2):235-240.

38. Ramadan W, et al. Oil of bitter orange: new topical antifungal agent. *Int J Dermatol.*1996 Jun;35(6):448-449.

39. Alderman GG, Elmer EH. Inhibition of growth and aflatoxin production of *Aspergillus parasiticus* by citrus oils. *Z Leb Unters-Forsch* 1976; 160(4):353-358.

40. Wattenberg LW, et al. Inhibition of carcinogenesis by some minor dietary constituents. *Princess Takamatsu Symp.* 1985; 16:193-203.

41. Crowell PL. Prevention and therapy of cancer by dietary monoterpenes. *J Nutr.* 1999 Mar;129(3):775S-778S.

42. Aruna K, Sivaramakrishnan VM. Anticarcinogenic effects of the essential oils from cumin, poppy and basil. *Phytother Res* 1996;10:577-580.

43. Juergens UR, et al. Anti-inflammatory activity of 1,8-cineole (eucalyptol) in bronchial asthma: a double blind placebo-controlled trial. *Respir. Med* 2003; 97(3):250-256.

44. Nasel C, et al. Functional imaging of effects of fragrances on the human brain after prolonged inhalation. *Chem Senses* 1994 Aug;19(4):359-364.

45. Steinmetz M, et al. Transmission and scanning electronmicroscopy study of the action of sage and rosemary essential oils and eucalyptol on Candida albicans. *Mycoses.* 1988 Jan;31(1):40-51.

46. Ulmer WT, Schött D. Chronic obstructive bronchitis. Effect of *Gelomyrtol forte* in a placebo-controlled double-blind study. Fortschr Med 1991 Sep;109(27):547-550.

47. Horne D, et al. Antimicrobial Effects of Essential Oils on *Streptococcus pneumoniae. J Essent Oil Res 2001 Sep/Oct;*13(5):387-392.

48. Halliwell B, Gutteridge J. *Free Radicals in Biology and Medicine*, 2nd Edition. (1989), Oxford: Clarendon Press.

49. Recsan Z, et al. Effect of essential oils on the lipids of the retina in the aging rat: a possible therapeutic use. *J Essent Oil Res* 1997;9(1):53-56.

50. Youdim KA, Deans SG. Effect of thyme oil and thymol dietary supplementation on the antioxidant status and fatty acid composition of the ageing rat brain. *Br J Nutr.* 2000 Jan;83(1):87-93.

51. Stevens N. *Natural Synergy: Essential Oils in Cancer Research.* Master's Thesis, Brigham Young University/University of Nevada Las Vegas, August 2002.

52. Suhail M, Young DG, et al. *Boswellia sacra* essential oil induces tumor cell-specific apoptosis and suppresses tumor aggressiveness in cultured human breast cancer cells. *BMC Complement and Altern Med.* 2011, 11:129.

53. Ni X, Young DG, et al. Frankincense essential oil prepared from hydrodistillation of *Boswellia sacra* gum resins induces human pancreatic cancer cell death in cultures and in a xenograft murine model. *BMC Complement and Altern Med.* 2012 Dec 13;12:253.

54. Woolley CL, Young DG, et al. Chemical differentiation of *Boswellia sacra* and *Boswellia carterii* essential oils by gas chromatography and chiral gas chromatography-mass spectrometry. *J Chromatog A.* 2012 Oct 26;1261:158-63.

55. Fung KM, Young DG, et al. Management of basal cell carcinoma of the skin using frankincense (*Boswellia sacra*) essential oil: a case report. *OA Alternative Medicine.* 2013 Jun 01:1(2):14.

56. Dozmorov MG, Young DG, et al. Differential effects of selective frankincense (Ru Xiang) essential oil versus non-selective sandalwood (Tan Xiang) essential oil on cultured bladder cancer cells;: a microarray and bioinformatics study. *Chin Med.* 2014 Jul 2;9:18.

57. Boren KE, Young DG, et al. Detecting Essential Oil Adulteration. *J Environmental Analytical Chemistry.* 2015 2:2.

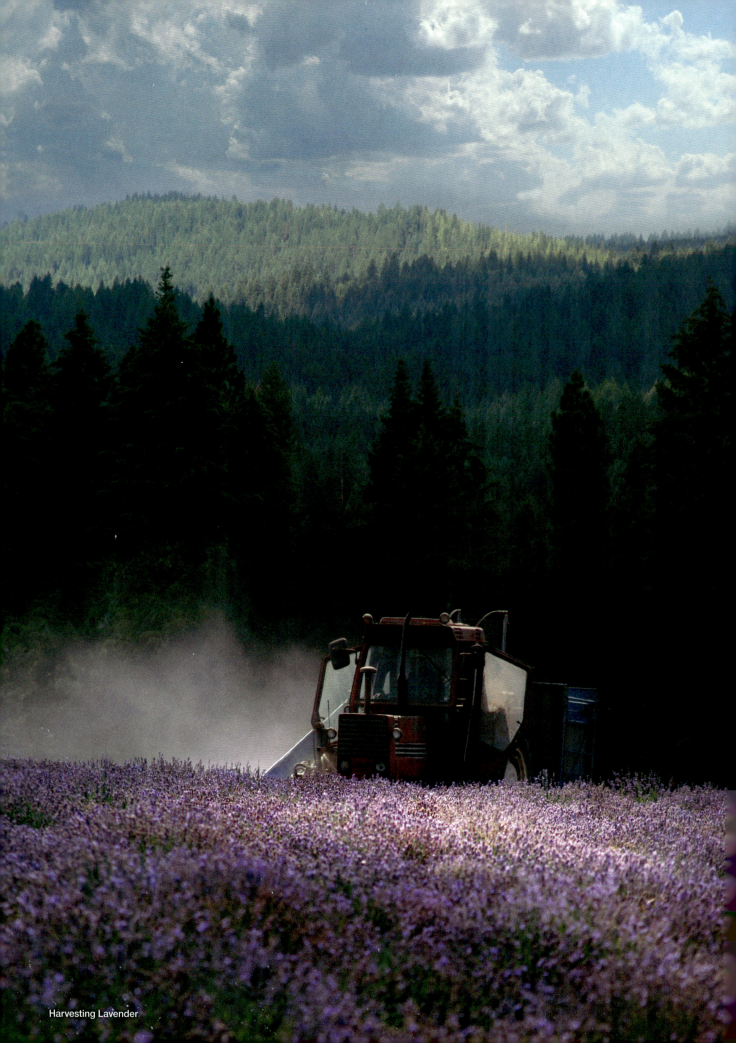
Harvesting Lavender

# Chapter 4
## Producing Therapeutic-Grade™ Essential Oils

## Therapeutic-Grade™ Essential Oils

As we begin to understand the power of essential oils in the realm of personal, holistic health care, we will appreciate the necessity for obtaining the purest essential oils possible. For this reason, the entire process of obtaining oils must be carefully watched over from the beginning to the end. No matter how costly pure essential oils may be, there can be no substitutes.

Just as chemists can synthetically "copycat" the constituents of a pure essential oil, many essential oil companies today label their oils "therapeutic," even though they buy from anonymous brokers and have no experience in meeting any standards. Young Living was the first to establish guidelines that define what a therapeutic essential oil is and to create oils that met or exceeded any known medicinal standard.

Synthetic or nature-identical oils are commonplace in the market and can be created cheaply and then sold in places like health food and drug stores or novelty and tourist shops for a very low price. They have no therapeutic efficacy and may even be harmful. For instance, fragrance-grade lavender may have a harmful effect instead of a healing effect on newly burned skin.

Extended or altered oils may have an essential oil base but are "enhanced" with certain lab-created constituents to increase volume or fragrance. Due to chemical impurities or an antagonistic balance among oil constituents, these oils may be either ineffective or even cause negative effects.

### USDA to Weaken the Purity of the Organic Label?

"Natural" and "organic" essential oils focus on growing in a natural, chemical-free environment but are not concerned with exactness of the time of harvest and the distillation to maximize the therapeutic potency of an essential oil. Such oils may be labeled "100% Pure Certified" or "Natural" but may have subtherapeutic values, and because of a 2011 decision to allow genetically modified alfalfa to be planted

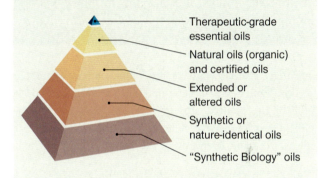

### Grades of Essential Oils

- Therapeutic-grade essential oils
- Natural oils (organic) and certified oils
- Extended or altered oils
- Synthetic or nature-identical oils
- "Synthetic Biology" oils

Five grades of essential oils are produced today:

1. **"Synthetic Biology:"**
In this new adulteration: high value molecules like esters, terpenoids, and aldehydes are recreated from synthetic DNA and then fermented by bioengineered yeasts, fungi, and enzymes. These flavors and fragrances are considered "natural" because they come from yeast, according to FDA and European regulations, and can be used to enhance cheaper oils.

2. **Synthetic or nature-identical oils:**
Created in a laboratory

3. **Extended or altered oils:**
Fragrance grade

4. **Natural oils and certified oils:**
Pass oil-standard tests but may not contain any or just a few therapeutic compounds

5. **Therapeutic-grade essential oils:**
Pure, medicinal, steam-distilled essential oils containing all desired therapeutic compounds

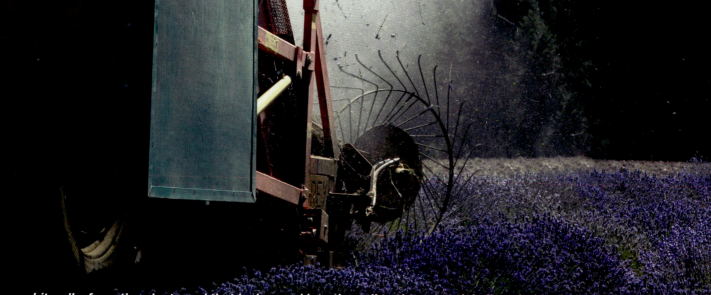

*Literally, from the plant seed that is dropped into the soil to the essential oil sealed in the amber bottle in Young Living's state-of-the-art bottling facility, the Seed to Seal® process is carefully supervised from beginning to end to ensure quality and purity of Young Living pure, therapeutic-grade™ essential oils.*

anywhere,[1] the very word "organic" may soon not guarantee freedom from GMO contamination. In the U.S., by 2014, 94% of the planted area of soybeans, 96% of cotton, and 93% of corn were genetically modified varieties.[2] If one GMO plant is approved, the door has been opened.

## Seed to Seal®

Young Living Essential Oils is the only company dedicated to the medicinal use and application of essential oils that is able to guarantee essential oil quality from seed to seal.

The oils that Young Living provides to consumers are extracted through steam distillation from a wide variety of plants, roots, bushes, trees, and resins and are as powerful and pure as the botanicals from which they are derived.

The life-giving energy of the essential oils that is carefully distilled from nature cannot be duplicated in a sterile laboratory. Synthetic constituents may be similar in structure but have none of the living plant energy that holds the God-given medicinal value of the oil that is released from the plant itself.

In *The Living Energy Universe*[3] by Gary Schwartz, PhD, and Linda Russek, PhD, the authors discuss the theory of "systemic memory." They note that the aromatic compounds contained in roses, for example, will have a different systemic memory than the very same aromatic compounds created chemically in a laboratory. "This implication may help explain why aromatherapy and other natural remedies such as herbs work. When the distiller extracts the 'essential' oils from a plant, he or she may be extracting the 'essential' systemic memories that reflect the wholeness of the plants themselves in addition to the unique combination of physical components that comprise the individual plants."

This is why Young Living takes so much care to capture the pure energy of the plants and guard the entire Seed to Seal process.

Years of experience have resulted in knowing the optimum species with the most therapeutic potential and the optimal time and manner to cultivate and harvest them.

Equally important, the freshly distilled oil is filtered, and stringent laboratory testing verifies the potency of the oil and desired chemical structure. The oil is then poured into bottles in Young Living's clean-room facility and shipped.

Young Living's Seed to Seal process guarantees a genuine, pure essential oil that has the highest therapeutic efficacy. This guarantee includes oils distilled from plants grown on Young Living's own farms, sourced from experienced distillers of many generations, or purchased from distillers who have been directed and taught distilling techniques by D. Gary Young. Young Living's essential oils continue to be used worldwide in more clinical and university studies than any other essential oils today.

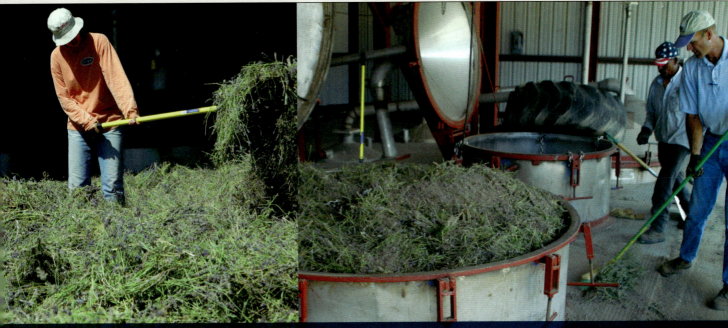

*Curing melissa - Predistillation*

*Young Living Lavender Farms' distillation chambers hold thousands of pounds of plant material.*

### Seed

Herbs are selected for the proper genus, species, and chemotype. Whether seeking Clove oil from Madagascar, Cistus oil from Spain, or Helichrysum oil from Croatia, Young Living experts constantly travel across the globe to verify plant, cultivation, and extraction quality to ensure absolute integrity of the essential oil.

For example, a huge increase in demand for helichrysum and a similar increase in illegal harvesting from poachers spurred Gary Young to purchase a two-story commercial building in Split, Croatia, and build a new distillery with four 4,000-liter and one 6,000-liter boilers, which began distilling helichrysum from Young Living's Croatian partner farm in June 2015.

### Cultivation

Young Living's essential oils are extracted from both wildcrafted and cultivated herbs, from established partnerships with growers and distillers all over the world. Some oils come from herbs cultivated in rural areas of countries such as Taiwan, Australia, Madagascar, Indonesia, and Brazil, harvested by indigenous peoples, who have untold years of experience with the plants and their growing conditions. Other oils come from Young Living farms in Ecuador, France, Canada, Croatia, and the United States, where organic growing practices are adhered to with great care and exactness.

### Organic Herb Farming

The key to producing oils with genuine therapeutic quality starts with the proper cultivation of the herbs in the field.

- Plants should be grown on virgin land uncontaminated by chemical fertilizers, pesticides, fungicides, or herbicides. They should also be grown away from nuclear plants, factories, interstates, highways, and heavily-populated cities, if possible.

- Because robust, healthy plants produce higher quality essential oils, the soil should be nourished with enzymes, minerals, and organic mulch. The mineral content of the soil is crucial to the proper development of the plant, and soils that lack minerals result in plants that produce inferior oils.

- Land and crops should be watered with deep-well, reservoir, or water-shed water. Mountain stream water is best because of its purity and high mineral content. Municipally treated water or secondary run-off water from residential and commercial areas can introduce undesirable chemical residues into the plant and the essential oil.

- Different varieties of plants produce different qualities of oils. Only those plants that produce the highest quality essential oil should be selected.

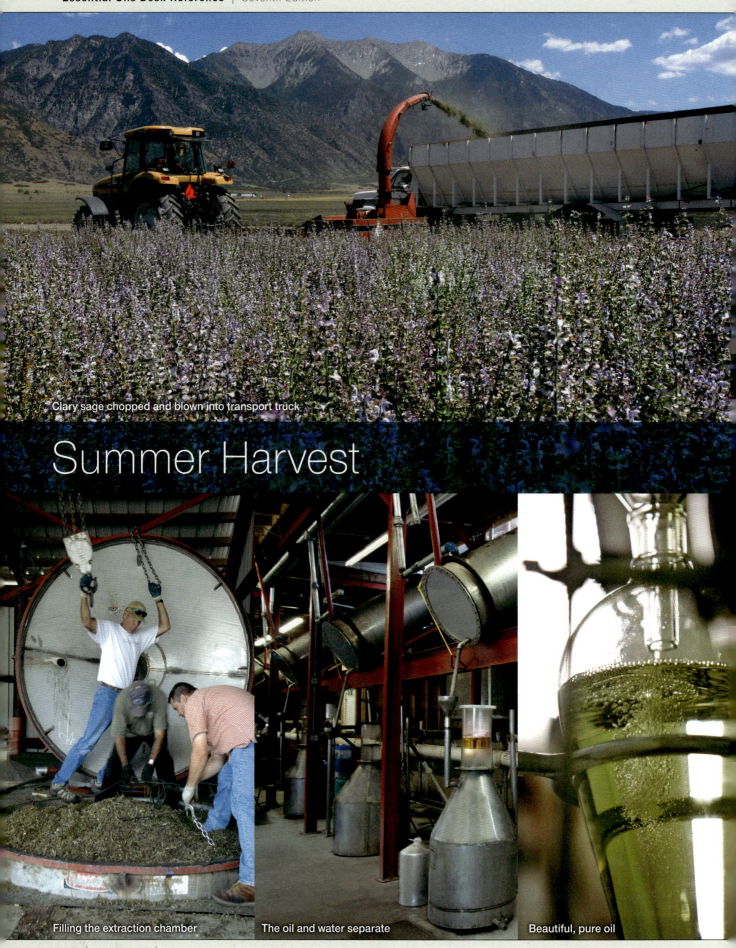

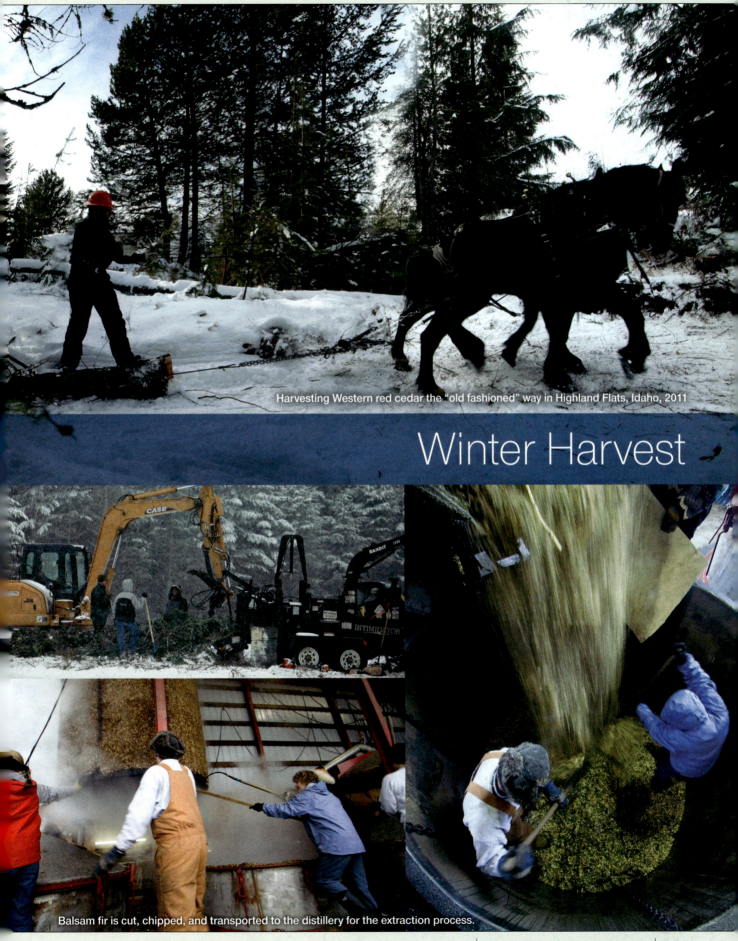

Producing Therapeutic-Grade Essential Oils | Chapter 4

Harvesting Western red cedar the "old fashioned" way in Highland Flats, Idaho, 2011

# Winter Harvest

Balsam fir is cut, chipped, and transported to the distillery for the extraction process.

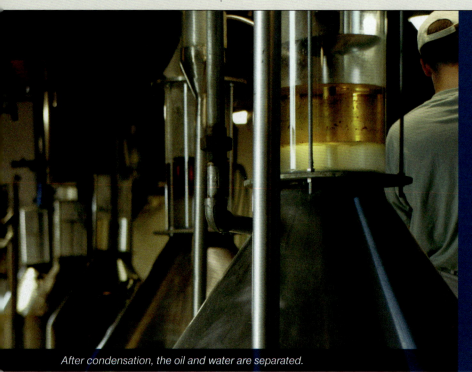
*After condensation, the oil and water are separated.*

## Different Forms of Essential Oil Production

**STEAM DISTILLATION** is a separation process for materials that are temperature sensitive like essential oils. Three methods of steam distillation are simple, hydro, and traditional.

In each of these processes as the steam rises, it carries the released oil vapor into the condenser, where the water and oil vapor convert to a

### Harvesting

The timing of the harvest is one of the most important factors in the production of therapeutic-grade oils. If the plants are harvested at the wrong time of the season or even at the incorrect time of day, they may distill into a substandard essential oil. In some instances, changing harvest time, by even a few hours, can make a huge difference. For example, German Chamomile harvested in the morning will produce oil with far more azulene (a powerful anti-inflammatory compound) than if it is harvested in the late afternoon.

Other factors that should be taken into consideration during the harvest include the amount of dew on the leaves, the percentage of plant in bloom, and weather conditions during the two weeks prior to harvest.

To prevent herbs from drying out prior to being distilled, distillation facilities should be located as close to the field as possible. Transporting herbs to distillation facilities hundreds or thousands of miles away heightens the risk of exposure to pollutants, dust, mold, and petrochemical residues.

Young Living continues to expand and develop strategic partnerships with growers and distillers throughout the world.

### Distillation

A master distiller must oversee the entire process by harvesting at just the right time for the plant maturity and distilling with the proper temperature, pressure, and time, which varies with different plant material. Young Living often experiments with innovative distillation techniques on its farms to maximize therapeutic potency of the oils. Other oils are distilled traditionally, using techniques that have been passed down through generations from father to son.

### Steam Distillation

Steam distillation is a separation process for materials that are temperature sensitive, like essential oils.
**Following are three methods of steam distillation.**

*Simple distillation.* The plant material is loaded into the extraction chamber filled with water, which is heated to soften the plant fiber so that the oil molecules can be released.

As steam begins to rise, the oil molecules are released as vapors, which are carried with the steam into the condenser. The cooling water in the condenser converts the steam to water and the vapors to oil.

The oil and water mixture continues to flow into the separator, where the oil rises to the top of the water so that it can be drained off into containers. Clove and nutmeg are distilled this way.

## Different Forms of Essential Oil Production (continued)

liquid and flow into the separator so that the oil can rise to the top of the water and be drained off.

Steam distillation has many variables. Subtle differences in equipment design and processing conditions can translate into huge differences in essential oil quality. The size and material of the extraction chamber, the type of condenser and separator, and the temperature and pressure can all have a huge impact on the oil quality.

**EXPRESSED OILS** are pressed from the rind of fruits such as grapefruit, lemon, lime, mandarin, orange, and tangerine. Rich in terpene alcohols, expressed oils are not technically "essential oils," even though they are highly regarded for their therapeutic properties and used in the same way as lavender, melaleuca, and other essential oils. Expressed oils should be sourced only from organically grown crops, since pesticide residues can become highly concentrated in the oil.

**ABSOLUTES** are technically not "essential oils" but are "essences." They are obtained from the grain alcohol extraction of a concrete, which is the solid, waxy residue derived from the extraction of plant materials, usually flower petals. This method of extraction is used primarily for botanicals where the fragrance and therapeutic parts of the plant can be unlocked only by using a solvent. Jasmine is extracted this way.

*Hydrodistillation.* Resinous material like frankincense and myrrh are extracted through the method of hydro-distillation.

The resin is immersed in boiling water that is in constant motion while steam is injected into the chamber.

The resinous gas is then released into the steam, which carries it to the condenser, where the steam and vapor are gradually cooled to a liquefied form.

The water and oil mixture travels into the separator so that the oil can flow to the top of the water and be poured off into containers.

*Traditional distillation.* Today, the traditional method of steam distillation is still used around the world.

Plant material is loaded into the extraction chamber and tightly compacted. As the boiler heats the water, steam is released into the bottom of the chamber and starts to travel upward, saturating the material.

The steam impregnates the plant fiber, causing it to release the oil molecule as a gas from the oil glands of the plant. Then the steam carries the gas to the condenser, where it goes through a phase-change condensation as it passes through the cooling process in the swan neck and liquefies into water and oil.

The water and oil mixture then flows into the separator, where the oil can rise to the top of the water to be poured off into containers.

In each of these processes as the steam rises, it carries the released oil vapor into the condenser, where the

water and oil vapor convert to a liquid and flow into the separator so that the oil can rise to the top of the water and be drained off.

### The Art of Distillation

Distillation is as much a science as it is an art. If the pressure or temperature is too high, or if the cooking chambers are constructed from reactive materials, the oil may not be therapeutic grade.

Vertical steam distillation offers the greatest potential for protecting the therapeutic benefits and quality of essential oils. In ancient distillation, low pressure (5 pounds or lower) and low temperature were extremely important to produce the therapeutic benefits. The late Marcel Espieu, who was president of the Lavender Growers Association in Southern France for 20 years, maintained that the best oil quality can be produced only when the pressure is zero pounds during distillation.

Temperature also has a distinct effect. At certain temperatures, the oil fragrance and chemical constituents become altered. High pressures and high temperatures seem to cause harshness in the oil. Even the oil pH and the polarity are greatly affected.

For example, cypress requires a minimum of 24 hours of distillation at 265°F and 5 pounds of pressure to extract most of the therapeutically active constituents. If distillation time is cut by only 2 hours, 18 to 20 constituents will be missing from the resulting oil.

**Essential Oils Desk Reference** | Seventh Edition

# The Distillation Process

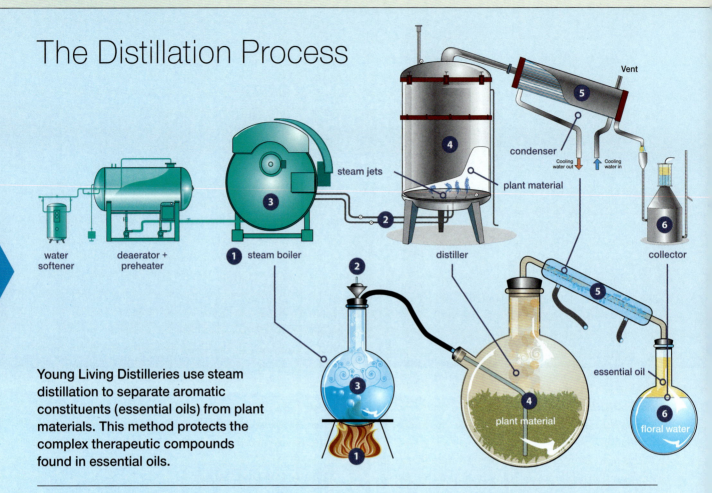

Young Living Distilleries use steam distillation to separate aromatic constituents (essential oils) from plant materials. This method protects the complex therapeutic compounds found in essential oils.

1. **Heat Source:** A hot plate heats the water and converts it into steam.

   At Young Living distilleries, the correct temperature of the steam is crucial, and the degree of heat is determined by the plant being distilled. Gas heaters warm the water, which is stored in massive holding tanks.

2. **Thermometer:** A thermometer is placed inside the heated flask, measuring the temperature of the steam.

   Young Living distillers use a valve to control steam temperature and pressure for extracting essential oils.

3. **Water Flask:** The water is boiled to produce steam, and the steam is routed to and forced below the plant material. As the steam rises, the aromatic oils are removed.

   Water tanks hold gallons of water. As water is turned to steam, it is piped to the bottom of the stainless steel chambers.

4. **Distillation Chamber:** The "cooking" chamber is filled with plant material. As the steam rises through the plants, the aromatic essential oils are released.

   Young Living distilleries have large, stainless steel chambers to produce essential oils. Distilling lavender can take as much as 12,500 liters of lavender stems and flowers to produce 4–5 gallons of essential oil.

5. **Condenser:** Steam with essential oils rises to the top of the chamber, where it is channeled into a cooling area called the condenser. Cold water surrounds the condenser tube, causing the steam with the volatile plant essences to turn back into liquid.

6. **Collecting Flask:** The newly condensed essential oil and water drip into a collecting flask. Because oil is lighter than water, the oil will float to the top of the flask, where it is collected for use.

   The collecting flasks at Young Living distilleries are located one floor below the stills. There, the essential oils are protected from sunlight exposure and kept cool. This protects the therapeutic qualities until the oil is collected and stored in dark glass or stainless steel containers.

Producing Therapeutic-Grade Essential Oils | Chapter 4

# Plant Parts Used to Distill Essential Oils

**Flower**
Amazonian Ylang
   Ylang
Ishpingo
Jasmine
Neroli
Rose
White Lotus
Ylang Ylang

**Flowering Tops**
Blue Tansy
Clary Sage
Clove (Bud and Stem)
Davana
Geranium
German Chamomile
Goldenrod
Helichrysum
Lavandin
Lavender
Ledum
Roman Chamomile
Yarrow

**Fruit/Rind/Berries**
Bergamot
Black Pepper
Coriander
Fennel
Grapefruit

Juniper
Lemon
Jade Lemon
Lime
Mandarin
Orange
Tangerine
Yuzu

**Grasses**
Lemongrass
Xiang Mao

**Gum/Resin**
Biblical Sweet Myrrh
Copaiba
Elemi
Frankincense
Frereana Frankincense
Myrrh
Sacred Frankincense
Onycha

**Leaves/Stems**
Basil
Canadian Fleabane
Cassia
Cistus
Citronella
Citrus Hystrix/
   Combava

Dill
Dorado Azul
Elemi
Eucalyptus Blue
Eucalyptus Citriodora
Eucalyptus Dives
Eucalyptus Globulus
Eucalyptus Polybractea
Eucalyptus Radiata
Eucalyptus Staigeriana
Geranium
Hyssop
Idaho Tansy
Juniper
Kaffir Lime
   (*Citrus hystrix*)
Laurus Nobilis
   (Bay Laurel)
Ledum
Lemon Myrtle
Manuka
Marjoram
Melaleuca Cajuput
Melaleuca Ericifolia
Melaleuca Quinque-
   nervia (Niaouli)
Melissa
Micromeria
Mountain Savory
Myrtle
Ocotea

Oregano
Palmarosa
Patchouli
Peppermint
Petitgrain
Plectranthus Oregano
Ravintsara
Rosemary
Ruta
Sage
Spanish Sage
Spearmint
Tarragon
Tea Tree
Thyme
Vitex
Wintergreen

**Root**
Angelica
Calamus
Ginger
Mugwort
Patchouli
Valerian
Vetiver

**Seed**
Anise
Cardamom
Carrot Seed

Celery Seed
Cumin
Nutmeg

**Wood/Bark/
Twigs/Needles**
Blue Cypress
Cassia
Cedar
Cedarwood
Cinnamon Bark
Cypress
Emerald Cypress
Hinoki
Hong Kuai
Idaho Balsam Fir
Idaho Blue Spruce
Idaho Ponderosa Pine
Lemon Myrtle
Manuka
Northern Lights
   Black Spruce
Palo Santo
Pine
Rosewood
Sandalwood
Spruce
Tsuga
Western Red Cedar
White Fir

However, most commercial cypress oil is distilled for only 2 hours and 15 minutes! This short distillation time allows the producer to cut costs and produces cheaper oil, since money is saved on the fuel needed to generate the steam. It also causes less wear and tear on equipment. Sadly, it results in oil with little or no therapeutic value.

In France, lavender produced commercially is often distilled for only 15 to 20 minutes at 155 pounds of pressure with a steam temperature approaching 350ºF. Although this high-temperature, high-pressure oil costs less to produce and is easily marketed, it is of poor quality. It retains few, if any, of the therapeutic properties of high-grade lavender distilled at zero pounds of pressure for a minimum of 1 hour and 15 minutes.

In many large commercial operations, distillers introduce chemicals into the steam-distillation process to increase the volume of oil produced. Chemical trucks may even pump solvents directly into the boiler water. This expands oil production by as much as 18 percent. These chemicals inevitably leach into the distilling water and mix with the essential oil, fracturing the molecular structure of the oil and altering both its fragrance and therapeutic value. These chemicals remain in the oil after it is sold because it is impossible to completely separate them from the oil.

Another way that essential oil producers increase the quantity of the oil extracted is through redistillation. This refers to the repeated distillation of the plant material to maximize the volume of oil by using second, third, and fourth stages of steam distillation. Each successive distillation generates a weaker and less potent essential oil. Such essential oils are also degraded due to prolonged exposure to water and heat used

Seventh Edition | **Essential Oils Desk Reference** | 43

in the redistillation process. Hydrolysis and/or oxidation of the essential oil occur(s) due to the water and/or heat, and the constituents responsible for its aroma and therapeutic properties begin to chemically break down.

## Combining Traditional Steam Distillation with Modern Technology

Few people appreciate how chemically complex essential oils are. They are rich tapestries of literally hundreds of chemical components, some of which—even in small quantities—contribute important therapeutic benefits. The key to preserving as many as possible of these delicate aromatic constituents is to steam-distill plant material in small batches using low pressure and low heat. This is the traditional method of distillation that has been used for centuries in Europe but is being abandoned in favor of high-volume pressure cookers designed to operate at over 400°F and use over 50 pounds of pressure. More importantly, the cooking chamber where the plants are distilled should be constructed of a nonreactive metal, preferably stainless steel, to reduce the possibility of the essential oil being chemically altered by more reactive metals such as aluminum or copper.

No solvents or synthetic chemicals should be used or added to the water used to generate steam because they might jeopardize the integrity of the essential oil. Even the addition of chemicals to water used in a closed-loop, heat-exchange system of the condenser can be risky, since there is no guarantee that they will be completely isolated from the essential oil. It is unfortunate that many essential oils distilled commercially are processed using boiler water laden with chemicals and descaling agents.

Absolutely no pesticides, herbicides, fungicides, or agricultural chemicals of any kind should be used in the cultivation of herbs earmarked for distillation. These chemicals—even in minute quantities—can react with the essential oil and degrade its purity and quality and render it therapeutically less effective. During distillation, pesticide residue leaches out of the plant material with the extracted essential oil.

## Young Living, the World Leader in Essential Oils and Distillation

During its 20-plus-year history, Young Living Essential Oils has proven again and again to be the world leader in essential oils. With the installation in January 2014 of a state-of-the-art distillery at its Highland Flats Tree Farm in Naples, Idaho, D. Gary Young ushered in a new era in distillation for the production of essential oils and proved that obstacles are no match for his illuminated vision.

### Innovation in Distillery Technology

The distilleries in Highland Flats, Idaho, and Mona, Utah, are the latest innovation in distillery technology, including an advanced computer program that monitors the distillation chamber and condenser and separator temperatures and pressures, starting with the steam injection flow into the extraction chamber to the steam exit and flow temperature levels through the condenser to the separator.

**The first critical factor** is the steam flow volume, which determines the temperature and ability to ramp the steam flow at the precise time to maintain sufficient temperature increase as the oil molecules travel up through the chamber for proper extraction without creating homogenization or reflux that will result in loss of oil, which will compromise the quality. The steam-injection rate and volume are very critical during the entire process.

**The second critical factor** is to make sure the condenser temperature is not too hot or too cold as it descends through 200 12-foot-long tubes to prevent fracturing of the molecules, which could change the chemistry and aroma.

**The third critical factor** is to be sure the temperature of the separator is right because many plants require a different separation temperature. If the temperature is wrong, many of the fine molecules that are important for therapeutic application are lost, although this is unimportant to the fragrance and food flavoring industry.

With Gary Young's new, innovative changes, up to 80 percent more of the fine molecules that are lost in normal distilling practices are now being captured.

The computer monitors all systems and makes changes instantly when needed. Manually, the operator may be monitoring, loading, or unloading a chamber and may not be able to make adjustments immediately, which could take several minutes to correct.

Cameras installed inside the swan neck enable the operator to watch the steam as it leaves the plant material carrying the oil into the condenser.

These two automated, state-of-the-art oil-extracting facilities are the most advanced distilling systems in the world today.

### Highland Flats Tree Farm, Naples, Idaho

- For the first time on January 4, 2014, semitrucks were able to drive inside the heated distillery building at the Highland Flats Tree Farm. There the chips are unloaded and then packed into the two 21,000-liter extraction chambers.

Producing Therapeutic-Grade Essential Oils | Chapter 4

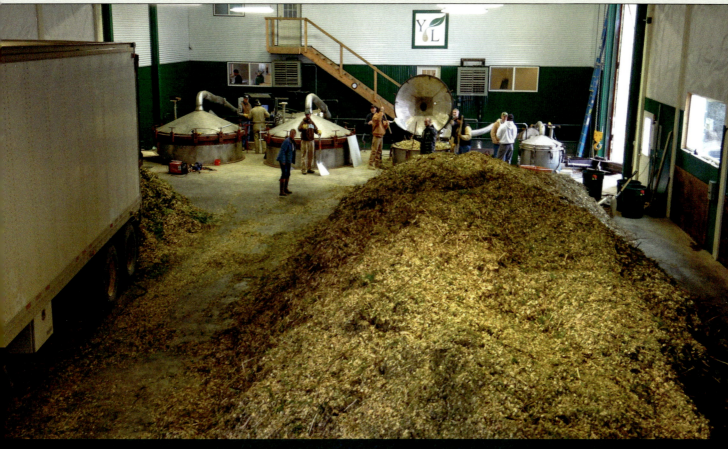

*The world's first fully automated, state-of-the-art distillery was installed in 2014 at the Young Living Highland Flats Tree Farm in Naples, Idaho.*

- Later in 2014, two more extraction chambers were installed. One was another 21,000-liter chamber for conifer distillation. The other was an 8,500-liter chamber for the distillation of Idaho Tansy, for a total of four extraction chambers.

- The Highland Flats distillery completely eliminates Gary's previous nightly drives of 125 miles in the semi-truck pulling two trailers over the treacherous, winding roads covered with snow and ice to the distillery in St. Maries. Gary and his workers are safer, the distillation process is infinitely faster, and the oil production is spectacular. **It is a dream come true.**

The Highland Flats farm is an amazing place to visit. From distilling, to separating, to decanting/filtering, to bottling, the oils are transferred from stainless steel to glass containers and never touch hands before they are sealed and packaged for shipping.

## Two More New Distilleries

After the Highland Flats distillery was finished, two additional distilleries were built, one in Canada and one in Croatia.

### Northern Lights Farm, Fort Nelson, British Columbia, Canada

In 2014 Gary broke ground for a new distillery located 8 miles outside of Fort Nelson in British Columbia, Canada, at Mile 308 on the Alcan Highway to answer the growing demand for more Black Spruce essential oil.

- The Northern Lights Farm has five extraction chambers: two 12,000-liter, one 20,000-liter, one 10,000-liter, and one 3,500-liter, bringing the total distilling capacity to 57,500 liters. The first distillation of black spruce trees took place on March 9, 2015.

Seventh Edition | Essential Oils Desk Reference | 45

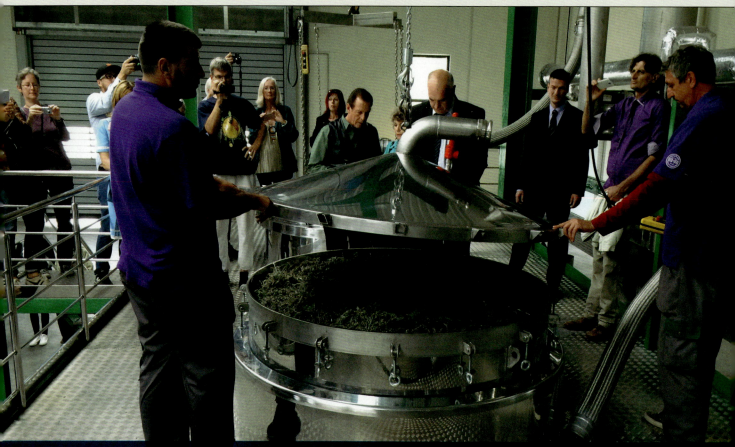

Members from around the world attended the ribbon cutting and official opening of the distillery in Split, October 6, 2015.

- The range of liters extracted from a single distillation is between 21 and 42 liters. The volume of oil depends on the age of the tree and the branch growth. Older trees with less branch growth and more hard wood naturally produce less oil, and different conifer trees differ in their production. Chips from the entire tree, not just branches, are distilled.

- The new extraction chambers use 30 percent less fuel than the older extraction chambers. The new condenser system reduces the water consumption by 20 percent, and all water in the distillation process is recycled and never leaves the holding reservoir again, thus preserving the eco system.

- The large, heated truck bay is fully insulated, with heated floors to melt snow and ice and remove the water in the chips for a better and greater distillation.

- Additional crops to be distilled currently include white fir, a new species of balsam fir, yarrow, German chamomile, goldenrod, ledum, and Canadian fleabane.

### Split, Croatia, Farm

In May 2015 Young Living purchased a two-story commercial building in Split, Croatia, totaling 16,580 square meters, which includes several offices; conference rooms; warehouse space; two large bays for the distillery; an enclosed boiler room; decanting, bottling, and labeling rooms; and a laboratory with a GC instrument for testing the oils.

In an amazing accomplishment, distilling of the much-needed helichrysum began on June 19, exactly 19 days from when Gary and his crew started to assemble everything for the distillery and refit the building, which enabled them to distill during the short 55-day time period allowed by the government for distilling helichrysum.

- The distillery has four 4,000-liter, one 6,000-liter, and four 1,000-liter extraction chambers, bringing the total distilling capacity to 26,000 liters.

- After crops are harvested, they are trucked to the new facility, where the Seed to Seal process continues with distilling, laboratory testing, filtering, and decanting.

Producing Therapeutic-Grade Essential Oils | Chapter 4

- Some of the oil goes to another area of the building, where it is bottled, labeled, and shipped to our European distribution center.

- Bulk oils are shipped to the warehouse in Utah for bottling, additional testing, labeling, and distributing to members in the U.S. and other countries throughout the world.

- Our new partner farm is growing 78 hectares (192 acres) of helichrysum and contracting with many other farmers who have small acreages of helichrysum.

- Croatia is a country very rich with aromatic plants that will be cultivated with other partner and cooperative farms and that will be distilled in the new facility.

Distillery operators say that distilling is both an art and a science. D. Gary Young combines research and science with more than 25 years of experience in engineering, designing, building, and operating nine existing distilleries and five partner distilleries in different countries. All of the distilleries that Gary Young has built throughout the world on five continents are bringing forth great discoveries in modern-day distillation, making him the only person in history to distill on such a worldwide scale. Consistency and increased control allow Young Living to further ensure the purity and quality of its world-class products.

The Seed to Seal process is Young Living's trademark and was developed by D. Gary Young at his first farm in St. Maries more than 20 years ago. Gary then took distilling to a higher level with the new distillery at Highland Flats and the upgrading of the distillery in Mona. Gradually, all of the Young Living distilleries will be upgraded to match the new operation. With the new automation and the most advanced technology available, modernizing the production process will be more efficient and effective than ever.

Young Living has again raised the bar of excellence in the essential oil industry; and with its Seed to Seal process, it is without question the world leader in essential oils.

## Essential Oil Production

Producing pure essential oils is very costly. It often requires several hundred or even thousands of pounds of raw plant material to produce a single pound of essential oil. For example, it can take 2–3 tons of melissa plant material to produce 1 pound of Melissa oil. This extremely low yield explains why it sells for $9,000 to $15,000 per kilo. It takes 5,000 pounds of rose petals to produce approximately 1 pint of Rose oil. It is easy to understand why these oils cost so much.

The vast majority of oils are produced for the perfume industry, which is interested only in their aromatic qualities.

High pressures, high temperatures, and chemical solvents are used in this distillation process to produce greater quantities of oil in a shorter time. To most people, these oils carry a pleasant aroma, but they lack true therapeutic properties. Many of the important chemical constituents necessary to produce therapeutic results are either flashed off with the high heat or are not released from the plant material.

## Testing

At Young Living, each essential oil must pass extensive testing to ensure an optimal bioactive profile. Young Living uses its own internal labs, as well as third-party testing from essential oil experts in other countries, to validate the purity and potency of essential oils.

### Routine Tests Done by the Quality Control Lab

Each raw oil is sent to our Quality Control lab for identity, composition, purity, and Safety Data Sheet (SDS) testing. This is done by first performing organoleptic testing such as appearance, color, and odor.

### Identity Testing

Identity testing is done using FTIR, refractive index, optical rotation, and specific gravity.

- **FTIR Spectroscopy:** Fourier transform infrared spectroscopy (FTIR) characterizes an essential oil by its functional components such as ketones, aldehydes, alcohols, etc.

- **Refractive Index:** Measures the bending of light as it passes through the essential oil. It gives an index of refraction for biochemical constituents in the essential oil.

- **Optical Rotation:** Measures how much polarized light rotates through an essential oil, which indicates the overall chirality of the oil and helps determine if there is adulteration.

- **Specific Gravity:** A measurement that indicates how dense a substance is by comparing it to the density of water.

### Composition Testing

Composition testing is done by GC and compared to a library containing 400,000+ components based on retention time and peak area. Young Living then uses a proprietary retention index database created by Dr. Hervé Casabianca at CRNS in France via GC-MS and provides firm identification of individual molecules in each essential oil.

- **Gas Chromatography (GC):** Using polar and nonpolar columns, a GC is able to separate components of an essential oil by the composition of the functional components of the oil.

Seventh Edition | **Essential Oils Desk Reference** | 47

- **GC/IRMS** (Gas Chromatography, Isotope Ratio, and Mass Spectrometry). This technology identifies ratios of isotopes and determines if those ratios are natural (created by plant metabolism) or synthetic (created in a lab). By this method, the IRMS can identify samples as either natural or synthetic.

### Purity Testing

Purity is determined by GC, Optical Rotation, ICP-MS, microbiological, and Peroxide Value testing. Using these tests, Young Living ensures that the purity of the essential oil is held to the high standard.

- **ICP-MS:** Inductively Coupled Plasma-Mass Spectroscopy (ICP-MS) is used to identify heavy metal contaminants that may occur naturally or be man-made. These include, but are not limited to, arsenic, cadmium, lead, and mercury. The ICP-MS is able to detect these heavy metals down to the part-per-billion (ppb) level.

- **Microbiological Testing:** Each new oil is tested to ensure that no microbial components are present. Although essential oils are not conducive to microbial growth, Young Living tests for the following: aerobic plate count, coliforms, yeast, mold, *Staphylococcus aureus*, *E. coli*, *Salmonella sp.*, and *Pseudomonas aeruginosa*.

- **Peroxide Value:** The determination of peroxides will give an initial evidence of rancidity in oils. This method is the most widely used to determine if primary oxidation has occurred in the oil.

### Safety Data Sheet Testing

Young Living also provides testing to create Safety Data Sheets (SDS), which include flash point and combustibility.

- **Flash Point:** A test that determines the temperature at which an oil will vaporize and ignite in air.

- **Combustibility:** A test that determines the flammability of an oil.

### Final Product Testing

Once each raw oil is approved by Quality, it is given to Production, where it is bottled. The final product is then sent again to the Quality Control Lab. Oils are then retested in their final packaging using the same tests done on the raw oil. This is done to verify that no contamination or adulteration has occurred in the production process.

### Sealing

The final step in Young Living's Seed to Seal process is carefully sealing each bottle of essential oil in Young Living's own clean-room facility and shipping it to members worldwide.

Literally, from the plant seed that is dropped into the soil to the essential oil sealed in the amber bottle in Young Living's clean room, the Seed to Seal process is carefully supervised from beginning to end to ensure the quality and purity of Young Living's therapeutic-grade essential oils.

---

ENDNOTES

1. Estabrook B. "Genetically Modified Alfalfa Officially on the Way," *The Atlantic*, January 28, 2011.

2. https://en.wikipedia.org/wiki/Genetically_modified_crops.

3. Schwartz G, Russek L. *The Living Energy Universe*, Hampton Roads Publishing Company, 1st edition, Charlottesville, VA, 1999:146.

# Chapter 5
## How to Safely Use Essential Oils

# Basic Guidelines for Safe Use

Guidelines are important to follow when using essential oils, especially if you are unfamiliar with the oils and their benefits. Many guidelines are listed below and are elaborated on throughout the chapter. However, no list of do's and don'ts can ever replace common sense. It is foolish to dive headlong into a pond when you do not know the depth of the water. The same is true when using essential oils. Start gradually and patiently find what works best for you and your family members.

**Storage**

1. Always keep a bottle of a pure carrier oil (e.g., V-6 Vegetable Oil Complex, olive oil, almond oil, coconut oil, or more fragrant massage oils such as Sensation, Relaxation, Ortho Ease, or Ortho Sport) handy when using essential oils. Carrier oils will dilute essential oils if the essential oils cause discomfort or skin irritation.

2. Keep bottles of essential oils tightly closed and store them in a cool location away from light. If stored properly, essential oils will maintain their potency for many years.

3. Keep essential oils out of reach of children. Treat the oils as you would any product for therapeutic use. Children love the oils and will often go through an entire bottle in a very short time. They want to give massages and do the same things they see you do.

**Usage**

4. Essential oils rich in menthol (such as Peppermint) should not be used on the throat or neck area of children under 18 months of age.

5. Angelica, Bergamot, Bitter Orange, Grapefruit, Lemon, Ruta, Tangerine, and other citrus oils are photosensitive and may cause a rash or dark pigmentation on skin exposed to direct sunlight or UV rays within 1–2 days after application.

6. Keep essential oils away from the eye area and never put them directly into ears. Do not handle contact lenses or rub eyes with essential oils on your fingers. Even in minute amounts, many essential oils may damage contacts and will irritate eyes.

7. Pregnant women should consult a health care professional when starting any type of health program. Oils are safe to use, but one needs to use common sense. Follow the directions and dilute with V-6 Vegetable Oil Complex until you become familiar with the oils you are using.

   Many pregnant women have said that they feel a very positive response from the unborn child when the oils are applied on the skin, but that is each woman's individual experience.

8. Epileptics and those with high blood pressure should consult their health care professional before using essential oils. Use extra caution with high ketone oils such as Basil, Rosemary, Sage, and Idaho Tansy oils.

9. People with allergies should test a small amount of oil on an area of sensitive skin, such as the inside of the upper arm, for 30 minutes before applying the oil on other areas of the body.

10. The bottoms of feet are safe locations to apply essential oils topically.

11. Direct inhalation of essential oils can be a deep and intensive application method, particularly for respiratory congestion and illness. However, this method should not be used more than 10–15 times throughout the day without consulting a health professional. Also, inhalation of essential oils is NOT recommended for those with asthmatic conditions.

12. Before taking essential oils internally, test your reactions by diluting 1 drop of essential oil in 1 teaspoon of an oil-soluble liquid like Blue Agave,

Seventh Edition | **Essential Oils Desk Reference** | 49

# Essential Oils Certified as GRAS

## (Generally Regarded as Safe), or as food additives, by the FDA

| Single Oils | | | | | Single Oils (cont.) | | | | | | | | |
|---|---|---|---|---|---|---|---|---|---|---|---|---|---|
| Anise | GS | FA | | | Lavender | GS | FA | | | Wintergreen | | FA | |
| Angelica | GS | FA | | | Lavandin | GS | FA | | | Yarrow | | FA | |
| Basil | GS | FA | | | Lemon | GS | FA | | | Ylang Ylang | GS | FA | |
| Bergamot | GS | FA | | | Lemongrass | GS | FA | | | | | | |
| Cajuput | | FA | | | Lime | GS | FA | | | | | | |
| Cardamom | | FA | | | Mandarin | GS | FA | | | | | | |
| Carrot Seed | | FA | | | Marjoram | GS | FA | | | | | | |
| Cassia | GS | FA | | | Mountain Savory | | FA | | | | | | |
| Cedarwood | | FA | | | Melissa | GS | FA | | | | | | |
| Celery Seed | GS | FA | | | Myrrh | GS | FA | FL | | | | | |
| Cinnamon Bark & Leaf | GS | FA | | | Myrtle | GS | FA | | | | | | |
| Cistus | | FA | | | Neroli | GS | FA | | | | | | |
| Citronella | GS | FA | | | Nutmeg | GS | FA | | | | | | |
| Citrus Rinds | GS | FA | | | Onycha | GS | FA | | | | | | |
| Clary Sage | GS | FA | | | Orange | GS | FA | | | | | | |
| Clove | GS | FA | | | Oregano | GS | FA | | | | | | |
| Copaiba | GS | FA | | | Palmarosa | GS | FA | | | | | | |
| Coriander | GS | FA | | | Patchouli | GS | FA | FL | | | | | |
| Cumin | GS | FA | | | Pepper | GS | FA | | | | | | |
| Dill | GS | FA | | | Peppermint | GS | FA | | | | | | |
| Eucalyptus Globulus | GS | FA | FL | | Petitgrain | GS | FA | | | | | | |
| Elemi | GS | FA | FL | | Pine | GS | FA | FL | | | | | |
| Fennel | GS | FA | | | Roman Chamomile | GS | FA | | | | | | |
| Frankincense | GS | FA | FL | | Rose | GS | FA | | | | | | |
| Geranium | GS | FA | | | Rosemary | GS | FA | | | | | | |
| German Chamomile | GS | FA | | | Savory | GS | FA | | | | | | |
| Ginger | GS | FA | | | Sage | GS | FA | | | | | | |
| Goldenrod | GS | | | | Sandalwood | GS | FA | FL | | | | | |
| Grapefruit | GS | FA | | | Spearmint | GS | FA | | | | | | |
| Helichrysum | GS | FA | | | Spruce | GS | FA | FL | | | | | |
| Hyssop | GS | FA | | | Tangerine | GS | FA | | | | | | |
| Idaho Balsam Fir | | FA | | | Tarragon | GS | FA | | | | | | |
| Jade Lemon | GS | FA | | | Tea Tree | | FA | | | | | | |
| Jasmine | GS | FA | | | Thyme | GS | FA | | | | | | |
| Juniper | GS | FA | | | Tsuga | GS | FA | FL | | | | | |
| Laurus Nobilis | GS | FA | | | Valerian | GS | FA | FL | | | | | |
| | | | | | Vetiver | GS | FA | | | | | | |

**Note:** Please also see the single oils listed as Vitality supplements in Chapter 6.

## Blends

| | | |
|---|---|---|
| Abundance | GS | |
| Believe | | FA |
| Citrus Fresh | GS | |
| Christmas Spirit | GS | |
| DiGize | GS | |
| EndoFlex | GS | |
| Gratitude | | FA |
| Joy | GS | |
| JuvaCleanse | GS | |
| JuvaFlex | GS | |
| Longevity | GS | |
| Thieves | GS | |
| M-Grain | GS | |
| Purification | GS | |
| Relieve It | GS | |
| Sacred Mountain | GS | |
| White Angelica | GS | |

**Note:** Please also see the blends listed as Vitality supplements in Chapter 7.

### CODE:

| | |
|---|---|
| GS | Generally regarded as safe (GRAS) |
| FA | FDA-approved food additive |
| FL | Flavoring agent |

**CAUTION:** Essential oils may sting if applied in or around the eyes. Some oils may be painful on mucous membranes unless diluted properly. Immediate dilution is strongly recommended if skin becomes painfully irritated or if oil accidentally gets into eyes. Flushing the area with a carrier oil should minimize discomfort almost immediately.

**DO NOT** flush with water! Essential oils are oil-soluble, not water-soluble. Water will only spread the oils over a larger surface, possibly worsening the problem. Use V-6 Vegetable Oil Complex, coconut oil, olive oil, or other carrier oil to flush the essential oils. Keep eyes closed, be patient, and the sting will quickly dissipate.

Yacon Syrup, olive oil, coconut oil, or rice or almond milk. If you intend to consume more than a few drops of diluted essential oil per day, we recommend first consulting a health care professional.

13. Be aware that reactions to essential oils, both topically and orally, can be delayed as long as 2–3 days.

14. Add 1–3 drops of undiluted essential oils directly to bath water. If more essential oil is desired, mix the oil first into bath salts or a bath gel base before adding to the bath water. Generally, never use more than 10 drops of essential oils in one bath. When essential oils are put directly into bath water without a dispersing agent, they can cause serious discomfort on sensitive skin because the essential oils tend to float, undiluted, on top of the water.

## Chemical Sensitivities and Allergies

Occasionally, individuals beginning to use quality essential oils will suffer rashes or allergic reactions. This may be due to using an undiluted spice, conifer, or citrus oil; or it may be caused by an interaction of the oil with residues of synthetic, petroleum-based, personal care products that have leached into the skin.

When using essential oils on a daily basis, it is imperative to avoid personal care products containing ammonium or hydrocarbon-based chemicals. These include quaternary compounds such as quaternariums and polyquaternariums. These chemicals can be fatal if ingested, especially benzalkonium chloride, which, unfortunately, is used in many personal care products on the market.

Other chemicals such as aluminum compounds, FD&C colors, formaldehyde, all parabens, talc, thimerosal, mercury, and titanium dioxide, just to name a few, are all toxic to the body and should be avoided. These compounds are commonly found in a variety of hand creams, mouthwashes, shampoos, antiperspirants, after-shave lotions, and hair care products.

Other compounds that present concerns are sodium lauryl sulfate, propylene glycol—extremely common in everything from toothpaste to shampoo—and aluminum salts found in many deodorants.

Of particular concern are the potentially hazardous preservatives and synthetic fragrances that abound in virtually all modern personal care products. Some of these include methylene chloride, methyl isobutyl ketone, and methyl ethyl ketone. These are not only toxic, but they can also react with some compounds in natural essential oils. The result can be a severe case of dermatitis or even septicemia (blood poisoning).

A classic case of a synthetic fragrance causing widespread damage occurred in the 1970s. AETT (acetyl ethyl tetra-methyl tetralin) appeared in numerous brands of personal care products throughout the United States. Even after a series of animal studies revealed that it caused significant brain and spinal cord damage, the FDA refused to ban the chemical. Finally, the cosmetic industry voluntarily withdrew AETT after allowing it to be distributed for years.

How many other toxins masquerading as preservatives or fragrances are currently being used in personal care products?

Many chemicals are easily absorbed through the skin due to its permeability. One study found that 13 percent of BHT (butylated hydroxytoluene) and 49 percent of DDT (a carcinogenic pesticide that was banned in 1972 but is still used in disease vector control) can be absorbed into the skin upon topical contact.[1]

Once absorbed, many chemicals can become trapped in the fatty subdermal layers of skin, where they can leach into the bloodstream. They can remain trapped for several months or years until a topical substance like an essential oil starts to move them from their resting place and cause them to come out of the skin in an uncomfortable way. Besides skin irritation, you could experience nausea, headaches, and other slight, temporary effects during this detoxifying process. Even in small concentrations, these chemicals and synthetic compounds are toxic and can compromise one's health.

It is all about what chemicals were used, how much, how long, and perhaps the level of toxicity in your body.

Essential oils have been known to digest toxic substances; so when they come in contact with chemical residue on the skin, the oils start to work against them.

The user may mistakenly assume that the threat of an interaction between oils and synthetic cosmetics used months before is small. However, a case of dermatitis is always a possibility.

Essential oils do not cause skin problems, rashes, or eruptions on the skin; but they may, only indirectly, as they go after the chemicals. Do not make the mistake of blaming the essential oils. Just be glad this chemical residue is coming out of your body.

You can always reduce the amount of oil you are using or stop the use of any oil for a couple of days and then start again slowly. You can also use V-6 Vegetable Oil Complex, other carrier or massage oils, or natural creams to dilute the oils.

# Before You Start

Always skin test an essential oil before using it. Each person's body is different, so apply oils to a small area first. Apply one oil or blend at a time. When layering oils that are new to you, allow enough time (3-5 minutes) for the body to respond before applying a second oil.

Use a small amount when applying essential oils to skin that may carry residue from cosmetics, personal care products, soaps, and cleansers containing synthetic chemicals. Some of them—especially petroleum-based chemicals—can penetrate and remain in the skin and fatty tissues for days or even weeks after use.

Essential oils may work against such chemicals and toxins built up in the body from chemicals in food, water, and work environment. If you have this kind of an experience using essential oils, it may be wise to reduce or stop using them for a few days and start an internal cleansing program before resuming regular use of essential oils. In addition, double your water intake and keep flushing those toxins out of your body.

You may also want to try the following alternatives to a detoxification program to determine the cause of the problem:

- Dilute 1–3 drops of essential oil in 1/2 teaspoon of V-6 Vegetable Oil Complex, massage oil, or any pure carrier oil such as almond, coconut, or olive. More dilution may be needed.

- Reduce the number of oils used at any time.

- Use single oils or oil blends one at a time.

- Reduce the amount of oil used.

- Reduce the frequency of application.

- Drink more purified or distilled water.

- Ask your health care professional to monitor detoxification.

- Test the diluted essential oil on a small patch of skin for 30 minutes. If any redness or irritation results, dilute the area immediately with V-6 or other carrier oil and then cleanse with soap and water.

- If skin irritation or other uncomfortable side effects persist, discontinue using the oil on that location and apply the oils on the bottoms of the feet.

You may also want to avoid using products that contain the following ingredients to eliminate potential problems:

- Cosmetics, deodorants, and skin care products containing aluminum, petrochemicals, or other synthetic ingredients

- Perms, hair colors or dyes, hair sprays, or gels containing synthetic chemicals; shampoos, toothpastes, mouthwashes, and soaps containing synthetic chemicals such as sodium laurel sulfate, propylene glycol, or lead acetate

- Garden sprays, paints, detergents, and cleansers containing toxic chemicals and solvents

You can use many essential oils anywhere on the body except on the eyes and in the ears. Other oils may irritate certain sensitive tissues. See recommended dilution rates in the chapters for singles and blends.

Keep "hot" oils such as Oregano, Cinnamon, Thyme, Eucalyptus, Mountain Savory, Lemon, and Orange essential oils or blends such as Thieves, PanAway, Relieve It, and Exodus II out of reach of children. These types of oils should always be diluted for both children and adults.

Children need to be taught how to use the oils so that they understand the safety issue. If a child or infant swallows an essential oil, do the following:

- Seek immediate emergency medical attention, if necessary.

- Give the child milk, cream, yogurt, or another safe, oil-soluble liquid to drink.

**NOTE:** If your body pH is low, your body will be acidic; therefore, you could also have less of a response or perhaps a minimal negative reaction to the oils.

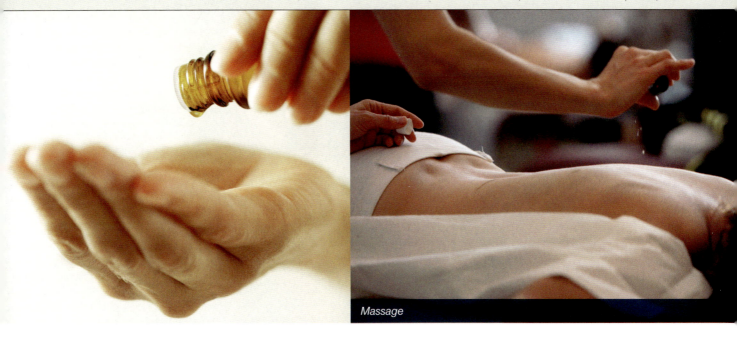
Massage

## Topical Application

Many oils are safe to apply directly to the skin without being diluted. Lavender is safe to use on children without dilution. However, you must be sure the essential oil you are using is not lavandin labeled as lavender or genetically altered lavender. When applying most other essential oils on children, dilute the oils with carrier oil. For dilution, add 15–30 drops of essential oil to 1 oz. of quality carrier oil, as mentioned previously.

Carrier oils such as V-6 Vegetable Oil Complex extend essential oils and provide more efficient use. When massaging, the carrier oil helps lubricate the skin.

When starting an essential oil application, depending on which oil you use, you may want to test for skin sensitivity by applying the oil first to the bottoms of the feet. See the Vita Flex foot charts to identify areas of best application. Start by applying 3–6 drops of a single oil or blend, spreading it over the bottom of each foot.

When applying essential oils to yourself, use 1–2 drops of oil on 2–3 locations 2 times a day. Increase to 4 times a day if needed. Apply the oil and allow it to absorb for 2–3 minutes before applying another oil or before getting dressed to avoid staining clothing.

As a general rule, when applying oils to yourself or another person for the first time, do not apply more than two single oils or blends at one time.

When mixing essential oil blends or diluting essential oils in a carrier oil, it is best to use containers made of glass or earthenware, rather than plastic. Plastic particles can leach into the oil and then into the skin once it is applied.

Before applying oils, wash hands thoroughly with soap and water.

### Massage

Start by applying 2 drops of a single oil or blend on the skin and massaging it in.

Dilute 1 drop with 15 drops of V-6 or other pure carrier oil such as jojoba, almond, coconut, olive, and/or grape seed for body massage if you are working on a large area, such as the back.

Keep in mind that many massage oils such as olive, almond, jojoba, or wheat germ oil may stain some fabrics.

### Acupuncture

Licensed acupuncturists can dramatically increase the effectiveness of acupuncture by using essential oils.

To start, place several drops of essential oil into the palm of your hand and dip the acupuncture needle tip into the oil before inserting it into the person. You can premix several oils in your hand if you wish to use more than one oil.

**Essential Oils Desk Reference** | Seventh Edition

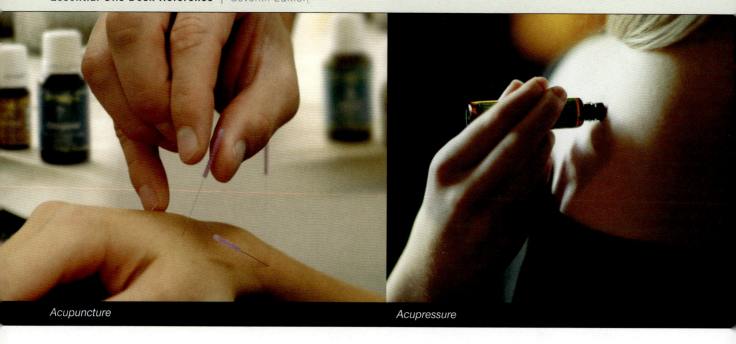

Acupuncture

Acupressure

## Acupressure

When performing an acupressure treatment, apply 1–3 drops of essential oil to the acupressure point with your finger. Using an auricular probe with a slender point to dispense oil may enhance the application.

Start by pressing firmly and then releasing. Avoid applying pressure to any particular pressure point too long. You may continue along the acupressure points and meridians or use the reflexology or Vita Flex points as well. Once you have completed small point stimulations, massage the general area with the essential oil.

## Warm Compress

For deeper penetration, use a warm compress after applying essential oils. Completely soak the cloth or towel by placing it in comfortably hot water. By the time you wring out the cloth and shake it, it will be a nice, warm temperature to be placed on the location. Then cover the cloth loosely with a dry towel or blanket to seal in the heat. Leave the cloth on for 15-30 minutes. Remove the cloth immediately if there is any discomfort.

## Cold Packs

Apply essential oils on the location, followed by cold water or ice packs, when treating inflamed or swollen tissues. Frozen packages of peas or corn make excellent ice packs that will mold to the contours of the body part and will not leak. Keep the cold pack on until the swelling diminishes.

For neurological problems, always use cold packs, never hot ones.

## Layering

This technique consists of applying multiple oils one at a time. For example, rub Marjoram over a sore muscle, massage it into the tissue gently until the area is dry, and then apply a second oil such as Peppermint until the oil is absorbed and the skin is dry. Then layer on the third oil, such as Basil, and continue massaging.

## Making a Compress

- Rub 1–3 drops on the location, diluted or neat, depending on the oil used and the skin sensitivity at that location.

- Cover the location with a hot, damp towel.

- Cover the moist towel with a dry towel for 10–30 minutes, depending on individual need.

As the oil penetrates the skin, you may experience a warming or even a burning sensation, especially in areas where the greatest benefits occur. If burning becomes uncomfortable, apply V-6 Vegetable Oil Complex, a massage oil, or any pure carrier oil such as olive, coconut, or almond to the location.

A second type of application is very mild and is suitable for children or those with sensitive skin.

- Place 5-15 drops of essential oil into a basin filled with warm water.

- Water temperature should be approximately 100ºF (38ºC), unless the patient suffers neurological conditions; in that case, use cool water.

54 | Chapter 5 | How to Safely Use Essential Oils

How to Safely Use Essential Oils | **Chapter 5**

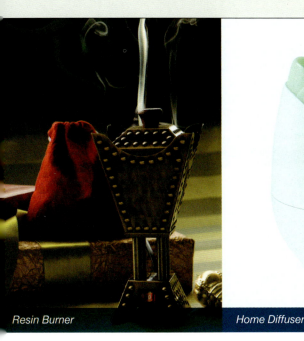
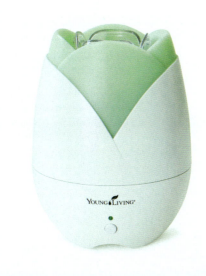
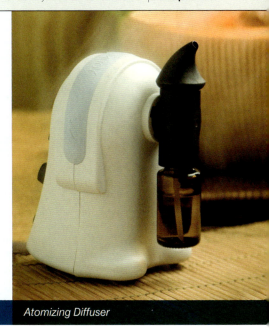

Resin Burner | Home Diffuser | Atomizing Diffuser

- Vigorously agitate the water and let it stand for 1 minute.
- Place a dry face cloth on top of the water to soak up oils that have floated to the surface.
- Wring out the water and apply the cloth on location. To seal in the warmth, cover the location with a thick towel for 15–30 minutes.

## Bath

Adding essential oils to bath water is challenging because oil does not mix with water. For even dispersion, mix 5–10 drops of essential oil in 1/4 cup of Epsom salts or bath gel base and then put the cup under a running faucet and gradually add water. This method will help the oils disperse in the bath evenly and prevent stronger oils from stinging sensitive areas.

You can also use premixed bath gels and shampoos containing essential oils as a liquid soap in the shower or bath. Lather down with the bath gel, let it soak in, and then rinse. To maximize benefits, leave the soap or shampoo on the skin or scalp for several minutes to allow the essential oils to penetrate.

You can create your own aromatic bath gels by placing 5–15 drops of essential oil in 1/2 oz. of an unscented bath gel base and then add to the bath water as described above.

## Shower

Essential oils can be added to Epsom salts and used in the shower. There are special shower heads containing an attached receptacle that can be filled with the essential oil/salts mixture. This allows essential oils to not only make contact with the skin but also diffuses the fragrance of the oils into the air. The shower head receptacle can hold approximately 1/4 to 1/2 cup of bath salts.

Start by adding 5–10 drops of essential oil to 1/4 cup of bath salt. Fill the shower head receptacle with the oil/salt mixture. Make sure neither oils nor salts come in contact with the plastic seal on top of the receptacle. This should provide enough salt material for about 2–3 showers. Some shower heads have a bypass feature that allows the user to switch from aromatic salt water to regular tap water.

## How to Enhance the Benefits of Topical Application

The longer essential oils stay in contact with the skin, the more likely they are to be absorbed. The ART Light Moisturizer, ART Renewal Serum, ART Sheerlumé Brightening Cream, Boswellia Wrinkle Cream, or Sandalwood Moisture Cream may be layered on top of the essential oils to reduce evaporation of the oils and enhance penetration. This may also help seal and protect cuts and wounds.

Do not use ointments on burns until they are at least three days old; however, LavaDerm Cooling Mist spray may be used immediately to provide comforting relief for minor burns, abrasions, dryness, and other skin irritations.

Seventh Edition | *Essential Oils Desk Reference* | 55

**Essential Oils Desk Reference** | Seventh Edition

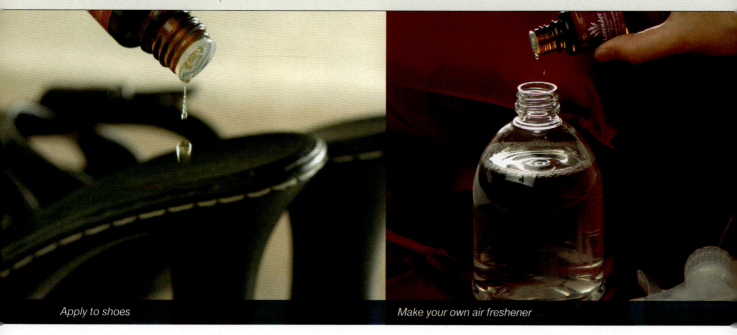

Apply to shoes

Make your own air freshener

# Diffusing

Diffused oils alter the structure of molecules that create odors, rather than just masking them. They also increase oxygen availability, produce negative ions, and release natural ozone. Many essential oils such as Eucalyptus Globulus and Radiata, Frankincense, Grapefruit, Lavender, Lemon, Lemongrass, Orange, and Tea Tree (Melaleuca Alternifolia), along with essential oil blends like Melrose, Purification, and Thieves, are extremely effective for eliminating and destroying airborne germs and bacteria.

A cold-air diffuser is designed to atomize a microfine mist of essential oils into the air, where they can remain suspended for several hours. Unlike aroma lamps or candles, a diffuser disperses essential oils without heating or burning, which can render the oil therapeutically less beneficial and even create toxic compounds. Research shows that cold-air diffusing certain oils may:

- Reduce bacteria, fungus, mold, and unpleasant odors
- Relax the body, relieve tension, and clear the mind
- Help with weight management
- Improve concentration, alertness, and mental clarity
- Stimulate neurotransmitters
- Stimulate secretion of endorphins
- Stimulate growth hormone production and receptivity
- Improve the secretion of IgA antibodies that fight candida
- Improve digestive function
- Improve hormonal balance
- Relieve headaches

## Guidelines for Diffusing

- Check the viscosity or thickness of the oil you want to diffuse. If the oil has too much natural wax and is too thick, it could plug the diffuser and make cleaning difficult.
- Start by diffusing oils for 15–30 minutes a day. As you become accustomed to the oils and recognize their effects, you may increase the diffusing time to 1–2 hours per day.
- By connecting your diffuser to a timer, you can gain better control over the length and duration of diffusing. For some respiratory conditions, you may diffuse the oils the entire night.
- Do not use more than one blend at a time in a diffuser, as this may alter the smell and the therapeutic benefit. However, a single oil may be added to a blend when diffusing.
- Place the diffuser high in the room so that the oil mist falls through the air and removes the odor-causing substances.

How to Safely Use Essential Oils | **Chapter 5**

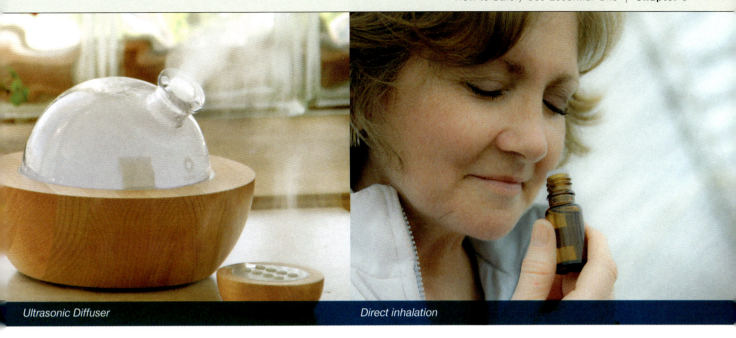

Ultrasonic Diffuser | Direct inhalation

- If you want to wash the diffuser before using a different oil blend, use Thieves Household Cleaner with warm water or any natural soap and warm water.

- If you do not have a diffuser, you can add several drops of essential oil to a spray bottle with 1 cup purified water and shake. You can use this to mist your entire house, workplace, or car.

- Air Freshener Oil Recipe:
  - 20 drops Lavender
  - 10 drops Lemon
  - 6 drops Bergamot
  - 5 drops Lime
  - 5 drops Grapefruit

  Diffuse neat or mix with 1 cup of distilled water in a spray bottle; shake well before spraying.

## Other Ways to Diffuse Oils

- Add your favorite essential oils to cedar chips to make your own potpourri.

- Put scented cedar chips in your closets or drawers to deodorize them.

- Sprinkle a few drops of conifer essential oils such as Spruce, Fir (all varieties), Cedar, or Pine onto logs in the fireplace. As the logs burn, they will disperse an evergreen smell. This method has no therapeutic benefit, however.

- Add 2 drops to a wet cloth and put in the clothes dryer.

- Put essential oils on cotton balls or tissues and place them in your car, home, work, or hotel heating or air conditioning vents.

- Put a few drops of oil in a bowl or pan of water and set it on a warm stove.

- On a damp cloth, sprinkle a few drops of one of your purifying essential oils and place the cloth near an intake duct of your heating and cooling system so that the air can carry the aroma throughout your home.

- Splash a few drops on your paper vacuum cleaner bag for an uplifting and happy feeling while cleaning the house.

## Humidifier and Vaporizer

Essential oils make ideal additions to humidifiers or vaporizers. Always check the viscosity of the oil; if it is too thick, it could plug the humidifier or make it difficult to clean. The following singles and blends are great to diffuse.

**Singles:** Idaho Balsam Fir, Frankincense, Sacred Frankincense, Peppermint, Lemon, Eucalyptus Radiata, Tea Tree (Melaleuca Alternifolia), Lavender, Ylang Ylang, and many others of your choice

**Blends:** Purification, Thieves, Raven, Melrose, Joy, RutaVaLa, The Gift, White Angelica, Sacred Mountain, and many others of your choice

**NOTE:** Test the oil before diffusing it in the vaporizer or humidifier; some essential oils may damage the plastic parts of vaporizers.

# Other Uses

## Direct Inhalation

- Place 2 or more drops into the palm of your left hand and rub clockwise with the flat palm of your right hand. Cup your hands together over your nose and mouth and inhale deeply. Do not touch your eyes!

- Add several drops of an essential oil to a bowl of hot (not boiling) water. Inhale the steaming vapors that rise from the bowl. To increase the intensity of the oil vapors inhaled, drape a towel over your head and the bowl before inhaling.

- Inhale directly from the bottle.

## Indirect or Subtle Inhalation
(Wearing as a perfume or cologne)

- Rub 2 or more drops of oil on your chest, neck, upper sternum, wrists, or under your nose and ears, and enjoy the fragrance throughout the day.

- There are many necklaces with different types of vessels hanging on them into which you can pour a particular oil to use throughout the day.

- Clay-type medallions may be hung around your neck or fastened with a clip on your clothing onto which you can put a few oil drops to give off a gentle fragrance the entire day.

## Vaginal Retention

For systemic health problems such as Candida or vaginitis, vaginal retention is one of the best ways for the body to absorb essential oils.

- Mix 20–30 drops of essential oil in 2 tablespoons of carrier oil.

- Apply this mixture to a tampon (for internal infection) or sanitary pad (for external lesions). Insert the tampon and retain for 8 hours or overnight. Use tampons or sanitary pads made with organic cotton.

## Rectal Retention

A retention enema is the most efficient way to deliver essential oils to the urinary tract and reproductive organs. Always use a sterile syringe.

- Mix 15–20 drops of essential oil in a tablespoon of carrier oil.

- Place the mixture in a small syringe and inject into the rectum.

- Retain the mixture through the night (or longer for best results).

- Clean and disinfect the applicator after each use.

---

ENDNOTE:

1. Bronaugh RL, et al. Extent of cutaneous metabolism during percutaneous absorption of xenobiotics. *Toxicol. Appl. Pharmacol.* 1989 Jul;99(3):534-43.

# Section 2
## Products

**PRODUCT DIRECTORY** . . . . . . . . . . . . . . . . . . . . . . . . . . . . . . . . . 60

**CHAPTER 6** Single Oils. . . . . . . . . . . . . . . . . . . . . . . . . . . . . . . . . . 65

**CHAPTER 7** Essential Oil Blends. . . . . . . . . . . . . . . . . . . . . . . . . . 143

**CHAPTER 8** Nutritional Support . . . . . . . . . . . . . . . . . . . . . . . . . . 167

**CHAPTER 9** Ningxia Wolfberry . . . . . . . . . . . . . . . . . . . . . . . . . . . 193

**CHAPTER 10** Hormones and Vibrant Health . . . . . . . . . . . . . . . . . . 207

**CHAPTER 11** Personal Care . . . . . . . . . . . . . . . . . . . . . . . . . . . . . 217

**CHAPTER 12** Healthy Choices for Children . . . . . . . . . . . . . . . . . . 247

**CHAPTER 13** Fortifying Your Home with Essential Oils . . . . . . . . 251

**CHAPTER 14** Animal Care . . . . . . . . . . . . . . . . . . . . . . . . . . . . . . . 257

# Product Directory

## Chapter 6—Single Oils

Amazonian Ylang Ylang . . . . . . . 68
Angelica . . . . . . . . . . . . . . . . . . 68
Anise . . . . . . . . . . . . . . . . . . . . 69
Basil . . . . . . . . . . . . . . . . . . . . . 69
Basil Vitality . . . . . . . . . . . . . . . 70
Bergamot . . . . . . . . . . . . . . . . . 70
Bergamot Vitality . . . . . . . . . . . 70
Biblical Sweet Myrrh . . . . . . . . 71
Black Pepper . . . . . . . . . . . . . . . 71
Black Pepper Vitality . . . . . . . . 71
Black Spruce . . . . . . . . . . . . . . . 72
Blue Cypress . . . . . . . . . . . . . . . 72
Blue Tansy . . . . . . . . . . . . . . . . 73
Calamus . . . . . . . . . . . . . . . . . . 73
Canadian Fleabane . . . . . . . . . . 73
Cardamom . . . . . . . . . . . . . . . . 74
Cardamom Vitality . . . . . . . . . . 74
Carrot Seed . . . . . . . . . . . . . . . . 74
Carrot Seed Vitality . . . . . . . . . 75
Cassia . . . . . . . . . . . . . . . . . . . . 75
Cedarwood . . . . . . . . . . . . . . . . 76
Celery Seed . . . . . . . . . . . . . . . . 76
Celery Seed Vitality . . . . . . . . . 76
Cinnamon Bark . . . . . . . . . . . . . 77
Cinnamon Bark Vitality . . . . . . 77
Cistus . . . . . . . . . . . . . . . . . . . . 78
Citronella . . . . . . . . . . . . . . . . . 78
Citrus Hystrix/Combava . . . . . . 79
Clary Sage . . . . . . . . . . . . . . . . . 79
Clove . . . . . . . . . . . . . . . . . . . . 80
Clove Vitality . . . . . . . . . . . . . . 80
Copaiba (Balsam Copaiba) . . . . 81
Copaiba Vitality . . . . . . . . . . . . 81
Coriander . . . . . . . . . . . . . . . . . 82
Coriander Vitality . . . . . . . . . . . 82
Cumin . . . . . . . . . . . . . . . . . . . 83
Cypress . . . . . . . . . . . . . . . . . . . 83
Dalmatia Bay Laurel . . . . . . . . . 84

Dalmatia Juniper . . . . . . . . . . . 84
Dalmatia Sage . . . . . . . . . . . . . 84
Davana . . . . . . . . . . . . . . . . . . . 84
Dill . . . . . . . . . . . . . . . . . . . . . 85
Dill Vitality . . . . . . . . . . . . . . . 86
Dorado Azul . . . . . . . . . . . . . . . 86
Douglas Fir . . . . . . . . . . . . . . . . 87
Elemi . . . . . . . . . . . . . . . . . . . . 87
Eucalyptus Blue . . . . . . . . . . . . 87
Eucalyptus Citriodora . . . . . . . . 88
Eucalyptus Globulus . . . . . . . . . 89
Eucalyptus Radiata . . . . . . . . . . 89
Eucalyptus Staigeriana . . . . . . . 90
Fennel . . . . . . . . . . . . . . . . . . . 90
Fennel Vitality . . . . . . . . . . . . . 90
Frankincense . . . . . . . . . . . . . . 91
Frankincense Vitality . . . . . . . . 91
Frereana Frankincense . . . . . . . 92
Galbanum . . . . . . . . . . . . . . . . 93
Geranium . . . . . . . . . . . . . . . . . 93
German Chamomile . . . . . . . . . 94
German Chamomile Vitality . . . 94
Ginger . . . . . . . . . . . . . . . . . . . 95
Ginger Vitality . . . . . . . . . . . . . 95
Goldenrod . . . . . . . . . . . . . . . . 95
Grapefruit . . . . . . . . . . . . . . . . 96
Grapefruit Vitality . . . . . . . . . . 96
Helichrysum . . . . . . . . . . . . . . . 97
Hinoki . . . . . . . . . . . . . . . . . . . 97
Hong Kuai . . . . . . . . . . . . . . . . 98
Hyssop . . . . . . . . . . . . . . . . . . . 98
Idaho Balsam Fir
    (Balsam Canada) . . . . . . . . . . 99
Idaho Blue Spruce . . . . . . . . . . 99
Idaho Ponderosa Pine . . . . . . . 100
Idaho Tansy . . . . . . . . . . . . . . 101
Ishpingo . . . . . . . . . . . . . . . . . 101
Jade Lemon . . . . . . . . . . . . . . . 101

Jade Lemon Vitality . . . . . . . . 102
Jasmine . . . . . . . . . . . . . . . . . . 102
Juniper . . . . . . . . . . . . . . . . . . 103
Laurus Nobilis (Bay Laurel) . . . 103
Laurus Nobilis Vitality
    (Bay Laurel) . . . . . . . . . . . . 103
Lavandin . . . . . . . . . . . . . . . . 104
Lavender . . . . . . . . . . . . . . . . . 104
Lavender Vitality . . . . . . . . . . . 105
Ledum . . . . . . . . . . . . . . . . . . 105
Lemon . . . . . . . . . . . . . . . . . . 105
Lemon Vitality . . . . . . . . . . . . 106
Lemongrass . . . . . . . . . . . . . . . 106
Lemongrass Vitality . . . . . . . . 107
Lemon Myrtle . . . . . . . . . . . . . 107
Lime . . . . . . . . . . . . . . . . . . . . 108
Lime Vitality . . . . . . . . . . . . . . 108
Mandarin . . . . . . . . . . . . . . . . 108
Manuka . . . . . . . . . . . . . . . . . 109
Marjoram . . . . . . . . . . . . . . . . 110
Marjoram Vitality . . . . . . . . . . 110
Mastrante . . . . . . . . . . . . . . . . 111
Melaleuca Alternifolia
    (Tea Tree) . . . . . . . . . . . . . . 133
Melaleuca Ericifolia . . . . . . . . 111
Melaleuca Quinquenervia
    (Niaouli) . . . . . . . . . . . . . . . 112
Melissa . . . . . . . . . . . . . . . . . . 112
Micromeria . . . . . . . . . . . . . . . 113
Mountain Savory . . . . . . . . . . 113
Mountain Savory Vitality . . . . 114
Myrrh . . . . . . . . . . . . . . . . . . . 114
Myrtle . . . . . . . . . . . . . . . . . . 115
Neroli (Bitter Orange) . . . . . . . 115
Northern Lights Black Spruce . 116
Nutmeg . . . . . . . . . . . . . . . . . 116
Nutmeg Vitality . . . . . . . . . . . 117
Ocotea . . . . . . . . . . . . . . . . . . 117

**Section 2**

| | | |
|---|---|---|
| Orange . . . . . . . . . . . . . . . . . . 118 | Rosemary . . . . . . . . . . . . . . . . 126 | Tarragon Vitality . . . . . . . . . . 133 |
| Orange Vitality . . . . . . . . . . . 118 | Rosemary Vitality . . . . . . . . . . 127 | Tea Tree . . . . . . . . . . . . . . . . 133 |
| Oregano . . . . . . . . . . . . . . . . . 118 | Rosewood . . . . . . . . . . . . . . . . 127 | Thyme . . . . . . . . . . . . . . . . . 134 |
| Oregano Vitality . . . . . . . . . . . 119 | Royal Hawaiian Sandalwood . . 128 | Thyme Vitality . . . . . . . . . . . . 135 |
| Palmarosa . . . . . . . . . . . . . . . . 119 | Ruta . . . . . . . . . . . . . . . . . . . 128 | Tsuga . . . . . . . . . . . . . . . . . . 135 |
| Palo Santo . . . . . . . . . . . . . . . 120 | Sacred Frankincense . . . . . . . . 128 | Valerian . . . . . . . . . . . . . . . . . 135 |
| Patchouli . . . . . . . . . . . . . . . . 120 | Sage . . . . . . . . . . . . . . . . . . . 129 | Vanilla . . . . . . . . . . . . . . . . . 136 |
| Peppermint . . . . . . . . . . . . . . . 121 | Sage Vitality . . . . . . . . . . . . . . 130 | Vetiver . . . . . . . . . . . . . . . . . 137 |
| Peppermint Vitality . . . . . . . . 122 | Sandalwood . . . . . . . . . . . . . . 130 | Western Red Cedar . . . . . . . . 137 |
| Petitgrain . . . . . . . . . . . . . . . . 122 | Spanish Sage . . . . . . . . . . . . . . 130 | White Fir . . . . . . . . . . . . . . . 138 |
| Pine . . . . . . . . . . . . . . . . . . . 123 | Spearmint . . . . . . . . . . . . . . . 131 | White Lotus . . . . . . . . . . . . . . 138 |
| Plectranthus Oregano . . . . . . . 123 | Spearmint Vitality . . . . . . . . . . 131 | Wintergreen . . . . . . . . . . . . . . 139 |
| Ravintsara . . . . . . . . . . . . . . . 124 | Spikenard . . . . . . . . . . . . . . . . 131 | Xiang Mao . . . . . . . . . . . . . . . 140 |
| Roman Chamomile . . . . . . . . 125 | Tangerine . . . . . . . . . . . . . . . . 132 | Yarrow . . . . . . . . . . . . . . . . . 140 |
| Rose . . . . . . . . . . . . . . . . . . . 125 | Tangerine Vitality . . . . . . . . . . 132 | Ylang Ylang . . . . . . . . . . . . . . 141 |
| Rose of Sharon (Cistus) . . . . . . 78 | Tarragon . . . . . . . . . . . . . . . . . 133 | Yuzu . . . . . . . . . . . . . . . . . . . 142 |

# Chapter 7—Essential Oil Blends

| | | |
|---|---|---|
| 3 Wise Men . . . . . . . . . . . . . . 143 | EndoFlex . . . . . . . . . . . . . . . . 149 | JuvaFlex . . . . . . . . . . . . . . . . . 154 |
| Abundance . . . . . . . . . . . . . . . 143 | EndoFlex Vitality . . . . . . . . . . 149 | JuvaFlex Vitality . . . . . . . . . . . 154 |
| Acceptance . . . . . . . . . . . . . . . 145 | En-R-Gee . . . . . . . . . . . . . . . . 149 | Lady Sclareol . . . . . . . . . 155, 215 |
| Amoressence . . . . . . . . . . . . . . 145 | Envision . . . . . . . . . . . . . . . . . 149 | Light the Fire . . . . . . . . . . . . . 155 |
| Aroma Ease . . . . . . . . . . . . . . 145 | Evergreen Essence . . . . . . . . . . 150 | Live with Passion . . . . . . . . . . 155 |
| Aroma Life . . . . . . . . . . . . . . . 145 | Exodus II . . . . . . . . . . . . . . . . 150 | Live Your Passion . . . . . . . . . . 155 |
| Aroma Siez . . . . . . . . . . . . . . . 145 | Forgiveness . . . . . . . . . . . . . . . 150 | Longevity . . . . . . . . . . . . . . . . 155 |
| Aroma Sleep . . . . . . . . . . . . . . 145 | Freedom . . . . . . . . . . . . . . . . . 150 | Longevity Vitality . . . . . . . . . . 155 |
| Australian Blue . . . . . . . . . . . . 146 | Gathering . . . . . . . . . . . . . . . . 150 | Magnify Your Purpose . . . . . . 155 |
| Awaken . . . . . . . . . . . . . . . . . 146 | GeneYus . . . . . . . . . . . . . 151, 250 | Melrose . . . . . . . . . . . . . . . . . 156 |
| Believe . . . . . . . . . . . . . . . . . . 146 | Gentle Baby . . . . . . . . . . . . . . 151 | M-Grain . . . . . . . . . . . . . . . . . 156 |
| Bite Buster . . . . . . . . . . . 146, 250 | GLF . . . . . . . . . . . . . . . . . . . . 151 | Mister . . . . . . . . . . . . . . 156, 215 |
| Brain Power . . . . . . . . . . . . . . 146 | GLF Vitality . . . . . . . . . . . . . . 151 | Motivation . . . . . . . . . . . . . . . 156 |
| Breathe Again Roll-On . . . . . . 147 | Gratitude . . . . . . . . . . . . . . . . 151 | Oola Balance . . . . . . . . . . . . . 156 |
| Build Your Dream . . . . . . . . . 147 | Grounding . . . . . . . . . . . . . . . 152 | Oola Faith . . . . . . . . . . . . . . . 157 |
| Christmas Spirit . . . . . . . . . . . 147 | Harmony . . . . . . . . . . . . . . . . 152 | Oola Family . . . . . . . . . . . . . . 157 |
| Citrus Fresh . . . . . . . . . . . . . . 147 | Highest Potential . . . . . . . . . . 152 | Oola Field . . . . . . . . . . . . . . . 157 |
| Citrus Fresh Vitality . . . . . . . . 147 | Hope . . . . . . . . . . . . . . . . . . . 152 | Oola Finance . . . . . . . . . . . . . 157 |
| Clarity . . . . . . . . . . . . . . . . . . 147 | Humility . . . . . . . . . . . . . . . . 152 | Oola Fitness . . . . . . . . . . . . . . 157 |
| Common Sense . . . . . . . . . . . . 147 | ImmuPower . . . . . . . . . . . . . . 153 | Oola Friends . . . . . . . . . . . . . . 157 |
| Cool Azul . . . . . . . . . . . . . . . . 148 | Inner Child . . . . . . . . . . . . . . . 153 | Oola Fun . . . . . . . . . . . . . . . . 158 |
| Deep Relief Roll-On . . . . . . . . 148 | Inner Harmony . . . . . . . . . . . . 153 | Oola Grow . . . . . . . . . . . . . . . 158 |
| DiGize . . . . . . . . . . . . . . . . . . 148 | Inspiration . . . . . . . . . . . . . . . 153 | Owie . . . . . . . . . . . . . . . 158, 250 |
| DiGize Vitality . . . . . . . . . . . . 148 | Into the Future . . . . . . . . . . . . 153 | PanAway . . . . . . . . . . . . . . . . 158 |
| Divine Release . . . . . . . . . . . . 148 | InTouch . . . . . . . . . . . . . . . . . 154 | Peace & Calming . . . . . . . . . . 158 |
| Dragon Time . . . . . . . . 148, 215 | Joy . . . . . . . . . . . . . . . . 154, 215 | Peace & Calming II . . . . . . . . 158 |
| Dream Catcher . . . . . . . . . . . . 149 | JuvaCleanse . . . . . . . . . . . . . . 154 | Present Time . . . . . . . . . . . . . 159 |
| Egyptian Gold . . . . . . . . . . . . 149 | JuvaCleanse Vitality . . . . . . . . 154 | Purification . . . . . . . . . . . . . . 159 |

Seventh Edition | **Essential Oils Desk Reference** | 61

**Essential Oils Desk Reference** | Seventh Edition

Raven. . . . . . . . . . . . . . . . 159
R.C.. . . . . . . . . . . . . . . . . 159
Reconnect . . . . . . . . . . . . . 159
Red Shot . . . . . . . . . . . . . . 160
Release. . . . . . . . . . . . . . . . 160
Relieve It . . . . . . . . . . . . . . 160
RutaVaLa . . . . . . . . . . . . . . 160
RutaVaLa Roll-On . . . . . . . . . 160
Sacred Mountain . . . . . . . . . . 160
SARA. . . . . . . . . . . . . . . . . 161
SclarEssence. . . . . . . . . . 161, 215

SclarEssence Vitality. . . . . . . . 161
Sensation . . . . . . . . . . . . . . 161
Shutran . . . . . . . . . . . . 161, 224
SleepyIze . . . . . . . . . . . . 161, 250
Slique Essence . . . . . . . . . . . 162
SniffleEase . . . . . . . . . . 162, 250
Stress Away. . . . . . . . . . . . . . 162
Stress Away Roll-On. . . . . . . . . 162
Surrender . . . . . . . . . . . . . . 162
The Gift . . . . . . . . . . . . . . . 163
Thieves. . . . . . . . . . . . . . . . 163

Thieves Vitality. . . . . . . . . . . 163
Tranquil Roll-On . . . . . . . . . . 163
Transformation. . . . . . . . . 163, 215
Trauma Life . . . . . . . . . . . . . 164
T.R. Care . . . . . . . . . . . . . . 164
TummyGize. . . . . . . . . . 164, 250
Valor . . . . . . . . . . . . . . . . . 164
Valor II. . . . . . . . . . . . . . . . 165
Valor Roll-On . . . . . . . . . . . . 165
White Angelica. . . . . . . . . . . . 165
White Light . . . . . . . . . . . . . 165

# Chapter 8—Nutritional Support

AgilEase . . . . . . . . . . . . . . . 169
AlkaLime . . . . . . . . . . . . . . . 169
Allerzyme. . . . . . . . . . . . . . . 169
Balance Complete
  Vanilla Cream Meal
   Replacement. . . . . . . . 169, 201
BLM (Bones, Ligaments,
  and Muscles) Capsules . . . . . 170
BLM (Bones, Ligaments, and
  Muscles) Powder. . . . . . . . . 170
Blue Agave . . . . . . . . . . . . . . 171
ComforTone . . . . . . . . . . . . . 171
CortiStop. . . . . . . . . . . . 171, 212
Detoxzyme. . . . . . . . . . . . . . 172
Digest & Cleanse. . . . . . . . . . . 172
Ecuadorian Dark
  Chocolessence. . . . . . . . . . . 172
Einkorn Grain (Wheat) . . . . . . 175
EndoGize. . . . . . . . . . . . 173, 212
Essentialzyme. . . . . . . . . . . . . 173
Essentialzymes-4. . . . . . . . . . . 174
Estro . . . . . . . . . . . . . . . . . 174
FemiGen . . . . . . . . . . . . 174, 213
Gary's True Grit
  Chocolate-Coated
   Wolfberry Crisp Bars 176, 201
  Einkorn Flour. . . . . . . . . . . 176
  Einkorn Granola. . . . . . 176, 201
  Einkorn Pancake
   and Waffle Mix. . . . . . . . 176
  Einkorn Rotini Pasta. . . . . . . 177

Einkorn Spaghetti . . . . . . . . . 177
  Gluten-Free
   Pancake and Waffle Mix . . . . 177
   NingXia Berry Syrup. . . 177, 201
ICP . . . . . . . . . . . . . . . . . . 177
ImmuPro . . . . . . . . 178, 201, 213
Inner Defense. . . . . . . . . . . . . 178
JuvaPower. . . . . . . . . . . . . . . 178
JuvaSpice . . . . . . . . . . . . . . . 179
JuvaTone . . . . . . . . . . . . . . . 179
K&B . . . . . . . . . . . . . . . . . 179
KidScents. . . . . . . . 180, 201, 249
  MightyVites Orange
   Cream Flavor . . 180, 201, 249
  MightyVites Wild
   Berry Flavor . . . 180, 201, 249
  MightyZyme. . . . . . . . 180, 249
Life 9 . . . . . . . . . . . . . . . . . 181
Longevity (Softgels) . . . . . . . . . 181
Master Formula . . . . . . . 181, 201
MegaCal. . . . . . . . . . . . . . . . 182
MindWise . . . . . . . . . . . . . . 182
Mineral Essence . . . . . . . . . . . 183
MultiGreens. . . . . . . . . . . . . . 183
NingXia Nitro . . . . . . . . 183, 203
NingXia Red . . . . . . . . . 184, 203
Ningxia Wolfberries
  (Organic Dried) . . . . . . 184, 203
NingXia Zyng . . . . . . . . 184, 203
OmegaGize3 . . . . . . . . . . . . . 184
ParaFree . . . . . . . . . . . . . . . . 185

PD 80/20. . . . . . . . . . . 185, 213
PowerGize . . . . . . . . . . . . . . 185
Power Meal . . . . . . . . . . . . . . 185
Prostate Health. . . . . . . . . 186, 214
Pure Protein Complete
  Chocolate Deluxe . . . . . . . . 186
  Vanilla Spice . . . . . . . . . . . 187
Rehemogen . . . . . . . . . . . . . 187
SleepEssence. . . . . . . . . . . . . . 188
Slique Bars
  Chocolate-Coated. . . . . 188, 203
  Tropical Berry Crunch . 188, 203
Slique CitraSlim. . . . . . . . . . . 188
Slique Gum . . . . . . . . . . 189, 234
Slique Shake. . . . . . . . . . 189, 203
Slique Tea. . . . . . . . . . . . . . . 189
Sulfurzyme Capsules
  and Powder. . . . . . . . . 190, 204
Super B . . . . . . . . . . . . . . . . 190
Super C . . . . . . . . . . . . . . . . 190
Super C Chewable . . . . . . . . . . 191
SuperCal . . . . . . . . . . . . . . . 191
Thieves Cough Drops. . . . 191, 234
Thieves Hard Lozenges. . . 191, 234
Thieves Mints. . . . . . . . . 191, 234
Thyromin. . . . . . . . . . . . . . . 191
Ultra Young . . . . . . . . . . . . . 192
Wolfberry Crisp Bars,
  Chocolate-Coated. . . . . . . . 204
Yacon Syrup. . . . . . . . . . . . . . 192

Product Directory | **Section 2**

# Chapter 9—NingXia Wolfberry

Balance Complete Vanilla
Meal Replacement. . . . . 169, 201
Boswellia Wrinkle Cream . 204, 239
Copaiba Vanilla Moisturizing
Conditioner . . . . . . . . . 204, 221
Copaiba Vanilla Moisturizing
Shampoo. . . . . . . . . . . 204, 221
Essential Beauty Serum
(Dry Skin). . . . . . . . . . 204, 219
Gary's True Grit
Chocolate-Coated
Wolfberry Crisp Bars. . . 176, 201
Einkorn Granola. . . . . . 176, 201
NingXia Berry Syrup. . . 177, 201
ImmuPro . . . . . . . . . 178, 201, 213
KidScents MightyVites. . . . . . . 201
Lavender Bath &
Shower Gel . . . . . . . . . 205, 217

Lavender Hand &
Body Lotion . . . . . . . . . 205, 218
Lavender Mint Invigorating
Conditioner . . . . . . . . . 205, 221
Lavender Mint Invigorating
Shampoo. . . . . . . . . . . 205, 221
Lip Balm, Cinnamint. . . . . . . . 205
Lip Balm, Grapefruit . . . . . . . . 205
Lip Balm, Lavender . . . . . . . . . 205
Master Formula . . . . . . . . 181, 201
NingXia Nitro . . . . . . . . . 183, 203
NingXia Red . . . . . . . . . . 184, 203
Ningxia Wolfberries
(Organic Dried) . . . . . 184, 203
NingXia Zyng . . . . . . . . . 184, 203
Orange Blossom
Facial Wash. . . . . . . . . 205, 240

Prenolone +
Body Cream . . . . . 205, 213, 223
Regenolone Moisturizing
Cream. . . . . . . . . . 205, 214, 223
Sandalwood Moisture
Cream. . . . . . . . . . . . . 205, 240
Slique Bars—Chocolate-
Coated . . . . . . . . . . . 188, 203
Slique Bars—Tropical
Berry Crunch . . . . . . . 188, 203
Slique Shake. . . . . . . . . . 189, 203
Sulfurzyme Capsules
and Powder. . . . . . . . . 190, 204
Wolfberry Eye Cream. . . . 205, 241
Wolfberry Crisp . . . . . . . . . . . 204
Wolfberry Crisp Bars,
Chocolate-Coated. . . . . . . . 204

# Chapter 10—Hormones and Vibrant Health

CortiStop. . . . . . . . . . . . 171, 212
Dragon Time . . . . . . . . . 148, 215
EndoGize. . . . . . . . . . . . 173, 212
FemiGen . . . . . . . . . . . . 174, 213
ImmuPro . . . . . . . . . 178, 201, 213
Joy . . . . . . . . . . . . . . . . 154, 215

Lady Sclareol . . . . . . . . . 155, 215
Mister . . . . . . . . . . . . . . 156, 215
PD 80/20. . . . . . . . . . . . 185, 213
Prenolone +
Body Cream . . . . . 205, 213, 223
Progessence Plus. . . . . . . 214, 223

Prostate Health. . . . . . . . 186, 214
Protec. . . . . . . . . . . . . . 214, 223
Regenolone Moisturizing
Cream. . . . . . . . . . 205, 214, 223
SclarEssence . . . . . . . . . . 161, 215
Transformation. . . . . . . . 163, 215

# Chapter 11—Personal Care

AromaGuard Meadow
Mist Deodorant . . . . . . . . . 220
AromaGuard Mountain
Mint Deodorant . . . . . . . . . 220
ART Beauty Masque . . . . . . . 237
ART Chocolate Masque. . . . . . 237
ART Creme Masque. . . . . . . . 237
ART Gentle Cleanser. . . . . . . 238
ART Intensive Moisturizer . . . . 238
ART L'Brianté –
Neutral/Winter Scent . . . . . 224
Pink/Summer Scent . . . . . . 224
Red/Amoressence Scent . . . . 225
ART Light Moisturizer. . . . . . 238
ART Refreshing Toner . . . . . . 238

ART Renewal Serum . . . . . . . 239
ART Sheerlumé
Brightening Cream . . . . . . . 239
Bath & Shower Gel Base . . . . . 217
Boswellia Wrinkle Cream . 204, 239
Cel-Lite Magic Massage Oil . . . 225
Cinnamint Lip Balm . . . . . . . 224
ClaraDerm. . . . . . . . . . . . . . 239
Cool Azul Pain Relief Cream . . 235
Cool Azul Sports Gel . . . . . . . 235
Copaiba Vanilla Moisturizing
Conditioner . . . . . . . . . 204, 221
Copaiba Vanilla Moisturizing
Shampoo. . . . . . . . . . . 204, 221
Dragon Time Bath &

Shower Gel . . . . . . . . . . . . . 217
Dragon Time Massage Oil . . . . 225
Essential Beauty Serum
(Dry Skin). . . . . . . . . . 204, 219
Evening Peace Bath &
Shower Gel . . . . . . . . . . . . . 217
Genesis Hand & Body Lotion . 218
Grapefruit Lip Balm. . . . . . . . 224
Háloa Áina Royal Hawaiian
Sandalwood* Soap Collection. . 243
KidScents Slique Toothpaste. . . 231
LavaDerm Cooling Mist. . . . . . 240
Lavender Bath &
Shower Gel . . . . . . . . . 205, 217
Lavender Conditioner . . . . . . 222

Seventh Edition | **Essential Oils Desk Reference** | 63

Lavender Foaming Hand Soap . 245
Lavender Hand &
    Body Lotion . . . . . . . . 205, 218
Lavender Lip Balm. . . . . . . . . 224
Lavender Mint Invigorating
    Conditioner . . . . . . . . 205, 221
Lavender Mint Invigorating
    Shampoo. . . . . . . . . . . 205, 221
Lavender-Oatmeal Bar Soap. . . 243
Lavender Shampoo. . . . . . . . . 222
Lemon-Sandalwood
    Cleansing Soap . . . . . . . . . . 243
Melaleuca-Geranium
    Moisturizing Soap. . . . . . . . 243
Mirah Shave Oil. . . . . . . . . . . 235
Morning Start Bath &
    Shower Gel . . . . . . . . . . . . 218
Morning Start
    Moisturizing Soap. . . . . . . . 244
Orange Blossom Facial
    Wash. . . . . . . . . . . . . . 205, 240
Ortho Ease Massage Oil. . . . . . 225

Ortho Sport Massage Oil . . . . . 225
Peppermint-Cedarwood
    Moisturizing Soap. . . . . . . . 244
Prenolone + Body
    Cream. . . . . . . . . 205, 213, 223
Progessence Plus. . . . . . . 214, 223
Protec. . . . . . . . . . . . . . . 214, 223
Regenolone Moisturizing
    Cream. . . . . . . . . 205, 214, 223
Relaxation Massage Oil . . . . . . 226
Rose Ointment. . . . . . . . . . . . 240
Royal Hawaiian Sandalwood Soap
    with Frankincense Oil. . . . . . 243
    with Lavender Oil. . . . . . . . . 243
    with Ylang Ylang Oil. . . . . . 243
Sacred Mountain
    Moisturizing Soap. . . . . . . . 244
Sandalwood Moisture
    Cream. . . . . . . . . . . . . . 205, 240
Satin Facial Scrub, Mint. . . . . . 241
Sensation Bath & Shower Gel. . . 218
Sensation Hand & Body Lotion. . 219

Sensation Massage Oil . . . . . . . 226
Shutran . . . . . . . . . . . . . 161, 224
Shutran Aftershave Lotion . . . . 235
Shutran Bar Soap . . . . . . . . . . 244
Shutran Shave Cream. . . . . . . . 236
Slique Gum . . . . . . . . . . . 189, 234
Thieves
    AromaBright Toothpaste. . . . 229
    Cleansing Soap . . . . . . . . . . 244
    Cough Drops . . . . . . . . 191, 234
    Dental Floss . . . . . . . . . . . . 231
    Dentarome Plus Toothpaste . 229
    Dentarome Ultra Toothpaste . . 229
    Foaming Hand Soap . . . 245, 252
    Fresh Essence Plus
        Mouthwash. . . . . . . . . . . 234
    Hard Lozenges . . . . . . . 191, 234
    Mints . . . . . . . . . . . . . 191, 234
    Waterless Hand Purifier . . 222, 253
V-6 Vegetable Oil Complex . . . 226
Valor Moisturizing Soap. . . . . . 244
Wolfberry Eye Cream. . . . 205, 241

# Chapter 12—Healthy Choices for Children

Bite Buster . . . . . . . . . . . 146, 250
GeneYus. . . . . . . . . . . . . 151, 250
KidScents
    Bath Gel . . . . . . . . . . . . . . 247
    Lotion. . . . . . . . . . . . . . . . 247
    MightyVites . . . . . 180, 201, 249

MightyVites Orange
    Cream Flavor . . 180, 201, 249
MightyVites Wild
    Berry Flavor . . . 180, 201, 249
MightyZyme. . . . . . . . . 180, 249
Shampoo. . . . . . . . . . . . . . . 247

Slique Toothpaste . . . . . 231, 247
Tender Tush . . . . . . . . . . . . 248
Owie . . . . . . . . . . . . . . . 158, 250
SleepyIze . . . . . . . . . . . 161, 250
SniffleEase . . . . . . . . . . . 162, 250
TummyGize. . . . . . . . . . 164, 250

# Chapter 13—Fortifying Your Home with Essential Oils

Thieves
    Automatic Dishwasher
        Powder . . . . . . . . . . . . . 251
    Dish Soap . . . . . . . . . . . . . 252

Foaming Hand Soap . . . 245, 252
Fruit & Veggie Soak . . . . . . . 253
Fruit & Veggie Spray. . . . . . . 253
Household Cleaner . . . . . . . . 253

Laundry Soap . . . . . . . . . . . 253
Spray. . . . . . . . . . . . . . . . . 253
Waterless Hand Purifier  222, 253
Wipes . . . . . . . . . . . . . . . . 254

# Chapter 14—Animal Care

Animal Scents
    Dental Pet Chews . . . . . . . . 265
    Ointment . . . . . . . . . . . . . 265
    Shampoo. . . . . . . . . . . . . . 265

Gary's Equine Essentials
    Massage Oil . . . . . . . . . . . . 270
    Shampoo. . . . . . . . . . . . . . 270
    Tail & Mane Sheen . . . . . . . 270
Infect Away . . . . . . . . . . . . . 266

Mendwell. . . . . . . . . . . . . . . 266
ParaGize. . . . . . . . . . . . . . . . 266
PuriClean. . . . . . . . . . . . . . . 266
RepelAroma . . . . . . . . . . . . . 266
T-Away. . . . . . . . . . . . . . . . . 266

# Chapter 6
## Single Oils

# Quality Assurance

This section describes over 80 single essential oils, including botanical information, therapeutic and traditional uses, chemical constituents of each oil, extraction method, cautions, and application instructions.

### How to Be Sure Your Essential Oils Are Pure, Therapeutic Grade

How can you be sure that your essential oils are pure, therapeutic grade? Start by asking the following questions from your essential oil supplier:

- Are the fragrances delicate, rich, and organic? Do they "feel" natural? Do the aromas vary from batch to batch as an indication that they are painstakingly distilled in small batches rather than industrially processed on a large scale?

- Does your supplier subject each batch of essential oils through multiple chemical analyses to test for purity and therapeutic quality? Are these tests performed by independent labs?

- Does your supplier grow and distill organically grown herbs?

- Are the distillation facilities part of the farm where the herbs are grown (so oils are freshly distilled), or do herbs wait days to be processed and lose potency?

- Does your supplier use low pressure and low temperature to distill essential oils so as to preserve all of their fragile chemical constituents? Are the distillation cookers fabricated from costly, food-grade stainless steel alloys to reduce the likelihood of the oils chemically reacting with metal?

- Does your supplier personally inspect the fields and distilleries where the herbs are grown and distilled? Do they verify that no synthetic or harmful solvents or chemicals are being used?

- How many years has your supplier been doing all of this?

### How to Maximize the Shelf Life of Your Essential Oils

The highest quality essential oils are bottled in dark glass. The reason for this is two-fold. First, glass is more stable than plastic and does not "breathe" the same way plastic does. Second, the darkness of the glass protects the oil from light that may chemically alter or degrade it over time.

After using an essential oil, keep the lid tightly sealed. Bottles that are improperly sealed can result in the loss of some of the lighter, lower-molecular-weight parts of the oil. In addition, over time oxygen in the air reacts with and oxidizes the oil.

Essential oils should be stored away from light, especially sunlight—even if they are already stored in amber glass bottles. The darker the storage conditions, the longer your oil will maintain its original chemistry and quality.

Store essential oils in a cool location. Excessive heat can derange the molecular structure of the oil the same way ultraviolet light can.

### Diluting Essential Oils

Most essential oils require dilution with a vegetable oil when being used either internally or externally. The amount of dilution depends on the essential oil. For example, oregano will require four times as much dilution as that of Roman Chamomile. Vegetable oils such as V-6 Vegetable Oil Complex are specifically formulated to dilute essential oils and have a long shelf life (over two years) without going rancid. For more information on specific usage instructions for each essential oil, please see the "Personal Usage Guide."

Seventh Edition | **Essential Oils Desk Reference** | 65

Essential Oils Desk Reference | Seventh Edition

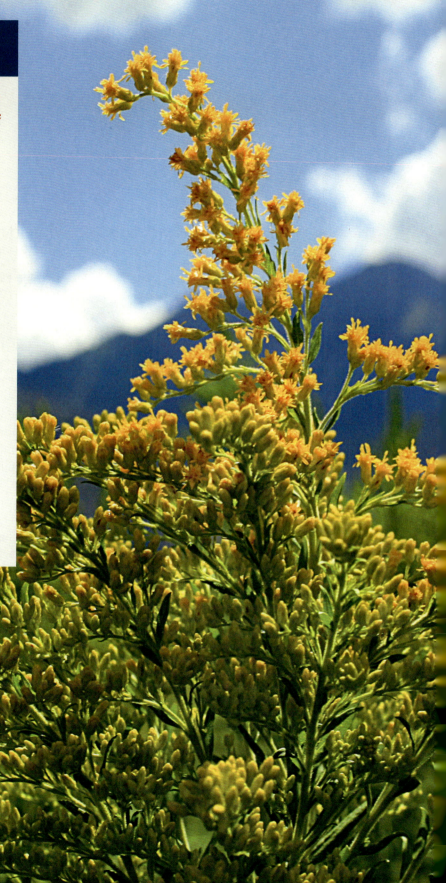

## Guidelines

**Please see Chapter 5 for additional details on how to use essential oils and follow the directions on the product labels.**

**Common uses:** Almost all single oils can be diffused, directly inhaled, and/or applied topically.

**Full body massage:** Dilute 1 drop essential oil with 15 drops of V-6 or other pure carrier oil.

**Possible skin sensitivity:** Test for sensitivity on small location of skin on underside of arm.

**Possible sun sensitivity:** Avoid direct sunlight or UV rays for up to 12 hours after applying product.

**Dietary and/or culinary use:** Vitality™ dietary essential oil singles can be added to food for delicious, concentrated flavor or used in capsules for their supporting properties. Follow the directions on the labels.

**Found-in list:** A list of the products containing each oil can be found in Appendix B.

Goldenrod *(Solidago Canadensis)*

Single Oils | **Chapter 6**

# Single Essential Oil Application Codes

**Neat = Straight, undiluted**

Dilution usually NOT required; suitable for all but the most sensitive skin. Safe for children over 2 years old.

**50-50 = Dilute 50-50**

Dilution recommended at 50-50 (1 part essential oils to 1 part V-6 Vegetable Oil Complex) for topical and internal use, especially when used on sensitive areas — face, neck, genital area, underarms, etc. Keep out of reach of children.

**20-80 = Dilute 20-80**

Always dilute 20-80 (1 part essential oils to 4 parts V-6 Vegetable Oil Complex) before applying to the skin or taking internally. Keep out of reach of children.

**PH = Photosensitizing**

Avoid using on skin exposed to direct sunlight or UV rays (e.g., sunlamps, tanning beds, etc.)

| | | | | | | | |
|---|---|---|---|---|---|---|---|
| Amazonian Ylang Ylang | | 50-50 | Frereana Frankincense | **20-80** | Nutmeg | | 50-50 |
| Angelica | PH | 50-50 | Galbanum | 50-50 | Ocotea | | **20-80** |
| Anise | | 50-50 | Geranium | Neat | Orange | PH | 50-50 |
| Basil | | **20-80** | German Chamomile | Neat | Oregano | | **20-80** |
| Bergamot | PH | 50-50 | Ginger | 50-50 | Palmarosa | | Neat |
| Biblical Sweet Myrrh | | 50-50 | Goldenrod | 50-50 | Palo Santo | | 50-50 |
| Black Pepper | | 50-50 | Grapefruit | PH 50-50 | Patchouli | | Neat |
| Black Spruce | | 50-50 | Helichrysum | Neat | Peppermint | | **20-80** |
| Blue Cypress | | Neat | Hinoki | 50-50 | Petitgrain | | Neat |
| Blue Tansy | | Neat | Hong Kuai | 50-50 | Pine | | 50-50 |
| Calamus | | 50-50 | Hyssop | 50-50 | Plectranthus Oregano | | **20-80** |
| Canadian Fleabane | | 50-50 | Idaho Balsam Fir | 50-50 | Ravintsara | | 50-50 |
| Cardamom | | 50-50 | Idaho Blue Spruce | Neat | Roman Chamomile | | Neat |
| Carrot Seed | | 50-50 | Idaho Ponderosa Pine | 50-50 | Rose | | Neat |
| Cassia | | **20-80** | Idaho Tansy | 50-50 | Rosemary | | 50-50 |
| Cedarwood | | Neat | Ishpingo | **20-80** | Rosewood | | Neat |
| Celery Seed | | 50-50 | Jade Lemon | PH 50-50 | Royal Hawaiian Sandalwood | | Neat |
| Cinnamon Bark | | **20-80** | Jasmine | Neat | Ruta | | 50-50 |
| Cistus | | Neat | Juniper | 50-50 | Sacred Frankincense | | Neat |
| Citronella | | 50-50 | Laurus Nobilis | 50-50 | Sage | | 50-50 |
| Citrus Hystrix | | 50-50 | Lavandin | Neat | Sandalwood | | Neat |
| Clary Sage | | 50-50 | Lavender | Neat | Spanish Sage | | 50-50 |
| Clove | | **20-80** | Ledum | 50-50 | Spearmint | | 50-50 |
| Copaiba | | Neat | Lemon | PH 50-50 | Spikenard | | Neat |
| Coriander | | 50-50 | Lemongrass | **20-80** | Tangerine | PH | 50-50 |
| Cumin | PH | **20-80** | Lemon Myrtle | **20-80** | Tarragon | | 50-50 |
| Cypress | | 50-50 | Lime | PH 50-50 | Thyme | | **20-80** |
| Dalmatia Bay Laurel | | 50-50 | Mandarin | PH 50-50 | Tsuga | | 50-50 |
| Dalmatia Juniper | | 50-50 | Manuka | Neat | Valerian | | Neat |
| Dalmatia Sage | | **20-80** | Marjoram | 50-50 | Vanilla | | Neat |
| Davana | | 50-50 | Mastrante | 50-50 | Vetiver | | Neat |
| Dill | | 50-50 | Melaleuca Alternifolia | 50-50 | Vitex | | 50-50 |
| Dorado Azul | | 50-50 | Melaleuca Cajuput | 50-50 | Western Red Cedar | | 50-50 |
| Douglas Fir | | 50-50 | Melaleuca Ericifolia | 50-50 | White Fir | | Neat |
| Elemi | | Neat | Melaleuca Quinquenervia | 50-50 | White Lotus | | 50-50 |
| Eucalyptus Blue | | 50-50 | Melissa | Neat | Wintergreen | | **20-80** |
| Eucalyptus Citriodora | | 50-50 | Micromeria | **20-80** | Xiang Mao | | Neat |
| Eucalyptus Dives | | 50-50 | Mountain Savory | 50-50 | Yarrow | | Neat |
| Eucalyptus Globulus | | 50-50 | Mugwort | 50-50 | Ylang Ylang | | 50-50 |
| Eucalyptus Radiata | | 50-50 | Myrrh | Neat | Yuzu | | Neat |
| Eucalyptus Staigeriana | | 50-50 | Myrtle | 50-50 | | | |
| Fennel | | Neat | Neroli | Neat | | | |
| Frankincense | | Neat | Northern Lights Black Spruce | 50-50 | | | |

Seventh Edition | **Essential Oils Desk Reference** | 67

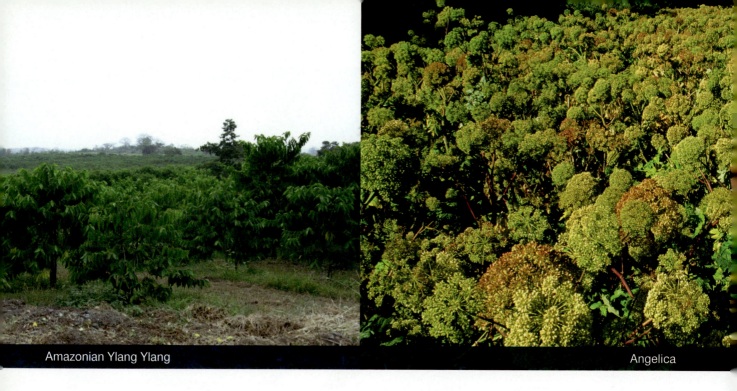

Amazonian Ylang Ylang

Angelica

## Amazonian Ylang Ylang
### (Cananga odorata Equitoriana)

The flowering ylang ylang tree is often found in the Philippines, Indonesia, and Madagascar. Now Gary Young has also translocated trees to the Young Living Ecuador Farm, where the aromatic flowers from thousands of trees bloom every day.

**Uses:** While renowned for its calming effect, several studies show it brings relief for the depressed and stressed, while it increases attentiveness and alertness, causing researchers to say it is "harmonizing."

**Fragrant Influence:** Balances male-female energies, enhances spiritual attunement, combats anger and low self-esteem, increases focus of thoughts, filters out negative energy, restores confidence and peace

**Directions: Aromatic:** Diffuse up to 1 hour 3 times daily or directly inhale. **Topical:** Dilute 1 drop essential oil with 1 drop V-6 or other pure carrier oil and apply 2-4 drops on location, chakras, and/or Vita Flex points.

**Technical Data: Botanical Family:** Annonaceae; **Plant Origin:** Ecuador; **Extraction Method:** Steam distilled from flowers; **Key Constituents:** Benzyl Acetate (15-29%), Germacrene D (10-20%), Linalool (10-25%), Benzyl Benzoate (4-12%), p-Cresyl Methyl Ether (2-10%)

### Selected Research

Tan LT, et al. Traditional Uses, Phytochemistry, and Bioactives of *Cananga odorata* (Ylang-Ylang). *Evid Based Complement Alternat Med.* 2015;2015 [Epub ahead of print].

Gnatta JR, et al. [Aromatherapy with ylang ylang for anxiety and self-esteem: a pilot study]. *Rev Esc Enferm USP.* 2014 Jun;48(3):492-9.

Moss M, et al. Modulation of cognitive performance and mood by aromas of peppermint and ylang ylang. *Int J Neurosci.* 2008 Jan;118(1):59-77.

Hongratanaworakit T, Buchbauer G. Relaxing effect of ylang ylang oil on humans after transdermal absorption. *Phytother Res.* 2006 Sep;20(9):758-763.

## Angelica (Angelica archangelica)

Known as the "holy spirit root" or the "oil of angels" by the Europeans, angelica's healing powers were so strong that it was believed to be of divine origin. From the time of Paracelsus, it was credited with the ability to protect from the plague. The stems were chewed during the plague of 1660 to prevent infection. When burned, the seeds and roots were thought to purify the air.

**Medical Properties:** Anticoagulant, relaxant, antispasmodic

**Uses:** Throat/lung infections, indigestion, menstrual problems/PMS, symptoms of dementia

**Fragrant Influence:** Assists in the release of pent-up negative feelings and restores memories to the point of origin before trauma or anger was experienced

**Directions: Aromatic:** Diffuse up to 30 minutes 3 times daily or directly inhale. **Dietary:** Dilute 1 drop essential oil with 1 drop V-6 or other pure carrier oil of choice, put in a capsule, and take up to 3 times daily or as needed. **Topical:** Dilute 1 drop essential oil with 1 drop V-6 or other pure carrier oil and apply 1-2 drops on location, chakras, and/or Vita Flex points.

**Caution:** Possible sun sensitivity.

**Technical Data: Botanical Family:** Apiaceae; **Plant Origin:** Belgium, France; **Extraction Method:** Steam distilled from seed/root; **Key Constituents:** Beta-Phellandrene (60-80%), Limonene (1-4%), Alpha-Pinene (5-10%)

### Selected Research

Prakash B, et al. Efficacy of *Angelica archangelica* essential oil, phenyl ethyl alcohol and α-terpineol against isolated molds from walnut and their antiaflatoxigenic and antioxidant activity. *J Food Sci Technol.* 2015 Apr;52(4):2220-8.

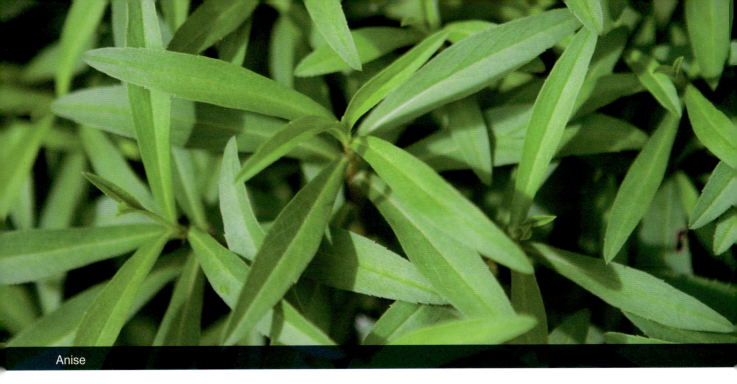

Fraternale D, et al. Essential Oil Composition and Antimicrobial Activity of *Angelica archangelica* L. (Apiaceae) Roots. *J Med Food.* 2014 Sep;17(9):1043-7.

Kumar D, et al. Coumarins from *Angelica archangelica* Linn. and their effects on anxiety-like behavior. *Prog Neuropsychopharmacol Biol Psychiatry.* 2013 Jan 10;40:180-6.

Bhat ZA, et al. *Angelica archangelica* Linn. is an angel on earth for the treatment of diseases. *Int J Nutr Pharmacol Neurol Dis.* 2011;1(1):36-50.

Kimura T, et al. Effect of ferulic acid and *Angelica archangelica* extract on behavioral and psychological symptoms of dementia in frontotemporal lobar degeneration and dementia with Lewy bodies. *Geriatr Gerontol Int.* 2011 Jul;11(3):309-314.

## Anise (Pimpinella anisum)

Listed in Dioscorides' *De Materia Medica* (AD 78), Europe's first authoritative guide to medicines, which became the standard reference work for herbal treatments for over 1,700 years.

**Medical Properties:** Digestive stimulant, anticoagulant, anesthetic/analgesic, antioxidant, diuretic, antitumoral, anti-inflammatory

**Uses:** Arthritis/rheumatism, cancer

**Directions: Aromatic:** Diffuse up to 30 minutes 3 times daily or directly inhale. **Dietary:** Put in a capsule and take up to 3 times daily or as needed. **Topical:** Dilute 1 drop essential oil with 1 drop V-6 or other pure carrier oil and apply on location, chakras, and/or Vita Flex points.

**Fragrant Influence:** Opens emotional blocks and recharges vital energy

**Technical Data: Botanical Family:** Apiaceae; **Plant Origin:** Turkey; **Extraction Method:** Steam distilled from the seeds (fruit); **Key Constituents:** Trans-Anethole (85-95%): Methyl Chavicol (2-4%); **ORAC:** 333,700 µTE/100g

## Selected Research

Koriem KM, et al. The Productive role of Anise Oil in Oxidative Stress and Genotoxicity Produced in Favism. *J Diet Suppl.* 2016 Jan 8:1-17.

Jamshidzadeh A, et al. An in vivo and in vitro investigation on hepatoprotective effects of *Pimpinella anisum* seed essential oil and extracts against carbon tetrachloride-induced toxicity. *Iran J Basic Med.* 2015 Feb;18(2):205-11.

Gradinaru AC, et al. Screening of antibacterial effects of anise essential oil alone and in combination with conventional antibiotics against *Streptococcus pneumoniae* clinical isolates. *Rev Med Chir Soc Med Nat Iasi.* 2014 Apr-Jun;118(2):537-43.

Lee JB, et al. Antiviral and immunostimulating effects of lignan-carbohydrate-protein complexes from *Pimpinella anisum*. *Biosci Biotechnol Biochem.* 2011 Mar;75(3):459-465.

## Basil (Ocimum basilicum)

Used extensively in traditional Asian Indian medicine, basil's name is derived from "basileum," the Greek name for king. In the 16th century, the powdered leaves were inhaled to treat migraines and chest infections. The Hindu people put basil sprigs on the chests of the dead to protect them from evil spirits. Italian women wore basil to attract possible suitors. It was listed in Hildegard's Medicine, a compilation of early German medicines by highly regarded Benedictine herbalist Hildegard of Bingen (1098-1179).

**Medical Properties:** Powerful antispasmodic, antiviral, antibacterial, anti-inflammatory, muscle relaxant

**Uses:** Migraines, throat/lung infections, insect bites

**Fragrant Influence:** Fights mental fatigue

**Directions: Aromatic:** Diffuse up to 30 minutes 3 times daily or directly inhale. **Topical:** Dilute 1 drop essential oil with 4 drops V-6 or other pure carrier oil

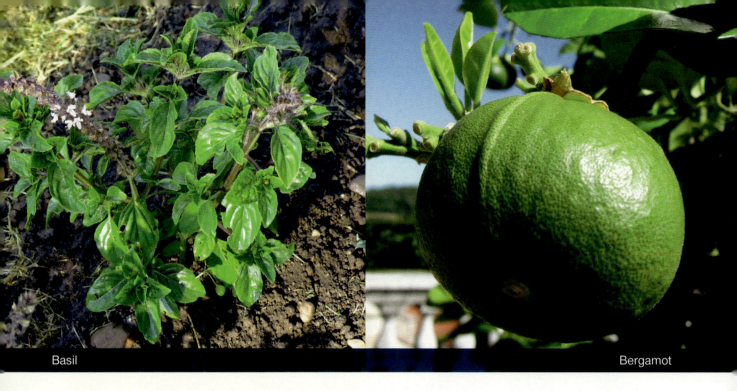

Basil

Bergamot

and apply 2-4 drops on location, temples, neck, or on chakras and/or Vita Flex points (crown of head, forehead, heart, and navel). Apply around ear for earache.

**Cautions:** Avoid use if epileptic. Do not pour oil into the ear.

### Basil Vitality™ *(Ocimum basilicum)*

**Directions: Dietary:** Dilute 1 drop with 4 drops of carrier oil. Put in a capsule and take 1 daily.

**Technical Data: Botanical Family:** Lamiaceae; **Plant Origin:** India, Utah, France; **Extraction Method:** Steam distilled from leaves, stems, and flowers; **Key Constituents:** Methylchavicol (estragol) (70-90%), Linalol (1-20%), 1,8-Cineole (Eucalyptol) (1-7%); **ORAC:** 54,000 µTE/100g

### Selected Research

Snoussi M, et al. Chemical composition and antibiofilm activity of *Petroselinum crispum* and *Ocimum basilicum* essential oils against Vibrio spp. strains. *Microb Pathog.* 2016 Jan;90:13-21.

Ogaly HA, et al. Hepatocyte Growth Factor Mediates the Antifibrogenic Action of *Ocimum basilicum* Essential Oil against CCl4-Induced Liver Fibrosis in Rats. *Molecules.* 2015 Jul 23;20(8):13518-35.

Shirazi MT, et al. Chemical composition, antioxidant, antimicrobial and cytotoxic activities of *Tagetes minuta* and *Ocimum basilicum* essential oils. *Food Sci Nutr.* 2014 Mar;2(2):146-55.

Siddiqui BS, et al. Evaluation of the antimycobacterium activity of the constituents from *Ocimum basilicum* against *Mycobacterium tuberculosis*. *J Ethnopharmacol.* 2012 Oct 31;144(1):220-2.

Kristinsson KG, et al. Effective treatment of experimental acute otitis media by application of volatile fluids into the ear canal. *J Infect. Dis.* 2005 Jun 1;191(11):1876-80.

### Bergamot *(Citrus aurantium bergamia)*
(also found in literature as *Citrus bergamia*)

Christopher Columbus is believed to have brought bergamot to Bergamo in Northern Italy from the Canary Islands. A mainstay in traditional Italian medicine, bergamot has been used in the Middle East for hundreds of years for skin conditions associated with an oily complexion. Bergamot is responsible for the distinctive flavor of the renowned Earl Grey Tea and was used in the first genuine eau de cologne.

**Medical Properties:** Calming, hormonal support, antibacterial, antidepressant

**Uses:** Agitation, depression, anxiety, intestinal parasites, insomnia, viral infections (herpes, cold sores)

**Fragrant Influence:** Relieves anxiety; mood-lifting qualities

**Directions: Aromatic:** Diffuse up to 1 hour 3 times daily or directly inhale. **Topical:** Dilute 1 drop essential oil with 1 drop V-6 or other pure carrier oil and apply 1-2 drops on location, chakras, and/or Vita Flex points.

**Caution:** Possible sun sensitivity.

### Bergamot Vitality™ *(Citrus aurantium bergamia)*

**Directions: Dietary:** Dilute 1 drop with 1 drop of carrier oil. Put in a capsule and take up to 3 times daily.

**Technical Data: Botanical Family:** Rutaceae; **Plant Origin:** Italy, Morocco; **Extraction Method:** Cold pressed from the rind. Also produced by vacuum distillation. Furocoumarin-free bergamot oil is specially distilled to minimize the concentration of sun-sensitizing compounds in the oil; **Key Constituents:** Limonene (30-45%), Linalyl Acetate (22-36%), Linalol (3-15%), Gamma-Terpinene (6-10%), Beta-Pinene (5.5-9.5%)

Single Oils | Chapter 6

## Selected Research

Rombolà L, et al. Rational Basis for the Use of Bergamot Essential Oil in Complementary Medicine to Treat Chronic Pain. *Mini Rev Med Chem.* 2016 Mar 21. [Epub ahead of print]

Toth PP, et al. Bergamot Reduces Plasma Lipids, Atherogenic Small Dense LDL, and Subclinical Atherosclerosis in Subjects with Moderate Hyperchloesterolemia: A 6 Months Prospective Study. *Front Pharmacol.* 2016 Jan 6;6:299. [Epub ahead of print]

Watanabe E, et al. Effects of bergamot (*Citrus bergamia* (Risso) Wright & Arn.) essential oil aromatherapy on mood states, parasympathetic nervous system activity, and salivary cortisol levels in 41 healthy females. *Forsch Komplementmed.* 2015;22(1):43-9.

Cosentino M, et al. The essential oil of bergamot stimulates reactive oxygen species production in human polymorphonuclear leukocytes. *Phytother Res.* 2014 Aug;28(8):1232-9.

Chen MC, et al. The effects of aromatherapy in relieving symptoms related to job stress among nurses. *Int J Nurs Pract.* 2013 Nov 15.

Saiyudthong S, Marsden CA. Acute effects of bergamot oil on anxiety-related behaviour and corticosterone level in rats. *Phytother Res.* 2011 Jun;25(6):858-62.

Borgatti M, et al. Bergamot (*Citrus bergamia* Risso) fruit extracts and identified components alter expression of interleukin 8 gene in cystic fibrosis bronchial epithelial cell lines. *BMC Biochem.* 2011;12:15.

## Biblical Sweet Myrrh (Commiphora erythraea)

A close cousin to the more well-known *Commiphora myrrha*, Biblical Sweet Myrrh is also called Opoponax. Used in dozens of perfumes to impart sweet balsamic notes, this myrrh species is found in Chanel's Coco Mademoiselle and Dior's Poison. Biblical Sweet Myrrh comes from myrrh resin gathered on the island of Socotra, off the coast of Yemen, and is distilled at the Young Living farm in Salalah, Oman. Like other frankincense species, it is highly anti-inflammatory, antimicrobial, and an antioxidant.

**Medical Properties:** Analgesic, antioxidant, anti-inflammatory, antimicrobial, antifungal, antiviral

**Uses:** Arthritis, digestive problems, nerve/muscle pain, fungal infections

**Fragrant Influence:** Promotes spiritual awareness and is uplifting. It contains sesquiterpenes, which stimulate the limbic system of the brain (the center of memory and emotions) and the hypothalamus, pineal, and pituitary glands. The hypothalamus is the master gland of the human body, producing many vital hormones, including thyroid and growth hormone.

**Directions: Aromatic:** Diffuse up to 30 minutes 3 times daily or directly inhale. **Topical:** Dilute 1 drop essential oil with 1 drop V-6 or other pure carrier oil and apply on location, chakras, and/or Vita Flex points.

**Technical Data: Botanical Family:** Burseraceae; **Plant Origin:** Socotra Island, Yemen; **Extraction Method:** Steam distilled from resin; **Key Constituents:** Trans-Beta-Ocimene (45-65%), Cis-Alpha-Bisabolene (10-15%), Alpha-Santalene (12-20%), Trans-Alpha-Bergamotene (3-8%), Cis-Alpha-Bergamotene (1-4%)

## Selected Research

Santoro S, et al. Agarsenone, a Cadinane Sesquiterpenoid from *Commiphora erythraea. J Nat Prod.* 2013 Jul 26;76(7):1254-9.

Bellezza I, et al. Furanodien-6-one from *Commiphora erythraea* inhibits the NF-kB signaling and attenuates LPS-induced neuroinflammation. *Mol Immunol.* 2013 Jul;54(3-4):347-54.

Shen T, et al. The genus *Commiphora*: a review of its traditional uses, phytochemistry and pharmacology. *J Ethnopharmacol.* 2012 Jul 13;142(2):319-30.

Cenci E, et al. Antiviral furanosesquiterpenes from *Commiphora erythraea. Nat Prod Commun.* 2012 Feb;7(2):143-4.

Marcotullio MC, et al. Protective effects of *Commiphora erythraea* resin constituents against cellular oxidative damage. *Molecules.* 2011 Dec 14;16(12):10357-69.

Fraternale D, et al. Anti-inflammatory, antioxidant and antifungal furanosesquiterpenoids isolated from *Commiphora erythraea* (Ehrenb.) Engl. resin. *Fitoterapia.* 2011 Jun;82(4):654-61.

## Black Pepper (Piper nigrum)

Used by the Egyptians in mummification, as evidenced by the discovery of black pepper in the nostrils and abdomen of Ramses II. Indian monks ate several black peppercorns a day to give them endurance during their arduous travels. In ancient times pepper was as valuable as gold or silver. When the barbarian Goth tribes of Europe vanquished Rome in 410 AD, they demanded 3,000 pounds of pepper as well as other valuables as a ransom. Traditional Chinese healers used pepper to treat cholera, malaria, and digestive problems.

**Medical Properties:** Analgesic, stimulates metabolism, antifungal

**Uses:** Obesity, arthritis, digestive problems, fatigue, nerve/muscle pain, fungal infections, tobacco cessation

**Fragrant Influence:** Stimulating, energizing, and empowering. A 2002 study found that fragrance inhalation of pepper oil induced a 1.7-fold increase in plasma adrenaline concentration (Haze, et al.).

**Directions: Aromatic:** Diffuse up to 30 minutes 3 times daily or directly inhale. **Topical:** Dilute 1 drop essential oil with 1 drop V-6 or other pure carrier oil and apply on location, chakras, and/or Vita Flex points.

## Black Pepper Vitality™ (Piper nigrum)

**Directions: Dietary:** Dilute 1 drop with 1 drop of carrier oil. Put in a capsule and take up to 3 times daily.

**Technical Data: Botanical Family:** Piperaceae; **Plant Origin:** Madagascar, Sri Lanka, England, India; **Extraction Method:** Steam distilled from fruit/berries; **Key Constituents:** Beta-Caryophyllene (12-29%), Limonene (10-17%), Sabinene (6-15%), Delta-3-Carene (3-15%), Alpha-Pinene (3-12%), Beta-Pinene (5-12%); **ORAC:** 79,700 µTE/100g

Seventh Edition | **Essential Oils Desk Reference** | 71

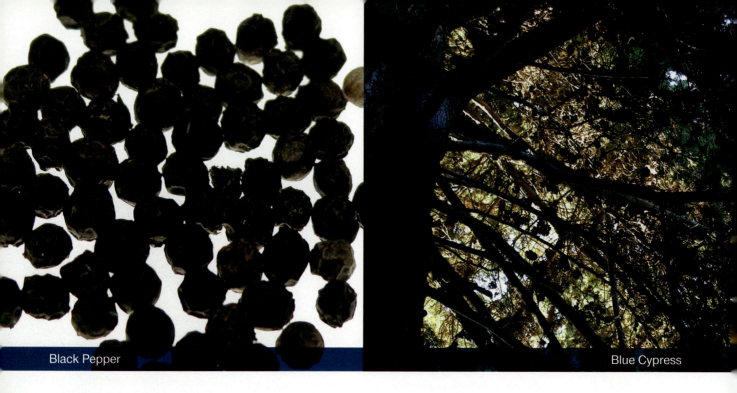

Black Pepper

Blue Cypress

### Selected Research

Chavarria D, et al. Lessons from black pepper: piperine and derivatives thereof. *Expert Opin Ther Pat.* 2016 Feb;26(2):245-64.

Cordell B, Buckle J. The effects of aromatherapy on nicotine craving on a U.S. campus: a small comparison study. *J Altern Complement Med.* 2013 Aug;19(8):709-13.

Kristiniak S, et al. Black pepper essential oil to enhance intravenous catheter insertion in patients with poor vein visibility: a controlled study. *J Altern Complement Med.* 2012 Nov;18(11):1003-7.

Kapoor IP, et al. Chemistry and in vitro antioxidant activity of volatile oil and oleoresins of black pepper (*Piper nigrum*). *J Agric Food Chem.* 2009 Jun 24;57(12):5358-64.

## Black Spruce *(Picea mariana)*

The Lakota Indians used black spruce to strengthen their ability to communicate with the Great Spirit. Traditionally, it was believed to possess the frequency of prosperity.

**Medical Properties:** Antispasmodic, antiparasitic, antiseptic, anti-inflammatory, hormone-like, cortisone-like, immune stimulant, antidiabetic

**Uses:** Arthritis/rheumatism, fungal infections (candida), sinus/respiratory infections, sciatica/lumbago

**Fragrant Influence:** Releases emotional blocks, bringing about a feeling of balance and grounding

**Directions: Aromatic:** Diffuse up to 30 minutes 3 times daily or directly inhale. **Dietary:** Take as a dietary supplement. **Topical:** Dilute 1 drop essential oil with 1 drop V-6 or other pure carrier oil and apply 2-4 drops on location, chakras, and/or Vita Flex points.

**Technical Data: Botanical Family:** Pinaceae; **Plant Origin:** Canada; **Extraction Method:** Steam distilled from branches, needles, and twigs; **Key Constituents:** Bornyl Acetate (24-35%), Camphene (14-26%), Alpha-Pinene (12-19%), Beta-Pinene (2-10%), Delta-3-Carene (4-10%), Limonene (3-6%), Myrcene (1-5%), Santene (1-5%), Tricyclene (1-4%)

### Selected Research

Prunier J, et al. From genotypes to phenotypes: expression levels of genes encompassing adaptive SNPs in black spruce. *Plant Cell Rep.* 2015 Aug 11 [Epub ahead of print]

Garcia-Pérez ME, et al. *Picea mariana* polyphenolic extract inhibits phlogogenic mediators produced by TNF-α-activated psoriatic keratinocytes: Impact on NF-κB pathway. *J Ethnopharmacol.* 2014;151(1):265-78.

Garcia-Pérez ME, et al. *Picea mariana* bark: a new source of trans-resveratrol and other bioactive polyphenols. *Food Chem.* 2012 Dec 1; 135(3):1173-82.

Tam TW, et al. Cree antidiabetic plant extracts display mechanism-based inactivation of CYP3A4. *Can J Physiol Pharmacol.* 2011 Jan;89(1):13-23.

## Blue Cypress *(Callitris intratropica)*

Blue cypress in ancient times was used for incense, perfume, and embalming.

**Medical Properties:** Anti-inflammatory, antiviral

**Uses:** Viral infections (herpes simplex, herpes zoster, cold sores, human papilloma virus, genital warts, etc.)

**Directions: Aromatic:** Diffuse up to 1 hour 3 times daily or directly inhale. **Topical:** Apply 2-4 drops on location, chakras, and/or Vita Flex points. Dilution not required except for the most sensitive skin.

**Technical Data: Botanical Family:** Cupressaceae; **Plant Origin:** Australia; **Extraction Method:** Steam distillation from the leaves and wood of the tree; **Key Constituents:** Gamma-Eudesmol (5-12%), Guaiol (10-20%), Bulnesol (5-11%), Dihydrocolumellarin (10-25%); **ORAC:** 73,100 μTE/100g

### Selected Research

Wanner J, et al. *Callitris intratropica* R.T. Baker & H.G. Smith as a Novel Rich Source of Deoxypodophyllotoxin. *Current Bioactive Compounds.* 2015, Aug;11, 73-77.

Horak S, et al. Use-dependent block of voltage-gated Cav2.1 Ca2+ channels by petasins and eudesmol isomers. *J Pharmacol Exp Ther.* 2009 Jul;330(1):220-6.

Zhao Q, et al. Antioxidant activities of eleven Australian essential oils. *Nat Prod Comm.* 2008;3(5):837-842.

Doimo L. Azulenes, Costols and γ-Lactones from Cypress-Pines (*Callitris columellaris, C. glaucophylla* and *C. intratropica*) Distilled Oils and Methanol Extracts. *J Essent Oil Res.* 2001 Jan/Feb 13:25-29.

Oyedeji AO, et al. Eudesma-1,4(15),11-triene from the essential oil of *Callitris intratropica. Phytochemistry.* 1998 48(4):657-660.

## Blue Tansy *(Tanacetum annuum)*

Moroccan Blue Tansy receives its lovely blue color from the constituent chamazulene.

**Medical Properties:** Anti-inflammatory, analgesic/anesthetic, antifungal, anti-itching, relaxant, hormone-like

**Directions: Aromatic:** Diffuse up to 1 hour 3 times daily or directly inhale. **Topical:** Apply 2-4 drops on location, chakras, and/or Vita Flex points. Dilution not required except for the most sensitive skin.

**Technical Data: Botanical Family:** Asteraceae or Compositae (daisy); **Plant Origin:** Morocco; **Extraction Method:** Steam distilled from flowering plant; **Key Constituents:** Camphor (10-17%), Sabinene (10-17%), Beta-Pinene (5-10%), Myrcene (7-13%), Alpha-Phellandrene (5-10%), Para-Cymene (3-8%), Chamazulene (3-6%); **ORAC:** 68,800 µTE/100g

### Selected Research

Zaim A, et al. Chemical Composition and Acridicid Properties of the Moroccan *Tanacetum annum* L. Essential Oils, Int J Engineering and Science 2015 May, 13-19.

Greche H, et al. Chemical Composition and Antifungal Properties of the Essential Oil of *Tanacetum annuum. J Essen Oil Res.* 2000 12(1):122-24.

Alejandro F, et al. Homoditerpenes from the essential oil of *Tanacetum annuum. Phytochem.* 1992 May 31(5):1727-30.

Alejandro F, et al. Gualianolides from *Tanacetum annuum. Phytochem.* 1990 29(11):2575-80.

## Calamus *(Acorus calamus)*

Commonly known as sweet flag, this plant may have been the biblical calamus of Exodus 30:23 used in the holy anointing oil. It seems to have originated in India or Arabia but now is found in many places throughout the world. Native Americans used calamus as a medicine and a stimulant, but low doses are also believed to be calming and to induce sleep. The Penobscot people have a tradition that it saved their people from a serious illness.

**Medical Properties:** Antibacterial, sedative, carminative, expectorant, antispasmodic, bronchodilator, hepatoprotective

**Uses:** Relaxes spasms, lung infections, agitation

**Fragrant Influence:** Believed to induce and promote positive thoughts

**Directions: Aromatic:** Diffuse up to 1 hour 3 times daily or directly inhale. **Topical:** Dilute 1 drop essential oil with 1 drop V-6 or other pure carrier oil. Apply 2-4 drops on location, chakras, and/or Vita Flex points.

**Caution:** Use only oil from the diploid species that does not contain β-asarone.

**Technical Data: Botanical Family:** Acoraceae; **Plant Origin:** India, Nepal, Brazil; **Extraction Method:** Steam extracted from roots; **Key Constituents:** Cis-Methyl Isoeugenol (13-21%), Syobunone (7-16%), Acorenone (5-15%), Calamuscenone (5-11%)

### Selected Research

Reddy S, et al. Effects of *Acorus calamus* Rhizome Extract on the Neuromodulatory System in Restraint Stress Male Rats. *Turk Neurosurg.* 2015;25(3):425-31.

Sharma V, et al. *Acorus calamus* (The Healing Plant): a review on its medicinal potential, micropropagation and conservation. *Nat Prod Res.* 2014;28(18):1454-66.

Muthuraman A, Singh N. Neuroprotective effect of saponin-rich extract of *Acorus calamus* L. in rat model of chronic constriction injury (CCI) of sciatic nerve-induced neuropathic pain. *J Ethnopharmacol.* 2012 Aug 1;142(3):723-31.

Ilaiyaraja N, Khanum F. Amelioration of alcohol-induced hepatotoxicity and oxidative stress in rats by *Acorus calamus. J Diet Suppl.* 2011 Dec;8(4):331-45.

Shah AJ, et al. Bronchodilatory effect of Acorus calamus (Linn.) is mediated through multiple pathways, *J Ethnopharmacol.* 2010 Sep 15;131(2):471-7.

## Canadian Fleabane *(Conyza canadensis)*

When bothered by rhinitis, the Zuni people inserted the crushed flowers of conyza in their nostrils for the relief of a good sneeze.

**Medical Properties:** Stimulates liver and pancreas, antiaging (stimulates growth hormone), antirheumatic, antispasmodic, vasodilating, reduces blood pressure, antifungal, antimicrobial

**Uses:** Hypertension, hepatitis, accelerated aging

**Directions: Aromatic:** Diffuse up to 1 hour 3 times daily or directly inhale. **Dietary:** Take as a dietary supplement. **Topical:** Dilute 1 drop essential oil with 1 drop V-6 or other pure carrier oil. Apply 2-4 drops on location, chakras, and/or Vita Flex points.

**Technical Data: Botanical Family:** Compositae; **Plant Origin:** Canada; **Extraction Method:** Steam distilled from stems, leaves, and flowers (aerial parts); **Key Constituents:** Limonene (60-80%), Trans-Alpha-Bergamotene (1-10%), Trans-Beta-Ocimene (2-6%), Gamma-Curcumene (1-8%); **ORAC:** 26,700 µTE/100g

### Selected Research

Banday JA, et al. Conyzagenin-A and B, two new epimerica lanostane triterpenoids from *Conyza canadensis. Nat Prod Res.* 2013;27(11):975-81.

Veres K, et al. Antifungal activity and composition of essential oils of *Conyza canadensis* herbs and roots. *Scientific World Journal.* 2012;489646.

Shakirullah M, et al. Antimicrobial activities of Conyzolide and Conysoflavone from *Conyza Canadensis. J Enzyme Inhib Med Chem.* 2011 Aug;26(4):468-71.

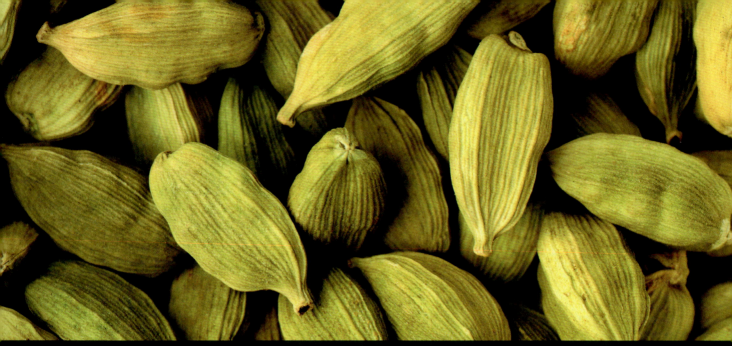
Cardamom

## Cardamom *(Elettaria cardamomum)*

Called "Grains of Paradise" since the Middle Ages, it has been used medicinally by Indian healers for millennia. One of the most prized spices in ancient Greece and Rome, cardamom was cultivated by the king of Babylon around the 7th century BC.

It is mentioned in one of the oldest known medical records, the Ebers Papyrus (dating from 16th century BC), an ancient Egyptian list of 877 prescriptions and recipes.

**Medical Properties:** Antispasmodic (neuromuscular), expectorant, antiparasitic (worms), antioxidant, antimicrobial

**Uses:** Lung/sinus infection, indigestion, senility, headaches

**Fragrant Influence:** Uplifting, refreshing, and invigorating

**Directions: Aromatic:** Diffuse up to 30 minutes 3 times daily or directly inhale. **Dietary:** Dilute 1 drop essential oil with 1 drop V-6 or other pure carrier oil, put in a capsule, and take up to 3 times daily as a dietary supplement. **Topical:** Dilute 1 drop essential oil with 1 drop V-6 or other pure carrier oil and apply on location, stomach, solar plexus, thighs, or on chakras and/or Vita Flex points.

## Cardamom Vitality™ *(Elettaria cardamomum)*

**Directions: Dietary:** Dilute 1 drop with 1 drop of carrier oil. Put in a capsule and take up to 3 times daily or as needed.

**Technical Data: Botanical Family:** Zingiberaceae; **Plant Origin:** Guatemala, Sri Lanka; **Extraction Method:** Steam distilled from seeds; **Key Constituents:** Alpha-Terpinyl Acetate (45-55%), 1,8-Cineole (Eucalyptol) (16-36%), Linalol (4-7%), Linalyl Acetate (3-7%); **ORAC:** 36,500 µTE/100g

### Selected Research

Nitasha Bhat GM, et al. Comparison of the efficacy of cardamom (*Elettaria cardamomum*) with pioglitazone on dexamethasone-induced hepatic steatosis, dyslipidemia, and hyperglycemia in albino rats. *J Adv Pharm Technol Res.* 2015 Jul-Sep;6(3):136-40.

Kumari S, Dutta A. Histological and ultrastructural studies on the toxic effect of pan masala and its amelioration by *Elettaria cardamomum*. *Chin J Nat Med.* 2014 Mar;12(3):199-203.

Qiblawi S. et al. Chemopreventive effects of cardamom (*Elettaria cardamomum* L.) on chemically induced skin carcinogenesis in Swiss albino mice. *J Med Food.* 2012 Jun;15(6):576-80.

Singh G, et al. Antioxidant and antimicrobial activities of essential oil and various oleoresins of *Elettaria cardamomum* (seeds and pods). *J Sci Food Agric.* 2008 Jan;88(2):280-289.

## Carrot Seed *(Daucus carota)*

Carrot seed oil is traditionally used for kidney and digestive disorders and to relieve liver congestion.

**Medical Properties:** Antiparasitic, antiseptic, purgative, diuretic, vasodilatory, antifungal

**Uses:** Skin conditions (eczema, oily skin, psoriasis, wrinkles), water retention, liver problems

**Directions: Topical:** Dilute 1 drop essential oil with 1 drop V-6 or other pure carrier oil and apply 1-2 drops on location, chakras, and/or Vita Flex points.

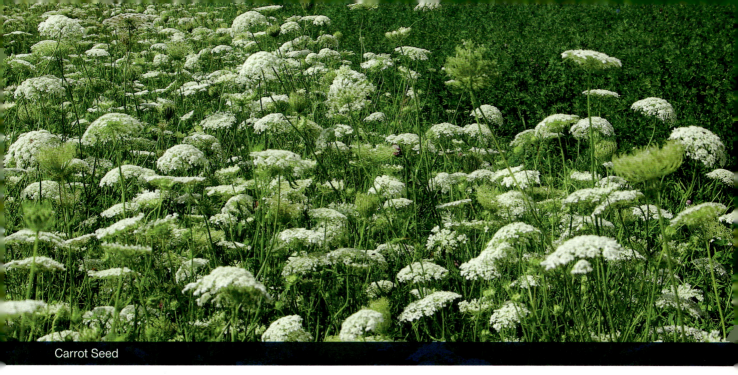

Carrot Seed

## Carrot Seed Vitality™ (Daucus carota)

**Directions: Dietary:** Put 4 drops in a capsule. Take 3 times daily or as needed.

**Technical Data: Botanical Family:** Apiaceae; **Plant Origin:** France; **Extraction Method:** Steam distilled from dried seeds; **Key Constituents:** Carotol (30-40%), Alpha-Pinene (12-16%), Trans-Beta-Caryophyllene (6-10%), Caryophyllene Oxide (3-5%)

### Selected Research

Alves-Silva JM, et al. New Claims for Wild Carrot (*Daucus carota* subsp. carota) Essential Oil. *Evid Based Complement Alternat Med.* 2016;2016:9045196. [Epub ahead of print]

Shebaby WN, et al. Antioxidant and hepatoprotective activities of the oil fractions from wild carrot (*Daucus carota* ssp. carota). *Pharm Biol.* 2015 Sep;53(9):1258-94.

Rokbeni N, et al. Variation of the chemical composition and antimicrobial activity of the essential oils of natural populations of Tunisian *Daucus carota* L. (Apiaceae). *Chem Biodivers.* 2013 Dec;10(12):2278-90.

Afzal M, et al. Comparison of protective and curative potential of *Daucus carota* root extract on renal ischemia reperfusion injury in rats. *Pharm Biol.* 2013 Jul;51(7):856-62.

Singh K, et al. In vivo antioxidant and hepatoprotective activity of methanolic extracts of *Daucus carota* seeds in experimental animals. *Asian Pac J Trop Biomed.* 2012 May;2(5):385-8.

## Cassia (Cinnamomum aromaticum) (Syn. C. cassia)

Cassia is rich in biblical history and is mentioned in one of the oldest known medical records, the Ebers Papyrus (dating from 16th century BC), an ancient Egyptian list of 877 prescriptions and recipes.

**Note:** While its aroma is similar to cinnamon, cassia is chemically and physically quite different.

**Medical Properties:** Anti-inflammatory (COX-2 inhibitor), antifungal, antibacterial, antiviral, anticoagulant

**Uses:** Cataracts, fungal infections (ringworm, candida), atherosclerosis, anxiolytic, diabetes, arteriosclerosis

**Directions: Aromatic:** Diffuse up to 1 hour 3 times daily. **Dietary:** Dilute 1 drop essential oil with 4 drops V-6 or other pure carrier oil. Put in a capsule and take 1 daily or as directed by a health care professional. **Topical:** Dilute 1 drop essential oil with 4 drops V-6 or other pure carrier oil and apply 1-2 drops on location, chakras, and/or Vita Flex points,

**Caution:** May irritate the nasal membranes if inhaled directly from diffuser or bottle

**Technical Data: Botanical Family:** Lauraceae; **Plant Origin:** China; **Extraction Method:** Steam distilled from branches, leaves, and petioles; **Key Constituents:** Trans-Cinnamaldehyde (70-88%), Trans-O, Methoxycinnamaldehyde (3-15%), Coumarine (1.5-4%), Cinnamyl Acetate (0-6%); **ORAC:** 15,170 µTE/100g

### Selected Research

Chang WL, et al. *Cinnamomum cassia* essential oil and its major constituent cinnamaldehyde induced cell cycle arrest and apoptosis in human oral squamous cell carcinoma HSC-3 cells. *Eviron Toxicol.* 2016 Feb 25.

Trinh NT, et al. Effect of a Vietnamese *Cinnamomum cassia* essential oil and its major component trans-cinnamaldehyde on the cell viability, membrane integrity, membrane fluidity, and proton motive force of *Listeria innocua. Can J Microbiol.* 2015 Apr;61(4):263-71.

Yu C, et al. Cinnamaldehyde/chemotherapeutic agents interaction and drug-metabolizing genes in colorectal cancer. *Mol Med Rep.* 2014 Feb;9(2):669-76.

Luo Q, et al. Identification of compounds from the water soluble extract of *Cinnamomum cassia* barks and their inhibitory effects against high-glucose-induced mesangial cells. *Molecules.* 2013 Sep 5;18(9):10930-43.

Hoehn AN, Stockert AL. The Effects of *Cinnamomum cassia* on Blood Glucose Values are Greater than those of Dietary Changes Alone. *Nutr Metab Insights.* 2012 Dec 13;5(77-83).

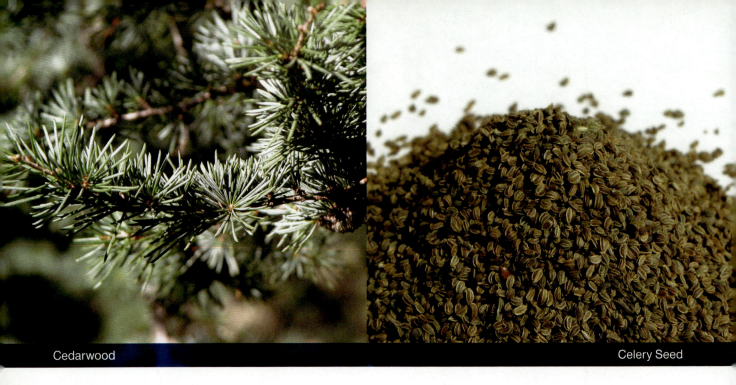
Cedarwood | Celery Seed

## Cedarwood (Cedrus atlantica)

Throughout antiquity, cedarwood has been used in medicines. The Egyptians used it for embalming the dead. It was used as both a traditional medicine and incense in Tibet.

**Medical Properties:** Combats hair loss (alopecia areata), antibacterial, lymphatic stimulant

**Uses:** Hair loss, arteriosclerosis, ADHD, skin problems (acne, eczema)

**Fragrant Influence:** Stimulates the limbic region of the brain (the center of emotions), stimulates the pineal gland, which releases melatonin. Terry Friedmann, MD, found in clinical tests that this oil may treat ADD and ADHD (attention deficit disorders) in children. It is recognized for its calming, purifying properties.

**Directions: Aromatic:** Diffuse up to 1 hour 3 times daily or directly inhale. **Dietary:** Take as a dietary supplement. **Topical:** Apply 2-4 drops directly to desired area or apply on chakras and/or Vita Flex points. Dilution not needed except for the most sensitive skin.

**Technical Data: Botanical Family:** Pinaceae; **Plant Origin:** Morocco, USA; Cedrus atlantica is the species most closely related to the biblical Cedars of Lebanon; **Extraction Method:** Steam distilled from bark; **Key Constituents:** Alpha-Himachalene (10-20%), Beta-Himachalene (35-55%), Gamma-Himachalene (8-15%), Delta-Cadinene (2-6%); **ORAC:** 169,000 µTE/100g

### Selected Research

Martins DF, et al. Inhalation of *Cedrus atlantica* essential oil Alleviates pain behavior through activation of descending pain modulation pathways in a mouse model of postoperative pain. *J Ethnopharmacol.* 2015 Sep 3. [Epub ahead of print]

Saab Am, et al. In vitro evaluation of the anti-proliferative activities of the wood essential oils of three Cedrus species against KI562 human chronic myelogenous leukemia cells. *Nat Prod Res.* 2012;26(23):2227-31.

Friedmann T. Attention deficit and hyperactivity disorder (ADHD). 2002. (Unpublished study) http://files.meetup.com/1481956/ADHD%20Research%20by%20Dr.%20Terry%20Friedmann.pdf.

## Celery Seed (Apium graveolens)

Long recognized as helpful in digestion, liver cleansing, and urinary tract support. It is also said to increase milk flow in nursing mothers.

**Medical Properties:** Antibacterial, antioxidant, antirheumatic, digestive aid, diuretic, liver protectant

**Uses:** Arthritis/rheumatism, digestive problems, liver problems/hepatitis

**Directions: Aromatic:** Diffuse up to 1 hour 3 times daily or directly inhale. **Topical:** Dilute 1 drop essential oil with 1 drop V-6 or other pure carrier oil and apply 1-2 drops on location, chakras, and/or Vita Flex points.

## Celery Seed Vitality™ (Apium graveolens)

**Directions: Dietary:** Dilute 2 drops with 2 drops of carrier oil. Put in a capsule and take up to 3 times daily or as needed.

**Technical Data: Botanical Family:** Apiaceae; **Plant Origin:** Europe; **Extraction Method:** Steam distilled from dried seeds; **Key Constituents:** Limonene (60-75%), Alpha and Beta Selinene (14-20%), Sednenolide (4-7%); **ORAC:** 30,300 µTE/100g

### Selected Research

Si Y, et al. Celery Seed Extract Blocks Peroxide Injury in Macrophages via Notch1/NF-κB Pathway. *Am J Chin Med.* 2015;43(3):443-55.

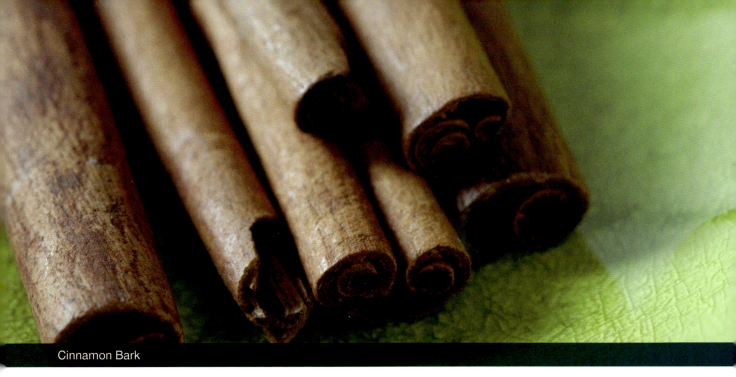

Cinnamon Bark

Kumar S, et al. Larvicidal, Repellent, and Irritant Potential of the Seed-Derived Essential oil of *Apium graveolens* Against Dengue Vector, *Aedes aegypti* L. (Diptera: Culicidae). *Front Public Health.* 2014 Sep 18;2:147.

Li P, et al. In vitro and in vivo antioxidant activities of a flavonoid isolated from celery (*Apium graveolens* L. var. dulce). *Food Funct.* 2014 Jan;5(1):50-6.

Moghadam MH, et al. Antihypertensive effect of celery seed on rat blood pressure in chronic administration. *J Med Food.* 2013 Jun;16(6):558-63.

Baananou S, et al. Antiulcergenic and antibacterial activities of *Apium graveolens* essential oil and extract. *Nat Prod Res.* 2013;27(12):1075-83.

## Cinnamon Bark
### (Cinnamomum zeylanicum) (Syn. C. verum)

Listed in Dioscorides' *De Materia Medica* (AD 78), Europe's first authoritative guide to medicines, which became the standard reference work for herbal treatments for over 1,700 years.

**Medical Properties:** Anti-inflammatory (COX-2 inhibitor), powerfully antibacterial, antiviral, antifungal, anticoagulant, circulatory stimulant, stomach protectant (ulcers), antiparasitic (worms)

**Uses:** Cardiovascular disease, infectious diseases, viral infections (herpes, etc.), digestive complaints, ulcers, and warts

**Fragrant Influence:** Thought to attract wealth

**Directions: Aromatic:** Diffuse up to 1 hour 3 times daily. **Topical:** Dilute 1 drop essential oil with 4 drops V-6 or other pure carrier oil and apply 1-2 drops on location, chakras, and/or Vita Flex points.

**Caution:** May irritate the nasal membranes if inhaled directly from diffuser or bottle.

## Cinnamon Bark Vitality™
### (Cinnamomum zeylanicum) (Syn. C. verum)

**Directions: Dietary:** Dilute 1 drop with 4 drops of carrier oil. Put in a capsule and take1 daily.

**Technical Data: Botanical Family:** Lauraceae; **Plant Origin:** Sri Lanka, Madagascar, Ceylon; **Extraction Method:** Steam distilled from bark; **Key Constituents:** Trans-Cinnamaldehyde (50-75%), Eugenol (4-7%), Beta-Caryophyllene (3-8%), Linalol (3-9%); **ORAC:** 10,340 µTE/100g

## Selected Research

Yang SM, et al. Molecular Mechanisms of *Cinnamomum verum* Component Cuminaldehyde Inhibits Cell Growth and Induces Cell Death in Human Long Squamous Cell Carcinoma NCI-H520 Cells In Vitro and In Vivo. *J Cancer.* 2016 Jan 5;7(3):251-61.

Cui H, et al. Liposome containing cinnamon oil with antibacterial activity against methicillin-resistant *Staphylococcus aureus* biofilm. *Biofouling.* 2016 Feb;32(2):215-25.

Yap PS, et al. Antibacterial Mode of Action of *Cinnamomum verum* Bark Essential Oil, Alone and in Combination with Piperacillin, Against a Multi-Drug-Resistant *Escherichia coli* Strain. *J Microbiol Biotechnol.* 2015 Aug 28;25 (8);1299-306.

Malik J, et al. Attenuating effect of standardized lyophilized *Cinnamomum zeylanicum* bark extract against streptozotocin-induced experimental dementia of Alzheimer's type. *J Basic Clin Physiol Pharmacol.* 2014 Oct 10. [Epub ahead of print]

Azeredo CM, et al. In vitro biological evaluation of eight different essential oils against *Trypanosoma cruzi*, with emphasis on *Cinnamomum verum* essential oil. *BMC Complement Altern Med.* 2014 Aug 22;14:309.

Sartorius T, et al. Cinnamon extract improves insulin sensitivity in the brain and lowers liver fat in mouse models of obesity. *PLoS One.* 2014 Mar 18;9(3):e92358.

Yüce A, et al. Effectiveness of cinnamon (*Cinnamomum zeylanicum*) bark oil in the prevention of carbon tetrachloride-induced damages on the male reproductive system. *Andrologia.* 2014 Apr;46(3):263-72.

Ghosh V, et al. Cinnamon oil nanoemulsion formulation by ultrasonic emulsification: investigation of its bacteriacidal activity. *J Nanosci Nanotechnol.* 2013 Jan;13(1):114-22.

Davis PA, et al. Cinnamon lowers fasting blood glucose: meta-analysis. *J Med Food.* 2011 Sep;14(9):884-9.

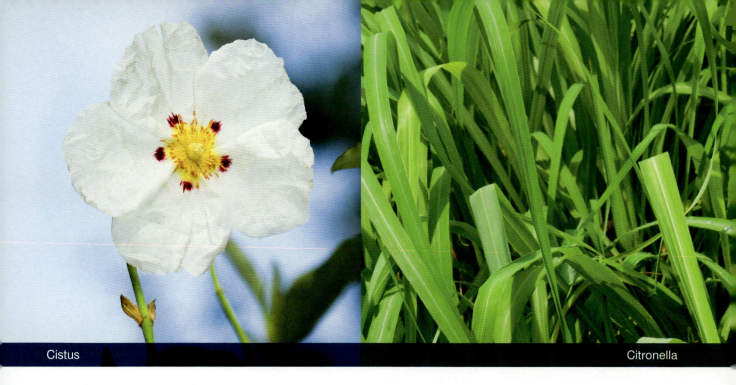

Cistus | Citronella

### Cistus *(Cistus ladanifer/ladaniferus)*
(also known as *Labdanum*)

Cistus is also known as "rock rose" and Rose of Sharon and has been studied for its effects on the regeneration of cells.

**Medical Properties:** Antiviral, antibacterial, antihemorrhagic, anti-inflammatory, supports sympathetic nervous system, immune stimulant

**Uses:** Hemorrhages, arthritis

**Fragrant Influence:** Calming to the nerves, elevates the emotions

**Directions: Aromatic:** Diffuse up to 1 hour 3 times daily or directly inhale. **Dietary:** Take 4 drops as dietary supplement. **Topical:** Apply 2-4 drops on location, chakras, and/or Vita Flex points. Dilution not needed except for the most sensitive skin.

**Technical Data: Botanical Family:** Cistaceae; **Plant Origin:** Spain; **Extraction Method:** Steam distilled from leaves and branches; **Key Constituents:** Alpha-Pinene (40-60%), Camphene (2-5%), Bornyl Acetate (3-6%), Trans-Pinocarveol (3-6%); **ORAC:** 3,860 µTE/100g

### Selected Research

El Hamsas El Youbi A, et al. In Vivo Anti-Inflammatory and Analgesic Effects of Aqueous Extract of *Cistus ladanifer* L. from Morocco. *Am J Ther.* 2016 Mar 1. [Epub ahead of print]

Loizzo MR, et al. Chemistry and functional properties in prevention of neurodegenerative disorders of five Cistus species essential oils. *Food Chem Toxicol.* 2015 Sep;59:586-94.

Papaefthimiou D, et al. Genus Cistus: a model for exploring labdane-type diterpenes' biosynthesis and a natural source of high value products with biological, aromatic, and pharmacological properties. *Front Chem.* 2014 Jun 11;2:35.

Tomás-Menor L, et al. Correlation between the antibacterial activity and the composition of extracts derived from various Spanish Cistus species. *Food Chem Toxicol.* 2013 May;55:313-22.

### Citronella *(Cymbopogon nardus)*

Used by various cultures to treat intestinal parasites, menstrual problems, and as a stimulant. Historically used to sanitize and deodorize surfaces. Enhanced insect repelling properties when combined with cedarwood.

**Medical Properties:** Powerful antioxidant, antibacterial, antifungal, insect repellent, anti-inflammatory, antispasmodic, antiparasitic (worms), relaxant

**Uses:** Respiratory infections, muscle/nerve pain, digestive/intestinal problems, anxiety, skin problems (acne, eczema, oily skin), skin-penetration enhancer

**Fragrant Influence:** Refreshing and uplifting

**Directions: Aromatic:** Diffuse up to 30 minutes 3 times daily or directly inhale. **Dietary:** Dilute 1 drop essential oil with 1 drop V-6 or other carrier oil, put in a capsule, and take up to 3 times daily or as needed as a dietary supplement. **Topical:** Dilute 1 drop essential oil with 1 drop V-6 or other pure carrier oil and apply on location, chakras, and/or Vita Flex points.

**Technical Data: Botanical Family:** Poaceae; **Plant Origin:** Sri Lanka; **Extraction Method:** Steam distilled from aerial parts and leaves; **Key Constituents:** Geraniol (18-30%), Limonene (5-10%), Trans-Methyl Isoeugenol (4-10%), Geranyl Acetate (5-10%), Borneol (3-8%); **ORAC:** 312,000 µTE/100g

### Selected Research

Batubara I, et al. Effects of inhaled citronella oil and related compounds on rat body weight and brown adipose tissue sympathetic nerve. *Nutrients.* 2015 Mar 12;7(3):1859-70.

Trindade LA, et al. Inhibition of adherence of *C. albicans* to dental implants and cover screws by *Cymbopogon nardus* essential oil and citronellal. *Clin Oral Investig.* 2015 Mar 26. [Epub ahead of print]

Wei LS, Wee W. Chemical composition and antimicrobial activity of *Cymbopogon nardus* citronella essential oil against systematic bacteria of aquatic animals. *Iran J Microbiol.* 2013 Jun;5(2):147-52.

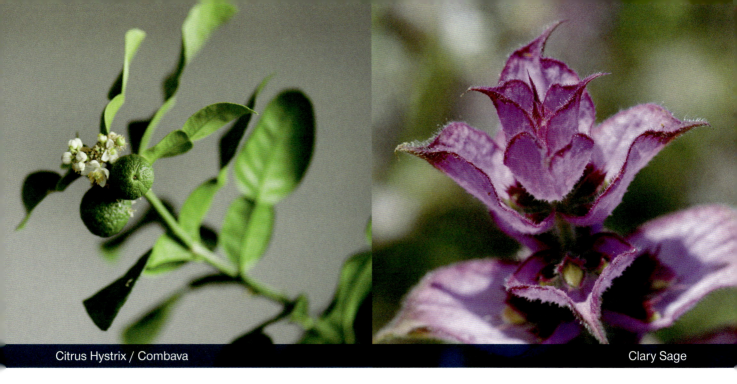

Citrus Hystrix / Combava

Clary Sage

Li WR, et al. Antifungal effects of citronella oil against *Aspergillus niger* ATCC 16404. *Appl Microbiol Biotechnol.* 2013 Aug;97(16):7483-92.

## Citrus Hystrix/Combava *(Citrus hystrix)*
(Also known as Kaffir lime)

Used as a flavorant and as a nausea, fainting, and headache treatment. Also used for stomachaches and dyspepsia.

**Medical Properties:** Anti-inflammatory, antimicrobial, antidepressant, relaxant, antitumoral, antioxidant, rich in citronellal, which possesses calmative properties

**Uses:** Stress, anxiety, trauma

**Directions: Aromatic:** Diffuse up to 30 minutes 3 times daily or directly inhale. **Dietary:** Take as a dietary supplement. **Topical:** Dilute 1 drop essential oil with 1 drop V-6 or other pure carrier oil and apply on location, chakras, and/or Vita Flex points.

**Technical Data: Botanical Family:** Rutaceae; **Plant Origin:** Indochina, Malaysia; **Extraction Method:** Steam distilled from leaves; **Key Constituents:** Citronnellal (65-80%), Linalol (3-6%), Citronnellol (2-5%), Isopulegol (2-4%); **ORAC:** 69,200 µTE/100g

### Selected Research

Wongsariya K, et al. Synergistic interaction and mode of action of *Citrus hystrix* essential oil against bacteria causing periodontal diseases. *Pharm Biol.* 2014 Mar;53(3):273-80.

Putri H, et al. Cardioprotective and hepatoprotective effects of *Citrus hystrix* peels extract on rats model. *Asian Pac J Trop Biomed.* 2013 May;3(5):371-5.

Panthong K, et al. Benzene, coumarin and quinolinone derivatives from the roots of *Citrus hystrix*. *Phytochemistry.* 2013 Apr;88:79-84.

Waikedre J, et al. Chemical composition and antimicrobial activity of the essential oils from New Caledonian *Citrus macroptera* and *Citrus hystrix*. *Chem Biodivers.* 2010 Apr;7(4):871-7.

## Clary Sage *(Salvia sclarea)*

Clary sage seeds were historically used by soaking the seeds and using the mucilage as an eye-wash and to draw thorns or splinters from the skin. It was also used to treat skin infections, acne, digestive disorders, women's ailments, and soothe and calm the skin. Aromatically, clary sage was used to enhance the immune system, calm digestive disorders, reduce inflammation such as eczema, calm muscle spasms, and for respiratory conditions.

**Medical Properties:** Anticoagulant, antioxidant, antidiabetic, estrogen-like, antifungal, antispasmodic, relaxant, cholesterol-reducing, antitumoral, anesthetic

**Uses:** Leukemia, menstrual discomforts/PMS, hormonal imbalance, insomnia, circulatory problems, high cholesterol, insect repellant

**Fragrant Influence:** Enhances one's ability to dream and is very calming and stress relieving

**Directions: Aromatic:** Diffuse up to 30 minutes 3 times daily or directly inhale. **Dietary:** Take as a dietary supplement. **Topical:** Dilute 1 drop essential oil with 1 drop V-6 or other pure carrier oil and apply on location, (feet, ankles, wrists) or apply on chakras and/or Vita Flex points. Rub 6-8 drops on lower back during PMS.

**Technical Data: Botanical Family:** Lamiaceae; **Plant Origin:** Utah, France; **Extraction Method:** Steam distilled from flowering plant; **Key Constituents:** Linalyl Acetate (56-78%), Linalol (7-24%), Germacrene D (2-12%), Sclareol (.4-3%); **ORAC:** 221,000 µTE/100g

### Selected Research

Chovanová R, et al. Modulation of mecA gene Expression by Essential Oil from *Salvia sclerea* and synergism with Oxacillin in Methicillin Resistant *Staphylococcus epidermis* Carrying Different Types of *Staphylococcal* Chromosomal Cassette mec. *Int J Microbiol.* 2016;2016:6475837.

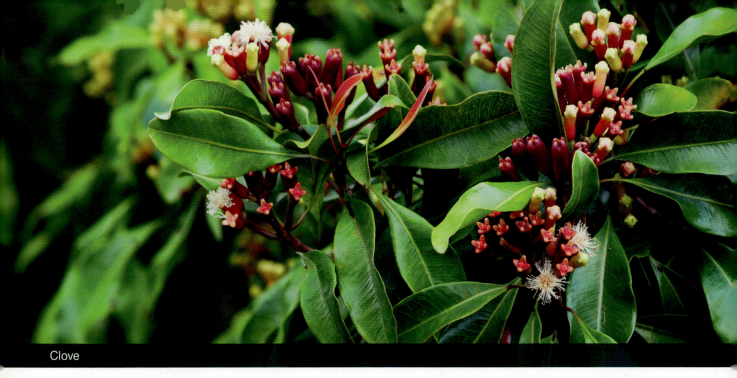
Clove

Sienkiewicz M, et al. The effect of clary sage oil on staphylococci responsible for wound infections. *Postepy Dermatol Alergol.* 2015 Feb;32(1):21-6.

Yuce E, et al. Essential oil composition, antioxidant and antifungal activities of *Salvia sclarea* L. from Munzur Valley in Tunceli, Turkey. *Cell Mol Biol* (Noisy-le-grand). 2014 Jun 15;60(2):1-5.

Lee KB, et al. Changes in 5-hydroxytryptaine and Cortisol Plasma Levels in Menopausal Women After Inhaltion of Clary Sage Oil. *Phytother Res.* 2014 May 7. [Epub ahead of print]

Seol GH, et al. Antidepressant-like effect of *Salvia sclarea* is explained by modulation of dopamine activities in rats. *J Ethnopharmacol.* 2010 Jul 6;130(1):187-90.

## Clove
### *(Syzygium aromaticum) (Syn. Eugenia caryophyllus)*

The people on the island of Ternate were free from epidemics until the 16th century, when Dutch conquerors destroyed the clove trees that flourished on the islands. Many of the islanders died from the epidemics that followed.

Cloves were reputed to be part of the "Marseilles Vinegar" or "Four Thieves Vinegar" that bandits who robbed the dead and dying used to protect themselves during the 15th century plague.

Clove was listed in Hildegard's *Medicine,* a compilation of early German medicines by highly regarded Benedictine herbalist Hildegard of Bingen (1098-1179).

Healers in China and India have used clove buds since ancient times as part of their treatments.

Eugenol, clove's principal constituent, was used in the dental industry for years to numb gums.

**Medical Properties:** Antiaging, antitumoral, antimicrobial, antifungal, antiviral, analgesic/anesthetic, antioxidant, anticoagulant, anti-inflammatory, stomach protectant (ulcers), antiparasitic (worms), anticonvulsant, bone preserving

**Uses:** Antiaging, cardiovascular disease, diabetes, arthritis/rheumatism, hepatitis, intestinal parasites/infections, for numbing all types of pain, throat/sinus/lung infections, cataracts, ulcers, lice, toothache, acne

**Fragrant Influence:** A mental stimulant; encourages sleep, stimulates dreams, and creates a sense of protection and courage

**Directions: Aromatic:** Diffuse up to 1 hour 3 times daily or directly inhale. **Topical:** Dilute 1 drop essential oil with 4 drops V-6 or other pure carrier oil and apply 2-4 drops on location, gums, mouth or on chakras and/or Vita Flex points. For tickling cough, put a drop on back of tongue.

**Caution:** Anticoagulant properties can be enhanced when combined with Warfarin, aspirin, etc.

## Clove Vitality™
### *(Syzygium aromaticum) (Syn. Eugenia caryophyllus)*

**Directions: Dietary:** Dilute 1 drop with 1 drop of carrier oil. Put in a capsule and take up to 3 times daily.

**Technical Data: Botanical Family:** Myrtaceae; **Plant Origin:** Madagascar, Spice Islands; **Extraction Method:** Steam distilled from flower bud and stem; **Key Constituents:** Eugenol (75-87%), Eugenol Acetate (8-15%), Beta-Carophyllene (2-7%); **ORAC:** 1,078,700 µTE/100g

### Selected Research

Issac A, et al. Safety and anti-ulcerogenic activity of a novel polyphenol-rich extract of clove buds (*Syzygium aromaticum* L.). *Food Funct.* 2015 Mar;6(3):842-52.

Kumar PS, et al. Anticancer potential of *Syzygium aromaticum* L. in MCF-7 human breast cancer cell lines. *Pharmacognosy Res.* 2014 Oct;6(4):350-4.

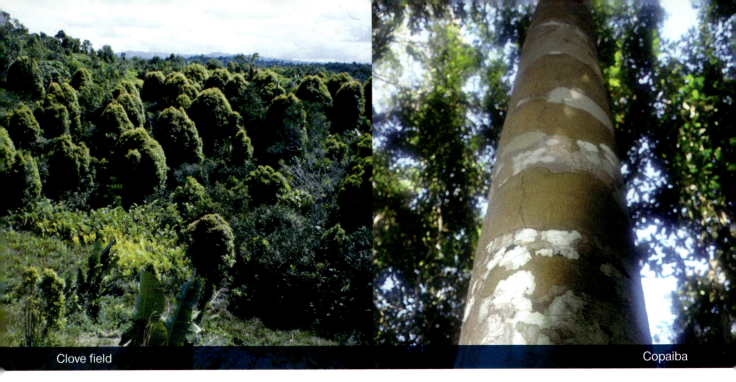

Clove field | Copaiba

Islamuddin M, et al. Apoptosis-like death in *Leishmania donovani promastigotes* induced by eugenol-rich oil of *Syzygium aromaticum*. J Med Microbiol. 2014 Jan;63(Pt 1):74-85.

Sultana B, et al. In vitro antimutagenic, antioxidant activities and total phenolics of clove (*Syzygium aromaticum* L.) seed extracts. Pak J Pharm Sci. 2014 Jul;27(4):893-9.

Khathi A, et al. Effects of *Syzygium aromaticum*-derived triterpenes on postprandial blood glucose in streptozotocin-induced diabetic rats following carbohydrate challenge. PLoS One. 2013 Nov 22;8(11):e816323.

Gupta A, et al. Comparative evaluation of antimicrobial efficacy of *Syzygium aromaticum, Ocimum sanctum* and *Cinnamomum zeylanicum* plant extracts against *Enterococcus faecalis*: a preliminary study. Int Edod J. 2013 Aug;46(8):775-83.

## Copaiba (Balsam Copaiba)
*(Copaifera officinalis, C. reticulata)*

Healers and *curanderos* in the Amazon use copaiba resin for all types of pain and inflammatory disorders, both internal (stomach ulcers and cancer) and external (skin disorders and insect bites).

In Peruvian traditional medicine, three or four drops of the resin are mixed with a spoonful of honey and taken as a natural sore throat remedy. It is also employed in Peruvian and Brazilian herbal medicine systems as an anti-inflammatory and antiseptic for the urinary tract (cystitis, bladder, and kidney disorders) and in the treatment of urinary problems, stomach ulcers, syphilis, tetanus, bronchitis, and tuberculosis.

In Brazilian herbal medicine, the resin is highly regarded as a strong antiseptic and expectorant for the respiratory tract (including bronchitis and sinusitis) and as an antiseptic gargle. It is a popular home remedy in Brazil for sore throats and tonsillitis (1/2 teaspoon of resin is added to warm water).

**Note:** The word "Copal" is derived from the Spanish word for incense (copelli) and can refer to any number of different resinous gums or exudates from trees in Malaysia and South America. Copals are known as black (*Protium copal*), white (*blanco*) (*Bursera bipinnata*), gold (*oro*) (*H. courbaril*), and Brazilian (*Copaifera langsdorfii or reticulata*). Only the Brazilian copal or copaiba has a GRAS distinction in the U.S. and has the most published research on its anti-inflammatory effects.

**Medical Properties:** Anti-inflammatory (powerful), neuroprotective, antimicrobial, anxiolytic, mucolytic, antiulcer, anticancer, antiseptic, kidney stone preventative

**Uses:** Pain relief (strong anti-inflammatory), arthritis, rheumatism, cancer, skin disorders (psoriasis), insect bites, stomach distress, urinary disorders, sore throat, anxiety

**Directions: Aromatic:** Diffuse up to 1 hour 3 times daily or directly inhale. **Dietary:** Put 2 drops in a capsule and take 3 times daily or as needed. As an alternative, add to food or rice milk, etc., as a dietary supplement. **Topical:** Apply on location or apply on chakras and/or Vita Flex points. Dilution not needed except for the most sensitive skin.

**Safety Data:** Approved as a food additive in the U.S.

## Copaiba Vitality *(Copaifera officinalis)*

**Directions: Dietary:** Put 2 drops in a capsule. Take 3 times daily or as needed.

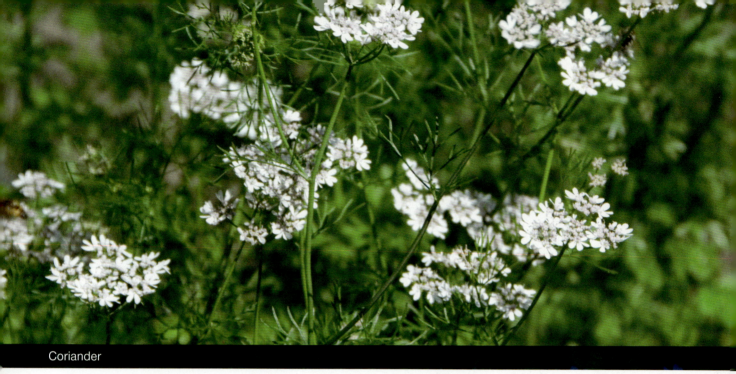

Coriander

**Technical Data: Botanical Family:** Fabaceae; **Plant Origin:** Brazil; **Extraction Method:** Steam distilled (vacuum distilled) from gum resin exudate from tapped trees; **Key Constituents:** Alpha-Copaene (2-5%), Alpha-Humulene (6-10%), Beta-Caryophyllene (39-72%), Delta-Cadinene (2-3%), Delta-Elemene (2-3%), Gamma-Elemene (1-8%), Germacrene D (4-6%), Trans-Alpha-Bergamotene (3-11%)

### Selected Research

Batista ÂG, et al. Polyphenols, antioxidants, and antimutagenic effects of *Copaifera langsdorffii* fruit. *Food Chem.* 2016 Apr 15;197 Pt B:1153-9.

Santiago KB, et al. Immunomodulatory action of Copaifera spp. oleoresins on cytokine production by human moncytes. *Biomed Pharmacother.* 2015 Mar;70:12-8.

Guimarães-Santos A, et al. Copaiba oil-resin treatment is neuroprotective and reduces neutrophil recruitment and microglia activation after motor cortex excitotoxic injury. *Evid Based Complement Alternat Med.* 2012;2012:918174.

Santos AO, et al. Antimicrobial activity of Brazilian copaiba oils obtained from different species of the Copaifera genus. *Mem Inst Oswaldo Cruz.* 2008 May;103(3):277-81.

Veiga Junior VF, et al. Chemical composition and anti-inflammatory activity of copaiba oils from *Copaifera cearensis* Huber ex Ducke, *Copaifera reticulata* Ducke and *Copaifera multijuga* Hayne—a comparative study. *J Ethnopharmacol.* 2007 Jun 13;112(2):248-54.

## Coriander *(Coriandrum sativum)*

Coriander seeds were found in the ancient Egyptian tomb of Ramses II. This oil has been researched at Cairo University for its effects in lowering glucose and insulin levels and supporting pancreatic function. It has also been studied for its effects in strengthening the pancreas.

**Medical Properties:** Anti-inflammatory, antioxidant, sedative, analgesic, antimicrobial, antifungal, liver protectant

**Uses:** Diabetes, arthritis, intestinal problems, skin conditions

**Fragrant Influence:** Soothing and calming

**Directions: Aromatic:** Diffuse up to 30 minutes 3 times daily or directly inhale. **Dietary:** Take as a dietary supplement. **Topical:** Dilute 1 drop essential oil with 1 drop V-6 or other pure carrier oil and apply to location or apply on chakras and/or Vita Flex points.

## Coriander Vitality™ *(Coriandrum sativum)*

**Directions: Dietary:** Dilute 1 drop with 1 drop of carrier oil. Put in a capsule and take up to 3 times daily or as needed.

**Technical Data: Botanical Family:** Apiaceae; **Plant Origin:** Russia; **Extraction Method:** Steam distilled from seeds (fruit); **Key Constituents:** Linalol (65-78%), Alpha-Pinene (3-7%), Camphor (4-6%), Gamma-Terpinene (2-7%), Limonene (2-5%), Geranyl Acetate (1-3.5%), Geraniol (0.5-3%); **ORAC:** 298,300 µTE/100g

### Selected Research

Alves S, et al. Study of the major essential oils compounds of *Coriandrum sativum* against *Acinetobacter baumannii* and the effect of linalool on adhesion, biofilms and quorum sensing. *Biofouling.* 2016 Feb;32(2):155-65.

Cioanca O, et al. Cognitive-enhancing and antioxidant activities of inhaled coriander volatile oil in amyloid β-(142) rat model of Alzheimer's disease. *Physiol Behav.* 2013 Aug 15;120:193-202.

Casetti F, et al. Antimicrobial activity against bacteria with dermatological relevance and skin tolerance of the essential oil from *Coriandrum sativum* L. fruits. *Phytother Res.* 2012 Mar;26(3):420-4.

Mahendra P, Bisht S. Anti-anxiety activity of *Coriandrum sativum* assessed using different experimental anxiety models. *Indian J Pharmacol.* 2012 Sep;43(5):574-7.

Aissaoui A, et al. Hypoglycemic and hypolipidemic effects of *Coriandrum sativum* L. in Meriones shawi rats. *J Ethnopharmacol.* 2011 Sep 1;137(1):652-61.

Pandey A, et al. Pharmacological screening of *Coriandrum sativum* Linn. for hepatoprotective activity. *J Pharm Bioallied Sci.* 2011 Jul;3(3):435-41.

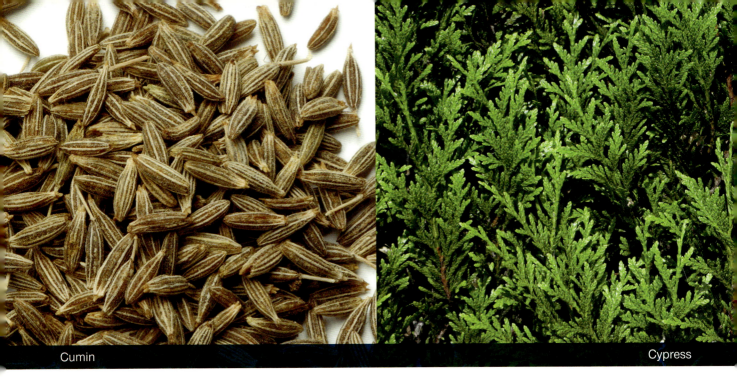

Cumin | Cypress

## Cumin *(Cuminum cyminum)*

The Hebrews used cumin as an antiseptic for circumcision. In ancient Egypt, cumin was used for cooking and mummification.

**Medical Properties:** Antitumoral, anti-inflammatory, antioxidant, antiviral, antifungal, antimicrobial, digestive aid, liver protectant, immune stimulant

**Uses:** Cancer, infectious disease, digestive problems

**Directions: Aromatic:** Diffuse up to 30 minutes 3 times daily or directly inhale. **Dietary:** Dilute as described under topical, put in a capsule, and take 1 daily or as directed by a health professional. **Topical:** Dilute 1 drop with 4 drops olive oil. Apply on chakras and/or Vita Flex points.

**Caution:** Possible sun/skin sensitivity.

**Technical Data: Botanical Family:** Apiaceae; **Plant Origin:** Egypt; **Extraction Method:** Steam distilled from seeds; **Key Constituents:** Cuminaldehyde (16-22%), Gamma-Terpinene (16-22%), Beta-Pinene (12-18%), Para-Mentha-1,3 + 1,4-dien-7-al (25-35%), Para-Cymene (3-8%); **ORAC:** 82,400 µTE/100g

### Selected Research

Khosravi AR, et al. Efficacy of *Cuminum cyminum* essential oil on the FUM1 gene expression of fumonsin-producing *Fusarium verticillioides* strains. *Avicenna J Phytomed.* 2015 Jan-Feb;5(1):34-42.

Tomy MJ, et al. Cuminaldehyde as a lipoxygenase inhibitor: in vitro and in silico validation. *Appl Biochem Biotechnol.* 2014 Sep;174(1):388-97.

Patil SB, et al. Insulinotropic and β-cell protective action of cuminaldehyde, cuminol and an inhibitor isolated from *Cuminum cyminum* in streptozotocin-induced diabetic rats. *Br J Nutr.* 2013 Oct;110(8):1434-43.

Kalaivani P, et al. *Cuminum cyminum,* a Dietary Spice, Attenuates Hypertension via Endothelial Nitric Oxide Synthesis and NO Pathway in Renovascular Hypertensive Rats. *Clin Exp Hypotens.* 2013;35(7):534-42.

## Cypress *(Cupressus sempervirens)*

The Phoenicians and Cretans used cypress for building ships and bows, while the Egyptians made sarcophagi from the wood. The Greeks used cypress to carve statues of their gods. The Greek word "sempervivens," from which the botanical name is derived, means "live forever." The tree shares its name with the island of Cypress, where it is used for worship. Cypress wood is noted for its durability, as it was used most famously for the original doors of St. Peter's Basilica at the Vatican that legends say lasted over 1,000 years.

**Medical Properties:** Improves circulation; is anti-infectious, antispasmodic, and an antioxidant; discourages fluid retention; improves respiration; promotes liver health

**Uses:** Diabetes, circulatory disorders, grounding, stabilizing

**Fragrant Influence:** Eases the feeling of loss and creates a sense of security and grounding. Also helps heal emotional trauma, calms, soothes anger, and helps life flow better. Can help soothe irritating coughs and minor chest discomfort.

**Directions: Aromatic:** Diffuse up to 1 hour 3 times daily or directly inhale. **Dietary:** Take as a dietary supplement. **Topical:** Dilute 1 drop essential oil with 1 drop V-6 or other pure carrier oil and apply 2-4 drops on location, massaging toward center of body. Can also apply on chakras and/or Vita Flex points.

**Technical Data: Botanical Family:** Cupressaceae; **Plant Origin:** France, Spain; **Extraction Method:** Steam distilled from branches; **Key Constituents:** Alpha-Pinene (40-65%), Beta-Pinene (0.5-3%), Delta-3-Carene (12-25%), Limonene (1.8-5%), Cedrol (0.8-7%), Myrcene (1-3.5%); **ORAC:** 24,300 µTE/100g

## Selected Research

Senol FS, et al. In vitro cholinesterase inhibitory and antioxidant effect of selected coniferous tree species. *Asian Pac J Trop Med.* 2015 Apr;8(4):269-75.

Selim SA, et al. Chemical composition, antimicrobial and antibiofilm activity of the essential oil and methanol extract of the Mediterranean cypress (*Cupressus sempervirens* L.). *BMC Complement Altern Med.* 2014 Jun 2;14:179.

Nejia H, et al. Extraction of essential oil from *Cupressus sempervirens*: comparison of global yields, chemical composition and antioxidant activity obtained by hydrodistillation and supercritical extraction. *Nat Prod Res.* 2013 Jan 14. [Epub ahead of print]

Ali SA, et al. Protective role of *Juniperus phoenicea* and *Cupressus sempervirens* against CCl(4) [induced hepotoxicity]. *World J Gastrointest Pharmacol Ther.* 2010 Dec 6;1(6):123-31.

## Dalmatia Bay Laurel *(Laurus nobilis) (Bay Laurel)*

The coastal region of Dalmatia, Croatia, is home to Dalmatia Bay Laurel. With its rich eucalyptol scent, Dalmatia Bay Laurel encourages healthy skin and enlivens massage oils when applied to the feet.

**Directions: Aromatic:** Diffuse up to 30 minutes 3 times daily. **Topical:** Dilute 1 drop with 1 drop V-6™ or olive oil and apply to desired area as needed.

**Technical Data: Botanical Family:** Lauraceae; **Plant Origin:** Croatia; **Extraction Method:** Steam distilled from leaves and twigs; **Key Constituents:** 1,8-Cineole (Eucalyptol) (40-50%), Alpha-Terpenyl Acetate (7-14%), Alpha-Pinene (4-8%), Beta-Pinene (3-6%), Sabinene (6-11%), Linalol (2-7%); **ORAC:** 98,900 µTE/100g

## Selected Research

Merghni A, et al. Antibacterial and antibiofilm activities of *Laurus nobilis* L. essential oil against *Staphylococccus aureus* strains associated with oral infections. *Pathol Biol* (Paris). 2015 Dec 4. Epub ahead of print.

Sahin Basak S, Candan F. Effect of *Laurus nobilis* L. Essential Oil and its Main Components on α-glucosidase and Reactive Oxygen Species Scavaging Activity. *Iran J Pharm Res.* 2013 Spring;12(2):367-79.

Lee T, et al. Effects of magnolialide isolated from the leaves of *Laurus nobilis* L. (Lauraceae) on immunoglobulin E-mediated type I hypersensitivity in vitro. *J Ethnopharmacol.* 2013 Sep 16;149(2):550-6.

## Dalmatia Juniper *(Juniperus oxycedrus)*

The juniper native to the Dalmatia region of Croatia is known for its skin supporting benefits. Thriving in Croatia's rocky soil, Dalmatia Juniper was traditionally used for intestinal complaints.

**Directions: Aromatic:** Diffuse up to 30 minutes 3 times daily. **Topical:** Dilute 1 drop with 1 drop V-6™ or olive oil and apply to desired area as needed.

**Technical Data: Botanical Family:** Cupressaceae; **Plant Origin:** Croatia; **Extraction Method:** Steam distilled from needles and branches; **Key Constituents:** Alpha-Pinene (36-56%), Limonene (10-25%), Myrcene (2-8%), Beta-Pinene (1-5%), Germacrene D (1-3.5%); Delta-Cadinene (0.8-3%); **ORAC:** 250 µTE/100g

## Selected Research

Loizzo MR, et al. Comparative chemical composition, antioxidant and hypoglycaemic activities of *Juniperus oycedrus* ssp. Oxycedrus L. berry and wood oils from Lebanon. *Food Chem.* 2007 105(2):572-8.

Bello R, et al. Effects on Arterial Blood Pressure of Methanol and Dichloromethanol Extracts from *Juniperus oycedrus* L. *Phytother Res.* 1996 11:161-2.

## Dalmatia Sage *(Salvia officinalis)*

Although it now grows elsewhere, sage is native to the Mediterranean area and its rich history was documented by Theophrastus and Pliny the Elder. It flourishes in the Dalmatia region of Croatia. The traditional uses of sage range from reducing fever and as a diuretic, while modern-day studies show improved cognitive function.

**Directions: Aromatic:** Diffuse up to 30 minutes 3 times daily. **Topical:** Dilute 1 drop with 4 drops V-6 or olive oil. Test on small area of skin on the underside of arm and apply to desired area as needed.

**Technical Data: Botanical Family:** Lamiaceae; **Plant Origin:** Croatia; **Extraction Method:** Steam distilled from leaves; **Key Constituents:** Alpha-Thujone (18-43%), Beta-Thujone (3-8.5%), 1,8-Cineole (Eucalyptol) (5.5-13%), Camphor (4.5-24.5%), Camphene (1.5-7%), Alpha-Pinene (1-6.5%), Alpha-Humulene (trace-12%); **ORAC:** 14,800 µTE/100g

## Selected Research

Garcia CS, et al. Pharmacological perspectives from Brazilian *Salvia officinalis* (Lamiaceae): antioxidant, and antitumor in mammalian cells. *An Acad Bras Cienc.* 2016 Feb 2. [Epub ahead of print]

Chovanová R, et al. The inhibition of the Tet(K) efflux pump of tetracycline resistant *Staphylococcus epidermis* by essential oils from three Salvia species. *Lett Appl Microbiol.* 2015 Jul;61(1):58-62.

Martins N, et al. Evaluation of bioactive properties and phenolic compounds in different extracts prepared from *Salvia officinalis* L. *Food Chem.* 2015 Mar 1;170:378-85.

Miroddi M, et al. Systematic review of clinical trials assessing pharmacological properties of Salvia species on memory, cognitive impairment and Alzheimer's disease. *CNS Neurological Ther.* 2014 Jun;20(6):485-95.

Zare Shahneh F, et al. Inhibitory and cytoxic activities of *Salvia officinalis* L. extract on human lymphoma and leukemia cells by induction of apoptosis. *Adv Pharm Bull.* 2013;3(1):51-5.

Kozics K, et al. Effects of *Salvia officinalis* and *Thymus vulgaris* on oxidant-induced DNA damage and antioxidant status in Hep22 cells. *Food Chem.* 2013 Dec 1;141(3):2198-206.

Rahte S, et al. *Salvia officinalis* for Hot Flushes: Towards Determination of Mechanism of Activity and Active Principles. *Planta Med.* 2013 Jun;79(9):753-60.

Kennedy, DO, Wightman EL. Herbal Extracts and Phytochemicals: Plant Secondary Metabolites and the Enhancement of Human Brain Function. *Advan Nutr* 2011). **2** (1): 32–50.

## Davana *(Artemisia pallens)*

Davana grows in the same areas of India as sandalwood. It has been used in India for diabetes, digestive problems (expels parasites), fighting infections, and calming anger. It has been recommended as an aphrodisiac and is often used

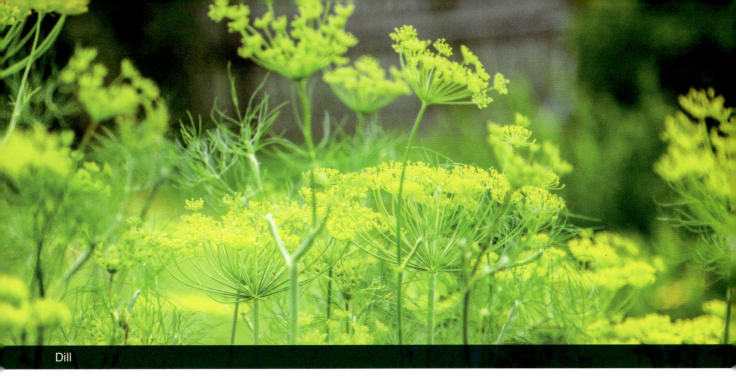

Dill

in perfumery. It has a very rich, concentrated aroma, is usually used in only very small quantities, and is usually used as a complement in very small amounts in essential oil blends. Davana should always be diluted because it is high in ketones. The aroma tends to develop differently, depending on the individual chemistry of the person wearing the oil.

**Medical Properties:** Anti-infectious, antiviral, aphrodisiac, anthelmintic, calmative, analgesic, anti-inflammatory

**Uses:** Skin infections, headaches, emotional stress, worm infestations, sugar metabolism

**Directions: Topical:** Dilute 1 drop essential oil with 1 drop V-6 or other pure carrier oil and apply 1-2 drops on location, chakras, or Vita Flex points.

**Technical Data: Botanical Family:** Asteraceae; **Extraction Method:** Steam distilled from flowers and leaves; **Key Constituents:** Davanone 1-2 (40-60%), Davana Ether 1-3 (5-10%), Ethyl Cinnamate (1-6%), Bicyclogermacrene (5-14%)

**Selected Research**

Honmore V, et al. *Artemisia pallens* alleviates acetaminiphen induced toxicity via modulation of endogenous biomarkers. *Pharm Biol.* 2015 Apr;3(4):571-81.

Ruikar AD, et al. Sesquiterpene lactone, a potent drug model from *Artemisia pallens* Wall with anti-inflammatory activity. *Arzneimittelforschung.* 2011;61(9):510-4.

Ruikar AD, et al. Studies on aerial parts of *Artemisia pallens* Wall for phenol, flavonoid and evaluation of antioxidant activity. *J Pharm Bioallied Sci.* 2011 Apr;3(2):302-5.

Ashok P, Upadhaya K. Analgesic and anti-inflammatory properties of Artemisia pallens Wall ex. DC. *The Pharma Research.* 2010;3(01):249-256.

## Dill *(Anethum graveolens)*

The dill plant is mentioned in the Papyrus of Ebers from Egypt (1550 BC). Roman gladiators rubbed their skin with dill before each match. Listed in Dioscorides' *De Materia Medica* (AD 78), Europe's first authoritative guide to medicines, which became the standard reference work for herbal treatments for over 1,700 years. It was listed in Hildegard's *Medicine,* a compilation of early German medicines by highly regarded Benedictine herbalist Hildegard of Bingen (1098-1179).

**Medical Properties:** Antidiabetic, antispasmodic, antifungal, antibacterial, expectorant, pancreatic stimulant, insulin/blood sugar regulator

**Uses:** Diabetes, digestive problems, liver deficiencies

**Fragrant Influence:** Calms the autonomic nervous system and, when diffused with Roman Chamomile, combats ADHD.

**Directions: Aromatic:** Diffuse up to 1 hour 3 times daily or directly inhale. **Topical:** Dilute 1 drop essential oil with 1 drop V-6 or other pure carrier oil and apply 2-4 drops on location or abdomen. Can also apply on chakras and/or Vita Flex points.

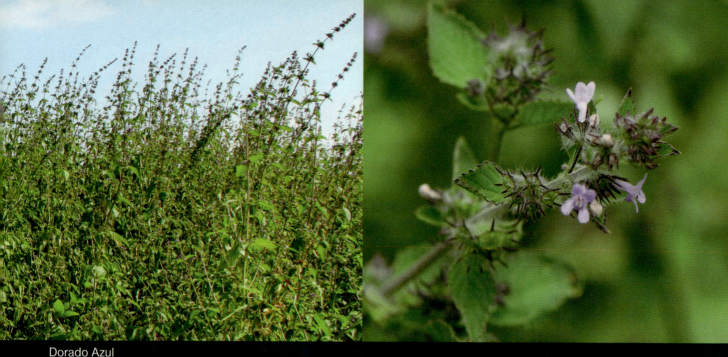
Dorado Azul

### Dill Vitality™ *(Anethum graveolens)*

**Directions: Dietary:** Dilute 1 drop with 1 drop of carrier oil. Put in a capsule and take up to 3 times daily.

**Technical Data: Botanical Family:** Apiaceae; **Plant Origin:** Austria, Hungary; **Extraction Method:** Steam distilled from whole plant; **Key Constituents:** Carvone (30-45%), Limonene (15-25%), Alpha- and Beta-Phellandrene (20-35%); **ORAC:** 35,600 µTE/100g

### Selected Research

Kaemi M. Phenolic profile, antioxidant capacity and anti-inflammatory activity of *Anethum graveolens* L. essential oil. *Nat Prod Res.* 2015;29(6):551-3.

Chen Y, et al. Dill (*Anethum graveolens* L.) essential oil induces *Candida albicans* apoptosis in a metacaspase-dependent manner. *Fungal Biol.* 2014 Apr;118(4):394-401.

Kazemi M. Phenolic profile, antioxidant capacity and anti-inflammatory activity of *Anethum graveolens* L. essential oil. *Nat Prod Res.* 2014 Aug 26:1-3.

Setorki M, et al. Suppressive impact of *Anethum graveolens* consumption on biochemical risk factors of atherosclerosis in hypercholesterolemic rabbits. *Int J Prev Med.* 2013 Aug;4(8):889-95.

### Dorado Azul *(Dorado azul guayfolius officinalis)* *(INCI: Hyptis suaveolens)*

Until about 2006, Dorado Azul was recognized in Ecuador as only a weed. It did not even have a botanical name until D. Gary Young distilled and analyzed it for the first time and gave it its identity. It is a red liquid when distilled, and the natives use it to reverse cancer.

**Medical Properties:** Anti-inflammatory, antioxidant, antimicrobial, antiseptic, antihyperglycemic, gastroprotective, liver protectant, respiratory stimulant

**Uses:** Colds, coughs, flu, bronchitis, asthma, allergic reactions that cause constriction and compromised breathing, any compromise to the respiratory tract, hormone balancer, diabetes, vascular dilator, circulatory stimulant, arthritic and rheumatoid-type pain, reducing candida and other intestinal tract problems, digestion, hygienic action for the mouth, enhances mood

**Directions: Aromatic:** Diffuse up to 30 minutes 3 times daily or directly inhale. **Dietary:** Take as a dietary supplement: 1-10 drops in a capsule or 1-2 drops under the tongue or add to drinking water. **Topical:** Dilute 1 drop essential oil with 1 drop V-6 or other pure carrier oil. Apply 2-4 drops on location, the abdomen, chakras, and/or Vita Flex points.

**Technical Data: Botanical Family:** Lamiaceae; **Plant Origin:** Ecuador; **Extraction Method:** Steam distilled from stems/leaves/flowers (aerial parts); **Key Constituents:** Alpha-Fenchol (4-12%), Beta-Pinene (7-12%), Bicyclogermacrene (4-8%), 1,8-Cineole (Eucalyptol) (23-46%), Limonene (3-7%), Sabinene (7-18%)

### Selected Research

Salini R, et al. Inhibition of quorum sensing mediated biofilm development and virulence in uropathogens by *Hyptis suaveolens*. *Antonie Van Leeuwenhoek.* 2015 Apr;107(4):107(4):1095-106.

Ghaffari H, et al. Antioxidant and neuroprotective activities of *Hyptis suaveolens* (L.) Poit. against oxidative stress-induced neurotoxicity. 2014 Apr;34(3):323-31.

Jesus NZ, et al. *Hyptis suaveolens* (L.) Poit. (Lamiaceae), a medicinal plant protects the stomach against several gastric ulcer models. *J Ethnopharmacol.* 2013 Dec. 12;150(3):982-8.

Ghaffari H, et al. Hepatoprotective and cytoprotective properties of *Hyptis suaveolens* against oxidative stress-induced damage by CCl(4) and H(2)O(2). *Asian Pac J Trop Med.* 2012 Nov;5(11):868-74.

Mishra SB, et al. Anti-hyperglycemic activity of leaves extract of *Hyptis suaveolens* L. Poit in streptozotocin induced diabetic rats. *Asian Pac J Trop Med.* 2011 Sep;4(9):689-93.

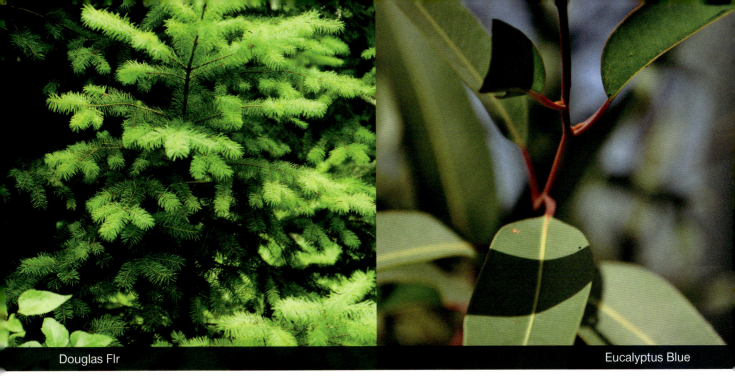

Douglas Fir | Eucalyptus Blue

## Douglas Fir *(Pseudotsuga menziesii)*

American Indians not only used Douglas fir for building and basketry but medicinally for ailments like headaches, stomachaches, the common cold, and rheumatism.

**Medical Properties:** Antitumoral, antioxidant, antifungal, pain relieving

**Uses:** Respiratory/sinus infections

**Directions: Aromatic:** Diffuse up to 1 hour 3 times daily or directly inhale. **Topical:** Dilute 1 drop essential oil with 1 drop V-6 or other pure carrier oil and apply 2-4 drops on location, chakras, and/or Vita Flex points.

**Technical Data: Botanical Family:** Pinaceae; **Plant Origin:** Idaho; **Extraction Method:** Steam distilled from wood/bark/twigs/needles; **Key Constituents:** Alpha-Pinene (25-40%), Beta-Pinene (7-15%), Limonene (6-11%), Bornyl Acetate (8-15%); **ORAC:** 69,000 µTE/100g

### Selected Research

Krauze-Baranowska M, et al. Flavonoids from *Pseudotsuga menziesii*. *Z Naturforsch C.* 2013 Mar-Apr;68(3-4):87-96.

Johnston WH, et al. Antimicrobial activity of some Pacific Northwest woods against anaerobic bacteria and yeast. *Phytother Res.* 2001 Nov;15(7):586-8.

## Elemi *(Canarium luzonicum)*

Elemi has been used in Europe for hundreds of years in salves for skin and is included in celebrated healing ointments such as baum paralytique. Used by a 17th century physician, J. J. Wecker on the battle wounds of soldiers, elemi belongs to the same botanical family as frankincense (*Boswellia carterii*) and myrrh (*Commiphora myrrha*). The Egyptians used elemi for embalming, and subsequent cultures (particularly in Europe) used it for skin care and for reducing fine lines, wrinkles, and improving skin tone.

**Medical Properties:** Antispasmodic, anti-inflammatory, antimicrobial, antiseptic, anticancer

**Uses:** Muscle/nerve pain, skin problems (scars, acne, wrinkles)

**Fragrant Influence:** Its spicy, incense-like fragrance is very conducive toward meditation. Can be grounding and used to clear the mind.

**Directions: Aromatic:** Diffuse up to 1 hour 3 times daily or directly inhale. **Dietary:** Use as a dietary supplement: put 1 drop in a capsule and take or put 1 drop in 4 fl. oz. of liquid (rice milk, etc.). **Topical:** Apply 2-4 drops on location, chakras, and/or Vita Flex points. Dilution not needed except for the most sensitive skin.

**Technical Data: Botanical Family:** Burseraceae; **Plant Origin:** Philippines; **Extraction Method:** Steam distilled from the gum/resin of the tree; **Key Constituents:** Limonene (40-72%), Alpha-Phellandrene (10-24%), Sabinene (3-8%), Elemol (1-25%)

### Selected Research

Mogana R, Wiart C. *Canarium* L.: A Phytochemical and Pharmacological Review. *J Pharm Res.* 2011 Aug 4(8):2482-89.

Hernández-Váquez L, et al. Valuable medicinal plants and resins: Commercial phytochemicals with bioactive properties. *Ind Crop Prod.* May 2010 Vol. 31 Issue 3:476-80.

Adewale MA. (-)-*trans*-β-Elemene and related compounds: occurrence, synthesis, and anticancer activity. *Tetrahedron.* 65 (2009):5145-59.

## Eucalyptus Blue *(Eucalyptus bicostata)*

Eucalyptus blue is grown and distilled on Young Living's farm in Ecuador. It is called blue gum, a tree that has been crossbred over 250 years in the wilds of the Andean Mountains in Ecuador and is a cross between Eucalyptus

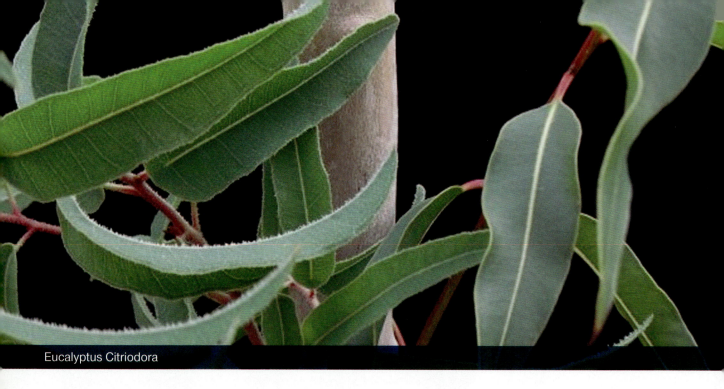

Eucalyptus Citriodora

citriodora and Eucalyptus globulus. The native people of Ecuador have used the disinfecting leaves to cover wounds and repel insects.

Although it contains a high percentage of eucalyptol, because of its balanced chemical constituents within the eucalyptus, it is the only eucalyptus that has been found in the world today that does not cause an allergic reaction in people who have allergies to eucalyptol. Eucalyptus Blue is preferred over many of the eucalyptus species, simply because of its well-balanced chemistry and its non-allergen effect for all types of respiratory conditions. In a recent study of eight eucalyptus species, Eucalyptus bicostata had the best antiviral activity. It is a great companion to Dorado Azul.

**Medical Properties:** Expectorant, diaphoretic, insecticidal, oestrogenic, antifungal, antiviral, antibacterial

**Uses:** Supports respiratory function to promote normal breathing, relieves sore muscles, calming, invigorating

**Fragrant Influence:** Has a fresh, balanced, invigorating aroma

**Directions: Aromatic:** Diffuse in diffuser or humidifier up to 30 minutes 3 times daily or directly inhale. **Topical:** Dilute 1 drop essential oil with 1 drop V-6 or other pure carrier oil and apply 2-4 drops on location or abdomen. Can also apply on chakras and/or Vita Flex points.

**Cautions:** Do not use Eucalyptus Blue as a dietary supplement. Large amounts of any eucalyptus oil may be toxic. Keep out of reach of children.

**Technical Data: Botanical Family:** Myrtaceae; **Plant Origin:** Ecuador; **Extraction Method:** Steam distilled from the leaves; **Key Constituents:** 1,8-Cineole (Eucalyptol) (40-80%), Alpha-pinene (10-30%), Aromadendrene (≤ 7%), Limonene (4-8%)

### Selected Research

Sebei K, et al. Chemical and antibacterial activities of seven Eucalyptus species essential oils leaves. *Biol Res.* 2015 Jan 19;48(1):7. [Epub ahead of print]

Elaissi A, et al. Chemical composition of 8 eucalyptus species' essential oils and the evaluation of their antibacterial, antifungal and antiviral activities. *BMC Complement Alternat Med.* 2012 Jun 28;12:81.

Elaissi A, et al. Antibacterial activity and chemical composition of 20 Eucalyptus species' essential oils. *Food Chem.* 2011 Dec 15;129(4):1427-34.

## Eucalyptus Citriodora
### (Eucalyptus citriodora)

Traditionally used to perfume linen closets and as an insect repellent.

**Medical Properties:** Analgesic, antiviral, antibacterial, antifungal, anticancer, liver protectant, expectorant, insecticidal

**Uses:** Fungal infections (ringworm, candida), respiratory infections, viral infections (herpes, shingles)

**Directions: Aromatic:** Diffuse up to 30 minutes 3 times daily or directly inhale. **Topical:** Dilute 1 drop essential oil with 1 drop V-6 or other pure carrier oil and apply 2-4 drops on location, chakras, and/or Vita Flex points.

**Technical Data: Botanical Family:** Myrtaceae; **Plant Origin:** China; **Extraction Method:** Steam distilled from leaves; **Key Constituents:** Citronellal (75-85%), Neo-Isopulegol + Isopulegol (0-10%); **ORAC:** 83,000 µTE/100g

### Selected Research

Lin L, et al. Nanoliposomes containing *Eucalyptus citriodora* as antibiotic with specific antimicrobial activity. *Chem Commun (Camb).* 2015 Feb 14;51(13):2653-5.

Al-Sayed E, El-Naga RN. Protective role of ellagitannins from *Eucalyptus citriodora* against ethanol-induced gastric ulcer in rats: impact on oxidative stress, inflammation and calcitonin-gene related peptide. *Phytomedicine.* 2015 Jan 15;22(1):5-15.

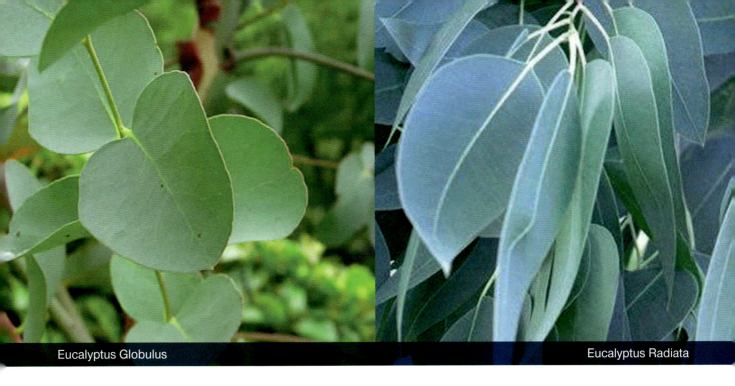

Eucalyptus Globulus | Eucalyptus Radiata

Ramos Alvarenga RF, et al. Airborne antituberculosis activity of *Eucalyptus citriodora* essential oil. *J Nat Prod.* 2014 Mar 28;77(3):603-10.

Siddique YH, et al. GC-MS analysis of *Eucalyptus citriodora* leaf extract and its role on the dietary supplementation in transgenic Drosphila model of Parkinson's disease. *Food Chem Toxicol.* 2013 May;55:29-35.

Bhagat M, et al. Anti-proliferative effect of leaf extracts of *Eucalyptus citriodora* against human cancer cells in vitro and in vivo. *Indian J Biochem Biophys.* 2012 Dec;49(6):451-7.

## Eucalyptus Globulus *(Eucalyptus globulus)*

For centuries, Australian Aborigines used the disinfecting leaves to cover wounds. Shown by laboratory tests to be a powerful antimicrobial agent, *E. globulus* contains a high percentage of eucalyptol (a key ingredient in many antiseptic mouth rinses). It is often used for the respiratory system. Eucalyptus has also been investigated for its powerful insect repellent effects (Trigg, 1996). Eucalyptus trees have been planted throughout parts of North Africa to successfully block the spread of malaria. According to Jean Valnet, MD, a solution of 2 percent eucalyptus oil sprayed on the skin will kill 70 percent of ambient staph bacteria. Some doctors still use solutions of eucalyptus oil in surgical dressings.

**Medical Properties:** Expectorant, mucolytic, antimicrobial, antibacterial, antifungal, antiviral, antiaging, antiulcer, antidiabetic

**Uses:** Respiratory/sinus infections, decongestant, rheumatism/arthritis, soothe sore muscles

**Fragrant Influence:** Promotes health, well-being, purification, and healing

**Directions: Aromatic:** Diffuse up to 30 minutes 3 times daily or directly inhale. **Dietary:** Take as a dietary supplement. **Topical:** Dilute 1 drop essential oil with 1 drop V-6 or other pure carrier oil and apply 2-4 drops on location, chakras, and/or Vita Flex points.

**Technical Data: Botanical Family:** Myrtaceae; **Plant Origin:** China; **Extraction Method:** Steam distilled from leaves; **Key Constituents:** 1,8-Cineole (Eucalyptol) (70-90%), Alpha-Pinene (1-5%), Limonene (6-9%), Para-Cymene (1-5%); **ORAC:** 2,400 µTE/100g

### Selected Research

Mekonnen A, et al. In Vitro Activity of Essential Oil of *Thymus schimperi, Matricaria chamomilla, Eucalyptus globulus,* and *Rosmarinus officinalis. Int J Microbiol.* 2016;2016:9545693. [Epub ahead of print]

Mota Vde S, et al. Antimicrobial activity of *Eucalyptus globulus* oil, xylitol and papain: a pilot study. *Rev Esc Enferm USP.* 2015 Mar-Apr;49(2):216-20.

Juergens UR. Anti-inflammatory Properties of the Monoterpene 1.8-cineole: Current Evidence for Co-medication in Inflammatory Airway Disease. *Drug Res* (Stuttg). 2014 May 15.

Dhibi S, et al. *Eucalyptus globulus* extract protects upon acetaminophen-induced kidney damage in male rat. *Bosn J Basic Med Sci.* 2014 May;14(2):99-104.

Esmaeili D, et al. Anti-*Helicobacter pylori* activities of shoya powder and essential oils of *Thymus vulgaris* and *Eucalyptus globulus*. *Open Microbiol J.* 2012;6:65-9.

Bachir RG, Benali M. Antibacterial activity of the essential oils from the leaves of *Eucalyptus globulus* against *Escherichia coli* and *Staphylococcus aureus. Asian Pac J Trop Biomed.* 2012 Sep;2(9):739-42.

## Eucalyptus Radiata *(Eucalyptus radiata)*

This eucalyptus species has been treasured in folk medicine. A 2011 study conducted at Heidelberg University found that *Eucalyptus radiata* has the second highest abundance of 1,8 cineole (Eucalyptol) after *E. globulus*.

**Medical Properties:** Antibacterial, antiviral, expectorant, anti-inflammatory

**Uses:** Respiratory/sinus infections, viral infections, fights herpes simplex when combined with bergamot

**Directions: Aromatic:** Diffuse up to 30 minutes up to 3 times daily or put in humidifier. Directly inhale. **Topical:** Dilute 1 drop essential oil with 1 drop V-6 or other pure carrier oil and apply 2-4 drops on location, chakras, and/or Vita Flex points.

**Technical Data: Botanical Family:** Myrtaceae; **Plant Origin:** Australia; **Extraction Method:** Steam distilled from leaves; **Key Constituents:** 1,8-Cineole (Eucalyptol) (60-75%), Alpha Terpineol (5-10%), Limonene (4-8%), Alpha Pine (2-6%)

### Selected Research

Sugumar S, et al. Ultrasonic emulsification of eucalyptus oil nanoemulsion: Antibacterial activity against *Staphylococcus aureus* and wound healing activity in Wister rats. *Ultrason Sonochem.* 2014 May;21(3):1044-9.

Murata S, et al. Antitumor effect of 1,8 cineole against colon cancer. *Oncol Rep.* 2013 Dec;30(6):2647-52.

Bendaoud H, et al. GC/MS analysis and antimicrobial and antioxidant activities of essential oil of *Eucalyptus radiata. J Sci Food Agric.* 2009 Jun;89(8):1292-1297.

## Eucalyptus Staigeriana
*(Eucalyptus staigeriana)*

This gentle eucalyptus species was valued by Australian Aborigines as a general cure-all. By 1788 it was introduced in Europe, where it was valued for treating respiratory conditions and for colic. Recent research documents staigeriana as a powerful antiparasitic as well as being highly antimicrobial.

**Medical Properties:** Antibacterial, diuretic, decongestant, expectorant, antiparasitic

**Uses:** Helps wounds, burns, and insect bites heal; suppresses coughs; relieves muscle aches

**Fragrant Influences:** Eucalyptus Staigeriana, also known as lemon iron bark, has a lemon-scented aroma, without the medicine-like scent of other eucalyptus oils. It can be used on people with sensitive skin.

**Directions: Aromatic:** Diffuse up to 30 minutes 3 times daily or put in humidifier. Directly inhale. **Topical:** Dilute 1 drop essential oil with 1 drop V-6 or other pure carrier oil and apply 2-4 drops on location, chakras, and/or Vita Flex points.

**Technical Data: Botanical Family:** Myrtaceae; **Plant Origin:** Australia, Brazil; **Extraction Method:** Steam distilled from leaves; **Key Constituents:** Alpha-Phellandrene (4-7%), Limonene (4-10%), 1,8 Cineole (Eucalyptol) (15-35%), Neral (7-15%), Geranial (10-20%)

### Selected Research

Ribeiro WL, et al. In vitro effects of *Eucalyptus staigeriana* nanoemulsion on *Haemonchus contortus* and toxicity in rodents. *Vet Parasitol.* 2015 Jul 26.

Nivea MS, et al. Contact and fumigant toxicity and repellency of

*Eucalyptus citriodora* Hook., *Eucalyptus staigeriana* F., *Cymbopogon winterianus* Jowitt and *Foeniculum vulgare* Mill. essential oils in the management of *Callosobruchus maculatus* (FABR.) (Coleoptera: Chrysomelidae, Bruchinae). *J Stored Prod Res.* 2013 Jul;54:41-7.

Gilles M, et al. Chemical composition and antimicrobial properties of essential oils of three Australian Eucalyptus species. *Food Chem.* 2010 15 Mar;119(2):731-37.

## Fennel *(Foeniculum vulgare)*

Fennel was believed to ward off evil spirits and to protect against spells cast by witches during medieval times. Sprigs were hung over doors to fend off evil phantasms. For hundreds of years, fennel seeds have been used as a digestive aid and to balance menstrual cycles. It is mentioned in one of the oldest known medical records, the Ebers Papyrus (dating from 16th century BC), an ancient Egyptian list of 877 prescriptions and recipes. It was listed in Hildegard's *Medicine*, a compilation of early German medicines by highly regarded Benedictine herbalist Hildegard of Bingen (1098-1179).

**Medical Properties:** Antidiabetic, anti-inflammatory, antitumoral, estrogen-like, digestive aid, antiparasitic (worms), antiseptic, antispasmodic, analgesic, increases metabolism

**Uses:** Diabetes, cancer, obesity, arthritis/rheumatism, urinary tract infection, fluid retention, intestinal parasites, menstrual problems/PMS, digestive problems

**Directions: Aromatic:** Diffuse up to 30 minutes 3 times daily or directly inhale. **Dietary:** Take as a dietary supplement. **Topical:** Apply 2-4 drops on location, chakras, and/or Vita Flex points. Dilution not required except for the most sensitive skin.

**Caution:** Avoid using if epileptic.

## Fennel Vitality™ *(Foeniculum vulgare)*

**Directions: Dietary:** Dilute 1 drop with 1 drop of carrier oil. Put in a capsule and take up to 3 times daily or as needed.

**Technical Data: Botanical Family:** Apiaceae; **Plant Origin:** Hungary; **Extraction Method:** Steam distilled from the crushed seeds (fruit); **Key Constituents:** Trans-Anethole (60-80%), Fenchone (8-20%), Alpha-Pinene (1-8%), Methyl Chavicol (2-6%); **ORAC:** 238,400 µTE/100g

### Selected Research

Mota AS, et al. Antimicrobial activity and chemical composition of the essential oils of Portuguese *Foeniculum vulgare* fruits. *Nat Prod Commun.* 2015 Apr;10(4):673-6.

Goswami N, Chatterjee S. Assessment of free radical scavenging potential and oxidative DNA damage preventive activity of *Trachyspermum ammi*

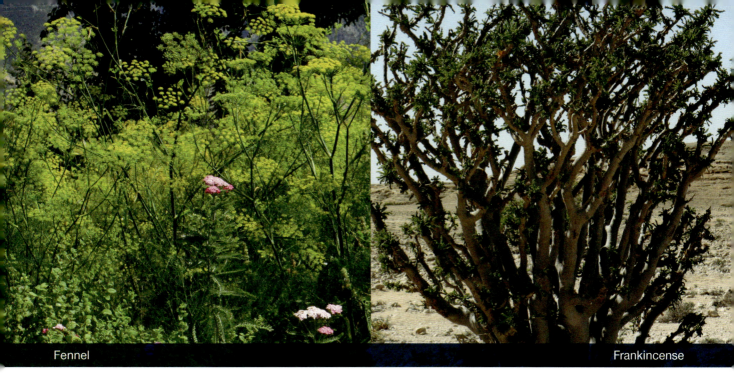

Fennel

Frankincense

L. (carom) and Foeniculum vulgare Mill. (fennel) seed extracts. *Biomed Res.* 2014;2014:582767.

Mesfin M, et al. Evaluation of anxiolytic activity of the essential oil of the aerial part of *Foeniculum vulgare* Miller in mice. *BMC Complement Altern Med.* 2014 Aug 23;14:310.

Senatore F, et al. Chemical composition, antimicrobial and antioxidant activities of anethole-rich oil from leaves of selected varieties of fennel [*Foeniculum vulgare* Mill. Ssp. Vulgare var. azoricum (Mill.) Thell]. *Fitoterapia.* 2013 Oct;90:214-9.

Omidvar S, et al. Effect of fennel on pain intensity in dysmenorrhea: A placebo-controlled trial. *Ayu.* 2012 Apr;33(2):311-3.

Qiu J, et al. Chemical composition of fennel essential oil and its impact on *Staphylococcus aureus* exotoxin production. *World J Microbiol Biotechnol.* 2012 Apr;28(4):1399-405.

## Frankincense (Boswellia carterii)

Also known as "olibanum," the name frankincense is derived from the Medieval French word for "real incense." Frankincense is considered the "holy anointing oil" in the Middle East and has been used in religious ceremonies for thousands of years. It was well known during the time of Christ for its anointing and healing powers and was one of the gifts given to Christ at His birth. "Used to treat every conceivable ill known to man," frankincense was valued more than gold during ancient times, and only those with great wealth and abundance possessed it. It is mentioned in one of the oldest known medical records, Ebers Papyrus (dating from 16th century BC), an ancient Egyptian list of 877 prescriptions and recipes.

**Medical Properties:** Antitumoral, immuno-stimulant, antidepressant, muscle relaxing

**Uses:** Depression, cancer, respiratory infections, inflammation, immune-stimulating

**Fragrant Influence:** Increases spiritual awareness, promotes meditation, improves attitude, and uplifts spirits

**Directions: Aromatic:** Diffuse up to 1 hour 3 times daily or directly inhale. **Topical:** Apply 2-4 drops on location, chakras, and/or Vita Flex points. Dilution not required except for the most sensitive skin.

## Frankincense Vitality™ (Boswellia carterii)

**Directions: Dietary:** Put 2 drops in a capsule. Take 3 times daily.

**Technical Data: Botanical Family:** Burseraceae; **Plant Origin:** Somalia; **Extraction Method:** Steam distilled from gum/resin; **Key Constituents:** Alpha-Pinene (30-65%), Limonene (8-20%), Sabinene (1-8%), Myrcene (1-14%), Beta-Caryophyllene (1-5%), Alpha-Thujene (1-15%), Incensole; **ORAC:** 630 µTE/100g

### Selected Research

Wang YG, et al. Hepatoprotective triterpenes from the gum resin of *Boswellia carterii. Fitoterapia.* 2016 Mar,109:266-73.

Mostafa DM, et al. Transdermal microemulsions of *Boswellia carterii* Bird: formulation, characterization and in vivo evaluation of anti-inflammatory activity. *Drug Deliv.* 2015 Sep;22(6):785-56.

Zaki AA, et al. Cardioprotective and antioxidant effects of oleogum resin "Olibanum" from *Boswellia carteri* Birdw. (Bursearaceae). *Chin J Nat Med.* 2014 May;12(5):345-50.

Woolley CL, et al. Chemical differentiation of *Boswellia sacra* and *Boswellia carterii* essential oils by gas chromatography and chiral gas chromatography-mass spectrometry. *J Chromatogr A.* 2012 Oct 26;1261:158-63.

Moussaieff A, et al. Incensole acetate, an incense component, elicits psychoactivity by activating TRPV3 channels in the brain. *FASEB J.* 2008 Aug;22(8):3024-34.

Moussaieff A, et al. Incensole acetate: a novel neuroprotective agent isolated from *Boswellia carterii. J Cereb Blood Flow Metab.* 2008 Jul;28(7):1341-52.

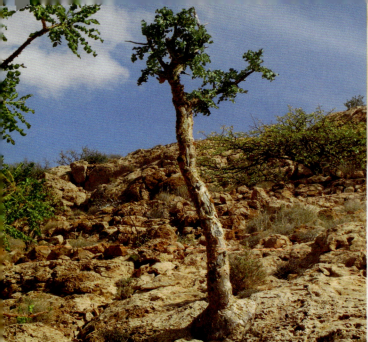
Frereana Frankincense

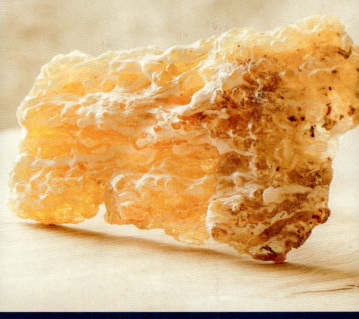
Frereana Frankincense resin

### Frereana Frankincense *(Boswellia frereana)*

This species of frankincense is native to northern Somalia, where the locals call it "Maydi" and the "King of Frankincense." Frereana incense has been a part of Eastern Orthodox and Catholic worship for hundreds of years.

Since *Boswellia carterii* also grows in Somalia, it is hard to explain why frereana has such a unique chemical composition, so different from *B. carterii* and other frankincense species. As shown by Frank and Unger, as well as E. J. Blain, frereana contains no boswellic acids. S. Hamm reports that frereana "is devoid of diterpenes of the incensole family." Now that a pure source can be guaranteed, it is hoped researchers will delve into the benefits of frereana.

There are unique constituents of frereana found in no other frankincense that have mostly been overlooked by researchers. Two frereana studies in 2010 and 2006 reported strong anti-inflammatory activity. Sadly, some trusting purchasers have received an amalgamation of cheaper frankincense resins rather than pure *Boswellia frereana*.

Political conditions in Somalia make it essential for a "feet on the ground" presence in order to secure contracts to obtain pure, high quality frereana resin. For this reason, D. Gary Young personally visited Somalia in November 2013 to contract with local clans of harvesters.

**Medical Properties:** Anti-inflammatory

**Uses:** Arthritis/rheumatism

**Fragrant Influence:** The aroma of frereana frankincense has a more lemony scent than carterii and is uplifting and cheering.

**Directions: Aromatic:** Diffuse up to 1 hour 3 times daily or directly inhale. **Dietary:** Dilute 1 drop of frankincense in 4 drops V-6 or other pure carrier oil, put in a capsule, and take 1 capsule before each meal or as desired. **Topical:** Apply 2-4 drops on location, chakras, and/or Vita Flex points. Dilution not required except for the most sensitive skin.

**Technical Data: Botanical Family:** Burseraceae; **Plant Origin:** Somalia; **Extraction Method:** Steam distilled from gum/resin; **Key Constituents:** Alpha-Thujene (23-45%), Alpha-Pinene (5-9%), Sabinene (1-8%), Para-Cymene (10-20%), Terpinen-4-ol (2-9%)

### Selected Research

Niebler J, Buettner A. Frankincense Revisited, Part I: Comparative Analysis of Volatiles in Commercially Relevant Boswellia Species. *Chem Biodivers.* 2016 May;12(5):613-29.

Blain EJ, et al. *Boswellia frereana* (frankincense) suppresses cytokine-induced matrix metalloproteinase expression and production of anti-inflammatory molecules in articular cartilage. *Phytother Res.* 2010 Jun;24(6):905-12.

Frank A, Unger M. Analysis of frankincense resin from various Boswellia species with inhibitory activity on human drug metabolizing cytochrome P450 enzymes using liquid chromatography mass spectrometry after automated on-line extraction. *J Chromatogr A.* 2006 Apr 21;1112(1-2):255-62.

Hamm S, et al. A chemical investigation by headspace SPME and GC-MS of volatile and semi-volatile terpenes in various olibanum samples. *Phytochemistry.* 2005 Jun;66(12):1499-514.

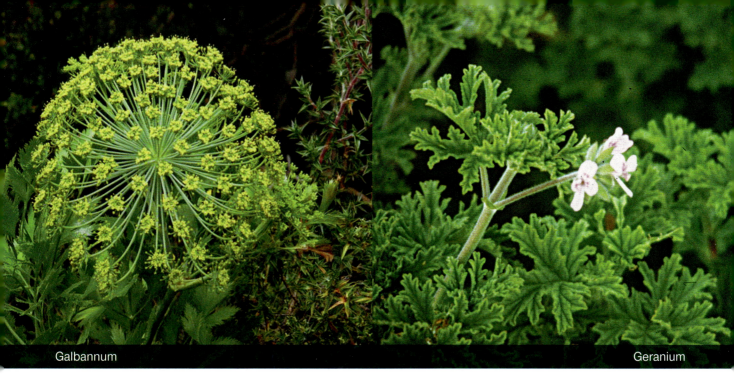

Galbannum

Geranium

## Galbanum *(Ferula galbaniflua)*

Mentioned in Egyptian papyri and the Old Testament (Exodus 30:34), it was esteemed for its medicinal and spiritual properties. Dioscorides, an ancient Roman historian, records that galbanum was used for its antispasmodic, diuretic, and pain-relieving properties.

**Medical Properties:** Antiseptic, analgesic, light antispasmodic, anti-inflammatory, circulatory stimulant, anticonvulsant

**Uses:** Digestive problems (diarrhea), nervous tension, rheumatism, skin conditions (scar tissue, wrinkles)

**Fragrant Influence:** Harmonic and balancing, amplifies spiritual awareness and meditation. When combined with Frankincense or Sandalwood, the frequency rises dramatically.

**Directions: Aromatic:** Diffuse up to 1 hour 3 times daily or directly inhale. **Dietary:** Put in a capsule, and take up to 3 times daily or as needed. **Topical:** Dilute 1 drop essential oil with 1 drop V-6 or other pure carrier oil and apply 2-4 drops on location, chakras, and/or Vita Flex points. Dilution not required except for the most sensitive skin.

**Technical Data: Botanical Family:** Apiaceae; **Plant Origin:** Persia; **Extraction Method:** Steam distilled from gum/resin derived from stems and branches; **Key Constituents:** Alpha-Pinene (5-21%), Beta-Pinene (40-70%), Delta-3-Carene (2-16%), Myrcene (2.5-3.5%), Sabinene (0.3-3%); **ORAC:** 26,200 µTE/100g

### Selected Research

Moosavi SJ, et al. Protective effect of *Ferula gummosa* hydroalcoholic extract against nitric oxide deficiency-induced oxidative stress and inflammation in rats renal tissues. *Clin Exp Hypertens.* 2015;37(2):136-41.

Gudarzi H, et al. Ethanolic extract of *Ferula gummosa* is cytotoxic against cancer cells by inducing apoptosis and cell cycle arrest. *Nat Prod Res.* 2015;29(6):546-50.

Abdollahi Fard M, Shojaii A. Efficacy of Iranian traditional medicine in the treatment of epilepsy. *Biomed Res Int.* 2013;2013:692751.

Gholitabar S, Roshan VD. Effect of treadmill exercise and *Ferula gummosa* on myocardial HSP72k, vascular function, and antioxidant defenses in spontaneously hypertensive rats. *Clin Exp Hypertens.* 2013;35(5):347-54.

Effekar F, et al. Antibacterial activity of the essential oil from *Ferula gummosa* seed. *Fitoterapia.* 2004 Dec;75(7-8):758-9.

## Geranium *(Pelargonium graveolens)*

Geranium has been used for centuries for regenerating and healing skin conditions.

**Medical Properties:** Antispasmodic, antioxidant, antitumoral, anti-inflammatory, anticancer, hemostatic (stops bleeding), antibacterial, antifungal, improves blood flow, liver and pancreas stimulant, dilates bile ducts for liver detoxification, helps cleanse oily skin; revitalizes skin cells

**Uses:** Hepatitis/fatty liver (Jean Valnet, MD), skin conditions (dermatitis, eczema, psoriasis, acne, vitiligo), fungal infections (ringworm), viral infections (herpes, shingles), hormone imbalances, circulatory problems (improves blood flow), menstrual problems/PMS

**Fragrant Influence:** Helps release negative memories and eases nervous tension; balances the emotions, lifts the spirit, and fosters peace, well-being, and hope

**Directions: Aromatic:** Diffuse up to 1 hour 3 times daily or directly inhale. **Dietary:** Dilute 1 drop of geranium in 4 drops V-6 or other pure carrier oil, put in a capsule, and take 1 capsule before each meal

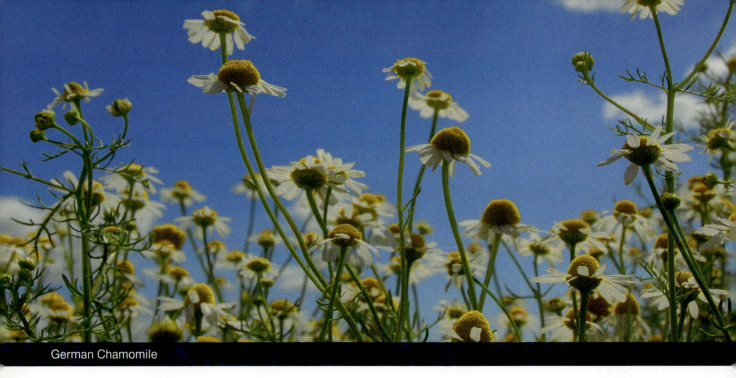
German Chamomile

or as desired. **Topical:** Apply 2-4 drops on location, chakras, and/or Vita Flex points. Dilution not required except for the most sensitive skin.

**Technical Data: Botanical Family:** Geraniaceae; **Plant Origin:** Egypt, India; **Extraction Method:** Steam distilled from the flowers and leaves; **Key Constituents:** Citronellol (25-36%), Geraniol (10-18%), Citronellyl Formate (5-8%), Linalol (4-8%).

### Selected Research

Rashidi Fakari F, Effect of Aroma of Geranium Essence on Anxiety and Physiological Parameters during First Stage of Labor in Nulliparous Women: a Randomized Clinical Trial. *J Caring Sci.* 2015 Jun 1;4(2):135-41.

Budzynska A, et al. Enzymatic profile, adhesive and invasive properties of *Candida albicans* under the influence of selected plant essential oils. *Acta Biochim Pol.* 2014;61(1):115-21.

Tabanaca N, et al. Bioactivity-Guided Investigation of Geranium Essential Oils as Natural Tick Repellents. *J Agric Food Chem.* 2013 Mar 25. [Epub ahead of print]

Bigos M, et al. Antimicrobial activity of geranium oil against clinical strains of *Staphylococcus aureus. Molecules.* 2012 Aug 28:17(9):10276-91.

Ben Hsouna A, Hamdi N. Phytochemical composition and antimicrobial activities of the essential oils and organic extracts from *Pelargonium graveolens* growing in Tunesia. *Lipids Health Dis.* 2012 Dec 5;11:167.

Malik T, et al. Potentiation of antimicrobial activity of ciprofloxacin by *Pelargonium graveolens* essential oil against selected uropathogens. *Phytother Res.* 2011 Aug;25(8):1225-8.

## German Chamomile
### (Chamomilla recutita) (Syn. Matricaria recutita)

Listed in Dioscorides' *De Materia Medica* (AD 78), Europe's first authoritative guide to medicines, which became the standard reference work for herbal treatments for over 1,700 years.

**Medical Properties:** Powerful antioxidant, inhibits lipid peroxidation, antitumoral, anti-inflammatory, relaxant, anesthetic; promotes digestion, liver, and gallbladder health.

**Uses:** Hepatitis/fatty liver, arteriosclerosis, insomnia, nervous tension, arthritis, carpal tunnel syndrome, skin problems such as acne, eczema, scar tissue

**Fragrant Influence:** Dispels anger, stabilizes emotions, and helps release emotions linked to the past. Soothes and clears the mind.

**Directions: Aromatic:** Diffuse up to 1 hour 3 times daily or directly inhale. **Topical:** Apply 2-4 drops on location, chakras, and/or Vita Flex points. Dilution not required except for the most sensitive skin.

## German Chamomile Vitality™
### (Chamomilla recutita) (Syn. Matricaria recutita)

**Directions: Dietary:** Put 2 drops in a capsule. Take 3 times daily or as needed.

**Technical Data: Botanical Family:** Asteraceae; **Plant Origin:** Utah, Idaho, Egypt, Hungary; **Extraction Method:** Steam distilled from flowers; **Key Constituents:** Chamazulene (2-5%), Bisabolol Oxide A (32-42%), Trans-Beta-Farnesene (18-26%), Bisbolol Oxide B (3-6%), Bisbolone Oxide A (3-6%), Cis Spiro Ether (4-8%); **ORAC:** 218,600 µTE/100g

### Selected Research

Sebai H, et al. Chemical composition, antioxidant properties and hepatoprotective effects of chamomile (*Matricaria recutita* L.) decoction extract against alcohol-induced oxidative stress in rat. *Gen Physiol Biophys.* 2015 Jul;34(3):263-75.

Capuzzo A, et al. Antioxidant and radical scavenging activities of chamazulene. *Nat Prod Res.* 2014 Dec;28(24):2321-3.

Ranjbar A, et al. Ameliorative effect of *Matricaria chamomilla* L. on paraquat: Induced oxidative damage in lung rats [sic rat lungs]. *Pharmacognosy Res.* 2014 Jul;6(3):199-203.

Zargaran A, et al. Potential effect and mechanism of action of topical chamomile (*Matricaria chammomila* [sic] L.) on migraine headache: A medical hypothesis. *Med Hypotheses.* 2014 Sep 6. [Epub ahead of print]

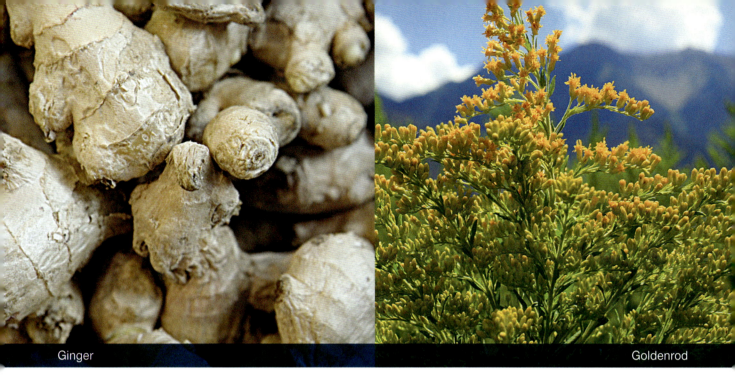

Ginger | Goldenrod

Tomić M, et al. Antihyperalgesic and Antiedematous Activities of Bisabool-Oxides-Rich Matricara Oil in a Rat Model of Inflammation. *Phytother Res.* 2013 Aug 27. [Epub ahead of print]

## Ginger *(Zingiber officinale)*

Traditionally used to combat nausea. Women in the West African country of Senegal weave belts of ginger root to restore their mates' sexual potency.

**Medical Properties:** Anti-inflammatory, anticoagulant, digestive aid, anesthetic, expectorant, antifungal

**Uses:** Rheumatism/arthritis, digestive disorders, respiratory infections/congestion, muscular aches/pains, nausea

**Fragrant Influence:** Gentle, stimulating, endowing physical energy, courage

**Directions: Aromatic:** Diffuse up to 1 hour 3 times daily or directly inhale. **Topical:** Dilute 1 drop essential oil with 1 drop V-6 or other pure carrier oil and apply 2-4 drops on location, chakras, and/or Vita Flex points.

**Caution:** Anticoagulant properties can be enhanced when combined with Warfarin, aspirin, etc.

## Ginger Vitality™ *(Zingiber officinale)*

**Directions: Dietary:** Dilute 1 drop with 1 drop of carrier oil. Put in a capsule and take up to 3 times daily.

**Technical Data: Botanical Family:** Zingiberaceae; **Plant Origin:** India, China; **Extraction Method:** Steam distilled from rhizomes/root; **Key Constituents:** Zingiberene (30-40%), Beta-Sesquiphellandrene (8-19%), 1,8-Cineole (Eucalyptol) + Beta-Phellandrene (4-10%), AR Curcumene (5-10%), Camphene (5-9%); **ORAC:** 99,300 µTE/100g

## Selected Research

Lai YS, et al. Ginger essential oil ameliorates hepatic injury and lipid accumulation in high fat diet-induced nonalcoholic fatty liver disease. *J Agric Food Chem.* 2016 Feb 21.

Gan Z, et al. Separation and preparation of 6-gingerol from molecular distillation residue of Yunnan ginger rhizomes by high-speed countercurrent chromatography and the antioxidant activity of ginger oils in vitro. *J Chromatogr B Analyt Technol Biomed Life Sci.* 2016 Jan 4;1011:99-107.

Lua PL, et al. Effects of inhaled ginger aromatherapy on chemotherapy-induced nausea and vomiting and health-related quality of life in women with breast cancer. *Complement Ther Med.* 2015 Jun;23(3):396-404.

Bartels EM, et al. Efficacy and safety of ginger in osteoarthritis patients: A meta-analysis of randomized placebo-controlled trials. *Osteoarthritis Cartilage.* 2014 Oct 6. Pii: S1063-4584(14)01276-X.

Khayat S, et al. Effect of treatment with ginger on the severity of premenstrual syndrome symptoms. *ISRN Obstet Gynecol.* 2014 May 4;2014:792708.

Kumar L, et al. Structural alternations in *Pseudomonas aeruginosa* by zingerone contribute to enhanced susceptibility to antibiotics, serum and phagocytes. *Life Sci.* 2014 Sep 30. S0024-3205(14)00766-8.

Lim S, et al. Ginger improves cognitive function via NGF-induced ERK/CREB activation in the hippocampus of the mouse. *J Nutr Biochem.* 2014 Oc;25(10):1058-65.

## Goldenrod *(Solidago canadensis)*

The genus name, *Solidago*, comes from the Latin solide, which means "to make whole." During the Boston Tea Party, when English tea was dumped into Boston Harbor, colonists drank goldenrod tea instead, which gave it the nickname "Liberty Tea."

**Medical Properties:** Diuretic, anti-inflammatory, antihypertensive, liver stimulant

**Uses:** Hypertension, liver congestion, hepatitis/fatty liver, circulatory conditions, urinary tract/bladder conditions

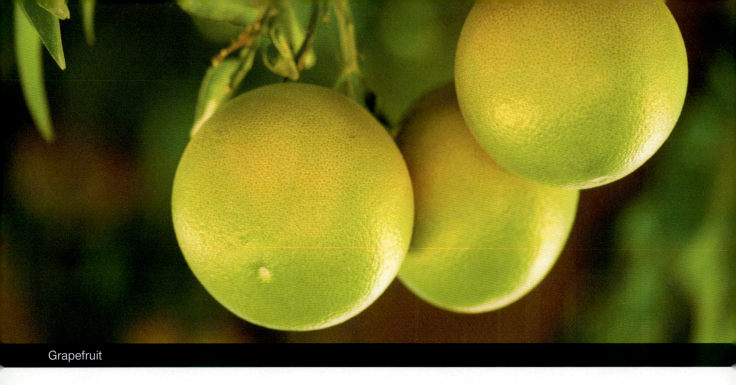

Grapefruit

**Directions: Aromatic:** Diffuse up to 30 minutes 3 times daily or directly inhale. **Dietary:** Take as a dietary supplement. **Topical:** Dilute 1 drop essential oil with 1 drop V-6 or other pure carrier oil and apply 2-4 drops on location, chakras, and/or Vita Flex points.

**Technical Data: Botanical Family:** Asteraceae; **Plant Origin:** Canada; **Extraction Method:** Steam distilled from flowering tops; **Key Constituents:** Alpha-Pinene (10-24%), Germacrene D (15-37%), Myrcene (4-10%), Sabinene (5-18%), Limonene (10-20%); **ORAC:** 61,900 µTE/100g

### Selected Research

Marksa M, et al. Development of an HPLC post-column antioxidant assay for *Solidago canadensis* radical scavengers. *Nat Prod Res.* 2015 Apr 2:1-8.

Huang Y, et al. Allelopathic effects of the extracts from an invasive species *Solidago canadensis* L. on *Microcystis aeruginosa. Lett Appl Microbiol.* 2013 Nov;57(5):451-8.

Huang Y, et al. Chemical constituents from *Solidago canadensis* with hypolipidemic effects in HFD-fed hamsters. *J Asian Nat Prod Res.* 2013;15(4):319-24.

Raghavendra BS, et al. Synergistic effect of *Eugenia jambolana* Linn. and *Solidago canadensis* Linn. leaf extracts with deltamethrin against the dengue vector *Aedes aegypti* Linn at Mysore. *Eviron Sci Pollut Res Int.* 2013 Jun;20(6):3830-5.

## Grapefruit *(Citrus paradisi)*

Grapefruit is believed to have originated in Barbados by an accidental crossing of sweet orange (*Citrus sinensis*) and pomelo (*Citrus maxima*). When it was discovered, it was called the "forbidden fruit."

**Medical Properties:** Antitumoral, metabolic stimulant, antiseptic, detoxifying, diuretic, fat-dissolving, cleansing for kidneys, lymphatic and vascular system; antidepressant, rich in limonene, which has been extensively studied in over 50 clinical studies for its ability to combat tumor growth

**Uses:** Alzheimer's, fluid retention, depression, obesity, liver disorders, anxiety, cellulite

**Fragrant Influence:** Refreshing and uplifting. A Mie University study found that citrus fragrances boosted immunity, induced relaxation, and reduced depression (Komori, et al., 1995).

**Directions: Aromatic:** Diffuse up to 1 hour 3 times daily or directly inhale. **Topical:** Dilute 1 drop essential oil with 1 drop V-6 or other pure carrier oil and apply 2-4 drops on location, chakras, and/or Vita Flex points.

**Caution:** Possible sun sensitivity.

## Grapefruit Vitality™ *(Citrus paradisi)*

**Directions: Dietary:** Put 2 drops in a capsule. Take 3 times daily.

**Technical Data: Botanical Family:** Rutaceae; **Plant Origin:** South Africa and California. (Grapefruit is a hybrid between Citrus maxima and Citrus sinensis.); **Extraction Method:** Cold pressed from rind; **Key Constituents:** Limonene (88-95%), Myrcene (1-4%); **ORAC:** 22,600 µTE/100g

### Selected Research

Onakpoya I, et al. The Effect of Grapefruit (*Citrus paradisi*) on Body Weight and Cardiovascular Risk Factors: A Systematic Review and Meta-analysis of Randomized Clinical Trials. *Crit Rev Food Sci Nutr.* 2015 Apr 16:0. [Epub ahead of print]

Gamboa-Gómez C, et al. Consumption of *Ocimum sanctum* L. and *Citrus paradise* infusions modulates lipid metabolism and insulin resistance in obese rats. *Food Funct.* 2014 May;5(5):927-35.

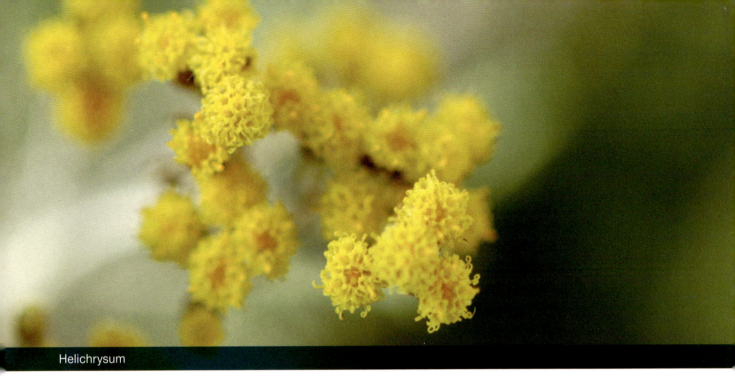

Helichrysum

Adukwu EC, et al. The anti-biofilm activity of lemongrass *(Cymbopogon flexuosus)* and grapefruit *(Citrus paradisi)* essential oils against five strains of *Staphylococcus aureus*. *J Appl Microbiol*. 2012 Nov;113(5):1217-27.

Flor-Weiler LB, et al. Susceptibility of four tick species, *Amblyomma americanum, Dermacentor variabilis, Ixodes scapularis*, and *Rhipicephalus sanguineus* (Acari: Ixodidae), to nootkatone from essential oil of grapefruit. *J Med Entomol*. 2011 Mar;48(2):322-6.

Murase T, et al. Nootkatone, a characteristic constituent of grapefruit, stimulates energy metabolism and prevents diet-induced obesity by activating AMPK. *Am J Physiol Endocrinol Metab*. 2010 Aug;299(2):E266-75.

## Helichrysum (Helichrysum italicum)

Helichrysum is also known by the names Immortelle and Everlasting. Helichrysum essential oil is renowned for its anti-inflammatory effects.

**Medical Properties:** Anticoagulant, anesthetic, antioxidant, antispasmodic, antiviral, liver protectant/detoxifier/stimulant, chelates chemicals and toxins, regenerates nerves

**Uses:** Herpes virus, arteriosclerosis, atherosclerosis, hypertension, blood clots, liver disorders, circulatory disorders, skin conditions (eczema, psoriasis scar tissue, varicose veins)

**Fragrant Influence:** Uplifting to the subconscious

**Directions: Aromatic:** Diffuse up to 1 hour 3 times daily or directly inhale. **Dietary:** Take as a dietary supplement. **Topical:** Apply 2-4 drops on location, temple, forehead, back of neck, outside of ear, chakras, and/or Vita Flex points. Dilution not required except for the most sensitive skin.

**Caution:** Anticoagulant properties can be enhanced when combined with Warfarin, aspirin, etc.

**Technical Data: Botanical Family:** Asteraceae; **Plant Origin:** Yugoslavia, Corsica, Croatia, Spain; **Extraction Method:** Steam distilled from flower; **Key Constituents:** Neryl Acetate (3-35%), Gamma-Curcumene (10-28%), Alpha-Pinene (15-32%), Beta-Caryophyllene (2-9%), Beta-Selinene (4-8%); **ORAC:** 1,700 µTE/100g

### Selected Research

Ćavar Zelijković S, et al. Volatiles of *Helichrysum italicum* (Roth) G. Don from Croatia. *Nat Prod Res*. 2015 Oct;29(19):1874-7.

Antunes Viegas D, et al. *Helichrysum italicum*: from traditional use to scientific data. *J Ethnopharmacol*. 2014;151(1):54-65.

Rigano D, et al. Intestinal antispasmodic effects of *Helichrysum italicum* (Roth) Don ssp. italicum and chemical identification of the active ingredients. *J Ethnopharmacol*. 2013 Oct 16. S0378-874(13)00681-8.

Taglialatela-Scafati O, et al. Antimicrobial phenolics and unusual glycerides from *Helichrysum italicum* subsp. microphyllum. *J Nat Prod*. 2013 Mar 22;76(3):346-53.

Appendino G, et al. Arzanol, an anti-inflammatory and anti-HIV-1 phloroglucinol alpha-Pyrone from *Helichrysum italicum* ssp. microphyllum. *J Nat Prod*. 2007 Apr;70(4):608-12.

## Hinoki (Chamaecyparis obtusa)

Hinoki wood has been used to construct many holy temples in Japan, including Horyuji Temple and Osaka Castle, and is said to be the "tree where God stayed." Hinoki wood is resistant to decay and carries a symbolic reputation of being immortal.

**Medical Properties:** Contains tau-muurolene, a powerful antifungal compound; reduces agitation and hyperactivity

**Uses:** Antibacterial, antiviral, antidepressant, anti-inflammatory, astringent, odor eliminator, promotes hair growth, stimulates digestion, relieves pain

**Fragrant Influence:** Calming and centering

**Directions: Aromatic:** Diffuse up to 30 minutes 3 times daily. **Topical:** Dilute 1 drop essential oil with 1 drop V-6 or other pure carrier oil and apply 2-4 drops to desired location, temple, forehead, back of neck, or outside of ear.

**Technical Data: Botanical Family:** Cupressaceae; **Plant Origin:** Southern Japan; **Extraction Method:** Steam distilled from sustainably harvested, culled wood; **Key Constituents:** Alpha-Pinene (35-60%), Gamma-Cadinene (3-8%), Delta-Cadinene (7-14%), Tau-Cadinol (7-15%), Tau-Muurolol (6-12%)

## Selected Research

Park Y, et al. Anti-inflammatory effects of essential oils extracted from *Chamaecyparis obtusa* on murine models of inflammation and RAW 264.7 cells. *Mol Med Rep.* 2016 Apr;13(4):3335-41.

Kim ES, et al. *Chamaecyparis obtusa* Essential Oil Inhibits Methicillin-Resistant *Staphylococcus aureus* Biofilm Formation and Expression of Virulence Factors. *J Med Food.* 2015 Jul;18(7):810-7

Chien TC, et al. Chemical composition and anti-inflammatory activity of *Chamaecyparis obtusa* f. formosana wood essential oil from Taiwan. *Nat Prod Commun.* 2014 May;9(5):723-6.

Kasuya H, et al. Effect on emotional behavior and stress by inhalation of the essential oil from *Chamaecyparis obtusa. Nat Prod Commun.* 2013 Apr;8(4):515-8.

Bae D, et al. Inhaled essential oil from *Chamaecyparis obtusa* ameliorates the impairments of cognitive function induced by injection of β-amyloid in rats. *Pharm Bull.* 2012 Jul;50(7):900-10.

Lee GS, et al. The essential oil of *Chamaecyparis obtusa* promote[s] hair growth through the induction of vascular endothelial growth factor gene. *Fitotherpia.* 2010 Jan;81(1):17-24.

## Hong Kuai *(Chamaecyparis formosensis)*

Hong Kuai trees grow up to 55-60 meters tall in high altitude areas of Taiwan and can live over 1,000 years. The wood of these trees is highly resistant to decay and valued for building temples. The highly scented oil was known for supporting respiratory health.

**Medical Properties:** Antifungal, anticancer, immune support

**Uses:** Fungal infections (ringworm), cancer, respiratory problems

**Fragrant Influence:** Calming and centering

**Directions: Aromatic:** Diffuse up to 30 minutes 3 times daily. **Topical:** Dilute 1 drop essential oil with 4 drops V-6 or other pure carrier oil and apply 2-4 drops to desired location, temple, forehead, back of neck, or outside of ear. Test on small area of skin on underside of arm.

**Technical Data: Botanical Family:** Cupressaceae; **Plant Origin:** Taiwan; **Extraction Method:** Steam distilled from sustainably harvested, culled wood; **Key Constituents:** Alpha-Pinene (4-6%), Myrtenal (3-7%), Myrtenol (11-18%), Myrtanol (13-19%), Delta-Cadinene (7-10%), Alpha-Elemol (1-4%), Tau-Muurolol (3-6%)

## Selected Research

Chen YJ, et al. Rapid discrimination and feature extraction of three Chamaecyparis species by static-HS/GC-MS. *J Agric Food Chem.* 2015 Jan 28;63(3):810-20.

Ho CL, et al. Composition and antipathogenic activities of the twig essential oil of *Chamaecyparis formosensis* from Taiwan. *Nat Prod Commun.* 2012 Jul;7(7):933-6.

Chen TH, et al. Isolation and cytotoxicity of the lignanoids from *Chamaecyparis formosensis. Planta Med.* 2008 Dec;74(15):1806-11.

Hsieh YH, et al. Effects of *Chamaecyparis formosensis* Matasumura extractives on lipopolysaccharide-induced release of nitrous oxide. *Phytomedicine.* 2007 Oct;14(10):675-80.

## Hyssop *(Hyssopus officinalis)*

While there is some uncertainty that *Hyssopus officinalis* is the same species of plant as the hyssop referred to in the Bible, there is no question that *H. officinalis* has been used medicinally for almost a millennium for its antiseptic properties. It has also been used for opening the respiratory system.

**Medical Properties:** Mucolytic, decongestant, anti-inflammatory, regulates lipid metabolism, antiviral, antibacterial, and antiparasitic

**Uses:** Respiratory infections/congestion, parasites (expelling worms), viral infections, and circulatory disorders

**Fragrant Influence:** Stimulates creativity and meditation

**Directions: Aromatic:** Diffuse up to 10 minutes 3 times daily or directly inhale. **Dietary:** Take as a dietary supplement. **Topical:** Dilute 1 drop essential oil with 1 drop V-6 or other pure carrier oil and apply 2-4 drops on location, chakras, and/or Vita Flex points.

**Caution:** Avoid use if epileptic.

**Technical Data: Botanical Family:** Lamiaceae; **Plant Origin:** France, Hungary, Utah; **Extraction Method:** Steam distilled from stems and leaves; **Key Constituents:** Beta-Pinene (13.5-23%), Sabinene (2-3%), Pinocamphone (5.5-17.5%), Iso-Pinochamphone (34.5-50%), Gemacrene D (2-3%), Limonene (1-4%); **ORAC:** 20,900 µTE/100g

## Selected Research

Stappen I, et al. Chemical composition and biological activity of essential oils of *Dracocephalum heterophyllum* and *Hyssopus officinais* from Western Himalaya. *Nat Prod Commun.* 2015 Jan;10(1):133-8.

Ma X, et al. Effect of *Hyssopus officinalis* L. on inhibiting airway inflammation and immune regulation in a chronic asthmatic mouse model. *Exp Ther Med.* 2014 Nov;8(5):1371-1374.

Vlase L, et al. Evaluation of antioxidant and antimicrobial activities and phenolic profile for *Hyssopus officinalis, Ocimum basilicum* and *Teucrium chamedrys. Molecules.* 2014 Apr 28;19(5):5490-507.

Miyazaki H, et al. Inhibitory effects of hyssop (*Hyssopus officinalis*) extracts on intestinal alpha-glucosidase activity and postprandial hyperglycemia. *J Nutr Sci Vitaminol* (Tokyo). 2003 Oct;49(5):346-9.

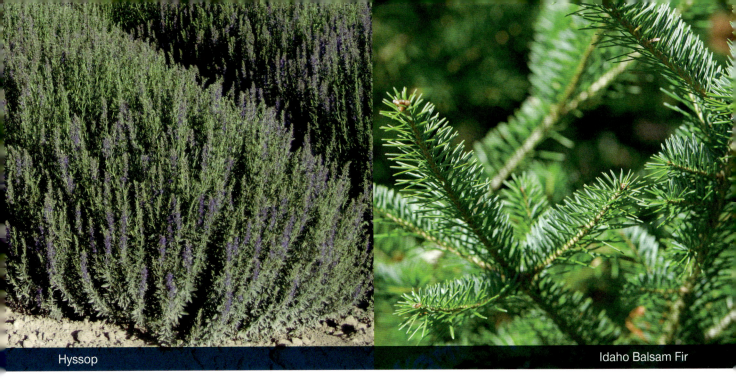

Hyssop | Idaho Balsam Fir

## Idaho Balsam Fir (Balsam Canada)
*(Abies balsamea)*

The balsam fir tree—a tree commonly used as a Christmas tree today—has been prized through the ages for its medicinal effects and ability to heal respiratory conditions and muscular and rheumatic pain.

**Medical Properties:** Anticoagulant, antibacterial, antiinflammatory, antitumoral

**Uses:** Throat/lung/sinus infections, fatigue, arthritis/rheumatism, urinary tract infections, scoliosis/lumbago/sciatica

**Fragrant Influence:** Grounding, stimulating to the mind, and relaxing to the body

**Directions: Aromatic:** Diffuse up to 1 hour 3 times daily or directly inhale. **Dietary:** Take as a dietary supplement. **Topical:** Dilute 1 drop essential oil with 1 drop V-6 or other pure carrier oil and apply 2-4 drops on location, chakras, and/or Vita Flex points. May use neat in Raindrop Technique. Dilution not required except on the most sensitive skin.

**Technical Data: Botanical Family:** Pinaceae; **Plant Origin:** Highland Flats in Naples, Idaho; **Extraction Method:** Steam distilled from leaves (needles) and branches; **Key Constituents:** Alpha-Pinene (6-9%), Beta-Pinene (14-24%), Camphene (10-15%), Limonene (1-5%); **ORAC:** 20,500 µTE/100g

### Selected Research

Nachar A, et al. Regulation of liver cell glucose homeostasis by dehydroabietic acid, abietic acid and squalene isolated from balsam fir (*Abies balsamea* L. Mill.) a plant of the Eastern James Bay Cree traditional pharmacopeia. *Phytochemistry.* 2015 Sep;177:373-9.

Lavoie S, et al. Lanostane- and cycloartane-type triterpenoids from *Abies balsamea* oleoresin. *Beilstein J Org Chem.* 2013 Jul 4;9:1333-9.

Pichette A, et al. Composition and antibacterial activity of *Abies balsamea* essential oil, *Phytother Res.* 2006 May;20(5):371-3.

Legault J, et al. Antitumor activity of balsam fir oil: production of reactive oxygen species induced by alpha-humulene as possible mechanism of action, *Planta Med.* 2003 May;69(5):402-7.

## Idaho Blue Spruce *(Picea pungens)*

Northwestern Native Americans considered the Idaho blue spruce to be a sacred tree and used it for smudging/purification rites. Spruce leaves, inner bark, gum, and twigs have been used historically by Native Americans for a variety of functions. Leaves were used as inhalants, fumigators, and revivers. The inner bark of the spruce was used for lung and throat troubles, inward troubles, in a poultice applied to wounds and for cuts and swelling, as a medicinal salt, applied to areas of inflammation, and in an antiscorbutic drink for scurvy and colds. Spruce gum was also used for caulking canoes. Various parts of the tree were also combined and used for stomach troubles, scabs, sores, as a salve for cuts and wounds, and in a tea for scurvy and as a cough remedy.

**Medical Properties:** Antinociceptive (analgesic; reduces sensitivity to pain), antioxidative, antibacterial, relaxant, possibly anticancerous

**Uses:** Antibacterial, pain relief, insecticide, antioxidant, expectorant, induces relaxation, nAChR (nicotinic acetylcholine receptor) inhibitor, prevents oxidation of LDL, GABA agonist, antimicrobial

**Fragrant Influence:** Releases emotional blocks, bringing about a feeling of balance and grounding

**Directions: Aromatic:** Diffuse up to 1 hour 3 times daily or directly inhale. **Dietary:** Take 2 drops in a

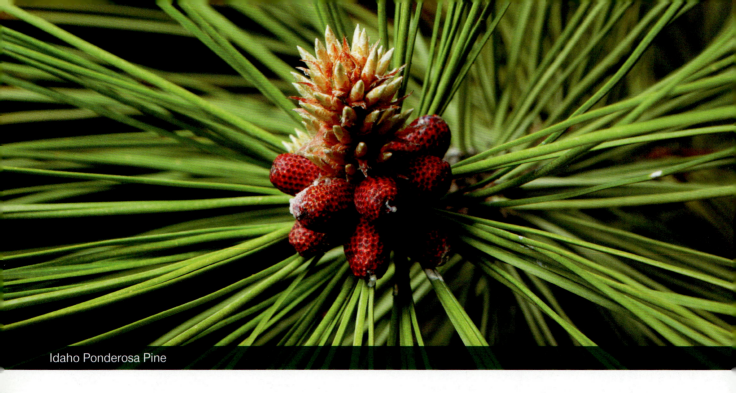

Idaho Ponderosa Pine

capsule daily as a dietary supplement. **Topical:** Apply 2-4 drops directly to desired location, chakras, and/or Vita Flex points. No dilution required except for the most sensitive skin.

**Technical Data: Botanical Family:** Pinaceae; **Plant Origin:** Idaho; **Extraction Method:** Steam distilled from all tree parts; **Key Constituents:** Alpha-Pinene (15-40%), Camphene (6-8%), Beta-Pinene (6-11%), Myrcene (3-7%), Limonene (18-25%), Bornyl Acetate (3-10%); **ORAC:** 575 µTE/g

### Selected Research

Pack JA, et al. Physical and Emotional Effects of Idaho Blue Spruce, unpublished Young Living Essential Oils study, 2013.

Matsubara E, et al. Bornyl acetate induces autonomic relaxation and reduces arousal level after visual display terminal work without any influences of task performance in low-dose condition. 2011. *Biomed Research* 32(2):151-157.

Tiwari M, Kakkar P. Plant derived antioxidants—Geraniol and camphene protect rat alveolar macrophages against t-BHP. *Toxicology in Vitro* 2009 Mar;23(2):295-301.

Him A, et al. Antinociceptive activity of alpha-pinene and fenchone. *Pharmacologyonline* 2008 3:363-369.

Leite AM, et al. Inhibitory effect of β-pinene, α-pinene, and eugenol on the growth of potential infectious endocartitis causing Gram-positive bacteria. *Brazilian J of Pharmaceut Sci* 2007 43(1):121-126.

Pacheco A, Lindner S. Effects of alpha-pinene and trichloroethylene on oxidation potentials of methanotrophic bacteria. *Bull Environ Contam Toxicol* 2005 74:133-140.

### Idaho Ponderosa Pine *(Pinus ponderosa)*

This large pine tree is native to western North America but grows throughout the temperate world. The official state tree of Montana, the ponderosa pine, gains its fragrant scent from an abundance of terpenes, including Delta-3-Carene, Beta-Pinene, Alpha-Pinene, and Limonene, listed above. A measurement by Ascending the Giants in 2011 landed a ponderosa pine in the record books as the tallest known pine (268.29 feet tall). Native Americans used the ponderosa pine to reduce coughs and fevers, while the pitch was used as an ointment for skin conditions. In sweat lodges, the tree boughs were used for muscular pain, and the pollen and needles were used in healing ceremonies.

**Medical Properties:** Antimicrobial, antifungal

**Uses:** Respiratory ailments, arthritis, rheumatism

**Fragrant Influence:** Relaxing, calming, and restorative; also emotionally uplifting

**Directions: Aromatic:** Diffuse up to 30 minutes 3 times daily or directly inhale. **Topical:** Dilute 1 drop essential oil with 1 drop V-6 or other pure carrier oil and apply 2-4 drops on location, chakras, and/or Vita Flex points.

**Cautions:** Do not take if pregnant or planning on becoming pregnant. Not for use on children.

**Technical Data: Botanical Family:** Pinus; **Plant Origin:** Idaho; **Extraction Method:** Steam distilled from all tree parts; **Key Constituents:** Delta-3-Carene (35-50%), Beta-Pinene (16-30%), Alpha-Pinene (7-10%), Limonene (5-8%)

### Selected Research

Lans C. Possible similarities between the folk medicine historically used by First Nations and American Indians in North America and the ethnoveterinary knowledge currently used in British Columbia, Canada. *J. Ethnopharmacol.* 2016 Jul 6. Epub ahead of print.

Baker B, Sinnott M. Analysis of sesquiterpene emissions by plants using solid phase microextraction. *J Chromatogr A.* 2009 Nov 27;1216(48):8442-51.

Krauze-Baranowska M, et al. Antifungal activity of the essential oils from some species of the genus Pinus. *Z Naturforsch C.* 2002 May-Jun;57(5-6):478-82.

Johnston WH, et al. Antimicrobial activity of some Pacific Northwest woods against anaerobic bacteria and yeast. *Phytother Res.* 2001 Nov;15(7):586-8.

## Idaho Tansy *(Tanacetum vulgare)*

This antimicrobial oil has been used extensively as an insect repellent. According to F. Joseph Montagna's herbal desk reference, it may tone the entire system (Montagna, 1990).

**Medical Properties:** Analgesic, antioxidant, antiviral, anticoagulant, immune stimulant, insect repellent

**Uses:** Arteriosclerosis, hypertension, arthritis/rheumatism

**Directions: Aromatic:** Diffuse up to 30 minutes 3 times daily or directly inhale. **Topical:** Dilute 1 drop essential oil with 1 drop V-6 or other pure carrier oil and apply on location, chakras, and/or Vita Flex points.

**Caution:** Do not use if pregnant.

**Technical Data: Botanical Family:** Asteraceae; **Plant Origin:** Idaho; **Extraction Method:** Steam distilled from leaves and stems; **Key Constituents:** Beta-Thujone (65-80%), Camphor (3-8%), Sabinene (1-4%), Germacrene D (3-7%)

### Selected Research

Álvarez ÁL, et al. A spiroketal-enol ether derivative from *Tanacetum vulgare* selectively inhibits HSV-1 and HSV-2 glycoprotein accumulation in Vero cells. *Antiviral Res.* 2015 Jul;119:8-18.

Piras A, et al. Chemical composition and antifungal activity of supercritical extract and essential oil of *Tanacetum vulgare* growing wild in Lithuania. *Nat Prod Res.* 2014 Nov;28(21):1906-9.

Alvarez AL, et al. In vitro anti HSV-1 and HSV-2 activity of *Tanacetum vulgare* extracts and isolated compounds: an approach to their mechanisms of action. *Phytother Res.* 2011 Feb;25(2):296-301.

Juan-Badaturuge M, et al. Antioxidant principles of *Tanacetum vulgare* L. aerial parts. *Nat Prod Commun.* 2009 Nov;4(11):1561-4.

Palsson K, et al. Tick repellent substances in the essential oil of *Tanacetum vulgare*. *J Med Entomol.* 2008 Jan;45(1):88-93.

## Ishpingo *(Ocotea quixos)*

*Ishpingo* is a Hispanic name for Ocotea, which is distilled from the flower and fruit of a tree found in the Amazon wilderness on the ranges of the west side of the Andes Mountains. It is commonly referred to by the native people throughout Ecuador as false canilla or false cinnamon. The tree grows to a very large size, reaching up to 48 inches in diameter and over 60 feet tall, making a large canopy top. Historical usage of ocotea dates back more than 500 years, when it was used to aromatize sweets and cakes. Of 79 ocotea species' studies on PubMed, only two refer to the properties of ocotea essential oil distilled from flowers or fruit rather than the leaves and bark of the tree.

**Medical Properties:** Antimicrobial, antioxidant, antifungal

**Directions: Aromatic:** Diffuse up to 1 hour 3 times daily or inhale directly. Dietary: Dilute 1 drop essential oil with 4 drops V-6 or other pure carrier oil, put in a capsule, and take 1 daily or as directed by a health care professional. **Topical:** Dilute 1 drop essential oil with 2 drops V-6 or other pure carrier oil and apply 1-2 drops on location, chakras, and/or Vita Flex points. Test on a small, inconspicuous area of skin to observe sensitivity.

**Technical Data: Botanical Family:** Lauraceae; **Plant Origin:** Ecuador; **Extraction Method:** Steam distillation from flower/fruit; **Key Constituents:** Trans-Cinnamaldehyde (10-3%), Methyl Cinnamate (7-25%), Cinnamyl Acetate (5-18%), Alpha-Pinene (3-9%)

### Selected Research

Guerrini A, et al. Composition of the volatile fraction of *Ocotea bofo* Kunth (Lauraceae) calyces by GC-MS and NMR fingerprinting and its antimicrobial and antioxidant activity. *J Agric Food Chem.* 2006 Oct 4;54(20):7778-88.

Bruni R, et al. Chemical composition and biological activities of Ishpingo essential oil, a traditional Ecuadorian spice from *Octotea quixos* (Lam.) Kosterm. (Lauraceae) flower calices. *Food Chem.* 2004 May;85(3):415-421.

## Jade Lemon
### *(Citrus limon Eureka var. formosensis)*

Taiwan and China are home to this exquisitely scented lemon variety. Unique among lemons, when fully mature it is a lovely green color, hence the name Jade Lemon. Not only is the color of this lemon unique, this essential oil has a tantalizing lemon-lime scent. Introduced at the 2014 YL convention, it has become a most beloved essential oil. Jade Lemon contains the same major constituents as Lemon essential oil but in slightly different percentages.

**Medical Properties:** Antitumoral, antiseptic, improves microcirculation, immune stimulant (may increase white blood cells), improves memory, relaxation; rich in limonene, which has been extensively studied in over 50 clinical studies for its ability to combat tumor growth.

**Uses:** Used to uplift and stimulate the mind and body. Can be used in household cleaning or mixed with Citronella essential oil for a pleasant, citrus-scented insect repellant.

**Directions: Aromatic:** Diffuse up to 1 hour 3 times daily or directly inhale. **Topical:** Dilute 1 drop essential oil with 1 drop with V-6 or other carrier oil and apply on location or on chakras and or Vita Flex points. Combine 10-15 drops with lotions and shampoos to energize the spirit.

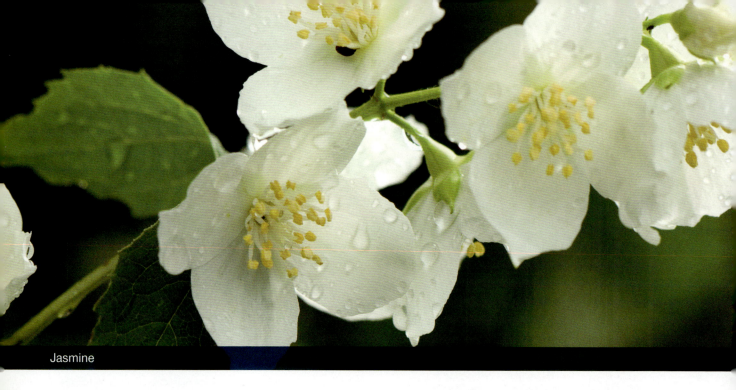
Jasmine

## Jade Lemon Vitality™
*(Citrus limon Eureka var. formosensis)*

**Directions: Dietary:** Put 2 drops in a capsule. Take 3 times daily.

**Technical Data: Botanical Family:** Rutaceae; **Plant Origin:** Taiwan; **Extraction Method:** Cold pressed from rind; it takes 3,000 lemons to produce 1 kilo of oil; **Key Constituents:** Limonene (59-73%), Gamma-Terpinene (6-12%), Beta-Pinene (7-16%), Alpha-Pinene (1.5-3%), Sabinene (1.5-3%); **ORAC:** 660 µTE/100g

### Selected Research

Khan RA, Riaz A. Behavioral effects of *Citrus limon* in rats. *Metab Brain Dis.* 2015 Apr;30(2):589-96.

Vandresen F, et al. Novel R-(+)-limonene-based thiosemicarbazones and their antitumor activity against human tumor cell lines. *Eur J Med Chem.* 2014 May 22;79:110-6.

Yavari Kia P, et al. The effect of lemon inhalation aromatherapy on nausea and vomiting of pregnancy: a double-blinded, randomized, controlled trial. *Iran Red Crescent Med J.* 2014 Mar;16(3):e14360.

Oliveira SA, et al. The antimicrobial effects of *Citrus limon* and *Citrus aurantium* essential oils on multi-species biofilms. *Braz Oral Res.* 2014 Jan-Feb;28(1) 22-7.

Guerra FQ, et al. Increasing antibiotic activity against a multidrug-resistant Acinetobacter spp by essential oils of *Citrus limon* and *Cinnamomum zeylandicum*. *Nat Prod Res.* 2012;26(23):2235-8.

Valgimigli L, et al. Lemon (*Citrus limon* Burm.f.) essential oil enhances the trans-epidermal release of lipid-(A, E) and water-(B6, C) soluble vitamins from topical emulsions in reconstructed human epidermis. *Int J Cosmet Sci.* 2012 Aug;34(4):347-56.

## Jasmine *(Jasminum officinale)*

Jasmine is nicknamed the "queen of the night" and "moonlight of the grove." For centuries, women have treasured jasmine for its beautiful, seductive fragrance. It is an absolute, or essence, rather than an essential oil.

**Note:** One pound of jasmine oil requires about 1,000 pounds of jasmine or 3.6 million fresh, unpacked blossoms. The blossoms must be collected before sunrise, or much of the fragrance will have evaporated. The quality of the blossoms may also be compromised if they are crushed. A single pound of pure jasmine oil may cost between $1,200 and $4,500. In contrast, synthetic jasmine oils can be obtained for $3.50 per pound, but they do not possess the therapeutic qualities as the pure oil.

**Medical Properties:** Uplifting, antidepressant, stimulating, antibacterial, antiviral

**Uses:** Anxiety, depression, menstrual problems/PMS, skin problems (eczema, wrinkles, greasy), frigidity

**Fragrant Influence:** Uplifting, counteracts hopelessness, nervous exhaustion, anxiety, depression, indifference, and listlessness.

**Directions: Aromatic:** Diffuse up to 1 hour 3 times daily or directly inhale. **Topical:** Apply 2-4 drops on location, chakras, and/or Vita Flex points. Dilution not required except for the most sensitive skin.

**Technical Data: Botanical Family:** Oleaceae; **Plant Origin:** India; **Extraction Method:** Absolute extraction from flower. Jasmine is actually an "essence" not an essential oil. The flowers must be picked at night to maximize fragrance; **Key Constituents:** Benzyl Acetate (18-28%), Benzyl Benzoate (14-21%), Linalol (3-8%), Phytol (6-12%), Isophytol (3-7%), Squalene (3-7%)

### Selected Research

Kaviani M, et al. Comparison of the effect of aromatherapy with *Jasminum officinale* and *Salvia officinale* on pain severity and labor outcome in nulliparous women. *Iran J Nurs Midwifery Res.* 2014 Nov;19(6):666-72.

Uniyal V, et al. Screening of some essential oils against Trichosporon species. *J Environ Biol.* 2013 Jan;34(1):17-22.

Zhao G, et al. Antiviral efficacy against hepatitis B virus replication of oleuropein isolated from *Jasminium officinale* L. var. grandiflorum. *J Ethnopharmacol.* 2009 Sep 7;125(2):265-8.

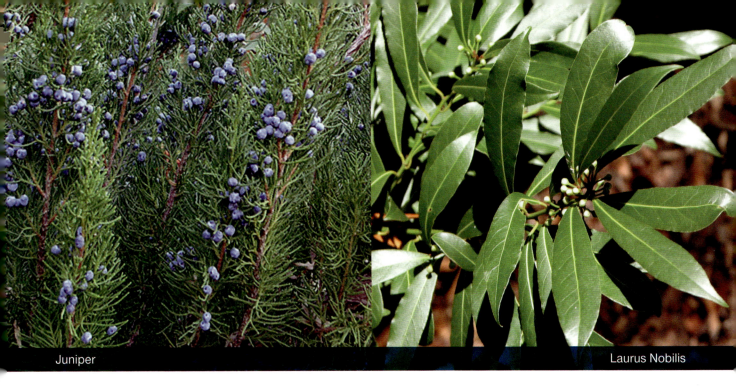
Juniper

Laurus Nobilis

## Juniper *(Juniperus osteosperma)*

Bundles of juniper berries were hung over doorways to ward off witches during medieval times. Juniper has been used for centuries as a diuretic. Until recently, French hospital wards burned sprigs of juniper and rosemary to protect from infection.

**Medical Properties:** Antiseptic, digestive cleanser/stimulant, purifying, detoxifying, increases circulation through the kidneys and promotes excretion of toxins, promotes nerve regeneration

**Uses:** Skin conditions (acne, eczema), liver problems, urinary/bladder infections, fluid retention

**Fragrant Influence:** Evokes feelings of health, love, and peace and may help to elevate one's spiritual awareness

**Directions: Aromatic:** Diffuse up to 30 minutes 3 times daily or directly inhale. **Dietary:** Take as a dietary supplement. **Topical:** Dilute 1 drop essential oil with 1 drop V-6 or other pure carrier oil and apply 2-4 drops on location, chakras, and/or Vita Flex points.

**Technical Data: Botanical Family:** Cupressaceae; **Plant Origin:** Utah; **Extraction Method:** Steam distilled from stems and leaves (aerial parts); **Key Constituents:** Alpha-Pinene (20-40%), Sabinene (3-18%), Myrcene (1-6%), Camphor (10-18%), Limonene (3-8%), Bornyl Acetate (12-20%), Terpinen-4-ol (3-8%); **ORAC:** 250 µTE/100g

### Selected Research

Acuña UM, et al. Antioxidant capacities of ten edible North American plants. *Phytother Res.* 2002 Jan 16(1):63-65.

Takacsova M, et al. Study of the antioxidative effects of thyme, sage, juniper and oregano. *Nahrung.* 1995;39(3):241-3.

## Laurus Nobilis (Bay Laurel) *(Laurus nobilis)*

Both the leaves and the black berries were used to alleviate indigestion and loss of appetite. During the Middle Ages, *Laurus nobilis* was used for angina, migraine, heart palpitations, and liver and spleen complaints.

**Medical Properties:** Antimicrobial, expectorant, mucolytic, antibacterial (staph, strep, *E. coli*), antifungal (candida), anticoagulant, anticonvulsant

**Uses:** Nerve regeneration, arthritis (rheumatoid), oral infections (gingivitis), respiratory infections, viral infections

**Directions: Aromatic:** Diffuse up to 30 minutes 3 times daily or directly inhale. **Topical:** Dilute 1 drop essential oil with 1 drop V-6 or other pure carrier oil and apply 2-4 drops on location, abdomen, chakras, and/or Vita Flex points.

## Laurus Nobilis Vitality™ (Bay Laurel) *(Laurus nobilis)*

**Directions: Dietary:** Dilute 1 drop with 1 drop of carrier oil. Put in a capsule and take up to 3 times daily or as needed.

**Technical Data: Botanical Family:** Lauraceae; **Plant Origin:** Croatia; **Extraction Method:** Steam distilled from leaves and twigs; **Key Constituents:** 1,8-Cineole (Eucalyptol) (40-50%), Alpha-Terpenyl Acetate (7-14%), Alpha-Pinene (4-8%), Beta-Pinene (3-6%), Sabinene (6-11%), Linalol (2-7%); **ORAC:** 98,900 µTE/100g

### Selected Research

Merghni A, et al. Antibacterial and antibiofilm activities of *Laurus nobilis* L. essential oil against *Staphylococccus aureus* strains associated with oral infections. *Pathol Biol* (Paris). 2015 Dec 4. Epub ahead of print.

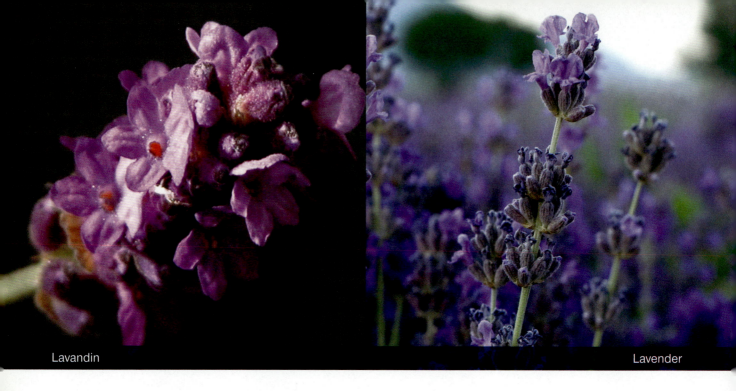

Lavandin

Lavender

Sahin Basak S, Candan F. Effect of *Laurus nobilis* L. Essential Oil and its Main Components on α-glucosidase and Reactive Oxygen Species Scavaging Activity. *Iran J Pharm Res.* 2013 Spring;12(2):367-79.

Lee T, et al. Effects of magnolialide isolated from the leaves of *Laurus nobilis* L. (Lauraceae) on immunoglobulin E-mediated type I hypersensitivity in vitro. *J Ethnopharmacol.* 2013 Sep 16;149(2):550-6.

## Lavandin *(Lavandula intermedia)*

Also known as *Lavandula* x *intermedia*, lavandin is a hybrid plant developed by crossing true lavender with spike lavender or aspic (*Lavandula latifolia*). It has been used to sterilize the animal cages in veterinary clinics and hospitals throughout Europe.

**Medical Properties:** Antibacterial, antifungal

**Uses:** Lavandin is a stronger antiseptic than lavender (*Lavandula angustifolia*). Its greater penetrating qualities make it well suited to help with respiratory, circulatory, and muscular conditions. However, its camphor content invalidates its use to soothe burns.

**Fragrant Influence:** Similar calming effects as lavender

**Directions: Aromatic:** Diffuse up to 1 hour 3 times daily or directly inhale. **Topical:** Apply 2-4 drops on location, chakras, and/or Vita Flex points. Dilution not required except for the most sensitive skin.

**Caution:** Avoid using for burns; instead, use pure lavender (*Lavandula angustifolia*).

**Technical Data: Botanical Family:** Lamiaceae; **Plant Origin:** France; **Extraction Method:** Steam distilled from the flowering top; **Key Constituents:** Linalyl acetate (25-38%), Linalol (24-37%), Camphor (6-8.5%), 1,8-Cineole (Eucalyptol) (4-8%), Borneol (1.5-3.5%), Terpinen-4-ol (1.5-5%), Lavandulyl Acetate (1.5-3.5%)

### Selected Research

Carrasco A, et al. Lavandin (*Lavandula x intermedia* Emeric ex Loiseleur) essential oil from Spain: determination of aromatic profile by gas chromatography-mass spectrometry, antioxidant and lipoxygenase inhibitory bioactivities. *Nat Prod Res.* 2015 Jun 24:1-8.

Végh A, et al. Composition and antipseudomonal effect of essential oils isolated from different lavender species. *Nat Prod Commun.* 2012 Oct;7(10):1393-6.

Blazeković B, et al. Evaluation of antioxidant potential of *Lavandula x intermedia* Emeric ex Loisel. 'Budrovka': a comparative study with *L. angustifolia* Mill. *Molecules.* 2010 Aug 30;15(9):5971-87.

Braden R, et al. The use of the essential oil lavandin to reduce preoperative anxiety in surgical patients. *J Perianesth Nurs.* 2009 Dec;24(6):348-355.

## Lavender *(Lavandula angustifolia)*

The French scientist René Gattefossé was the first to discover lavender's ability to promote tissue regeneration and speed wound healing when he severely burned his arm in a laboratory explosion. Today, lavender is one of the few essential oils to still be listed in the British Pharmacopoeia.

**Medical Properties:** Antiseptic, antifungal, analgesic, antitumoral, anticonvulsant, vasodilating, relaxant, anti-inflammatory, reduces blood fat/cholesterol, combats excess sebum on skin

**Uses:** Respiratory infections, high blood pressure, arteriosclerosis, menstrual problems/PMS, skin conditions (perineal repair, acne, eczema, psoriasis, scarring, stretch marks), burns, hair loss, insomnia, nervous tension

**Fragrant Influence:** Calming, relaxing, and balancing, both physically and emotionally. Lavender has been documented to improve concentration and mental acuity.

104 | Chapter 6 | Single Oils

Single Oils | **Chapter 6**

University of Miami researchers found that inhalation of lavender oil increased beta waves in the brain, suggesting heightened relaxation. It also reduced depression and improved cognitive performance (Diego MA, et al., 1998). A 2001 Osaka Kyoiku University study found that lavender reduced mental stress and increased alertness (Motomura, 2001).

**Directions: Aromatic:** Diffuse up to 1 hour 3 times daily or directly inhale. **Topical:** Apply 2-4 drops on location, chakras, and/or Vita Flex points. Dilution not required except for the most sensitive skin.

**Caution:** True lavender is often adulterated with hybrid lavender (lavandin), synthetic linalol and linalyl acetate, or synthetic fragrance chemicals like ethyl vanillin.

## Lavender Vitality™ *(Lavandula angustifolia)*

**Directions: Dietary:** Put 2 drops in a capsule. Take 3 times daily.

**Technical Data: Botanical Family:** Lamiaceae; **Plant Origin:** Utah, Idaho, France; **Extraction Method:** Steam distilled from flowering top; **Key Constituents:** Linalyl Acetate (21-47%), Linalol (23-46%), Cis-Beta-Ocimene (1-8%), Trans-Beta-Ocimene (1-5%), Terpinen-4-ol (1-8%); **ORAC:** 360 μTE/100g

### Selected Research

Dyer J, et al. The use of aromasticks to help with sleep problems: A patient experience survey. *Complement Ther Clin Pract.* 2016 Feb;22:51-8.

Giovannini D, et al. *Lavandula angustifolia* Mill. Essential Oil Exerts Antibacterial and Anti-Inflammatory Effect in Macrophage Mediated Immune Response to *Staphylococcus aureus. Immunol Invest.* 2016 Jan;45(1):11-28.

Hashemi SH, et al. The Effect of Massage with Lavender Oil on Restless Leg Syndrome in Hemodialysis Patients: A Randomized Controlled Trial. *Nurs Midwifery Stud.* 2015 Dec;4(4):29617. [Epub ahead of print]

Prusinowska R, et al, Hydrolytes from lavender (*Lavender angustifolia*)—their chemical composition as well as aromatic, antimicrobial and antioxidant properties. *Nat Prod Res.* 2015 Mar 4:1-8.

Tayarani-Najaran Z, et al. Comparative studies of cytotoxic and apoptotic properties of different extracts and essential oil of *Lavandula angustifolia* on malignant and normal cells. *Nutr Cancer.* 2014;66(3):424-34.

Yap PS, et al. Membrane disruption and anti-quorum sensing effects of synergistic interaction between *Lavandula angustifolia* (lavender oil) in combination with antibiotic against plasmid-conferred multi-drug-resistant *Escherichia coli. J Applied Microbiol.* 2014 May;116(5):1119-28.

Vakili A, et al. Effect of lavender oil (*Lavandula angustifolia*) on cerebral edema and its possible mechanisms in an experimental model of stroke. *Brain Res.* 2014 Feb 22;1548:56-62.

Raisi Dehkordi Z, et al. Effect of lavender inhalation on the symptoms of primary dysmenorrhea and the amount of menstrual bleeding: A randomized clinical trial. *Complement Ther Med.* 2014 Apr;22(2):212-9.

O'Conner DW, et al. A randomized, controlled cross-over trial of dermally-applied lavender (*Lavandula angustifolia*) as a treatment of agitated behaviour in dementia. *BMC Complement Altern Med.* 2013 Nov 13;13:315.

## Ledum *(Rhododendrum groenlandicum)*

Known colloquially as "Labrador tea," ledum has been reclassified from the genus Ledum and is now classified as *Rhododendrum groenlandicum.* It is a strongly aromatic herb that has been used for centuries in folk medicine. The native people of Eastern Canada used this herb for tea, as a general tonic, and to treat a variety of kidney-related problems. Ledum has helped protect the native people of North America against scurvy for more than 5,000 years. The Cree used it for fevers and colds.

**Medical Properties:** Anti-inflammatory, antitumoral, antibacterial, diuretic, liver-protectant

**Uses:** Liver problems/hepatitis/fatty liver, obesity, water retention

**Directions: Aromatic:** Diffuse up to 30 minutes 3 times daily or directly inhale. **Dietary:** Take as a dietary supplement. **Topical:** Dilute 1 drop essential oil with 1 drop V-6 and apply on location, chakras, and/or Vita Flex points.

**Technical Data: Botanical Family:** Ericaceae; **Plant Origin:** North America (Canada); **Extraction Method:** Steam distilled from flowering tops; **Key Constituents:** Limonene (10-40%), Cis-Para-Mentha-1(7),8-dien-8-ol (1-12%), Trans-Para-Mentha-1(7),8-dien-8-ol (2-8%), Alpha-Selinene (4-20%), Trans-Para-Mentha-1,3,8-Triene (2-7%)

### Selected Research

*Rhododendron groenlandicum* (Labrador tea), an antidiabetic plant from the traditional pharmacopoeia of the Canadian Eastern James Bay Cree, improves rental integrity in the diet-induced obese mouse model. *Pharm Biol.* 2016 Feb 26:1-9.

Ouchfoun M, et al. Labrador tea (*Rhodendron groenlandicum*) attenuates insulin resistance in a diet-induced obesity mouse model. *Eur J Nutr.* 2015 Apr 28. [Epub ahead of print]

Dampc A, Luczkiewicz M. Labrador tea—the aromatic beverage and spice: a print review of origin, processing and safety. *J Sci Food Agric.* 2014 Aug 25. [Epub ahead of print]

Dufour D, et al. Antioxidant, anti-inflammatory and anticancer activities of methanolic extracts from *Ledum groenlandicum* Retzius. *J Ethnopharm.* 2007 Apr 111(1):22-28.

## Lemon *(Citrus limon)*

Lemon oil has been widely used in skin care to cleanse skin, reduce wrinkles, and combat acne. Lemon peel was used as an antiseptic, carminative, diuretic, eupeptic, a vascular stimulant and protector, and as a vitaminic (Arias, et al., 2005). It is also used as a flavorant for cleaning, cooking, and treating scurvy and a variety of other ailments.

**Medical Properties:** Antitumoral, antiseptic, improves microcirculation, immune stimulant (may increase white blood cells), improves memory, relaxation; rich

Seventh Edition | **Essential Oils Desk Reference** | **105**

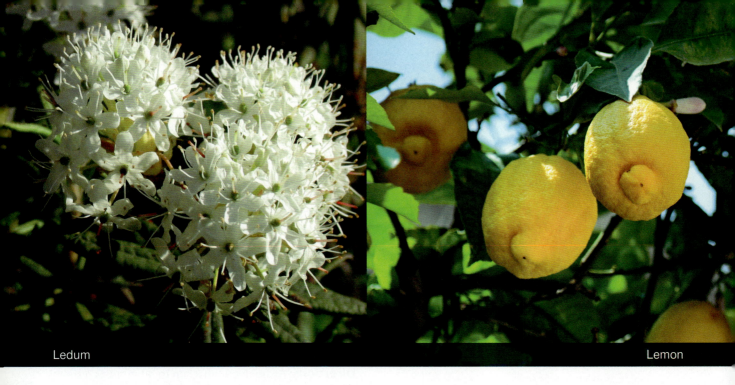

Ledum | Lemon

in limonene, which has been extensively studied in over 50 clinical studies for its ability to combat tumor growth

**Uses:** Circulatory problems, arteriosclerosis, obesity, parasites, urinary tract infections, varicose veins, anxiety, hypertension, digestive problems, acne

**Fragrant Influence:** It promotes clarity of thought and purpose with a fragrance that is invigorating, enhancing, and warming.

A Mie University study found that citrus fragrances boosted immunity, induced relaxation, and reduced depression (Komori, et al., 1995).

**Directions: Aromatic:** Diffuse up to 1 hour 3 times daily or directly inhale. **Topical:** Dilute 1 drop essential oil with 1 drop V-6 or other pure carrier oil and apply 2-4 drops on location, chakras, and/or Vita Flex points.

**Caution:** Possible sun sensitivity.

## Lemon Vitality™ (Citrus limon)

**Directions: Dietary:** Put 2 drops in a capsule. Take 3 times daily or as needed.

**Technical Data: Botanical Family:** Rutaceae; **Plant Origin:** California, Italy; **Extraction Method:** Cold pressed from rind. It takes 3,000 lemons to produce 1 kilo of oil; **Key Constituents:** Limonene (59-73%), Gamma-Terpinene (6-12%), Beta-Pinene (7-16%), Alpha-Pinene (1.5-3%), Sabinene (1.5-3%); **ORAC:** 660 µTE/100g

### Selected Research

Khan RA, Riaz A. Behavioral effects of *Citrus limon* in rats. *Metab Brain Dis.* 2015 Apr;30(2):589-96.

Vandresen F, et al. Novel R-(+)-limonene-based thiosemicarbazones and their antitumor activity against human tumor cell lines. *Eur J Med Chem.* 2014 May 22;79:110-6.

Yavari Kia P, et al. The effect of lemon inhalation aromatherapy on nausea and vomiting of pregnancy: a double-blinded, randomized, controlled trial. *Iran Red Crescent Med J.* 2014 Mar;16(3):e14360.

Oliveira SA, et al. The antimicrobial effects of *Citrus limon* and *Citrus aurantium* essential oils on multi-species biofilms. Braz Oral Res. 2014 Jan-Feb;28(1) 22-7.

Guerra FQ, et al. Increasing antibiotic activity against a multidrug-resistant Acinetobacter spp by essential oils of *Citrus limon* and *Cinnamomum zeylandicum*. *Nat Prod Res.* 2012;26(23):2235-8.

Valgimigli L, et al. Lemon (*Citrus limon* Burm.f.) essential oil enhances the trans-epidermal release of lipid-(A, E) and water-(B6, C) soluble vitamins from topical emulsions in reconstructed human epidermis. *Int J Cosmet Sci.* 2012 Aug;34(4):347-56.

## Lemongrass (Cymbopogon flexuosus)

Lemongrass is used for purification and digestion. Historically it was used for hypertension, inflammation, as a sedative, and for treatment of fevers and digestion. In a 2008 study, 91 single essential oils were tested against MRSA (Methicillin-resistant *Staphylococcus aureus*) and lemongrass. The study found that "Remarkably, lemongrass essential oil completely inhibited all MRSA growth on the plate" (Chao S, et al., 2008).

**Medical Properties:** Antifungal, antibacterial, antiparasitic, anti-inflammatory, regenerates connective tissues and ligaments, dilates blood vessels, improves circulation, promotes lymph flow, anticancerous. Several research articles document strong antifungal and antibacterial properties of lemongrass.

**Uses:** Bladder infection, respiratory/sinus infection, digestive problems, parasites, torn ligaments/muscles, fluid retention, varicose veins, salmonella, candida

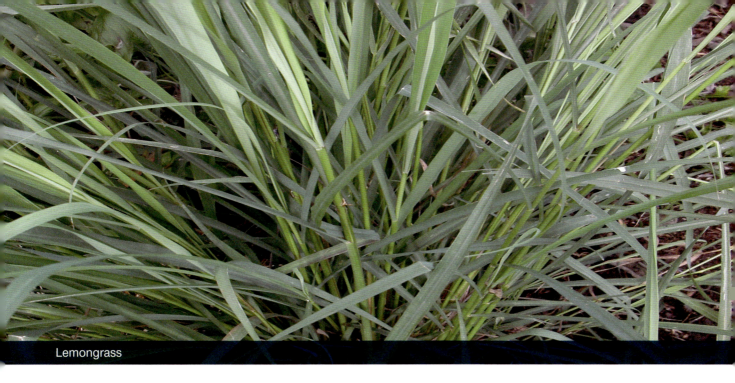

Lemongrass

**Fragrant Influence:** Promotes psychic awareness and purification

**Directions: Aromatic:** Diffuse up to 1 hour 3 times daily or directly inhale. **Topical:** Dilute 1 drop essential oil with 4 drops V-6 or other pure carrier oil and apply 1-2 drops on location, chakras, and/or Vita Flex points.

## Lemongrass Vitality™
*(Cymbopogon flexuosus)*

**Directions: Dietary:** Dilute 1 drop with 1 drop of carrier oil. Put in a capsule and take up to 3 times daily.

**Technical Data: Botanical Family:** Poaceae; **Plant Origin:** India, Guatemala; **Extraction Method:** Steam distilled from herb/grass; **Key Constituents:** Geranial (35-47%), Geraniol (1.5-8%), Neral (25-35%), Geranyl Acetate (1-6%); **ORAC:** 1,780 µTE/100g

### Selected Research

Bustos C RO, et al. Edible antimicrobial films based on microencapsulated lemongrass oil. *J Food Sci Technol.* 2016 Jan;53(1):832-9.

Goes TC, et al. Effect of Lemongrass Aroma on Experimental Anxiety in Humans. *J Altern Complement Med.* 2015 Dec;21(12):766-73.

Ahmad A, Viljoen A. The in vitro antimicrobial activity of *Cymbopogon* essential oil (lemon grass) and its interaction with silver ions. *Phytomedicine.* 2015 Jun 1;22(6):657-65.

Vázquez-Sánchez D, et al. Antimicrobial activity of essential oils against *Staphylococcus aureus* biofilms. *Food Sci Technol Int.* 2014 Oct 3.

Katsukawa M, et al. Citral, a component of lemongrass oil, activates PPAR α and γ and suppresses COX-2 expression. *Biochim Biophys Acta.* 2010 Nov;1801(11):1214-1220.

Sharma PR, et al. Anticancer activity of an essential oil from *Cymbopogon flexuosus. Chem Biol Interact.* 2009 May;179(2-3):160-168.

Chao SC, et al. Inhibition of methicillin-resistant *Staphylococcus aureus* (MRSA) by essential oils. *Flavour Fragr J.* 2008; 2:444-449.

## Lemon Myrtle *(Backhousia citriodora)*

The aboriginal people of Australia valued lemon myrtle's flavor in cooking, calling it "bush food." It is also known as the "queen of lemon herbs." Lemon myrtle can replace lemon in milk-based foods, as it does not have lemon's curdling problems. Lemon myrtle was also widely used as a healing plant. It is the highest natural source of the constituent citral. Since citral, consisting of isomers geranial and neral, has a strong and sweet lemon scent, lemon myrtle continues to be valued in perfumery. It is used in health care and cleaning products such as soaps, shampoos, and lotions. Lemon myrtle is cultivated in Queensland and the north coast of New South Wales, Australia.

**Medical Properties:** Antiseptic, antimicrobial, antifungal, anti-inflammatory, central nervous system stimulant

**Uses:** Weight loss, respiratory/sinus infection, treatment of MCV (molluscum contagiosum virus) in children

**Fragrant Influences:** Uplifting and invigorating, lemon myrtle's fresh and sweet lemon scent encourages follow-through with goals.

**Directions: Aromatic:** Diffuse up to 30 minutes 3 times daily or directly inhale. **Topical:** Dilute 1 drop essential oil with 4 drops V-6 or other pure carrier oil and apply on location, chakras, and/or Vita Flex points.

**Technical Data: Botanical Family:** Myrtaceae; **Plant Origin:** Australia; **Extraction Method:** Steam distilled from leaves; **Key Constituents:** Geranial (45-60%), Neral (30-45%); **ORAC:** 2368 µmole TE/gram

### Selected Research

Sakulnarmrat K, et al. Cytoprotective and pro-apoptotic activities of native Australian herbs polyphenolic-rich extracts. *Food Chem.* 2013 Jan 1;136(1):9-17.

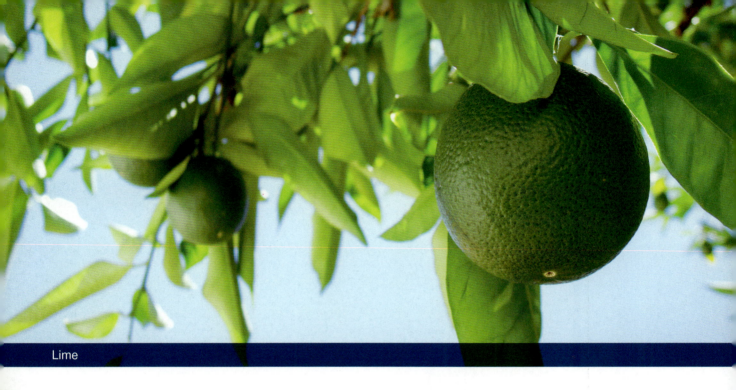

Lime

Modak T, et al. Effects of citral, a naturally occurring antiadipogenic molecule, on an energy-intense diet model of obesity. *Indian J Pharmacol.* 2011 May-Jun; 43(3):300-305.

Burke BE, et al. Essential oil of Australian lemon myrtle (*Backhousia citriodora*) in the treatment of mulluscum contagiosum in children. *Biomed Pharmacother.* 2004 May;58(4):245-7.

Wilkinson JM, et al. Bioactivity of *Backhousia citriodora*: antibacterial and antifungal activity. *J. Agric Food Chem.* 2003 Jan 1;51(1):76-81.

## Lime (Citrus latifolia or C. aurantifolia)

Primarily used in skin care and in supporting and strengthening the respiratory and immune systems.

**Medical Properties:** Antirheumatic, antiviral, antibacterial

**Uses:** Skin conditions (acne, herpes), insect bites, respiratory problems, decongests the lymphatic system, weight loss

**Directions: Aromatic:** Diffuse up to 30 minutes 3 times daily or directly inhale. **Topical:** Dilute 1 drop essential oil with 1 drop V-6 or other pure carrier oil and apply on location, chakras, and/or Vita Flex points.

**Caution:** Possible sun sensitivity.

## Lime Vitality™ (Citrus aurantifolia)

**Directions: Dietary:** Dilute 1 drop with 1 drop of carrier oil. Put in a capsule and take up to 3 times daily.

**Technical Data: Botanical Family:** Rutaceae; **Plant Origin:** *C. latifolia*: Mexico, *C. aurantifolia Swingle*: Southeast Asia; **Extraction Method:** Cold expression from the rind of the unripe fruit; **Key Constituents:** Limonene (42-50%), Gamma-Terpinene (8-11%), Beta-Pinene (18-24%); **ORAC:** 26,200 µTE/100g

### Selected Research

Ruiz-Pérez NJ, et al. Antimycotic Activity and Genotoxic Evaluation of *Citrus sinensis* and *Citrus latifolia* Essential Oils. *Sci Rep.* 2016 May 3;6:25371.

Kummer R, et al. Evaluation of Anti-Inflammatory Activity of *Citrus latifolia* Tanaka Essential Oil and Limonene in Experimental Mouse Models. *Evid Based Complement Alternat Med.* 2013;2013:859083.

Meiyanto E, et al. Natural products for cancer-targeted therapy: citrus flavonoids as potent chemopreventive agents. *Asian Pac J Cancer Prev.* 2012;13(2):427-436.

Bonaccorsi I, et al. Multidimensional enantio gas chromatography/mass spectrometry and gas chromatography-combustion-isotope ratio mass spectrometry for the authenticity assessment of lime essential oils (*C. aurantifolia* Swingle and *C. latifolia* Tanaka. *J Chromatogr A.* 2012 Feb 24:1226:87-95.

## Mandarin (Citrus reticulata)

This fruit was traditionally given to Imperial Chinese officials named the Mandarins.

**Medical Properties:** Light antispasmodic, digestive tonic (digestoid), antifungal, and stimulates the gallbladder; rich in limonene, which has been extensively studied in over 50 clinical studies for its ability to combat tumor growth

**Uses:** Digestive problems, fluid retention, insomnia, anxiety, intestinal problems, skin problems (congested and oily skin, scars, acne), stretch marks (when combined with either Jasmine, Lavender, Sandalwood, and/or Frankincense)

**Fragrant Influence:** Appeasing, gentle, promotes happiness. A Mie University study found that citrus fragrances boosted immunity, induced relaxation, and reduced depression (Komori, et al., 1995).

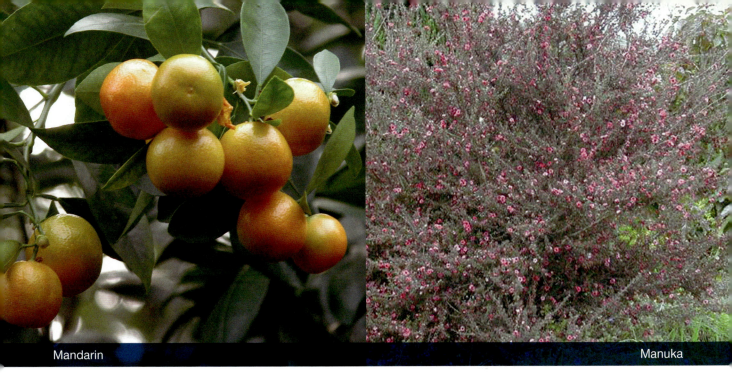

Mandarin | Manuka

**Directions: Aromatic:** Diffuse up to 1 hour 3 times daily or directly inhale. **Dietary:** Take as a dietary supplement. **Topical:** Dilute 1 drop essential oil with 1 drop V-6 or other pure carrier oil and apply 2-4 drops on location, chakras, and/or Vita Flex points.

**Caution:** Possible sun sensitivity.

**Technical Data: Botanical Family:** Rutaceae; **Plant Origin:** Madagascar, Italy; **Extraction Method:** Cold pressed from rind; **Key Constituents:** Limonene (65-75%), Gamma-Terpinene (16-22%), Alpha-Pinene (2-3%), Beta-Pinene (1.2-2%), Myrcene (1.5-2%); **ORAC:** 26,500 µTE/100g

### Selected Research

Apraj VD, Pandita NS. Evaluation of Skin Anti-aging Potential of *Citrus reticulata* Blanco Peel. *Pharmacognosy Res.* 2016 Jul-Sep;8)3):160-8.

Tao N, et al. Anti-fungal activity of *Citrus reticulata* Blanco essential oil against *Penicillium italicum* and *Penicillium digatum*. *Food Chem.* 2014 Jun 15;153:265-7.

El-Khadragy MF, et al. Neuroprotective effects of *Citrus reticulata* in scopoline-induced dementia oxidative stress in rats. *CNS Neurol Disord Drug Targets.* 2014;13(4):684-90.

Zhang Y, et al. Phenolic compositions and antioxidant capacities of Chinese wild mandarin (*Citrus reticulata* Blanco) fruits. *Food Chem.* 2014 Feb 15;145:674-80.

Manassero CA, et al. In vitro comparative analysis of antiproliferative activity of essential oil from mandarin peel and its principle component limonene. *Nat Prod Res.* 2013;27(6):1475-8.

Kawahata I, et al. Potent activity of nobiletin-rich *Citrus reticulata* peel extract to facilitate cAMP/PKA/ERK/CREB signaling associated with learning and memory in cultured hippocampal neurons: identification of the substances responsible for the pharmacological action. *J Neural Transm.* 2013 Oct;120(10):1397-409.

## Manuka *(Leptospermum scoparium)*

Similar to tea tree oil but warmer, richer, and milder, manuka oil has long been used in treatment of skin, foot, and hair problems. Like tea tree oil, it is antibacterial, antiviral, and antifungal, so it can help in eliminating a wide variety of problems. Some research suggests that manuka may be more potent in fighting bacteria and fungi than tea tree oil. "Manuka" is the Maori name for the bushy tree from which the oil is produced.

**Medical Properties:** Antibacterial, antifungal, anti-inflammatory, anti-acne. Although research is ongoing, many believe manuka has potential in fighting antibiotic-resistant organisms, such as MRSA. A leading German aromatherapist reports that the manuka aroma is psychologically very beneficial for people who suffer from stress and anxiety. Its skin-healing properties are exceptional.

**Uses:** Skin infections, acne, bedsores, mild sunburn, fungal infections, itching, respiratory infections, sore throats, pain relief in muscles and joints, athletes foot and ringworm, dandruff, body odor, cold sores, dermatitis, rhinitis, tonsillitis, stress relief, sleep aid

**Directions: Aromatic:** Diffuse up to 30 minutes 3 times daily. **Topical:** Apply 2-4 drops on desired area 1-3 times daily. Dilution not required except for the most sensitive skin.

**Technical Data: Botanical Family:** Myrtaceae; **Plant Origin:** New Zealand and Australia; **Extraction Method:** Steam distillation of chopped leaves and small stems; **Key Constituents:** Leptospermone (16-19%), Trans-Calamenene (12-16%), Flavesone (2-8%), Isoleptospermone (4-7%), Alpha-Copaene (3-6%), Cadena-3,5-diene (3-7%), Alpha-Selinene (2-5%); **ORAC:** 106,200 µTE/100g

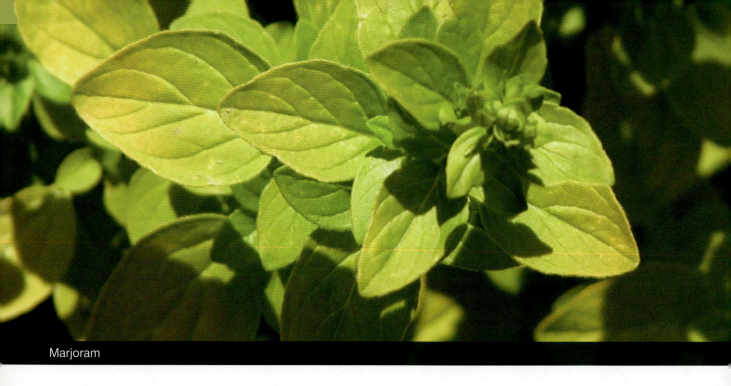

Marjoram

## Selected Research

Killeen DP, et al. Nortriketones: Antimicrobial Trimethylated Acylphloroglucinols from Mānuka (*Leptospermum scoparium*). *J Nat Prod.* 2016 Jan 5. [Epub ahead of print]

Hammond EN, Donkor ES. Antibacterial effect of Manuka honey on *Clostridium difficile*. *BMC Res Notes.* 2013 May 7;6(1):188.

Song CY, et al. In vitro efficacy of the essential oil from *Leptospermum scoparium* (manuka) on antimicrobial susceptibility and biofilm formation in *Staphylococcus pseudintermedius* isolates from dogs. *Vet Dermatol.* 2013 Aug;24(4):404-8.

Cooke A, Cooke MD. An investigation into the antimicrobial properties of manuka and kanuka oil. *Cawthorn Report.* 1994 Sep;No. 263.

## Marjoram *(Origanum majorana)*

Marjoram was known as the "herb of happiness" to the Romans and "joy of the mountains" to the Greeks. It was believed to increase longevity. Listed in Dioscorides' *De Materia Medica* (AD 78), Europe's first authoritative guide to medicines, which became the standard reference work for herbal treatments for over 1,700 years. It was listed in Hildegard's *Medicine,* a compilation of early German medicines by highly regarded Benedictine herbalist Hildegard of Bingen (1098-1179).

**Medical Properties:** Its muscle-soothing properties help relieve body and joint discomfort. May also help soothe the digestive tract and is a general relaxant. Antibacterial, antifungal, vasodilator, lowers blood pressure, promotes intestinal peristalsis, expectorant, mucolytic.

**Uses:** Arthritis/rheumatism, muscle/nerve pain, headaches, circulatory disorders, respiratory infections, menstrual problems/PMS, fungal infections, ringworm, shingles, sores, spasms, and fluid retention

**Fragrant Influence:** Assists in calming the nerves

**Directions: Aromatic:** Diffuse up to 30 minutes 3 times daily or directly inhale. **Dietary:** Take as a dietary supplement. **Topical:** Dilute 1 drop essential oil with 1 drop V-6 or other pure carrier oil and apply 2-4 drops on location, chakras, and/or Vita Flex points.

## Marjoram Vitality™ *(Origanum majorana)*

**Directions: Dietary:** Dilute 1 drop with 1 drop of carrier oil. Put in a capsule and take up to 3 times daily or as needed.

**Technical Data: Botanical Family:** Lamiaceae; **Plant Origin:** France, Egypt; **Extraction Method:** Steam distilled from leaves; **Key Constituents:** Terpinen-4-ol (20-33%), Gamma-Terpinene (10-17%), Linalol + Cis-4-Thujanol (4-26%), Alpha-Terpinene (6-10%), Alpha-Terpineol (2-7%), Sabinene (4-9%); **ORAC:** 130,900 µTE/100g

### Selected Research

Soliman AM, et al. *Origanum majorana* Attenuates Nephrotoxicity of Cisplatin Anticancer Drug through Ameliorating Oxidative Stress. *Nutrients.* 2016 May 5;8(5). pii: E264 doi: 10.3390/nu8050264.

Erenler R, et al. Isolation and identification of chemical constituents of *Origanum majorana* and investigation of antiproliferative and antioxidant activities. *J Food Agric.* 2015 Feb 27. [Epub ahead of print]

Rafaie AA, et al. Oxidative damage and nephrotoxicity induced by pralletrin in rat and the protective effect of *Origanum majorana* essential oil. *Asian Pac J Trop Med.* 2014 Sep;7S1:S506-13.

Al Dhaheri Y, et al. Anti-metastatic and anti-tumor growth effects of *Origanum majorana* on highly metastatic human breast cancer cells: inhibition of NFκB signaling and reduction of nitric oxide production. *PLoS One.* 2013 Jul 10;8(7):e68808.

Srivatstava A, et al. Evaluation of the properties of a tissue containing origanum oil as an antifungal additive. *J Prosthet Dent.* 2013 Oct;110(4):313-9.

Gutierrez RMP. Inhibition of Advanced Glycation End-Product Formation by *Origanum majorana* L. In Vitro and in Streptozotocin-Induced Diabetic Rats. *Evid Based Complement Alternat Med.* 2012;2012.

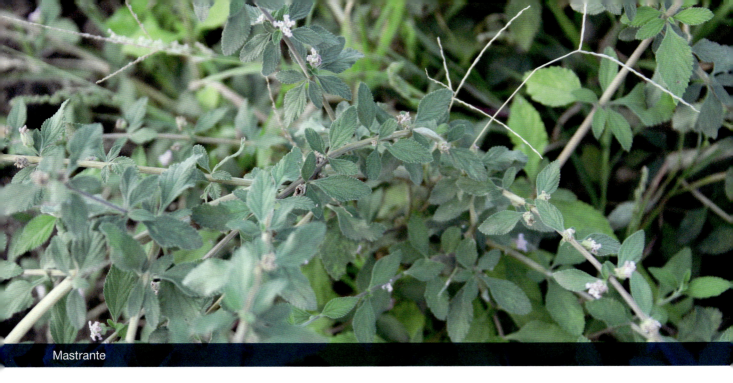
Mastrante

## Mastrante *(Lippia alba)*

The plant Mastrante *(Lippia alba)* was given its botanical name by the Scottish botanist Philip Miller (1691-1771) and the British plant taxonomist N.E. Brown (1849-1934). As a result, in scientific literature it is listed as: *"Lippia alba* (Miller or Mill.) N.E. Brown." In Brazil, it is called *"erva cidreira do campo,"* which means "lemon balm of the field." The aromatic shrub grows in southern Texas, Mexico, the Caribbean, and Central and South America.

The leaves of Mastrante are used to flavor foods, most notably molé sauces from Oaxaca, Mexico. In folk medicine it is known as a sedative, an antidepressant, and has pain-relieving properties.

**Medical Properties:** Antioxidant, analgesic, antibacterial, antiviral, antifungal, antispasmodic

**Uses:** Anti-candida agent, coughs, bronchitis, migraine headaches in women, vasorelaxant for heart disease

**Fragrant Influence:** This earthy aroma is grounding and calming.

**Directions: Aromatic:** Diffuse up to 30 minutes 3 times daily or directly inhale. **Topical:** Dilute 1 drop essential oil with 1 drop V-6 or other pure carrier oil and apply on location, chakras, and/or Vita Flex points.

**Technical Data: Botanical Family:** Verbenaceae; **Plant Origin:** Ecuador; **Extraction Method:** Steam distilled from leaves; **Key Constituents:** Carvone (35-50%), Limonene (20-30%), Germacrene D (10-17%), Alpha-Bourbonene (1-3%), Camphor (0.5-2%)

## Selected Research

Sousa DG, et al. Essential oil of *Lippia alba* and its main constituent citral block the excitability of rat sciatic nerves. *Braz J Med Biol Res.* 2015 Aug;48(8):697-702.

Machado TF, et al. The antimicrobial efficacy of *Lippia alba* essential oil and its interaction with food ingredients. *Braz J Microbiol.* 2014 Aug 29;45(2):699-705.

Chies CE, et al. Antioxidant Effect of *Lippia alba* (Miller) N.E. Brown. *Antioxidants.* 2013 2(4):194-205.

Carmona F, et al. *Lippia alba* (Mill.) N.E. Brown hydroethanolic extract of the leaves is effective in the treatment of migraine in women. *Phytomedicine.* 2013 Jul;20(10):947-50.

Gómez LA, et al. Comparative study on in vitro activities of citral, limonene and essential oils from *Lippia citriodora* and *L. alba* on yellow fever virus. *Nat Prod Commun.* 2013 Feb;8(2):249-52.

Blanco MA, et al. Antispasmodic effects and composition of the essential oils from two South American chemotypes of *Lippia alba*. *J Ethnopharmacol.* 2013 Oct 7;149(3):803-9.

Heldwein CG, et al. Participation of the GABAergic system in the anesthetic effect of *Lippia alba* (Mill.) N.E. Brown essential oil. *Braz J Med Biol Res.* 2012 May;45(5):436-43.

## Melaleuca Alternifolia
(See Tea Tree)

## Melaleuca Ericifolia *(Melaleuca ericifolia)*

The Aboriginal people of Australia used the bark of Melaleuca Ericifolia as roofing for their shelters and for blankets and paintings. Oil from the leaves was used for medicine.

**Medical Properties:** Powerful antibacterial, antifungal, antiviral, antiparasitic, anti-inflammatory

**Uses:** Herpes virus, respiratory/sinus infections

**Directions: Aromatic:** Diffuse up to 1 hour 3 times daily or directly inhale. **Dietary:** Take as a dietary supplement. **Topical:** Dilute 1 drop essential oil with 1 drop V-6 or other pure carrier oil and apply 2-4 drops on location, temples, wrists, throat, face, chest, chakras, and/or Vita Flex points.

**Technical Data: Botanical Family:** Myrtaceae; **Plant Origin:** Australia; **Extraction Method:** Steam distilled from leaves and branches; **Key Constituents:** Alpha-Pinene (5-10%), 1,8-Cineole + Beta-Phellandrene (18-28%), Alpha-Terpineol (1-5%), Para-Cymene (1-6%), Linalol (34-45%), Aromadendrene (2-6%); **ORAC:** 61,100 µTE/100g

### Selected Research

Abuznait AH, et al. Induction of expression and functional activity of P-glycoprotein efflux transporter by bioactive plant natural products. *Food Chem Toxicol.* 2011 Nov;49(11):2765-72.

Abdel Bar FM, et al. Design and pharmacophore of biaryl methyl eugenol analogs as breast cancer invasion inhibitors. *Bioorg Med Chem.* 2010 Jan 15;18(2):496-507.

Abdel Bar FM, et al. Antiproliferative triterpenes from *Melaleuca ericifolia. J Nat Prod.* 2008 Oct;71(10):1787-90.

## Melaleuca Quinquenervia (Niaouli)
### (Melaleuca viridiflora)

A brew from the bruised leaves of *Melaleuca quinquenervia* was used by Aboriginal people in Australia for colds, headaches, and other sicknesses.

**Medical Properties:** Male hormone-like, anti-inflammatory, antibacterial, antiviral, and antiparasitic (amoeba and parasites in the blood), vasodilating, skin penetration enhancer (hormones)

**Uses:** Hypertension, urinary tract/bladder infections, respiratory/sinus infections, allergies

**Directions: Aromatic:** Diffuse up to 1 hour 3 times daily or directly inhale. **Topical:** Dilute 1 drop essential oil with 1 drop V-6 or other pure carrier oil and apply on location, chakras, and/or Vita Flex points.

**Technical Data: Botanical Family:** Myrtaceae; **Plant Origin:** Australia, New Caledonia; **Extraction Method:** Steam distilled from leaves and twigs; **Key Constituents:** 1,8-Cineole (Eucalyptol) (55-75%), Alpha-Pinene (5-12%), Limonene (1-9%), Beta-Pinene (1-5%), Viridiflorol (2-6%); **ORAC:** 18,600 µTE/100g

### Selected Research

Cock IE, et al. The potential of selected Australian medicinal plants with anti-Proteus activity for the treatment and prevention of rheumatoid arthritis. *Pharmacogn Mag.* 2015 May;11(Suppl 1):S190-208.

Park HM, et al. Larvicidal activity of Myrtaceae essential oils and their components against *Aedes aegypti*, acute toxicity on *Daphnia magna* and aqueous residue. *J Med Entomol.* 2011 Mar;48(2):405-19.

Monti D, et al. Niaouli oils from different sources: analysis and influence on cutaneous permeation of estradiol in vitro. *Drug Deliv.* 2009 Jul;16(5):237-42.

Nam SY, et al. Essential oil of niaouli preferentially potentiates antigen-specific cellular immunity and cytokine production by macrophages. *Immunopharmacol Immunotoxicol.* 2008;30(3):459-74.

## Melissa (Melissa officinalis)
### (Also known as lemon balm)

Anciently, melissa was used for nervous disorders and many different ailments dealing with the heart or the emotions. It was also used to promote fertility. Melissa was the main ingredient in Carmelite water, distilled in France since 1611 by the Carmelite monks.

The University of Maryland Medical Center writes that Melissa "was used as far back as the Middle Ages to reduce stress and anxiety, promote sleep, improve appetite, and ease pain and discomfort from indigestion."

An old Arabian proverb states, "Balm makes the heart merry and joyful," which may be why Avicenna advocated the use of lemon balm in treating depression and anxiety.

Recent studies document its antiviral activities and memory and learning benefits.

**Medical Properties:** Anti-inflammatory, antiviral, relaxant, hypotensive, anti-oxidative, antitumoral

**Uses:** Viral infections (herpes, etc.), depression, anxiety, insomnia

**Fragrant Influence:** Brings out gentle characteristics within people. It is calming and uplifting and balances emotions. It removes emotional blocks and instills a positive outlook on life.

**Directions: Aromatic:** Diffuse up to 1 hour 3 times daily or directly inhale. **Dietary:** Put 2 drops in a capsule and take 3 times daily or as needed. **Topical:** Apply 2-4 drops directly to affected area as needed or on chakras and/or Vita Flex points. Dilution not required except for extremely sensitive skin.

**Technical Data: Botanical Family:** Lamiaceae; **Plant Origin:** Utah, Idaho, France; **Extraction Method:** Steam distilled from aerial parts before flowering; **Key Constituents:** Geranial (25-35%), Neral (18-28%), Beta-Caryophyllene (12-19%); **ORAC:** 134,300 µTE/100g

### Selected Research

Pourghanbari G, et al. Antiviral activity of the oseltamivir and *Melissa officinalis* essential oil against avian influenza A virus (H9N2). *Virusdisease.* 2016 Jun;27(2):170-8.

Shojaii A, et al. Medicinal Herbs in Iranian Traditional Medicine for Learning and Memory. *Iran J Med Sci.* 2016 May;41(3):S43.

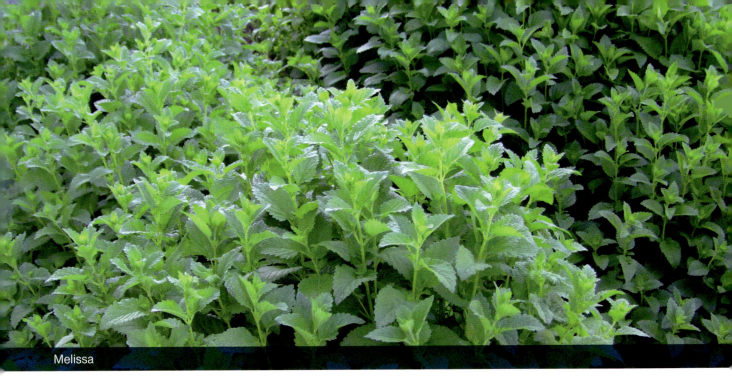
Melissa

Ozarowski M, et al. Influence of the *Melissa officinalis* Leaf Extract on Long-Term Memory in Scopolamine Animal Model with Assessment of Mechanism of activity. *Evid Based Complement Alternat Med.* 2016;2016:9729818. [Epub ahead of print]

Akbarzadeh M, et al. Effect of *Melissa officinalis* Capsule on the Intensity of Premenstrual Syndrome Symptoms in High School Girl Students. *Nurs Midwifery Stud.* 2015 Jun;4(2):e27001. [Epub ahead of print]

Jahanban-Esfahlan A, et al. Anti Proliferative Properties of *Melissa officinalis* in Different Human Cancer Cells. *Asian Pac J Cancer Prev.* 2015;16(14):5703-7.

Astani A, et al. Attachment and Penetration of Acyclovir-resistant *Herpes simplex* Virus are Inhibited by *Melissa officinalis* Extract. *Phytother Res.* 2014 Oct;28(10):147-52.

Joukar S, et al. Efficacy of *Melissa officinalis* in suppressing ventricular arrhythmias following ischemia-reperfusion of the heart: a comparison with amiodarone. *Med Princ Pract.* 2014;23(4):340-5.

**Technical Data: Botanical Family:** Lamiaceae; **Plant Origin:** Israel; **Extraction Method:** Steam distilled from leaf, stem, and flower; **Key Constituents:** Pulegone (50-65%), Menthol (7-12%), Beta-Caryophyllene (3-9%), Isopulegol (3-6%), Menthone (1-5%), Neomenthol (1-5%)

## Selected Research

Abu-Gharbieh E, et al. Anti-inflammatory and gastroprotective activities of the aqueous extract of *Micromeria fruticosa* (L.) Druce ssp Serpyllifolia in mice. *Pak J Pharm Sci.* 2013 Jul;26(4):799-803.

Shehab NG, Abu-Gharbieh E. Constituents and biological activity of the essential oil and the aqueous extract of *Micromeria fruticosa* (L.) Druce subsp. serpyllifolia. *Pak J Pharm Sci.* 2012 Jul;25(3):687-92.

Ali-Shtayeh MS, et al. Traditional knowledge of wild edible plants used in Palestine (Northern West Bank): a comparative study. *J Ethnobiol Ethnomed.* 2008 May 12;4:13.

## Micromeria *(Micromeria fruticosa)*

Micromeria is found in Israel and in the eastern Mediterranean. It is known in folk medicine as having anti-inflammatory properties and for digestive support.

**Medical Properties:** Anti-inflammatory, gastroprotective

**Uses:** Stomach upsets

**Fragrant Influence:** Revitalizes and refreshes the mind

**Directions: Topical:** Dilute 1 drop essential oil with 4 drops V-6 or other pure carrier oil and apply 2-4 drops on location, chakras, and/or Vita Flex points.

**Caution:** Contains high levels of pulegone. Do not use if pregnant or trying to conceive.

## Mountain Savory *(Satureja montana)*

Mountain savory has been used historically as a general tonic for the body.

**Medical Properties:** Strong antibacterial, antifungal, antiviral, antiparasitic, immune stimulant, anti-inflammatory action

**Uses:** Viral infections (herpes, HIV, etc.), scoliosis/lumbago/back problems

**Fragrant Influence:** Revitalizes and stimulates the nervous system. It is a powerful energizer and motivator.

**Directions: Aromatic:** Diffuse up to 10 minutes 3 times daily or directly inhale. **Topical:** Dilute 1 drop essential oil with 1 drop V-6 or other pure carrier oil and apply on location, chakras, and/or Vita Flex points.

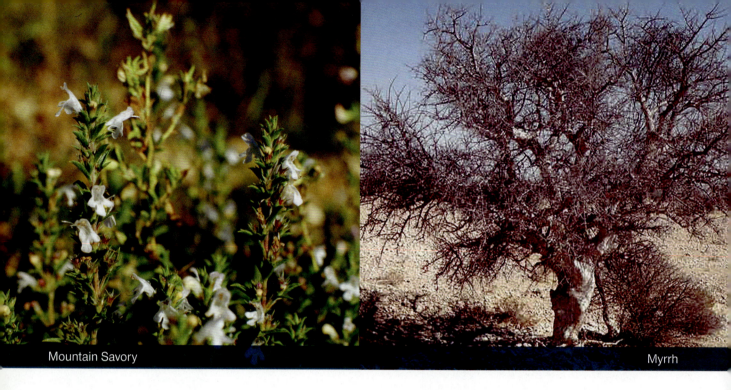

Mountain Savory

Myrrh

## Mountain Savory Vitality™ (Satureja montana)

**Directions:** Dietary: Dilute 1 drop with 4 drops of carrier oil. Put in a capsule and take 1 daily or as needed.

**Technical Data: Botanical Family:** Lamiaceae; **Plant Origin:** France; **Extraction Method:** Steam distilled from flowering plant; **Key Constituents:** Carvacrol (22-35%), Thymol (14-24%), Gamma-Terpinene (8-15%), Carvacrol Methyl Ether (4-9%), Beta-Caryophyllene (3-7%); **ORAC:** 11,300 µTE/100g

### Selected Research

Miladi H, et al. Antibiofilm formation and anti-adhesive property of three Mediterranean essential oils against a foodborne pathogen *Salmonella* strain. *Microb Pathog.* 2016 Jan 21;93:22-31.

Kundaković T, et al. Cytotoxicity and antimicrobial activity of the essential oil from *Satureja montana* subsp. pisidica (Lamiceae). *Nat Prod Commun.* 2014 Apr;9(4):569-72.

Dunkić V, et al. Chemotaxic and micromorphological traits of *Satureja montana* L. and S. subspicata Vis. (Lamiaceae). *Chem Biodivers.* 2012 Dec;9(12):2825-42.

Serrano C, et al. Antioxidant and antimicrobial activity of *Satureja montana* L. extracts. *J Sci Food Agric.* 2011 Jul;91(9):1554-60.

Zavatti M, et al. Experimental study on *Satureja montana* as a treatment for premature ejaculation. *J Ethnopharmacol.* 2011 Jan 27;133(2):629-33.

## Myrrh (Commiphora myrrha)

It is mentioned in one of the oldest known medical records, the Ebers Papyrus (dating from 16th century BC), an ancient Egyptian list of 877 prescriptions and recipes. The Arabian people used myrrh for many skin conditions such as chapped and cracked skin and wrinkles. It was listed in Hildegard's *Medicine*, a compilation of early German medicines by highly regarded Benedictine herbalist Hildegard of Bingen (1098-1179).

**Medical Properties:** Powerful antioxidant, antitumoral, anti-inflammatory, antibacterial, antiviral, antiparasitic, analgesic/anesthetic

**Uses:** Diabetes, cancer, hepatitis, fungal infections (candida, ringworm), tooth/gum infections, skin conditions (eczema, chapped, cracked, wrinkles, stretch marks)

**Fragrant Influence:** Promotes spiritual awareness and is uplifting. It contains sesquiterpenes, which stimulate the limbic system of the brain (the center of memory and emotions) and the hypothalamus, pineal, and pituitary glands. The hypothalamus is the master gland of the human body, producing many vital hormones, including thyroid and growth hormone.

**Directions: Aromatic:** Diffuse up to 1 hour 3 times daily or directly inhale. **Topical:** Apply 2-4 drops on location, chakras, and/or Vita Flex points. Dilution not required except for the most sensitive skin.

**Technical Data: Botanical Family:** Burseraceae; **Plant Origin:** Somalia; **Extraction Method:** Steam distilled from gum/resin; **Key Constituents:** Lindestrene (7-16%), Curzerene (9-32%), Furanoendesma-1,3-diene (25-50%), 2-Methoxy Furanogermacrene (1-10%), Beta-Elemene (1-9%); **ORAC:** 379,800 µTE/100g

### Selected Research

Huang C, et al. Z-guggulsterone Negatively Controls Microglia-Mediated Neuroinflammation Via Blocking IκB-α-NK-κB Signals. *Neurosci Lett.* 2016 Feb 12. [Epub ahead of print]

Ahmad A, et al. Hepatoprotective effect of *Commiphora myrrha* against d-GaIN/LPS-induced hepatic injury in a rat model through attenuation of pro inflammatory cytokines and related genes. *Pharm Biol.* 2015 Dec;53(12):1759-67.

Gao W, et al. Cycloartan-24-ene-1α,2α,3β-triol, a clycloartane-type triterpenoid from the resinous exudates of *Commiphora myrrha*, induces apoptosis in human prostatic cancer PC-3 cells. *Oncol Rep.* 2015 Mar;33(3):1107-14.

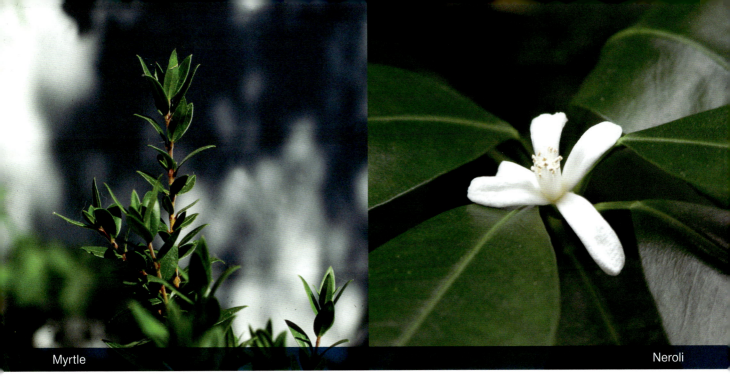

Myrtle

Neroli

Lee K, et al. Anti-biofilm, anti-hemolysis, and anti-virulence activities of black pepper, cananga, myrrh oils, and nerolidol against *Staphylococcus aureus. Appl Microbiol Biotechnol.* 2014 July 16. [Epub ahead of print]

Chen Y, et al. Composition and potential anticancer activities of essential oils obtained from myrrh and frankincense. *Oncol Lett.* 2013 Oct;6(4):1140-1146.

Xu J, et al. Four new sesquiterpenes from *Commiphora myrrha* and their neuroprotective effects. *Fitoterapia.* 2012 Jun;83(4):801-5.

Su S, et al. Evaluation of the anti-inflammatory and analgesic properties of individual and combined extracts from *Commiphora myrrha* and *Boswellia carterii. J Ethnopharmacol.* 2012 Jan 31;139(2):649-56.

## Myrtle *(Myrtus communis)*

Myrtle has been researched by Dr. Daniel Pénoël for normalizing hormonal imbalances of the thyroid and ovaries, as well as balancing the hypothyroid. It has also been researched for its soothing effects on the respiratory system.

**Medical Properties:** Antimutagenic, liver stimulant, prostate and thyroid stimulant, sinus/lung decongestant, antispasmodic, antihyperglycemic, anti-inflammatory, antinociceptive

**Uses:** Thyroid problems, throat/lung/sinus infections, prostate problems, skin irritations (acne, blemishes, bruises, oily skin, psoriasis, etc.), muscle spasms

**Fragrant Influence:** Elevating and euphoric

**Directions: Aromatic:** Diffuse up to 30 minutes 3 times daily or put in humidifier. Directly inhale. **Dietary:** Take as a dietary supplement. **Topical:** Dilute 1 drop essential oil with 1 drop V-6 or other pure carrier oil and apply 2-4 drops on location, chakras, and/or Vita Flex points.

**Technical Data: Botanical Family:** Myrtaceae; **Plant Origin:** Tunisia, Morocco; **Extraction Method:** Steam distilled from leaves; **Key Constituents:** Alpha-Pinene (15-60%), 1,8-Cineole (Eucalyptol) (15-40%), Limonene (4-18%), Myrtenyl Acetate (trace-20%); **ORAC:** 25,400 µTE/100g

## Selected Research

Kordali S, et al. Antifungal and Herbicidal Effects of Fruit Essential Oils of Four *Myrtus communis* Genotypes. *Chem Biodivers.* 2016 Jan;13(1):77-84.

Ebrahimabadi EH, et al. Combination of GC/FID/Mass spectrometry fingerprints and multivariate calibration techniques for recognition of antimicrobial constituents of *Myrtus communis* L. essential oil. *J Chromatog B Analyt Technol Biomed Life Sci.* 2016 Jan 1;1008:50-7.

Bouzabata A, et al. *Myrtus communis* L. as a source of a bioactive and safe essential oil. *Food Chem Toxicol.* 2015 Jan;75:166-72.

Aleksic V, et al. Synergistic effect of *Myrtus communis* L. essential oils and conventional antibiotics against multi-drug resistant *Acinetobacter baumannii* wound isolates. *Phytomedicine.* 2014 Oct 15;21(12):1666-74.

Ogur R. Studies with *Myrtus communis* L.: Anticancer properties. *J Intercult Ethnopharmacol.* 2014 Oct-Dec;3(4):135-7.

Alipour G, et al. Review of pharmacological effects of *Myrtus communis* L. and its active constituents. *Phytother Res.* 2014 Aug;28(8):1125-36.

Janbaz KH, et al. Broncodilator, vasodilator and spasmolytic activities of methanolic extract of *Myrtus communis* L. *J Physiol Pharmacol.* 2013 Aug;64(4):479-84.

Choudhary MI, et al. New inhibitors of ROS generation and T-cell proliferation from *Myrtus communis. Org Lett.* 2013 Apr 19;15(8):1862-5.

## Neroli (Bitter Orange) *(Citrus aurantium amara)*

Highly regarded by the ancient Egyptians for its ability to heal the mind, body, and spirit.

**Medical Properties:** Antiparasitic, digestive tonic, antidepressive, hypotensive (lowers blood pressure)

**Uses:** Hypertension, anxiety, depression, hysteria, insomnia, skin conditions (scars, stretch marks, thread veins, wrinkles)

**Fragrant Influence:** A natural relaxant used to treat depression and anxiety. It strengthens and stabilizes the emotions and uplifts and inspires the hopeless, encouraging confidence, courage, joy, peace, and sensuality. It brings everything into focus at the moment.

**Directions: Aromatic:** Diffuse up to 1 hour 3 times daily or directly inhale. **Dietary:** Dilute 1 drop essential oil with 1 drop V-6 or other pure carrier oil, put in a capsule, and take up to 3 times daily or as needed. **Topical:** Apply 2-4 drops on location, chakras, and/or Vita Flex points. Dilution not required except for the most sensitive skin.

**Technical Data: Botanical Family:** Rutaceae; **Plant Origin:** Tunisia; **Extraction Method:** Steam distilled from flowers of the bitter orange tree; **Key Constituents:** Linalol (28-44%), Limonene (9-18%), Beta-Pinene (7-17%), Linalyl Acetate (3-15%), Trans-Ocimene (3-8%), Alpha-Terpineol (2-5.5%), Trans-Nerolidol (1-5%), Myrcene (1-4%)

### Selected Research

Pimenta FC, et al. Anxiolytic Effect of *Citrus aurantium* L. in Patients with Chronic Myeloid Leukemia. *Phytother Res.* 2016 Jan 20. [Epub ahead of print]

Metoui N, et al. Activity antifungal of the essential oils; aqueous and ethanol extracts from *Citrus aurantium* L. *Nat Prod Res.* 2015 Jul 24:1-4.

Khodabakhsh P, et al. Analgesic and anti-inflammatory activities of *Citrus aurantium* L. blossoms essential oil (neroli): involvement of the nitric oxide/cyclic-guanosine monophosphate pathway. *J Nat Med.* 2015 Jul;69(3):324-31.

Bonamin F, et al. The effect of a minor constituent of essential oil from *Citrus aurantium:* The role of β-myrcene in preventing peptic ulcer disease. *Chem Biol Interact.* 2014 Apr 5;212:11-9.

Choi S, et al. Effects of Inhalation of Essential Oil of *Citrus aurantium* L. var. amara on Menopausal Symptoms, Stress, and Estrogen in Postmenopausal Women: A Randomized Controlled Trial. *Evid Based Complement Alternat Med.* 2014;2014:796518.

Ullah N, et al. Nephroprotective potentials of *Citrus aurantium:* a prospective pharmacological study on experimental models. *Pak J Pharm Sci.* 2014 May;27(3):505-10.

## Northern Lights Black Spruce
### (Picea mariana)

The Lakota Indians used black spruce to strengthen their ability to communicate with the Great Spirit. Traditionally, it was believed to possess the frequency of prosperity.

**Medical Properties:** Antispasmodic, antiparasitic, antiseptic, anti-inflammatory, hormone-like, cortisone-like, immune stimulant, antidiabetic

**Uses:** Arthritis/rheumatism, fungal infections (candida), sinus/respiratory infections, sciatica/lumbago

**Fragrant Influence:** Releases emotional blocks, bringing about a feeling of balance and grounding

**Directions: Aromatic:** Diffuse 1 hour up to 3 times daily or directly inhale. **Topical:** Dilute 1 drop essential oil with 1 drop V-6 or other pure carrier oil and apply 2-4 drops on location, chakras, and/or Vita Flex points.

**Technical Data: Botanical Family:** Pinaceae; **Plant Origin:** Canada; **Extraction Method:** Steam distilled from entire tree; **Key Constituents:** Bornyl Acetate (24-35%), Camphene (14-26%), Alpha-Pinene (12-19%), Beta-Pinene (2-10%), Delta-3-Carene (4-10%), Limonene (3-6%), Myrcene (1-5%), Santene (1-5%), Tricyclene (1-4%)

### Selected Research

Prunier J, et al. From genotypes to phenotypes: expression levels of genes encompassing adaptive SNPs in black spruce. *Plant Cell Rep.* 2015 Aug 11 [Epub ahead of print]

Garcia-Pérez ME, et al. *Picea mariana* polyphenolic extract inhibits phlogenic mediators produced by TNF-α-activated psoriatic keratinocytes: Impact on NF-κB pathway. *J Ethnopharmacol.* 2014;151(1):265-78.

Garcia-Pérez ME, et al. *Picea mariana* bark: a new source of trans-resveratrol and other bioactive polyphenols. *Food Chem.* 2012 Dec 1; 135(3):1173-82.

Tam TW, et al. Cree antidiabetic plant extracts display mechanism-based inactivation of CYP3A4. *Can J Physiol Pharmacol.* 2011 Jan;89(1):13-23.

## Nutmeg (Myristica fragrans)

Nutmeg was listed in Hildegard's *Medicine,* a compilation of early German medicines by highly regarded Benedictine herbalist Hildegard of Bingen (1098-1179).

**Medical Properties:** Anti-inflammatory, anticoagulant, antiseptic, antiparasitic, analgesic, liver protectant, stomach protectant (ulcers), circulatory stimulant, adrenal stimulant, muscle relaxing, increases production of growth hormone/melatonin

**Uses:** Rheumatism/arthritis, cardiovascular disease, hypertension, hepatitis, ulcers, digestive disorders, antiparasitic, nerve pain, fatigue/exhaustion, neuropathy

**Directions: Aromatic:** Diffuse up to 30 minutes 3 times daily or directly inhale. **Topical:** Dilute 1 drop essential oil with 1 drop V-6 or other pure carrier oil and apply on location, chakras, and/or Vita Flex points.

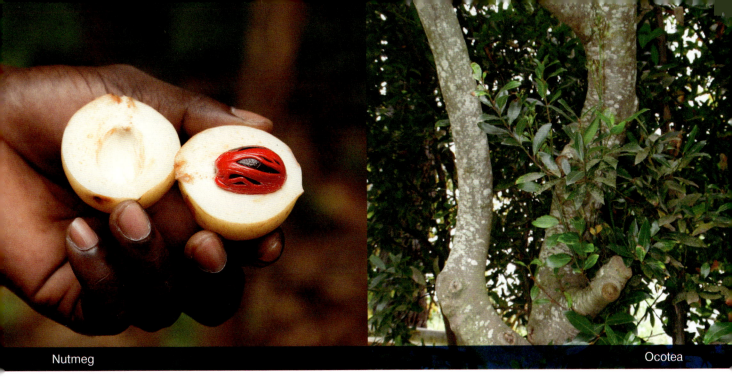

Nutmeg | Ocotea

## Nutmeg Vitality™ (Myristica fragrans)

**Directions: Dietary:** Dilute 1 drop with 1 drop of carrier oil. Put in a capsule and take up to 3 times a day or as needed.

**Technical Data: Botanical Family:** Myristicaceae; **Plant Origin:** Tunisia, Indonesia; **Extraction Method:** Steam distilled from fruits and seeds; **Key Constituents:** Sabinene (14-29%), Beta-Pinene (13-18%), Alpha-Pinene (15-28%), Limonene (2-7%), Gamma-Terpinene (2-6%), Terpinene-4-ol (2-6%), Myristicine (5-12%); **ORAC:** 158,100 µTE/100g

### Selected Research

Muñoz Acuña U, et al. New acyclic bis phenylpropanoid and neolignans, from *Myristica fragrans* Houtt., exhibiting PARP-1 and NF-κB inhibitory effects. *Food Chem.* 2016 Jul 1;202:269-75.

Cuong TD, et al. Potent acetylcholinesterase inhibitory compounds from *Myristica fragrans. Nat Prod Commun.* 2014 Apr;9(4):499-502.

Piaru SP, et al. Antioxidant and antiangiogenic activities of the essential oils of *Myristica fragrans* and *Morinda citrifolia. Asian Pac J Trop Med.* 2012 Apr;5(4):294-8.

Piras A, et al. Extraction and separation of volatile and fixed oils from seeds of *Myristica fragrans* by supercritical $CO_2$: chemical composition and cytotoxic activity on Caco-2 cancer cells. *J Food Sci.* 2012 Apr;77(4):C498-53.

Wajab A, et al. Anticonvulsant activities of nutmeg oil of *Myristica fragrans. Phytother Res.* 2009 Feb;23(2):153-8.

Morita T, et al. Hepatoprotective effect of myristicin from nutmeg (*Myristica fragrans*) on lipopolysaccharide/d-galactosamine-induced liver injury. *J Agric Food Chem.* 2003 Mar 12;51(6):1560-1565.

## Ocotea (Ocotea quixos)

Ocotea is distilled from a tree found in the Amazon wilderness, on the ranges of the west side of the Andes Mountains. It is commonly referred to by the native people throughout Ecuador as *Ishpingo* and is considered to be a false canilla or false cinnamon. The tree grows to a very large size, reaching up to 48 inches in diameter and over 60 feet tall, making a large canopy top. Historical usage of ocotea dates back more than 500 years, when it was used to aromatize sweets and cakes.

**Medical Properties:** Antifungal, disinfectant, anti-inflammatory

**Uses:** Hypertension, high blood pressure, anxiety, internal irritation, may lower insulin needs for diabetics and reduce blood sugar fluctuations, infection, digestive support

**Fragrant Influence:** Has a complex aroma, which may increase feelings of fullness; related to the cinnamon species but has an aroma that is different from any common cinnamon

**Directions: Aromatic:** Diffuse up to 1 hour 3 times daily or inhale directly. **Dietary:** Dilute 1 drop essential oil with 4 drops V-6 or other pure carrier oil, put in a capsule, and take 1 daily or as directed by a health care professional. **Topical:** Dilute 1 drop essential oil with 4 drops V-6 or other pure carrier oil and apply 1-2 drops on location, chakras, and/or Vita Flex points. Test on a small, inconspicuous area of skin to observe sensitivity.

**Technical Data: Botanical Family:** Lauraceae; **Plant Origin:** Ecuador, Central and South America; **Extraction Method:** Steam distilled from the leaves; **Key Constituents:** Beta-Caryophyllene (10-35%), Cinnamyl Acetate (1-24%), Methyl Cinnamate (4-24%), Alpha-Humulene (1-17%), Trans-Cinnamaldehyde (trace-12%)

### Selected Research

Ballabeni V, et al. *Ocotea quixos* Lam. essential oil: in vitro and in vivo investigation on its anti-inflammatory properties, *Fitoterapia*, 2010 Jun;81(4):289-95.

Tognolini M, et al. Comparative screening of plant essential oils: phenylpropanoids moiety as basic core for antiplatelet activity. *Life Sci.* 2006 Feb 23;78(13):1419-32.

Sacchetti, G, et al. Essential oil of wild *Octotea quixos* (lam.) Kosterm. (Lauraceae) leaves from Amazonian Ecuador. *Flav Fragr J.* 2006 21:674-76.

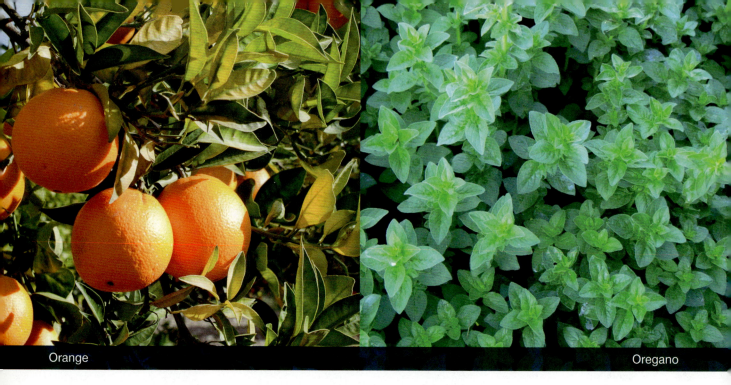

Orange | Oregano

## Orange *(Citrus sinensis)*

Beloved for its clean, fresh scent, Orange essential oil was also shown to reduce anxiety in children awaiting dental treatment. Salivary cortisol levels were lowered as were pulse rates (Jafarzadeh, 2013).

**Medical Properties:** Antitumoral, relaxant, anticoagulant, circulatory stimulant. Rich in limonene, which has been extensively studied in over 50 clinical studies for its ability to combat tumor growth.

**Uses:** Arteriosclerosis, hypertension, cancer, insomnia, and complexion (dull and oily), fluid retention, wrinkles

**Fragrant Influence:** Uplifting and antidepressant. A Mie University study found that citrus fragrances boosted immunity, induced relaxation, and reduced depression (Komori, et al., 1995).

**Directions: Aromatic:** Diffuse up to 1 hour 3 times daily or directly inhale. **Topical:** Dilute 1 drop essential oil with 1 drop V-6 or other pure carrier oil and apply 2-4 drops on location, chakras, and/or Vita Flex points.

**Caution:** Possible sun sensitivity.

## Orange Vitality™ *(Citrus sinensis)*

**Directions: Dietary:** Put 2 drops in a capsule. Take 3 times daily.

**Technical Data: Botanical Family:** Rutaceae; **Plant Origin:** USA, South Africa, Italy, China; **Extraction Method:** Cold pressed from rind; **Key Constituents:** Limonene (85-96%), Myrcene (0.5-3%); **ORAC:** 1,890 µTE/100g

### Selected Research

Shetty SB, Antimicrobial effects of *Citrus sinensis* peel extracts against dental caries bacteria: An in vitro study. *J Clin Exp Dent.* 2016 Feb 1,8(1):e71-e77.

Hussain KA, et al. Antimicrobial effects of *Citrus sinensis* peel extracts against periodontopathic bacteria: an in vitro study. *Rocz Panstw Zaki Hig.* 2015:66(2):173-8.

Hasheminia D, et al. Can ambient orange fragrance reduce patient anxiety during surgical removal of impacted mandibular third molars? *J Oral Maxillofac Surg.* 2014 Sep;72(9):1671-6.

D'Alessio PA, et al. Oral administration of d-limonene controls inflammation in rat colitis and displays anti-inflammatory properties as diet supplementation in humans. *Life Sci.* 2013 Jul 10;92(24-26):1151-6.

Miller JA, et al. Human breast cancer tissue disposition and bioactivity of limonene in women with early-stage breast cancer. *Cancer Prev Res (Phila).* 2013 Jun;6(6):577-84.

Polo CM, et al. Gastric Ulcers in Middle-Aged Rats: The Healing Effect of Essential Oils from *Citrus aurantium* L. (Rutaceae). *Evid Based Complement Alternat Med.* 2012;2012:509451. [Epub ahead of print]

## Oregano *(Origanum vulgare) (Syn. O. majorana)*

Listed in Hildegard's *Medicine,* a compilation of early German medicines by highly regarded Benedictine herbalist Hildegard of Bingen (1098-1179).

**Medical Properties:** Antiaging, powerful antiviral, antibacterial, antifungal, antiparasitic, anti-inflammatory, antioxidant, immune stimulant, antinociceptive, radioprotective, liver protectant

**Uses:** Arthritis, rheumatism, respiratory infectious diseases, infections, tuberculosis, digestive problems

**Fragrant Influence:** Creates a feeling of security.

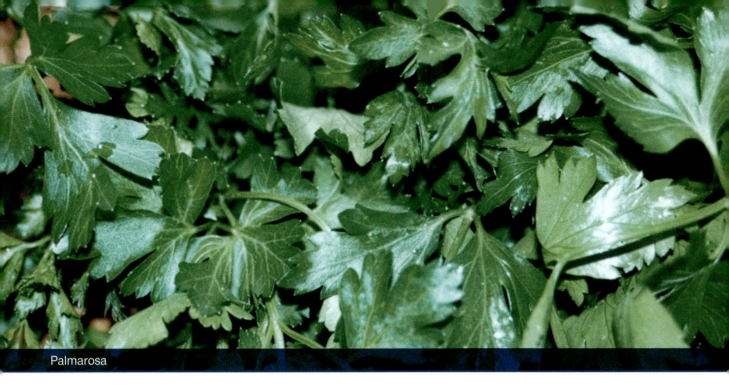
Palmarosa

**Directions: Topical:** Dilute 1 drop essential oil with 4 drops V-6 or other pure carrier oil and test on a small area of skin on the underside of arm. Apply 1-2 drops on location, chakras, and/or Vita Flex points. May use neat in Raindrop Technique.

**Caution:** High in phenols, Oregano may irritate the nasal membranes or skin if inhaled directly from diffuser or bottle or applied neat.

## Oregano Vitality™
*(Origanum vulgare) (Syn. O. majorana)*

**Directions: Dietary:** Dilute 1 with 1 drop of carrier oil. Put in a capsule and take up to 3 times daily.

**Technical Data: Botanical Family:** Lamiaceae; **Plant Origin:** USA, France, Germany, Turkey; **Extraction Method:** Steam distilled from leaves; **Key Constituents:** Carvacrol (60-75%), Gamma-Terpinene (3.5-8.5%), Para-Cymene (5.5-9%), Beta-Caryophyllene (2-5%), Myrcene (1-3%), Thymol (0-5%); **ORAC:** 15,300 µTE/100g

### Selected Research

Kubatka P, et al. Oregano demonstrates distinct tumour-suppressive effects in breast carcinoma model. *Eur J Nutr.* 2016 Feb 23.

Gomes Neto NJ, et al. Influence of general stress-response alternative sigma factors σ(S) (RpoS) and σ(B) (SigB) on bacterial tolerance to the essential oils from *Origanum vulgare* L. and *Rosmarinus officinalis* L. and pulsed electric fields. *Int J Food Microbiol.* 2015 Oct 15;211:32-7.

Begnini KR, et al. Composition and Antiproliferative Effect of Essential Oil of *Origanum vulgare* Against Tumor Cell Lines. *J Med Food.* 2014 Oc;17(10):1129-33.

Afarineshe Khaki MR, et al. Antinociceptive Effect of Aqueous Extract of *Origanum vulgare* L. in male Rats: Possible Involvement of the GABAergic System. *Iran J Pharm Res.* 2013 Spring;12(2):407-13.

Schillaci D, et al. *Origanum vulgare* subsp. hirtum essential oil prevented biofilm formation and showed antibacterial activity against planktonic and sessile bacterial cells. *J Food Prod.* 2013 Oct;76(10):1747-52.

## Palmarosa *(Cymbopogon martini)*

A relative of lemongrass, palmarosa was used in temple incense by the ancient Egyptians.

**Medical Properties:** Antibacterial, antifungal, antiviral, supports heart and nervous system, reduces blood sugar fluctuations, stimulates new skin cell growth, regulates sebum production in skin

**Uses:** Fungal infections/candida, neuroprotective, cardiovascular/circulatory diseases, digestive problems, skin problems (acne, eczema)

**Fragrant Influence:** Creates a feeling of security. It also helps to reduce stress and tension and promotes recovery from nervous exhaustion.

**Directions: Aromatic:** Diffuse up to 1 hour 3 times daily or directly inhale. **Dietary:** Dilute 1 drop essential oil with 1 drop V-6 or other pure carrier oil, put in a capsule, and take up to 3 times daily. **Topical:** Apply 2-4 drops on location, chakras, and/or Vita Flex points. Dilution not required except for the most sensitive skin.

**Technical Data: Botanical Family:** Poaceae; **Plant Origin:** India; **Extraction Method:** Steam distilled from leaves; **Key Constituents:** Geraniol (70-85%), Geranyl Acetate (6-10%), Linalol (3-7%); **ORAC:** 127,800 µTE/100g

### Selected Research

Janbaz KH, et al. Bronchodilator, vasodilator and spasmolytic activities of *Cymbopogon martini. J Physiol Pharmacol.* 2014 Dec;65(6):859-66.

Murbach Teles Andrade BF, et al. *Cymbopogon martini* essential oil and geraniol at noncytotoxic concentrations exerted immunomodulatory/anti-inflammatory effects in human monocytes. *J Pharm Pharmacol.* 2014 Oct;66(10):1491-1496.

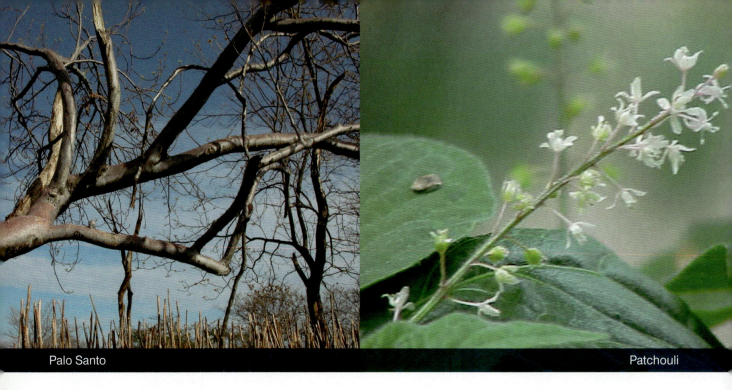

Palo Santo

Patchouli

Ghadyale V, et al. Effective Control of Postprandial Glucose Level through Inhibition of Intestinal Alpha Glucosidase by *Cymbopogon martinii* (Roxb.). *Evid Based Complement Alternat Med.* 2012;2012:372909.

Buch P, et al. Neuroprotective activity of *Cymbopogon martinii* against cerebral ischemia/reperfusion-induced oxidative stress in rats. *J. Ethnopharmacol.* 2012 Jun 26;142(1):35-40.

Gacche RN, et al. Kinetics of Inhition of Monamine Oxidase Using *Cymbopogon martinii* (Roxb.) Wats.: A Potential Antidepressant Herbal Ingredient with Antioxidant Activity. *Indian J Biochem.* 2011 Jul;26(3):303-8.

## Palo Santo *(Bursera graveolens)*

Palo Santo comes from the same botanical family as Frankincense, although it is found in South America. Like Frankincense, Palo Santo is known as a spiritual oil, with a deep-rooted tradition in which it was used by the Incas to purify and cleanse the air of negative energies and for good luck. It is used in South America to repel mosquitoes, for fevers, infections, and skin diseases. It is currently used by shamans of the Andes in curing ceremonies. Even its Spanish name reflects how highly this oil was regarded: *palo santo* means "holy or sacred wood."

**Note:** Constituents can vary depending on whether the wood is harvested from coastal or inland areas and if the trunk is red or white.

**Medical Properties:** Anticancerous, antiblastic, anti-inflammatory, antibacterial, antifungal, antiviral

**Uses:** Inflammation, regrowth of knee cartilage, joints, arthritis, rheumatism, gout, respiratory problems, reduces airborne contaminants when diffused

**Directions: Aromatic:** Diffuse up to 1 hour 3 times daily or directly inhale. **Dietary:** Put 10-15 drops in a capsule and take 1 or 2 times a day. Can also put 1-6 drops under the tongue or in a glass of water. **Topical:** Dilute 1 drop essential oil with 1 drop V-6 or other pure carrier oil and apply on location, chakras, and/or Vita Flex points.

**Cautions:** If pregnant or under a doctor's care, consult your physician. Should not be used on children under 18 months old.

**Technical Data: Botanical Family:** Burseraceae; **Plant Origin:** Ecuador; **Extraction Method:** Steam distilled from the sawdust of the dead bark, wood, and branches; **Key Constituents:** Limonene (45-80%), Alpha-Terpineol (4-18%), Para-Cymene (1-6%), Carvone (0.5-6%), Beta-Bisabolene (0.5-7), Fonenol (0.5-4%)

### Selected Research

Monzote L, et al. Chemical composition and anti-proliferative properties of *Bursera graveolens* essential oil, *Nat Prod Commun.* 2012 Nov;7(11):1531-4.

Nakanishi T, et al. A new and known cytotoxic aryltetralin-type lignans from stems of *Bursera graveolens*. *Chem Pharm Bull* (Tokyo). 2005 Feb;53(2):229-231.

## Patchouli *(Pogostemon cablin)*

While Patchouli oil is known as an all-purpose insect repellent, it is also highly prized in the perfumery industry. Patchouli has many benefits for chapped and wrinkled skin.

**Medical Properties:** Relaxant, antitumoral, digestive aid that combats nausea, anti-inflammatory, antimicrobial, antifungal, insecticidal, prevents wrinkles and chapped skin, relieves itching

**Uses:** Hypertension, inflammatory bowel disease, skin conditions (eczema, acne), fluid retention, Listeria infection, insect repellent

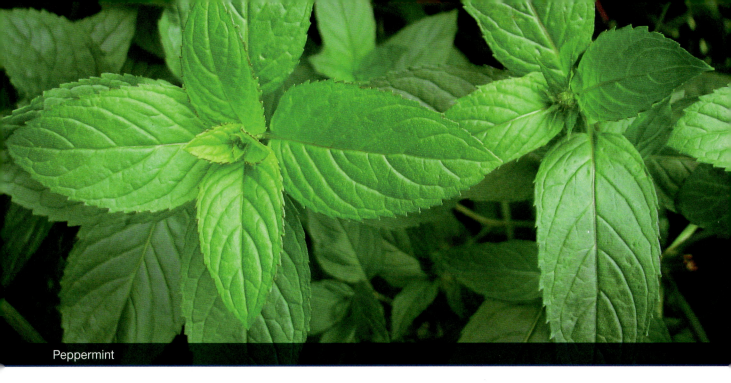
Peppermint

**Directions: Aromatic:** Diffuse up to 1 hour 3 times daily or directly inhale. **Dietary:** Take as a dietary supplement. **Topical:** Apply 2-4 drops on location, chakras, and/or Vita Flex points. Dilution not required except for the most sensitive skin.

**Fragrant Influence:** A relaxant that clarifies thoughts, allowing the discarding of jealousies, obsessions, and insecurities.

**Technical Data: Botanical Family:** Lamiaceae; **Plant Origin:** Indonesia; **Extraction Method:** Steam distilled from leaves and stems; **Key Constituents:** Patchoulol (27-35%), Bulnesene (13-21%), Alpha-Guaiene (11-16%), Beta-Patchoulene (1.8-3.5%), Beta-Caryophyllene (2-5%), Pogostol (1-2.5%), Norpatchoulenol (0.35-1%), Copaene (trace-1%); **ORAC:** 49,400 µTE/100g

### Selected Research

Yoon SC, et al. Anti-allergic and anti-inflammatory effects of aqueous extract of *Pogostemon cablin*. *Int J Mol Med.* 2016 Jan;37(1):217-24.

Swamy MK, Sinniah UR. A Comprehensive Review on the Phytochemical Constituents and Pharmacological Activities of *Pogostemon cablin* Benth: An Aromatic Medicinal Plant of Industrial Importance. *Molecules.* 2015 May 12;20(5):8521-47.

Lin RF, et al. Prevention of UV radiation-induced cutaneous photoaging in mice by topical administration of patchouli oil. *J Ethnopharmacol.* 2014 Jun 11;154(2):408-18.

Kocevski D, et al. Antifungal effect of *Allium tuberosum*, *Cinnamomum cassia*, and *Pogostemon cablin* essential oils and their components against population of *Aspergillus* species. *J Food Sci.* 2013 May;78(5):M731-7.

Jeong JB, et al. Patchouli alcohol, an essential oil of *Pogostemon cablin*, exhibits anti-tumorigenic activity in human colorectal cancer cells. *Int Immunopharmacol.* 2013 Jun;16(2):184-90.

Yu J, et al. Extraction and analysis of the essential oil in *Pogostemon cablin* by enzymatic hydrolysis and inhibitory activity against Hela cell proliferation. *Zhong Yao Cai.* 2012 May;35(5):796-9.

Yang Y, et al. Anti-emetic principles of *Pogostemon cablin* (Blanco) Benth. *Phytomedicine.* 1999 May;6(2):89-93.

## Peppermint (Mentha piperita)

Peppermint is one of the oldest and most highly regarded herbs for soothing digestion. Jean Valnet, MD, studied peppermint's effect on the liver and respiratory systems. Alan Hirsch, MD, studied peppermint's ability to directly affect the brain's satiety center (the ventromedial nucleus of the hypothalamus), which triggers a sensation of fullness after meals. A highly regarded digestive stimulant.

**Medical Properties:** Anti-inflammatory, antitumoral, antiparasitic (worms), antibacterial, antiviral, antifungal, gallbladder/digestive stimulant, pain relieving, curbs appetite

**Uses:** Rheumatism/arthritis, respiratory infections (pneumonia, tuberculosis, etc.), obesity, viral infections (herpes simplex, herpes zoster, cold sores, human papilloma virus, etc.), fungal infections/candida, digestive problems, headaches, nausea, skin conditions (itchy skin, varicose veins, eczema, psoriasis, dermatitis), scoliosis/lumbago/back problems

**Fragrant Influence:** Purifying and stimulating to the conscious mind. Research indicates that peppermint aroma, inhaled during mental tasks, may help attention, performance, and focus (Barker, et al., 2003). Peppermint may also be an effective appetite suppressant when inhaled (Hirsch and Gomez, 1995). University of Kiel researchers found that peppermint lessened headache pain in a double-blind, placebo-controlled, cross-over study.

**Directions: Aromatic:** Diffuse up to 1 hour 3 times daily or directly inhale. Inhale 5-10 times a day to curb appetite. **Topical:** Dilute 1 drop essential oil

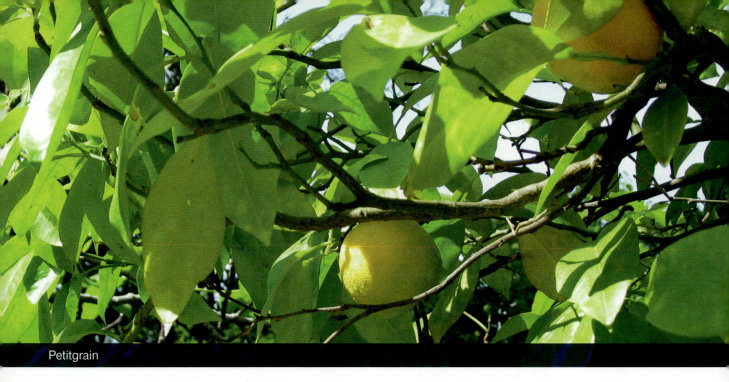

Petitgrain

with 4 drops V-6 or other pure carrier oil and apply 1-2 drops on location, abdomen, temples, chakras, and/or Vita Flex points. To improve concentration, alertness, and memory, place 1-2 drops on the tongue.

**Cautions:** Avoid contact with eyes, mucus membranes, sensitive skin, or fresh wounds or burns. Do not apply on infants younger than 18 months of age.

## Peppermint Vitality™ *(Mentha piperita)*

**Directions: Dietary:** Put 2 drops in a capsule. Take 3 times daily.

**Technical Data: Botanical Family:** Lamiaceae; **Plant Origin:** North America, Mediterranean area, Great Britain; **Extraction Method:** Steam distilled from leaves and stems; **Key Constituents:** Menthol (25-50%), Menthone (12-44%), Menthofuran (0.5-5%), 1.8-Cineole (Eucalyptol) (1-8%), Isomenthone (1-7%), Neomenthol (1.5-7%), Pulegone (0.5-3%), Menthyl Acetate (1-18%); **ORAC:** 37,300 µTE/100g

### Selected Research

Haber SL, El-Ibiary SY. Peppermint oil for treatment of irritable bowel syndrome. *Am J. Health Syst. Pharm.* 2016 Jan 15;73(2):22-31.

Husain FM, et al. Sub-MICs of *Mentha piperita* essential oil and menthol inhibits AHL mediated quorum sensing and biofilm of Gram-negative bacteria. *Front Microbiol.* 2015 May 13;6:420. [Epub ahead of print]

Ferreira P, et al. *Mentha piperita* essential oil induces apoptosis in yeast associated with both cytosolic and mitochondrial ROS-mediated damage. *FEMS Yeast Res.* 2014 Jul 26. [Epub ahead of print]

Meamarbashi A. Instant effects of peppermint essential oil on the physiological parameters and exercise performance. *Avicenna J Phytomed.* 2014 Jan;4(1):72-8.

Rozza AL, et al. Effect of menthol in experimentally induced ulcers: Pathways of gastroprotection. *Chem Biol Interact.* 2013 Oct 9;206(2):272-278.

Tayarani-Najaran Z, et al. Antiemetic activity of volatile oil from *Mentha spicata* and *Mentha x piperita* in chemotherapy-induced nausea and vomiting. *Ecancermedicalscience.* 2013;7:290.

Lane BS, et al. Examination of the effectiveness of peppermint aromatherapy on nausea in women post C-section. *J Holist Nurs.* 2012 Jun;30(2):90-104.

Barker S, et al. Improved performance on clerical tasks associated with administration of peppermint odor. *Percept Mot Skills.* 2003 Dec;97(3 pt.1):1007-1010.

## Petitgrain *(Citrus aurantium amara)* *(Syn. Citrus sinensis)*

Petitgrain derives its name from the extraction of the oil, which at one time was from the green, unripe oranges when they were still about the size of a cherry.

**Medical Properties:** Antispasmodic, anti-inflammatory, relaxant, reestablishes nerve equilibrium

**Uses:** Insomnia, anxiety, muscle spasms, skin conditions, antitumoral

**Fragrant Influence:** Uplifting and refreshing to the senses; clears confusion, reduces mental fatigue and depression; stimulates the mind and improves memory.

**Directions: Aromatic:** Diffuse up to 30 minutes up to 3 times daily or directly inhale. **Dietary:** Take as a dietary supplement. **Topical:** Apply 2 drops on location, chakras, and/or Vita Flex points. Dilution not required except for the most sensitive skin.

**Technical Data: Botanical Family:** Rutaceae; **Plant Origin:** Paraguay; **Extraction Method:** Steam distilled from leaves and twigs; **Key Constituents:** Linalyl Acetate (40-55%), Linalol (15-30%), Alpha-Terpineol (3.5-7.5%), Geranyl Acetate (2-5%), Geraniol (2-4.5%); **ORAC:** 73,600 µTE/100g

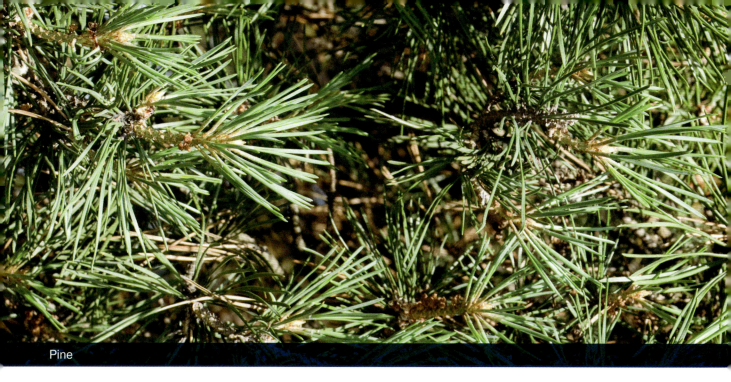
Pine

### Selected Research

Zou Z, et al. Antioxidant activity of Citrus fruits. *Food Chem.* 2016 Apr 1;196:885-96.

Activity of antifungal of the essential oils; aqueous and ethanol extracts from *Citrus aurantium* L. *Nat Prod Res.* 2015 Jul 24:1-4.

Choi SY, et al. Effects of Inhalation of Essential Oil of *Citrus aurantium* L. var. amara on Menopausal Symptoms, Stress, and Estrogen in Postmenopausal Women: A Randomized Controlled Study. *Evid Based Complement Alternat Med.* 2014;2014:796518. [Epub ahead of print]

Soudani N, et al. Oxidative stress-related lung dysfunction by chromium (VI): alleviation by *Citrus aurantium* L. *J Physiol Biochem.* 2013 Jun;69(2):239-53.

## Pine *(Pinus sylvestris)*

Pine was first investigated by Hippocrates, the father of Western medicine, for its benefits to the respiratory system. In 1990, Dr. Pénoël and Dr. Franchomme described pine oil's antiseptic properties in their medical textbook. Pine is also used in massage for stressed muscles and joints. It shares many of the same properties as *Eucalyptus globulus*, and the action of both oils is enhanced when blended. Native Americans stuffed mattresses with pine needles to repel lice and fleas. It was used to treat lung infections and even added to baths to revitalize those suffering from mental or emotional fatigue.

**Medical Properties:** Hormone-like, antidiabetic, cortisone-like, antiseptic, lymphatic stimulant

**Uses:** Throat/lung/sinus infections, rheumatism/arthritis, skin parasites, urinary tract infection, anticancer

**Fragrant Influence:** Relieves anxiety and revitalizes mind, body, and spirit. It also has an empowering, yet grounding fragrance.

**Directions: Aromatic:** Diffuse up to 30 minutes 3 times daily or directly inhale. **Topical:** Dilute 1 drop essential oil with 1 drop V-6 or other pure carrier oil and apply on location, chakras, and/or Vita Flex points.

**Caution:** Beware of pine oils adulterated with turpentine, a low-cost, but potentially hazardous, filler.

**Technical Data: Botanical Family:** Pinaceae (pine); **Plant Origin:** Austria, USA, Canada; **Extraction Method:** Steam distilled from needles; **Key Constituents:** Alpha-Pinene (55-70%), Beta-Pinene (3-8%), Limonene (5-10%), Delta-3-Carene (6-12%)

### Selected Research

Hoai NT, et al. Selectivity of *Pinus sylvestris* extract and essential oil to estrogen-insensitive breast cancer cells *Pinus sylvestris* against cancer cells. *Pharmacogn Mag.* 2015 Oct;11(Suppl 2):S290-5.

Amalinei RL, et al. Polyphenol-rich extract from *Pinus sylvestris* L. bark—chemical and antitumor studies. *Rev Med Chir Soc Med Nat Iasi.* 2014 Apr-Jun;118(2):551-7.

Fayemiwo KA, et al. Lavicidal efficacies and chemical composition of essential oils of *Pinus sylvestris* and *Syzygium aromaticum* against mosquitoes. *Asian Pac J Trop Biomed.* 2014 Jan;4(1):30-4.

Süntar I, et al. Appraisal on the wound healing and anti-inflammatory activities of the essential oils obtained from the cones and needles of Pinus species by *in vivo* and *in vitro* experimental models. *J Ethnopharmacol.* 2012 Jan;139(2):533-540.

## Plectranthus Oregano *(Plectranthus amboinicus)*

The leaves of this plant have been used in traditional medicine for coughs, sore throats, and nasal congestion. Also used for infections and rheumatism, Plectranthus Oregano's flavor makes it popular for cooking, especially in soups.

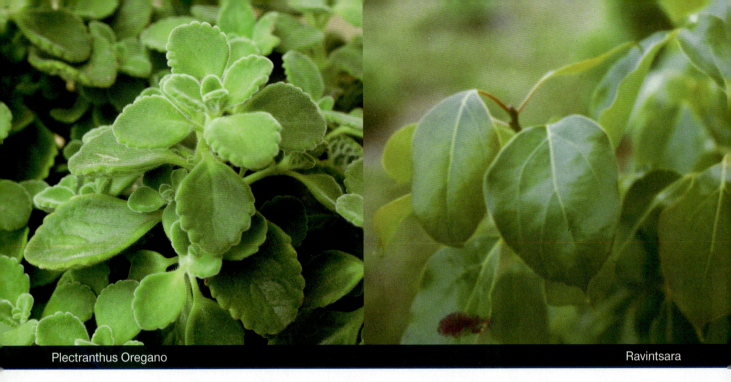

Plectranthus Oregano

Ravintsara

**Medical Properties:** Antitumoral, antibacterial, antioxidant, analgesic, anti-inflammatory, antihyperlipodemic, liver protectant

**Uses:** Infections, cancer, arthritis, diabetes, rheumatism

**Directions: Aromatic:** Diffuse up to 1 hour 3 times daily or directly inhale. **Topical:** Dilute 1 drop essential oil with 4 drops V-6 or other pure carrier oil and apply 2-4 drops on location, chakras, and/or Vita Flex points.

**Technical Data: Botanical Family:** Lamiaceae; **Plant Origin:** Ecuador; **Extraction Method:** Steam distilled from leaves; **Key Constituents:** Para-Cymene (14-27%), Gamma-Terpinene (16-24%), Carvacrol (25-45%), Beta-Caryophyllene (4-11%), Alpha-Bergamotene (2-6%)

### Selected Research

Arumugam G, et al. *Plectranthus amboinicus* (Lour,) Spreng: Botanical, Phytochemical, Pharmacological and Nutritional Significance. *Molecules.* 2016 Mar 30;21(4). Pii: E369.

Santos NO, et al. Assessing the Chemical Composition and Antimicrobial Activity of Essential Oils from Brazilian Plants—*Eremanthus erythropappus* (Asteraceae) *Plectranthus barbatus,* and *P. amboinicus* (Lamoaceae). *Molecules.* 2015 May 11;20(5):8440-52.

Manjamalai A, Grace VM. The chemotherapeutic effect of essential oil of *Plectranthus amboinicus* (Lour) on lung metastasis developed by B16F-10 cell line in C57BL/6 mice. *Cancer Invest.* 2013 Jan;31(1):74-82.

de Oliveira FF, et al. Efficacy of *Plectranthus amboinicus* (Lour.) Spreng in a Murine Model of Methicillin-Resistant *Staphylococcus aureus* Skin Abscesses. *Evid Based Complement Alternat Med.* 2013;2013:291592.

Gonçalves TB, et al. Effect of subinhibitory and inhibitory concentrations of *Plectranthus amboinicus* (Lour.) Spreng essential oil on *Klebsiella pneumoniae. Phytomedicine.* 2012 Aug 15;19(11):962-8.

Viswanathaswamy AH, et al. Antihyperglycemic and antihyperlipidemic activity of *Plectranthus amboinicus* on normal and alloxan-induced diabetic rats. *Indian J Pharm Sci.* 2011 Mar;73(2):139-45.

## Ravintsara *(Cinnamomum camphora)*

Ravintsara is referred to by the people of Madagascar as "the oil that heals." It is antimicrobial and supporting to the nerves and respiratory system. It is also known to be clarifying, stimulating, and purifying. It also helps to clear brain fog and strengthen motivation.

**Medical Properties:** Antitumoral, antiviral, antibacterial

**Uses:** Herpes virus/viral infections (including colds, respiratory infections), throat/lung infections, hepatitis, shingles, pneumonia

**Directions: Aromatic:** Diffuse up to 30 minutes 3 times daily or directly inhale. **Topical:** Dilute 1 drop essential oil with 1 drop V-6 or other pure carrier oil and apply on location, chakras, and/or Vita Flex points.

**Technical Data: Botanical Family:** Lauraceae; **Plant Origin:** Madagascar; **Extraction Method:** Steam distilled from branches and leaves; **Key Constituents:** 1,8-Cineole (Eucalyptol) (50-65%), Sabinene (9-16%), Alpha-Terpineol (5-10%), Alpha-Pinene (4-6%); **ORAC:** 890 µTE/100g

### Selected Research

Jiang H, et al. GCxGC-TOFMS Analysis of Essential Oils Composition from Leaves, Twigs and Seeds of *Cinnamomum camphora* L. Presl and Their Insecticidal and Repellent Activities. *Molecules.* 2016 Mar 28;21(4) pii; E423.

Marasini BP, et al. Evaluation of antibacterial activity of some traditionally used medicinal plants against human pathogenic bacteria. *Biomed Res Int.* 2015;2015:265425. [Epub ahead of print]

Yang F, et al. Linalool, derived from *Cinnamomum camphora* (L.) Presl leaf extracts, possesses molluscicidal activity against *Oncomelania hupensis* and inhibits infection of *Schistosoma japonicum. Parasit Vectors.* 2014 Aug 29;7:407 [Epub ahead of print]

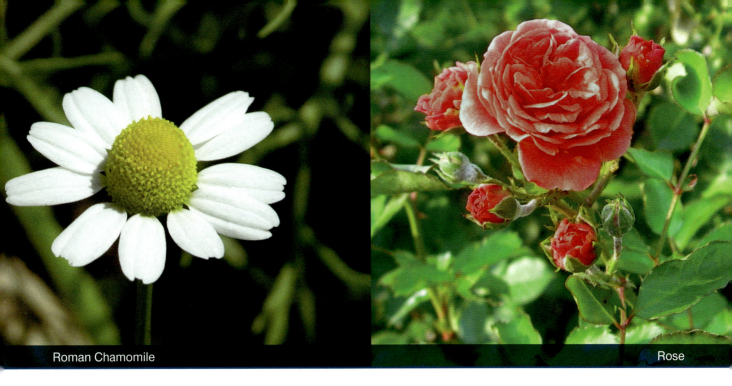

Roman Chamomile

Rose

Li H, et al. [Study on anti-inflammatory effect of different chemotype of *Cinnamomum camphora* on rat arthritis model induced by Freund's adjuvant]. *Zhongguo Zhong Za Zhi.* 2009 Dec;34(24):3251-4.

Lee HJ, et al. In vitro anti-inflammatory and anti-oxidative effects of *Cinnamomum camphora* extracts. *J. Ethnopharmacol.* 2006 Jan;103(2):208-216.

## Roman Chamomile
### (Anthemis nobilis) (Syn. Chamaemelum nobile)

Used in Europe for skin regeneration. For centuries, mothers have used chamomile to calm crying children, combat digestive and liver ailments, and relieve toothaches.

**Medical Properties:** Relaxant, antispasmodic, anti-inflammatory, antiparasitic, antibacterial, anesthetic

**Uses:** Relieves restlessness, anxiety, ADHD, depression, insomnia, skin conditions (acne, dermatitis, eczema)

**Fragrant Influence:** Because it is calming and relaxing, it can combat depression, insomnia, and stress. It minimizes anxiety, irritability, and nervousness. It may also dispel anger, stabilize the emotions, and help to release emotions that are linked to the past.

**Directions: Aromatic:** Diffuse up to 30 minutes 3 times daily or directly inhale. **Topical:** Apply 2-4 drops on location, chakras, and/or Vita Flex points. Dilution not required except for the most sensitive skin.

**Technical Data: Botanical Family:** Asteraceae; **Plant Origin:** Utah, France; **Extraction Method:** Steam distilled from flowering top; **Key Constituents:** Isobutyl Angelate + Isamyl Methacrylate (30-45%), Isoamyl Angelate (12-22%), Methyl Allyl Angelate (6-10%), Isobutyl n-butyrate (2-9%), 2-Methyl Butyl Angelate (3-7%); **ORAC:** 240 µTE/100g

## Selected Research

Guimarães R, et al. Wild Roman chamomile extracts and phenolic compounds: enzymatic assays and molecular modelling studies with VEGFR-2 tyrosine kinase. *Food Funct.* 2016 Jan 20;7(1):79-83.

Kazemian H, et al. Antibacterial, anti-swarming and anti-biofilm formation activities of *Chamaemelum nobile* against *Pseudomonas aeruginosa*. *Rev Soc Bras Med Trop.* 2015 Aug;48(4):432-6.

Zhao J, et al. Octulosonic acid derivatives from Roman chamomile (*Chamaemelum nobile*) with activities against inflammation and metabolic disorder. *J Nat Prod.* 2014 Mar 28;77(3):509-15.

Zeggwagh NA, et al. Vascular effects of aqueous extract of *Chamaemelum nobile*: in vitro pharmacological studies in rats. *Clin Exp Hypertens.* 2013;35(3):300-6.

Srivastava JK, et al. Chamomile: A herbal medicine of the past with bright future. *Mol Med Res.* 2010 Nov 1;3(6):895-901.

Eddouks M, et al. Potent hypoglycemic activity of the aqueous extract of *Chamaemelum nobile* in normal and streptozotocin-induced rats. *Diabetes Res Clin Pract.* 2005 Mar;67(3):189-95.

## Rose (Rosa damascena)

Rose has been used for the skin for thousands of years. The Arab physician, Avicenna, was responsible for first distilling rose oil, eventually authoring an entire book on the healing attributes of the rose water derived from the distillation of rose. Throughout much of ancient history, the oil was produced by enfleurage, a process of pressing the petals along with a vegetable oil to extract the essence. Today, however, almost all rose oils are solvent extracted.

**Note:** The Bulgarian *Rosa damascena* (high in citronellol) is very different from Moroccan *Rosa centifolia* (high in phenyl ethanol). They have different colors, aromas, and therapeutic actions.

**Medical Properties:** Anti-inflammatory, anti-HIV, antioxidant, anxiolytic, hepatoprotective, relaxant, reduces scarring, antiulcer, immunomodulating, cancer chemopreventive, DNA damage prevention

**Uses:** Hypertension, heart strengthening, anxiety, viral infections (herpes simplex), skin conditions (scarring, wrinkles, acne), ulcers

**Fragrant Influence:** Its beautiful fragrance is intoxicating and aphrodisiac-like. It helps bring balance and harmony, allowing one to overcome insecurities. The effect of rose on the heart brings good cheer with calming and a lightness of spirit.

**Directions: Aromatic:** Diffuse up to 1 hour 3 times daily or directly inhale. **Dietary:** Take as a dietary supplement. **Topical:** Apply 2-4 drops on location, chakras, and/or Vita Flex points. Dilution not required except for the most sensitive skin.

**Technical Data: Botanical Family:** Rosaceae; **Plant Origin:** Bulgaria, Turkey; **Extraction Method:** Therapeutic-grade oil is steam distilled from flowers (a two-part process); **Key Constituents:** Citronellol (24-50%), Geraniol (10-22%), Nerol (5-12%), Beta-Phenylethyl Alcohol (0.5-5%); **ORAC:** 160,400 µTE/100g

**Selected Research**

Mahboubi M. *Rosa damascena* as holy ancient herb with novel applications. *J Tradit Complement Med.* e-Collection 2016 Jan.

Esfandiary E, et al. Novel effects of *Rosa damascena* extract on memory and neurogenesis in a rat model of Alzheimer's disease. *Adv Biomed Res* 2015 Jul 27. [Epub ahead of print]

Mohammadpour T, et al. Protection against brain tissues oxidative damage as a possible mechanism for the beneficial effects of *Rosa damascena* hydroalcoholic extract on scopolamine induced memory impairment in rats. *Nutr Neurosci.* 2014 Jun 29. [Epub ahead of print]

Bani S, et al. The Effect of *Rosa Damascena* Extract on Primary Dysmenorrhea: A Double-blind Cross-over Clinical Trial. *Iran Red Crescent Med J.* 2014 Jan;16(1):e14643.

Abbasi Maleki N, et al. Suppressive effects of *Rosa damascena* essential oil on naloxone-precipitated morphine withdrawal signs in male mice. *Iran J Pharm Res.* 2013 Summer;12(3):357-61.

Naziroğlu M, et al. Rose oil (from *Rosa x damascena* Mill.) vapor attenuates depression-induced oxidative toxicity in rat brain. *J Nat Med.* 2013 Jan;67(1):152-8.

Hongratanaworakit T. Relaxing effect of rose oil on humans. *Nat Prod Commun.* 2009 Feb;4(2):291-296.

## Rose of Sharon *(Cistus ladaniferus)*

(See Cistus)

## Rosemary *(Rosmarinus officinalis)*

Rosemary was part of the "Marseilles Vinegar" or "Four Thieves Vinegar" that bandits who robbed the dead and dying used to protect themselves during the 15th century plague. The name of the oil is derived from the Latin words for dew of the sea (ros + marinus). According to folklore history, rosemary originally had white flowers; however, they turned red after the Virgin Mary laid her cloak on the bush.

At the time of ancient Greece (about 1,000 BC), rosemary was burned as incense. Later cultures believed that it warded off devils, a practice that eventually became adopted by the sick, who then burned rosemary to protect against infection.

It was listed in Hildegard's *Medicine,* a compilation of early German medicines by highly regarded Benedictine herbalist Hildegard of Bingen (1098-1179).

Until recently, French hospitals used rosemary to disinfect the air.

**Medical Properties:** Liver-protecting, anti-inflammatory, antitumoral, antifungal, antibacterial, anticancer, antidepressant, hypertension moderator (high blood pressure), enhances mental clarity/concentration

**Uses:** Infectious disease, liver conditions/hepatitis, throat/lung infections, hair loss (alopecia areata), acne, impaired memory/Alzheimer's, weight loss

**Fragrant Influence:** Helps overcome mental fatigue and improves mental clarity and focus. University of Miami scientists found that inhaling rosemary boosted alertness, eased anxiety, and amplified analytic and mental ability.

**Directions: Aromatic:** Diffuse up to 1 hour 3 times daily or directly inhale. **Topical:** Dilute 1 drop essential oil with 1 drop V-6 or other pure carrier oil and apply 2-4 drops on location, chakras, and/or Vita Flex points.

**Cautions:** Do not use on children under 4 years of age. Do not use Rosemary for high blood pressure if already taking ACE inhibitor prescription drugs.

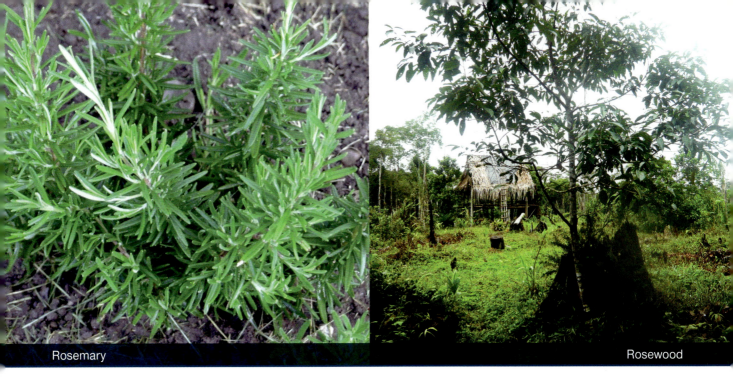

Rosemary | Rosewood

## Rosemary Vitality™ (Rosmarinus officinalis)

**Directions: Dietary:** Dilute 1 drop with 4 drops of carrier oil. Put in a capsule and take 1 daily.

**Technical Data: Botanical Family:** Lamiaceae; **Plant Origin:** Tunisia, Morocco, Spain; **Extraction Method:** Steam distilled from leaves; **Key Constituents:** 1,8-Cineole (Eucalyptol) (38-55%), Camphor (5-15%), Alpha-Pinene (9-14%), Beta-Pinene (4-9%), Camphene (2.5-6%), Borneol (1.5-5%), Limonene (1-4%); **ORAC:** 330 µTE/100g

### Selected Research

Tomi K, et al. Enantioselective GC-MS analysis of volatile components from rosemary (*Rosmarinus officinalis*) essential oils and hydrosols. *Biosci Biotechnol Biochem.* 2016 Feb 29:1-8.

El-Naggar SA, et al. Efficacy of *Rosmarinus officinalis* leaves extract against cyclophosphamide-induced hepatotoxicity. *Pharm Biol.* 2016 Feb 1:1-10.

Raskovic A, et al. Analgesic effects of rosemary essential oil and its interactions with codeine and paracetamol in mice. *Eur Rev Med Pharmacol Sci.* 2015 Jan;19(1):165-72.

da Silva Bomfim N, et al. Antifungal activity and inhibition of fumonisin production by *Rosmarinus officinalis* L. essential oil in *Fusarium verticillioides* (Sacc.) Nirenberg. *Food Chem.* 2015 Jan 1;166:330-6.

Sebai H, et al. Protective Effect of *Lavandula stoechas* and *Rosmarinus officinalis* Essential Oils Against Reproductive Damage and Oxidative Stress in Alloxan-Induced Diabetic Rats. *J Med Food.* 2014 Aug 8. [Epub ahead of print]

Gauch LM, et al. Effects of *Rosmarinus officinalis* essential oil on germ tube formation by *Candida albicans* isolated from denture wearers. *Rev Soc Bras Med Trop.* 2014 May-Jun;47(3):389-91.

Rašković A, et al. Antioxidant activity of rosemary (*Rosmarinus officinalis* L.) essential oil and its hepatoprotective potential. *BMC Complement Altern Med.* 2014 Jul 7;14:225.

Petiwala SM, et al. Rosemary (*Rosmarinus officinalis*) extract modulates CHOP/GADD153 to promote androgen receptor degradation and decreases xenograft tumor growth. *PLoS One.* 2014 Mar 5;9(3):e89772.

Petrolini FV, et al. Evaluation of the antibacterial potential of *Petroselinum crispin* and *Rosmarinus officinalis* against bacteria that cause urinary tract infections. *Braz J Microbiol.* 2013 Dec 17;44(3):829-34.

## Rosewood (Aniba rosaeodora)

Rosewood essential oil is antibacterial and antiviral, but it is most well-known for improving the skin. In France, it is used for natural skin rejuvenation.

**Medical Properties:** Antibacterial, antiviral, antiparasitic, antifungal, antimutagenic, anxiolytic, improves skin elasticity.

**Uses:** Fungal infections/candida, skin conditions (eczema, psoriasis)

**Fragrant Influence:** Empowering and emotionally stabilizing

**Directions: Aromatic:** Diffuse up to 1 hour 3 times daily or directly inhale. **Dietary:** Take as a dietary supplement. **Topical:** Apply 2-4 drops on location, chakras, and/or Vita Flex points. Dilution not required except for the most sensitive skin.

**Technical Data: Botanical Family:** Lauraceae; **Plant Origin:** Brazil; **Extraction Method:** Steam distilled from wood; **Key Constituents:** Linalol (70-90%), Alpha-Terpineol (2-7%), Alpha-Copaene (trace-3%), 1,8-Cineole (Eucalyptol) (trace-3%), Geraniol (0.5-2.5%); **ORAC:** 113,200 µTE/100g

### Selected Research

de Siqueira RJ, et al. Linalool-rich rosewood oil induces vago-vagal bradycardiac and depressor reflex in rats. *Phytother Res.* 2013 Jan;28(1):42-8.

Kohn LK, et al. In vitro activity of Brazilian plants (*Maytenus ilicifolia* and *Aniba rosaeodora*) against bovine herpesvirus type 5 and avian metapneumovirus. *Pharm Biol.* 2012 Oct;50(10):1269-75.

Seour J, et al. Selective cytotoxicity of *Aniba rosaeodora* essential oil towards epidermoid cancer cells through induction of apoptosis. *Mutat Res.* 2011 Jan 10;718(102):24-32.

Linck VM, et al. Effects of inhaled linalool in anxiety, social interaction and aggressive behavior in mice. *Phytomedicine.* 2010 Jul;17(8-9):679-683.

de Almeida RN, et al. Rosewood oil induces sedation and inhibits compound action potential in rodents. *J Ethnopharmacol.* 2009 Jul 30;124(3):440-3.

## Royal Hawaiian Sandalwood™*
### (Santalum paniculatum)

Used for centuries in Ayurvedic medicine for skin revitalization, yoga, and meditation. Listed in Dioscorides' *De Materia Medica* (AD 78), Europe's first authoritative guide to medicines, which became the standard reference work for herbal treatments for over 1,700 years.

Research at Brigham Young University in Provo, Utah, documented the oil's ability to inhibit several types of cancerous cells (Stevens).

**Medical Properties:** Antitumoral, antibacterial, antiviral, immune stimulant

**Uses:** Cancer, viral infections (herpes simplex, herpes zoster, cold sores, human papilloma virus, etc.), skin conditions (acne, wrinkles, scars, etc.)

**Fragrant Influence:** Enhances deep sleep and may help remove negative programming from the cells. It is high in sesquiterpenes that stimulate the pineal gland and the limbic region of the brain, the center of emotions. The pineal gland is responsible for releasing melatonin, a powerful immune stimulant and antitumoral agent. Can be grounding and stabilizing.

**Directions: Aromatic:** Diffuse up to 1 hour 3 times daily or directly inhale. **Dietary:** Take as a dietary supplement. **Topical:** Apply 2-4 drops on location, chakras, and/or Vita Flex points. Dilution not required except for the most sensitive skin.

**Technical Data: Botanical Family:** Santalaceae; **Plant Origin:** Hawaii; **Extraction Method:** Steam distilled from wood; **Key Constituents:** Alpha-Santalol (41-55%), Beta-Santalol (16-24%); **ORAC:** 160 µTE/100g

### Selected Research

Teixeira da Silva JA, et al. Sandalwood: basic biology, tissue culture, and genetic transformation. *Planta.* 2016 Jan 8. [Epub ahead of print]

Santha S, Dwivedi C. Anticancer Effects of Sandalwood (*Santalum album*). *Anticancer Res.* 2015 Jun;35(6):3137-45.

Dozmorov MG, et al. Differential effects of selective frankincense (Ru Xiang) essential oil versus non-selective sandalwood (Tan Xiang) essential oil on cultured bladder cancer cells: a microarray and bioinformatics study. *Chin Med.* 2014 Jul 2;9:18. [Epub ahead of print]

Paulpandi M, et al. In vitro anti-viral effect of β-santalol against influenza viral replication. *Phytomedicine.* 2012 Feb 15;19(3-4):231-5.

Kulkarni CR, et al. Antihyperglycemic and antihyperlipidemic effect of *Santalum album* in streptozotocin induced diabetic rats. *Pharm Biol.* 2012 Mar;50(3):360-5.

*Royal Hawaiian Sandalwood is a trademark of Jawmin, LLC.

## Ruta (Ruta graveolens)

Commonly known as rue. In traditional medicine it was used as a magic herb and a protection against evil. It was used to treat nervous afflictions, digestive problems, hysterics, and as an abortifacient. Formerly used to treat menstrual disorders and hysteria. Anecdotal reports suggest it has sleep-inducing properties.

**Medical Properties:** Anti-inflammatory, anti-diabetic, antimicrobial, hypotensive, anxiolytic, sleep promoting

**Uses:** Hysteria, stress, nervousness, digestion

**Fragrant Influence:** Calming and relaxing

**Directions: Aromatic:** Diffuse up to 1 hour 3 times daily or directly inhale. **Topical:** Dilute 1 drop essential oil with 1 drop V-6 or other pure carrier oil and apply 2-4 drops on location, chakras, and/or Vita Flex points.

**Caution:** Possible sun sensitivity.

**Technical Data: Botanical Family:** Rutaceae; **Plant Origin:** Ecuador; **Extraction Method:** Steam distilled from aerial parts of the herb; **Key Constituents:** 2-Nonanone (40-53%), 2-Undecanone (35-48%), 2-Nonyl Acetate (0.5-2%), Geijerene (1-3%), 2-Decanone (1-3%)

### Selected Research

Schelz Z, et al. Antiproliferative Effects of Various Furanoacridones Isolated from *Ruta graveolens* on Human Breast Cancer Cell Lines. *Anticancer Res.* 2016 Jun;36(6):2751-8.

Arora S, Tandon S. DNA fragmentation and cell cycle arrest: a hallmark of apoptosis induced by *Ruta graveolens* in human cancer cells. *Homeopathy.* 2015 Jan;104(1):36-47.

Ghosh S, et al. Graveoline isolated from ethanolic extract of *Ruta graveolens* triggers apoptosis and autophagy in skin melanoma cells: a novel apoptosis independent autophagic signaling pathway. *Phytother Res.* 2014 Aug;28(8):1153-62.

Sivakamavalli J, et al. Discrete nanoparticles of *Ruta graveolens* induces the bacterial and fungal biofilm inhibition. *Cell Commun Adhes.* 2014 Aug;21(4):229-38.

Ratheesh M, Helen A. Oral administration of alkaloid fraction from *Ruta graveolens* inhibits oxidative stress and inflammation in hypercholesterolemic rabbits. *Pharm Biol.* 2013 Dec;51(12):1552-8.

## Sacred Frankincense (Boswellia sacra)

Young Living's Sacred Frankincense oil is the first Omani Frankincense to be available to those outside of Saudi royals or the privileged of Oman. It is regarded the world over as the rarest, most sought-after aromatic in existence.

After 15 years of research, 15 trips to Oman, and numerous meetings and negotiations with Omani officials, D. Gary Young was granted the first export permit in the modern history of Oman for the release and export of the oil and permission to build a Young Living distillery in the country and to export the resulting essential oil out of Oman. Gary Young was on-site to supervise the build-

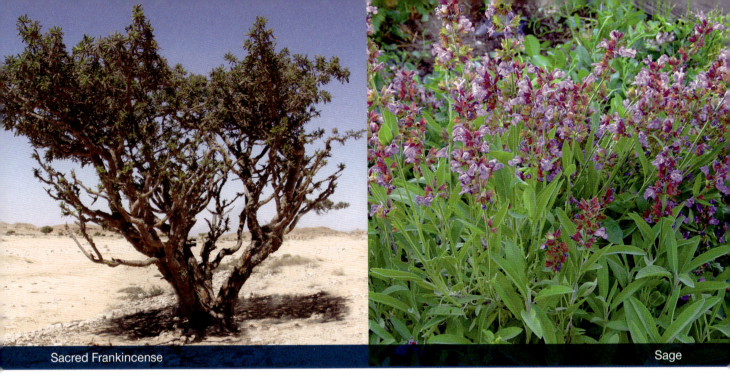

ing of Young Living's Omani distillery, and Young Living has contracted with local harvesters to secure our supply of Omani resin. This marks the first time any Westerners have been able to experience the unique spiritual properties of Sacred Frankincense essential oil.

Omani Frankincense is highly regarded as the Frankincense of the ancients and the traditional spiritual oil of biblical times. Historically, it is believed that this beautiful, white hojari resin produced the Frankincense that was taken to the Christ Child.

Science continues to document the oil's immense healing properties, which users of this oil already know.

**Medical Properties:** Frankincense has been tested as an anticancer agent (Ni, et al., 2012; Suhail, et al., 2011). Therapeutic-grade Frankincense oil contains boswellic acids, which are potent anti-inflammatory agents against rheumatoid arthritis and osteoporosis.

**Traditional Uses:** It supports skin health and treats stomach disorders, ulcers, cancer, dental and gum diseases, bad blood, infections, mental disorders, and insect bites. It is calming, meditative, relaxing, and promotes higher states of spiritual awareness and higher levels of consciousness and sensitivity.

**Directions: Aromatic:** Diffuse up to 1 hour 3 times daily or directly inhale. **Dietary:** Put 2 drops in a capsule and take 3 times daily or as needed or put 1-2 drops in water and drink. **Topical:** Apply 2-4 drops on location, chakras, and/or Vita Flex points. Dilution is not required except for the most sensitive skin.

**Complement to:** *Boswellia carterii*, traditional frankincense

**Technical Data: Botanical Family:** Burseraceae; **Plant Origin:** Oman; **Extraction Method:** Steam distilled from gum/resin; **Key Constituents:** Alpha-pinene (53-90%), Camphene (1-4%), Sabinene (1-7%), Para-cymene (0.4-4%), Limonene (2-7.5%)

**Selected Research**

Grover AK, Samson SE. Benefits of antioxidant supplements for knee osteoarthritis: rationale and reality. *Nutr. J.* 2016 Jan 5;15(1):1. [Epub ahead of print]

Niebler J, Buettner A. Identification of odorants in frankincense (*Boswellia sacra* Fleuck.) by aroma extract dilution analysis and two-dimensional gas chromatography-mass spectrometry/olfactometry. *Phytochemistry.* 2015 Jan;109:66-75.

Al-Harrasi A, et al. Analgesic effects of crude extracts and fractions of Omani frankincense obtained from traditional medicinal plant *Boswellia sacra* on animal models. *Asian Pac J Trop Med.* 2014 Sep;7S1:S485-90.

Ni X, et al. Frankincense essential oil prepared from hydrodistillation of *Boswellia sacra* gum resins induces human pancreatic cancer cell death in cultures and in a xenograft murine model. *BMC Complement Alternat Med.* 2012 Dec 13;12:253.

Woolley CL, et al. Chemical differentiation of *Boswellia sacra* and *Boswellia carterii* essential oils by gas chromatography and chiral gas chromatography-mass spectrometry. *J Chromatogr A.* 2012 Oct 26;1261:158-63.

Suhail MM, et al. *Boswellia sacra* essential oil induces tumor cell-specific apoptosis and suppresses tumor aggressiveness in cultured human breast cancer cells. *BMC Complement Alternat Med.* 2011 Dec;11:129.

## Sage *(Salvia officinalis)*

Known as "herba sacra" or sacred herb by the ancient Romans, sage's name, *Salvia,* is derived from the word for "salvation." Sage has been used in Europe for oral infections and skin conditions. It has been recognized for its benefits of strengthening the vital centers and supporting metabolism.

**Medical Properties:** Antibacterial, antifungal, antioxidant, antitumoral, anti-inflammatory, anxiolytic, hormone regulating, estrogen-like, antiviral, circulatory stimulant, gallbladder stimulant

**Uses:** Menstrual problems/PMS, estrogen, progesterone, and testosterone deficiencies, liver problems

**Fragrant Influence:** Mentally stimulating, anxiety-reducing, and helps combat despair and mental fatigue. Sage strengthens the vital centers of the body, balancing the pelvic chakra, where negative emotions from denial and abuse are stored.

**Directions: Aromatic:** Diffuse up to 1 hour 3 times daily or directly inhale. **Dietary:** Dilute 1 drop essential oil with 4 drops V-6 or other pure carrier oil. Put in a capsule and take 1 daily or as directed by a health care professional. **Topical:** Dilute 1 drop essential oil with 1 drop V-6 or other pure carrier oil and apply 2-4 drops on location, chakras, and/or Vita Flex points.

**Cautions:** Avoid if epileptic. Avoid use on persons with high blood pressure.

## Sage Vitality™ (Salvia officinalis)

**Directions: Dietary:** Dilute 2 drops with 4 drops of carrier oil. Put in a capsule and take 1 daily.

**Cautions:** Avoid if epileptic. Avoid use by persons with high blood pressure.

**Technical Data: Botanical Family:** Lamiaceae; **Plant Origin:** Spain, Croatia, France; **Extraction Method:** Steam distilled from leaves; **Key Constituents:** Alpha-Thujone (18-43%), Beta-Thujone (3-8.5%), 1,8-Cineole (Eucalyptol) (5.5-13%), Camphor (4.5-24.5%), Camphene (1.5-7%), Alpha-Pinene (1-6.5%), Alpha-Humulene (trace-12%); **ORAC:** 14,800 µTE/100g

### Selected Research

Garcia CS, et al. Pharmacological perspectives from Brazilian *Salvia officinalis* (Lamiaceae): antioxidant, and antitumor in mammalian cells. *An Acad Bras Cienc.* 2016 Feb 2. [Epub ahead of print]

Chovanová R, et al. The inhibition of the Tet(K) efflux pump of tetracycline resistant *Staphylococcus epidermis* by essential oils from three Salvia species. *Lett Appl Microbiol.* 2015 Jul;61(1):58-62.

Martins N, et al. Evaluation of bioactive properties and phenolic compounds in different extracts prepared from *Salvia officinalis* L. *Food Chem.* 2015 Mar 1;170:378-85.

Miroddi M, et al. Systematic review of clinical trials assessing pharmacological properties of Salvia species on memory, cognitive impairment and Alzheimer's disease. *CNS Neurological Ther.* 2014 Jun;20(6):485-95.

Zare Shahneh F, et al. Inhibitory and cytoxic activities of *Salvia officinalis* L. extract on human lymphoma and leukemia cells by induction of apoptosis. *Adv Pharm Bull.* 2013;3(1):51-5.

Kozics K, et al. Effects of *Salvia officinalis* and *Thymus vulgaris* on oxidant-induced DNA damage and antioxidant status in Hep22 cells. *Food Chem.* 2013 Dec 1;141(3):2198-206.

Rahte S, et al. *Salvia officinalis* for Hot Flushes: Towards Determination of Mechanism of Activity and Active Principles. *Planta Med.* 2013 Jun;79(9):753-60.

## Sandalwood (Santalum album)
(See also Royal Hawaiian Sandalwood)

**Technical Data: Botanical Family:** Santalaceae; **Plant Origin:** Australia; **Extraction Method:** Steam distilled from wood; **Key Constituents:** Alpha-Santalol (41-55%), Beta-Santalol (16-24%); ORAC: 160 µTE/100g

## Spanish Sage (Salvia lavandulifolia)
(Also referred to as Sage Lavender)

The sage plant has been highly praised throughout history for its powers of longevity and healing. Pliny the Elder said that sage (called "salvia" by the Romans) was used as a local anesthetic for the skin and as a diuretic, in addition to other uses. It was considered a sacred herb to the Romans and was harvested by a person wearing a white tunic, who had well-washed, bare feet.

During the Middle Ages, the plant was prized throughout Europe because of its exceptional healing effects and was used in a mixture with other herbs designed to ward off the plague.

In Spain, Spanish sage is used in cooking. It has a stronger aroma and flavor than common sage (*S. officinalis*).

**Medical Properties:** Antiseptic, astringent, chemopreventive, expectorant, reduces mucous, reduces fevers, purifies the blood, eliminates toxins, aids digestion, lowers blood sugar levels without affecting insulin levels, acts as a tonic to improve general health

**Uses:** Age-related memory loss, cuts, acne, arthritis, dandruff, colds, flu, eczema, hair loss, sweating, anxiety, headaches, asthma, laryngitis, coughs, muscular aches and pains, depression, epilepsy, soothing agent, menstrual disorders, digestive disorders. In food it is used as a spice; in manufacturing it is used as a fragrance component in soaps and cosmetics

**Fragrant Influence:** Camphoraceous, herbaceous, similar to rosemary

**Directions: Aromatic:** Diffuse up to 1 hour 3 times daily or directly inhale. **Dietary:** Take as a dietary supplement. **Topical:** Dilute 1 drop essential oil with 1 drop V-6 or other pure carrier oil and apply 2-4 drops on location, chakras, and/or Vita Flex points.

**Cautions:** Avoid if epileptic. Avoid use on persons with high blood pressure.

**Technical Data: Botanical Family:** Lamiaceae; **Plant Origin:** Central Europe and Asia Minor, esp. Spain; **Extraction Method:** Steam distilled from the leaves; **Key Constituents:** 1,8-cineole (Eucalyptol) (10-30%), Alpha-Pinene (4-11%), Limonene (2-6%), Camphor (11-36%), Linalol (0.3-4%), Alpha-Terpinyl Acetate (0.5-9%), Linalyl Acetate (0.1-5%)

130 | Chapter 6 | Single Oils

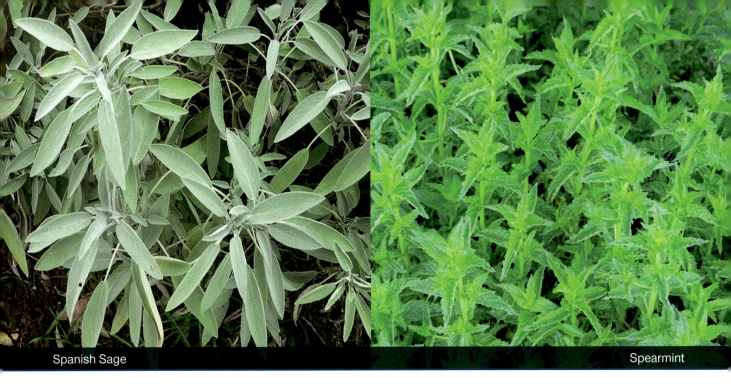

Spanish Sage | Spearmint

### Selected Research

Porres-Martinez M, et al. Protective properties of *Salvia lavandulifolia* Vahl. essential oil against oxidative stress-induced neuronal injury. *Food Chem Toxicol.* 2015 Jun;80:154-62.

Miroddi M, et al. Systematic review of clinical trials assessing pharmacological properties of Salvia species on memory, cognitive impairment and Alzheimer's disease. *CNS Neurological Ther.* 2014 Jun;20(6):485-95.

Kennedy DO, et al. Monoterpenoid extract of sage (*Salvia lavandulaefolia*) with cholinesterase inhibiting properties improves cognitive performance and mood in healthy adults. *J Psychopharmacol.* 2011 Aug;25(8):1088-100.

Ramos AA, et al. Protection by *Salvia* extracts against oxidative and alkylation damage to DNA In human HCT15 and CO115 cells. *J Toxicol Environ Health A.* 2012;75(13-15):765-75.

## Spearmint (Mentha spicata)

Spearmint is gentler than peppermint yet is beneficial for headaches and migraines, fatigue, nervous disorders, and digestive problems.

**Medical Properties:** Increases metabolism, antibacterial, antispasmodic, anti-inflammatory, antiseptic, mucolytic, gallbladder stimulant, digestive aid, antitumor

**Uses:** Obesity, intestinal/digestive disorders, nausea, hepatitis

**Fragrant Influence:** Opens and releases emotional blocks and brings about a feeling of balance and a lasting sense of well-being

**Directions: Aromatic:** Diffuse up to 1 hour 3 times daily or directly inhale. **Topical:** Dilute 1 drop essential oil with 1 drop V-6 or other pure carrier oil and apply 2-4 drops on location, chakras, and/or Vita Flex points.

## Spearmint Vitality™ (Mentha spicata)

**Directions: Dietary:** Dilute 1 drop with 1 drop of carrier oil. Put in a capsule and take up to 3 times daily.

**Technical Data: Botanical Family:** Lamiaceae; **Plant Origin:** Utah, China; **Extraction Method:** Steam distilled from leaves; **Key Constituents:** Carvone (45-80%), Limonene (10-30%), Cis-Dihydrocarvone (1-8%); **ORAC:** 540 µTE/100g

### Selected Research

Nogoceke FP, et al. Antimanic-like effects of (R)-(-)-carvone and (S)-(+)-carvone in mice. *Neurosci Lett.* 2016 Mar 9. [Epub ahead of print]

Shahbazi Y. Chemical Composition and In Vitro Antibacterial Activity of *Mentha spicata* Essential Oil against Common Food-Borne Pathenogenic Bacteria. *J Pathog.* 2015:2015. [Epub ahead of print]

Snoussi M, et al. *Mentha spicata* Essential Oil: Chemical Composition, Antioxidant and Antibacterial Activities against Planktonic and Biofilm Cultures of *Vibrio* pp. Strains. *Molecules.* 2015 Aug 7;20(8):14402-24.

Tayarani-Najaran Z, et al. Antiemetic activity of volatile oil from *Mentha spicata* and *Mentha x piperita* in chemotherapy-induced nausea and vomiting. *Ecancermedicalscience.* 2013;7:290.

Mousavi NS, et al. Effects of Subinhibitory Concentrations of Essential Oils of *Mentha spicata* and *Cuminum cyminum* on Virulence Factors of *Pseudomonas aeruginosa. J Med Plants.* Vol. 9, Suppl. No. 6, Winter 2010.

## Spikenard (Nardostachys jatamansi)

Highly regarded in India as a medicinal herb. It was the one of the most precious oils in ancient times, used only by priests, kings, or high initiates. References in the New Testament describe how Mary of Bethany used spikenard oil to anoint the feet of Jesus before the Last Supper (John 12:3).

**Medical Properties:** Antibacterial, antifungal, anti-inflammatory, antioxidant, relaxant, immune stimulant

**Uses:** Insomnia, menstrual problems/PMS, heart arrhythmias, nervous tension

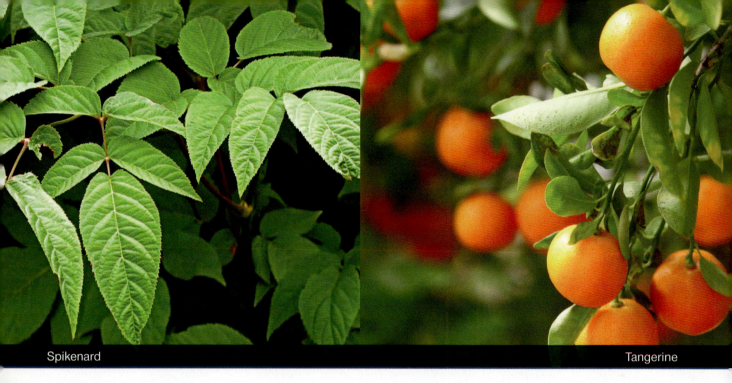

Spikenard                                                                                          Tangerine

**Fragrant Influence:** Relaxing, soothing, helps nourish and regenerate the skin

**Directions**: **Aromatic:** Diffuse up to 1 hour 3 times daily or directly inhale. **Dietary:** Take as a dietary supplement. **Topical:** Apply 2-4 drops on location, chakras, and/or Vita Flex points. Dilution not required except for the most sensitive skin.

**Technical Data:** **Botanical Family:** Valerianaceae; **Plant Origin:** India; **Extraction Method:** Steam distilled from roots; **Key Constituents:** Calarene (10-35%), Beta-Maaliene (4-13%), Alpha-Copaene (5-14%), Aristolene (2-9%), Seychellene (1-5%), Patchouli Alcohol (2-7%), 9-Aristolen-1-ol (1-5%); **ORAC:** 54,800 µTE/100g

### Selected Research

Chaudhary S, et al. Evaluation of antioxidant and anticancer activity of extract and fractions of *Nardostachys jatamansi* DC in breast carcinoma. *BMC Complement Altern Med.* 2015 Mar 10;15:50.

Bae GS, et al. Beneficial Effects of Fractions of *Nardostacys jatamansi* on Lipopolysaccharide-Induced Inflammatory Response. *Evid Based Complement Alternat Med.* 2014;2014837835. [Epub ahead of print]

Dhuna K, et al. Cytoprotective effect of methanolic extract of *Nardostacys jatamansi* against hydrogen peroxide induced oxidative damage I C6 glioma cells. *Acta Biochem Pol.* 2013;60(1):21-31.

Lyle N, et al. Stress modulating antioxidant effect of *Nardostachys jatamansi*. *Indian J Biochem Biophys.* 2009 Feb;46(1):93-98.

## Tangerine *(Citrus reticulata)*

Because of Tangerine essential oil's high limonene content, it is a great booster for the immune system.

**Medical Properties:** Antitumoral, relaxant, antispasmodic, digestive aid, and circulatory enhancer; rich in limonene, which has been extensively studied in over 50 clinical studies for its ability to combat tumor growth.

**Uses:** Obesity, anxiety, insomnia, irritability, lung health, learning and memory support, Alzheimer's, liver problems, digestive problems, parasites, fluid retention

**Fragrant Influence:** Promotes happiness, calming, helps with anxiety and nervousness. A Mie University study found that citrus fragrances boosted immunity, induced relaxation, and reduced depression (Komori, et al., 1995).

**Directions:** **Aromatic:** Diffuse up to 1 hour 3 times daily or directly inhale. **Topical:** Dilute 1 drop essential oil with 1 drop V-6 or other pure carrier oil and apply 2-4 drops on location, chakras, and/or Vita Flex points.

**Caution:** Possible sun sensitivity.

## Tangerine Vitality™ *(Citrus reticulata)*

**Directions:** **Dietary:** Put 2 drops in a capsule. Take 3 times daily.

**Technical Data:** **Botanical Family:** Rutaceae; **Plant Origin:** Brazil; **Extraction Method:** Cold pressed from rind; **Key Constituents:** Limonene (90-97%), Gamma-Terpinene (0.3-3%), Myrcene (1-3%)

### Selected Research

Fomani M, et al. Oxidative burst inhibition, cytotoxicity and antibacterial acriquinoline alkaloids from *Citrus reticulata* (Blanco). *Bioorg Med Chem Lett.* 2016 Jan 15;26(2):306-9.

Tao N, et al. Anti-fungal activity of *Citrus reticulata* Blanco essential oil against *Penicillium italicum* and *Penicillium digitatum*. *Food Chem.* 2014 Jun 15;153:265-71.

Zhang Y, et al. Phenolic compositions and antioxidant capacities of Chinese wild mandarin (*Citrus reticulata* Blanco) fruits. *Food Chem.* 2014 Feb 15;145:674-80.

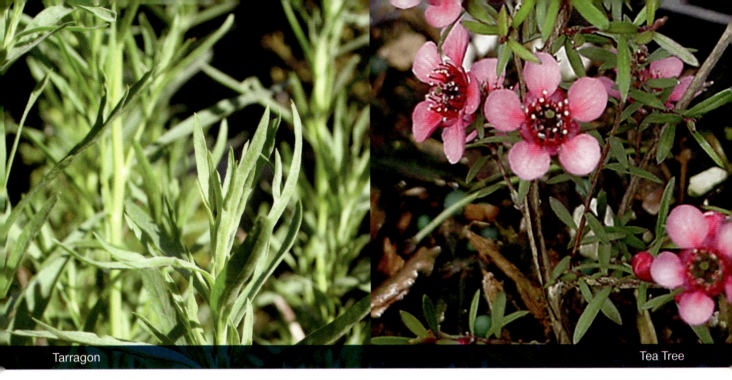

Tarragon

Tea Tree

Kawahata I, et al. Potent activity of nobiletin-rich *Citrus reticulata* peel extract to facilitate cAMP/ERK/CREB-signaling associated with learning and memory in cultured hippocampal neurons: identification of the substances responsible for pharmacological action. *J Neural Transm.* 2013 Apr 16. [Epub ahead of print]

Seki T, et al. Nobiletin-rich *Citrus reticulata* peels, a kampo medicine for Alzheimer's disease: a case series. *Geriatr Gerontol Int.* 2013 Jan;13(1):236-8.

Kim MJ, et al. *Citrus reticulata* Blanco induces apoptosis in human gastric cancer cells SNU-668. *Nutr Cancer.* 2005;51(1):78-82.

## Tarragon (Artemisia dracunculus)

Tarragon's botanical name is from the Greek and Latin. Artemisia is for the Greek goddess Artemis, and dracunculus is derived from the Latin for "little dragon." However intimidating the name, tarragon was recommended by the Arab healer Avicenna for bad digestion. Tarragon may have been introduced to Europe by the Crusaders returning from the Middle East.

**Medical Properties:** Antispasmodic, antibacterial, anti-inflammatory, antiparasitic, digestive aid, anticonvulsant, enhances insulin sensitivity

**Uses:** Intestinal disorders, urinary tract infection, nausea, menstrual problems/PMS

**Fragrant Influence:** May help alleviate deep depression

**Directions: Aromatic:** Diffuse up to 30 minutes 3 times daily or directly inhale. **Topical:** Dilute 1 drop essential oil with 1 drop V-6 or other pure carrier oil and apply 2-4 drops on location, chakras, and/or Vita Flex points.

**Caution:** Avoid use if epileptic.

## Tarragon Vitality™ (Artemisia dracunculus)

**Directions: Dietary:** Dilute 1 drop with 4 drops of carrier oil. Put in a capsule and take 1 daily or as needed.

**Caution:** Avoid use if epileptic.

**Technical Data: Botanical Family:** Asteraceae; **Plant Origin:** Italy; **Extraction Method:** Steam distilled from leaves; **Key Constituents:** Methyl Chavicol (Estragole) (68-80%), Trans-Beta-Ocimene (6-12%), Cis-Beta-Ocimene (6-12%), Limonene (2-6%); **ORAC:** 37,900 µTE/100g

### Selected Research

Talbi M, et al. Two natural compounds—a benzofuran and a phenylpropane—from *Artemisia dracunculus*. *J Asian Nat Prod Res.* 2016 Mar 16. [Epub ahead of print]

Mohammad Reza S, et al. The Nociceptive and Anti-Inflammatory Effects of *Artemisia dracunculus* L. Aqueous Extract on Fructose Fed Male Rats. *Evid Based Complement Alternat Med.* 2015;2015. [Epub ahead of print]

Maham M, et al. Antinociceptive effect of the essential oil of tarragon (*Artemisia dracunculus*). *Pharm Biol.* 2014 Feb;52(2):208-12.

Obanda DN, et al. Bioactives of *Artemisia dracunculus* L. enhance insulin sensitivity by modulation of ceramide metabolism in rat skeletal muscle cells. *Nutrition.* 2014 Jul-Aug;30(7-8 Suppl):S59-66.

Hong L, Ying SH. Ethanol Extract and Isolated Constituents from *Artemisia dracunculus* Inhibit Esophageal Squamous Cell Carcinoma and Induce Apoptotic Cell Death. *Drug Res* (Stuttg). 2014 Jul 30.

## Tea Tree (Melaleuca alternifolia)

Highly regarded as an antimicrobial and antiseptic essential oil. It has high levels of terpinen-4-ol.

**Medical Properties:** Powerful antibacterial, antifungal, antiviral, antiparasitic, anti-inflammatory action

**Uses:** Fungal infections (candida, ringworm), sinus/lung infections, tooth/gum disease, water retention/hypertension, skin conditions (acne, sores)

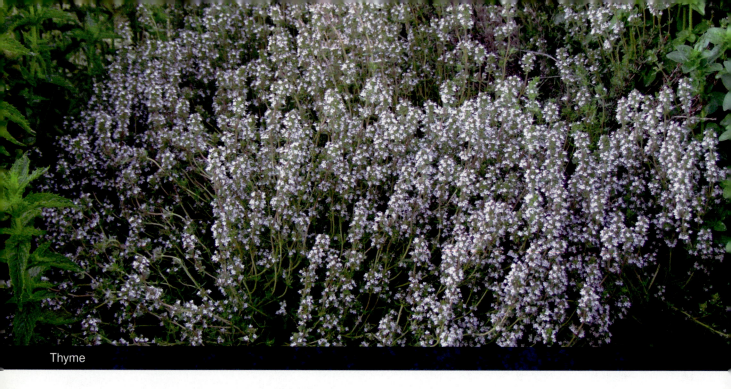

Thyme

**Fragrant Influence:** Promotes cleansing and purity

**Directions: Aromatic:** Diffuse up to 30 minutes 3 times daily or directly inhale. **Topical:** Dilute 1 drop essential oil with 1 drop V-6 or other pure carrier oil and apply 2-4 drops on location, chakras, and/or Vita Flex points.

**Technical Data: Botanical Family:** Myrtaceae; **Plant Origin:** Australia, France; **Extraction Method:** Steam distilled from leaves; **Key Constituents:** Terpinen-4-ol (30-45%), Gamma-Terpinene (10-28%), Alpha-Terpinene (5-13%), 1,8-Cineole (Eucalyptol) (0-15%), Alpha-Terpineol (1.5-8%), Para-Cymene (0.5-12%), Limonene (0.5-4%), Aromadendrene (trace-7%), Delta-Cadinene (trace-8%), Alpha-Pinene (1-6%)

### Selected Research

Li M, et al. Tea tree oil nanoemulsions for inhalation therapies of bacterial and fungal pneumonia. *Colloids Surf B Biointerfaces*. 2016 Feb 9;141:408-416.

Comin VM, et al. Influence of *Melaleuca alternifolia* oil nanoparticles on aspects of *Pseudomonas aeruginosa* biofilm. *Microb Pathog*. 2016 Jan 25. [Epub ahead of print]

Mertas A, et al. The influence of tea tree oil (*Melaleuca alternifolia*) on fluconazole activity against fluconazole-resistant *Candida albicans*. *Biomed Res. Int*. 2015;2015:590470. [Epub ahead of print]

Hammer KA. Treatment of acne with tea tree oil (melaleuca) products; a review of efficacy, tolerability and potential modes of action. *Int J Antimicrob Agents*. 2015 Feb;45(2):106-10.

Li X, et al. *Melaleuca alternifolia* Concentrate Inhibits in Vitro Entry of Influenza Virus into Host Cells. *Molecules*. 2013 Aug 9;18(8):9550-66.

Chin KB, Cordell B. The Effect of Tea Tree Oil (*Melaleuca alternifolia*) on Wound Healing Using a Dressing Model. *J Altern Complement Med*. 2013 Jul 13.

Cuaron JA, et al. Tea tree oil-induced transcriptional alterations in *Staphylococcus aureus*. *Phytother Res*. 2013 Mar;27(3):390-6.

## Thyme (Thymus vulgaris)

Also known as Red Thyme. It is mentioned in one of the oldest known medical records, the Ebers Papyrus (dating from 16th century BC), an ancient Egyptian list of 877 prescriptions and recipes. The Egyptians used thyme for embalming. Listed in Dioscorides' *De Materia Medica* (AD 78), Europe's first authoritative guide to medicines, which became the standard reference work for herbal treatments for over 1,700 years.

Thyme was listed in Hildegard's *Medicine,* a compilation of early German medicines by highly regarded Benedictine herbalist Hildegard of Bingen (1098-1179).

**Medical Properties:** Antiaging, antioxidant, anti-inflammatory, antispasmodic, highly antimicrobial, antifungal, antiviral, antiparasitic. A solution of thyme's most active ingredient, thymol, is used in many over-the-counter products such as mouthwash and vapor rubs because of its purifying agents.

**Uses:** Infectious diseases, cardiovascular disease, Alzheimer's disease, hepatitis

**Fragrant Influence:** It may be beneficial in helping to overcome fatigue and exhaustion after illness.

**Directions: Aromatic:** Diffuse up to 10 minutes 3 times daily. **Topical:** Dilute 1 drop essential oil with 4 drops V-6 or other pure carrier oil. Test on small area on the underside of arm. Apply on location, chakras, and/or Vita Flex points.

**Caution:** May irritate the nasal membranes or skin if inhaled directly from diffuser or bottle or applied neat.

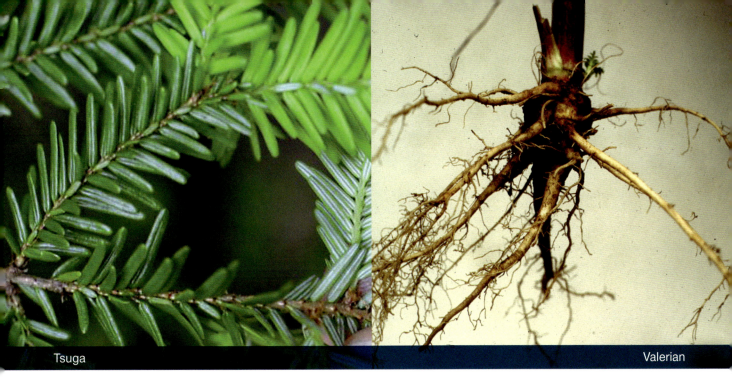

Tsuga | Valerian

### Thyme Vitality™ *(Thymus vulgaris)*

**Directions: Dietary:** Dilute 1 drop with 1 drop of carrier oil. Put in a capsule and take up to 3 times daily.

**Technical Data: Botanical Family:** Lamiaceae; **Plant Origin:** Mediterranean area; **Extraction Method:** Steam distilled from leaves, stems, flowers; **Key Constituents:** Thymol (37-55%), Para-cymene (14-28%), Gamma-Terpinene (4-11%), Linalol (3-6.5%), Carvacrol (0.5-5.5%), Myrcene (1-2.8%); **ORAC:** 15,960 µTE/100g

### Selected Research

Rudolph K, et al. Expression, crystallization and structure elucidation of γ-terpinene synthase from *Thymus vulgaris*. *Acta Crystallogr F Struct Biol Commun*. 2016 Jan 1;72(Pt 1):16-23.

Perina FJ, et al. *Thymus vulgaris* essential oil and thymol against *Alternaria alternata* (Fr.) Keissler: effects on growth, viability, early infection and cellular mnode of action. *Pest Manag Sci*. 2015 Oct;71(10):1371-8.

Ahmad A, et al. Unraveling the complex antimicrobial interactions of essential oils—the case of *Thymus vulgaris* (thyme). *Molecules*. 2014 Mar 6;19(3):2896-910.

Salmalian H, et al. Comparative effect of *Thymus vulgaris* and ibuprofen on primary dysmenorrhea: A triple-blind clinical study. *Caspiam J Intern Med*. 2014 Spring;5(2):82-8.

Grespan R, et al. Hepatoprotective Effect of Pretreatment with *Thymus vulgaris* Essential Oil Experimental Model of Acetaminophen-Induced Injury. *Evid Based Complement Alternat Med*. 2014;2014:954136.

Fachini-Queiroz FC, et al. Effects of Thymol and Carvacrol, Constituents of *Thymus vulgaris* L. Essential Oil, on the Inflammatory Response. *Evid Based Complement Alternat Med*. 2012;2012:657026.

### Tsuga *(Tsuga canadensis)*

Several North American Indian tribes used Tsuga for a number of complaints. To this day, it is used in modern herbalism for its antiseptic and astringent properties. Diarrhea, colitis, cystitis, and diverticulitis are treated by a tsuga tea; it can also be used as a poultice to cleanse wounds.

**Medical Properties:** Analgesic, antirheumatic, blood cleanser, stimulant, cell regenerating

**Uses:** Respiratory conditions, kidney/urinary infections, skin conditions, venereal diseases

**Directions: Aromatic:** Diffuse up to 30 minutes 3 times daily or directly inhale. **Topical:** Dilute 1 drop essential oil with 1 drop V-6 or other pure carrier oil and apply on location, chakras, and/or Vita Flex points.

**Technical Data: Botanical Family:** Pinaceae; **Plant Origin:** Canada; **Extraction Method:** Steam distilled from needles and twigs of the conifer tree commercially known as eastern hemlock; **Key Constituents:** Alpha-Pinene (18-25%), Beta-Pinene (1-3%), Camphene (13-17%), Limonene (3-5%), Bornyl Acetate (27-40%), Tricyclene (5-7%), Myrcene (2-5%); **ORAC:** 7,100 µTE/100g

### Selected Research

Torres A, et al. Pro-apoptotic and anti-angiogenic properties of the α/β-thujone fraction from *Thuja occidentalis* on glioblastoma cells. *J Neurooncol*. 2016 Feb 22. [Epub ahead of print]

Feucht W, et al. Nuclei of *Tsuga Canadensis:* a role of flavonols in chromatin organization. *Int J Mol Sci*. 2011;12(10):6834-55.

Feucht W, et al. Flavanol binding of nuclei from tree species. *Plant Cell Rep*. 2004;22(6):430-436.

### Valerian *(Valeriana officinalis)*

During the last three decades, valerian has been clinically investigated for its tranquilizing properties. Researchers have pinpointed the sesquiterpenes valerenic acid and valerone as the active constituents that exert a calming effect on the central nervous system. The German Commission E has pronounced valerian to be an effective treatment for restlessness and for sleep disturbances resulting from nervous conditions.

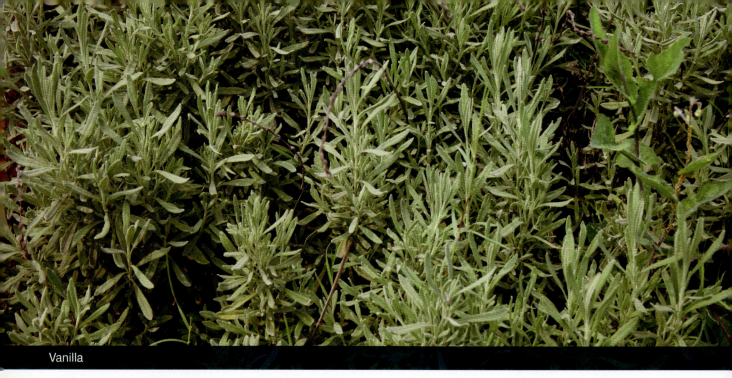
Vanilla

**Medical Properties:** Sedative and tranquilizing to the central nervous system, antispasmodic

**Uses:** Insomnia, anxiety, dysmenorrhea

**Fragrant Influence:** Calming, relaxing, grounding, emotionally balancing

**Directions: Aromatic:** Diffuse up to 1 hour 3 times daily or directly inhale. **Dietary:** Put 2 drops in a capsule and take 3 times daily or as needed. **Topical:** Apply 2-4 drops on location, chakras, and/or Vita Flex points. Dilution not required except for the most sensitive skin.

**Technical Data: Botanical Family:** Valerianaceae; **Plant Origin:** Belgium, Croatia; **Extraction Method:** Steam distilled from root; **Key Constituents:** Bornyl Acetate (35-43%), Camphene (22-31%), Alpha-Pinene (5-8%), Beta-Pinene (3-6%), Limonene (1-3%), Valerenal (2-8%), Myrtenyl Acetate (2-5%); **ORAC:** 6,200 µTE/100g

### Selected Research

Chen HW, et al. Sesquiterpenes and a monoterpenoid with acetylcholinesterase (AchE) inhibitory activity from *Valeriana officinalis* var. latiofolia in vitro and in vivo. *Fitoterapia*. 2016 Mar 11. [Epub ahead of print]

Hassani S, et al. Can *Valeriana officinalis* root extract prevent early postoperative cognitive dysfunction after CABG [coronary artery bypass graft] surgery? A randomized, double-blind, placebo-controlled study. *Psychopharmacology* (Berl). 2015 Mar;232(5):843-50.

Jung HY, et al. Valerenic Acid Protects Against Physical and Psychological Stress by Reducing the Turnover of Serotonin and Norpinephrine in Mouse Hippocampus-Amygdala Region. *J Med Food*. 2015 Jul 15. [Epub ahead of print]

Becker A, et al. The anxiolytic effects of a Valerian extract is based on valerenic acid. *BMC Complement Altern Med*. 2014 Jul 28;14:267.

Gromball J, et al. Hyperactivity, concentration difficulties and impulsiveness improve during seven weeks' treatment with valerian root and lemon balm extracts in primary school children. *Phytomedicine*. 2014 Jul-Aug;21(8-9):1098-103.

Hassani S, et al. Can *Valeriana officinalis* root extract prevent early postoperative cognitive dysfunction after CABG surgery? A randomized, double-blind, placebo-controlled trial. *Psychopharmacolog* (Berlin). 2014 Aug 31. [Epub ahead of print]

## Vanilla *(Vanilla planifolia)*

Vanilla essential oil, created for the first time by Young Living Essential Oils, is the highest known oil in vanillin, which is similar in chemical structure to the aromatic compound eugenol, found in cloves. Recent tests conducted at independent laboratories found that the vanilla content of this vanilla oil is over 10 times higher than commercially available super-concentrated vanilla extracts. The same way that eugenol in clove oil numbs dental tissue, vanillin numbs stress and food cravings.

The importance of vanillin is now being investigated by scientists who are researching the ways in which activating vanilloid-type brain receptors can enhance well-being and combat depression.

**Medical Properties:** Mood elevating; weakens or numbs stress and food cravings

**Uses:** Appetite control, depression

**Fragrant Influence:** Uplifts mood through vanilloid receptor action in brain

**Directions: Aromatic:** Diffuse up to 1 hour 3 times daily or inhale directly. **Dietary:** Take as a dietary supplement. **Topical:** Apply 2-4 drops on location, chakras, and/or Vita Flex points. Dilution not required except for the most sensitive skin.

**Technical Data: Botanical Family:** Orchidaceae; **Plant Origin:** Brazil; **Extraction Method:** Proprietary vacuum distillation; **Key Constituents:** Vanillin (85-95%)

### Selected Research

Bilcu M, et al. Efficiency of vanilla, patchouli and ylang ylang essential oils stabilized by iron oxide@C14 nanostructures against bacterial adherence and biofilms formed by *Staphylococcus aureus* and *Klebsiella pneumoniae* clinical strains. *Molecules*. 2014 Nov 4;19(11):17943-56.

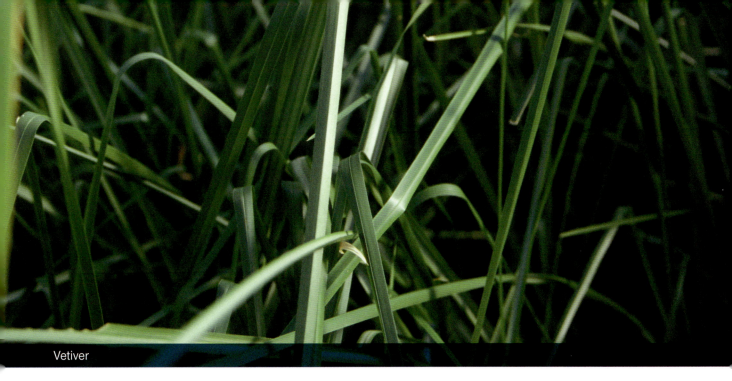
Vetiver

Kundu A, Mitra A. Flavoring Extracts of *Hemidesmus indicus* Roots and *Vanilla planifolia* Pods Exhibit In Vitro Acetylcholinesterase Inhibitory Activities. *Plant Foods Hum Nutr.* 2013 May 29. [Epub ahead of print]

Moussaieff A, et al. Incensole acetate, an incense component, elicits psychoactivity by activating TRPV3 channels in the brain, *FASEB J.* 2008 Aug;22(8):3024-34.

Widiez T, et al. Functional characterization of two new members of the caffeoyl CoA O-methyltransferase-like gene family from *Vanilla planifolia* reveals a new class of plastid-localized O-methyltransferase. *Plant Mol Biol.* 2011 Aug;76(6):475-88.

## Vetiver *(Vetiveria zizanoides) (Syn. V. zizanioides)*

It is well known for its anti-inflammatory properties and is traditionally used for arthritic symptoms.

**Medical Properties:** Antiseptic, antispasmodic, relaxant, circulatory stimulant

**Uses:** ADHD, anxiety, rheumatism/arthritis, depression (including postpartum), insomnia, skin care (oily, aging, acne, wrinkles)

**Fragrant Influence:** Psychologically grounding, calming, and stabilizing. It helps us cope with stress and recover from emotional trauma. Terry Friedmann, MD, found in preliminary clinical tests that vetiver may be successful in the treatment of ADD and ADHD (attention deficit disorders) in children (Friedmann 2002).

**Directions: Aromatic:** Diffuse up to 1 hour 3 times daily or directly inhale. **Dietary:** Take as a dietary supplement. **Topical:** Apply 2-4 drops on location, chakras, and/or Vita Flex points. Dilution not required except for the most sensitive skin. **Oral:** Gargle with mouthwash.

**Technical Data: Botanical Family:** Poaceae; **Plant Origin:** Haiti, Ecuador; **Extraction Method:** Steam distilled from root; **Key Constituents:** Isovalencenol (1-16%), Khusimol (7-21%), Alpha-Vetivone (2-7%), Beta-Vetivone (4-14%), Beta-Vetivenene (1-8%); **ORAC:** 74,300 µTE/100g

### Selected Research

Ethyl 4-(4-methylphenyl)-4 pentenoate from *Vetiver zisanioides* Inhibits Dengue NS2B-NS3 Protease and Prevents Viral Assembly: A Computational Molecular Dynamics and Docking Study. *Cell Biochem Biophys.* 2016 June 21. Epub ahead of print.

Saiyudthong S, et al. Anxiety-like behaviour and c-fos expression in rats that inhaled vetiver essential oil. *Nat Prod Res.* 2015 Nov;29(22):2141-4.

Peng HY, et al. Effect of *Vetiveria zizanioides* essential oil on melanogenesis in melanoma cells: downregulation of tyrosinase expression and suppression of oxidative stress. *ScientificWorldJournal.* 2014 Mar 19;2014:2014. [Epub ahead of print]

Gupta R, et al. Anticonvulsant activity of ethanol extracts of *Vetiveria zizanoides* roots in experimental mice. *Pharm Biol.* 2013 Dec;51(12):1521-4.

Dwivedi GR. et al. Tricyclic sesquiterpenes from *Vetiveria zizanoides* (L.) Nash as antimycobacterial agents. *Chem Biol Drug Des.* 2013 Nov;82(5):587-94.

Matsubara E, et al. Volatiles emitted from the roots of *Vetiveria zizanoides* suppress the decline in attention during a visual display task. *Biomed Res.* 2012;33(5):299-308.

Friedmann T. Attention deficit and hyperactivity disorder (ADHD). 2002. (Unpublished study) http://files.meetup.com/1481956/ADHD%20Research%20by%20Dr.%20Terry%20Friedmann.pdf.

## Western Red Cedar *(Thuja plicata)*

This oil is different from Canadian Red Cedar, which is distilled from the bark of the same plant, *Thuja plicata*. This oil is not red in color, because it is derived from needles and branches.

**Medical Properties:** Antiseptic, antimicrobial

**Uses:** Throat/lung infections, urinary tract infections

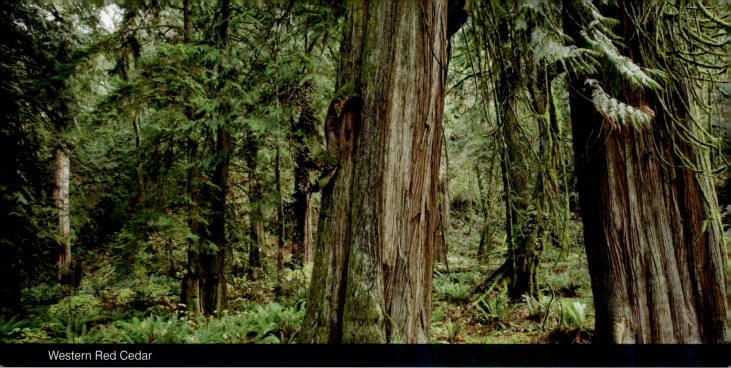
Western Red Cedar

**Fragrant Influences:** recognized for its calming, purifying properties and helping a person cope with stress and emotional traumas

**Directions: Aromatic:** Diffuse up to 1 hour 3 times daily or directly inhale. **Topical:** Dilute 1 drop essential oil with 1 drop V-6 or other pure carrier oil and apply 1-2 drops on location, chakras, and/or Vita Flex points. **Other:** Add to woodchips and place in closets and dressers to repel insects.

**Technical Data: Botanical Family:** Cupressaceae; **Plant Origin:** Utah, Idaho, Canada; **Extraction Method:** Steam distilled from needles and branches; **Key Constituents:** Alpha-Thujone (60-80%), Beta-Thujone (4-7%), Alpha-Pinene (2-20%), Sabinene (2-4%)

### Selected Research

Foster AJ, et al. Identification of genes in *Thuja plicata* foliar terpenoid defenses. *Plant Physiol.* 2013 Apr;161(4):1993-2004.

Hudson J, et al. The antimicrobial properties of cedar leaf (*Thuja plicata*) oil; a safe and efficient decontamination agent for buildings. *Int J Environ Res Public Health.* 2011 Dec;8(12):4477-4487.

Tsiri D, et al. Chemosystematic value of the essential oil composition of Thuja species cultivated in Poland—antimicrobial activity. *Molecules.* 2009 Nov 19;14(11):4707-15.

## White Fir (Abies concolor)

A white fir infusion of the needles was used as a bath by the Acoma and Laguna Indians to help with rheumatism. The Tewa Indians used the sap from the main stem and larger branches for cuts.

**Medical Properties:** Antitumoral, anticancerous, antioxidant, pain relieving

**Uses:** Respiratory infections, antifungal

**Directions: Aromatic:** Diffuse up to 1 hour 3 times daily or directly inhale. **Dietary:** Put 2 drops in a capsule. Take 3 times daily or as needed. **Topical:** Apply 2-4 drops on location, chakras, and/or Vita Flex points. Dilution not required except for the most sensitive skin.

**Technical Data: Botanical Family:** Pinaceae; **Plant Origin:** Idaho; **Extraction Method:** Steam distilled from wood/bark/twigs/needles; **Key Constituents:** Alpha-Pinene (8-12%), Beta-Pinene (20-30%), Camphene (7-15%), Bornyl Acetate (11-16%), Delta-Cadinene (2-7%); **ORAC:** 47,900 µTE/100g

### Selected Research

Bağci E, Diğrak M, Antimicrobial Activity of Essential Oils from some *Abies* (Fir) Species from Turkey. *Flavour Fragr J.* 1996 11:251-56.

Ulubelen A, et al. Phytochemical investigation of *Abies concolor. J Pharm Sci.* 1996 Nov;55(11):1308-10.

## White Lotus (Nymphaea lotus)

In ancient Egypt the lotus was used widely as a religious and ceremonial icon. In 400 AD, the Christian church of Ephesus designated Mary as "The Bearer of God." The numerous churches dedicated to Mary that were built thereafter incorporated the image of the lotus, including one image of lotus leaves, flowers, and fruits surrounding a golden cross.

**Medical Properties:** Anticancerous, anti-inflammatory, immune supporting

**Traditional Uses:** White lotus was traditionally used by the Egyptians for spiritual, emotional, and physical application. Research in China found that white lotus contains anticancerous and strong immune supporting properties.

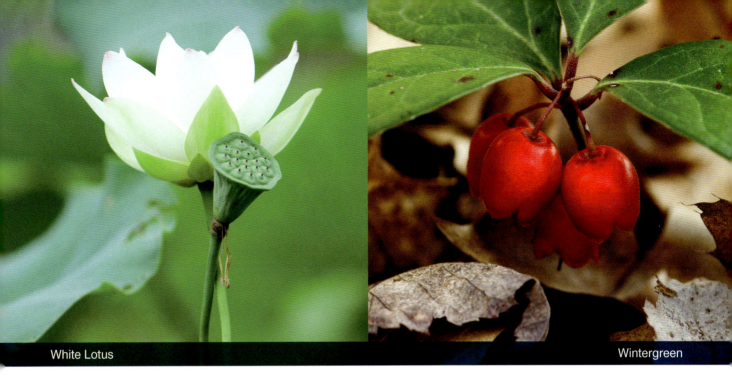

White Lotus

Wintergreen

**Other Uses:** Inflamed eyes, jaundice, kidneys, liver spots, menstruation (promotes), palpitations, rheumatism, sciatica, sprains, sunburn, toothaches, tuberculosis, vomiting

**Fragrant Influence:** Stimulates a positive attitude and a general feeling of well-being

**Directions: Topical:** Dilute 1 drop essential oil with 1 drop V-6 or other pure carrier oil and apply 1-2 drops on location, chakras, and/or Vita Flex points.

**Technical Data: Botanical Family:** Nymphaeaceae; **Plant Origin:** Egypt; **Extraction Method:** Steam distilled from the flowers; **Key Constituents:** Tetradecene (7-9%), Pentadecane (8-11%), Heptadecadiene (9-11%), Pentadecene (6-9%), Octadecene (7-10%), Ethyl-9-Hexadecenoate (9-12%), Ethyl Hexadecanoate (17-22%), Ethyl Linoleate (8-11%)

### Selected Research

Bello FH, et al. The effect of methanol rhizome extract on *Nymphaea lotus* Linn. (Nymphaeaceae) in animal modes of diarrhoea. *J Ethnopharmacol.* 2016 May 20;190:13-21.

Debnath S, et al. Inhibitory effect of *Nymphaea pubescens Willd.* [syn. *Nymphaea lotus* L.] flower extract on carrageenan-induced inflammation and CCl-induced hepatotoxicity in rats. *Food Chem Toxicol.* 2013 Jul 1. S0278-6915(13):00415-8.

Zhu M, et al. Relationship between the Composition of Flavonoids and Flower Color Variation in Tropical Water Lily (*Nymphaea*) Cultivars. *PLoS One.* 2012;7(4):e34335.

### Wintergreen (Gaultheria procumbens)

Leaves have been chewed to increase respiratory capacity by Native Americans when running long distances and performing difficult labor. Settlers in early America had their children chew the leaves for several weeks each spring to prevent tooth decay. Wintergreen was used as a substitute for black tea during the Revolutionary War.

**Medical Properties:** Anticoagulant, antispasmodic, highly anti-inflammatory, vasodilator, analgesic/anesthetic, reduces blood pressure and all types of pain. Methyl salicylate, the principal constituent of wintergreen oil, has been incorporated into numerous liniments and ointments for musculoskeletal problems. The oil is also used as a flavoring agent in candies and chewing gums.

**Uses:** Arthritis/rheumatism, muscle/nerve pain, hypertension, arteriosclerosis, hepatitis/fatty liver

**Fragrant Influence:** It stimulates and increases awareness in all levels of the sensory system.

**Directions: Aromatic:** Diffuse up to 10 minutes 3 times daily or directly inhale. **Dietary:** Take as a dietary supplement. **Topical:** Dilute 1 drop essential oil with 4 drops V-6 or other pure carrier oil. Apply 1-2 drops on location, chakras, and/or Vita Flex points.

**Cautions:** Avoid use if epileptic. Anticoagulant properties can be enhanced when used with Warfarin or aspirin.

**Technical Data: Botanical Family:** Ericaceae; **Plant Origin:** China, North America; **Extraction Method:** Steam distilled from leaves and bark; **Key Constituent:** Methyl Salicylate (90+%); **ORAC:** 101,800 µTE/100g

### Selected Research

Michel P, et al. Polyphenolic Profile, Antioxidant and Anti-Inflammatory Activity of Eastern Teaberry (*Gaultheria procumbens* L.) Leaf Extracts. *Molecules.* 2014 Dec 8;19(2):20498-20520.

Salleh FM, et al. Wintergreen oil: a novel method in Wheatley's trichrome staining technique. *J Microbiol Methods.* 2012 Oct;91(1):174-8.

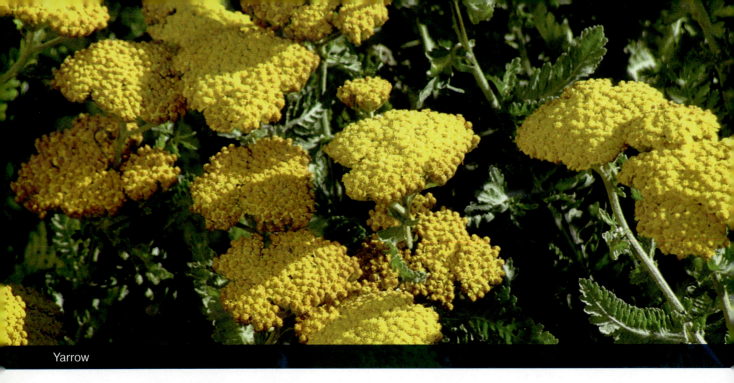
Yarrow

Tanen DA, et al. Comparison of oral aspirin versus topical applied methyl salicylate for platelet inhibition. *Ann Pharmacother.* 2008 Oct;42(10):1396-1401.

Charles CH, et al. Effect of an essential oil-containing dentifrice on dental plaque microbial composition. *Am J Dent.* 2000 Sep;13(Spec No):26C-30C.

Joss JD, LeBlond RF. Potentiation of warfarin anticoagulation associated with topical methyl salicylate. *Ann Pharmacother.* 2000 Jun;34(6):729-33.

## Xiang Mao (Cymbopogon citratus)

This aromatic grass is sometimes called red lemongrass and has been used in folk medicine as a calming agent. It was also used to keep air in the home fresh.

**Medical Properties:** Chemopreventive, antimicrobial, anxiolytic, renal protective, gastroprotective, antifungal, antiparasitic, cholesterol reducer

**Uses:** Bladder infection, respiratory/sinus infection, digestive problems, parasites, torn ligaments/muscles, fluid retention, varicose veins, Salmonella, *Candida albicans*

**Fragrant Influence:** Like its close cousin, *Cymbopogon flexuosus,* this lemongrass species sharpens awareness and is a purifier

**Directions: Aromatic:** Diffuse up to 1 hour 3 times daily or directly inhale. **Topical:** Apply 1-2 drops on location, chakras, and/or Vita Flex points. Dilution not required except on the most sensitive skin.

**Technical Data: Botanical Family:** Poaceae; **Plant Origin:** Taiwan; **Extraction Method:** Steam distilled from grasses; **Key Constituents:** Limonene (3-7%), Citronellal (40-50%), Citronellol (11-16%), Geraniol (15-18%), Germacrene-D (1-3%), Alpha-Elemol (1-2%)

### Selected Research

Leite CJ, et al. Inactivation of *Escherichia coli, Listeria monocytogenes,* and *Salmonella enteritidis* by *Cymbopogn citratratus* D.C. Stapf. Essential Oil in Pineapple Juice. *J Food Prot.* 2016 Feb;79(2):213-9.

Goes TC, et al. Effect of lemongrass aroma on Experimental Anxiety in Humans. *J Altern Complement Med.* 2015 Sept 14. [Epub ahead of print]

Sagradas J, et al. Ethnopharmacological communication gastroprotective effect of *Cymbopogon citratus* infusion on acute ethanol-induced gastric lesions in rats. *J Ethnopharmacol.* 2015 Jul 6. [Epub ahead of print]

Bao XL, et al. Polysaccharides from *Cymbopogon citratus* with antitumor and immunomodulatory activity. *Pharm Biol.* 2015 Jan;53(1):117-24.

Boukhatem MN, et al. Lemon grass (*Cymbopogon citratus*) essential oil as a potent anti-inflammatory and antifungal drug. *Libyan J Med.* 2014 Sep 19;9:25431. [Epub ahead of print]

Korenblum E, et al. Antimicrobial action and anti-corrosion effect against sulfate reducing bacteria by lemongrass *(Cymbopogon citratus)* essential oil and its major component, the citral. *AMB Express.* 2013 Aug 10;3(1):44.

Fernandes C, et al. Investigation of the mechanisms underlying the gastroprotective effect of *Cymbopogon citratus* essential oil. *J Young Pharm.* 2012 Jan;4(1):28-32.

Machado M, et al. Monoterpenic aldehydes as potential anti-Leishmania agents: activity of *Cymbopogon citratus* and citral on *L. infantum, L. tropica* and *L. major. Exp Parasitol.* 2012 Mar;130(3):223-31.

## Yarrow (Achillea millefolium)

The Greek Achilles, hero of the Trojan War, was said to have used the yarrow herb to help cure the injury to his Achilles tendon. Yarrow was considered sacred by the Chinese, who recognized the harmony of the Yin and Yang energies within it. It has been said that the fragrance of yarrow makes possible the meeting of heaven and earth. Yarrow was used by Germanic tribes for the treatment of battle wounds.

**Medical Properties:** Anti-inflammatory, hormone-like, combats scarring, supports prostate

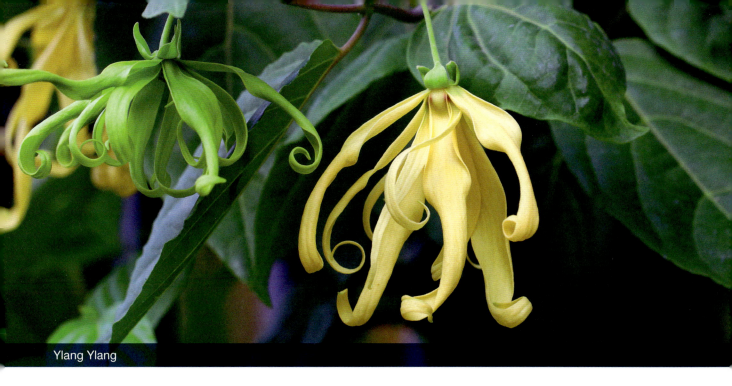
Ylang Ylang

**Uses:** Prostate problems, menstrual problems/PMS, varicose veins

**Fragrant Influence:** Balancing highs and lows, both external and internal, yarrow simultaneously inspires and grounds us. Useful during meditation and supportive to intuitive energies. Reduces confusion and ambivalence.

**Directions: Aromatic:** Diffuse up to 1 hour 3 times daily or directly inhale. **Dietary:** Put 2 drops in a capsule and take 3 times daily or as needed. **Topical:** Apply 2-4 drops on location, chakras, and/or Vita Flex points. Dilution not required except for the most sensitive skin.

**Technical Data: Botanical Family:** Asteraceae; **Plant Origin:** North America, Europe, Asia; **Extraction Method:** Steam distilled from flowers, leaves, and stems; **Key Constituents:** Chamazulene (5-18%), Trans-Beta-Caryophyllene (5-13%), Germacrene D (8-25%), Sabinene (5-15%), Beta-Pinene (4-10%), 1,8-Cineole (Eucalyptol) (2-10%); **ORAC:** 55,900 µTE/100g

### Selected Research

Freysdottir J, et al. A polysaccharide fraction from *Achillea millefolium* increases cytokine secretion and reduces activation of Akt, ERK and NF-κB in THP-1 monoccytes. *Carbohyd Polym.* 2016 Jun 5;143:131-8.

Shahani S, et al. Radioprotective Effect of *Achillea millefolium* L. Against Genotoxicity Induced by Ionizing Radiation in Human Normal Lymphocytes. *Dose Response.* 2015 Apr 29;13(1):1559325815583761.

Jenabi E, Fereidoony B. Effect of *Achillea millefolium* on Relief of Primary Dysmenorrhea: A Double-Blind Randomized Trial. *J Pediatr Adolesc Gynecol.* 2015 Oct;28(5):402-4.

Peng HY, et al. The melanogenesis alteration effects of *Achillea millefolium* L. essential oil and linalyl acetate: involvement of oxidative stress and the other JNK and ERK signaling pathways in melanoma cells. *PLoS One.* 2014 Apr 17;9(4):e95186. [Epub ahead of print]

## Ylang Ylang (Cananga odorata)

Ylang ylang means "flower of flowers." The flowers have been used to cover the beds of newlywed couples on their wedding night. Traditionally used in hair formulas to promote thick, shiny, lustrous hair.

Flowers are picked early in the morning to maximize oil yield. The highest quality oil is drawn from the first distillation and is known as ylang ylang complete.

**Medical Properties:** Antispasmodic, vasodilating, antidiabetic, anti-inflammatory, antiparasitic, regulates heartbeat

**Uses:** Cardiac arrhythmia, cardiac problems, anxiety, hypertension, depression, hair loss, intestinal problems

**Fragrant Influence:** Balances male-female energies, enhances spiritual attunement, combats anger, combats low self-esteem, increases focus of thoughts, filters out negative energy, restores confidence and peace

**Directions: Aromatic:** Diffuse up to 1 hour 3 times daily or directly inhale. **Dietary:** Take as a dietary supplement. **Topical:** Dilute 1 drop essential oil with 1 drop V-6 or other pure carrier oil and apply 2-4 drops on location, chakras, and/or Vita Flex points.

**Caution:** Use sparingly if you have low blood pressure

**Technical Data: Botanical Family:** Annonaceae; **Plant Origin:** Madagascar, Ecuador; **Extraction Method:** Steam distilled from flowers; **Key Constituents:** Germacrene D (14-27%), (E,E)-Alpha-Farnesene (5-23%), Benzyl Acetate (1-15%), Geranyl Acetate (2-11%), Beta-Caryophyllene (2-19%), Benzyl Benzoate (4-8%), Linalol (2-16%), Para-Cresyl Methyl Ether (0.5-9%), Methyl Benzoate (1-5%), Benzyl Salicyclate (1-5%); **ORAC:** 130,000 µTE/100g

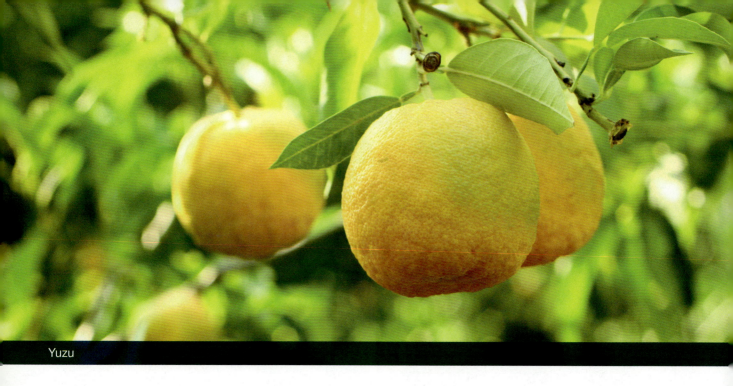

Yuzu

### Selected Research

Soonwera M. Efficacy of essential oil from *Cananga odorata* (Lamk.) Hook.f. & Thomson (Annonaceae) against three mosquito species *Aedes aegypti* (L.), *Anapheles dirus* (Peyton and Harrisoh), and *Culex quinquefasciatus* (Say). *Parasitol Res.* 2015 Sept 4. [Epub ahead of print]

Tan LT, et al. Traditional Uses, Phytochemistry, and Bioactives of *Cananga odorata* (Ylang-Ylang). *Evid Based Complement Alternat Med.* 2015;2015:896314. [Epub ahead of print]

Gnatta JR, et al. [Aromatherapy with ylang ylang for anxiety and self-esteem: a pilot study.] *Rev Esc Eferm USP.* 2014 Jun;48(3):492-9.

Moss M, et al. Modulation of cognitive performance and mood by aromas of peppermint and ylang ylang. *Int J Neurosci.* 2008 Jan;118(1):59-77.

Hongratanaworakit T, Buchbauer G. Relaxing effect of ylang ylang oil on humans after transdermal absorption. *Phytother Res.* 2006 Sep;20(9):758-763.

Hongratanaworakit T, Buchbauer G. Evaluation of the harmonizing effect of ylang-ylang oil on humans after inhalation. *Planta Med.* 2004 Jul;70(7):632-6.

### Yuzu *(Citrus junos)*

Thought to be a hybrid between Ichang papeda and Satsuma mandarin. Commonly used in cooking and for enhancing flavors due to the fragrant rind. There are a few reports on the use of yuzu essential oil for cosmetics and aromatherapy.

**Medical Properties:** Anti-inflammatory, anticancer, antidiabetic, asthma

**Uses:** Flavorant, inflammation, brain protection, stress

**Fragrant Influence:** High levels of limonene positively affect mood and heighten senses.

**Directions: Aromatic:** Diffuse up to 1 hour 3 times daily or directly inhale. **Dietary:** Put 2 drops in a capsule. Take 3 times daily or as needed. **Topical:** Apply 2-4 drops on location, chakras, and/or Vita Flex points. Dilution not required except on the most sensitive skin.

**Caution:** Possible sun sensitivity.

**Technical Data: Botanical Family:** Rutaceae; **Plant Origin:** China; **Extraction Method:** Cold-pressed from rind; **Key Constituents:** Limonene (60-85%), Beta-Phellandrene (1-5%), Gamma-Terpinene (5-15%), Linalool (0.5-3%); **ORAC:** 620 μmole TE/gram

### Selected Research

Yoo KM, Moon B. Comparative carotenoid compositions during maturation and their antioxidant capacities of three citrus varieties. *Food Chem.* 2016 Apr 1;196:544-09.

Kim TH, et al. Inhibitory effects of yuzu and its components on human platelet aggregation. *Biomol Ther* (Seoul). 2015 Mar;23(2):149-55.

Matsumoto T, et al. Effects of olfactory stimulation from the fragrance of the Japanese citrus fruit yuzu (*Citrus junos* Sieb. ex Tanaka) on mood states and salivary chromogranin A as an endocrinologic stress marker. *J Altern Complement Med.* 2014 Jun;20(6):500-6.

Kim SH, et al. *Citrus junos* Tanaka Peel Extract Exerts Antidiabetic Effects via AMPK and PPAR-γ both In Vitro and In Vivo in Mice Fed a High-Fat Diet. *Evid Based Complement Alternat Med.* 2013;2013;921012.

Yang HJ, et al. Yuzu Extract Prevents Cognitive Decline and Impaired Glucose Homeostasis in β-Amyloid-Infused Rats. *J Nutr.* 2013 Jul;143(7):1093-9.

Hirota R, et al. Anti inflammatory effects on limonene from Yuzu (*Citrus junos* Tanaka) essential oil on eosinophils. *J Food Sci.* 2010 Apr;75(3):H87-92.

# Chapter 7
## Oil Blends

## Formulating Essential Oil Blends

This section describes specific blends that were formulated after years of research for both physical and emotional health. Each of these blends is formulated to maximize the synergistic effect between various oil chemistries and harmonic frequencies. When chemistry and frequency coincide, noticeable physical, spiritual, and emotional benefits can be attained.

Remember that some essential oils may be irritating to those with sensitive skin, and remember to avoid getting them in your eyes. In case you accidentally do get oil in an eye, dilute it quickly with a few drops of V-6 Vegetable Oil Complex, olive oil, or any other vegetable oil that is readily available, and call your doctor if necessary. Do not use water to rinse the eye, as water drives the oil into the tissues and creates more burning and pain.

All essential oils should be stored in a cool, dark place to preserve their fragile constituents that may dissipate over time or be damaged by harmful sunlight.

## Guidelines

**Please see Chapter 5 for additional details on how to use essential oils and follow the directions on the product labels.**

**Common uses:** Almost all blends can be diffused, directly inhaled, and/or applied topically.

**Full body massage:** Dilute 1 drop essential oil blend with 15 drops of V-6 or other pure carrier oil.

**Possible skin sensitivity:** Test for sensitivity on small location of skin on underside of arm.

**Possible sun sensitivity:** Avoid direct sunlight or UV rays for up to 12 hours after applying product.

**Dietary and/or culinary use:** Vitality™ dietary essential oil blends can be added to food for delicious, concentrated flavor or used in capsules for their supporting properties. Follow the directions on the labels.

**Found-in list:** A list of the single oils contained in each blend can also be found in Appendix C.

## Essential Oil Blends

### 3 Wise Men™

This blend of 3 Wise Men promotes feelings of reverence and spiritual awareness combined with the power of therapeutic-grade essential oils that open the subconscious. It enhances emotional equilibrium as it soothes and uplifts the heart.

**Ingredients:** sweet almond oil, Royal Hawaiian Sandalwood*, Juniper, Frankincense, Black Spruce, Myrrh

**Directions: Aromatic:** Diffuse up to 1 hour 3 times daily or directly inhale. **Topical:** Dilute 1 drop with 1 drop of V-6 or other pure carrier oil. Add 2 drops on crown of head, behind ears, over eyebrows, on chest, over thymus, at back of neck, or on desired location as needed.

### Abundance™

This blend exemplifies the true power of synergy. Together, all of its component oils are magnified in vibration, creating the law of attraction and the energy and frequency of prosperity and plentitude.

Seventh Edition | **Essential Oils Desk Reference** | 143

**Essential Oils Desk Reference** | Seventh Edition

# Essential Oil Blend Application Codes

**Neat = Straight, undiluted**
Dilution usually NOT required; suitable for all but the most sensitive skin. Safe for children over 2 years old.

**50-50 = Dilute 50-50**
Dilution recommended at 50-50 (1 part essential oils to 1 part V-6 Vegetable Oil Complex) for topical and internal use, especially when used on sensitive areas — face, neck, genital area, underarms, etc. Keep out of reach of children.

**20-80 = Dilute 20-80**
Always dilute 20-80 (1 part essential oils to 4 parts V-6 Vegetable Oil Complex) before applying to the skin or taking internally. Keep out of reach of children.

**PH = Photosensitizing**
Avoid using on skin exposed to direct sunlight or UV rays (e.g., sunlamps, tanning beds, etc.).

| | | | |
|---|---|---|---|
| 3 Wise Men | **50-50** | GLF | **PH** **20-80** | PanAway | **20-80** |
| Abundance | **50-50** | Gratitude | **Neat** | Peace & Calming | **PH** **50-50** |
| Acceptance | **Neat** | Grounding | **PH** **50-50** | Peace & Calming II | **PH** **50-50** |
| Amoressence | **Neat** | Harmony | **PH** **Neat** | Present Time | **PH** **Neat** |
| Aroma Ease | **50-50** | Highest Potential | **PH** **50-50** | Purification | **Neat** |
| Aroma Life | **Neat** | Hope | **Neat** | Raven | **50-50** |
| Aroma Siez | **50-50** | Humility | **PH** **Neat** | R.C. | **50-50** |
| Aroma Sleep | **Neat** | ImmuPower | **20-80** | Reconnect | **PH** **Neat** |
| Australian Blue | **Neat** | Inner Child | **PH** **50-50** | Release | **PH** **Neat** |
| Awaken | **PH** **Neat** | Inner Harmony | **Neat** | Relieve It | **PH** **50-50** |
| Believe | **50-50** | Inspiration | **PH** **Neat** | RutaVaLa | **PH** **50-50** |
| Bite Buster | **Neat** | Into The Future | **PH** **20-80** | RutaVaLa Roll-On | **Neat** |
| Brain Power | **Neat** | InTouch | **PH** **Neat** | Sacred Mountain | **PH** **50-50** |
| Breathe Again Roll-On | **Neat** | Joy | **PH** **Neat** | SARA | **PH** **20-80** |
| Build Your Dream | **50-50** | JuvaCleanse | **50-50** | SclarEssence | **PH** **50-50** |
| Christmas Spirit | **PH** **20-80** | JuvaFlex | **Neat** | Sensation | **Neat** |
| Citrus Fresh | **PH** **50-50** | Lady Sclareol | **PH** **Neat** | Shutran | **PH** **Neat** |
| Clarity | **PH** **50-50** | Light the Fire | **PH** **20-80** | SleepyIze | **Neat** |
| Common Sense | **Neat** | Live with Passion | **PH** **50-50** | Slique Essence | **Neat** |
| Cool Azul | **PH** **Neat** | Live Your Passion | **50-50** | SniffleEase | **Neat** |
| Deep Relief Roll-On | **PH** **Neat** | Longevity | **PH** **20-80** | Stress Away | **PH** **Neat** |
| DiGize | **PH** **50-50** | Magnify Your Purpose | **50-50** | Stress Away Roll-On | **PH** **Neat** |
| Divine Release | **PH** **Neat** | Melrose | **50-50** | Surrender | **PH** **Neat** |
| Dragon Time | **PH** **50-50** | M-Grain | **50-50** | The Gift | **50-50** |
| Dream Catcher | **PH** **50-50** | Mister | **Neat** | Thieves | **PH** **20-80** |
| Egyptian Gold | **PH** **20-80** | Motivation | **50-50** | Tranquil Roll-On | **PH** **Neat** |
| EndoFlex | **50-50** | Oola Balance | **50-50** | Transformation | **PH** **50-50** |
| En-R-Gee | **20-80** | Oola Faith | **PH** **Neat** | Trauma Life | **50-50** |
| Envision | **50-50** | Oola Family | **PH** **Neat** | T.R. Care | **PH** **Neat** |
| Evergreen Essence | **50-50** | Oola Field | **PH** **Neat** | TummyGize | **PH** **Neat** |
| Exodus II | **PH** **20-80** | Oola Finance | **PH** **Neat** | Valor | **Neat** |
| Forgiveness | **PH** **Neat** | Oola Fitness | **Neat** | Valor Roll-On | **Neat** |
| Freedom | **Neat** | Oola Friends | **Neat** | White Angelica | **PH** **Neat** |
| Gathering | **Neat** | Oola Fun | **PH** **Neat** | White Light | **50-50** |
| GeneYus | **PH** **Neat** | Oola Grow | **PH** **Neat** | | |
| Gentle Baby | **50-50** | Owie | **Neat** | | |

**Ingredients:** Orange, Frankincense, Patchouli, Clove, Ginger, Myrrh, Cinnamon Bark, Black Spruce

**Directions: Aromatic:** Diffuse up to 30-45 minutes daily or directly inhale. Avoid contact with eyes. **Topical:** Dilute 1 drop with 1 drop V-6 or other pure carrier oil. Apply 1-2 drops over heart or on wrists, neck, temples, or desired location as needed. Use Release first to release emotions that prevent us from receiving abundance. Follow with one or several blends such as Acceptance, Believe, Envision, Into the Future, The Gift, Joy, Magnify Your Purpose, Motivation, or Valor.

## Acceptance™

Acceptance stimulates the mind, compelling us to open and accept new things, people, or relationships in life, allowing one to reach a higher potential. It also helps us to overcome procrastination and denial.

**Ingredients:** sweet almond oil, Coriander, Geranium, Bergamot, Frankincense, Royal Hawaiian Sandalwood, Bitter Orange (Neroli), Grapefruit, Tangerine, Spearmint, Lemon, Blue Cypress, Davana, Kaffir Lime, Ocotea, Jasmine, Matricaria (German Chamomile)

**Directions: Aromatic:** Diffuse up to 1 hour 3 times daily or directly inhale. **Topical:** Dilution not required, except for the most sensitive skin. Apply 2-4 drops over heart and thymus, on wrists, behind ears, on neck and temples, or on desired location as needed.

## Amoressence™

A limited-edition blend available only at a Young Living Beauty School event.

**Ingredients:** Vetiver, Idaho Blue Spruce, Jasmine, Davana, Ocotea, Ylang Ylang, Roman Chamomile, Vanilla, Geranium

**Directions: Aromatic:** Diffuse up to 1 hour 3 times daily or directly inhale. **Topical:** Dilute as needed and apply to desired area.

## Aroma Ease™

This comforting blend has a cool, minty aroma that contains powerful essential oil constituents. Use Aroma Ease to reduce the effects of nausea and other sensations of digestive discomfort.

**Ingredients:** Peppermint, Spearmint, Ginger, Cardamom, Fennel

**Directions: Aromatic:** Diffuse up to 30 minutes 3 times daily or directly inhale. **Topical:** Dilute 1 drop with 1 drop of V-6 or other pure carrier oil and apply on desired location as needed.

## Aroma Life™

Aroma Life improves cardiovascular, lymphatic, and circulatory systems; lowers high blood pressure; and reduces stress.

**Ingredients:** sesame seed oil, Cypress, Marjoram, Ylang Ylang, Helichrysum

**Directions: Aromatic:** Diffuse up to 1 hour 3 times daily or directly inhale. **Topical:** Dilution not required, except for the most sensitive skin. Apply 2-4 drops on the abdomen, in conjunction with Raindrop Technique, or on desired location as needed. Apply 1-2 drops over heart and along spine from first to fourth thoracic vertebrae (which correspond to the cardiopulmonary nerves).

## Aroma Siez™

Aroma Siez is an advanced complex of anti-inflammatory, muscle-relaxing essential oils that promote circulation and relieve headaches and tight, inflamed, aching muscles resulting from injury, fatigue, or stress.

**Ingredients:** Basil, Marjoram, Lavender, Peppermint, Cypress

**Directions: Topical:** Dilute 1 drop with 1 drop of V-6 or other pure carrier oil and apply on sore muscles, ligaments, locations of poor circulation, or desired location as needed.

**Caution:** Possible skin sensitivity.

## Aroma Sleep™

AromaSleep provides a relaxing aroma to re-establish a positive energy flow to the body, helping calm your mind and feelings prior to bedtime.

**Ingredients:** Lavender, Geranium, Roman Chamomile, Bergamot, Tangerine, Sacred Frankincense, Valerian, Ruta

**Directions: Aromatic:** Diffuse up to 1 hour 3 times daily or directly inhale. **Topical:** Dilution not required, except for the most sensitive skin. Apply 2-4 drops directly on desired location as needed.

## Australian Blue™

This blend includes a rare Australian aromatic called blue cypress, a part of the aboriginal pharmacopoeia for thousands of years. It is distilled from the wood of *Callitris intratropica*, the northern cypress pine, which has antiviral properties. Its aromatic influence uplifts and inspires while simultaneously grounds and stabilizes.

**Ingredients:** Blue Cypress, Ylang Ylang, Cedarwood, White Fir, Geranium, Grapefruit, Tangerine, Spearmint, Davana, Kaffir Lime, Lemon, Ocotea, Jasmine, Matricaria (German Chamomile), Blue Tansy, Rose

**Directions: Aromatic:** Diffuse up to 1 hour 3-4 times daily or directly inhale. **Topical:** Dilution not required, except for the most sensitive skin. Apply 1-2 drops on wrists, neck, temples, foot Vita Flex points, or desired location as needed.

## Awaken™

Five specific blends combine to awaken and enhance inner self-awareness that strengthens the desire to reach one's highest potential. It stimulates right brain creativity, amplifying the function of the pineal and pituitary glands in balancing the energy centers of the body and helps us identify our true desires and how best to pursue them.

**Ingredients:** Joy, Forgiveness, Present Time, Dream Catcher, Harmony

**Directions: Aromatic:** Diffuse up to 1 hour 3 times daily or directly inhale. **Topical:** Dilution not required, except for the most sensitive skin. Apply 2-4 drops over heart, on wrists, neck, temples, forehead, foot Vita Flex points, or desired location as needed. For clearing allergies, rub over sternum.

**Caution:** Possible sun sensitivity.

## Believe™

Believe helps release the unlimited potential everyone possesses. It restores feelings of hope, making it possible to more fully experience health, happiness, and vitality.

**Ingredients:** Balsam Canada (Idaho Balsam Fir), Coriander, Bergamot, Frankincense, Idaho Blue Spruce, Ylang Ylang, Geranium

**Directions: Aromatic:** Diffuse up to 1 hour 3 times daily or directly inhale. **Topical:** Dilution not required, except for the most sensitive skin. Apply 2-4 drops over heart, on wrists, neck, temples, forehead, foot Vita Flex points, or desired location as needed.

**Caution:** Possible skin sensitivity.

## Bite Buster™

Bite Buster is an excellent insect repellant formulated especially for kids.

**Ingredients:** caprylic/capric glycerides, Idaho Tansy, Citronella, Palo Santo

**Directions: Aromatic:** Diffuse up to 1 hour 3 times daily. **Topical:** Recommended application is for children ages 2-12. To be applied only by a trusted adult or under adult supervision. Dilution not required, except for the most sensitive skin. Apply 2-4 drops directly on desired location as needed.

## Brain Power™

Brain Power promotes deep concentration and channels physical energy into mental energy. It also increases mental potential and clarity, and long-term use may retard the aging process. Many of the oils in this blend are high in sesquiterpene compounds that increase activity in the pineal, pituitary, and hypothalamus glands and thereby increase output of growth hormone and melatonin.

The oils also help dissolve petrochemicals that congest the receptor sites, clearing the "brain fog" that people experience due to exposure to synthetic petrochemicals in food, skin, hair care products, and air.

**Ingredients:** Royal Hawaiian Sandalwood, Cedarwood, Frankincense, Melissa, Blue Cypress, Lavender, Helichrysum

**Directions: Aromatic:** Diffuse up to 1 hour 3 times daily or directly inhale. **Topical:** Dilution not required, except for the most sensitive skin. Apply 2-4 drops on back of neck, throat, temples, under nose, or on desired location as needed. Apply 1 or 2 drops with a finger on insides of cheeks in mouth.

**Caution:** Possible skin sensitivity.

Oil Blends | Chapter 7

## Breathe Again™ Roll-On

This supercharged version of the R.C. blend is packaged in a convenient dispenser for easy use when air pollution makes it difficult to breathe, or throat and nasal congestion strike. Contains four different eucalyptus oils and five additional essential oils, all known for their ability to relax airways, make breathing easier, and reduce coughing. In addition, these oils have anti-inflammatory characteristics.

**Ingredients:** caprylic/capric triglyceride, Eucalyptus Staigeriana, Eucalyptus Globulus, Laurus Nobilis (Bay Laurel), Rose Hip Seed Oil, Peppermint, Eucalyptus Radiata, Copaiba, Myrtle, Blue Cypress, Eucalyptus Blue

**Directions: Topical:** Apply generously to throat, neck, or chest as desired for relief of symptoms related to colds, coughs, or sinus/lung congestion.

## Build Your Dream™

A unique blend, Build Your Dream is designed to empower and give clarity to your thoughts and purpose when used aromatically.

**Ingredients:** Lavender, Sacred Frankincense, Melissa, Blue Cypress, Hong Kuai, Idaho Blue Spruce, Ylang Ylang, Dream Catcher, Believe, Blue Lotus

**Directions: Aromatic:** Diffuse up to 30 minutes 3 times daily or directly inhale. **Topical:** Dilute 1 drop with 1 drop V-6 or other pure carrier oil and apply on desired location as needed.

## Christmas Spirit™

Christmas Spirit is a purifying blend of evergreen, citrus, and spice, reminiscent of winter holidays, and brings joy, peace, happiness, and security.

**Ingredients:** Orange, Cinnamon Bark, Black Spruce

**Directions: Aromatic:** Diffuse up to 30 minutes 3 times daily or directly inhale. **Topical:** Dilute 1 drop with 4 drops of V-6 or carrier oil. Apply 1-2 drops over heart, on wrists, neck, temples, foot Vita Flex points, or desired location as needed.

**Caution:** Possible sun/skin sensitivity.

## Citrus Fresh™

Citrus Fresh stimulates the right brain to amplify creativity and well-being, eradicates anxiety, and works well as an air purifier. When diffused, it adds a clean, fresh scent to any environment.

**Ingredients:** Orange, Tangerine, Grapefruit, Lemon, Mandarin, Spearmint

**Directions: Aromatic:** Diffuse up to 1 hour 3 times daily or directly inhale. **Topical:** Dilute 1 part to 1 part V-6 or other pure carrier oil and apply 1-2 drops on edge of ears, wrists, neck, temples, foot VitaFlex points, or desired location as needed.

**Caution:** Possible sun/skin sensitivity.

## Citrus Fresh Vitality™

**Ingredients:** Orange, Tangerine, Grapefruit, Lemon, Mandarin, Spearmint

**Directions: Dietary:** Put 2 drops in a capsule and take 3 times daily. Great for culinary use.

## Clarity™

Clarity promotes a clear mind and amplifies mental alertness and vitality. It increases energy when overly tired and brings greater focus to the spirit and mind.

**Ingredients:** Basil, Cardamom, Rosemary, Peppermint, Coriander, Geranium, Bergamot, Lemon, Ylang Ylang, Jasmine, Roman Chamomile, Palmarosa

**Directions: Aromatic:** Diffuse up to 1 hour 3 times a day or directly inhale. **Topical:** Dilute 1 drop with 1 drop of V-6 or pure carrier oil and apply 1-2 drops on edge of ears, wrists, neck, forehead, temples, foot VitaFlex points (brain and large toe), or desired location as needed. Clarity works well with Brain Power, Palo Santo, Lemon, or Peppermint, as they enhance its effects.

**Caution:** Possible sun/skin sensitivity.

## Common Sense™

Common Sense is a proprietary blend of pure Young Living essential oils especially formulated by D. Gary Young to increase mental acuity, improve decision-making abilities, and strengthen everyday thinking skills.

**Ingredients:** Frankincense, Ylang Ylang, Ocotea, Goldenrod, Ruta, Dorado Azul, Lime

Seventh Edition | **Essential Oils Desk Reference** | 147

**Directions: Aromatic:** Diffuse up to 30 minutes 3 times daily, directly inhale, or wear as a fragrance. **Topical:** Dilute 1 drop with 4 drops of V-6 or carrier oil and apply to desired area as needed.

**Caution:** Possible sun sensitivity.

## Cool Azul™

Cool Azul may be applied topically after physical activities to relieve sore or stressed muscles or for a cooling, aromatic sensation.

**Ingredients:** Wintergreen, Peppermint, Sage, Copaiba, Oregano, Melaleuca Quinquenervia (Niaouli), Plectranthus Oregano, Lavender, Blue Cypress, Elemi, Vetiver, Caraway, Dorado Azul, Matricaria (German Chamomile)

**Directions: Topical:** Dilute with V-6 or other pure carrier oil as needed and apply topically.

**Caution:** Possible sun sensitivity.

## Deep Relief Roll-On™

This convenient roll-on relieves muscle soreness and tension, soothes sore joints and ligaments, helps calm stressed nerves, and reduces inflammation. This powerful blend contains nine essential oils, most of which are known for their anti-inflammatory and pain-relieving characteristics.

This highly portable roll-on with its no-mess application is easy to carry in your pocket, purse, briefcase, etc. It also passes through airport security for "easy breathing" while flying high.

**Ingredients:** Peppermint, caprylic/capric triglyceride, Lemon, Balsam Canada (Idaho Balsam Fir), Clove, Copaiba, coconut oil, Wintergreen, Helichrysum, Vetiver, Dorado Azul

**Directions: Topical:** Apply generously on location. For head tension, apply on temples, back of neck, and forehead.

**Caution:** Possible sun sensitivity.

## DiGize™

This blend relieves digestive problems, including indigestion, heartburn, gas, and bloating. It helps fight candida as it kills and digests parasite infestation.

**Ingredients:** Tarragon, Ginger, Peppermint, Juniper, Fennel, Lemongrass, Anise, Patchouli

**Directions: Aromatic:** Diffuse up to 30 minutes 3 times daily or directly inhale. **Topical:** Dilute 1 drop with 1 drop of V-6 or other pure carrier oil and apply to Vita Flex points on feet and ankles for stomach and intestinal relief or on desired location as needed. Massage or use as a compress on the stomach.

**Caution:** Possible sun sensitivity.

## DiGize Vitality™

**Ingredients:** Tarragon, Ginger, Peppermint, Juniper, Fennel, Lemongrass, Anise, Patchouli

**Directions: Dietary:** Dilute 1 drop with 4 drops of carrier oil. Put in a capsule and take 1 daily.

## Divine Release™

Divine Release is an elevating blend that helps release feelings of anger and promotes forgiveness to encourage the gentle characteristics within oneself for a positive outlook on life.

**Ingredients:** Royal Hawaiian Sandalwood, Roman Chamomile, Frankincense, Melissa, Geranium, Grapefruit, Blue Cypress, Hinoki, Helichrysum, Bergamot, Rose, Ledum, Angelica

**Directions: Aromatic:** Diffuse up to 1 hour 3 times daily or directly inhale. **Topical:** Dilution not required, except for the most sensitive skin. Apply 2-4 drops directly on desired location as needed.

**Caution:** Possible sun sensitivity.

## Dragon Time™

This blend relieves PMS symptoms and menstrual discomforts, including cramping and irregular periods. It helps balance emotions, alleviating mood swings and headaches caused by hormonal imbalance.

**Ingredients:** Fennel, Clary Sage, Marjoram, Lavender, Yarrow, Jasmine

**Directions: Aromatic:** Diffuse up to 30 minutes 3 times daily or directly inhale. **Topical:** Dilute 1 drop with 1 drop V-6 or other pure carrier oil and apply 1-2 drops on wrists, neck, temples, foot Vita Flex points, or desired location as needed. Apply with a hot compress or directly over lower abdomen, across lower back, or on location of pain. Use on both sides of ankles and feet.

**Caution:** Possible sun sensitivity.

Oil Blends | Chapter 7

## Dream Catcher™

This blend stimulates the emotional centers of the brain, awakening creative thoughts and enhancing dreams and visualizations, promoting greater potential for realizing your dreams and staying on your path. It also protects from negative thoughts and dreams that might cloud your vision.

**Ingredients:** Royal Hawaiian Sandalwood, Tangerine, Ylang Ylang, Black Pepper, Bergamot, Anise, Juniper, Geranium, Blue Cypress, Davana, Citrus Hystrix, Jasmine, Matricaria (German Chamomile), Blue Tansy, Rose, Grapefruit, Spearmint

**Directions: Aromatic:** Diffuse up to 1 hour 3 times daily (most effective before and during sleep) or directly inhale. **Topical:** Dilute 1 drop with 1 drop V-6 or other pure carrier oil and apply on forehead, ears, throat, eyebrows, base of neck, under nose, or on desired location as needed. Use during meditation, in saunas, or just before sleeping.

**Caution:** Possible sun/skin sensitivity.

**Note:** If unpleasant dreams occur, continue to use, since subconscious memories and thoughts will still need to be resolved. Hold on to your dreams and visualize the problems being solved. It may be helpful to write down the dreams upon arising.

## Egyptian Gold™

This is a very unique blend that combines the most valuable essences of the Middle East and Central Europe. It offers a truly enchanting aromatic effect that stimulates the central nervous system and the immune and respiratory systems.

**Ingredients:** Frankincense, Balsam Canada (Idaho Balsam Fir), Lavender, Myrrh, Hyssop, Northern Lights Black Spruce, Cedarwood, Vetiver, Rose, Cinnamon Bark

**Directions: Aromatic:** Diffuse up to 10 minutes 3 times daily or directly inhale. **Dietary:** Dilute 1 drop with 4 drops of V-6 or pure carrier oil and put in a capsule; take 1 capsule before each meal or as desired. **Topical:** Dilute 1 drop with 4 drops of V-6 or other pure carrier oil and apply 1-2 drops over heart, on wrists, neck, temples, foot Vita Flex points, or desired location as needed.

**Caution:** Possible sun sensitivity.

## EndoFlex™

This blend amplifies metabolism and vitality and creates hormonal balance.

**Ingredients:** Spearmint, Sesame Seed Oil, Sage, Geranium, Myrtle, Matricaria (German Chamomile), Nutmeg

**Directions: Aromatic:** Diffuse up to 30 minutes 3 times daily or directly inhale. **Topical:** Dilute 1 drop with 1 drop of V-6 or other pure carrier oil and apply over lower back, thyroid, kidneys, liver, feet, glandular locations, foot Vita Flex points, or desired location as needed.

## EndoFlex Vitality™

**Ingredients:** Spearmint, sesame seed oil, Sage, Geranium, Myrtle, Matricaria (German Chamomile), Nutmeg

**Directions: Dietary:** Dilute 1 drop with 1 drop of carrier oil. Put in a capsule and take up to 3 times daily.

## En-R-Gee™

This blend increases vitality, circulation, and alertness.

**Ingredients:** Rosemary, Juniper, Lemongrass, Nutmeg, Balsam Canada (Idaho Balsam Fir), Clove, Black Pepper

**Directions: Aromatic:** Diffuse up to 30 minutes 3 times daily or directly inhale. **Topical:** Dilute 1 drop with 4 drops of V-6 or other pure carrier oil. Apply on temples, back of neck, forehead, chakras, foot Vita Flex points, or desired location as needed. It may also be used with Raindrop Technique. Rub En-R-Gee on feet and Awaken on temples for intensified effect.

**Caution:** Possible skin sensitivity. Avoid contact with mucous membranes or sensitive skin.

## Envision™

This blend renews focus and stimulates creative and intuitive abilities needed to achieve goals and dreams. It helps to reawaken internal drive and independence and to overcome fears and emotional blocks.

**Ingredients:** Black Spruce, Geranium, Orange, Lavender, Sage, Rose

**Directions: Aromatic:** Diffuse up to 30 minutes 3 times daily or directly inhale. **Topical:** Dilute 1 drop

Seventh Edition | **Essential Oils Desk Reference** | 149

**Essential Oils Desk Reference** | Seventh Edition

with 1 drop of V-6 or other pure carrier oil and apply 1-2 drops on forehead, edge of ears, wrists, neck, temples, foot Vita Flex points, or desired location as needed.

## Evergreen Essence™

Evergreen Essence essential oil blend has a refreshing, crisp scent that is invigorating and emotionally strengthening. With an arrangement of popular evergreen trees, the scents of pine, fir, and spruce complement one another and may assist in the release of occasional emotional blocks. Refreshing to the senses, Evergreen Essence brings a feeling of balance, peace, and security. The relaxing scent may also help clear the mind for a calming sense of meditation and reflection.

**Ingredients:** Idaho Blue Spruce, Ponderosa Pine, Scotch Pine, Red Fir, Western Red Cedar, White Fir, Black Pine, Pinyon Pine, Lodgepole Pine

**Directions: Aromatic:** Diffuse up to 1 hour 3 times daily or directly inhale. **Topical:** Dilute 1 part to 1 part V-6 or other pure carrier oil. Apply 1-2 drops over heart, on wrists, neck, temples, foot Vita Flex points, or desired location as needed.

**Caution:** Possible skin sensitivity.

## Exodus II™

Some researchers believe that these aromatics were used by Aaron, the brother of Moses, to protect the Israelites from a plague. Modern science shows that these oils contain immune-stimulating and antimicrobial compounds. Because of the complex chemistry of essential oils, it is very difficult for viruses and bacteria to mutate and acquire resistance to them.

**Ingredients:** olive oil, Myrrh, Cassia, Cinnamon Bark, Calamus, Northern Lights Black Spruce, Hyssop, Vetiver, Frankincense

**Directions: Aromatic:** Diffuse up to 10 minutes 3 times daily or directly inhale. **Topical:** Dilute 1 drop with 4 drops of V-6 or other pure carrier oil. Apply 1-2 drops on ears, wrists, foot Vita Flex points, along spine as in Raindrop Technique, or desired location as needed.

**Caution:** Possible sun/skin sensitivity. Not intended for children under 12 years of age, unless directed by a health care professional.

## Forgiveness™

This blend helps to release hurt feelings and negative emotions. It also helps release negative memories, allowing one to move past emotional barriers and attain higher awareness, assisting the person to forgive and let go.

**Ingredients:** sesame seed oil, Melissa, Geranium, Frankincense, Royal Hawaiian Sandalwood, Coriander, Angelica, Lavender, Bergamot, Lemon, Ylang Ylang, Jasmine, Helichrysum, Roman Chamomile, Palmarosa, Rose

**Directions: Aromatic:** Diffuse up to 1 hour 3 times daily or directly inhale. **Topical:** Dilution not required, except for the most sensitive skin. Apply 2-4 drops behind ears, on wrists, neck, temples, navel, solar plexus, heart, or desired location as needed.

**Caution:** Possible sun/skin sensitivity.

## Freedom™

This liberating blend was created to help re-establish a positive energy flow through the body to promote a sense of balance. It is part of the Freedom Collection Bundle.

**Ingredients:** Copaiba, Sacred Frankincense, Idaho Blue Spruce, Vetiver, Lavender, Peppermint, Palo Santo, Valerian, Ruta

**Directions: Aromatic:** Diffuse up to 1 hour 3 times daily or directly inhale. **Topical:** Dilution not required, except for the most sensitive skin. Apply 2-4 drops directly on desired location as needed.

## Gathering™

This blend is created to help us overcome the bombardment of chaotic energy that alters our focus and takes us off our path toward higher achievements. Northern Lights Black Spruce and Vetiver have a strong effect when blended with Frankincense and Sandalwood in gathering our emotional and spiritual thoughts, helping us to achieve our potential. These oils help increase the oxygen around the pineal and pituitary glands, bringing greater harmonic frequency to receive the communication we desire.

This blend helps bring people together on a physical, emotional, and spiritual level for greater focus and clarity. It helps one stay focused, grounded, and clear in gathering motivation for self-improvement.

**Ingredients:** Lavender, Northern Lights Black Spruce, Geranium, Royal Hawaiian Sandalwood, Ylang Ylang, Vetiver, Cinnamon Bark, Rose

**150** | Chapter 7 | Oil Blends

**Directions: Aromatic:** Diffuse up to 1 hour 3 times daily or directly inhale. **Topical:** Dilution not required, except for the most sensitive skin. Apply 1-2 drops on edge of ears, wrists, neck, temples, or along the spine as in Raindrop Technique. Use Forgiveness on the navel; The Gift and Sacred Mountain on the crown (to clear negative attitudes); Valor on the crown or feet; 3 Wise Men on the crown; Clarity on the temples; and Dream Catcher on the forehead, ears, throat, eyebrows, base of neck, and under the nose.

**Caution:** Possible skin sensitivity.

## GeneYus™

Diffuse GeneYus to help young minds focus and concentrate on projects.

**Ingredients:** fractionated coconut oil, Sacred Frankincense, Blue Cypress, Cedarwood, Idaho Blue Spruce, Palo Santo, Melissa, Northern Lights Black Spruce, almond oil, Bergamot, Myrrh, Vetiver, Geranium, Royal Hawaiian Sandalwood, Ylang Ylang, Hyssop, Coriander, Rose

**Directions: Aromatic:** Diffuse up to 1 hour 3 times daily. **Topical:** Recommended application is for children ages 2-12. To be applied only by a trusted adult or under adult supervision. Dilution not required, except for the most sensitive skin. Apply 2-4 drops directly on desired location as needed.

**Caution:** Possible sun sensitivity.

## Gentle Baby™

This blend is comforting, soothing, relaxing, and beneficial for reducing stress during pregnancy. It helps reduce stretch marks and scar tissue, rejuvenates the skin, improves elasticity, and helps to reduce wrinkles.

It is particularly soothing to babies with dry, chapped skin and diaper rash. Skin issues improve when using Gentle Baby with Rose Ointment on the top of it. Gentle Baby is calming and brings a feeling of peace for tiny babies, children, and adults.

**Ingredients:** Coriander, Geranium, Palmarosa, Lavender, Ylang Ylang, Roman Chamomile, Bergamot (furocoumarin-free), Lemon, Jasmine, Rose

**Directions: Aromatic:** Diffuse up to 30 minutes 3 times daily or directly inhale. **Topical:** Dilute 1 part essential oil to 1 part V-6 or other pure carrier oil for body massage and for applying on baby's skin. Apply over mother's abdomen, on feet, lower back, face, and neck locations; apply on location for dry, chapped skin or diaper rash. Use as needed. **For Pregnancy and Delivery:** Use for massage throughout entire pregnancy for relieving stress and anxiety, creating serenity, and preventing scarring. Massage on the perineum to help it stretch for easier birthing.

**Caution:** Possible sun sensitivity.

## GLF™

The initials of this essential oil blend stand for **G**allbladder and **L**iver **F**lush. It is formulated with oils that help to cleanse and restore liver and gallbladder function when taken in capsules as a dietary supplement.

**Ingredients:** Grapefruit, Ledum, Helichrysum, Celery Seed, Hyssop, Spearmint

**Directions: Dietary:** Dilute 1 part oil with 4 parts V-6 or other pure carrier oil and take 1-3 capsules daily to support a detoxification and cleansing routine focused on the liver and gallbladder. **Topical:** Dilute 1 drop with 1 drop of V-6 or other pure carrier oil and apply on desired location as needed.

**Caution:** Possible sun sensitivity.

## GLF™ Vitality™

**Ingredients:** Grapefruit, Ledum, Helichrysum, Celery Seed, Hyssop, Spearmint

**Directions: Dietary:** Dilute 1 drop with 4 drops of carrier oil. Put in a capsule and take 1 before each meal or as desired.

## Gratitude™

This delightful blend is designed to elevate, soothe, and bring relief to the body while helping to foster a grateful attitude. It is also nourishing and supportive to the skin. The New Testament tells us that on one occasion, Christ healed 10 lepers (Luke 17:12-19), but only one returned to express his thanks. This blend embodies the spirit of that grateful leper.

**Ingredients:** Balsam Canada (Idaho Balsam Fir), Frankincense, Coriander, Myrrh, Ylang Ylang, Bergamot (furocoumarin-free), Northern Lights Black Spruce, Vetiver, Geranium

**Directions: Aromatic:** Diffuse up to 1 hour 3 times daily or directly inhale. **Topical:** Dilution not required, except for the most sensitive skin. Apply 2-4 drops behind ears, over heart, on wrists, base of neck, temples, base of spine, or desired location as needed.

## Grounding™

This blend creates a feeling of solidarity and balance. It stabilizes and grounds us so we can cope constructively with reality. When we're hurting emotionally, we resort to avoidance. When this happens, it is easy to make poor choices that lead to unhealthy relationships and unwise business decisions. We seek to escape because we do not have anchoring or awareness to know how to deal with our emotions.

**Ingredients:** White Fir, Black Spruce, Ylang Ylang, Pine, Cedarwood, Angelica, Juniper

**Directions: Aromatic:** Diffuse up to 30 minutes 3 times daily or directly inhale. **Topical:** Dilute 1 drop with 1 drop V-6 or other pure carrier oil and apply 1-2 drops behind ears, on wrists, base of neck, temples, base of spine, or desired location as needed.

**Caution:** Possible sun/skin sensitivity.

## Harmony™

This blend promotes physical and emotional healing by creating a harmonic balance for the energy centers of the body. It brings us into harmony with all things, people, and cycles of life. It is beneficial in reducing stress, amplifying well-being, and dissipating feelings of discord. It is also uplifting and elevating to the mind, creating a positive attitude.

**Ingredients:** Royal Hawaiian Sandalwood, Lavender, Ylang Ylang, Frankincense, Orange, Angelica, Geranium, Hyssop, Spanish Sage, Black Spruce, Coriander, Bergamot, Lemon, Jasmine, Roman Chamomile, Palmarosa, Rose

**Directions: Aromatic:** Diffuse up to 1 hour 3 times daily or directly inhale. **Topical:** Dilution not required, except for the most sensitive skin. Apply 2-4 drops on edge of ears, wrists, neck, temples, over heart, on chakras, on foot Vita Flex points, or desired location as needed.

**Caution:** Possible sun/skin sensitivity.

## Highest Potential™

This blend elevates the mind as you gather your thoughts and mental energy to achieve your highest potential. It harmonizes several grounding, calming, inspiring, and empowering essential oils into one intoxicating blend.

Biochemist R. W. Moncrieff wrote that Ylang Ylang "soothes and inhibits anger born of frustration," which removes roadblocks and opens new vistas. The uplifting fragrance of Jasmine spurs creativity, while Lavender clears the thought processes for focused intentions.

**Ingredients:** Blue Cypress, Ylang Ylang, Jasmine, Cedarwood, Geranium, Lavender, Northern Lights Black Spruce, Frankincense, Royal Hawaiian Sandalwood, White Fir, Vetiver, Cinnamon Bark, Davana, Citrus Hystrix, Rose, German Chamomile, Blue Tansy, Grapefruit, Tangerine, Spearmint, Lemon, Ocotea

**Directions: Aromatic:** Diffuse up to 30 minutes 3 times daily or directly inhale. **Topical:** Dilution not required, except for the most sensitive skin. Apply 2-4 drops on edge of ears, wrists, neck, temples, or desired location as needed.

**Caution:** Possible sun/skin sensitivity.

## Hope™

Hope is essential for moving forward in life. Hopelessness can cause a loss of vision, goals, and dreams. This blend helps you reconnect with a feeling of strength and grounding, restoring hope for tomorrow. It has helped many overcome suicidal depression.

**Ingredients:** sweet almond oil, Melissa, Juniper, Myrrh, Black Spruce

**Directions: Aromatic:** Diffuse up to 1 hour 3 times daily or directly inhale. **Topical:** Dilution not required, except for the most sensitive skin. Apply 2-4 drops on edge of ears, wrists, neck, temples, over heart, on chakras, foot Vita Flex points, or desired location as needed.

**Caution:** Possible skin sensitivity.

## Humility™

Having humility and forgiveness helps us heal ourselves and our earth (2 Chronicles 7:14). Humility is an integral component in obtaining forgiveness and is needed for a closer relationship with God. Through the frequency and fragrance of this blend, you may arrive at a place where healing can begin.

**Ingredients:** caprylic/capric triglyceride, Coriander, Ylang Ylang, Bergamot (furocoumarin-free), Geranium, Melissa, Frankincense, Myrrh, Northern Lights Black Spruce, Vetiver, Bitter Orange (Neroli), Rose

Oil Blends | **Chapter 7**

**Directions: Aromatic:** Diffuse up to 1 hour 3 times daily or directly inhale. **Topical:** Dilution not required, except for the most sensitive skin. Apply 2-4 drops over heart, on neck, forehead, temples, or desired location as needed.

**Caution:** Possible sun/skin sensitivity.

## ImmuPower™

This blend strengthens immunity and DNA repair in the cells. It is strongly antiseptic and anti-infectious.

**Ingredients:** Hyssop, Mountain Savory, Cistus, Camphor (Ravintsara), Frankincense, Oregano, Clove, Cumin, Dorado Azul

**Directions: Aromatic:** Diffuse up to 30 minutes 3 times daily or directly inhale. Alternate the diffused oils with Thieves and Exodus II. To enhance effects, add Melissa, Palo Santo, Clove, Cistus, or Dorado Azul. **Topical:** Dilute 1 drop with 4 drops of V-6 or other pure carrier oil and apply around navel, chest, temples, wrists, under nose, on foot Vita Flex points, or desired location as needed. Use with Raindrop Technique.

**Caution:** Possible skin sensitivity. This blend needs to be well-diluted before using on children.

## Inner Child™

When children have been abused, they become disconnected from their inner child, or identity, which causes confusion. This fractures the personality and creates problems that tend to surface in the early- to mid-adult years, often mislabeled as a midlife crisis. This fragrance stimulates memory response and helps one reconnect with the inner self or identity. This is one of the first steps to finding emotional balance.

**Ingredients:** Orange, Tangerine, Ylang Ylang, Royal Hawaiian Sandalwood, Jasmine, Lemongrass, Black Spruce, Bitter Orange (Neroli)

**Directions: Aromatic:** Diffuse up to 1 hour 3 times daily or directly inhale. **Topical:** Dilute 1 drop with 1 drop of V-6 or other pure carrier oil and apply 1-2 drops on edge of ears, wrists, neck, temples, or desired location as needed.

**Caution:** Possible sun sensitivity.

## Inner Harmony™

Inner Harmony is a calming formula that can be used to promote emotional clearing and self-renewal.

**Ingredients:** Geranium, Lavender, Royal Hawaiian Sandalwood, Ylang Ylang, Idaho Blue Spruce, Sacred Frankincense, Roman Chamomile, Tangerine, Orange, Northern Lights Black Spruce, Myrrh, Rose, Angelica, Vetiver, Melissa

**Directions: Aromatic:** Diffuse up to 1 hour 3 times daily or directly inhale. **Topical:** Dilution not required, except for the most sensitive skin. Apply 2-4 drops directly on desired location as needed.

## Inspiration™

This blend is formulated to help find a calm space in our minds and bring us closer to that creative center where our higher intuition operates. These oils were traditionally used by the Native Americans to enhance spirituality, prayer, and inner awareness.

**Ingredients:** Cedarwood, Black Spruce, Myrtle, Coriander, Royal Hawaiian Sandalwood, Frankincense, Bergamot (furocoumarin-free), Vetiver, Ylang Ylang, Geranium

**Directions: Aromatic:** Diffuse up to 1 hour 3 times daily or directly inhale. **Topical:** Dilution not required, except for the most sensitive skin. Apply 2-4 drops on edge of ears, wrists, neck, temples, forehead, crown of head, bottoms of feet, along spine, or desired location as needed.

**Caution:** Possible sun/skin sensitivity.

## Into the Future™

This blend helps one leave the past behind in order to progress with vision and excitement. So many times we find ourselves settling for mediocrity and sacrificing our own potential and success because of fear of the unknown and the future. This blend inspires determination and a pioneering spirit and creates a strong emotional feeling of being able to reach one's potential.

**Ingredients:** sweet almond oil, Clary Sage, Ylang Ylang, White Fir, Idaho Blue Spruce, Jasmine, Juniper, Frankincense, Orange, Cedarwood, White Lotus

**Directions: Aromatic:** Diffuse up to 1 hour 3 times daily or directly inhale. **Topical:** Dilute 1 drop with 4 drops of V-6 or other pure carrier oil and apply 1-2 drops on edge of ears, over heart, on wrists, neck, temples, or desired location as needed.

**Caution:** Possible sun/skin sensitivity.

Seventh Edition | **Essential Oils Desk Reference** | 153

**Essential Oils Desk Reference** | Seventh Edition

## InTouch™

This uplifting blend can help support mood by encouraging positive energy in times of restlessness and unease and to help ground and unite the body, mind, and spirit.

**Ingredients:** caprylic/capric triglyceride, Vetiver, Melissa, Royal Hawaiian Sandalwood, Cedarwood, Idaho Blue Spruce

**Directions: Aromatic:** Diffuse up to 1 hour 3 times daily or directly inhale. **Topical:** Dilution not required, except for the most sensitive skin. Apply 2-4 drops directly on desired location as needed. For children: to be applied only by a trusted adult or under adult supervision.

**Caution:** Possible sun sensitivity.

## Joy™

This beautiful blend produces a magnetic energy that brings joy to the heart, mind, and soul. It inspires romance and helps overcome deep-seated grief and depression.

**Ingredients:** Bergamot, Ylang Ylang, Geranium, Lemon, Coriander, Tangerine, Jasmine, Roman Chamomile, Palmarosa, Rose

**Directions: Aromatic:** Diffuse up to 1 hour 3 times daily or directly inhale. **Topical:** Dilution not required, except for the most sensitive skin. Apply 2-4 drops over the heart, thymus, temples, wrists, or desired location as needed. It may also be massaged on the lower back, abdomen, and heart and brain Vita Flex points.

**Caution:** Possible sun/skin sensitivity.

## JuvaCleanse®

The liver is the body's largest internal organ and major detoxifier. Even the toxins in the air we breathe are filtered by the liver, including chemicals from aerosol cleaners, paint, insect sprays, etc.; but eventually those filters need to be cleaned. The essential oils of Ledum, Celery Seed, and Helichrysum have long been known for their liver cleansing properties. JuvaCleanse was clinically tested in 2003 for removing mercury from body tissues.

In 2003 a study conducted by Roger Lewis, MD, at the Young Life Research Clinic in Springville, Utah, evaluated the efficacy of Helichrysum, Ledum, and Celery Seed in treating cases of advanced Hepatitis C.

In one case a 20-year-old male diagnosed with Hepatitis C had a viral count of 13,200. After taking two capsules (approx. 750 mg each) of JuvaCleanse per day for one month with no other intervention, the patient's viral count dropped more than 80 percent to 2,580.

**Ingredients:** Helichrysum, Ledum, Celery Seed

**Directions: Aromatic:** Diffuse up to 30 minutes 3 times daily or directly inhale. **Dietary:** Take 1 capsule 2 times daily as a dietary supplement. **Topical:** Dilute 1 drop with 1 drop of V-6 or other pure carrier oil and apply over the liver, on the liver and kidney Vita Flex points on the foot, or desired location as needed. Use with Raindrop Technique.

## JuvaCleanse® Vitality™

**Ingredients:** Helichrysum, Ledum, Celery Seed

**Directions: Dietary:** Dilute 1 drop with 4 drops of carrier oil. Put in a capsule and take 1 daily or as needed.

## JuvaFlex™

This blend helps with liver and lymphatic detoxification. The emotions of anger and hate create toxins that are stored in the liver that can lead to sickness and disease. JuvaFlex helps break addictions to coffee, alcohol, drugs, and tobacco.

**Ingredients:** sesame seed oil, Fennel, Geranium, Rosemary, Roman Chamomile, Blue Tansy, Helichrysum

**Directions: Aromatic:** Diffuse up to 30 minutes 3 times daily or directly inhale. **Topical:** Dilution not required, except for the most sensitive skin. Apply 2-4 drops over liver location, massage 3-4 drops on the Vita Flex points on the foot and along the spine as in Raindrop Technique, or apply on desired location as needed. Use a warm compress with 3-4 drops of oils with Ortho Sport or Ortho Ease massage oils.

## JuvaFlex® Vitality™

**Ingredients:** sesame seed oil, Fennel, Geranium, Rosemary, Roman Chamomile, Blue Tansy, Helichrysum

**Directions: Dietary:** Put 2 drops in a capsule. Take 3 times daily or as needed.

Oil Blends | Chapter 7

## Lady Sclareol™

This oil, rich in phytoestrogens, is designed to be worn as an exquisite fragrance. It enhances the feminine nature by improving mood and raising estrogen levels. It may also provide relief for PMS symptoms.

**Ingredients:** Geranium, Coriander, Vetiver, Orange, Clary Sage, Bergamot, Ylang Ylang, Royal Hawaiian Sandalwood, Spanish Sage, Jasmine, Idaho Blue Spruce, Spearmint, Hinoki

**Directions: Aromatic:** Diffuse up to 1 hour 3 times daily or directly inhale. **Topical:** Dilution not required, except for the most sensitive skin. Apply 2-4 drops to Vita Flex points on the ankles, at the clavicle notch, to the abdomen for relief of premenstrual discomfort, or on desired location as needed. Use as a fragrance.

**Caution.** Possible sun sensitivity.

## Light the Fire™

Light the Fire is an inspiring blend with a warm, spicy aroma that can encourage feelings of power and ambition.

**Ingredients:** Nutmeg, Cassia, Mastrante, Ocotea, Canadian Fleabane, Lemon, Hinoki, Black Pepper, Northern Lights Black Spruce

**Directions: Aromatic:** Diffuse up to 10 minutes 3 times daily or directly inhale. **Topical:** Dilute 1 drop with 4 drops of V-6 or other pure carrier oil and apply on desired location as needed.

**Caution:** Possible sun/skin sensitivity.

## Live with Passion™

This blend revives the zest for life and improves internal energy with a combination of essential oils formulated specifically to help people attain an optimistic attitude.

**Ingredients:** Royal Hawaiian Sandalwood, Clary Sage, Ginger, Jasmine, Angelica, Patchouli, Cedarwood, Helichrysum, Melissa, Bitter Orange (Neroli)

**Directions: Aromatic:** Diffuse up to 30 minutes 3 times daily or directly inhale. **Topical:** Dilute 1 drop with 1 drop of V-6 or other pure carrier oil before using on sensitive locations such as the face, neck, genital location, etc. Apply on wrists, temples, chest, forehead, or desired location as needed. Mix 2-4 drops of oil with 2 tablespoons of a bath and shower gel or mix with ½ cup bath salts water and pour into the tub. Soak for 20-30 minutes or until water cools.

**Caution:** Possible sun/skin sensitivity.

## Live Your Passion™

Live Your Passion enhances the zest for life and improves internal energy to specifically help people go forward with motivation and excitement.

**Ingredients:** Orange, Royal Hawaiian Sandalwood, Nutmeg, Lime, Idaho Blue Spruce, Northern Lights Black Spruce, Ylang Ylang, Frankincense, Peppermint

**Directions: Aromatic:** Diffuse up to 30 minutes 3 times daily. **Topical:** Mix 1 drop of oil with 1 drop of carrier oil and apply as needed.

## Longevity™

This oil contains the highest antioxidant and DNA-protecting essential oils. When taken as a dietary supplement, this blend promotes longevity and prevents premature aging (see Longevity Softgels in the Nutritional Support chapter).

**Ingredients:** Thyme, Orange, Clove, Frankincense

**Directions: Aromatic:** Diffuse up to 10 minutes 3 times daily or directly inhale. **Dietary:** As a dietary supplement, put a few drops of oil diluted with V-6 or pure carrier oil in a capsule and swallow or put 2-3 drops in Blue Agave, Yacon Syrup, or maple syrup in a spoon; mix and swallow; or mix in about 4 fl. oz. of NingXia Red, goat milk, or rice milk, etc. **Topical:** Dilute 1 drop with 4 drops of V-6 or other pure carrier oil and apply on desired location as needed.

**Caution:** Possible sun/skin sensitivity.

## Longevity Vitality™

**Ingredients:** Thyme, Orange, Clove, Frankincense

**Directions: Dietary:** Dilute 1 drop with 4 drops of carrier oil. Put in a capsule and take 1 daily or as needed.

## Magnify Your Purpose™

This blend stimulates the endocrine system for greater energy flow to the right hemisphere of the brain, activating creativity, motivation, and focus. This helps strengthen commitment to purpose, desire, and intentions until you realize your goals.

Seventh Edition | **Essential Oils Desk Reference** | 155

**Ingredients:** Royal Hawaiian Sandalwood, Sage, Coriander, Patchouli, Nutmeg, Bergamot, Cinnamon Bark, Ginger, Ylang Ylang, Geranium

**Directions: Aromatic:** Diffuse up to 30 minutes 3 times daily or directly inhale. **Topical:** Dilute 1 drop with 1 drop of V-6 or other pure carrier oil and apply on heart, solar plexus, thymus, temples, ears, wrists, or desired location as needed.

**Caution:** Possible skin sensitivity.

## Melrose™

This is a blend of four essential oils that have strong antiseptic properties to cleanse and disinfect cuts, scrapes, burns, rashes, and bruised tissue. These oils help regenerate damaged tissue and reduce inflammation. It is powerful when diffused to dispel odors, purify the air, and protect against daily radiation bombardment.

**Ingredients:** Rosemary, Tea Tree, Clove, Melaleuca Quinquenervia (Niaouli)

**Directions: Aromatic:** Diffuse up to 30 minutes 3 times daily or directly inhale. **Topical:** Dilute 1 drop with 1 drop of V-6 or other pure carrier oil and apply to broken skin, cuts, scrapes, burns, rashes, infection, or desired location as needed. Follow with Rose Ointment to keep oils sealed in wound. Put 1-2 drops on a piece of cotton and place in the ear for earaches.

**Caution:** Possible skin sensitivity.

## M-Grain™

This blend helps relieve pain from slight headaches to severe migraine headaches. It is anti-inflammatory and antispasmodic.

**Ingredients:** Basil, Marjoram, Lavender, Roman Chamomile, Peppermint, Helichrysum

**Directions: Aromatic:** Diffuse up to 30 minutes 3 times daily or directly inhale. **Topical:** Dilute 1 drop with 1 drop of V-6 or other pure carrier oil and apply on brain stem, forehead, crown of head, shoulders, back of neck, temples, foot Vita Flex points, or desired location as needed.

**Caution:** Possible skin sensitivity.

## Mister™

This blend helps to decongest the prostate and promote greater male hormonal balance.

**Ingredients:** sesame seed oil, Sage, Fennel, Lavender, Myrtle, Yarrow, Peppermint

**Directions: Aromatic:** Diffuse up to 30 minutes 3 times daily or directly inhale. **Topical:** Dilution not required, except for the most sensitive skin. Apply 2-4 drops to ankle Vita Flex points, lower pelvis, or locations of concern as needed. Use in a hot compress.

## Motivation™

Motivation stimulates feelings of action and accomplishment, providing positive energy to help overcome feelings of fear and procrastination.

**Ingredients:** Roman Chamomile, Black Spruce, Ylang Ylang, Lavender

**Directions: Aromatic:** Diffuse up to 30 minutes 3 times daily or directly inhale. **Topical:** Dilute 1 drop with 1 drop of V-6 or other pure carrier oil and apply on feet (big toe), chest, nape of the neck, behind ears, wrists, around navel, or desired location as needed.

## Oola®** Balance™

Oola Balance is designed to align and balance your center, giving you an increase in concentration with a positive outlook. As mind and body are balanced, the ability to focus on passions, behaviors, and health are amplified for the better.

**Ingredients:** fractionated coconut oil, Lavender, Ylang Ylang, Frankincense, Ocotea, Idaho Blue Spruce, Royal Hawaiian Sandalwood, Balsam Canada (Idaho Balsam Fir), Sacred Frankincense, Jasmine, Northern Lights Black Spruce, Orange, Angelica, Geranium, Hyssop, Spanish Sage, Myrrh, Vetiver, Cistus, Coriander, Bergamot, Lemon, Roman Chamomile, Palmarosa, Rose

**Directions: Aromatic:** Diffuse up to 30 minutes 3 times daily or directly inhale. **Topical:** Apply 1-2 drops on edge of ears, wrists, neck, temples, or other locations as desired.

Oil Blends | Chapter 7

## Oola®** Faith™

This blend can awaken feelings of spirituality and humility. Inhaling the aroma may promote deeper meditation and create a greater sense of connection.

**Ingredients:** caprylic/capric triglyceride, Sacred Frankincense, Balsam Canada (Idaho Balsam Fir), Myrrh, Juniper, Hyssop, Cedarwood, Sage, Hinoki, Rose, Geranium, Palo Santo, Coriander, Bergamot, Lemon, Ylang Ylang, Jasmine, Roman Chamomile, Palmarosa

**Directions: Aromatic:** Diffuse up to 30 minutes 3 times daily or directly inhale. **Topical:** Apply on desired location as needed.

**Caution:** Possible sun sensitivity.

## Oola®** Family™

This is a powerful blend that is formulated to support feelings of unconditional love, patience, and respect. It may help uplift emotions and release negative feelings to provide balance and clarity.

**Ingredients:** caprylic/capric triglyceride, Ylang Ylang, Lavender, Orange, Geranium, Cardamom, Tangerine, Frankincense, Cedarwood, Coriander, Pine, Royal Hawaiian Sandalwood, Lemongrass, Bergamot, Xiang Mao, Lemon, Black Spruce, Lime, Roman Chamomile, Palmarosa

**Directions: Aromatic:** Diffuse up to 30 minutes 3 times daily or directly inhale. **Topical:** Apply on desired location as needed.

**Caution:** Possible sun sensitivity.

## Oola®** Field™

This blend encourages feelings of self-worth and strength to help you overcome barriers and reach your true, unlimited potential.

**Ingredients:** caprylic/capric triglyceride, Cardamom, Frankincense, Ylang Ylang, sweet almond oil, Nutmeg, Ginger, Bitter Orange (Neroli), Balsam Canada (Idaho Balsam Fir), Coriander, Black Spruce, Bergamot, Idaho Blue Spruce, Geranium

**Directions: Aromatic:** Diffuse up to 30 minutes 3 times daily or directly inhale. **Topical:** Apply on desired location as needed.

**Caution:** Possible sun sensitivity.

## Oola®** Finance™

This Oola blend is designed to encourage positive emotions and increased feelings of abundance. Its uplifting aroma promotes a sense of clarity and alertness to help you focus on and realize financial objectives.

**Ingredients:** fractionated coconut oil, Frankincense, Orange, Ocotea, Balsam Canada (Idaho Balsam Fir), Royal Hawaiian Sandalwood, Basil, Geranium, Lavender, Cardamom, Coriander, Ylang Ylang, Northern Lights Black Spruce, Rosemary, Citronella (nardus), Citronella (winterianus), Bergamot (furocoumarin-free), Vetiver, Peppermint, Melissa, Myrrh, Cinnamon Bark, Lemon, Jasmine, Roman Chamomile, Palmarosa, Bitter Orange (Neroli), Rose

**Directions: Aromatic:** Diffuse up to 30 minutes 3 times daily or directly inhale. **Topical:** Apply on desired location as needed.

**Caution:** Possible sun sensitivity.

## Oola®** Fitness™

This energizing blend is formulated to empower and promote discipline and inspiration to set and achieve fitness goals.

**Ingredients:** caprylic/capric triglyceride, Cypress, Copaiba, Basil, Cistus, Marjoram, Peppermint, Clary Sage, Idaho Blue Spruce, Balsam Canada (Idaho Balsam Fir), Nutmeg, Black Pepper

**Directions: Aromatic:** Diffuse up to 30 minutes 3 times daily or directly inhale. **Topical:** Apply on desired location as needed.

## Oola®** Friends™

A welcoming blend, Oola Friends helps bring harmonic balance to the energy centers of the body to encourage feelings of self-worth, confidence, and awareness.

**Ingredients:** caprylic/capric triglyceride, Lavender, Frankincense, Blue Cypress, Orange, Royal Hawaiian Sandalwood, Palo Santo, Xiang Mao, Ylang Ylang, Mandarin, Angelica, Geranium, Hyssop, Spanish Sage, Black Spruce, Jasmine, Lemongrass, Bitter Orange (Neroli), Coriander, Bergamot, Lemon, Roman Chamomile, Palmarosa, Rose

**Directions: Aromatic:** Diffuse up to 30 minutes 3 times daily or directly inhale. **Topical:** Apply on desired location as needed.

Seventh Edition | **Essential Oils Desk Reference** | 157

## Oola®** Fun™

This uplifting and revitalizing essential oil blend promotes euphoric emotions. The cheerful aroma boosts self-confidence and encourages the mind to enjoy life's simple pleasures.

**Ingredients:** caprylic/capric triglyceride, Spearmint, Cedarwood, Myrtle, Lemon, Grapefruit, Tangerine, Jasmine, Nutmeg

**Directions: Aromatic:** Diffuse up to 30 minutes 3 times daily or directly inhale. **Topical:** Apply on desired location as needed.

**Caution:** Possible sun sensitivity.

## Oola®** Grow™

Oola Grow is designed to help you reach unlimited potential and growth in many aspects of life. Whether it's emotional, spiritual, or mental, Oola Grow gives you courage to focus on the task at hand and helps you move forward toward positive advancements and progression.

**Ingredients:** fractionated coconut oil, White Fir, Blue Cypress, Ylang Ylang, Roman Chamomile, almond oil, Northern Lights Black Spruce, Coriander, Geranium, Jasmine, Cedarwood, Lavender, Frankincense, Bergamot (furocoumarin-free), Clary Sage, Royal Hawaiian Sandalwood, Grapefruit, Tangerine, Spearmint, Vetiver, Lemon, Neroli, Idaho Blue Spruce, Ocotea, Juniper, Orange, Cinnamon Bark, Citrus Hystrix, Rose, White Lotus

**Directions: Aromatic:** Diffuse up to 30 minutes 3 times daily or directly inhale. **Topical:** Apply 1-2 drops on edge of ears, wrists, neck, temples, or desired location as needed.

**Caution:** Possible sun sensitivity.

## Owie™

Apply Owie topically to improve the appearance of your child's skin and to help heal a wound.

**Ingredients:** caprylic/capric glycerides, Balsam Canada (Idaho Balsam Fir), Tea Tree, Helichrysum, Elemi, Cistus, Hinoki, Clove

**Directions: Topical:** Recommended application is for children ages 2-12. To be applied only by a trusted adult or under adult supervision. Dilution not required, except for the most sensitive skin. Apply 2-4 drops directly on desired location as needed.

## PanAway®

This very popular blend reduces pain and inflammation, increases circulation, and accelerates healing. It relieves swelling and discomfort from arthritis, sprains, muscle spasms, cramps, bumps, and bruises.

**Ingredients:** Wintergreen, Helichrysum, Clove, Peppermint

**Directions: Topical:** Dilute 1 drop with 4 drops of V-6 or other pure carrier oil. Apply on temples, back of neck, forehead, or desired location as needed. Use as a compress or for a Raindrop Technique-style massage along the spine. Use for relief of deep tissue pain. Add additional Helichrysum to enhance the effect. When the pain is bone related, more Wintergreen may be added. May be diluted with Ortho Ease or Ortho Sport massage oils.

**Caution:** Possible skin sensitivity. Not intended for children under the age of 6 without the advice of a health care professional.

## Peace & Calming®

This blend promotes relaxation and a deep sense of peace and emotional well-being, helping to dampen tensions and uplift spirits. When massaged on the bottoms of feet, it can be a wonderful prelude to a peaceful night's rest. It may calm overactive and hard-to-manage children. It also reduces depression, anxiety, stress, and insomnia. Many people use it for relief from restless leg syndrome.

**Ingredients:** Tangerine, Orange, Ylang Ylang, Patchouli, Blue Tansy

**Directions: Aromatic:** Diffuse up to 1 hour 3 times daily or directly inhale. **Topical:** Dilute 1 drop with 1 drop of V-6 or other pure carrier oil and apply to wrists, edge of ears, foot Vita Flex points, or desired location as needed. Combine with Lavender for insomnia and Matricaria (German Chamomile) for calming.

**Caution:** Possible sun/skin sensitivity.

## Peace & Calming II™

Peace & Calming II has a relaxing and pleasant aroma that may contribute to calming the mind and giving a sense of overall well-being.

**Ingredients:** Tangerine, Orange, Ylang Ylang, Patchouli, Northern Lights Black Spruce, Matricaria (German Chamomile), Vetiver, Cistus, Bergamot, Cassia, Davana

**Directions: Aromatic:** Diffuse up to 1 hour 3 times daily or directly inhale. **Topical:** Dilute 1 drop with 1 drop of V-6™ or other pure carrier oil and apply on desired location as needed.

**Caution:** Possible sun sensitivity.

## Present Time™

This blend is an empowering fragrance that creates a feeling of being in the moment. Disease develops when we live in the past and with regret. Being in the present time is the key to progressing and moving forward.

**Ingredients:** sweet almond oil, Bitter Orange (Neroli), Black Spruce, Ylang Ylang

**Directions: Aromatic:** Diffuse up to 30 minutes 3 times daily or directly inhale. **Topical:** Dilution not required, except for the most sensitive skin. Apply to sternum and thymus area, neck, forehead, or desired location as needed.

**Caution:** Possible sun sensitivity.

## Purification®

This purifying blend cleanses and disinfects the air and neutralizes mildew, cigarette smoke, and disagreeable odors. It disinfects and cleans cuts, scrapes, and bites from spiders, bees, hornets, and wasps.

**Ingredients:** Citronella, Rosemary, Lemongrass, Tea Tree, Lavandin, Myrtle

**Directions: Aromatic:** Diffuse up to 30 minutes 3 times daily or directly inhale. **Topical:** Dilution not required, except for the most sensitive skin. Apply on location to cuts, sores, bruises, or wounds as needed.

## Raven™

The oils of this blend fight against respiratory disease and infections such as tuberculosis, influenza, and pneumonia. It is highly antiviral and antiseptic.

**Ingredients:** Camphor (Ravintsara), Lemon, Wintergreen, Peppermint, Eucalyptus Radiata

**Directions: Aromatic:** Diffuse up to 30 minutes 3 times daily or directly inhale. **Topical:** Dilute 1 drop with 1 drop of V-6 or other pure carrier oil and apply to throat and lung location, foot Vita Flex points, or desired location as needed. Use as a hot compress over lungs or with Raindrop Technique. To use in suppository, dilute with V-6 1:10 and retain during the night.

**Caution:** For external use only. Possible sun/skin sensitivity. Not intended for children under the age of 6 without the advice of a health care professional.

## R.C.™

R.C. gives relief from colds, bronchitis, sore throats, sinusitis, coughs, and respiratory congestion. It decongests sinus passages, combats lung infections, and relieves allergy symptoms.

**Ingredients:** Eucalyptus Globulus, Myrtle, Marjoram, Pine, Eucalyptus Radiata, Eucalyptus Citriodora, Lavender, Cypress, Black Spruce, Peppermint

**Directions: Aromatic:** Diffuse up to 30 minutes 3 times daily or directly inhale. To combat sinus and lung congestion, add R.C., Raven, Dorado Azul, or Eucalyptus Blue to a bowl of steaming hot water. Place a towel over your head and inhale the steam from the mixture. Combine with Raven and Thieves (alternating morning and night) to enhance effects. **Topical:** Dilute 1 drop with 1 drop of V-6 or other pure carrier oil and apply on chest, neck, throat, over sinus location, or on desired location as needed. Use as a hot compress or with Raindrop Technique.

## Reconnect™

Apply Reconnect to help the mind to react positively and to help you reconnect to your surroundings.

**Ingredients:** fractionated coconut oil, Sacred Frankincense, Lavender, Blue Cypress, Cedarwood, Melissa, Idaho Blue Spruce, Palo Santo, Northern Lights Black Spruce, almond oil, Bergamot, Myrrh, Vetiver, Geranium, Royal Hawaiian Sandalwood, Ylang Ylang, Hyssop, Rose

**Directions: Aromatic:** Diffuse up to 1 hour 3 times daily or directly inhale. **Topical:** To be applied only by a trusted adult or under adult supervision. Dilution not required, except for the most sensitive skin. Apply 2-4 drops directly on desired location as needed.

**Caution:** Possible sun sensitivity.

# Red Shot™

Red Shot is a limited-time-only blend that adds a delicious variation to NingXia Red.

**Ingredients:** Tangerine, Mandarin, Lime, Grapefruit, Cassia, Spearmint

**Directions: Dietary:** Add 1-2 drops to 2 ounces of NingXia Red or put 2 drops in a capsule and take 3 times daily or as needed.

# Release™

This is a helpful blend to release anger and memory trauma from the liver in order to create emotional well-being. It helps open the subconscious mind through pineal stimulation to release deep-seated trauma. It is one of the most powerful of the emotionally supporting essential oil blends.

**Ingredients:** Ylang Ylang, olive oil, Lavandin, Geranium, Royal Hawaiian Sandalwood, Grapefruit, Tangerine, Spearmint, Lemon, Blue Cypress, Davana, Kaffir Lime, Ocotea, Jasmine, Matricaria (German Chamomile), Blue Tansy, Rose

**Directions: Aromatic:** Diffuse up to 1 hour 3 times daily or directly inhale. **Topical:** Dilution not required, except for the most sensitive skin. Apply over liver, anywhere trauma has occurred, or use as a compress. Massage on bottoms of feet and behind ears as needed.

**Caution:** Possible sun sensitivity.

# Relieve It™

This blend is high in anti-inflammatory compounds that relieve deep tissue pain and muscle soreness.

**Ingredients:** Black Spruce, Black Pepper, Hyssop, Peppermint

**Directions: Topical:** Dilute 1 drop with 1 drop of V-6 or other pure carrier oil and apply on location to relieve pain as needed. Use as a cold or hot compress.

**Caution:** Possible skin sensitivity.

# RutaVaLa™

RutaVaLa is a proprietary blend of *Ruta graveolens* (Ruta), Lavender, and Valerian essential oils that promotes relaxation of the body and mind, soothes stressed nerves, and induces sleep. Ruta has long been used in South America to promote the relaxation of body and mind, relieve and soothe stressed nerves, and revitalize passion.

**Ingredients:** Lavender, Valerian, Ruta

**Directions: Aromatic:** Diffuse up to 30 minutes 3 times daily or directly inhale. **Topical:** Dilute 1 drop with 1 drop of V-6 or other pure carrier oil. Apply several drops to wrists, temples, neck, or desired location as needed. Apply to the bottoms of feet; children love it.

# RutaVaLa™ Roll-On

RutaVaLa Roll-On is a proprietary blend of *Ruta graveolens* (Ruta), Lavender, and Valerian essential oils that promotes relaxation of the body and mind, soothes stressed nerves, and induces sleep. Ruta has long been used in South America to promote the relaxation of body and mind, relieve and soothe stressed nerves, and revitalize passion.

**Ingredients:** caprylic/capric triglyceride, Lavender, Valerian, Ruta

**Directions: Topical:** Apply generously to wrists, temples, neck, or any desired location as needed. Apply to the bottoms of feet; children love it.

# Sacred Mountain™

Mountain aromas instill strength, empowerment, grounding, and protection with the spiritual feeling of being in a sacred environment.

**Ingredients:** Black Spruce, Ylang Ylang, Balsam Canada (Idaho Balsam Fir), Cedarwood

**Directions: Aromatic:** Diffuse up to 30 minutes 3 times daily or directly inhale. **Topical:** Dilute 1 drop with 1 drop of V-6 or other pure carrier oil. Apply to crown of head, back of neck, behind ears, on thymus and wrists, or desired location as needed.

**Caution:** Possible sun/skin sensitivity.

Oil Blends | Chapter 7

## SARA™

This very specific blend enables one to relax into a mental state to facilitate the release of trauma from sexual and/or ritual abuse. SARA also helps unlock other traumatic experiences such as physical and emotional abuse.

**Ingredients:** sweet almond oil, Ylang Ylang, Geranium, Lavender, Orange, Cedarwood, Blue Cypress, Davana, Citrus Hystrix, Jasmine, Rose, Matricaria (German Chamomile), Blue Tansy, Grapefruit, Tangerine, Spearmint, Lemon, Ocotea, White Lotus

**Directions: Topical:** Dilute 1 drop with 4 drops of V-6 or other pure carrier oils. Apply over energy centers and locations of abuse, on navel, lower abdomen, temples, nose, Vita Flex points on the feet, or desired location as needed.

**Caution:** Possible sun/skin sensitivity.

## SclarEssence™

This blend balances hormones naturally using essential oil phytoestrogens. It helps to increase estrogen levels by supporting the body's own production of hormones. It combines the soothing effects of Peppermint with the balancing power of Fennel and Clary Sage and the calming action of Spanish Sage for an extraordinary topical and aromatic blend and Vitality dietary supplement.

**Ingredients:** Clary Sage, Peppermint, Spanish Sage, Fennel

**Directions: Aromatic:** Diffuse up to 30 minutes 3 times daily or directly inhale. **Topical:** Dilute 1 drop with 1 drop of V-6 or other pure carrier oil and apply on desired location as needed.

**Caution:** Possible sun sensitivity. Do not use in conjunction with any other hormone products.

## SclarEssence Vitality™

**Ingredients:** Clary Sage, Peppermint, Spanish Sage, Fennel

**Directions: Dietary:** Dilute 1 drop with 1 drop of carrier oil. Put in a capsule and take up to 3 times daily or as needed.

## Sensation™

This beautiful smell is profoundly romantic, refreshing, and arousing. It amplifies the excitement of experiencing new heights of self-expression and awareness.

Sensation is also nourishing and hydrating for the skin and is beneficial for many skin problems.

**Ingredients:** Coriander, Ylang Ylang, Bergamot (furocoumarin-free), Jasmine, Geranium

**Directions: Aromatic:** Diffuse up to 1 hour 3 times daily or directly inhale. **Topical:** Dilution not required, except for the most sensitive skin. Apply 2-4 drops on location, neck, or wrists as needed. Use as a compress over abdomen.

## Shutran™

Shutran is an empowering essential oil blend that is specifically designed for men to boost feelings of masculinity and confidence.

**Ingredients:** Idaho Blue Spruce, Ylang Ylang, Ocotea, Hinoki, Davana, Cedarwood, Lavender, Coriander, Lemon, Northern Lights Black Spruce

**Directions: Topical:** Apply 2-4 drops 2 times daily or as needed.

**Caution:** Possible sun sensitivity.

## SleepyIze™

SleepyIze calms and relaxes the mind and body prior to children's bedtime.

**Ingredients:** caprylic/capric glycerides, Lavender, Geranium, Roman Chamomile, Tangerine, Bergamot, Sacred Frankincense, Valerian, Ruta

**Directions: Aromatic:** Diffuse up to 1 hour 3 times daily or directly inhale. **Topical:** Recommended application is for children ages 2-12. To be applied only by a trusted adult or under adult supervision. Dilution not required, except for the most sensitive skin. Apply 2-4 drops directly on desired location as needed.

**Caution:** Possible sun sensitivity.

Seventh Edition | Essential Oils Desk Reference | 161

# Slique™ Essence

Slique Essence combines powerful essential oils and stevia extract to support healthy weight-management goals. It suppresses food cravings, especially when used in conjunction with Slique Tea or any of the Slique products. The oils in this blend add a flavorful and uplifting element to any day, with the added support of Spearmint to aid proper digestion. Ocotea essential oil was chosen for its irresistible cinnamon-esque aroma, which can help trigger feelings of fullness and reduce the number of unexpected cravings. Slique Essence is antibacterial, antifungal, a lipid regulator, and a glucose regulator.

Stevia is added as an all-natural sweetener that provides a pleasant, sweet taste with no added calories.

**Ingredients:** Grapefruit, Tangerine, Spearmint, Lemon, Ocotea, Stevia Extract

**Directions: Aromatic:** Direct inhalation preferred. **Note:** The Stevia extract in this formula may impede diffuser performance. **Dietary:** Shake vigorously before use. Add 2-4 drops to 4-6 oz. of your favorite beverage, Slique Tea, or water. Use between and during meals regularly throughout the day whenever hunger feelings occur. **Topical:** Dilution not required, except for the most sensitive skin. Shake well and apply liberally to temples, back of neck, or wrists as needed.

# SniffleEase™

SniffleEase is a refreshing, rejuvenating blend formulated just for kids for when they have congestion.

**Ingredients:** caprylic/capric glycerides, Eucalyptus Blue, Palo Santo, Lavender, Dorado Azul, Ravintsara, Myrtle, Eucalyptus Globulus, Marjoram, Pine, Eucalyptus Citriodora, Cypress, Eucalyptus Radiata, Black Spruce, Peppermint

**Directions: Aromatic:** Diffuse up to 1 hour 3 times daily or directly inhale. **Topical:** Recommended application is for children ages 2-12. To be applied only by a trusted adult or under adult supervision. Dilution not required, except for the most sensitive skin. Apply 2-4 drops directly on desired location as needed.

# Stress Away™

This is a gentle, fragrant blend that brings a feeling of peace and tranquility to both children and adults and helps relieve daily stress and nervous tension. It helps with normal, everyday stress, improves mental response, restores equilibrium, promotes relaxation, and lowers hypertension.

**Ingredients:** Copaiba, Lime, Cedarwood, Vanilla, Ocotea, Lavender

**Directions: Aromatic:** Diffuse up to 1 hour 3 times daily or directly inhale. **Topical:** Dilution not required, except for the most sensitive skin. Shake well and apply liberally to temples, back of neck, or wrists as needed.

**Caution:** Possible sun/skin sensitivity.

# Stress Away™ Roll-On

This is a gentle, fragrant blend that brings a feeling of peace and tranquility to both children and adults and helps relieve daily stress and nervous tension. It helps with normal, everyday stress, improves mental response, restores equilibrium, promotes relaxation, and lowers hypertension.

**Ingredients:** Copaiba, Lime, Cedarwood, Vanilla, Ocotea, Lavender

**Directions: Topical:** Shake well and apply liberally to temples, back of neck, or wrists as needed.

**Caution:** Possible sun/skin sensitivity

# Surrender™

This inviting oil helps one surrender aggression and a controlling attitude. Stress and tension are released quickly when we surrender willfulness.

**Ingredients:** Lavender, Lemon, Black Spruce, Roman Chamomile, Angelica, Mountain Savory

**Directions: Aromatic:** Diffuse up to 1 hour 3 times daily or directly inhale. **Topical:** Dilution not required, except for the most sensitive skin. Apply 2-4 drops directly on forehead, solar plexus, along ear rim, chest, nape of neck, and desired location as needed.

**Caution:** Possible sun/skin sensitivity.

Oil Blends | **Chapter 7**

## The Gift™

The Gift is the very "essence of Arabia," blending the oils of antiquity into a most unique and exotic fragrance. It combines seven ancient therapeutic oils to capture the spirit of Arabia.

This oil blend represents Mary's gift to Gary in honor of Shutran's noble journey through the book *The One Gift*, a historical novel depicting the wit, intrigue, sorrow, and romance of the ancient frankincense and myrrh caravans.

Out of the writings and legends of antiquity, healing mysteries unfold as we discover powerful uses for herbs and oils in healing the injuries of war, accidents, scorpion stings, and snakebites and in sacred rituals for attaining greater spiritual attunement for healing and protecting the body.

Present-day science is now documenting the properties of these oils that augment the immune system, stimulate healing, and overcome depression. Myrrh and Frankincense are being touted for their anticancer, anti-infectious, antibacterial, and antiviral abilities, as well as being a topical anesthesia and having the ability to regenerate bone and cartilage. They are the oldest known substances for their immune stimulating and healing powers to ever come out of the ancient world.

**Ingredients:** Balsam Canada (Idaho Balsam Fir), Sacred Frankincense, Jasmine, Northern Lights Black Spruce, Myrrh, Vetiver, Cistus

**Directions: Aromatic:** Diffuse up to 30 minutes 3 times daily or directly inhale. **Topical:** Dilute 1 drop with 1 drop of V-6 or other pure carrier oil and apply on desired location as needed. Wear as a fragrance. Massage on the bottoms of feet.

## Thieves®

This is a most amazing blend of highly antiviral, antiseptic, antibacterial, and anti-infectious essential oils.

It was created from research based on legends about a group of 15th-century thieves who rubbed botanicals on themselves to avoid contracting the plague while they robbed the bodies of the dead and dying. When apprehended, the thieves were forced to tell what their secret was and disclosed the formula of the herbs, spices, and oils they used to protect themselves in exchange for more lenient punishment.

Studies conducted at Weber State University (Ogden, UT) during 1997 demonstrated the killing power of these amazing oils against airborne microorganisms. The analysis showed that after 10 minutes of Thieves diffusion in the air, there was an 82 percent reduction in the gram positive *Micrococcus luteus* organism bioaerosol, a 96 percent reduction in gram negative *Pseudomonas aeruginosa* organism bioaerosol, and a 44 percent reduction in *S. aureus* bioaerosol (Chao SC, et al., 1998).

**Ingredients:** Clove, Lemon, Cinnamon Bark, Eucalyptus Radiata, Rosemary

**Directions: Aromatic:** Diffuse up to 10 minutes 3 times daily or directly inhale. **Topical:** Dilute 1 drop with 4 drops V-6 or other pure carrier oil. Apply on desired location as needed. For headaches, put 1 drop on tongue and push against roof of mouth. Apply neat to bottoms of feet.

**Caution:** Possible sun/skin sensitivity.

## Thieves Vitality™

**Ingredients:** Clove, Lemon, Cinnamon Bark, Eucalyptus Radiata, Rosemary

**Directions: Dietary:** Dilute 1 drop with 4 drops of carrier oil. Put in a capsule and take 1 daily.

## Tranquil™ Roll-On

This proprietary blend of Lavender, Cedarwood, and Roman Chamomile essential oils, packaged in a roll-on applicator, provides convenient and portable relaxation and stress relief. All three of these oils have been well documented as being effective in reducing restlessness, decreasing anxiety, and inducing a calming feeling to mind and body. Their combined effect is uplifting as well as relaxing and can be useful in promoting sleep as well as reducing stress.

**Ingredients:** Lavender, Cedarwood, caprylic/capric triglyceride, Roman Chamomile, coconut oil

**Directions: Topical:** Apply liberally to temples, back of neck, or wrists as needed for relaxation.

**Caution:** Possible sun sensitivity.

## Transformation™

Repressed trauma and tragedy from the past may be out of sight, but they are definitely not out of mind. Memories are imprinted in our cells for better or worse. Stored negative emotions need to be replaced with joy, hope, and courage.

Transformation blend radiates with the purifying oils of Lemon and Peppermint, along with the revitalizing power of sesquiterpenes from Sandalwood and Frankincense. Idaho Blue Spruce anchors new mental programming.

Reaching into the deepest recesses of memory, Transformation empowers and upholds the changes you want to make in your belief system. Positive, uplifting beliefs are foundational for the transformation of behavior.

**Ingredients:** Lemon, Peppermint, Royal Hawaiian Sandalwood, Clary Sage, Sacred Frankincense, Idaho Blue Spruce, Cardamom, Ocotea, Palo Santo

**Directions: Aromatic:** Diffuse up to 1 hour 3 times daily for most effective use or directly inhale. **Topical:** Dilute 1 drop with 1 drop of V-6 or other pure carrier oil and apply topically on appropriate Vita Flex points or desired location as needed.

**Caution:** Possible sun sensitivity.

## Trauma Life™

The emotional trauma from accidents, death of loved ones, assault, abuse, etc., can implant its devastation deep within the hidden recesses of the mind, causing life-long problems that seem endless.

Being able to release such burdens can bring about a new "lease on life" with a return to motivation and vitality.

This blend combats stress and uproots trauma that cause insomnia, anger, restlessness, and a weakened immune response.

**Ingredients:** Royal Hawaiian Sandalwood, Frankincense, Valerian, Black Spruce, Davana, Lavender, Geranium, Helichrysum, Citrus Hystrix, Rose

**Directions: Aromatic:** Diffuse up to 1 hour 3 times daily or directly inhale. **Topical:** Dilute 1 drop with 1 drop of V-6 or other pure carrier oil and apply to bottoms of feet, chest, forehead, back of neck, behind ears, along spine as in Raindrop Technique, or on desired location as needed.

## T.R. Care™

This unique blend is designed to restore confidence and uplift emotions by reducing stress and calming the mind, body, and spirit.

**Ingredients:** Roman Chamomile, Tangerine, Lavender, Bergamot, Royal Hawaiian Sandalwood, Ylang Ylang, Frankincense, Valerian, Blue Cypress, Orange, Geranium, Northern Lights Black Spruce, Davana, Ruta, Jasmine, Angelica, Cedarwood, Helichrysum, Hyssop, Spanish Sage, Patchouli, Citrus Hystrix, White Fir, Blue Tansy, Vetiver, Coriander, Bergamot (furocoumarin-free), Rose, Lemon, Cinnamon Bark, Palmarosa, Matricaria (German Chamomile), Grapefruit, Spearmint, Ocotea

**Directions: Aromatic:** Diffuse up to 1 hour 3 times daily or directly inhale. **Topical:** Dilution not required, except for the most sensitive skin. Apply 2-4 drops directly on desired location as needed.

**Caution:** Possible sun sensitivity.

## TummyGize™

TummyGize is a quieting, relaxing blend that can be applied to little tummies that are upset. It also supports proper digestion.

**Ingredients:** caprylic/capric glycerides, Spearmint, Peppermint, Tangerine, Fennel, Anise, Ginger, Cardamom

**Directions: Aromatic:** Diffuse up to 1 hour 3 times daily or directly inhale. **Topical:** Recommended application is for children ages 2-12. To be applied only by a trusted adult or under adult supervision. Dilution not required, except for the most sensitive skin. Apply 2-4 drops directly on desired location as needed.

**Caution:** Possible sun sensitivity.

## Valor®

This blend was formulated to balance energies and instill courage, confidence, and self-esteem. It helps the body self-correct its balance and alignment.

**Ingredients:** caprylic/capric triglyceride, Black Spruce, Rosewood, Blue Tansy, Frankincense

**Directions: Aromatic:** Diffuse up to 1 hour 3 times daily or directly inhale. **Topical:** Dilution not required, except for the most sensitive skin. Apply 2-4 drops to wrists, chest, and back of neck, bottoms of feet, along spine as in Raindrop Technique, or on desired location as needed. When using a series of oils, apply Valor first and wait 5 to 10 minutes before applying other oils.

Oil Blends | **Chapter 7**

## Valor II™

This formula offers an inspiring and calming aroma that can promote empowerment and uplift the soul.

**Ingredients:** caprylic/capric triglyceride, Ylang Ylang, Coriander, Bergamot, Northern Lights Black Spruce, Matricaria (German Chamomile), Idaho Blue Spruce, Frankincense, Vetiver, Cistus, Cassia, Davana, Geranium

**Directions: Aromatic:** Diffuse up to 1 hour 3 times daily or directly inhale. **Topical:** Apply 2-4 drops on desired location. Apply to wrists, chest, back of neck, bottoms of feet, along spine as in Raindrop Technique, or on desired location as needed. When using a series of oils, apply Valor II first and wait 5 to 10 minutes before applying other oils.

## Valor® Roll-On

Valor Essential Oil Roll-On is an empowering combination of therapeutic-grade essential oils that works with both the physical and spiritual aspects of the body to increase feelings of strength, courage, and self-esteem in the face of adversity. Renowned for its strengthening qualities, Valor enhances an individual's internal resources. It has also been found to help energy alignment in the body.

This has become a very popular blend, now offered in a portable, convenient, roll-on application.

**Ingredients:** caprylic/capric triglyceride, Black Spruce, Rosewood, Frankincense, Blue Tansy

**Directions: Topical:** Apply generously on feet, wrists, shoulders, back of neck to ease tension, or desired area as needed. Wear as a fragrance.

## White Angelica™

Increases and strengthens the aura around the body to bring a renewed sense of strength and protection, creating a feeling of wholeness in the realm of one's own spirituality. Its frequency neutralizes negative energy and gives a feeling of security.

**Ingredients:** sweet almond oil, Bergamot, Myrrh, Geranium, Royal Hawaiian Sandalwood, Ylang Ylang, Coriander, Black Spruce, Melissa, Hyssop, Rose

**Directions: Aromatic:** Diffuse up to 30 minutes 3 times daily or directly inhale. **Topical:** Dilution not required except for the most sensitive skin. Apply to shoulders, along spine, on crown of head, on wrists, behind ears, on back of neck, on foot Vita Flex points, or on desired area as needed.

**Caution:** Possible sun sensitivity.

## White Light™

White Light is a balancing essential oil blend meant to elevate the mind, awaken the senses, and promote harmony with nature.

**Ingredients:** White Fir, White Cedar, White Spruce, White Pine

**Directions: Aromatic:** Diffuse up to 30 minutes 3 times daily or directly inhale. **Topical:** Dilute 1 drop with 1 drop of V-6 or other carrier oil and apply on desired location as needed.

---

**Notes**

\* Royal Hawaiian Sandalwood is a registered trademark of Jawmin, LLC
\*\* Oola is a registered trademark of OolaMoola, LLC

Seventh Edition | **Essential Oils Desk Reference** | **165**

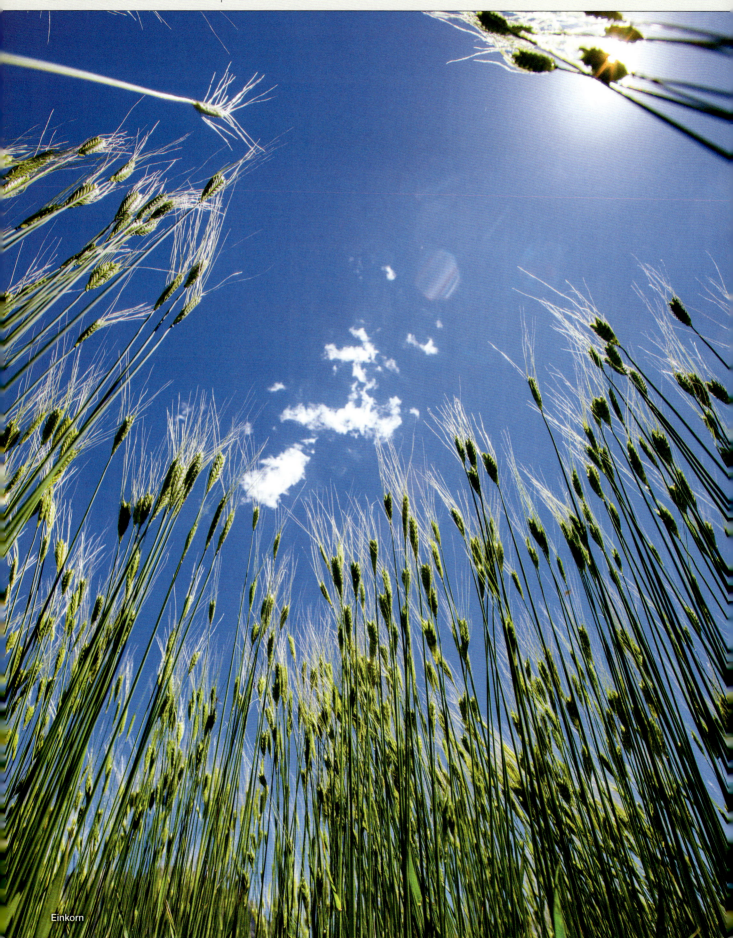
Einkorn

# Chapter 8
## Nutritional Support

## Nutrition Today

In today's world, it has become increasingly difficult to buy or grow food with all the nutrients that our bodies need. It is so sad that our water, air, and soil have become so polluted and devitalized that even the food grown in the best soils does not contain the same nutritional value that it did even 10 years ago.

Because of this, people are turning more and more to nutritional supplementation in the form of tablets, capsules, powders, liquids, and now even high-tech equipment and machines that are touted to perform miracles. The "Fountain of Youth" is still something "just around the corner." "Will it be found?" is a question that doubtfully will be answered, but people will always keep looking.

Supplementation with essential oils is continuing to grow. D. Gary Young formulated the first nutritionals with essential oils about 30 years ago. He began experimenting in the apothecary in his clinic, where he combined the herbs that he crushed with the few essential oils he had brought back with him from Europe. His first two successful products were VitaGreen (now MultiGreens) and ComforTone, which he formulated in 1984, and they are still as popular and effective as they were back then.

He saw tremendous, positive response with his patients, which began many years of formulating numerous products with essential oils. When he pioneered his products, he had no idea that this would become such a prominent way of delivering nutrients to the body and that many other companies would follow his lead.

Today at Young Living, he has formulated an outstanding line of wellness products that provide an unparalleled opportunity for children and adults of all ages to strengthen, invigorate, and protect the body while at the same time uplift and enlighten their mind and spirit.

Young Living provides some of the most potent nutritional supplements available to support health and well-being, combining herbs and various nutrients formulated with pure, therapeutic-grade essential oils, which act as catalysts to help with nutrient absorption as well as assist in removing cellular wastes.

Most Young Living supplements are dissolved and assimilated by the body within a couple of hours. Because of their purity and quality, they have a strength and efficacy unequaled in the marketplace. Taking them throughout the day will provide better nutrient assimilation than taxing the body with a handful of supplements to digest all at once.

As you begin your regimen, we recommend that you follow the directions on the labels as your body learns what it likes and needs. Choose products best suited to your metabolism, need, and physiological makeup.

For example, if you are on a cleansing program, you may want to use only those products designed to facilitate the cleansing for the first few days and then gradually add other products for building or balancing body systems. You may find it better to wait until after the cleansing is completed to add new products, which you will have to determine after you begin your program.

There are always guidelines to follow with each product, which is certainly advisable, especially when using the products for the first time. There is an old adage that says, "Only your body knows," which is very true when you use a natural product. Your body will tell you by how it responds and how you feel. If you are uncertain, then just follow the directions or ask your health care professional to help you.

It is often recommended that you stop taking your supplements for one day a week to allow the body to rest and engage its natural recuperative powers.

**Essential Oils Desk Reference** | Seventh Edition

# Enzyme Quick Reference Guide

*Please copy this page for a quick, daily reference. Keep it in the kitchen or carry it with you when traveling.*

## Open Capsules:

All capsules may be opened and enzymes sprinkled on any food or mixed in any liquid.

## Combinations:

If more than one enzyme is recommended, you may take just one or a combination and see how your body responds. Basically, any combination is acceptable.

## Key:

**Essentialzyme** (caplet)

**Essentialzymes-4** (two capsules):

**E-4 yellow capsule:** for proteins, carbohydrates, sugars, and starches

**E-4 white capsule:** for fats

## Example:

If for your evening meal you eat chicken, salad, vegetable, bread, juice, and apple pie, you will need more enzymes to digest during the night: 2 E-4 yellow, 2 Essentialzyme, 1 Allerzyme, and 6 Detoxzyme. If it seems like too many, just reduce the number. For children: 3 Mightyzyme, 1 E-4 yellow, 1 Detoxzyme

## Standard Dosages:

For each meal:
Adults: 2–4;
Children: 1–2;
Babies: ¼ to ½.

*Check with your health care professional regarding children younger than 2 years of age.*

## Choices:

The first enzyme listed is usually the first choice in combination with any others as desired.

---

**Start the Morning: Essentialzyme** (Adults: 2–4; Children: 1–2 or Mightyzyme 1–3; Babies: ¼ to ½)
Essentialzyme is an overall enzyme that supports the pancreas, which produces glucose the body needs throughout the day for energy.

---

## General Food Categories:

| | |
|---|---|
| Carbohydrates, fruits, vegetables . . . . . . . . . . . . . . . | **E-4 yellow**, Detoxzyme, Allerzyme, Mightyzyme |
| Fats . . . . . . . . . . . . . . . . . . . . . . . . . . . . . . . . . . | **E-4 white, E-4 yellow**, Essentialzyme, Mightyzyme |
| Protein of any kind . . . . . . . . . . . . . . . . . . . . . . | **E-4 yellow**, Detoxzyme, Mightyzyme |
| Sugars, starches . . . . . . . . . . . . . . . . . . . . . . . . . | **E-4 yellow**, Allerzyme, Essentialzyme, Mightyzyme |

## Specific Foods:

| | |
|---|---|
| Eggs, meat, fish . . . . . . . . . . . . . . . . . . . . . . . . . . | **E-4 yellow**, Essentialzyme, Detoxzyme, Mightyzyme |
| Grains, oatmeal, wheat toast . . . . . . . . . . . . . . . . . | **E-4 yellow**, Allerzyme, Detoxzyme, Mightyzyme |
| Meat with pasta, salad, cheese . . . . . . . . . . . . . . . . | **E-4 yellow**, Essentialzyme, Allerzyme |
| Meat with salad, bread, dessert . . . . . . . . . . . . . . . | **E-4 yellow**, Detoxzyme |
| Milk, yogurt, kefir . . . . . . . . . . . . . . . . . . . . . . . . | **E-4 white**, Allerzyme, Mightyzyme |
| Pasta, cheese, bread . . . . . . . . . . . . . . . . . . . . . . . | **Essentialzyme**, E-4 yellow, Detoxzyme |
| Rice, vegetables, fruit . . . . . . . . . . . . . . . . . . . . . | **Allerzyme**, E-4 yellow, Mightyzyme |
| Salad *(no meat)*, vegetables . . . . . . . . . . . . . . . . . | **E-4 yellow**, Allerzyme, Detoxzyme, Mightyzyme |
| Sweets *(ice cream, frozen Rice Dream, cookies, cake, candy bars, granola bars, apple pie)* . . . . . . . . . . | **E-4 yellow**, Allerzyme, Detoxzyme |

## Carbohydrate Categories:

| | |
|---|---|
| **Carbohydrates** *(simple: refined sugars, fruits)* . . . . . . . . | **Allerzyme**, Detoxzyme, E-4 yellow, Mightyzyme |
| **Carbohydrates** *(complex: vegetables, fruits, grains, beans, rice, bread, some milk products)* . . . . . . . | **E-4 yellow**, Allerzyme, Essentialzyme, E-4 white |

---

## Bedtime: . . . . . . . . . . . . . . . . . . . . . . . .   **Detoxzyme:** 5–15 as desired; Mightyzyme: 3–4

**168** | **Chapter 8** | Nutritional Support

Nutritional Support | **Chapter 8**

# Nutritional Supplements

Nutritional supplementation is a great blessing that modern technology has provided for our world today, but the value is determined by quality, quantity, and frequency. With those in place, you are certain to achieve great benefits to your health in our very busy world today.

## AgilEase™

Perfect for an active lifestyle, AgilEase supports the body's response to acute inflammation in healthy individuals, promotes healthy joint flexibility and mobility, and supports cartilage health.

**Ingredients:** frankincense resin powder, calcium fructoborate (from plant minerals), curcuminoids complex: [turmeric extract, piperine (from black pepper whole fruit extract)], collagen type II (chicken sternum extract), glucosamine sulfate, hyaluronic acid (as sodium hyaluronate), rice flour, hypromellose, silicon dioxide, potassium chloride

**Essential Oils:** Wintergreen, Copaiba, Clove, Northern Lights Black Spruce

**Directions:** Consume 2 capsules daily.

## AlkaLime®

This specially designed alkaline mineral powder contains an array of high-alkaline salts and other yeast- and fungus-fighting elements, such as citric acid and essential oils. This precisely balanced, acid-neutralizing mineral formulation helps preserve the body's proper pH balance, the cornerstone of health. By boosting blood alkalinity, yeast and fungus are deprived of the acidic terrain they require in which to flourish. When the blood and tissues of the body are already alkaline balanced, the effectiveness of the essential oils and other nutrients is even greater.

AlkaLime may help reduce the following signs of acid-based yeast and fungus dominance:

- Fatigue/low energy
- Unexplained aches and pains
- Overweight conditions
- Low resistance to illness
- Allergies
- Headaches
- Irritability/mood swings
- Indigestion
- Colitis/ulcers
- Diarrhea/constipation
- Urinary tract infections
- Rectal/vaginal itch
- Candida

**Ingredients:** sodium (as sodium bicarbonate, sodium phosphate, sodium sulfate), calcium (as calcium carbonate, calcium phosphate, calcium sulfate), magnesium (as magnesium phosphate), potassium (as potassium bicarbonate, potassium chloride, potassium phosphate, potassium sulfate), lemon powder, citric acid, tartaric acid, stevia (Reb. A), silica

**Essential Oils:** Lemon, Lime

**Directions:** Stir 1 teaspoon into 4-6 oz. of distilled or purified water; let sit for 20-25 seconds. Gently stir until thoroughly mixed and then drink immediately. Mix only with water. Take 1-3 times daily 1 hour before meals or before retiring to bed as an aid in alkalizing. As an antacid, AlkaLime may be taken as needed.

**Caution:** Not recommended for sodium-restricted diets or for individuals with high blood pressure.

## Allerzyme®

Allerzyme is a vegetarian enzyme complex blend of enzymes, complementary botanicals, Ginger, Peppermint, and other essential oils that support proper digestion, waste elimination, and nutrient utilization. This potent enzyme complex is formulated to combat allergies, gas, fermentation, fatigue, and irritable bowel syndrome. It also contains a powerful combination of sugar- and starch-splitting enzymes, as well as small amounts of fat- and protein-digesting enzymes.

**Ingredients:** plantain leaf, amylase, bromelain, peptidase, protease, invertase, phytase, barley grass, lipase, lactase, cellulase, alpha-galactosidase, diastase, hypromellose, water, silica

**Essential Oils:** Tarragon, Ginger, Peppermint, Juniper, Fennel, Lemongrass, Anise, Patchouli

**Directions:** Take 1 capsule 3 times daily just prior to meals or as needed.

## Balance Complete™
## Vanilla Cream Meal Replacement

Balance Complete is a super-food meal replacement that is high in fiber and protein, consisting of good fats, enzymes, vitamins, and minerals needed to form a nutritious, great-tasting protein drink that satisfies

Seventh Edition | **Essential Oils Desk Reference** | 169

the appetite. It is a powerful nutritive energizer and a cleanser, which helps to improve digestion and support colon health. The high antioxidant benefits of the Ningxia wolfberry (*Lycium barbarum*) powder, in combination with brown rice bran, barley grass, aloe vera, cinnamon powder, and whey protein blend, create the building blocks for strengthening the immune system and bringing back the renewed feelings of energy and vitality.

**Ingredients:** Proprietary V-Fiber™ Blend: [larch polysaccharides, Ningxia wolfberry fruit powder, brown rice bran, guar gum, konjac, xanthan gum, chicory root fiber extract (FOS), sodium alginate], whey protein concentrate, nonfat dry milk, medium-chain triglycerides, natural vanilla flavor, fructose, lecithin, calcium (as tricalcium phosphate), Proprietary Enzyme Complex: [lactase, lipase, bromelain, papain, amylase], xylitol, magnesium oxide, barley grass powder, neohesperidin derivative (flavor from natural citrus), cinnamon bark powder, mixed carotenoids (vitamin A), lo han kuo extract, cream flavor, barley grass juice, aloe vera, vitamin C (ascorbic acid), mixed tocopherols (vitamin E), vitamin B3 (niacinamide), zinc oxide, selenium (as selenomethionine), beta-carotene, molybdenum citrate; vitamin B5 (pantothenic acid from calcium pantothenate), vitamin B6 (pyridoxine HCI), chromium amino nicotinate, vitamin B1 (thiamine HCI), vitamin B2 (riboflavin), vitamin D3 (cholecalciferol), vitamin B12 (methylcobalamin, folic acid, biotin, iodine (as potassium iodide)

**Essential Oil:** Orange

**Directions:** Add 2 scoops of Balance Complete to 8 oz. of cold water. May be mixed with rice, almond, or other milk, etc. Shake, stir, or blend until smooth. For added flavor, add fruit or other essential oils.

For a delicious nutritional drink, mix 1-2 scoops of Balance Complete with ½ cup carrot juice, ½ cup coconut milk, 1 drop Orange oil, and ¼ cup added water (or equivalent amount of ice); blend; and enjoy nutrition at its best!

For a five-day cleanse, replace all three daily meals with Balance Complete and follow the recommended schedule. As part of a low-calorie diet, replace two daily meals with Balance Complete.

**Allergen Warning:** Contains ingredients derived from milk and soy.

## BLM™ (Bones, Ligaments, and Muscles) Capsules

BLM supports normal bone and joint health. This formula combines powerful, natural ingredients, such as type II collagen, MSM, glucosamine sulfate, and manganese citrate, enhanced with the anti-inflammatory and pain-relieving essential oils of Idaho Balsam Fir, Wintergreen, and Clove.

These ingredients support healthy cell function and encourage joint health and fluid movement.

This product is a highly effective arthritis treatment for building bones, ligaments, and muscles. The exclusive collagen and hyaluronic acid blend strengthens and rebuilds damaged joints and cartilage as it combats arthritis inflammation and bone pain.

**Ingredients:** sodium, manganese, Proprietary BLM Blend: [glucosamine sulfate, type II collagen (chicken sternum extract), MSM (methylsulfonylmethane)], gelatin, rice flour, magnesium stearate, silicon dioxide

**Essential Oils:** Idaho Balsam Fir (Balsam Canada), Wintergreen, Clove

**Directions:** Take 1 capsule 3 times daily if you weigh less than 120 lbs. Take 1 capsule 4 times daily if you weigh between 120 and 200 lbs. Take 1 capsule 5 times daily if you weigh over 200 lbs. Allow 4-8 weeks of daily use before expecting noticeable results.

**Allergen Warning:** Contains ingredients derived from shellfish.

## BLM™ (Bones, Ligaments, and Muscles) Powder

BLM supports normal bone and joint health. This formula combines powerful, natural ingredients such as type II collagen, MSM, glucosamine sulfate, and manganese citrate, enhanced with the anti-inflammatory and pain-relieving essential oils of Idaho Balsam Fir, Wintergreen, and Clove.

These ingredients support healthy cell function and encourage joint health and fluid movement.

This product is highly effective in helping to build bones, ligaments, and muscles and in relieving pain from arthritis and other related maladies. The exclusive collagen and hyaluronic acid blend strengthens and rebuilds damaged joints and cartilage as it combats arthritis inflammation and bone pain.

The powder is the same formula as found in BLM capsules, with the addition of Peppermint and bacteria-fighting xylitol to strengthen bones.

**Ingredients:** manganese, potassium (as potassium chloride), Proprietary BLM Powder Blend: [glucosamine sulfate, type II collagen (chicken), xylitol, MSM (methylsulfonylmethane)], rice bran

**Essential Oils:** Clove, Peppermint, Idaho Balsam Fir, Wintergreen

**Directions:** If you weigh less than 120 lbs., take ¼ teaspoon 3 times daily. If you weigh 120-200 lbs., take ¼ teaspoon 4 times daily. If you weigh more than 200 lbs., take ¼ teaspoon 5 times daily. Allow 4-8 weeks of daily use before expecting noticeable results.

**Allergen Warning:** Contains an ingredient derived from shellfish.

## Blue Agave

Considered the Mexican Tree of Life and Abundance, agave has been part of the Southwestern diet for centuries. A favorite food of the Aztecs, agave nectar was used in religious ceremonies and was labeled by some as the nectar of the gods. The natives of Mexico call the juice "honey water."

The blue agave cactus grows in Mexico, central and tropical South America, and southern and western United States. It produces a sweetener that is about 68 percent fructose, 22 percent glucose, and 4 percent fructooligosaccharides. Because of its heavy fructose concentration, Blue Agave is 32 percent sweeter than table sugar but has a low glycemic index of about 34. This means that when consumed, Blue Agave has a minimal impact on blood sugar levels following consumption. It is well suited for people with candida infections.

**Ingredients:** Blue Agave

**Directions:** Use as a supplemental sweetener, 1-2 drops per cup of liquid or as desired. In recipes use 1/2 to 3/4 cup in place of 1 cup of sugar.

## ComforTone®

ComforTone (capsules) is an effective combination of herbs and essential oils that supports the health of the digestive system by eliminating residues from the colon and enhancing its natural ability to function optimally. Because it supports normal peristalsis (the wave-like contractions that move food through the intestines),

ComforTone is ideal for strengthening the system that delivers nutrients to the rest of the body. This herbal formulation is combined with powerful essential oils that are antiparasitic, anti-inflammatory, ease intestinal cramps, help soothe the discomforts of the digestive tract, and aid in the elimination process.

The unique essential oil called Ocotea, produced from a plant that grows in the Amazon, is extremely powerful in combating candida, which is the foundation for many health concerns. The other essential oils in this complex formulation truly make it the overall best product for cleansing the colon while benefiting the liver, gall bladder, and overall process of digestion.

**Ingredients:** cascara sagrada bark, psyllium seed, barberry bark, burdock root, fennel seed, garlic, echinacea root, bentonite, diatomaceous earth, ginger root, German chamomile flower extract, apple pectin, licorice root, cayenne fruit, gelatin, water, silicon dioxide

**Essential Oils:** Tarragon, Ginger, Tangerine, Rosemary, Anise, Peppermint, Ocotea, German Chamomile

**Directions:** Take 1 capsule 3 times daily. Drink at least 64 ounces of water throughout the day for best results.

**Cautions:** Read and follow directions carefully. Do not use if you have or develop diarrhea, loose stools, or abdominal pain. Consult your health care professional if you have frequent diarrhea. During pregnancy, check with a health care professional before using. Do not exceed recommended dosage. Not for long-term use; do not exceed two weeks. Not to be used as a weight loss product.

## CortiStop®

CortiStop is a proprietary dietary supplement designed to help the body maintain its natural balance and harmony. When under stress, the body produces cortisol. When too much cortisol is produced, it can have negative health consequences such as feelings of fatigue, difficulty maintaining healthy weight, and difficulty maintaining optimal health of cardiovascular systems. CortiStop supports the glandular systems of women.

**Ingredients:** pregnenolone, L-a-phosphatidylserine, L-a-phosphatidylcholine, black cohosh extract, DHEA, rice flour, silica, gelatin

**Essential Oils:** Clary Sage, Canadian Fleabane (Conyza), Fennel, Frankincense, Peppermint

**Directions:** Take 2 capsules in the morning before breakfast. If desired, for extra benefits, take 2 more capsules before bedtime. Use daily for 8 weeks. Discontinue for 2-4 weeks before resuming.

**Cautions:** For adult use only.

**Allergen Warning:** Contains soy-derived ingredients.

## Detoxzyme®

Detoxzyme combines powerful and effective essential oils with a myriad of fast-acting enzymes that assist in the complete digestive process, helping to detoxify and promote cleansing, which is essential for maintaining and building health.

The enzymes in this product are designed to digest starches, sugars, proteins, and fats and along with the trace minerals help the body detoxify, reducing cholesterol and triglycerides. Detoxzyme helps in opening the gallbladder duct and cleansing the liver, preventing candida and yeast overgrowth while promoting detoxification and parasite cleansing.

Detoxzyme also contains phytase, an enzyme essential for unlocking the mineral content of many grains, nuts, seeds, and other foods that contain high levels of essential minerals that are unavailable to the human body because they are bound up in insoluble, indigestible phytate complexes. Thus, the phytase in Detoxzyme results in a huge boost in mineral absorption from diets high in nuts, seeds, and whole grains.

This important enzyme formula facilitates remarkable absorption of nutrients from foods and supplements, thus providing increased energy levels and optimal health.

**Ingredients:** amylase, cumin seed powder, invertase, protease 4.5, glucoamylase, bromelain, phytase, lipase, cellulase, lactase, alpha-galactosidase, vegetable cellulose, rice bran, water, silica,

**Essential Oils:** Cumin, Anise, Fennel

**Directions:** Take 1-2 capsules 3 times daily between meals or as needed.

**Warning:** Not for children under 12 years of age except under the supervision of a health care professional. If discomfort persists, discontinue use and consult your physician.

## Digest & Cleanse™

Digest & Cleanse is formulated with clinically proven and time-tested essential oils that work synergistically to help soothe gastrointestinal upset, prevent gas, and stimulate stomach secretions, supporting healthy digestion.

Essential oils are distilled from large amounts of fresh and/or dried herbs, plants, and trees. It often takes many pounds of plant material to make 1 ounce of an essential oil. Because the oils are so potent, it takes only a very few drops of the oil to achieve the desired digestive and cleansing effects.

The Digest & Cleanse softgels release their unique blend of essential oils in the intestines, the targeted area for optimal absorption.

Good health begins with a healthy bowel. Stress, overeating, and toxins can irritate the gastrointestinal system and cause cramps, gas, and nausea that interfere with the body's natural digestive and detoxification functions. Supplementing with Digest & Cleanse will soothe the bowel, prevent gas, and stimulate the liver, gall bladder, and stomach secretions, thus aiding digestion and absorption that is imperative for good health.

**Ingredients:** virgin coconut oil, fractionated coconut oil, gelatin, glycerin, aqueous coating solution (water, oleic acid, sodium alginate, medium-chain triglycerides, ethyl-cellulose, ammonium hydroxide, stearic acid)

**Essential Oils:** Peppermint, Caraway, Lemon, Ginger, Fennel, Anise

**Directions:** Take 1 softgel 1-3 times daily with water 30-60 minutes prior to meals.

## Ecuadorian Dark Chocolessence™

In his quest to bring healthful, natural products to the world, D. Gary Young recognized the power of cacao and set out to create and then refine a delicacy packed with cacao's nutritional goodness. The result is the newest Ecuadorian Dark Chocolessence. Complex, slightly acidic, and luxuriously dark, the small batch Ecuadorian chocolate brings together a mosaic of pure Young Living essential oils combined with the distinctive cocoa flavors of exclusively sourced Ecuadorian cocoa beans and is crafted with the expertise of an award-winning chocolatier for the richest experience possible.

Cacao has been sought throughout history for its rich flavor and high amounts of beneficial flavonoids and antioxidants. It was so precious that it was saved for royalty and the elite. Today cacao is considered one of the world's premier superfoods.

Ecuadorian Dark Chocolate Chocolessence is in a class by itself. The health benefits include cardiovascular support, mood support, skin support, immune support, weight-management support, and oral support.

**Ingredients:** Ecuadorian cocoa beans, cane sugar, cocoa butter

## Ecuadorian Dark Chocolessence with Cinnamon Bark, Nutmeg, and Clove

**Essential Oils:** Cinnamon Bark Vitality, Nutmeg Vitality, Clove Vitality

## Ecuadorian Dark Chocolessence with Tangerine and Ginger

**Essential Oils:** Tangerine Vitality, Ginger Vitality

**Directions:** Consume 1 bar or as desired.

## Einkorn Grain (Wheat)
(See Gary's True Grit Einkorn Products)

## EndoGize™

EndoGize helps women maintain a healthy endocrine system. With everyday worries and not taking care of ourselves nutritionally, the body becomes stressed and out of balance, which is particularly unhealthy for women. This can increase cortisol levels and decrease estrogen or testosterone, which can lead to a diminished libido and imbalanced metabolism that further leads to a decrease in energy and an increase in food consumption.

For a woman's body to maintain health and vitality, it is critical for her to maintain a healthy endocrine system. The endocrine system regulates several body systems by releasing hormones into the bloodstream. Once in the bloodstream, hormones travel to specific body systems such as the adrenals, pituitary, hypothalamus, thyroid, and ovaries. When the endocrine system is not balanced, each of these body systems is unable to function properly and can put undue stress on other systems within the body.

**Ingredients:** vitamin B6 (as pyridoxine HCI), zinc (as zinc aspartate), Proprietary EndoGize Blend: [ashwaganda root, muira puama bark, L-arginine, epimedium aerial parts, tribulus terrestris fruit extract, phosphatidylcholine, soy lecithin, black pepper fruit extract, glycoamylase, acid stable protease, eurycoma longifolia root extract, amylase, cellulase], DHEA, rice flour, gelatin

**Essential Oils:** Ginger, Myrrh, Cassia, Clary Sage, Canadian Fleabane

**Directions:** Take 1 capsule 2 times daily for 4 weeks. Discontinue use for 2 weeks before resuming.

**Allergen Warning:** Contains soy.

## Essentialzyme™

Essentialzyme is an advanced, multi-enzyme complex that promotes digestion and assists in the assimilation of nutrients. Enzyme supplementation is particularly important for people suffering from chronic pancreatitis, cystic fibrosis, or for any condition where the pancreas duct or common bile duct is blocked, thereby preventing enzymes from reaching the intestines.

Essentialzyme is a bilayer, Peppermint-coated caplet that combines pure essential oils, herbs, and pancreatic and plant-derived enzymes to support overall digestion. Its dual time-release technology increases its effect during digestion.

Essentialzyme helps re-establish proper enzyme balance in the digestive system and throughout the body, helps to improve intestinal flora, and may also help retard the aging process. This is a high-quality, complex enzyme formula created to help improve and aid digestion and elimination of toxic waste from the body, which in turn means more energy and vitality.

**Ingredients:** calcium (as di-calcium phosphate), Proprietary Delayed Release Blend (Light): [pancrealipase, pancreatin, trypsin], Proprietary Immediate Release Blend (Dark): [betaine (HCI), bromelain, thyme leaf powder, carrot powder, alfalfa sprout powder, alfalfa leaf powder, papain, cumin seed powder, Essential Oil Blend], microcrystalline cellulose, dicalcium phosphate, hydroxypropylcellulose, hydroxypropylmethylcellulose, stearic acid, silicon dioxide, croscarmellose sodium, **Coating:** sodium citrate, sodium carboxymethyl cellulose, dextrin, lecithin, dextrose, peppermint essential oil

**Essential Oils:** Essential Oil Blend: Anise, Fennel, Peppermint, Tarragon, Clove

**Directions:** Take 1 caplet, 1 hour before your largest meal of the day for best results.

**Warning:** Do not give to children under 6 years of age except under the supervision of a health care professional. If discomfort persists, discontinue use.

## Essentialzymes-4™

Essentialzymes-4 is a multispectral enzyme complex specially formulated to aid the digestion of dietary fats, proteins, fiber, and carbohydrates commonly found in the modern, processed diet. Essentialzymes-4 combines both animal- and plant-based enzymes into a single solution to help the body more completely break down problematic foods such as high fats and excessive starch. The dual time-release technology releases the animal- and plant-based enzymes at separate times within the digestive tract, allowing for optimal absorption of key nutrients and amino acids.

The plant-based enzymes capsule is designed to release immediately upon entering the stomach, where the pH environment is broad, acidic, and more conducive to plant-based enzyme breakdown and proper absorption.

The animal-based enzyme capsule is formulated to delay its release in the lower intestine region, where the environment is more alkaline, and the pH level is better suited for animal-based enzyme breakdown and proper absorption.

**Ingredients (Yellow Capsule):** protease (4.5, 6.0), amylase, cellulase, lipase, peptidase, phytase, bromelain, papain, rice flour, gelatin capsule, magnesium stearate, silicon dioxide

**Essential Oils:** Anise, Ginger, Rosemary, Tarragon, Fennel

**Ingredients (White Capsule):** bee pollen powder, pancreatin, lipase, rice flour, hypromellose capsule, magnesium stearate, silicon dioxide

**Essential Oils:** Ginger, Fennel, Tarragon, Anise, Lemongrass

**Directions:** Take 2 capsules (1 dual dose blister pack) 2 times daily with largest meals (4 capsules total).

**Allergen Warning:** Contains bee product.

## Estro™

Estro is an herbal tincture containing plant-derived phytoestrogens, such as black cohosh, which are widely used in Europe as safe alternatives to synthetic estrogen. Phytoestrogens have been researched for their ability to support the body during PMS without many of the side effects associated with estrogen-replacement therapies.

The essential oil of Clary Sage, containing natural sclareol, is a plant-based estrogen that is very calming and emotionally balancing. It helps ease the discomforts of menstrual cramps and assists in the transition of menopause, regulating hormonal imbalances.

Estro combines the wonderful benefits of royal jelly, rich in amino acids, minerals, and vitamins B5 and B6, and helps to provide immune-stimulating properties and energy.

Any woman will appreciate the great results from using and enjoying the wonderful responses this product gives.

**Ingredients:** black cohosh root, blue cohosh root, royal jelly, distilled water, ethanol

**Essential Oils:** Fennel, Lavender, Clary Sage

**Directions:** Take 3 half droppers (3 ml) 3 times daily in distilled water or as needed. Shake well before using. Refrigerate after opening.

**Allergen Warning:** Contains bee product.

## FemiGen™

FemiGen combines whole food herbs like wild yam, damiana, and dong quai with synergistic amino acids and select hormone-balancing essential oils to supply special nutritional support to the female systems. FemiGen acts as a natural estrogen and helps balance the hormones and the reproductive system from the developmental years all the way through menopause.

**Ingredients:** magnesium (magnesium carbonate), damiana leaf, *Epimedium sagittatum* aerial plant, wild yam root, dong quai root, muira puama root, ginseng root, licorice root extract, black cohosh root, L-carnitine, dimethylglycine HCI, cramp bark, squaw vine, L-phenylalanine, L-cystine, L-cysteine HCI, gelatin

**Essential Oils:** Fennel, Clary Sage, Sage, Ylang Ylang

**Directions:** Take 2 capsules with breakfast and 2 capsules with lunch.

Nutritional Support | **Chapter 8**

# Gary's True Grit Einkorn Grain Products

## Einkorn Grain (Wheat) and Those "Amber Waves of Grain"

In the 1950s, the American PhD plant pathologist Norman Borlaug went to Mexico to help fight stem rust, a fungus that infects wheat. For the next decade, he worked with colleagues to cross-breed wheat to be disease-resistant and to have higher yields. Because the first strains of this new wheat could not stand up with its abnormally large seed head, he crossed this wheat with Japanese dwarf wheat (with short, stockier stems), which resulted in semi-dwarf wheat that was more disease resistant; and wherever it was planted, yields soared.

The Green Revolution had started. Mexico, India, and Pakistan saw their yields *double.* Borlaug was awarded the Nobel Peace Prize in 1970, the Presidential Medal of Freedom (1977), and the Congressional Gold Medal (2006). He certainly had noble intentions. But for consumers, the results were *not* noble but decidedly unhealthy.

Mark Hyman, MD, writes that we now "eat dwarf wheat plants with much higher amounts of starch and gluten and many more chromosomes coding for all sorts of new odd proteins. The man who engineered this modern wheat won the Nobel Prize—it promised to feed millions of starving around the world. Well, it has, and it has made them **fat and sick**."[1] (Emphasis added)

Dr. Hyman warns that this new "Frankenfood" has three important ways to drive obesity, diabetes, heart disease, cancer, dementia, and more:

- It contains the Super Starch amylopectin A that is super fattening.
- It contains a form of Super Gluten that is super-inflammatory.
- It contains forms of a Super Drug that is super addictive and makes you crave and eat more.[2]

The author of the best-selling book *Wheat Belly,* Dr. William Davis, told CBS News that modern wheat is a "perfect, chronic poison." He says the wheat we eat today isn't the wheat our grandmothers had. "It's an 18-inch tall plant created by genetic research in the '60s and '70s. This thing has many new features nobody told you about, such as there's a new protein in this thing called gliadin. It's not gluten. I'm not addressing people with gluten sensitivities and celiac disease. I'm talking about everybody else. This thing binds into the opiate receptors in your brain and in most people stimulates appetite such that we consume 440 more calories per day, 365 days per year."[3]

The new dwarf wheat makes a lot of money for Big Agriculture, makes consumers fatter, and deprives them of the nutrition that the first wheat species (Emmer, Einkorn) had and still have in abundance.

Einkorn (*Triticum monococcum*) is the wheat (*chitta'im* in Hebrew) first mentioned in the Bible in Genesis 30:14: "And Reuben went in the days of wheat harvest, and found mandrakes in the field, and brought them unto his mother Leah." A website devoted to einkorn added, "Abraham and Sarah offered einkorn cakes to the three angels that visited them"[4] (Genesis 18:4).

Stan Ness of the website Einkorn.com explains the difference between Einkorn (cultivated about 7500 BC) and the 1950-60s dwarf wheat:

1. "Wheat gluten studies have found einkorn wheat may be non-toxic to sufferers of gluten intolerance.[5]
2. Modern wheats have 42 chromosomes while einkorn grain has just 14 (friendlier to the body's digestive system).
3. Einkorn contains 3 to 4 times more beta-carotene than modern wheats (boosts immunity, helps prevent cancer and heart disease).
4. Einkorn contains 2 times more Vitamin A (retinol equivalent) than modern wheats (healthy eyes, reproductive organs, and prevention of many cancers).
5. Einkorn contains 3 to 4 times more lutein than modern wheats (prevention of macular degeneration and cataracts).
6. Einkorn contains 4-5 times more riboflavin than modern wheats (used by the body to create energy and is an antioxidant that slows down aging)."[6]

Not mentioned in the above list of einkorn benefits is that einkorn is significantly higher in protein than hard red spring wheat.[7] Health educator Carol Kenny, PhD, quantified this: "Einkorn is nutrient-dense, with protein content equaling durum wheat and some 35%-50% higher than hard red wheat."[8]

Dr. Mark Hyman's fears about the "Super Gluten" in dwarf wheat were confirmed by the research of Dr. Alessio Fasano, a celiac expert from the University of Maryland School of Medicine. Dr. Hyman writes that Dr. Fasano "discovered a protein made in the intestine called 'zonulin' that is increased by exposure to gluten.[9] Zonulin breaks up the tight junctions or cement between the intestinal cells that normally protect your immune system from

Seventh Edition | **Essential Oils Desk Reference** | 175

bugs and foreign proteins in food leaking across the intestinal barrier. If you have a 'leaky gut,' you will get inflammation throughout your whole body and a whole list of symptoms and diseases."[10]

Dr. Hyman warns that hybridization of wheat led to the many more chromosomes of dwarf wheat, which codes for all sorts of odd new proteins. Truly what was meant to feed the world has turned out to be a real "Frankenfood."

Back to those "amber waves of grain." They are waving tall again! Einkorn cultivation is increasing in Canada and the U.S. because of the demand of health-conscious consumers who want the *original* "Staff of Life."

There are interesting and fun products made with einkorn wheat that can be consumed daily. Be sure to watch for them.

**See:** Gary's True Grit Chocolate-Coated Wolfberry Crisp Bars, Gary's True Grit Einkorn Flour, Gary's True Grit Einkorn Granola, Gary's True Grit Einkorn Pancake and Waffle Mix, Gary's True Grit Einkorn Rotini Pasta, and Gary's True Grit Einkorn Spaghetti.

## Gary's True Grit™ Chocolate-Coated Wolfberry Crisp™ Bars

The Chocolate-Coated Wolfberry Crisp bar is a delicious, convenient, whole-food, low-glycemic, super-nutrient bar, containing 6 grams of protein. It is rich in antioxidants and phytonutrients and does not significantly raise blood sugar levels. It is a great all-natural snack for when you are on the go, at work, at school, or even when you want a meal replacement.

**Ingredients:** whey cocoa protein crisps (whey protein isolate, whey protein concentrate, tapioca starch), dark chocolate (cane sugar, palm kernel oil, cocoa powder, calcium carbonate, sunflower lecithin, salt), isomalto-oligosaccharide (from tapioca), pea protein (pea protein, rice starch), ancient grain granola (whole rolled oats, evaporated cane juice, rice syrup, flax seed, coconut, puffed quinoa, amaranth, chia, vanilla, salt), organic brown rice syrup, shredded coconut, wolfberries, dried almonds, quinoa, honey, glycerin, einkorn flour, gum arabic, organic cane sugar, virgin coconut oil, natural chocolate flavor, salt, cocoa extract, mixed tocopherols

**Directions:** Eat as desired.

**Allergen Warning:** Contains milk (whey), wheat (einkorn), and tree nuts (cashews, coconut, walnuts). Manufactured in a facility that also processes other tree nuts, peanuts, soy, and eggs.

## Gary's True Grit™ Einkorn Flour

Einkorn Flour contains only unhybridized Einkorn grain that has been milled and packaged for use in all flour recipes. The flour is delicious and exceptionally easy to digest.

**Ingredients:** whole grain Einkorn Flour

**Allergen Warning:** Contains einkorn wheat. Manufactured in a facility that also processes tree nuts, peanuts, soy, milk, and eggs.

## Gary's True Grit™ Einkorn Granola

Einkorn Granola is a tasty combination of crunchy einkorn clusters and a variety of nuts, berries, and seeds packed with energy, a sophisticated flavor, and a symphony of textures. It is made with only the finest, carefully selected, and naturally derived ingredients.

- No added colors, flavors, or preservatives
- No high fructose corn syrup
- Non-GMO ingredients
- Made with whole grains
- Vegan recipe

**Ingredients:** oats, whole grain einkorn flour, syrup (from fruit juice and grain dextrin), sunflower oil, sunflower seeds, coconut sugar, cranberries, almonds, wolfberries, walnuts, pecans, cacao nibs, vanilla extract, sea salt, Saigon cinnamon

**Allergen Warning:** Contains einkorn wheat and tree nuts (coconut, almond, walnut, pecan). Manufactured in a facility that also processes tree nuts, soy, and milk.

## Gary's True Grit™ Einkorn Pancake and Waffle Mix

A unique mix for a healthy breakfast that combines ancient Einkorn wheat with other healthful grains and a special blend of ground legumes, added for a concentrated source of protein and fiber, making this a nutritious and tasty meal that will be enjoyed by the entire family.

The oldest known variety of grain, einkorn is nutritious and unhybridized, making it exceptionally easy for the body to digest.

**Ingredients:** whole grain Einkorn Flour, brown rice flour, amaranth flour, tapioca flour, sorghum flour (sorghum bicolor), dhokla flour (Indian flour made from chickpeas)

**Allergen Warning:** Contains einkorn wheat. Manufactured in a facility that also processes tree nuts, peanuts, soy, milk, and eggs.

Nutritional Support | **Chapter 8**

## Gary's True Grit™ Einkorn Rotini Pasta

This natural, delicious alternative to traditional pastas makes the oldest variety of grain new again with a fun, new spiral shape that will have the whole family wanting more. Einkorn is the oldest known variety of grain, and because it is unhybridized, it is exceptionally easy for the body to digest.

**Ingredients:** whole grain Einkorn Flour, water

**Directions:** Boil 3 quarts of water, add 2 teaspoons of salt, if desired. Add pasta to boiling water. Return to boil. Cook uncovered 8-10 minutes, stirring occasionally. Drain and serve as desired.

**Caution:** Choking hazard. Keep out of reach of children.

**Allergen Warning:** Contains einkorn wheat. Manufactured in a facility that also processes tree nuts, peanuts, soy, milk, and eggs.

## Gary's True Grit™ Einkorn Spaghetti

This is a natural, delicious alternative to traditional pastas that the whole family will love. Einkorn is the oldest known variety of grain, and because it is unhybridized, it is exceptionally easy for the body to digest.

**Ingredients:** whole grain Einkorn Flour, water

**Directions:** Boil 3 quarts of water; add 2 teaspoons of salt, if desired. Add pasta to boiling water. Return to boil. Cook uncovered 8-10 minutes, stirring occasionally. Drain and serve as desired.

**Allergen Warning:** Contains einkorn wheat. Manufactured in a facility that also processes tree nuts, peanuts, soy, milk, and eggs.

## Gary's True Grit™ Gluten-Free Pancake and Waffle Mix

A unique and delicious combination of ancient grain and bean flours, this gluten-free, all-purpose mix makes delicious pancakes and waffles and is the perfect flour replacement to use in many of your favorite recipes.

**Ingredients:** gluten-free oat flour, arrowroot flour, garbanzo bean flour, sorghum flour, amaranth flour

## Gary's True Grit™ NingXia Berry Syrup

NingXia Berry Syrup is a premium, all-purpose syrup that combines naturally delicious ingredients with pure Orange and Lemon essential oils for a perfect complement to your favorite pancake and waffle mix or desserts.

**Ingredients:** cane sugar, water, berry juice concentrate [blueberry, plum, sweet cherry, aronia, pomegranate], vanilla extract, xanthan gum, wolfberry seed oil

**Essential Oils:** Lemon, Orange

**Directions:** Use as desired on pancakes, waffles, and with your favorite desserts.

## ICP™

ICP is a great colon cleanser with an advanced mix of fibers that scours out residues.

A healthy digestive system is important for the proper functioning of all other systems because it absorbs nutrients that are used throughout the body. ICP provides ingredients such as psyllium, oat bran, and flax and fennel seeds to form a combination of soluble and insoluble fibers. Enhanced with a special blend of essential oils, the fibers work to decrease the buildup of wastes, dispel gas, improve nutrient absorption, and help maintain a healthy heart.

**Ingredients:** Proprietary ICP Blend: [psyllium seed, flax seed oil, oat bran, fennel powder, rice bran, guar gum, yucca root, cellulose], Proprietary ICP Enzyme Blend: [lipase, protease, phytase, peptidase, aloe vera leaf juice]

**Essential Oils:** Fennel, Anise, Tarragon, Ginger, Lemongrass, Rosemary

**Directions:** Mix 2 rounded teaspoons with at least 8 ounces of warm water or juice 1 time daily. ICP mixes better in warm water. If cleansing or eating a high-protein diet, drink 3 times daily. Drink immediately, as this product tends to thicken quickly when added to liquid.

For maintenance, mix 1 teaspoon in water or juice 1 time daily and drink 5 times a week.
For best results, take ComforTone for 2-3 days before ICP to ensure regular bowel movements. Once bowels are moving regularly, start taking ICP morning and night. ICP absorbs toxins and improves peristalsis, the wave-like movement of the intestinal walls as they move the waste matter through the intestinal tract. ICP will also help slow down the bowel movements when experiencing diarrhea.

Seventh Edition | **Essential Oils Desk Reference** | 177

**Essential Oils Desk Reference** | Seventh Edition

**Caution:** Using without enough liquid may cause choking. Do not use if you have difficulty swallowing.

**Allergen Alert:** May cause allergic reaction in people sensitive to inhaled or ingested psyllium.

## ImmuPro™

ImmuPro chewable tablets are packed with some of the most powerful immune stimulants known, including wolfberry polysaccharide and beta glucan (a polysaccharide from reishi, maitake, and *Agaricus blazei* mushrooms). Reishi, maitake, and *Agaricus blazei* organic mushrooms are the highest known sources of a rich variety of beta glucans, potent immune-stimulating polysaccharides that have been documented by numerous studies as having significant immune-boosting effects.

Numerous studies have documented the ability of these botanicals to reverse cancer and stimulate both cell-mediated and humoral immunity, dramatically boosting levels of macrophages, neutrophils, phagocytes, B-cells, T-cells, natural killer cells, interleukins, and interferons.

ImmuPro combines complex and potent, immune-boosting minerals such as zinc, copper, and selenium. It also contains melatonin, one of the most powerful immune stimulants known. Melatonin levels steadily decrease with age, which is a factor that contributes to accelerated aging.

**Ingredients:** calcium (as c. carbonate), zinc (as z. bisglycinate), selenium (as s. glycinate chelate), copper (c. glycinate chelate), strawberry powder, wolfberry fruit polysaccharide, raspberry fruit powder, Reishi whole mushroom powder, Maitake mushroom mycelia powder, larch tree wood extract, mushroom fruit powder, melatonin, dextrose (non-GMO), hydroxylpropyl cellulose, stevia, silicon dioxide, magnesium stearate, maltodextrin (non-GMO)

**Essential Oil:** Orange

**Directions:** Chew 1-2 tablets daily as needed. Do not exceed 2 tablets per day.

**Caution:** Do not drive or operate machinery when taking melatonin.

## Inner Defense®

Inner Defense is our defense and protection in today's toxic environment. It can be difficult to maintain a healthy, functioning immune system with constant exposure to harmful viruses, bacteria, poor diet, devitalized food, polluted water and air, and lack of sleep, which can negatively affect physical and emotional health.

Using a wide variety of antibacterial, antiviral, and antifungal essential oils like Oregano, Thyme, and the proprietary essential oil blend of Thieves helps protect our bodies and environment in many ways. Inner Defense strengthens the body systems by creating an unfriendly environment for yeast and fungus, improving digestion, supporting the respiratory system, and fighting against the invasion of destructive viruses and bacteria.

Because essential oils are so concentrated and potent, only a few drops are needed to support the body systems and maintain health and vitality. Easy-to-swallow, liquid softgels dissolve quickly in the stomach for maximum results.

**Ingredients:** virgin coconut oil, fish gelatin, glycerin, water

**Essential Oils:** Thieves Blend: [Clove, Lemon, Eucalyptus Radiata, Rosemary, Cinnamon Bark], O3 Super Blend: [Oregano, Thyme, Lemongrass]

**Directions:** Take 1-2 capsules daily (a.m.) or take 1 capsule 3-5 times daily when stressed or to eliminate bacterial and viral infections. For best results, take Life 9 probiotic 8 hours after taking Inner Defense.

**Allergen Warning:** Contains bee product.

## JuvaPower®

JuvaPower is a high-antioxidant, whole-food vegetable powder complex that is a rich source of acid-binding foods. It is formulated with powerful, liver-supporting nutrients with intestinal cleansing benefits. JuvaPower is one of the most important and supportive supplements to take on a daily basis. It is very cleansing to the colon and to the liver, which is the cleansing and filtering gland of our bloodstream, vitally important in today's world, where we are bombarded with toxins daily.

**Ingredients:** Proprietary JuvaPower Blend: [rice seed bran, spinach leaf, tomato fruit, beet root, flaxseed bran, oat bran, broccoli floret/stalk, cucumber, dill seed, barley sprout seed, ginger root and rhizome, slippery elm bark, L-taurine, psyllium seed husk, anise seed, fennel seed, aloe vera leaf extract, peppermint leaf

**178** | **Chapter 8** | Nutritional Support

**Essential Oils:** Anise, Fennel

**Directions:** Sprinkle 1 tablespoon on food or stir 4-8 oz. into purified drinking water or rice or almond milk and drink. Not to replace balanced meals. Use 3 times daily for maximum benefits as a supplement to the diet.

**Allergen Alert:** May cause allergic reaction in people sensitive to inhaled or ingested psyllium.

## JuvaSpice®

JuvaSpice is a delicious and extremely healthy spice to use as a seasoning on your foods on a daily basis. It is very similar to JuvaPower in its cleansing and supporting health benefits. JuvaSpice was formulated with powerful, liver-supporting nutrients and cleansing benefits.

JuvaSpice is a convenient, easy-to-use product. Just sprinkle it over your soups, salads, specially prepared meals, and even over popcorn. The health benefits of this product are of vital importance, especially in today's world.

**Ingredients:** Proprietary JuvaSpice Blend: [rice seed bran, spinach leaf, tomato fruit, beet root, flaxseed bran, oat bran, broccoli floret/stalk, cucumber, potassium (chloride), Redmond Real Salt®, dill seed, barley sprouted seed, cayenne pepper fruit, ginger root and rhizome, slippery elm bark, L-taurine, psyllium seed husk, anise seed, fennel seed, aloe vera leaf extract, peppermint leaf

**Essential Oils:** Anise, Fennel

**Directions:** Use 1 gram (1/3-1/2 teaspoon) 1 time daily or as needed.

**Allergen Alert:** May cause allergic reaction in people sensitive to inhaled or ingested psyllium.

## JuvaTone®

JuvaTone is a special herbal complex designed to support the liver with an excellent source of choline, a nutrient that is vital for proper liver function and necessary for those with high-protein diets. JuvaTone also contains inositol and dl-methionine, which help with the body's process of elimination. Methionine helps recycle glutathione, a natural antioxidant crucial for normal liver function. Other ingredients include Oregon grape root, a source of the liver-supporting compound berberine, and therapeutic-grade essential oils to enhance overall effectiveness.

The liver is one of the most important organs of the body. It purifies the blood and is a key to converting carbohydrates to energy. An overtaxed liver may affect our energy, digestion, and skin. Fats and bile within the liver may easily become oversaturated with oil-soluble toxins, synthetic chemicals, and heavy metals.

As toxins build, the liver becomes taxed and stressed, resulting in aggravating skin conditions, rashes, fatigue, headaches, muscle pain, digestive disturbances, pallor, dizziness, irritability, mood swings, and mental confusion.

The liver also plays a major role in helping the body detoxify. The final products of digestion are transported through the hepatic portal vein from the colon to the liver to be cleansed.

**Ingredients:** calcium (as dicalcium phosphate), iron (dicalcium phosphate, parsley leaf powder), copper (as copper citrate), sodium, choline (from c. bitartrate), DI-methionine, beet root, inositol, dandelion root, L-cysteine HCI, alfalfa sprout, Oregon grape root, parsley leaf powder, bee propolis, echinacea purpurea root, cellulose, silicon dioxide, magnesium stearate, cellulose film-coating

**Essential Oils:** Lemon, German Chamomile, Geranium, Rosemary, Myrtle, Blue Tansy

**Directions:** Take 2 tablets 2 times daily. Increase as needed up to 4 tablets 4 times daily. Best when taken between meals. For optimum results, use with ComforTone 1 hour apart.

## K&B™

K&B is formulated to nutritionally support normal kidney and bladder health. Juniper enhances the body's efforts to maintain proper fluid balance. Parsley supports kidney and bladder function and aids overall urinary health. Uva Ursi supports both urinary and digestive system health. The pure, therapeutic-grade essential oils added to the ingredients fortify the effectiveness of its overall use for kidney and bladder infections and other related conditions.

**Ingredients:** juniper berry extract, parsley leaf extract, uva-ursi leaf extract, dandelion root extract, German chamomile flower extract, royal jelly, water, ethyl alcohol

**Essential Oils:** Geranium, Fennel, Clove, Roman Chamomile, Sage, Juniper

**Directions:** Take 3 half droppers 3 times daily in distilled water or as needed.

**Allergen Warning:** Contains bee product.

# KidScents®

KidScents nutritional supplements provide a full spectrum of children's vitamin support with no sugar, artificial flavorings, or dyes. (See also the chapter on *Healthy Choices for Children*.)

## KidScents® MightyVites™

KidScents MightyVites is a whole food, multinutrient that contains super fruits, plants, and vegetables that deliver the full spectrum of vitamins, minerals, antioxidants, and phytonutrients, specifically designed for children's developing bodies.

Children's diets often need to bridge between what they are eating and what they should be eating. To fuel growth and normal activity levels, a child's diet must provide plenty of vitamins and minerals as well as support stores of nutrients in preparation for the accelerated growth spurts of the teenage years.

The Ningxia wolfberry fruit is the highest antioxidant food known, making it an excellent whole food with 18 amino acids; 21 trace minerals; vitamins B1, B2, B6, C, E; polyphenols; carotenoids; magnesium; and potassium.

This super-enriched, chewable vitamin is perfect for children to energize, build their bodies, and protect their entire system the way Mother Nature intended.

**Ingredients:** vitamin A, vitamin C (as ascorbic acid from orange), vitamin D (as cholecalciferol), vitamin E (as d-alpha tocopheryl acid succinate), vitamin K (phytonadione), thiamine (vitamin B1 as thiamine mononitrate), riboflavin (vitamin B2), niacin (as niacinamide), vitamin B6 (as pyridoxine HCI), vitamin B6 (as pyridoxal-5-phosphate), folate (as folic acid), vitamin B12 (methylcobalamin), biotin (vitamin H), pantothenic acid (as d-calcium pantothenate), iodine (as potassium iodide), magnesium (as magnesium oxide), zinc (from zinc yeast complex), selenium (from selenium yeast complex), copper (from copper yeast complex), chromium (from chromium yeast complex), sorbitol, fructose, natural flavors, lecithin (soy), citric acid, silica, magnesium stearate, di-calcium phosphate

**Allergen Warning:** Contains an ingredient derived from soy.

## MightyVites™ Wild Berry Proprietary Blend

**Ingredients:** grape skin powder, Ningxia wolfberry fruit, cherry juice powder, strawberry juice powder, malic acid, broccoli floret, methylsulfonylmethane, barley grass, curcumins, citrus flavonoids (from tangerine), spirulina algae, tocotrienols (from natural palm oil), olive leaf extract, boron (as boron AAC), lutein (from marigold flowers)

## MightyVites™ Orange Cream Proprietary Blend

**Ingredients:** orange juice powder, Ningxia wolfberry fruit, malic acid, broccoli floret, methylsulfonylmethane, barley grass, curcumins, citrus flavonoids (from tangerine), spirulina algae, grape skin powder, tocotrienols (from natural palm oil), olive leaf extract, boron (as boron AAC), lutein (from marigold flowers),

**Directions:** Children 4-12 years old, take 3 chewable tablets daily. Can be taken separately or in 1 daily dose.

## KidScents® MightyZyme™

KidScents MightyZyme is an all-natural, vegetarian, chewable tablet, designed to give children added enzyme nutrition to prevent any enzyme depletion, which is the precursor to body dysfunction that could impede growth and brain development. Children today face a world of fast foods and nutritionally depleted foods that are practically devoid of enzymes critical for the proper body function of everything from breathing, thinking, circulation, and digestion. MightyZyme combines nine different digestive enzymes with several other nutrients to support healthy digestion, relieving occasional symptoms, including stomach pressure, bloating, gas, pain, and minor cramping that may occur after eating.

MightyZyme chewable tablets address each of the digestive needs of growing bodies and assist with normal digestion of all foods, including proteins, carbohydrates, and fats. They energize, build, and protect your child's whole system, the way Mother Nature intended.

**Ingredients:** folate (as folic acid), calcium (from calcium carbonate), Proprietary MightyZyme Blend: [lipase, alfalfa leaf powder, protease 4.5, amylase, bromelain, carrot root powder, protease 6.0, peptidase, phytase, protease 3.0, cellulase], carnauba wax, fructose, maltodextrin, apple juice concentrate, coconut oil, silica

Nutritional Support | **Chapter 8**

**Essential Oil:** Peppermint

**Directions:** For children age 6 or older: chew 1 tablet 3 times daily prior to or with meals. For children ages 2-6 years of age: chew 1/2 to 1 tablet (crushed if needed and mixed with yogurt or applesauce).

## Life 9™

This high-potency probiotic builds and restores intestinal health. Probiotics are important because of their positive effect on the bowels. Many do not realize that the bowels are the source of health and vitality and where nutrients are absorbed into the bloodstream. They are also the command center of the immune system and eliminators of waste products. If the bowels are not working properly, optimal health is impossible and the body is vulnerable to myriad conditions.

For the bowels to work properly, probiotics are necessary for every intestinal function and to prevent the proliferation of harmful bacteria.

We may do many things that can increase the need for probiotic supplementation such as taking drugs and antibiotics, drinking chlorinated water, consuming sugar, eating a low-fiber diet, and undergoing stress.

Life 9 is a proprietary, high-potency combination of nine beneficial bacteria strains that promote natural digestive balance and support a healthy immune system.

Encapsulated in advanced, delayed-release capsules with a dual-sorbent desiccant in a bottle with a special cap to ensure product efficacy, Life 9's 17 billion* beneficial active cultures per serving bypass the stomach, which improves overall product efficacy.

Probiotics have been shown to assist the body in manufacturing B vitamins, improve nutrient absorption, support immune function, improve digestion, and reduce yeast growth. Life 9 may be taken by healthy children and adults to help maintain optimal well-being. Research indicates that those concerned about proper digestion will benefit from taking Life 9.

This product may be very helpful when taken intensively during or after illness to boost immunity and support recovery. It is especially important after taking antibiotics or suffering any gastrointestinal distress.

**Ingredients:** L. acidophilus, Bifidobacterium lactis, Lactobacillus plantarum, Lactobacillus rhamnosus, Lactobacillus salivarius, Streptococcus thermophilus, Bifidobacterium breve, Bifidobacterium bifidum/bif lactis, Bifidobacterium longum, calcium carbonate,

microcystalline cellulose, Hypromellose and gellan gum delayed-release capsule, rice bran, silica

**Directions:** Take 1 capsule every night following a meal or as needed for intestinal health and comfort and to strengthen immunity. Keep in a cool, dark place. Tightly secure special cap after use. Refrigerate after opening.

## Longevity™ (Softgels)

A daily antioxidant in your maintenance program is a tremendous support to the body. That is what makes Longevity Softgels so important. As a potent, proprietary blend of fat-soluble antioxidants, they are as essential as a multivitamin and should be taken daily to prevent the harmful effects of our modern lifestyle. One of the most powerful antioxidant supplements available, with an ORAC score of 150,000, this formula provides 700 times the antioxidant power of carrots.

It prevents the damaging effects of aging, diet, and the environment. It is formulated with the pure essential oils of Thyme, Orange, Frankincense, and in particular Clove, one of nature's strongest antioxidants, for ultra-antioxidant support.

Longevity protects DHA levels for brain function and cardiovascular health, promotes healthy cell regeneration, supports the liver, increases immune function, and strengthens the nervous system.

**Ingredients:** virgin coconut oil, fractionated coconut oil, gelatin, water, glycerin, aqueous coating solution: [oleic acid, sodium alginate, medium-chain triglycerides, ethylcellulose, ammonium hydroxide, stearic acid], mixed tocopherols (vitamin E)

**Essential Oils:** Thyme, Orange, Clove, Frankincense

**Directions:** Take 1 softgel 1 time daily with food or as needed.

## Master Formula™

Master Formula is a full-spectrum, premium multinutrient supplement, providing vitamins, minerals, and food-based nutriment to support general health and well-being for men and women. By using a Synergistic Suspension Isolation process (SSI Technology), ingredients are delivered in three distinct delivery forms. Collectively, these ingredients provide a premium, synergistic complex to support your body.

*Per serving at date of manufacture.

Seventh Edition | **Essential Oils Desk Reference** | 181

## Micronized Nutrient Capsules

Micronized Nutrient Capsules are an organic food blend of B vitamins along with chelated minerals to naturally support the body.

**Ingredients:** vitamin A (from beta carotene), thiamin (vitamin B1), riboflavin (vitamin B2), niacin (vitamin B3), vitamin B6 (pyridoxine), folate (vitamin B9), vitamin B12 (methylcobalamin), biotin, pantothenic acid (vitamin B5), iron (ferrous bisglycinate chelate), magnesium (magnesium glycinate chelate), zinc (zinc glycinate chelate), selenium (selenium glycinate chelate), copper (copper glycinate chelate), manganese (manganese glycinate chelate), chromium (chromium nicotinate glycinate chelate), molybdenum glycinate chelate, Proprietary Master Formula Capsule Blend: [Atlantic kelp, inositol, PABA (para amino benzoic acid), spirulina algae, barley grass, citrus bioflavonoids from lemon whole fruit powder, orange whole fruit powder, lime whole fruit powder, tangerine whole fruit powder, grapefruit whole fruit powder, Ningxia wolfberry fruit powder, olive leaf extract, boron citrate, lycopene], hypromellose, magnesium stearate (vegetable source), silicon dioxide, microcrystalline cellulose

## Phyto-Caplets

Phyto-Caplets are a trace mineral complex and supporting prebiotics; a powerful fruit, vegetable, and herb extract blend along with vitamin C to help scavenge free radicals in the body.

**Ingredients:** vitamin C (calcium ascorbate and acerola cherry), calcium (calcium carbonate), potassium (potassium chloride), choline (choline bitartrate), Proprietary Master Formula Tablet Blend: [fructooligosaccharides, trace minerals], Spectra™ Fruit, Vegetable, and Herb Blend: [coffea arabica fruit extract, broccoli sprout seed concentrate, camellia sinensis leaf extract, onion bulb extract, apple fruit skin extract, acerola fruit extract, camu camu fruit concentrate, quercetin flower extract, tomato fruit concentrate, broccoli floret and stem concentrate, acai fruit concentrate, turmeric root concentrate, garlic clove concentrate, basil leaf concentrate, oregano leaf concentrate, cinnamon branch/stem concentrate, elderberry fruit concentrate, carrot root concentrate, mangosteen fruit concentrate, black currant fruit extract, blueberry fruit extract, sweet cherry fruit concentrate, blackberry fruit concentrate, chokeberry fruit concentrate, raspberry fruit concentrate, spinach leaf concentrate, kale leaf concentrate, bilberry fruit extract, Brussels sprout head concentrate], microcrystalline cellulose, stearic acid, croscarmellose sodium, organic maltodextrin, silicon dioxide, organic sunflower lecithin, organic palm olein, organic guar gum

## Liquid Vitamin Capsule

Liquid Vitamin Capsules contain pure essential oils and fat soluble vitamins, which provide antioxidants and vitamins in a liquid delivery.

**Ingredients:** vitamin A (from beta carotene), vitamin D3 (cholecalciferol), vitamin E (d-alpha tocopheryl succinate), vitamin K (K2 as menaquinone-7), sunflower lecithin (non-GMO), hypromellose

**Essentials Oils:** Turmeric, Cardamom, Clove, Fennel, Ginger

**Directions:** Take 1 packet (1 liquid capsule, 1 caplet, 2 capsules) daily with water or NingXia Red. Do not take on an empty stomach.

## MegaCal™

This is a high-powered calcium and essential mineral complex with an almost 1/1 calcium to magnesium ratio. It contains elemental magnesium and calcium along with key quantities of zinc, manganese, and copper, balanced to scientific ratios to avoid mineral interactions and competition.

Calcium and magnesium are necessary not only for healthy bones and teeth but also for proper heart and blood function and to keep nerves and muscles working properly.

**Ingredients:** vitamin C, calcium (lactate, glycerophosphate, carbonate, and ascorbate), magnesium (as citrate, sulfate, and carbonate), zinc (as z. gluconate), manganese (as sulfate), xylitol, fractionated coconut oil

**Essential Oil:** Lemon

**Directions:** Take 1 teaspoon with 1 cup of water or juice daily, at least 1 hour after a meal or taking medication or an hour before bed. Do not exceed 3 servings daily.

## MindWise™

MindWise delivers the exotic sacha inchi nut oil and a proprietary blend of pure essential oils and more to support normal brain and cardiovascular function.

**Ingredients:** vitamin D, Proprietary MindWise Memory Blend: [pomegranate fruit extract, rhododendron leaf extract, GPC (L-alpha glycerylphosphorylcholine), ALCAR (acetyl-L-carnitine), CoQ10 (Kaneka Q10™) (as ubiquinone), turmeric root powder, lithium orotate, sacha inchi nut oil, fractionated coconut oil, water, pomegranate juice concentrate, acai puree, glycerin, gum acacia, fruit and vegetable juice for color, natural pomegranate acai flavor, stevia, natural oil flavor, natural acai oil flavor, organic guar gum]

**Essential Oils:** Peppermint, Fennel, Anise, Lemon, Lime

**Directions:** For optimal effect adults should follow initial dose schedule for 7-10 days followed by maintenance schedule. **Adult Initial Dose:** Take 2 tablespoons 1 time daily for the first 7-10 days. **Adult Maintenance Dose:** Take 1 tablespoon 1 time daily or as needed. **Children:** Take 1-2 teaspoons 1 time daily. Should be taken with a meal. Shake well before each use. Consume within 30 days of opening.

**Allergen Warning:** Contains tree nuts.

## Mineral Essence™

This product is a very balanced, organic, ionic mineral complex with more than 60 different minerals. Without minerals, vitamins cannot be properly assimilated or absorbed by the body. Mineral Essence has a natural electrolyte balance, helping to prevent disease and premature aging. Minerals are necessary for proper immune and metabolic functions, and essential oils enhance the bioavailability of minerals, which provides us with a superior product.

To demonstrate this, a group of volunteers consumed a teaspoon of liquid trace minerals without essential oils. Each volunteer experienced diarrhea within 24 hours. Following a cleansing period of several days, the same volunteers were given a double dosage of the same liquid trace minerals blended with essential oils. None experienced diarrhea. [Personal communication with D. Gary Young.]

According to two-time Nobel Prize winner Linus Pauling, PhD, "You can trace every sickness, every disease, and every ailment to a mineral deficiency." Ionic minerals are the most fully and quickly absorbed form of minerals available.

**Ingredients:** magnesium, chloride, trace mineral complex, honey, royal jelly

**Essential Oils:** Lemon, Cinnamon Bark, Peppermint

**Directions:** Take 5 half droppers (1 ml each) morning and evening or as needed for a mineral supplement. May be added to 4-8 oz. of distilled or purified water or juice before drinking.

**Allergen Warning:** Contains bee products.

## MultiGreens™

MultiGreens is a nutritious chlorophyll formula designed to boost vitality by working with the glandular, nervous, and circulatory systems. It is a natural, sustainable energy source with bioactive sea vegetables that increase vitality, nutrient-dense bee pollen, a purifying therapeutic-grade essential oil blend to increase assimilation, and an excellent source of choline, critical for energy production.

Clinical experience has shown that before putting essential oils in the MultiGreens formula, there was 42 percent blood absorption in 24 hours. After adding the essential oils to the formula, blood absorption increased to 64 percent in 30 minutes and 86 percent in 1 hour. The conclusion was that the cells were now receiving nutrients that they had previously not been able to assimilate. [Personal communication with D. Gary Young.]

**Ingredients**: Proprietary MultiGreens Blend: [bee pollen, barley grass juice concentrate, spirulina, choline (as choline bitartrate), eleuthero root, alfalfa, kelp], amino acid complex: [L-arginine, L-cysteine, L-tyrosine], gelatin, silica

**Essential Oils:** Rosemary, Lemon, Lemongrass, Melissa

**Directions:** Take 3 capsules 2 times daily.

## NingXia Nitro™

NingXia Nitro is an all-natural way to increase cognitive alertness, enhance mental fitness, promote energy, and support overall performance. Its benefits are derived from a wide range of powerful cognitive enhancers like wolfberry seed oil combined with therapeutic-grade essential oils. It improves physical performance, speeds up recovery, and increases overall energy reserves, while avoiding the typical caffeine crash.

Other supportive ingredients such as B vitamins, green tea extract (derived from the leaves of *Camilla sinensis* that are unfermented, a source of ECGC), choline, and Korean ginseng have been added to sharpen the mind and invigorate the senses. NingXia Nitro is a simple and convenient way to become more focused, support mental acuity, and enhance physical performance.

**Ingredients:** niacin (as niacinamide), vitamin B6 (as pyridoxine HCl), vitamin B12 (as methylcobalamin), iodine (as potassium iodide), Proprietary Nitro Energy Blend: [d-ribose, green tea leaf extract, choline (as choline bitartrate), mulberry leaf extract, Korean ginseng root extract], vanilla fruit oil, chocolate bean oil, yerba mate leaf oil, wolfberry seed oil, purified water, Nitro Fruit Juice Blend Concentrate: [sweet cherry, kiwi, blueberry, acerola, bilberry, black currant, raspberry, strawberry, cranberry], coconut nectar, natural flavors, pectin, xanthan gum

Contains 40 mg of naturally occurring caffeine.

**Essential Oils:** Spearmint, Peppermint, Nutmeg, Black Pepper

**Directions:** Consume directly from the tube or mix with 2-4 oz. NingXia Red, 1 can of NingXia Zyng, or 4 oz. water anytime you need a pick-me-up. Best served chilled. Shake well before use.

**Allergen Warning:** Contains milk and tree nut (coconut). Not recommended for children.

## NingXia Red® (Juice)

Ningxia wolfberries have long been treasured in the natural health community. Their phytochemical profile is legendary: amazing polysaccharides, calcium, 18 amino acids, 21 trace minerals, beta-carotene, vitamins B1, B2, B6, and E, along with polyphenols. Thanks to the power of synergy, this new formulation of NingXia Red juice is more powerful than ever with the addition of new and highly efficacious ingredients.

NingXia Red's new formula promotes free radical scavenging by providing high levels of powerful antioxidants while boosting energy. It supports brain and cognitive health as well as digestive health. The nutritive power of NingXia Red fortifies the cardiovascular system and supports healthy blood pressure levels while promoting restful sleep patterns. It aids the body's natural anti-inflammatory response and enhances immune function. It also provides nutrients needed for healthy insulin sensitivity and promotes a feeling of satiety if taken prior to meals. NingXia Red also supports proper muscle and joint health.

**Ingredients:** sodium, Proprietary NingXia Red Blend: [whole Ningxia wolfberry puree, blueberry juice from concentrate, plum juice from concentrate, cherry juice from concentrate, aronia juice from concentrate, pomegranate juice from concentrate], water, tartaric acid, natural blueberry flavoring, pure vanilla extract, malic acid, pectin, sodium benzoate (to maintain freshness), natural stevia extract

**Essential Oils:** Grape, Orange, Yuzu, Lemon, Tangerine

**Directions:** Drink 1-2 fl. oz. 1-2 times daily. Best served chilled. Shake well before use. Refrigerate after opening and consume within 30 days.

## Ningxia Wolfberry (Organic Dried)

The Ningxia wolfberry is one of earth's most powerful antioxidant fruits. It is rich in polysaccharides, with more vitamin C than oranges, more beta-carotene than carrots, and more calcium than broccoli. These little, red Ningxia wolfberries are delicious and make a great, healthy snack. They can be used in cooking, salads, desserts, etc. The people in Inner Mongolia, where the *Lycium barbarum* species grows, drink wolfberry tea throughout the day and consume no less than 1-2 oz. daily.

**Ingredients:** Ningxia Organic Dried Wolfberries

**Directions:** Chew them, add them to oatmeal and pancakes, mix them in salads, make jams and jellies with them, and mix them with nuts and other dried fruit to make your own trail mix. Keep in cool, dark place.

## NingXia Zyng™

NingXia Zyng is a light, sparkling beverage that delivers a splash of hydrating energy. It is fueled by a proprietary blend of pure Black Pepper and Lime essential oils, wolfberry puree, and white tea extract that is combined with vitamins to create a unique, delicious, and refreshing beverage.

**Ingredients:** carbonated water, organic evaporated cane juice, pear juice concentrate, wolfberry puree, citric acid, blackberry juice concentrate, natural flavor, white tea leaf extract, stevia rebaudiana leaf extract, d-calcium pantothenate, niacinamide, d-alpha-tocopherol acetate, pyridoxine hydrochloride, retinyl palmitate

Contains 35 mg of naturally occurring caffeine. Contains no artificial sweeteners, colors, or preservatives.

**Essential Oils:** Black Pepper, Lime

**Directions:** Invert can once before opening.

## OmegaGize³®

This formula blends the omega-3 fatty acids DHA and EPA with powerful CoQ10, a vitamin-like substance that powers energy in every cell in the body while performing as an impressive antioxidant. The fish oil complex in OmegaGize³ is derived from some of the cleanest water on the planet and is enhanced with essential oils and mixed carotenoids for stability. OmegaGize³ also contains vitamin D and vitamin E.

It is clinically proven that omega-3 (EPA, DHA, ALA) fatty acid nutrients added to one's diet fortify and strengthen the body. There are good fats and bad fats. Omega-3 essential fatty acids found in fish oil are among the best good fats. Volumes of research confirm that omega-3 fats reduce systemic inflammation and support cardiovascular, joint, eye, and brain health.

While eating more fish is one way to consume these essential fatty acids, it is important to note that fish are often polluted with mercury and other toxins, beside the fact that a person would have to consume a lot on a regular basis. While eating a lot of fish can be worrisome due to ocean pollutants, there are no worries with this formula, as OmegaGize[3] actually tests lower than the maximum-allowable standard set worldwide to limit environmental pollutants. Even the capsule of OmegaGize[3] is ocean-derived and ensures optimal omega-3 absorption with no fishy taste.

**Ingredients:** vitamin D (as cholecalciferol), vitamin E (as tocotrienols), Proprietary OmegaGize[3] Blend: [omega-3 fatty acids (from fish oil) [eicosapentaenoic acid (EPA), docosahexaenoic acid (DHA)], Coenzyme Q10 (as ubiquinone)], gelatin, silicon dioxide, purified water, vitamin A (from mixed carotenoids)

**Essential Oils:** Clove, German Chamomile, Spearmint

**Directions:** Take 2-4 capsules twice daily, 2 in the morning and 2 in the evening for daily maintenance. Take up to 8 capsules per day for greater health benefits.

## ParaFree™

ParaFree is formulated with an advanced blend of some of the strongest essential oils studied for their cleansing abilities and antiparasitic properties. This formula also includes the added benefits of sesame seed oil and olive oil.

**Ingredients:** sesame seed oil, olive oil, gelatin, glycerin, deionized water

**Essential Oils:** Cumin, Anise (fruit oil), Fennel, Vetiver, Bay Laurel, Nutmeg, Tea Tree, Thyme, Clove, Ocotea, Dorado Azul, Tarragon, Ginger, Peppermint, Juniper, Fennel, Lemongrass, Anise, Patchouli

**Directions:** Take 3 softgels 2 times daily or as needed. For best results, take for 21 consecutive days and discontinue for 7 days. Repeat cycle 3 times. Take on an empty stomach for maximum results.

**Note:** During pregnancy, check with a health care professional before using. A good parasite cleanse is recommended before conception. Consult your health care professional before starting a cleansing program.

## PD 80/20™

PD 80/20™ is a dietary supplement formulated to help maximize internal health and support the endocrine system. It contains pregnenolone and DHEA, two substances produced naturally by the body that decline with age. Pregnenolone is the key precursor for the body's production of estrogen, DHEA, and progesterone. It also has an impact on mental acuity and memory. DHEA is involved in maintaining the health of the cardiovascular and immune systems.

As hormone levels decline with age, maintaining adequate hormone reserves becomes vital for sustaining health and preventing premature aging.

**Ingredients:** pregnenolone, DHEA, rice flour, gelatin

**Directions:** Take 1 capsule daily.

## PowerGize™

PowerGize is an herbal supplement that sustains energy, boosts stamina, increases strength, and enhances physical performance.

**Ingredients:** ashwagandha root extract, longjack root powder, fenugreek seed extract, epimedium leaf powder, desert hyacinth root powder, tribulus fruit/leaf extract, muira puama bark powder, hypromellose, rice flour, silicon dioxide

**Essential Oils:** Idaho Blue Spruce, Goldenrod, Cassia

**Directions:** Consume 2 capsules daily.

## Power Meal™

A delicious, satisfying, rice-based vegetarian meal replacement that contains Ningxia wolfberries, Power Meal is rich in calcium and delivers an impressive 20 grams of protein per serving, plus a complete vitamin, mineral, and enzyme profile.

Benefits include:
- Builds lean muscle mass
- Contains antioxidants that strengthen immunity
- Supports bone health
- Includes amino acids that enhance digestive activity

Whole-grain, brown rice protein is one of the very best sources of protein available. Rich in selenium, manganese, and phenolics, brown rice contains powerful antioxidants that work in multiple ways to boost the immune system. A great alternative to whey or soy protein, brown rice protein is:

- Dairy-free
- Allergen-free
- Easily absorbed in the body
- Rich in amino acids

Whether used as a meal alternative or snack, Power Meal can serve as an excellent weight management tool. Power Meal provides the building blocks required for regeneration and energy.

**Ingredients:** vitamin A, vitamin C, vitamin D, vitamin E, thiamin, riboflavin, niacin, vitamin B6, folate, vitamin B12, biotin, calcium, iron, pantothenic acid, phosphorus, magnesium, zinc, selenium, copper, manganese, chromium, rice protein concentrate, rice bran and germ, Ningxia wolfberry fruit, fructose, natural flavors, apple fruit, chicory root fiber extract (FOS), medium-chain triglycerides, calcium (as tri-calcium phosphate), soy lecithin, guar gum, magnesium (from m. oxide), MSM (methylsulfonylmethane), xanthan gum, lo han kuo extract, cinnamon bark, lipase, protease 4.5, ginkgo biloba extract, protease 3.0, vitamin E (mixed tocopherols), manganese (from m. gluconate), ginger root, choline bitartrate, eleuthero root, PABA (para-aminobenzoic acid), zinc (from zinc lactate), vitamin C (as ascorbic acid), protease 6.0, phytase, vitamin A (as beta-carotene), talin, betaine HCl, peptidase, white pepper fruit, niacin (vitamin B3), selenium (from selenomethionine), clove flower bud, alpha-lipoic acid, vitamin A (from mixed carotenoids), kelp, nutmeg seed, fennel seed, copper (from copper gluconate), pantothenic acid (from calcium pantothenate) (vitamin B5), neohesperidin derivative (flavor from natural citrus), lycopene, cardamom seed, vitamin B6 (from pyridoxine HCl), thiamin HCl (vitamin B1), riboflavin (vitamin B2), lutein, chromium (from chromium aminonicotinate), zeaxanthin, astaxanthin, cholecalciferol, folic acid, biotin, vitamin B12 (from methylcobalamin)

**Essential Oils:** Orange, Lemon, Grapefruit, Anise, Fennel, Nutmeg

**Directions:** Take 2 scoops in water or rice or other milk. Shake, stir, or blend until smooth. Add fruit or essential oils to enhance flavor.

**Allergen Warning:** Contains ingredients derived from soy and tree nut (coconut).

## Prostate Health™

Prostate Health is uniquely formulated to support the male glandular system in maintaining healthy, normal prostate function. The ingredients of saw palmetto and pumpkin seed oil support a healthy prostate gland.

A proprietary blend of pure Geranium, Fennel, Myrtle, Lavender, and Peppermint essential oils contains the chemical compounds of citral, anethole, and linalool that are anti-inflammatory.

Precise vegetable softgels quickly release their nutrients to be absorbed into the system, helping to reduce inflammation, promote easy urination, and support normal male activities.

Prostate Health is beneficial to any male adult who wants to support a healthy sex life and urinary tract flow.

**Ingredients:** saw palmetto extract, pumpkin seed oil, non-GMO modified cornstarch, carrageenan, glycerin, sorbitol, purified water

**Essential Oils:** Geranium, Fennel, Lavender, Myrtle, Peppermint

**Directions:** Take 1 softgel 2 times daily. For maximum benefit, Prostate Health should be taken consistently over time.

**Caution:** If taking medication for a medical condition, consult a health care professional prior to use. Saw palmetto may possibly affect the blood's ability to clot and could interfere with any blood-thinning drug (Warfarin, Plavix, or even aspirin). This product is not for use by women or anyone under 18 years of age.

## Pure Protein Complete™ Chocolate Deluxe

Pure Protein Complete Chocolate Deluxe is a comprehensive protein powder in a delicious chocolate flavor that combines a proprietary 5-protein blend, a powerful B-vitamin blend, amino acids, ancient peat, and apple extract to deliver 25 grams of protein per serving.

**Ingredients:** thiamin (as thiamin hydrochloride), riboflavin, niacin, vitamin B6 (as pyridoxine hydrochloride), vitamin B12 (as methylcobalamin), biotin, pantothenic acid (as d-calcium pantothenate), calcium (as d-calcium pantothenate), zinc, Pure Protein Proprietary Blend: [rBGH-free whey protein concentrate, pea protein isolate, goat whey protein concentrate, egg albumin, organic hemp seed protein, ancient peat, apple extract], Enzyme Proprietary Complex: [alpha and beta amylase, protease, lipase, cellulase, lactase, L. acidophilus, papain, bromelain], organic evaporated cane juice crystals, cocoa powder, natural flavors, xanthan gum, Amino Acid Blend: [L-leucine, L-isoleucine, L-valine, L-methionine, L-lysine, L-glutamine], sodium chloride, stevia, lou han guo fruit extract

**Essential Oil:** Orange

**Directions:** Add 2 level scoops to 8 oz. of cold water or rice, almond, or coconut milk, etc., and blend until smooth. Add fruit or essential oils to enhance flavor. For a delicious nutritional drink, mix 1-2 scoops of Pure Protein Complete with ½ cup carrot juice, ½ cup coconut milk, 1 drop Orange oil, and ¼ cup added water (or equivalent amount of ice); blend; and enjoy nutrition at its best!

**Allergen Warning:** Contains milk- and egg-derived ingredients.

## Pure Protein Complete™ Vanilla Spice

Pure Protein Complete Vanilla Spice is the perfect-anytime protein boost. It is high in bioactive whey protein and low in carbohydrates, fats, and calories. Each serving of Pure Protein Complete provides 25 grams of a proprietary 5-protein blend supported by a specialized enzyme blend, a low-glycemic carbohydrate matrix, and generous amounts of complementary vitamins and minerals.

Pure Protein Complete can be used to help support a weight loss program, while it sustains energy, curbs appetite, enhances enzyme activity, and builds lean muscle mass. It mixes easily into liquids and tastes delicious.

**Ingredients:** thiamin (as thiamin hydrochloride), riboflavin, niacin, vitamin B6 (as pyridoxine hydrochloride), vitamin B12 (as methylcobalamin), biotin, pantothenic acid (as d-calcium pantothenate), calcium (as d-calcium pantothenate), zinc, Pure Protein Proprietary Blend: [rBGH-free whey protein concentrate, pea protein isolate, goat whey protein concentrate, egg albumin, organic hemp seed protein, ancient peat, apple extract], Enzyme Proprietary Complex: [alpha and beta amylase, protease, lipase, cellulase, lactase, L. acidophilus, papain, bromelain], organic evaporated cane juice crystals, natural flavors, xanthan gum, Amino Acid Blend: [L-leucine,

L-isoleucine, L-valine, L-methionine, L-lysine, L-glutamine], sodium chloride, stevia rebaudiana, organic ground nutmeg, lou han guo fruit extract

**Essential Oil:** Orange

**Directions:** Add 2 level scoops to 8 oz. of cold water or rice, almond, or coconut milk, etc., and blend until smooth. Add fruit or essential oils to enhance flavor. For a delicious nutritional drink, mix 1-2 scoops of Pure Protein Complete with ½ cup carrot juice, ½ cup coconut milk, 1 drop Orange oil, and ¼ cup added water (or equivalent amount of ice); blend; and enjoy nutrition at its best!

Mix 1 scoop of Power Meal and 1 scoop of Pure Protein Complete together to make a very tasty, nutritious protein drink.

**Allergen Warning:** Contains milk- and egg-derived ingredients.

## Rehemogen™

Rehemogen tincture contains herbs that were used by Native Americans to cleanse, purify, disinfect, and build the blood. It contains cascara sagrada, red clover, poke root, prickly ash bark, and burdock root, which have been historically used for their cleansing and building properties. Rehemogen is also formulated with essential oils to fortify digestion.

**Ingredients:** red clover blossom, licorice root, poke root, peach bark, Oregon grape root, stillingia root, sarsaparilla root, cascara sagrada bark, prickly ash bark, burdock root, buckthorn bark, royal jelly, distilled water, ethanol

**Essential Oils:** Roman Chamomile, Rosemary, Thyme, Tea Tree

**Directions:** Mix 3 ml in distilled water 3 times daily just prior to or with meals containing protein. Shake well before using. Refrigerate after opening.

**Caution:** Read and follow directions carefully. Do not use if you have or develop diarrhea, loose stools, or abdominal pain because cascara sagrada bark and buckthorn bark may worsen these conditions and be harmful to your health.

**Allergen Warning:** Contains bee product.

## SleepEssence™

Four powerful essential oils that have unique sleep-enhancing properties are combined into a softgel, vegetarian capsule for easy digestion. Lavender, Vetiver, Valerian, and Ruta essential oils mixed with the hormone melatonin create a peaceful, well-regarded sleep aid. SleepEssence is a natural way to enjoy a good night's sleep.

**Ingredients:** melatonin, lecithin, coconut meat oil, carrageenan, glycerin, modified cornstarch, sorbitol

**Essential Oils:** Lavender, Vetiver, Valerian, Mandarin, Rue

**Direction:** Take 1-2 softgel capsules 30-60 minutes before going to bed.

## Slique® Bars—Chocolate-Coated

Chocolate-Coated Slique Bars are safe, innovative, vegetarian weight-management bars that help you feel full sooner and longer, manage satiety, moderate cravings, and provide healthy calories and essential nutrition.

These unique, delicious bars are loaded with exotic baru nuts and wholesome almonds and deliver essential nutrients and antioxidants through the addition of three pure essential oils; goldenberries and wolfberries; and D. Gary Young's exclusive dehydrated cacao nibs, all covered with a swirl of organic Ecuadorian dark chocolate.

**Ingredients:** organic Ecuadorian dark chocolate (cane sugar, chocolate liquor, cocoa butter, soy lecithin, vanilla extract), baru nuts, almonds, honey, chicory root inulin, dates, coconut, cacao nibs, goldenberries, Bing cherries, wolfberries, quinoa crisps, chia seeds, potato skin extract, sea salt, sunflower lecithin

**Essential Oils:** Vanilla, Orange, Cinnamon Bark

**Directions:** Consume before or between meals with 12 oz. of water to help control hunger. As with any weight-management product, this formula is designed and intended for use with a sensible program of diet and exercise.

**Allergen Warning:** Contains baru nuts, almonds, coconut, and soy. Manufactured in a facility that also processes tree nuts, peanuts, soy, milk, and eggs. Contains bee product.

## Slique® Bars—Tropical Berry Crunch

Slique Bars are safe, innovative, vegetarian weight-management bars that help you feel full sooner and longer, manage satiety, moderate cravings, and provide healthy calories and essential nutrition.

These unique, delicious bars are loaded with exotic baru nuts and wholesome almonds and deliver essential nutrients and antioxidants through the addition of three pure essential oils; goldenberries and wolfberries; and D. Gary Young's exclusive dehydrated cacao nibs.

**Ingredients:** baru nuts, almonds, honey, chicory root inulin, dates, coconut, cacao nibs, goldenberries, Bing cherries, wolfberries, quinoa crisps, chia seeds, potato skin extract, sea salt, sunflower lecithin

**Essential Oils:** Vanilla, Orange, Cinnamon Bark

**Directions:** Consume before or between meals with 12 oz. of water to help control hunger. As with any weight-management product, this formula is designed and intended for use with a sensible program of diet and exercise.

**Allergen Warning:** Contains baru nuts, almonds, coconut, and soy. Manufactured in a facility that also processes tree nuts, peanuts, soy, milk, and eggs. Contains bee product.

## Slique CitraSlim™

Slique CitraSlim is formulated with naturally derived ingredients and seven citral-dense essential oils to help promote your healthy weight management goals when combined with a healthy diet and exercise.

The unique natural ingredients work with your body to achieve weight loss in a healthy manner, burn excess fat, increase antioxidant activity, support healthy energy levels, reduce oxidative stress, and support a healthy metabolism.

**Ingredients (Liquid Capsule):** Lemongrass essential oil, fractionated coconut oil (caprylic/capric glycerides), pomegranate seed oil, silicon dioxide, gelatin, water

**Essential Oils (Liquid Capsule):** Lemon Myrtle, Idaho Balsam Fir

**Ingredients (Powder Capsule):** cassia dried bark powder, orange whole fruit extract, grapefruit whole fruit extract, guarana whole fruit extract, pterostilbene, bitter orange unripened fruit extract, ocotea leaf powder, fenugreek seed extract, amylase, cellulase, lipase, protease, hypromellose

**Essential Oils (Powder Capsule):** Spearmint, Ocotea, Cassia, Fennel

**Directions:** Consume 2 powder capsules with 8 ounces of water in the morning. Consume 1 powder and 1 liquid capsule with 8 ounces of water in the afternoon, before 3 p.m. If morning capsules are missed, you may combine with afternoon dose, before 3 p.m.

**Cautions:** Use as directed.

**Allergen Warning:** Contains coconut.

## Slique® Gum

This unique chewing gum promotes good oral health and helps with appetite control. It is infused with *Boswellia frereana* frankincense resin, famous for its tooth and gum benefits. Natural sweeteners and the act of chewing alleviate snack cravings, making this gum a helpful tool in weight management. Peppermint and Spearmint essential oils in the formula invigorate and freshen the breath.

**Ingredients:** frankincense gum resin, gumbase, isomalt, sorbitol, natural flavors, calcium stearate, natural sweeteners, colors: [red cabbage juice, turmeric], xylitol

**Essential Oils:** Peppermint, Spearmint

**Directions:** Chew 1 tablet before or after meals.

**Allergen Warning:** Contains traces of soy.

## Slique® Shake

Slique Shake is a complete meal replacement high in protein that helps maintain lean muscle mass and promotes satiety to support your healthy weight-management goals when combined with a sensible diet and regular exercise.

This vegan-friendly shake is infused with the Slique essential oil blend and includes essential dietary fibers and essential proteins that combine satisfying nutrition with a great berry taste. It is best paired with almond milk, fruit, or your favorite Vitality essential oils. Slique Shake supports healthy digestion, is an excellent source of vitamins B1, B2, B6, C, and iron and contains no artificial colors, flavors, or preservatives.

**Ingredients:** pea protein isolate, isomalto-oligosaccharide, medium chain triglycerides, tapioca dextrose, organic coconut palm sugar, natural flavor, organic quinoa powder, organic pumpkin seed protein, xanthan gum, strawberry fruit powder, sodium citrate, malic acid, fruit & veg-

etable extract blend (green tea leaf extract, guarana seed extract, red & white grape extracts, grapefruit extract, black carrot extract, vitamin B3), alfalfa grass juice powder, organic wolfberry fruit powder, stevia leaf extract, vitamins and minerals: dipotassium phosphate, monosodium phosphate, magnesium oxide, zinc gluconate, organic B vitamin blend (guava extract, holy basil extract, citrus limon extract), ascorbic acid, molybdenum glycinate, niacin, copper gluconate, biotin, vitamin A acetate, sodium selenite, d-calcium pantothenate, chromium nicotinate glycinate chelate, riboflavin pyridoxine HCl, potassium iodide, methylcobalamin

**Essential Oils:** Slique Essence essential oil blend: Grapefruit, Tangerine, Spearmint, Lemon, Ocotea, Stevia leaf extract

**Directions:** Add one Slique Shake packet to 8 ounces of water or milk of your choice. Shake, stir, or blend until smooth. Fruit, vegetables, or essential oils may be added for additional variety or to enhance flavor.

## Slique® Tea

Slique Ocotea Oolong Cacao Slimming Spice Tea is a delicious, premium blend of wholesome and rare ingredients. It offers a natural alternative to sugar-laden fruit drinks from concentrates, sodas, and coffees and can be used as part of a healthy weight-management program. It contains Ecuadorian ocotea leaf (*Ocotea quixos*), a member of the cinnamon family traditionally used by natives for health and wellness. Amazonian cacao is then added, along with pure, proprietary Vanilla essential oil.

Slique Tea also contains jade oolong tea leaves, sought after for their rich aroma and powerful antioxidant content. These leaves are handpicked from the high mountain regions of Taiwan, known for producing some of the world's finest teas.

All of these ingredients are enriched with 100 percent pure, therapeutic-grade Arabian frankincense powder, an exclusive ingredient from Young Living's distillery in Salalah, Oman.

Delicious served hot or cold, Slique Tea is a guilt-free staple to any diet regimen.

**Ingredients:** jade oolong tea, inulin, ocotea leaf, Ecuadorian cacao powder, Sacred Frankincense powder, natural stevia extract

**Essential Oil:** Vanilla

**Directions:** Bring 8 oz. of water to a rolling boil; let cool for 3½ minutes. Place 1 pouch in a cup, mug, or filter and add water. Steep for at least 3 minutes. Use daily before and after workouts, with meals, or anytime you need a natural boost. Delicious served hot or cold. Add your favorite Young Living essential oils as desired.

**Caution:** Contains naturally occurring tea caffeine. Not recommended for children.

## Sulfurzyme® Capsules and Powder

Sulfurzyme is a unique combination of MSM (methyl-sulfonylmethane), the protein-building compound found in breast milk, fresh fruits and vegetables, and Ningxia wolfberry. Together, they create a new concept in balancing the immune system and supporting almost every major function of the body. MSM has the ability to equalize water pressure inside the cells, which is a considerable benefit for those plagued with bursitis, arthritis, and tendonitis.

Ningxia wolfberry supplies nutrients to enhance the proper assimilation and metabolism of sulfur.

**Ingredients (Capsules):** MSM, Ningxia wolfberry fruit powder, hypromellose, rice flour, magnesium stearate, silica

**Directions (Capsules):** Take 2 capsules 2 times daily or as needed 1 hour before or after meals.

**Ingredients (Powder):** MSM, FOS (fructooligosaccharides), Ningxia wolfberry fruit powder, stevia leaf extract, calcium silicate

**Directions (Powder):** Take ½ teaspoon with juice or distilled water 2 times daily 1 hour before or after meals.

## Super B™

Super B is a comprehensive source of the B vitamins essential for good health, including thiamine (vitamin B1), riboflavin (vitamin B2), niacin (vitamin B3), pyridoxine (vitamin B6), vitamin B12, biotin, folic acid, and PABA. It also includes minerals that aid in the assimilation and metabolism of B vitamins.

B vitamins are particularly important during times of stress when reserves are depleted. Although research has shown that mega doses of B vitamins are not healthy, it has been known that the diets of many Americans do not provide the recommended amounts of B vitamins essential for normal functions of immune response.

When many B vitamins are combined at once in the stomach, it can cause fermentation, resulting in stomach upset. To avoid this, Super B uses a special formulation process to isolate the various vitamins so that they are released at different times.

**Ingredients:** thiamin (vitamin B1)(as thiamine HCI), riboflavin (vitamin B2), niacin (vitamin B3) (as nicotinic acid and niacinamide), vitamin B6 (as pyridoxine HCI), folate (vitamin B9), vitamin B12 (as methylcobalamin), biotin (vitamin B7), pantothenic acid (vitamin B5)(as d-calcium pantothenate), calcium (as dicalcium phosphate), magnesium (as m. bisglycinate chelate), zinc (as z. bisglycinate chelate), selenium (as s. glycinate complex), manganese (as m. bisglycinate chelate), PABA (para amino benzoic acid), cellulose, stearic acid, diglycerides

**Essential Oil:** Nutmeg

**Directions:** Take 2 tablets daily with a meal. If taken on an empty stomach, a person may experience a temporary niacin flush/warming sensation, a normal reaction that may last up to an hour.

## Super C™

Physical stress, alcohol, smoking, and using certain medications may lower the blood levels of this essential vitamin. When citrus fruits are not readily available, diets may not contain enough vitamin C. Super C is properly balanced with rutin, biotin, bioflavonoids, and trace minerals to work synergistically, balance the electrolytes, and increase the absorption rate of vitamin C. Without bioflavonoids, vitamin C has a hard time getting inside cells, and without proper electrolyte balance and trace minerals, it will not stay there for long.

**Ingredients:** vitamin C (as ascorbic acid), calcium (as calcium carbonate and dicalcium phosphate), zinc (gluconate), manganese (as manganese sulfate), potassium (as potassium chloride), citrus bioflavonoids, rutin, cayenne pepper fruit, cellulose, stearic acid, magnesium stearate, vegetable food-grade coating, silica

**Essential Oils:** Orange, Tangerine, Grapefruit, Lemon, Lemongrass

**Directions:** For reinforcing immune strength, take 2 tablets daily. For maintenance, take 1 tablet daily. Best taken before meals.

Nutritional Support | Chapter 8

## Super C™ Chewable

Super C Chewable is the only vitamin C chewable in the world that combines citrus essential oils, citrus bioflavonoids, and whole-food, natural vitamin C in one tablet.

Super C Chewable is the most complete, biologically utilizable vitamin C supplement available that is derived from a whole-food source of acerola cherries. It is a delicious way to get your daily dose of vitamin C without having to swallow pills. Its tangy, citrus flavor goes down easily and starts working immediately. Both adults and children enjoy it.

**Ingredients:** vitamin C (as ascorbic acid), acerola cherry fruit extract, camu camu whole fruit powder, rose hips fruit powder, citrus bioflavonoids (from lemon whole fruit powder, orange whole fruit powder, lime whole fruit powder, tangerine whole fruit powder, grapefruit whole fruit powder), non-GMO tapioca dextrose, sorbitol, calcium ascorbate, stevia, hydroxypropyl cellulose, stearic acid, silicon dioxide, magnesium stearate

**Essential Oil:** Orange

**Directions:** Take 1 chewable tablet 3 times daily or as needed.

**Allergen Warning:** Contains milk or milk derivatives.

## SuperCal™

This is a high-powered calcium, potassium, and magnesium complex that restores proper electrolyte and hormonal balance and improves muscle and bone development.

**Ingredients:** calcium (from calcium citrate), magnesium (from magnesium citrate), zinc (from zinc citrate), potassium (from potassium citrate), boron (as sodium borate), gelatin, stearic acid, cellulose

**Essential Oils:** Marjoram, Wintergreen, Lemongrass, Myrtle

**Directions:** Take 1-2 capsules right before a meal or as needed.

## Thieves® Cough Drops

Thieves Cough Drops soothe sore throats, relieve coughs, and cool nasal passages. They are free from sugar, dyes, preservatives, and artificial flavors. With the Thieves blend, Lemon, and Peppermint essential oils, these sweet, spicy drops taste great and provide effective relief in combination with natural menthol.

**Ingredients:** menthol, isomalt, pectin, stevia leaf extract, water

**Essential Oils:** Cinnamon Bark, Clove, Eucalyptus Radiata, Lemon, Peppermint, Rosemary

**Directions:** Adults and children 5 years and over: dissolve 1 drop slowly in mouth and repeat every 2 hours as needed. Children under 5 years of age: ask a doctor.

## Thieves® Hard Lozenges

Infused with Peppermint and Lemon essential oils and powered by Thieves essential oil blend, Thieves Hard Lozenges provide extra strength and effectiveness for lasting results you can feel. Both adults and children have found it to ease the pain of a sore throat and help with dryness.

**Ingredients:** lemon rind, pectin, isomalt, stevia extract, water

**Essential Oils:** Lemon, Thieves blend: [Clove, Lemon, Cinnamon Bark, Eucalyptus Radiata, Rosemary], Peppermint

**Directions:** Dissolve 1 lozenge in mouth as needed.

## Thieves® Mints

A healthy alternative to freshening your breath, the natural, sugar-free ingredients in Thieves Mints include the power of Thieves essential oil blend and Peppermint.

**Ingredients:** sorbitol, calcium stearate, stevia rebaudiana extract

**Essential Oils:** Thieves blend: [Clove, Lemon, Cinnamon Bark, Eucalyptus Radiata, Rosemary], Peppermint

**Directions:** Dissolve 1 mint in mouth, as desired.

## Thyromin™

A well-functioning body needs a strong thyroid. Thyromin was developed to nourish the thyroid, balance metabolism, and reduce fatigue. It contains a combination of specially selected glandular nutrients, herbs, amino acids, minerals, and essential oils. All of the oils are therapeutic-grade quality and are perfectly balanced to bring about the most beneficial and nutritional support to the thyroid.

**Ingredients:** vitamin E (as mixed tocopherols), iodine (from kelp and potassium iodide), potassium (as potassium citrate and potassium iodide), Proprietary Thyromin Blend: [parsley leaf, thyroid powder, L-tyrosine, pituitary extract (from porcine), adrenal extract (from porcine), L-cystine, L-cysteine HCI], gelatin, magnesium carbonate, magnesium stearate

**Essential Oils:** Peppermint, Spearmint, Myrtle, Myrrh

**Directions:** Adults 19 years or older, take 1-2 capsules daily, immediately before going to sleep. If under 19 years, consult with a health care professional for dosage recommendations.

## Ultra Young®

Ultra Young is an oil-infused supplement that is rich in vitamin C and supports antioxidant activity for health and wellness.

**Ingredients:** vitamin C (as ascorbic acid), L-Arginine, GPC (glycerylphosphorylcholine), Canadian fleabane aerial parts, water, glycerin, sunflower lecithin, stevia, vitamin E (as mixed tocopherols)

**Essential Oils:** Ocotea, Spearmint, Tangerine, Grapefruit

**Directions: For oral use only:** Add 1 ml (full dropper) to a glass of water or directly into mouth once daily.

## Wolfberry Crisp™ Bars, Chocolate-Coated

(See Gary's True Grit™ Chocolate-Coated Wolfberry Crisp™ Bars)

## Yacon Syrup

The Peruvian yacon plant resembles a sweet potato but with a black skin. While deliciously sweet, Yacon Syrup contains inulin, the complex sugar that slowly breaks down into FOS (fructooligosaccharide). Inulin is not digestible so it passes through the body, with the result that it is half the calories of other sugars. FOS is well-known for its prebiotic effects and also supports microflora in the large intestine, while it promotes the absorption of calcium.

Growing in the Andes Mountains, yacon takes up valuable minerals from volcanic ash build-up, adding high mineral content to high amino acid and vitamin A content. Thus, yacon is similar to the Ningxia wolfberry in its nutrient profile.

**Ingredient:** Yacon Syrup

**Directions:** Yacon Syrup can be used like honey (in beverages, cooking, cereal, and baking). In recipes use 3/4 cup of Yacon Syrup in place of 1 cup of sugar. You may also need to reduce the liquid amounts as you would for honey.

ENDNOTES:
1. http://www.huffingtonpost.com/dr-mark-hyman/wheat-gluten_b_1274872.html.
2. Ibid.
3. http://www.cbsnews.com/news/modern-wheat-a-perfect-chronic-poison-doctor-says/.
4. http://organicconnectmag.com/wp-content/uploads/2012/06/einkorn.html.
5. Pizzuti D, et al. Lack of intestinal mucosal toxicity of *Triticum monococcum* in celiac disease patients. *Scand J Gastroenterol.* 2006 Nov; 41(11):1305-11.
6. http://www.einkorn.com/types-of-wheat-nutritional-content-health-benefits-comparison/.
7. Abdel-Aal, ES, et al. Compositional and nutritional characteristics of a spring einkorn and spelt wheats. *Cereal Chem.* 72:621-624.
8. http://pathways4health.org/2010/03/05/wheat-varieties-and-processing-methods/.
9. Drago S, Fasano A, et al., Gliadin, zonulin and gut permeability: Effects on celiac and non-celiac intestinal mucosa and intestinal cell lines. *Scand J Gastroenterol.* 2006 Apr;41(4):408-19.
10. http://www.huffingtonpost.com/dr-mark-hyman/wheat-gluten_b_1274872.html.

# Chapter 9
# Ningxia Wolfberry

## Chinese Wolfberry Comes to the Modern World

Wolfberry legends and records of ancient Chinese medicine reach back 5,000 years. *Ben Zao Gen Mo*, a physician's handbook written during the Ming Dynasty (1468-1664 AD), documents the ancient use of wolfberry.

The Ningxia wolfberry is still included in a number of Chinese herbal pharmacopoeias and is prescribed for patients with liver and kidney deficiencies, as well as with diabetes and vision problems.

For most of their long history, the people of the west elbow plateau of the Yellow River where the Ningxia wolfberry grows have been relatively isolated from the rest of civilization by deserts, mountains, and the enormous landmass of central China, which shielded them from outside influences and cultures.

This geographical isolation, in addition to China's political isolation, has contributed to the late discovery of this Chinese superfood by the West.

### Nutritional Profile

In the mid-1980's when biochemists at the Ningxia Institute of Nutrition analyzed the Ningxia wolfberry, they found that it is 15.6 percent protein (dry weight) and contains at least 21 essential minerals, as well as significant levels of vitamins such as thiamin (vitamin B1), niacin (vitamin B3), and vitamin C. In fact, the Ningxia wolfberry is one of the richest known whole-food sources of natural vitamin B1 or thiamin, which is essential for proper energy production, carbohydrate metabolism, and thyroid function.[1,2]

### Protein

With a total of 15.6 percent protein (dry weight), the Ningxia wolfberry contains as much protein as raw oats, one of the richest known sources of plant protein.[1,2] Just as important as the total protein content are the amino acids that are present, as amino acids are the building blocks of proteins. The wolfberry is rich in the essential amino acid leucine, as well as in the semi-essential amino acid L-arginine.

Protein is a vital building block of white blood cells and antibodies, which are some of the most prolifically reproducing cells in the body.

Protein also helps maintain a healthy thymus gland, which is vital for optimum cell-mediated immunity.

## Geography and Botany

Native to the Ningxia Hui Autonomous Region of northern China, *Lycium barbarum L.* is a small, red, medicinal berry that is known as *Lycii fructus* or wolfberry in the West and Gou qi zi (Goji) throughout China.

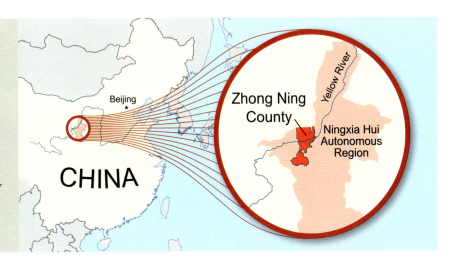

## Nutrients in 100 Grams of Ningxia Wolfberry

| Nutrient | Amount | % RDA |
|---|---|---|
| Protein | 15.6 g | 31.2 |
| Fiber | 21 g | 84 |
| Fat | 0.45 g | <1 |
| Sugar | 42 g | N/A |
| Vitamin A | 12,600 iu | 250 |
| Vitamin B-1 | 27 mg | 1800 |
| Vitamin B-3 | 88 mg | 440 |
| Vitamin B-5 | 88 mg | 440 |
| Vitamin C | 148 mg | 246 |
| Biotin | 28 µg | 9 |
| Calcium | 110 mg | 11 |
| Chromium | 79 mg | 65 |
| Copper | 1.1 mg | 55 |
| Iron | 11 mg | 61 |
| Magnesium | 130 mg | 32.5 |
| Manganese | 1.3 mg | 65 |
| Potassium | 1,600 mg | 102 |
| Zinc | 1.8 mg | 12 |

Source: Preliminary data from dried fruit of Ningxia wolfberry (*Lycium barbarum*) stored 1-3 years.

## Leucine

Since it is not possible for the body to synthesize leucine, it is critical that foods containing leucine be included in one's diet. Leucine is the only dietary protein that has the capacity to cause the growth of muscle tissue and as a dietary supplement has shown to slow muscle atrophy in aged mice.[3]

## Arginine

A semi-essential amino acid, L-arginine is considered an important nutrient for healthy immunity. L-arginine's ability to ramp up non-inflammatory immunity may be due to its use in the production of nitric oxide, which is used by the body to kill pathogens.[4,5] L-arginine also plays a key role in cell division, tissue regeneration, and wound healing. For that reason many hospitals add it to enteral and parenteral tube feedings for burn and trauma patients.

## Synergy of Arginine and Glutamine

L-arginine's stimulation of healthy immunity may be amplified when combined with another amino acid found in the Ningxia wolfberry: L-glutamine.

A medical group at Shanghai Medical University in China researched the use of an arginine and glutamine solution for tube feeding in gastrointestinal cancer patients, where adequate nutrition and amplified immunity is of life-or-death importance.

In this double-blind clinical trial, 48 patients were randomized into a control group with a standard diet and a treatment group supplemented with arginine and glutamine. The study lasted eight days.

Tolerance of both diets was excellent, according to the researchers, but with big differences in immune and inflammatory responses between the two groups.

Patients who received these two amino acids showed greater immunity and less inflammation than the control group.

The supplemented group had much higher levels of nitric oxide, total lymphocytes, T-lymphocytes, T-helper cells, and NK cells. They also exhibited lower levels of C-reactive protein, a marker for inflammation and heart disease.[6]

## Location, Location, Location: Silt Water and Minerals

The location where the Ningxia wolfberry crop is grown is a large, contributing factor to the rich mineral profile of the Ningxia wolfberry.

The Yellow River flood plain, where the Ningxia wolfberry crop is concentrated, derives its water from the foothills of the Bayan Har Mountains of the Himalayan range in Qinghai Provence.

As this water flows down through mountain gorges and valleys, it becomes charged with minerals. By the time it reaches the Ningxia province of Northern China, it is mineral-rich silt water. The silt concentration in the river is so high that the Yellow River is named for the coloration these minerals impart to the water.

## Vitamins and Minerals: Key to Long Life

Vitamins and minerals often work in pairs, such that many minerals cannot be assimilated into the body without the presence of a specific vitamin. It is interesting to note that the Ningxia wolfberry contains many of these vitamin-mineral pairs.

Some of the many functions that minerals perform in the body include electrolyte balance of our cells, nerve conduction for muscle contraction, bone and teeth formation, and enzyme activation. Minerals are so important that every process of the body depends on them.

## Potassium

The Ningxia wolfberry is one of the highest wholefood sources of potassium.

Potassium is an essential mineral micronutrient in human nutrition. The body does not make it; so, therefore, it must be found through dietary sources.

Potassium cations are important in neuron function (brain and nerve) and in influencing osmotic balance between cells.

The potassium ion channels modulate the release of GABA in the brain.[7] Researchers have found that the age-related decline in higher brain functions is due, in large part, to a lack of the inhibitory neurotransmitter, GABA. Higher brain functions, such as visual recognition and language comprehension, decline as people get older. This decline appears to be due to a reduction of GABA, which results in neurons with specific tasks being more easily fired by some other types of stimulus, slowing down processing of information in the brain.[8]

## Zinc

The Ningxia wolfberry is a rich vegetarian source of zinc, a mineral critical for healthy immunity. The dried berry has five times as much zinc as Brussels sprouts and more zinc than raw eggs.[1,2]

Zinc plays an essential role in the production of natural killer cells, IgG, gamma interferon, and tumor necrosis factor alpha. Zinc also enhances the microbe-killing activity of macrophages and increases levels of CD4 cytotoxic lymphocytes while lowering levels of CD8 immune-suppressing lymphocytes.[9]

According to Lothar Rink, an immunologist at the University of Lubeck School of Medicine in Germany, "The important role of zinc as an essential trace element for immune function has already been well established." He cited over 100 studies in support of this.[10]

Zinc deficiencies have been shown in both animal and human models to produce a variety of immune deficits, including T-lymphocyte depletion in the spleen and lymph nodes, impaired antibody response, shrinking of the thymus gland, and lower populations of cells associated with both humoral and cell-mediated immunity.[11]

Even more disconcerting is the fact that zinc deficiencies become more pronounced with advancing age as stomach acid declines, making it more difficult for the body to absorb zinc.

A Wayne State University study discovered that among a group of 180 randomly selected elderly subjects, the mean dietary intake of zinc was only 9 mg per day, which is 40 percent less than the recommended dietary allowance of 15 mg per day set by the Food and Nutrition Board.

Moreover, 36 percent of this group had depleted levels of zinc in two types of immune cells, granulocytes and lymphocytes, which correlated with depleted interleukin-1 (IL-1) production. Following zinc supplementation in a selected group, IL-1 jumped and lymphocyte activity surged.[12]

A September 2004 Case Western Reserve University review strongly indicates that zinc is effective for treating the common cold caused by the rhinovirus. "Clinical trial

## Amino Acids in 100 Grams of Ningxia Wolfberry

| | |
|---|---|
| Alanine . . . . . . . .720 mg | Lysine . . . . . . . . . 390 mg |
| Arginine . . . . . .930 mg | Methionine . . . . . 148 mg |
| Aspartate. . . . 2,100 mg | Phenylalanine . . . 380 mg |
| Glutamine. . . 1,400 mg | Proline. . . . . . . .1,030 mg |
| Glycine . . . . . . .430 mg | Serine. . . . . . . . . . 640 mg |
| Histidine. . . . . .270 mg | Thereonine. . . . . . 460 mg |
| Isoleucine . . . . .350 mg | Tyrosine. . . . . . . . 160 mg |
| Leucine . . . . . . .630 mg | Valine . . . . . . . .1,040 mg |

Source: Preliminary data from dried fruit of Ningxia wolfberry (*Lycium barbarum*) stored 1-3 years.

data support the value of zinc in reducing the duration and severity of symptoms of the common cold when administered within 24 hours of the onset of common cold symptoms," states Hulisz in the *Journal of the American Pharmaceutical Association.*[13]

The value of zinc was confirmed by a 2015 common cold study that showed "zinc acetate lozenges shortened the duration of nasal discharges by 34%, sneezing by 22%, scratchy throat by 33%, sore throat by 18%, hoarseness by 43%, and cough by 46%. Zinc lozenges shortened the duration of muscle ache by 54%, but there was no difference in the duration of headache and fever."[14]

Minerals such as zinc also constitute central components of some of the most powerful antioxidant compounds in the body. For instance, the mineral zinc is instrumental in the formation of superoxide dismutase (SOD), a key enzymatic antioxidant that declines with age. Antioxidants are discussed in further detail later.

## Fiber

With over 21 percent fiber by weight, the Ningxia wolfberry has more fiber than oat bran and double the fiber of buckwheat. In fact, the Ningxia wolfberry has one of the highest percentages of fiber of any whole food.[1,2]

The Ningxia wolfberry is also rich in soluble fiber, which is highly efficient in removing triglycerides and cholesterol from the blood and lowering the risk of heart disease. Numerous studies have linked a high intake of soluble fiber with lowered blood pressure and improved cardiovascular health.[15-18]

Cholesterol is one of the few compounds in the body that cannot be broken down into smaller components and excreted. The only mechanism by which cholesterol can be flushed from the body is through bile acids. However, if feces lack sufficient fiber, cholesterol is not sufficiently excreted, forcing the remainder to be recirculated in the gall bladder.

Besides lowering cholesterol, a diet high in fiber has been directly linked to a lower risk of cancer, increased stability of blood sugar levels, and a lowered risk of heart disease.

## More than Vitamins, Minerals, and Amino Acids

The Ningxia wolfberry is more than just a whole food high in minerals and vitamins; it also contains many unique phytonutrients that have been shown to protect the liver, eyes, heart, and cellular DNA from age-related degeneration and disease.

## Carotenoids

During the past five years, food scientists working for the state government in Germany have identified a number of carotenoids that can stimulate immunity without provoking inflammation that can worsen the symptoms of arthritis. Chief among these is beta cryptoxanthin, but other carotenoids have also been identified, including alpha carotene and lutein.

As one of the richest sources of carotenoids, the Ningxia wolfberry can provide significant immune-boosting potential.[19-20]

Some of these carotenoids are zeaxanthin, lutein, and beta-cryptoxanthin.

Zeaxanthin is a pigment concentrated in the eye.

Both zeaxanthin and lutein have been shown to protect against skin cancer and protect the eyes against diseases such as age-related macular degeneration, the most common cause of blindness in older people.[21] One study found that "lutein and zeaxanthin and foods rich in these carotenoids may decrease the risk of cataracts severe enough to require extractions."[22]

Beta-cryptoxanthin has been shown to inhibit cancer. It has also been researched for stimulating bone growth.[23-28]

## Cerebrosides and Pyrroles

In 1998 Korean researchers discovered special compounds in wolfberries that afford powerful protection for the most important organ in the human body: the liver.

Known as pyrroles and cerobrosides, these nutrients have been shown to protect against liver damage caused by both toxins and hepatitis.[29-31]

## Polysaccharides

The Ningxia wolfberry ranks high in a protein-sugar complex known as a polysaccharide. During the last 15 years, a number of studies have documented the cardioprotective, anticancerous, and immune-stimulating properties of the wolfberry polysaccharide. Studies show that polysaccharides in the Ningxia wolfberry positively affect natural killer cell function, which helps fight cancer.[32-34]

## Carotenoid (Xanthophyl) Content of 100 Grams of Ningxia Wolfberry

| | |
|---|---|
| Alpha carotene | 101 µg |
| Beta carotene | 23 µg |
| Lutein | 2.1 µg |
| Zeaxanthin | 278 µg |
| Beta crytoxanthin | 32 µg |

Source: Preliminary data from dried fruit of Ningxia wolfberry (Lycium barbarum) stored 1-3 years. Analysis by Eurofins Scientific, Petaluma, CA.

The first wolfberry polysaccharide was identified in 1994 when Chinese biochemists extracted a protein-carbohydrate complex (also known as a glycoprotein) from the wolfberry.[35]

Dubbing it "Lycium barbarum polysaccharide," researchers began learning that this low-glycemic, long-chain molecule could be responsible for many of the wolfberry's strong immune-boosting, anticancer, and cardiovascular protective benefits.

Lycium barbarum polysaccharide is a very large sugar-protein complex that occurs only in wolfberries. Of all the wolfberry species, *Lycium barbarum* L. contains the highest concentrations of Lycium barbarum polysaccharide.

The high polysaccharide and fiber content of the Ningxia wolfberry can promote the growth of beneficial bacteria in the gastrointestinal system. Diets high in protective, vegetable fibers, such as those in the wolfberry, result in higher levels of health-giving lactobacilli cultures and reduced populations of damaging cultures like *Clostridium perfringens*.

Beneficial bacteria may block cancer by producing short-chain fatty acids in the colon, which acidify the terrain.[36] This reduced pH in the colon is strongly associated with lower colon cancer risk.[37]

## Clinical Studies on Wolfberry Extracts

The Ningxia wolfberry's immune-boosting effect seems to be combined with an anti-inflammatory effect.[38] This means that the immune-supporting action of Ningxia wolfberry is less likely to trigger worsening of arthritis or other autoimmune diseases that are inflammatory in nature.

- A 2003 Institute of Medicinal Biotechnology study at the Peking Union Medical College in Beijing, China, found that Ningxia wolfberry polysaccharide stimulated production of interleukin-2, a non-inflammatory part of immunity that protects against cancer cells and microbial invasion.[39]

- A March 2003 study published in the *European Journal of Pharmacology* showed in vitro data that Ningxia wolfberry polysaccharide dramatically expanded output of interleukin-2 and tumor necrosis factor alpha from specialized human immune cells known as peripheral mononuclear cells (PMC).

  The surges in both interleukin-2 and tumor necrosis factor alpha hit a peak after 4 to 12 hours and remained well above baseline for 24 hours.[32]

- A 2014 Chinese study showed Lycium barbarum polysaccharides protect the epithelial cells in the human eye.[40]

- An August 2001 study by the State Key Laboratory of Bio-Organic Chemistry in Shanghai showed that the Ningxia wolfberry polysaccharide had an unusual combination of "good immunoactivity and antioxidative activity."

  The polysaccharide markedly spurred phagocyte immune cell activity and promoted lymphocyte upregulation.[41]

- A 2004 study at the Huazhong University of Science and Technology in Wuhan, China, documented the ability of wolfberry polysaccharide to enhance the proliferation of lymphocyte immune cells in the spleen.[42]

- A 2015 study in the journal *Food Nutrition Research* found that Lycium barbarum polysaccharides cause human hepatoma (malignant tumor of the liver) cells to self-destruct (induce apoptosis).[43]

- A 2004 Huazhong University of Science and Technology study found that mice treated with 10 mg/kg of wolfberry polysaccharide for 10 days showed improved macrophage phagocytosis, spleen lymphocyte proliferation, cytotoxic T-lymphocyte (CTL) activity, and interleukin-2 (IL-2) expression. Polysaccharide-fed animals could also resist the growth of transplanted cancer tumor cells (sarcoma S180).[44]

## All Sugars Are Not Equal

The dried wolfberries used extensively by the Ningxia people have been shown to have a very low glycemic index. A glycemic index is a measure of the impact a food has on blood sugar levels two hours after ingestion. The lower the rise in blood sugar levels, the lower the glycemic index.

The consumption of low glycemic foods is very important for minimizing the insidious degenerative damage caused by long-term, elevated blood sugar levels, which are strenuous to the heart, kidneys, pancreas, and circulatory system. Over time, the injury can become cumulative, shaving years off one's life.

## Synergy: 1 + 1 = 3

Ultimately, the synergy of all of these nutrients may be responsible for the Ningxia wolfberry's ability to support so many different functions of the body.

## Other Bioactive Components of Ningxia Wolfberry

| | | | |
|---|---|---|---|
| Cyclic diterpene glycosides[1] | Monomethyl succinate[2] | Beta cryptoxanthin[7,8] | Scopoletin[5,12] |
| Alpha carotene[7,8] | Monoterpene glycosides[2] | Cerobrosides[9] | Taurine[15] |
| Betaine[5,10] | P-coumaric acid[5] | Cyclic peptides[1] | Vanillic acid[12] |
| Beta-D-Glucopyranosyl ascorbate[3] | Polypheonols[14] | Daucosterol[5] | Withanolides[13] |
| | Polysaccharides[6,11] | Ellagic Acid[14] | Zeaxanthin dipalmitate[4,7,8] |
| Beta sitosterol[5] | Pyroles | Lutein[7,8] | |

1. Yahara S, et al. Cyclic peptides, acyclic diterpene glycosides and other compounds from Lycium chinense Mill. *Chem Pharm Bull* (Tokyo). 1993 Apr;41(4):703-9.

2. Hiserodt RD, et al. Identification of monomenthyl succinate, monomenthyl glutarate, and dimenthyl glutarate in nature by high performance liquid chromatography-tandem mass spectrometry. *J Agric Food Chem*. 2004 Jun 2;52(11):3536-41.

3. Toyoda-Ono Y, et al. 2-O-(beta-D-Glucopyranosyl) ascorbic acid, a novel ascorbic acid analogue isolated from Lycium fruit. *J Agric Food Chem*. 2004 Apr 7;52(7):2092-6.

4. Weller P, Breithaupt DE. Identification and quantification of zeaxanthin esters in plants using liquid chromatography-mass spectrometry. *J Agric Food Chem*. 2003 Nov 19;51(24):7044-9.

5. Xie C, et al. Studies on chemical constituents in fruit of Lycium barbarum L. *Zhongguo Zhong Yao Za Zhi*. 2001 May;26(5):323-4.

6. Huang LJ, Tian GY, Ji GZ. Structure elucidation of glycan of glycoconjugate LbGp3 isolated from the fruit of Lycium barbarum L. *J Asian Nat Prod Res*. 1999;1(4):259-67.

7. Li Z, Peng G, Zhang S. Separation and determination of carotenoids in Fructus lycii by isocratic non-aqueous reversed-phase liquid chromatography. *Se Pu*. 1998 Jul;16(4):341-3.

8. Analysis by Eurofins Scientific, Petaluma, CA.

9. Kim SY, et al. LCC, a cerebroside from Lycium chinense, protects primary cultured rat hepatocytes exposed to galactosamine. *Phytother Res*. 2000 Sep;14(6):448-51.

10. Shin YG, et al. Determination of betaine in Lycium chinense fruits by liquid chromatography-electrospray ionization mass spectrometry. *J Chromatogr A*. 1999 Oct 1;857(1-2):331-5.

11. Peng X, Tian G. Structural characterization of the glycan part of glycoconjugate LbGp2 from Lycium barbarum L. *Carbohydr Res*. 2001 Mar 9;331(1):95-9.

12. Hansel R, Huang JT. Lycium chinense, III: isolation of scopoletin and vanillic acid. *Arch Pharm (Weinheim)*. 1977 Jan;310(1):38-40.

13. Hansel R, Huang JT, Rosenberg D. Two withanolides from Lycium chinense. *Arch Pharm (Weinheim)*. 1975 Aug;308(8):653-4.

14. Brunswick Laboratories, Wareham, MA 2005.

15. Xie H, Zhang S. Determination of taurine in Lycium barbarum L. by high performance liquid chromatography with OPA-urea pre-column derivatization. *Se Pu*. 1997 Jan;15(1):54-6.

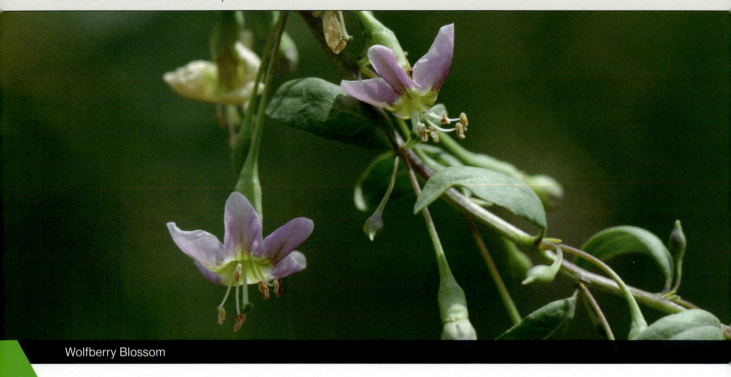

Wolfberry Blossom

According to Cornell University biochemist Riu Liu, PhD, "The additive and synergistic effects of phytochemicals in fruits and vegetables are responsible for their potent antioxidant and anticancer activities. . . . This partially explains why no single antioxidant can replace the combination of natural phytochemicals in fruits and vegetables in achieving the health benefits."[45]

## Protecting Cells from Oxidation

Each of the 3 trillion cells of the human body has a cell membrane composed primarily of fats that is susceptible to oxidative damage. The cell's energy is produced in mitochondria, where carbohydrates and oxygen are combined.

As this reaction takes place, free radical "sparks" shoot off that can damage the cell. Some of this damage occurs to the fats (lipids) that form the outer structure of both the mitochondria and the cell itself.

When these fats become oxidized or "rancid," malondialdehyde (MDA) starts to build up. The more of these "lipid peroxides" and MDA that form, the more brittle the cell membrane becomes, and the poorer the cell functions until eventually it self-destructs.

Protecting these fats from oxidative damage (or rancidity) is crucial for slowing down the damage that occurs with aging and keeping the machinery humming normally.

Oxidative stress to the body has been linked to diseases ranging from cancer to heart disease. This is why antioxidants are so important to the body. The simplest way to maximize antioxidant levels is with a diet high in antioxidant foods.

## ORAC Test Measures Antioxidant Levels of Common Foods

In 1994 Tufts University developed a powerful, new method of assaying the antioxidant capacity of common foods called the Oxygen Radical Absorbance Capacity assay (ORAC). A food's ORAC score is a measure of its free-radical fighting capacity.

The ORAC assay is currently the most sensitive and reliable method used for calculating a food's antioxidant potential against the free radical peroxyl. The peroxyl radical is the second most common in the human body.

### Sugars Found in Ningxia Wolfberry

| | |
|---|---|
| Rhamnose | 1.03% |
| Mannose | 14.8% |
| Galactose | 4.3% |
| Xylose | 13.3% |
| Glucose | 62.7% |

Source: Huang L, et al. Isolation, purification and physico-chemical properties of immunoactive constituents from the fruit of Lycium barbarum L. *Yao Xue Xue Bao.* 1998 Jul;33(7):512-6.

### Glycemic Index* of Selected Foods

| | |
|---|---|
| Glucose | 100 |
| Brown Rice | 66 |
| Millet | 72 |
| Buckwheat | 54 |
| Ningxia Wolfberry | 29 |

*Measures the speed with which a food raises blood sugar levels.

Ningxia Wolfberry | **Chapter 9**

## An Astounding Antioxidant

In 2000 Young Living Essential Oils commissioned an ORAC assay on the Ningxia wolfberry. The results were astonishing and showed that dried Ningxia wolfberries had 5 times the antioxidant capacity of prunes, 10 times that of oranges, 12 times that of raisins, and 55 times that of cauliflower. In fact, according to the published ORAC data, dried Ningxia wolfberries had one of the highest known ORAC score of any whole food (303 µmTE/g).[46]

## Protecting Against Superoxide and Other Free Radicals

While the peroxyl radical is the second most prevalent antioxidant in the body, the most prevalent and most damaging in the body is superoxide. A test has been developed that measures the superoxide-scavenging capacity of a food.

## Animal Studies on Reversing Aging

Other studies have confirmed that Ningxia wolfberry has strong activity against the superoxide radical. A 2003 investigation by the Chinese Academy of Science tested the ability of Ningxia wolfberry polysaccharide (LBP) to reverse the effects of aging in three-month-old female mice who were dosed with a chemical that vastly accelerates the aging process, D-galactose.[39]

D-galactose was used because it mimics the type of damage typically seen in the elderly and diabetics.

To measure the animals' ability to resist aging, lead researcher Hong-Bin Deng used a number of tests, including an immunological assay, a memory test, and an AGE (advanced glycosylated end products) test. He also assayed serum levels of superoxide dismutase (SOD), which is the most important free-radical deactivator, due to its function of quenching deadly superoxide radicals.

Hong-Bin Deng found that the wolfberry polysaccharide restored SOD levels in aging animals to that of more youthful levels. The polysaccharide also blunted the damaging effects of D-galactose on mental function and AGE levels in the tissues. In short, the wolfberry appeared to reverse aging in animals subjected to a chemical that hastened the onset of old age.

## Ningxia Wolfberry vs. High-altitude Stress

A related study at the Faculty of Preventive Medicine at Ningxia Medicine College in Yinchuan tested SOD and catalase activity in a group of 56 mice who were subjected to oxidative stress caused by lack of oxygen. These "hypoxic" conditions were similar to what you would find at high altitudes.

In a subgroup fed Ningxia wolfberry, both SOD and catalase activity jumped significantly compared with the control group.

## Top Antioxidant Foods

| Food | ORAC2 (µmTE/g) | Food | ORAC² (µmTE/g) |
|---|---|---|---|
| Ningxia Wolfberry (*Lycium barbarum*), dried[3] | 303 | Kale | 18 |
| Chinese wolfberry (*Lycium chinense*) | 202 | Raspberry | 16 |
| Acai, fresh | 184 | Apple | 14 |
| Black Raspberry | 164 | Peach | 13 |
| Pomegranate | 105 | Spinach | 12 |
| Ningxia Wolfberry (*Lycium barbarum*), fresh[4] | 95 | Red Grape | 11 |
| Prune | 57 | Brussels Sprouts | 9 |
| Blackberry | 51 | Alfalfa Sprouts | 9 |
| Boysenberry | 35 | Broccoli Florets | 9 |
| Blueberry | 32 | Kiwi | 9 |
| Plum | 28 | Beet | 8 |
| Red Raspberry | 27 | Onion | 4 |
| Strawberry | 26 | Cauliflower | 4 |
| Orange | 24 | Mango | 3 |
| Cherry | 21 | Cabbage | 3 |
| Raisin | 21 | Banana | 3 |
| Garlic | 19 | Apple | 3 |
| | | Tomato | 2 |
| | | Carrot | 2 |

1. All foods are fresh unless otherwise noted with "dried."
2. Oxygen Radical Absorbance Capacity
3. Data from dried fruit stored 1-3 years. Analysis performed by Brunswick Labs, Wareham, MA
4. Analysis performed by Brunswick Labs, Wareham, MA

The simultaneous elevation of both of these antioxidant enzymes is important because the two depend on each other to maximize their effectiveness. While SOD deactivates superoxide free radicals, catalase mops up hydrogen peroxide free radicals.

The combination of the two working together is vital because SOD actually produces hydrogen peroxide as a byproduct of defusing superoxide. Catalase is one of the few enzymes capable of neutralizing hydrogen peroxide.[47]

## Ningxia Wolfberry Extends Cell Life

Gerontologists at the Department of Cell Biology and Genetics at Peking University discovered that including a vanishingly small amount of wolfberry (0.025 percent) in the culture medium could extend the number of times human lung cells could divide from 49 times to 61 times.

Each time a cell divides, the chance of error creeps in, as well as the cumulative burden of oxidative damage. Using wolfberry in the nutrient broth, researchers effectively increased the lifespan of the lung tissue by 22 percent.[48]

An October 2002 study at the Department of Histology and Embryology at the Ningxia Medical College in Yinchuan tested the ability of Ningxia wolfberry to help

Seventh Edition | **Essential Oils Desk Reference** | 199

sperm-producing cells resist damage from excess cold (hyperthermic conditions) and ultraviolet sunlight radiation.

According to lead researcher, Wang, "We found that fructus lycii polysaccharide (FLPS) is a potent inhibitor of both of these reactions. Together, these results demonstrate the protective effect of FLPS on time and hyperthermia induced testicular degeneration in vitro."[49]

This study is significant not only because of its implications for increased fertility (yes, it is true that Ningxia wolfberry extracts have been used for centuries to boost reproductive success) but also as it pertains to the antioxidant protection that Ningxia wolfberry affords to cells that are most vulnerable to oxidative damage: testicle cells.

Reproductive cells are very easily damaged by cold stresses and UV radiation, so the ability of Ningxia wolfberry to effectively defend against these types of attacks helps to show the true measure of the berry's antioxidant potential.

### Healthy Immunity and Antiaging

As mentioned previously, the Ningxia wolfberry contains a polysaccharide that has been shown to positively affect natural killer cell function.[34]

During the past two decades, a number of clinical studies have shown a direct link between cancer, accelerated aging, and poor immune function. In particular, a key weapon in our nonspecific immunity called a "natural killer" cell is very adept at automatically destroying suspicious-looking cancer cells without requiring "education" in the immune glands of the body (e.g., thymus).[50-55]

A 2002 study at the University of Milan documented a direct link between stress and inflammation and lowered, natural killer cell activity and poorer outcomes in cancer cases.[56]

An earlier study published in the *International Journal of Cancer* showed that animals with higher levels of NK (natural killer) activity were able to suppress metastatic cancer growth by up to 7-fold in comparison with normal mice.[57]

Researchers at the Mount Sinai Medical Center in New York also showed a link between low immunity (natural killer cell activity) and poor outcomes in cancer survival.

After analyzing the survival data from 102 colorectal cancer patients, Tartter and Steinberg found that having a preoperative low NK cell function triggered a frightening jump in the danger of cancer recurrence.[58]

Similarly, a 2002 Chiba University study on 140 patients with colorectal cancer found that lowered NK cell activity was linked to a 50 percent risk of cancer colonization and spread compared to patients with normal or better NK cell function.

Lead researcher, Eisuke Kondo, stated that "the patient's own anticancer immunity, as well as the potent malignancy of the tumor, may play a role in the development of recurrence following curative surgery. . . . Preliminary data showed that among several immunological parameters examined . . . , preoperative natural killer (NK) cell activity was the only one associated with . . . distant metastasis following curative surgery for colorectal cancer."[59]

### Whole Wolfberry Clinical Trials

The first study conducted on the power of the wolfberry to protect against superoxide measured the ability of the body to produce the free-radical, enzymatic, antioxidant superoxide dismutase (SOD). SOD is the body's frontline defense against superoxide, and it is this enzymatic antioxidant that is so important in neutralizing the free radical superoxide.

In 1982 the following study was conducted in China. Fifty persons aged 64-80 were given 50 grams of wolfberries for 10 days.

Blood samples were taken before the study began and after 10 days of consuming a diet that included wolfberries. The blood samples at the end of 10 days showed that levels of SOD had increased by 48 percent. In addition, lipid peroxides had dropped by 65 percent.[60]

Another study published in December 2004 by Kaohsiung Medical University in Taiwan indicates that the Ningxia wolfberry may indeed have strong superoxide-neutralizing activity.

Researchers found that depending on its concentration, a water extract of wolfberry scavenged from 28.8 percent to 82.2 percent of superoxide radicals. The concentrations of wolfberry that inhibited 50 percent of the superoxide activity were tiny, ranging from 0.77 to 2.55 parts per million. This works out to 0.000077 and 0.00025 percent.

The minute concentrations used are indicative of the Ningxia wolfberry's exceptional superoxide-neutralizing power.[61]

For further reading, please see: Young DG, Lawrence R, Schreuder M. *Discovery of the Ultimate Superfood*. Lehi, UT: Life Science Publishing, 2005.

# Nutritional Products with Ningxia Wolfberry

*(See the "Nutritional Support" chapter for more information.)*

The Ningxia wolfberry is a fabulous source of nutrients for nutritional products.

All of the following products contain Ningxia wolfberry (*Lycium barbarum*), which is the highest antioxidant food known, making it an excellent whole food with 18 amino acids; 21 trace minerals; vitamins B1, B2, B6, C, E; polyphenols; carotenoids; magnesium; and potassium.

## Balance Complete™ Vanilla Cream Meal Replacement

Balance Complete is a super-food meal replacement that is high in fiber and protein, with the good fats, enzymes, vitamins, and minerals needed to form a nutritious, great tasting protein drink that satisfies the appetite. It is a powerful nutritive energizer and cleanser, which helps to improve digestion and support colon health.

The high antioxidant benefits of the Ningxia wolfberry powder, brown rice bran, barley grass, aloe vera, cinnamon powder, and whey protein blend create the building blocks for strengthening the immune system and bringing back the renewed feelings of energy and vitality.

## Gary's True Grit™ Chocolate-Coated Wolfberry Crisp™ Bars

The Chocolate-Coated Wolfberry Crisp bar is a delicious, convenient, whole-food, low-glycemic, super-nutrient bar, containing 6 grams of protein and is delightful coated in chocolate. It is rich in antioxidants and phytonutrients and does not significantly raise blood sugar levels. It is a great all-natural snack for when you are on the go, at work, at school, or even when you want a meal replacement.

## Gary's True Grit™ Einkorn Granola

The tasty combination of naturally sourced grains, nuts, berries, and seeds provides both simple and complex carbs to keep you going throughout the day. The crunchy clusters are mixed with Organic Dried Ningxia Wolfberries, cranberries, cacao nibs, coconut sugar, sunflower seeds, almonds, walnuts, and pecans, with just the right amount of sea salt.

## Gary's True Grit™ NingXia Berry Syrup

This premium all-purpose syrup combines natural, delicious ingredients, including wolfberry seed oil, with pure Orange and Lemon essential oils to create the perfect complement to Gary's True Grit Einkorn Pancakes and Waffle Mix or your favorite dessert.

## ImmuPro™

ImmuPro chewable tablets are packed with some of the most powerful immune stimulants known, including wolfberry polysaccharide and beta glucan (a polysaccharide from reishi, maitake, and *Agaricus blazei* mushrooms).

Numerous studies have documented the ability of these botanicals to reverse cancer and stimulate both cell-mediated and humoral immunity, dramatically boosting levels of macrophages, neutrophils, phagocytes, B-cells, T-cells, natural killer cells, interleukins, and interferons.

ImmuPro combines complex and potent, immune-boosting minerals such as zinc, copper, and selenium. It also contains melatonin, one of the most powerful immune stimulants known, shown to clinically reverse tumor growth. Melatonin levels steadily decrease with age and are a factor that contributes to accelerated aging.

## KidScents® MightyVites™

KidScents MightyVites is a whole-food multinutrient that contains wolfberry fruit and other super fruits, plants, and vegetables that deliver the full spectrum of vitamins, minerals, antioxidants, and phytonutrients, specifically designed for children's developing bodies.

Children's diets often need to bridge between what they are eating and what they should be eating. To fuel growth and normal activity levels, a child's diet must provide plenty of vitamins and minerals as well as store nutrients in preparation for the accelerated growth spurts of the teenage years.

This super enriched, chewable vitamin is perfect for children to energize, build their bodies, and protect their entire system the way Mother Nature intended.

## Master Formula™

Master Formula is a full-spectrum, premium multinutrient supplement that contains wolfberry fruit powder, providing vitamins, minerals, and food-based nutriment to support general health and well-being for men and women.

By using a Synergistic Suspension Isolation process (SSI Technology), ingredients are delivered in three distinct delivery forms. Collectively, these ingredients provide a premium, synergistic complex to support your body.

**Essential Oils Desk Reference** | Seventh Edition

## Ningxia Red® Recipes:

*These are great oils to add to a shot of NingXia Red Juice—have fun and bottoms up!*

### The Holy Cow
- 1 drop Peppermint
- 2 drops Frankincense
- 1 drop Lemon

### To Your Health
- 1 drop Orange
- 2 drops Tangerine
- 1 drop Thieves blend

### Oh, My Gosh
- 1 drop Ocotea
- 4 drops Peppermint
- 3 drops Tangerine
- 3 drops Lemon

### Oh, My Gosh, for Your Digestion
- 2 drops Tangerine
- 1 drop Frankincense
- 1 drop Fennel
- 1 drop Peppermint

### The Nuclear Explosion
- 1 drop Peppermint
- 1 drop Lavender
- 1 drop Frankincense
- 1 drop Lemon
- 1 drop Tangerine
- 1 drop Orange

### Who Let the Dogs Out?
- 1 drop Lemon
- 2 drops Tangerine
- 1 drop Frankincense
- 1 drop Cinnamon Bark

*(Take the shot; then go "woof, woof, woof, woof, woof.")*

Variation: Put 1 drop Cassia on the back of your hand and lick it off just before consuming the drink.

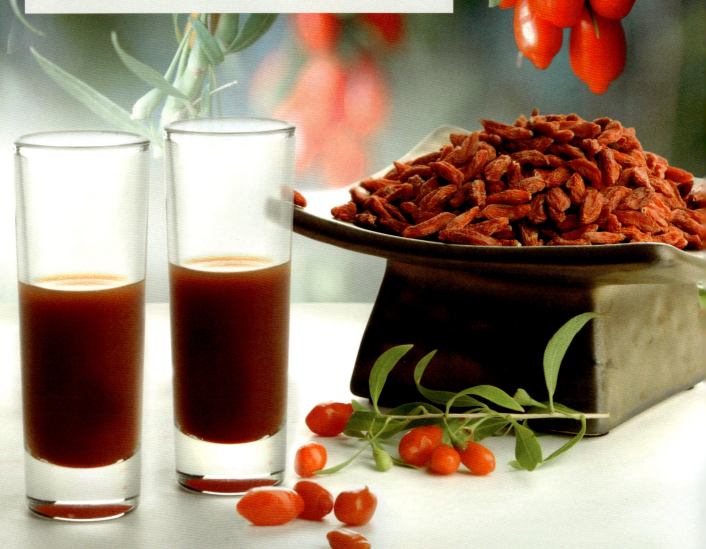

202 | Chapter 9 | Ningxia Wolfberry

Ningxia Wolfberry | Chapter 9

## NingXia Nitro™

NingXia Nitro is an all-natural way to increase cognitive alertness, enhance mental fitness, and support overall performance. It contains a wide range of powerful cognitive enhancers, including wolfberry seed oil and a proprietary blend of pure Black Pepper, Nutmeg, Vanilla, Chocolate, Yerba Mate, Spearmint, and Peppermint essential oils.

NingXia Nitro contains Bioenergy Ribose®, a form of D-Ribose that has been clinically tested for its ability to increase energy, endurance, and aerobic activity and is currently used by the Olympic athletes. This ingredient improves physical performance, speeds up recovery, and increases overall energy reserves.

Other supportive ingredients in NingXia Nitro, such as B vitamins, green tea extract, choline, and Korean ginseng, sharpen the mind and invigorate the senses.

## NingXia Red® (Juice)

NingXia Red is a powerful antioxidant supplement drink made from wolfberry juice, blueberry juice, pomegranate juice, apricot juice, raspberry juice, and Lemon and Orange essential oils.

NingXia Red supports immune function, liver function, and eye health and is reported to increase energy.

It is the highest known protection against the dangerous superoxide free radicals, as documented in the S-ORAC test conducted by Brunswick Laboratories. It is rich in ellagic acid, polyphenols, flavonoids, vitamins, and minerals. In addition, it has 18 amino acids, 21 trace minerals, beta-carotene, and vitamins B1, B2, B6, and E.

It is an excellent whole-food source of nutrients that gives energy and strength to the body without harmful stimulates. It also has an amazing low glycemic index of 11 that does not spike the blood sugar levels.

## Ningxia Wolfberries (Organic Dried)

The Ningxia wolfberry is one of earth's most powerful antioxidant fruits. It is rich in polysaccharides, with more vitamin C than oranges, more beta-carotene than carrots, and more calcium than broccoli.

These little, red Ningxia wolfberries are delicious and make a great, healthful snack. They can be used in cooking, salads, desserts, etc.

## NingXia Zyng™

NingXia Zyng is a light, sparkling beverage that delivers a splash of hydrating energy. Zyng is fueled by a proprietary blend of pure Black Pepper and Lime essential oils, wolfberry puree, and white tea extract, coupled with a blend of vitamins to create a unique and refreshing experience. Containing just 35 calories, 8.4 ounces of NingXia Zyng will invigorate your senses with no artificial flavors, colors, sweeteners, or preservatives.

## Slique® Bars—Tropical Berry Crunch

Slique Bars are safe, innovative weight-management tools that utilize a dual-target approach to help manage satiety. First, Slique Bars are loaded with exotic baru nuts and wholesome almonds that promote satiation when combined with protein and high levels of fiber. Second, Slique bars contain clinical amounts of Slendesta®, an all-natural ingredient derived from potato skin extract that when ingested triggers the release of cholecystokinin in the body, increasing the duration of feelings of fullness.

Slique Bars also deliver essential nutrients and antioxidants through the addition of pure Cinnamon Bark, Vanilla, and Orange essential oils; a dried-fruit blend featuring goldenberries and wolfberries; and D. Gary Young's exclusive dehydrated cacao nibs. Slique Bars' dual-targeted satiety approach and medley of exotic fruits, nuts, and science creates the perfect stimulant-free nutritious snack to help you feel fuller longer.

## Slique® Bars—Chocolate-Coated

Chocolate-Coated Slique Bars are a safe, delicious weight management snack loaded with exotic baru nuts and wholesome almonds. Slique Bars deliver essential nutrients from a unique superfruit blend of goldenberries and wolfberries, plus Cinnamon, Vanilla, and Orange essential oils.

## Slique® Shake

Slique Shake is a complete meal replacement that provides quick, satisfying, and delicious nutrition. It is sweetened with stevia, organic coconut palm sugar, wolfberries, and strawberries and uses pea protein, quinoa, wolfberry, pumpkin seed protein, and alfalfa grass juice, making it an excellent source of protein and dietary fiber. In a convenient single-serving size packet, it's great to take with you for a quick and easy meal.

Seventh Edition | **Essential Oils Desk Reference** | 203

**Essential Oils Desk Reference** | Seventh Edition

## Sulfurzyme® Capsules and Powder

Sulfurzyme is a unique combination of MSM, the protein-building compound found in breast milk, fresh fruits and vegetables, and Ningxia wolfberry. Together, they create a new concept in balancing the immune system and supporting almost every major function of the body.

Of particular importance is the ability of MSM to equalize water pressure inside the cells, a considerable benefit for those plagued with bursitis, arthritis, and tendonitis.

Ningxia wolfberry supplies nutrients to enhance the proper assimilation and metabolism of sulfur.

## Wolfberry Crisp™

Wolfberry Crisp is a delicious, convenient, whole-food, low-glycemic, super-nutrient bar, containing 16 grams of protein.

It is rich in antioxidants and phytonutrients and does not significantly raise blood sugar levels. It also contains soy and whey protein complex, organic Blue Agave nectar, wolfberry fruit, pumpkin seeds, cashews, walnuts, carob chips, vanilla bean extract, and natural banana flavoring.

It is a delicious meal replacement that is all natural and certified kosher.

## Wolfberry Crisp™ Bars, Chocolate Coated

*(See Gary's True Grit™ Chocolate-Coated Wolfberry Crisp™ Bars)*

# Personal Care Products with Ningxia Wolfberry

*(See the "Personal Body Care" chapter for more information.)*

For centuries, the Chinese living in Inner Mongolia have been using a very unusual oil with exceptional benefits for the skin: wolfberry seed oil.

This rare and expensive oil from Inner Mongolia is painstakingly extracted from the seeds of the Ningxia wolfberry. Not only is the oil rich in vitamin E and linoleic and linolenic acids, but it also has an unusual chemistry that makes it ideal for nourishing and hydrating the skin.

"The wolfberry seed oil is one of the best oils for the skin," according to researcher Sue Chao. "It is sought after throughout Asia and has some very unusual regenerative properties such as protecting aging skin and adding luster to skin."

All of the following personal body care products contain Ningxia wolfberry.

## Boswellia Wrinkle Cream™

Boswellia Wrinkle Cream contains the pure essential oils of Frankincense, Sandalwood, Myrrh, Ylang Ylang, and Geranium that moisturize while minimizing shine, relaxing facial tension, and reducing the effects of sun damage.

This wrinkle cream also contains wolfberry seed oil, which helps build collagen and when used daily will help minimize and prevent wrinkles.

## Copaiba Vanilla Moisturizing Conditioner

Plant-based, safe, and environmentally responsible, Copaiba Vanilla Moisturizing Conditioner is a rich, hydrating conditioner for dry or damaged hair.

Formulated with botanical extracts; vitamins; silk proteins; wolfberry fruit extract and berries; the benefits of pure Copaiba, Lavender, Geranium, and Lime essential oils; and vanilla absolute, this gentle conditioner protects and conditions for a soothing, revitalizing experience.

## Copaiba Vanilla Moisturizing Shampoo

Copaiba Vanilla Moisturizing Shampoo calms and moisturizes dry, irritated scalps and is a natural sealant that can help tame "flyaway" hair and lock in moisture.

Plant-based, safe, and environmentally responsible, this shampoo contains wolfberry fruit extract and berries and the essential oils of Copaiba, Lavender, Geranium, Lime, plus vanilla absolute and is a rich, hydrating cleanser for dry or damaged hair.

## Essential Beauty™ Serum (Dry)

Essential oils provide wonderful benefits when used on the skin. Lavender, Blue Cypress, and Royal Hawaiian Sandalwood™ are known for their ability to restore the skin's natural moisture balance. The fine lipid structure of essential oils enable them to penetrate deep into skin tissues, carrying many active ingredients that renew, balance, and build skin health.

**204** | **Chapter 9** | Ningxia Wolfberry

This serum has a wonderful skin-conditioning base of coconut, avocado, jojoba, rosehip seed, and wolfberry seed oils. Vitamin E and lecithin are added for a greater softening effect.

## Lavender Bath & Shower Gel

Infused with pure Lavender oil, Lavender Bath & Shower Gel will cleanse and rejuvenate your skin while it soothes and relaxes your mind.

It is free of chemicals and synthetic preservatives and contains plant-based ingredients like wolfberry fruit extract and berries and the essential oils of Lavender, Lemon, Myrrh, and Davana.

## Lavender Hand & Body Lotion

Infused with wolfberry seed oil; Lavender, Myrrh, Lemon, and Davana essential oils; and other plant-based ingredients, Lavender Hand & Body Lotion moisturizes and protects skin from overexposure for long-lasting hydration.

This formula is certified eco-friendly and all natural.

## Lavender Mint Invigorating Conditioner

Plant-based, safe, and environmentally responsible, Lavender Mint Invigorating Conditioner is an invigorating daily moisture blend suitable for all hair types.

Containing botanical extracts, vitamins, silk protein, wolfberry fruit extract and berries, and the benefits of pure Lavender and Peppermint essential oils, this conditioner provides a rejuvenating and invigorating experience suitable for all hair types.

## Lavender Mint Invigorating Shampoo

Lavender Mint Invigorating Shampoo contains wolfberry fruit extract and berries and Lavender essential oil to soothe the scalp and calm unmanageable hair and Peppermint essential oil to stimulate the blood flow to the hair follicle—allowing hair to better absorb nutrients.

Plant-based, safe, and environmentally responsible, this shampoo is an invigorating, daily cleansing blend suitable for all hair types.

## Lip Balm, Cinnamint™

This balm moisturizes and protects your lips by combining the nutritious wolfberry seed oil with MSM and pure Cinnamon Bark, Peppermint, Spearmint, and Orange essential oils. Cinnamint Lip Balm helps prevent skin dehydration for soft, smooth lips.

## Lip Balm, Grapefruit

This balm is infused with Grapefruit essential oil, wolfberry seed oil, and antioxidants that seal in moisture to prevent dehydration for smooth, supple lips.

## Lip Balm, Lavender

This balm soothes dry, chapped lips with gentle, protective Lavender essential oil and the moisturizing benefits of wolfberry seed oil, jojoba oil, and vitamin E.

## Orange Blossom Facial Wash™

This gentle, soap-free facial wash cleanses the skin without stripping natural oils. In addition to wolfberry seed oil, it contains MSM for softening, kelp to improve elasticity, and Lavender essential oil to soothe acne-prone skin and other problems.

## Prenolone® + Body Cream

Prenolone Plus Body Cream contains pregnenolone; DHEA; wolfberry seed oil; blue and black cohosh; and Ylang Ylang, Clary Sage, and other essential oils to nourish the skin and help maintain healthy estrogen levels.

## Regenolone Moisturizing Cream™

Regenolone is a natural moisturizer formulated to support proper estrogen levels in women.

In addition to wolfberry seed oil, it contains wild yam; black and blue cohosh; and Peppermint, Wintergreen, and other essential oils to invigorate the skin and enhance absorption.

## Sandalwood Moisture Cream™

Sandalwood Moisture Cream is an ultra-hydrating moisturizer infused with wolfberry seed oil and pure essential oils of Myrrh, Lavender, Sandalwood, and Rosemary. In addition, MSM—a naturally occurring, plant-based chemical—softens skin and promotes elasticity.

When used daily after cleansing and toning, this moisture cream promotes younger, healthier skin.

## Wolfberry Eye Cream™

Wolfberry Eye Cream is a natural, water-based moisturizer. Containing the antiaging properties of wolfberry seed oil and the essential oils of Lavender, Roman Chamomile, Frankincense, and Geranium, this cream soothes tired eyes and minimizes the appearance of bags, circles, and fine lines. Use in the morning and before bed.

## ENDNOTES

1. Young G, et al. *Ningxia wolfberry: the ultimate superfood.* Lehi: Life Science Publishing, 2006.

2. U.S. Department of Agriculture, Agricultural Research Service. 2011. USDA Nutrient Database for Standard Reference, Release 24. Nutrient Data Laboratory Home Page. http://www.ars.usda.gov/ba/bhnrc/ndl.

3. Combaret L, et al. A leucine-supplemented diet restores the defective post prandial inhibition of proteasome-dependent proteolysis in aged rat skeletal muscle. *J physiol.* 2005;569(2):489-499.

4. Bogdan C, et al. The role of nitric oxide in innate immunity. *Immunol Rev.* 2000 Feb;173:17-26.

5. Jyothi MD, Khar A. Induction of nitric oxide production by natural killer cells: its role in tumor cell death. *Nitric Oxide.* 1999 Oct;3(5):409-418.

6. Wu GH, et al. Modulation of postoperative immune and inflammatory response by immune-enhancing enteral diet in gastrointestinal cancer patients. *World J Gastroenterol.* 2001 Jun;7(3):357-362.

7. Chan O, et al. ATP-sensitive K(+) channels regulate the release of GABA in the ventromedial hypothalamus during hypoglycemia. *Diabetes.* 2007;56(4):1120-1126.

8. Leventhal AG, et al. GABA and its agonists improved visual cortical function in senescent monkeys. *Science.* 2003;300(5620):812.

9. Shankar AH, Prasad AS. Zinc and immune function: the biological basis of altered resistance to infection. *Am J Clin Nutr.* 1998 Aug;68(2 Suppl):447S-463S.

10. Rink L, Kirchner H. Zinc-altered immune function and cytokine production. *J Nutr.* 2000 May;130(5S Suppl):1407S-1411S.

11. Shankar AH, Prasad AS. Zinc and immune function: the biological basis of altered resistance to infection. *Am J Clin Nutr.* 1998 Aug;68(2 Suppl):447S-463S.

12. Prasad AS, et al. Zinc deficiency in elderly patients. *Nutrition.* 1993 May-Jun;9(3):218-24.

13. Hulisz D. Efficacy of zinc against common cold viruses: an overview. *J Am Pharm Assoc.* 2004 Sep-Oct;44(5):594-603.

14. Hemilä H, Chalker E. The effectiveness of high dose zinc acetate lozenges on various common cold symptoms: a meta-analysis. *BMC Fam Pract.* 2015 Feb 25;16:24.

15. Brown L, et al. Cholesterol-lowering effects of dietary fiber: A meta-analysis. *Am J Clin Nutr.*1999;69(1)30-42.

16. Romero AL, et al. Cookies enriched with psyllium or oat bran lower plasma LDL cholesterol in normal and hypercholesterolemic men from Northern Mexico. *J Am Coll Nutr.* 1998;17(6):601-608.

17. Mekki N, et al. Effects of lowering fat and increasing dietary fiber on fasting and postprandial plasma lipids in hypercholesterolemic subjects consuming a mixed Mediterranean-Western diet. *Am J Clin Nutr.* 1997;66(6):1443-1451.

18. Ullrich IH. Evaluation of a high-fiber diet in hyperlipidemia: A review. *J Am Coll Nutr.* 1987;6(1):19-25.

19. Watzl B, et al. Supplementation of a low-carotenoid diet with tomato or carrot juice modulates immune functions in healthy men. *Ann Nutr Metab.* 2003;47(6):255-261.

20. Watzl B, et al. Modulation of human T-lymphocyte functions by the consumption of carotenoid-rich vegetables. *Br J Nutr.* 1999 Nov;82(5):383-389.

21. Gale CR, et al. Lutein and zeaxanthin status and risk of age-related macular degeneration. *Invest Opthalmol Vis Sci.* 2003 Jun;44(6):2461-2465.

22. Chasen-Taber L, et al. A prospective study of carotenoid and vitamin A intakes and risk of cataract extraction in US women. *Am J Clin Nutr.* 1999 Oct;70(4):509-516.

23. Noguchi S, et al. Effects of oxygenated carotenoid beta-cryptoxanthin on morphological differentiation and apoptosis in Neuro2a neuroblastoma cells. *Biosci Biotechnol Biochem.* 2003 Nov;67(11):2467-2469.

24. Donaldson MS. Nutrition and cancer: A review of the evidence for an anti-cancer diet. *Nutr J.* 2004 Oct 20;3(1):19.

25. Nomura AM, et al. Serum vitamins and the subsequent risk of bladder cancer. *J Urol.* 2003 Oct;170(4 Pt 1):1146-1150.

26. Uchiyama S, Yamaguchi M. beta-Cryptoxanthin stimulates cell proliferation and transcriptional activity in osteoblastic MC3T3-E1 cells. *Int J Mol Med.* 2005 Apr;15(4):675-681.

27. Yamaguchi M, Uchiyama S. beta-Cryptoxanthin stimulates bone formation and inhibits bone resorption in tissue culture in vitro. *Mol Cell Biochem.* 2004 Mar;258(1-2):137-144.

28. Uchiyama S, et al. Oral administration of beta-cryptoxanthin induces anabolic effects on bone components in the femoral tissues of rats in vivo. *Biol Pharm Bull.* 2004 Feb;27(2):232-235.

29. Kim SY, et al. New antihepatotoxic cerebroside from Lycium chinense fruits. *J Nat Prod.* 1997 Mar;60(3):274-276.

30. Chin YW, et al. Hepatoprotective pyrrole derivatives of Lycium chinense fruits. *Bioorg Med Chem Lett.* 2003 Jan 6;13(1):79-81.

31. Kim HP, et al. Zeaxanthin dipalmitate from Lycium chinense fruit reduces experimentally induced hepatic fibrosis in rats. *Biol Pharm Bull.* 2002 Mar;25(3):390-392.

32. Gan L, et al. A polysaccharide-protein complex from Lycium barbarum upregulates cytokine expression in human peripheral blood mononuclear cells. *Eur J Pharmacol.* 2003 Jun 27;471(3):217-222.

33. Jia YX, et al. The effect of Lycium barbarum polysaccharide on vascular tension in two-kidney, one clip model of hypertension. *Sheng Li Xue Bao.* 1998 Jun;50(3):309-314.

34. Hu Q, et al. A study on the anti-cancer effect of ningxia wolfberry. *J Tradit Chin Med.* 1989 Jun;9(2):117-124.

35. Tian G, Wang C. Structure elucidation of a high MW glycan of a glycoprotein isolated from the fruit of Lycium barbarum L. *Acta Bioch Bioph Sin.* 1995;05. http://en.cnki.com.cn/Article_en/CJFDTOTAL-SHWL505.003.htm.

36. Goldin BR, Gorbach SL. The effect of milk and lactobacillus feeding on human intestinal bacterial enzyme activity. *Am J Clin Nutr.* 1984;39(5):756–761.

37. Aso Y, Akazan H. Prophylactic effect of a Lactobacillus casei preparation on the recurrence of superficial bladder cancer. BLP Study Group. *Urol Int.* 1992;49(3):125–129.

38. Xu Y, et al. Advances in immunopharmacological study of Lycium barbarum L. *Zhong Yao Cai.* 2000 May;23(5):295-298.

39. Deng HB, et al. Inhibiting effects of Achyranthes bidentata polysaccharide and Lycium barbarum polysaccharide on nonenzyme glycation in D-galactose induced mouse aging model. *Biomed Environ Sci.* 2003 Sep;16(3):267-275.

40. Qi B, et al. Lycium barbarum polysaccharides protect human lens epithelial cells against oxidative stress-induced apoptosis and senescence. *PLoS One.* 2014 Oct 15;9(10):e110275.

41. Peng XM, et al. Physico-chemical properties and activity of glycoconjugate LbGp2 from Lycium barbarum L. *Yao Xue Xue Bao.* 2001 Aug;36(8):599-602.

42. Du G, et al. Experimental study on the enhancement of murine splenic lymphocyte proliferation by Lycium barbarum glycopeptide. *J Huazhong Univ Sci Technolog Med Sci.* 2004;24(5):518-20, 527.

43. Zhang Q, et al. Composition of Lycium barbarum polysaccharides and their apoptosis-inducing effect on human hepatoma SMMC-7721 cells. *Food Nutr Res.* 2015 Nov 11;59:28696.

44. Gan L, et al. Immunomodulation and antitumor activity by a polysaccharide-protein complex from Lycium barbarum. *Int Immunopharmacol.* 2004 Apr;4(4):563-569.

45. Liu RH. Health benefits of fruit and vegetables are from additive and synergistic combinations of phytochemicals. *Am J Clin Nutr.* 2003 Sep;78(3 Suppl):517S-520S.

46. Data from dried fruit stored 1-3 years. Analysis performed by Brunswick Laboratories, Wareham, MA.

47. Li G, et al. Effect of Lycium barbarum L on defending free radicals of mice caused by hypoxia. *Wei Sheng Yan Jiu.* 2002 Feb;31(1):30-31.

48. Wu BY, et al. Effect of wolfberry fruit and epimedium on DNA synthesis of the aging-youth 2BS fusion cells. *Zhongguo Zhong Xi Yi Jie He Za Zhi.* 2003 Dec;23(12):926-928.

49. Wang Y, et al. Protective effect of Fructus lycii polysaccharides against time and hyperthermia-induced damage in cultured seminiferous epithelium. *J Ethnopharmacol.* 2002 Oct;82(2-3):169-175.

50. Krtolica A, et al. Senescent fibroblasts promote epithelial cell growth and tumorgenesis: a link between cancer and aging. *Proc Natl Acad Sci U S A.* 2001 Oct;98(21):12072-12077.

51. Talmadge J, et al. Role of NK cells in tumour growth and metastasis in beige mice. *Nature.* 1980 Apr;284(5757):622-624.

52. Wu J, Lanier LL. Natural killer cells and cancer. *Adv Cancer Res.* 2003;90:127-156.

53. Herberman RB, Ortaldo JR. Natural killer cells: their roles in defenses against disease. *Science.* 1981 Oct;214(4516):24-30.

54. Levy SM, et al. Prognostic risk assessment in primary breast cancer by behavioral and immunological parameters. *Health Psychol.* 1985;4(2):99-113.

55. Schantz SP, et al. Evidence for the role of natural immunity in the control of metastatic spread of head and neck cancer. *Cancer Immunol Immunother.* 1987;25(2):141-148.

56. Gaspani L, et al. The analgesic drug tramadol prevents the effect of surgery on natural killer cell activity and metastatic colonization in rats. *J Neuroimmunol.* 2002 Aug;129(1-2):18-24.

57. Gorelik E, et al. Role of NK cells in the control of metastatic spread and growth of tumor cells in mice. *Int J Cancer.* 1982 Jul 15;30(1):107-112.

58. Tartter PI, et al. The prognostic significance of natural killer cytotoxicity in patients with colorectal cancer. *Arch Surg.* 1987 Nov;122(11):1264-1268.

59. Kondo E, et al. Preoperative natural killer cell activity as a prognostic factor for distant metastasis following surgery for colon cancer. *Dig Surg.* 2003;20(5):445-451.

60. Li Xueru, et al. Clinical Experiment on Lycium. *Bulletin on Achievements in Scientific and Technological Research,* Serial 84, No. 4, 1988.

61. Wu SJ, et al. Antioxidant activities of some common ingredients of traditional Chinese medicine, Angelica sinensis, Lycium barbarum and Poria cocos. *Phytother Res.* 2004 Dec;18(12):1008-1012.

# Chapter 10
## Hormones and Vibrant Health

## Understanding Hormone Health

Hormones are critical to maintaining vibrant health, regulating numerous activities in the body. The pituitary gland sends hormone messages to your other glands and other areas of the body to signal them into action. Hormones help control blood pressure, fight against eye degeneration, and work to overcome or reduce various cancers.

Estrogen and progesterone need to be balanced in order to work together as counterparts. Together, they are responsible for balance in blood clotting and the storage or use of fat in the body. But the estrogen and progesterone balance can be upset, disrupting a positive attitude and normal feelings of well-being. Xenoestrogens (literally "foreign" estrogens) are chemically manufactured hormones that are used in pesticides and animal growth hormones. They are increasingly found in food and cause an overbalance of estrogen in the body with many adverse effects.

Progesterone and testosterone increase physical desire. Testosterone helps build muscle and decrease fat, while both estrogen and testosterone convert the bad cholesterol (LDL) to good cholesterol (HDL). Hormones help with good brain function in maintaining optimal body functions, and most important, they work to help keep us young.

### Hormonal Testing

Before starting any type of natural progesterone, pregnenolone, or DHEA program that targets the hormone system of the body, it is important to have your hormone levels tested by requesting a blood hormone panel taken in your doctor's office, hospital, clinic, or qualified laboratory. After the analysis is evaluated by your doctor or health care professional, you may ask for his or her help in determining the best program for you.

In order to have the most accurate type of testing, you have to be prepared to spend some money, and perhaps more than you were planning to spend; however, because of the complexity of hormone therapy, any deficiencies must be correctly identified before supplementation is begun.

A good hormone panel will cost between $300 and $400, as costs will vary from clinic to clinic. It is also much better to ask for a specialist, not just a general practitioner, who might tell you that your hormones are just fine for your age. Unfortunately, most health care practitioners know very little about hormone analysis, ranges, subsequent causes and effects, and solutions. To be able to determine your needs, you should have your hormone panel taken every week for four weeks to cover the complete cycle, thereby giving you the best results. Otherwise, you may have a single panel taken at the time when your estrogen is high and be told all is well, even when you may think and feel differently.

Other types of analyses are available that determine hormone levels such as saliva testing or hair analysis, but they are very unreliable and are not recommended. Naturopath D. Gary Young has found in 25 years of research that hormones and enzymes are two of the most critical needs of the human body and are among the least understood. Bringing balance takes a lot more than just taking natural progesterone.

The body ages faster when we do not eat live foods that are rich in natural enzymes and hormones. Our world today is a world of processed and prepackaged foods treated with all kinds of chemicals, sugars, and salt. Fruits and vegetables are sprayed with pesticides, insecticides, herbicides, and other growth and beautifying chemicals for our consumption. Animals are given synthetic growth hormones, which displace women's natural hormones. Our air is polluted and the water we drink is often contaminated or treated with chemicals for purification. Then we wonder why hormones start to decline at age 25, and strange, unexpected maladies start to show up in children and young adults. More men and women are becoming victims of sterility as young as 20 years of age. In addition, never in history have we seen young women between the ages of 25 and 30 experiencing bone density loss, which leads them into osteoporosis.

Why is this happening? Why are there more cancers, more heart disease, more diabetes, more respiratory failure, more viruses and mutations of bacteria, and more fungus? Why is there such increased disease and body dysfunction, not only in older people but in children and young adults as well? Why are so many babies being born with birth defects and diseases that seem unexplainable?

Lack of proper nutrients, hormone imbalance, and insufficient enzymes are key factors in the cause of overall diminishing health to a state of disease and malfunction of the body. Balancing hormones is one of the secrets to maintaining good health, and without proper enzymes, no hormone therapy program will be as effective as it could be for either women or men.

Natural estrogens are called steroid hormones and passively enter into the cells, where they bind to and activate the estrogen receptors. It is important to understand that there are different types of estrogens and three major hormones that the body naturally produces in women called oestrogens: estrone (E1), which is produced during menopause; estradiol (E2), which is predominant in nonpregnant females; and estriol (E3), which is predominant in pregnancy. All three are produced from androgens through enzyme activity, which produces testosterone. The conversion of testosterone to estradial and androstenedione to estrone is performed by the enzyme aromatase.

More than 50 percent of the body's estrogen is in the form of estrone, which is manufactured and stored as estrone sulphate in the fat cells and ovaries so that the body can call for it when needed, so it can be converted as the body dictates. However, estrone sulphate is a chemical compound that attracts breast cancer cells when too much is produced.

Oncologists for years have warned about estrogen therapy and its sensitivity to causing cancer, for which reason they tell women to stay away from products containing estrogen or products that stimulate estrogen production. Unfortunately, doctors do not tell you that there are two forms of estrone, which are good or bad, depending on the biological activity, or potency, of the estrogen. Estrogens are important in many cellular activities such as growth, strength, mental clarity, etc., in various target cells. This is normal and beneficial but too much estrogenic stimulation can have a negative effect. Therefore, proper metabolism and excretion of estrogens is crucial.

Estradiol converts to either 2-hydroxyestrone, a good estrone metabolite that prevents cancer,[1] or 16-alpha-hydroxyestrone that feeds cancer cells. If these estrogens are metabolized into the 2-hydroxylated estrone and estradiol, they lose much of their estrogenic activity

and cell proliferation and are termed "good" estrogen metabolites. Studies show that when the production of 2-hydroxyestrone increases, the body resists cancer; and when 2-hydroxyestrone decreases, cancer risk increases.[1] Research indicates that women who metabolize more estrogens down the C-16 pathway, as opposed to the C-2 pathway, have elevated breast cancer risk.[2]

. . . . . . . . . . . . . . . . . . . . . . . . . . . . . . . . . . . . .

The 16-alpha-hydroxyestrone, or bad estrone, is deemed carcinogenic and increases the risk with estrogen-sensitive cancers. All inorganic estrogen compounds will manufacture 16-alpha-hydroxyestrone.

Natural, organic compounds will metabolize to 2-hydroxyestrone, or good anticancer estrone, unless the liver is toxic and/or enzyme deficient.

. . . . . . . . . . . . . . . . . . . . . . . . . . . . . . . . . . . . .

Follow four simple rules to maintain good hormone production:

1. Keep the liver clean.

2. Consume enzyme-rich foods or add good quality, active, complex enzymes such as Essentialzyme and Essentialzymes-4 to give your digestive system a natural boost. Children who start early by consuming the supplement MightyZyme will have a head start on maintaining hormone balance and healthy body function as they grow older.

3. Eat a fiber-rich diet supplemented with ICP and JuvaPower.

4. Avoid processed foods, foods grown with chemicals, body and hair care products formulated with damaging chemicals, and the use of synthetic chemicals in all forms.

### Declining Hormones Signal Old Age

As we age, hormone imbalances can contribute to accelerated aging and heightened risk of cancer and other chronic diseases. Hormone replacement therapy using natural hormones (not synthetic compounds or look-alikes) in a cream application for transdermal absorption is one of the most common ways to address hormone imbalances. Natural hormone therapy is often very beneficial for combating a number of health problems such as sleep disturbance, depression, anxiety, obesity, as well as reducing the risk of cancer and helping to fight chronic diseases such as osteoporosis.

In the specific case of progesterone, Harvard University researcher, John R. Lee, MD, found that natural progesterone is very well absorbed through the skin, 20 to 40 times more efficiently than if taken by mouth.[3] Topical hormone creams with essential oils have a greater ability to penetrate through the skin and enter into the blood much more quickly than other hormone creams that do not have essential oils.

Hormones such as DHEA, melatonin, testosterone, and progesterone decrease with age. Estrogen (estradiol) also drops with age, although not as quickly as progesterone; but as progesterone drops, an estrogen-dominant condition is created that is common in women over 40.

## Melatonin: The Hormone of Darkness

Melatonin is a natural hormone that regulates sleep. During daylight, the pineal gland in the brain produces an important neurotransmitter called serotonin. A neurotransmitter is a chemical that relays messages between nerve cells.

At night, however, the pineal gland stops producing serotonin and instead makes melatonin, which when released causes drowsiness and lowers body temperature, inducing sleep. Your body produces melatonin when it's dark. The darker your sleeping environment, the more melatonin your body will produce. If you happen to sleep with a night light on, your body will produce less melatonin, which might account for why some people have difficulty falling asleep.

Children sleep far better in a completely dark room than with a light on somewhere to help them find the bathroom in the middle of the night or to ease their fears about the dark or being alone. With good melatonin production, children and adults alike will awake in the morning refreshed and positive for a new day.

At one time it was thought that melatonin levels declined with age; however, newer evidence suggests that melatonin levels do not decline with age after all. A decline of melatonin is most likely caused by foods devoid of sufficient nutrients and enzymes. Low melatonin levels seem to be directly linked to lowered immunity, resulting in disturbed sleep cycles, anxiousness, heightened cancer risk, etc. Some evidence suggests that individuals with cluster headaches have lower-than-average levels of the hormone melatonin.

Sufficient melatonin helps to reduce irritable bowel syndrome, anxiety, elevated blood pressure at night, and cluster headaches. Melatonin supplements appear to be helpful for people whose natural sleep cycle has been disturbed, such as travelers suffering from jet lag.

It has been suggested that melatonin might work through the nervous system to help in the digestive tract. A preliminary, double-blind study suggests that melatonin may decrease nocturnal seizure frequency for children with epilepsy, perhaps by improving sleep and reducing the side effects of medication.[4] One double-blind study suggests that topical application of melatonin may increase hair growth in women with thinning hair, for undiscovered reasons.[5] Additional research helps us to further understand the influence of melatonin on hair physiology.[6,7] Melatonin might also be helpful to individuals trying to quit using sleeping pills.

Melatonin has been used with conventional cancer therapy in more than a dozen clinical studies. Preliminary results have been surprisingly good. A double-blind study was conducted on 30 people with advanced brain tumors who had received standard radiation treatment. It was suggested that melatonin might prolong life and also improve the quality of life. These 30 participants were divided into two groups. One group received 20 mg daily of melatonin, and the other did not. After one year, 6 of 14 individuals in the melatonin group were still alive, but just 1 of 16 from the control group was alive.[8] The melatonin group also had fewer side effects from the radiation treatment—a notable improvement in their quality of life.[9]

Melatonin also works as a very powerful antioxidant at night while we are sleeping. It crosses through cell membranes and the blood brain barrier, working as a free radical scavenger. Interestingly enough, melatonin is sometimes referred to as a "suicidal antioxidant" because of its tremendous free-radical absorbent capacity. When melatonin reacts with free radicals, it oxidizes and cannot convert back to its former state because it forms several stable end products and can no longer function as an antioxidant.

Melatonin has shown remarkable benefits in preventing gallstones by converting cholesterol to bile and increasing the production of aromatase or increasing the mobility of stones and moving them out of the gallbladder. Aromatase is an enzyme found in the adrenal glands, brain, and many other tissues of the body. Its main function is to convert androstenedione to estrone and testosterone to estradiol, which is an important part of sexual development.

Recent research demonstrates the ability of melatonin to prevent DNA damage by some carcinogens and stops the mechanism by which cancer begins.[10] Melatonin appears to work by increasing levels of the body's own tumor-fighting proteins known as cytokines.

Recent research shows that melatonin enhances the effectiveness of standard therapy for breast cancer, prostate cancers, and Glioblastoma multiforme (GBM), which is the most common and aggressive type of primary brain tumor in humans.[11] Although it is the most prevalent, GBMs occur in only 2–3 cases per 100,000 people in Europe and North America. Glioblastomas are a common type of brain tumor of the canine, and research is ongoing to use this as a model for developing treatments in humans. Melatonin definitely shows possible benefits not only for humans but for animals as well in the fight against this terrible affliction.

Melatonin is helpful in regulating metabolism and increasing thermogenesis, as well as in increasing energy during the wake cycle, which could explain the weight loss in several case studies. Research has greatly increased since 2008 and will continue to help discover more benefits for the human body with this special hormone.

**DHEA: Vibrant Health**

The most common hormone in the body is 5-Dehydroepiandrosterone (5-DHEA). It is the most abundant circulating natural steroid hormone that is produced in the body by both men and women because it is the precursor to over 50 other hormones in the body. It is manufactured by enzymes from cholesterol and secreted by the adrenal glands, the gonads, adipose tissue, and the brain.

DHEA is converted by enzymes to pregnenolone and then to 170-Hydroxypregnenolone that helps regulate steroid hormones and directs them down their final metabolic pathway for further conversion to proper male and female hormones for normal body function.

DHEA has a broad range of biological effects in humans and other mammals. It acts on the androgen receptor both directly and through its metabolites, which include androstenediol and androstenedione, which further convert to the production of the male sex hormone androgen, which converts to testosterone and the female estrogens to estrone and estradiol.

Although DHEA is manufactured naturally in the body, it is also produced as a supplement, which can be made in a laboratory from a substance called diosgenin, found in soybeans and wild yam. Wild yam cream and supplements are a natural source of DHEA, but the body cannot convert wild yam to DHEA on its own. The conversion must be done in a laboratory.

Dehydroepiandrosterone sulfate (DHEAS) is the sulfate version of DHEA, which is primarily converted in the adrenals, liver, and small intestine. In the blood, most DHEA is found as DHEAS, with levels that are about 300 times higher than those of free DHEA. Orally ingested DHEA is converted to its sulfate when passing through intestines and liver. DHEA levels naturally reach their peak in the early morning hours, but DHEAS levels show no variation throughout the day. DHEAS may be viewed as a storage reservoir for the body to produce sex hormones on demand when needed to maintain normal body functions.

A decline in DHEA is directly correlated with lower energy and obesity. The greater the production and proper balance with DHEA, the greater sex life, energy, weight balance, normal sleep patterns, and a feeling of well-being. DHEA also strengthens the neurons in the brain for better memory retention with sharp, clear thinking.

Another benefit of DHEA is that it keeps cortisol levels in balance, which helps the immune system operate at an optimal level. This in turn helps to reduce the risk of Alzheimer's disease and premature aging, which are always associated with bone density loss.

DHEA produces hormones responsible for burning fat and converting fat to muscle. Instead of losing weight because of muscle breakdown and fluid loss, it actually helps build lean muscle tissue. It appears that DHEA blocks G6PD (glucose-6-phosphate-dehydrogenase), the major enzyme that produces fat tissue and cancer cells. G6PD redirects excess glucose from anabolic (growth) fat production into catabolic (breakdown) energy metabolism. This would seem to make man dependent upon diet for weight control.

DHEA seems to have many benefits to the well-being of the mind and body. It seems to have a positive effect on the mind, helping memory, decreasing mood swings, and protecting against degenerative disease such as Alzheimer's, various cancers, immune dysfunction, heart disease, blood platelet abnormality, weight gain, and the list goes on and on. This is a hormone that is well worth studying, as its value to the human body seems immense. There is much yet for research to discover and science to substantiate.

## The following shows the chain of conversion from cholesterol to estrogen.

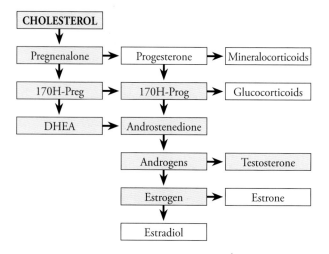

## Cortisol: The Death Hormone

Cortisol helps you handle ongoing and difficult stress situations. When stress levels continue, cortisol levels go up, which can lead to adrenal fatigue and burnout. Cortisol is important for normal function of the brain, immune system, muscle tone and strength, blood circulation, and sugar levels.

Although cortisol is a valuable hormone, when it is too high or too low, its being out of balance can be dangerous and even fatal. Cortisol is known not only as the death hormone but also as the stress hormone and the fight-or-flight hormone. Cortisol seems to increase with age, contributing to a number of problems such as high blood pressure, obesity, and blood sugar imbalances. Lowering cortisol levels not only decreases immunity but increases insulin sensitivity and enhances fat metabolism.

Cortisol is manufactured in the adrenal glands and secreted through the adrenal cortex when the body reacts to stress, triggering an immunological response to heighten the survival instincts. It gives us that burst of energy in the morning when we need to "jump start" the heart after a night of sleep-inducing melatonin. Cortisol also reduces sensitivity to pain, suppresses the immune system by stopping overproduction of white blood cells, aids in the breakdown of fat and protein to help metabolize and convert glucose in the liver to increase blood sugar, and stops the release of inflammatory substances in the body.

However, low cortisol levels can be risky and, therefore, need to be understood. Adrenal exhaustion can lead to dangerously low levels of cortisol that could bring on cardiac arrest or failure to wake up the heart in the morning. Keeping cortisol levels in balance is critical to life. High cortisol can lead to rapid weight gain and obesity. Low cortisol can cause chronic fatigue and low sex drive and lead to depression. It can also decrease thyroid function, which results in mental fatigue, digestive problems, lowered immune resistance, increased blood pressure, and muscle wasting. Cortisol increases because of stress and too much acid in the body. Coffee and other caffeine-containing drinks stimulate the production of cortisol.

A major key to healthy levels of cortisol is to keep the hormone system balanced. Higher levels of DHEA will lower cortisol levels as well as many other aspects of body functions. However, the foundation for a healthy body and balanced hormones is to eat live, unprocessed, nutritious foods; get enough rest and exercise; and maintain a balanced lifestyle that supports the needs of work, home, and family.

If your cortisol is too high or you are just concerned about having good balance, then the product CortiStop would be a supplement to add to your daily regimen.

# Dangers of Synthetic Hormones

Recent research has discredited many of the supposed benefits of synthetic hormones such as those made with horse urine, estrogens, medroxy-progesterone acetate, and other synthetic progestins. These patented synthetic hormones are very different biochemically from the natural hormones found in plants and the human body, and their effects can be hazardous to health. Long-term use of these synthetic hormones has been linked with dramatically higher risks of heart disease, stroke, ovarian cancer, breast cancer, and osteoporosis.

Natural hormones cannot be patented, which makes them not very popular with companies making synthetic products. Natural hormones found in the human body are some of the safest natural compounds used to prevent heart disease and cancer. It is interesting that when a woman reaches the later stage of pregnancy, her levels of progesterone rise to over 300 times that of normal, and both mother and child thrive. Obviously, the body knows what it needs, and the body's production of natural progesterone is totally safe and healthy. When the body receives "the right tools," or a natural substance, it usually knows what to do.

### Osteoporosis and Prostate Cancer

Natural progesterone has been used to successfully treat osteoporosis, heart disease, and breast cancer in women. Research by John R. Lee, MD, has shown that progesterone can be used to effectively treat prostate cancer and Benign Prostate Hyperplasia (BPH) in men.[12]

### Lowering Cancer Risk Naturally

As women grow older and approach menopause, between ages 40 and 50, they become increasingly susceptible to estrogen dominance, due to an increased frequency of ovulation and dramatically lowered production of progesterone. This shortage of progesterone can lead to osteoporosis, mood swings, depression, weight gain, and increased risk of breast, endometrial, cervical, and uterine cancers.

Premenopausal women can also suffer from an estrogen deficiency, which can markedly increase their risk of heart disease, which is one reason why heart disease in women reaches the equivalent of men after age 40. A simultaneous estrogen and progesterone deficiency is one of the most common and insidious conditions afflicting women over age 40 and can result in significant detrimental effects on both physical and mental health.

Transdermal hormone creams have revolutionized the way women can manage hormone control. Because natural progesterone, pregnenolone, and DHEA are readily absorbed through the skin and into the tissues, they are rapidly becoming the standard for convenient and economical hormone replacement therapy in the United States. Many transdermal hormone creams are available to balance progesterone, estrogen, and DHEA deficiencies in women. Women who are primarily progesterone deficient and estrogen dominant need progesterone support, and women who are deficient in both estrogen and progesterone need both pregnenolone and progesterone hormones. The body will convert pregnenolone into the amount of estrogen the body needs.

### Andropause: Menopause in Men

A cream containing DHEA and pregnenolone is a first line of defense for men with declining testosterone and DHEA. Men over 40 often begin to see various symptoms manifest that could indicate the beginning of a possible hormone imbalance. Such symptoms listed would suggest further investigation to perhaps start on a preventative program before conditions worsen.

- Loss of sexual desire
- Less strength and shrinking muscles
- Reduced energy
- Depression
- Increased anxiety
- Thinning hair
- Wrinkles and aging
- Prostate Problems: restricted urine flow, declining sexual performance, etc.

### Essential Oils: Enhanced Hormone Penetration of the Skin

A number of clinical studies have shown that essential oils greatly enhance the ability of hormones and other medical products to penetrate the skin and enter the blood stream. Studies conducted at Pisa University in 2002 found that essential oils such as cajuput, cardamom, melissa, myrtle, niaouli, and orange, containing essential oil chemical constituents such as 1,8-cineole, alpha-pinene, alpha-terpineol, and d-limonene, boosted estradiol hormone penetration through the skin and into the blood and body tissues.[13] A study at the China Pharmaceutical University in Nanjing similarly found a dramatic increase in drug absorption using formulations with eucalyptus and peppermint essential oils.[14]

# Products for Hormone Support

## CortiStop®

This capsule contains natural progesterone and hormone precursors, which help to support the female glandular system and balance cortisol production in the body.

**Ingredients:** Proprietary CortiStop Blend: [pregnenolone, L-a-phosphatidylserine, L-a-phosphatidylcholine black cohosh root extract], DHEA (derived from wild yam root), rice flour, silica, gelatin

**Essential Oils:** Clary Sage, Canadian Fleabane, Fennel, Frankincense, Peppermint

**Directions:** Take 2 capsules in the morning before breakfast, and if desired, take another 2 capsules before going to bed. Take daily for 8 weeks and then rest the body for 2-4 weeks before starting again.

## EndoGize™

This daily supplement was formulated to support and maintain a healthy and balanced endocrine system. Women can benefit greatly with strong support to the hormone activity of the body.

**Ingredients:** vitamin B6 (as pyridoxine HCl); zinc (as z. aspartate), Proprietary EndoGize Blend: [ashwagandha root powder, muira puama bark, L-arginine, epimedium aerial parts, tribulus terrestris fruit extract, phosphatidylcholine, lecithin (soy), black pepper fruit extract, glucoamylase, protease (acid stable), eurycoma longifolia root extract, amylase, cellulase], DHEA, rice flour, gelatin

**Essential Oils:** Ginger, Myrrh, Cassia, Clary Sage, Canadian Fleabane

**Directions:** Take 1 capsule 2 times daily for 4 weeks, rest for 2 weeks, and then start again.

**Allergen Warning:** contains soy

Hormones and Vibrant Health | **Chapter 10**

## FemiGen™

A good product to support a woman's reproductive system is always helpful in maintaining balance as a woman transitions into menopause.

**Ingredients:** magnesium; Proprietary FemiGen Blend [damiana leaf, epimedium aerial plant, wild yam root, dong quai root, muira puama root, ginseng root, licorice root extract, black cohosh root, L-carnitine, dimethylglycine HCl, cramp bark, squaw vine aerial parts, L-phenylalanine, L-cystine, L-cysteine HCl], gelatin

**Essential Oils:** Fennel, Clary Sage, Sage, Ylang Ylang

**Directions:** Take 2 capsules with breakfast and 2 capsules with midday meal.

## ImmuPro™

This tasty tablet boosts melatonin and T-lymphocyte immune cells. It is designed for people who have difficulty sleeping, shortened sleep cycles, low immunity, or high risk of cancer. It is a powerful antioxidant that provides energy and immune support. It is also helpful for children who are restless at night and have trouble getting to sleep. Chewing one-half of a tablet is often sufficient for children.

**Ingredients:** calcium (as c. carbonate), zinc (as z. citrate), selenium (as selenomethionine), copper (as c. chelate), Proprietary ImmuPro Blend: [strawberry fruit powder, fructose, raspberry juice concentrate, Ningxia wolfberry fruit polysaccharides, reishi mycelia, maitake mycelia, arabinogalactin extract, agaricus blazei mycelis], melatonin, virgin coconut oil, acacia stem/branch, melatonin, silica

**Essential Oil:** Orange

**Directions:** Chew 1 tablet before bed. If under stress, chew 1 tablet 2-4 times daily.

## PD 80/20™

Easy to take in a capsule, this product is designed to give natural, over-all hormone support.

**Ingredients:** pregnenolone, DHEA, rice flour, gelatin

**Directions:** Take 1 capsule daily.

## Prenolone® + Body Cream

This triple hormone cream contains pure pregnenolone derived from soy and DHEA derived from wild yam. Pregnenolone is the precursor hormone from which the body creates all other sex and adrenal hormones, including progesterone, estradiol, estrone, estriol, testosterone, DHEA, and aldosterone. Soy-derived progesterone works the same way as progesterone naturally produced in the human body and is easily absorbed and used by the body.

This cream is a broad-spectrum hormone supplement that helps boost insufficient levels of estrogen and progesterone in both men and women. It is formulated to help with symptoms of estrogen dominance, which include osteoporosis, depression, bloating, mood swings, weight gain, PMS, hot flashes, menstrual irregularity, cramps, increased risk of breast and endometrial cancer, and heart disease.

Studies have shown that topical application of progesterone creams have far better results than hormones taken orally.[3] Essential oils also increase the absorption of hormones through the skin into the blood stream. John Lee, MD, discusses in detail the benefits of topically applied progesterone in his book *What Your Doctor May Not Tell You About Menopause*. According to Dr. Lee, progesterone can actually reverse bone loss in older women as well as reduce the need for hormone replacement in women lacking ovaries or not ovulating.[12]

**Ingredients:** water, dimethyl sulfone (MSM), caprylic/capric triglyceride, sorbitol, lecithin, pregnenolone, wolfberry seed oil, shea butter, glyceryl stearate, Roman chamomile flower extract, rosebud flower extract, calendula flower extract, St. John's wort extract, gingko biloba leaf extract, grape seed extract, aloe vera leaf gel, green tea leaf extract, stearic acid, sodium PCA, algae extract, DHEA, wild yam root extract, black cohosh root, blue cohosh root, eleuthero root extract, retinyl palmitate (vitamin A), kelp extract, flax seed oil, trace mineral complex, tocopherol acetate (vitamin E), hydrolyzed wheat protein, tocopherol linoleate (vitamin E), wheat germ oil, allantoin, asorbic acid (vitamin C), locust bean gum

**Essential Oils:** Ylang Ylang, Clary Sage, Geranium, Fennel, Sage, Blue Yarrow, Bergamot

**Directions:** Begin using one day after menstrual cycle ends or as desired. Massage 1/4-1/2 teaspoon thoroughly into soft tissue areas of the body such as arms, thighs, abdomen, neck, etc., until absorbed. Rotate sites of application daily. Individual needs may vary. Apply for three weeks, rest for one week, and then start again.

**Allergen Warning:** contains wheat

Seventh Edition | **Essential Oils Desk Reference** | 213

## Progessence® Plus

With this first-ever pure progesterone serum to enter the market, many women are reporting excellent results in balancing and normalizing hormone levels. As women age, hormone levels drop, causing all kinds of maladies such as sleep and mood disorders and eventually the possibility of more critical ailments. This product was formulated by Dan Purser, MD, and D. Gary Young, ND, to balance and enhance the natural effects of progesterone. Pure, USP-grade, super-micronized progesterone from wild yam is infused into pure, therapeutic-grade essential oils, creating a smooth, revitalizing serum that is easily absorbed into the skin. Another great benefit is that there is no need to change application sites like progesterone creams. The serum is a clear, smooth liquid that easily penetrates the skin. It does not have a cream base.

**Ingredients:** coconut oil, tocopherol, wild yam extract

**Essential Oils:** Copaiba, Sacred Frankincense, Cedarwood, Bergamot (furocoumarin-free), Peppermint, Rosewood, Clove

**Directions:** Apply to skin during morning or evening routine. Do not exceed 2 applications per day.

## Prostate Health™

Contains high-powered herbal extracts such as saw palmetto that improve prostate function. It slows the body's production of DHT, a hormone that creates abnormal cell proliferation in the prostate. BPH (benign prostate hyperplasia), common in men over age 40, can eventually lead to prostate cancer, one of the most common forms of cancer in the United States. BPH symptoms include incontinence, restricted urine flow, and impotence.

**Ingredients:** saw palmetto, pumpkin seed oil
**Essential Oils:** Geranium, Fennel, Lavender, Myrtle, Peppermint
**Directions:** Take 1 softgel capsule 2 times daily.

## Protec™

Protec is a balancing blend of natural ingredients that supports health and hygiene for men and women. It is designed to be used in a night-long retention enema or douche.

**Ingredients:** grape seed oil, wheat germ oil, sweet almond oil, olive fruit oil
**Essential Oils:** Frankincense, Myrrh, Sage, Cumin
**Directions:** Insert ½-1 fl. oz. into the rectum to support prostate; or for women, use an implant vaginally for desired benefits.

## Regenolone Moisturizing Cream™

This muscle and joint pain cream is designed for people who suffer severe pain from inflammation or stiffness from arthritis, rheumatism, or other muscle and joint conditions. Formulated with pregnenolone, wolfberry seed oil, progesterone, MSM, plant and herb extracts, and essential oils, this product provides unmatched relief from all types of arthritic, muscle, and skeletal pain.

**Ingredients:** water, dimethyl sulfone (MSM), fractionated coconut/palm oil, sorbitol, pregnenolone, lecithin, shea butter, glyceryl stearate, aloe vera leaf, sodium PCA, stearic acid, calendula flower extract, Roman chamomile flower extract, rosebud flower extract, green tea leaf extract, St. John's wort extract, ginkgo biloba extract, grape seed extract, algae extract, tocopheryl acetate and linoleate (vitamin E), hydrolyzed wheat protein, locust bean gum, trace minerals, flaxseed oil, wheat germ oil, allantoin, wild yam root extract, eleuthero root extract, kelp extract, retinyl palmitate (vitamin A), black cohosh root extract, blue cohosh extract, ascorbic acid (vitamin C)

**Essential Oils:** Wintergreen, Peppermint, Douglas Fir, Oregano

**Directions:** Apply 1/8-1/4 teaspoon on location 3 times a day as needed to combat pain associated with arthritis, sciatica, back pain, and carpal tunnel syndrome. Do not exceed 5 applications per day.

**Allergen Warning:** contains wheat product

# Essential Oil Hormone Support

Many women ages 40-plus have found that essential oils effectively combat PMS and menopause problems. Oils with estrogen-like activity include Fennel, Anise, Clary Sage, and Sage. Fennel, Anise, and Clary Sage may be combined in equal proportions in a double 00 size capsule and ingested. Take 2 to 8 capsules daily to raise estrogen levels according to need.

It is recommended that you find an endocrinologist who can monitor your estrogen levels through blood testing every 30 days until you have reached optimal levels. Research conducted at the Young Life Research Clinic in Springville, Utah, showed that ingestion of these oils, up to 8 capsules per day, did not cause any side effects or toxicity in the human body.

# Essential Oil Blends

**Dragon Time™** contains natural phytoestrogens, which help to balance emotions, especially during the monthly cycle. It may be used by both young and mature women, depending on desire and need.

**Essential Oils:** Fennel, Clary Sage, Marjoram, Lavender, Yarrow, Jasmine

**Directions:** Inhale directly, put a drop on the skin underneath the nose, or apply topically with V-6 Vegetable Oil Complex.

**Joy™ and Transformation™** are two essential oil blends that are both uplifting and calming at the same time. They may help to replace negative thoughts with positive and motivating thoughts that may help change your general attitude, emotional well-being, and behavior.

**Essential Oils in Joy:** Bergamot (furocoumarin-free), Geranium, Lemon, Coriander, Tangerine, Jasmine, Roman Chamomile, Palmarosa, Rose

**Essential Oils in Transformation:** Lemon, Peppermint, Royal Hawaiian Sandalwood, Clary Sage, Sacred Frankincense, Idaho Blue Spruce, Cardamom, Ocotea, Palo Santo

**Directions:** Diffuse, inhale directly, wear topically as a perfume, or combine with V-6 Vegetable Oil Complex for a relaxing massage.

**Lady Sclareol™** helps balance emotions, promotes mental clarity, and supports the endocrine system while menstruating.

**Essential Oils:** Geranium, Coriander, Vetiver, Orange, Clary Sage, Bergamot (furocoumarin-free), Ylang Ylang, Royal Hawaiian Sandalwood, Spanish Sage, Jasmine, Idaho Blue Spruce, Spearmint, Hinoki

**Directions:** Diffuse, inhale directly from the bottle, put a drop on the skin underneath the nose, or apply topically with V-6 Vegetable Oil Complex directly on hips and navel areas.

**Mister™** is an essential oil blend for men that helps balance emotions and promotes mental stability during times of stress for men of all ages.

**Essential Oils:** Sage, Fennel, Lavender, Myrtle, Peppermint, Blue Yarrow

**Directions:** This essential oil blend supports the male reproductive system. It may be taken as a dietary supplement: 3-10 drops under tongue 2-3 times daily or 10-20 drops in water or in a capsule 2 times daily. Use for 7 days and then rest the body for 4 days. Massage on the Vita Flex points between scrotum and rectum.

**SclarEssence™** contains properties that may support the overall emotional health of women, bringing about a peaceful attitude with daily activities and accomplishments.

**Essential Oils:** Clary Sage, Peppermint, Spanish Sage, Fennel

**Directions:** Diffuse, apply topically with V-6 Vegetable Oil Complex, put 2-3 drops in water and take as needed.

For more information on the many regenerative abilities of pregnenolone, please refer to the publication *Pregnenolone: A Radical New Approach to Health, Long Life, and Emotional Well-Being* by D. Gary Young, ND.

---

ENDNOTES

1. Bradlow HL, et al. 2-Hydroxyestrone: the 'good' estrogen. *J Endocrinol.* 1996 Sep;150 Suppl:S259-265.

2. Muti P, et al. Estrogen metabolism and risk of breast cancer: A prospective study of the 2:16α-hydroxyestrone ratio in premenopausal and postmenopausal women. *Epidemiology.* 2000 Nov;11(6):635-640.

3. Lee JR. Topical progesterone. *Menopause.* 2003 Jul;10(4):374-379.

4. Fauteck J, et al. Melatonin in epilepsy: first results of replacement therapy and first clinical results. *Biol Signals Recept.* 1999;8(1-2):105-110.

5. Fischer TW, et al. Melatonin increases anagen hair rate in women with androgenetic alopecia or diffuse alopecia: results of a pilot randomized controlled trial. *Br J Dermatol.* 2004 Feb;150(2):341-345.

6. Fischer TW, et al. Melatonin and the hair follicle. *J Pineal Res.* 2008 Jan;44(1):1-15.

7. Fischer TW. The influence of melatonin on hair physiology. *Hautarzt.* 2009 Dec;60(12):962-972. [German]

8. Lissoni P, et al. Increased survival time in brain glioblastomas by a radioneuroendocrine strategy with radiotherapy plus melatonin compared to radiotherapy alone. *Oncology.* 1996 Jan;53(1):43-46.

9. Lissoni P, et al. Neuroimmunomodulation in medical oncology: application of psychoneuroimmunology with subcutaneous low-dose IL-2 and the pineal hormone melatonin in patients with untreatable metastatic solid tumors. *Anticancer Res.* 2008 Mar;28(2B):1377-1381.

10. Jung B, Ahmad N. Melatonin in cancer management: progress and promise. *Cancer Res.* 2006 Oct;15;66(20):9789-9793.

11. Sánchez-Hidalgo M, et al. Melatonin, a natural programmed cell death inducer in cancer. *Curr Med Chem.* 2012 May; Epub.

12. Lee JR, Hopkins V. *What your doctor may not tell you about™ menopause: the breakthrough on natural hormone balance.* New York: Grand Central Publishing, 2004.

13. Monti D, et al. Effect of different terpene-containing essential oils on permeation of estradiol through hairless mouse skin. *Int J Pharm.* 2002 Apr;237(1-2):209-214.

14. Abdullah D, et al. Enhancing effect of essential oils on the penetration of 5-fluorouracil through rat skin. *Yao Xue Xue Bao.* 1996;31(3):214-221.

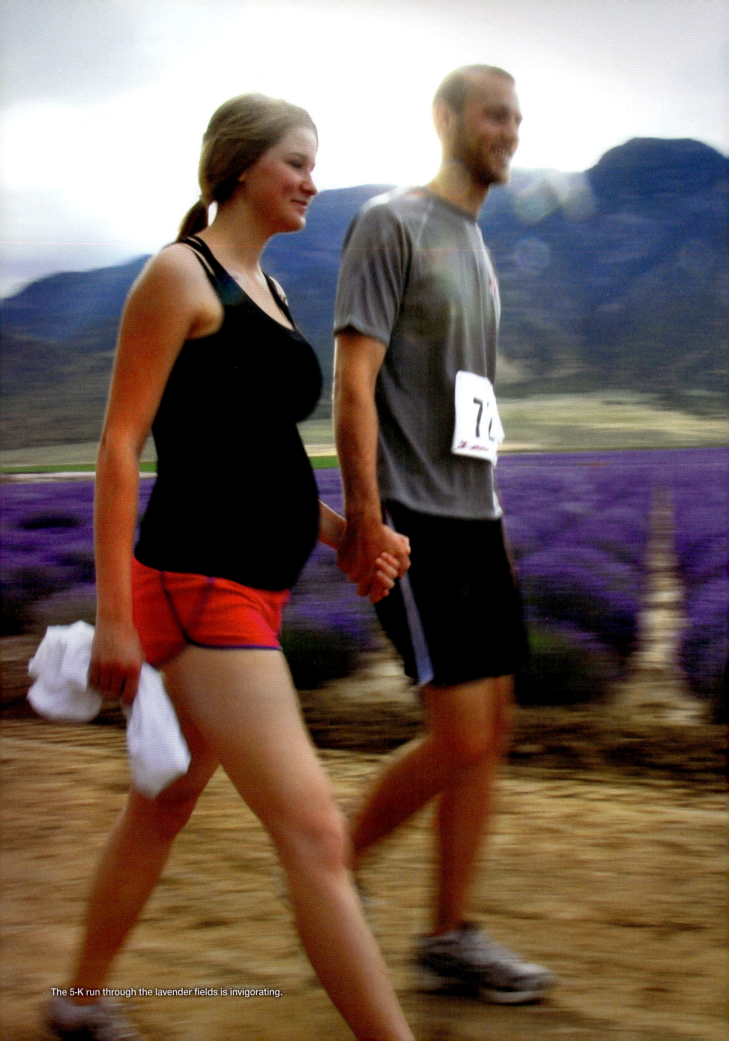

The 5-K run through the lavender fields is invigorating.

# Chapter 11
## Personal Care

## Safe, Natural Products

Being conscious of what you put in your body is very important. However, since your skin is your largest organ, being careful what you put on it is equally important. You will find our personal care products—including shower, moisturizing, soap, oral care, skin care, and deodorant products—free from chemicals, sulfates, toxins, synthetic colorants, dyes, artificial flavors, and preservatives. You can feel safe using these high quality, essential oil-infused products.

## Bath & Shower Gels

### Bath & Shower Gel Base

Bath & Shower Gel Base is the perfect way to create a customized aromatherapy bath. Add a few drops of a favorite essential oil single or blend for a fragrant and luxurious experience. Bath & Shower Gel Base contains only natural botanical ingredients that are perfect for cleansing the pores.

**Ingredients:** deionized water, decyl glucoside, coco betaine, lauryl glucoside, coco-glucoside, glyceryl oleate, citric acid, glycerin, levulinic acid, p-Anisic acid, xanthan gum, inulin, sodium phytate

**Directions:** Add 5-15 drops of one or more essential oils to 8 ounces of gel base. Mix well. Apply liberally to the body during bath or shower.

### Dragon Time™ Bath & Shower Gel

Dragon Time Bath & Shower Gel combines the soothing properties of essential oils with naturally moisturizing botanicals for a luxurious gel that leaves you feeling clean, relaxed, and uplifted.

Particularly comforting for women during their monthly cycle, this shower gel offers support both physically and emotionally.

**Ingredients:** deionized water, decyl glucoside, coco betaine, lauryl glucoside, coco-glucoside, glyceryl oleate, citric acid, glycerin, levulinic acid, p-Anisic acid, xanthan gum, inulin, sodium phytate

**Essential Oils:** Tangerine, Geranium, Fennel, Lavender, Sage, Marjoram, Clary Sage, Coriander, Bergamot (Furocoumarin-free), Lemon, Ylang Ylang, Jasmine, Roman Chamomile, Palmarosa, Blue Tansy

### Evening Peace™ Bath & Shower Gel

Evening Peace Bath & Shower Gel refreshes the skin and calms the mind. Designed to relax tired, fatigued muscles and help soothe away stress and tension at the end of the day, this shower gel invokes feelings of serenity and relaxation while nourishing the skin naturally.

**Ingredients:** deionized water, decyl glucoside, coco betaine, lauryl glucoside, coco-glucoside, glyceryl oleate, citric acid, glycerin, levulinic acid, p-Anisic acid, xanthan gum, inulin, sodium phytate

**Essential Oils:** Ylang Ylang, Royal Hawaiian Sandalwood, Coriander, Bergamot (Furocoumarin-free), Blue Tansy, Geranium, Clary Sage, Lemon, Jasmine, Roman Chamomile, Palmarosa

### Lavender Bath & Shower Gel

Infused with pure Lavender oil, Lavender Bath & Shower Gel will cleanse and rejuvenate your skin while it soothes and relaxes your mind. It is free of chemicals and synthetic preservatives and contains plant-based ingredients like coconut oil and star anise.

**Ingredients:** water, sodium methyl cocoyl taurate, sodium lauroamphoacetate, lauramidopropyl betaine, sodium chloride, glycerin, levulinic acid, p-Anisic acid, hydroxypropyl methylcellulose, citric acid, potassium sorbate, sodium astrocaryum murmururate, sea salt, rosemary extract, phytic acid

**Essential Oils:** Lavender, Lemon, Myrrh, Davana

## Morning Start® Bath & Shower Gel

Morning Start Bath & Shower Gel is an invigorating gel full of naturally cleansing and moisturizing botanicals to jumpstart your day with vigor and energy.

Peppermint, Lemongrass, and Rosemary essential oils uplift and energize the body and mind, while Juniper purifies and cleanses the skin.

**Ingredients:** deionized water, decyl glucoside, coco betaine, lauryl glucoside, coco-glucoside, glyceryl oleate, citric acid, glycerin, levulinic acid, p-Anisic acid, xanthan gum, inulin, sodium phytate

**Essential Oils:** Lemongrass, Rosemary, Juniper, Peppermint

# Body Lotions

## Genesis™ Hand & Body Lotion

Genesis Hand & Body Lotion is an ultra-moisturizing cream containing sweet almond oil and other natural botanicals to soothe and nourish dry, dehydrated skin.

Geranium, Jasmine, and other pure essential oils are included for their therapeutic, skin care benefits.

**Ingredients:** water, dimethyl sulfone (MSM), glyceryl stearate, stearic acid, glycerin, grape seed extract, sodium hyaluronate, sorbitol, rose hip seed oil, shea butter, mango seed butter, wheat germ oil, kukui seed oil, lecithin, safflower seed oil, apricot kernel oil, sweet almond oil, vitamin E (tocopheryl acetate), vitamin A (retinyl palmitate), jojoba seed oil, calendula flower extract, chamomile extract, green tea leaf extract, St. John's Wort extract, algae extract, aloe vera gel, vitamin C (ascorbic acid), gingko biloba extract

**Essential Oils:** Palmarosa, Coriander, Bergamot (Furocoumarin-free), Geranium, Jasmine, Lemon, Ylang Ylang, Roman Chamomile

**Allergen Warning:** Contains wheat product.

## Sensation™ Bath & Shower Gel

Sensation Bath & Shower Gel combines an enchantingly fragrant mix of oils purportedly used by Cleopatra to enhance love and increase desire. Containing the finest natural ingredients, this shower gel nourishes and refreshes the skin.

**Ingredients:** deionized water, decyl glucoside, coco betaine, lauryl glucoside, coco-glucoside, glyceryl oleate, citric acid, glycerin, levulinic acid, p-Anisic acid, xanthan gum, inulin, sodium phytate

**Essential Oils:** Coriander, Ylang Ylang, Bergamot (Furocoumarin-free), Jasmine, Geranium

## Lavender Hand & Body Lotion

Infused with Lavender essential oil and other plant-based ingredients, Lavender Hand & Body Lotion moisturizes and protects skin from overexposure to the elements for long-lasting hydration. This formula is certified eco-friendly and all natural.

**Ingredients:** water, sandalwood extract, phellodendron amurense bark extract, barley extract, cetearyl alcohol, glycerin, glyceryl stearate, sodium stearoyl lactylate, levulinic acid, p-Anisic acid, laminaria digitata, algae, xanthan gum, hydrolyzed silk, sorbic acid, astrocaryum murumuru seed butter, wolfberry seed oil, olive fruit unsaponifiables, rosemary leaf extract, vitamin E (tocopherol), sodium phytate, beeswax, aloe vera leaf extract

**Essential Oils:** Lavender, Lemon, Myrrh, Davana

Personal Body Care | **Chapter 11**

## Sensation™ Hand & Body Lotion

Sensation Hand & Body Lotion is an ultra-moisturizing cream that contains several pure essential oils purportedly revered by Cleopatra for enhancing feelings of love and romance. Ylang Ylang encourages relaxation, Jasmine balances female energy, and Geranium nourishes and refreshes the skin. This lotion leaves the skin soft and moist while protecting it from harsh weather, chemicals, and dry air.

**Ingredients:** deionized water, dimethyl sulfone (MSM), glyceryl stearate, stearic acid, glycerine, grape seed extract, sodium hyaluronate, sorbitol, rose hip seed oil, shea butter, mango seed butter, wheat germ oil, kukui seed oil, safflower seed oil, apricot kernel oil, sweet almond oil, vitamin E (tocopheryl acetate), vitamin A (retinyl palmitate), jojoba seed oil, sesame seed oil, calendula extract, chamomile extract, green tea leaf extract, St. John's Wort extract, algae extract, aloe vera gel, vitamin C (ascorbic acid), gingko biloba leaf extract

**Essential Oils:** Ylang Ylang, Coriander, Bergamot (Furocoumarin-free), Jasmine, Geranium

## Essential Beauty™ Serum (Dry Skin)

Wonderful benefits are seen when essential oils are used on the skin. The fine lipid structure of essential oils enable them to penetrate deep into skin tissues, carrying many active ingredients that renew, balance, and build skin health. Essential Beauty Serum for dry skin contains essential oils like Blue Cypress and Lavender, known for their ability to restore the skin's natural moisture balance.

**Ingredients:** coconut oil, avocado oil, blue cypress wood oil, rosehip seed oil, jojoba oil, vitamin E (tocopheryl), wolfberry seed oil, lecithin

**Essential Oils:** Cedarwood, Lavender, Myrrh, Clove, Royal Hawaiian Sandalwood

**Directions:** Add 3-5 drops to daily moisturizer and apply gently over face and neck. For spot treatment, apply serum directly onto desired area and rub gently into skin.

# Deodorants

Most deodorants today are loaded with toxic chemicals ranging from aluminum to antifreeze. As the chemicals leach through the skin into the blood and tissues, they can create a toxic buildup in the body that can lead to cancer, liver damage, and neurological diseases.

## Perils of Aluminum

Glen Scott, MD, of Cincinnati, and Patricia Saunders, a government microbiologist, warned of aluminum neurotoxicity, causing the FDA to require aluminum-bearing antiperspirants to carry a renal dysfunction warning (June 9, 2003).

According to the *Antiperspirant Products Final Monograph*, the FDA is "concerned that people with renal dysfunction may not be aware that the daily use of antiperspirant products containing aluminum may put them at higher risk because of exposure to aluminum in the product." Young children are "at higher risk resulting from exposure to aluminum." Parents and others "must keep these products away from children and seek professional assistance if accidental ingestion occurs."

## Sources of Aluminum Exposure and Contamination

Many over-the-counter deodorants, antiperspirants, baby wipes, skin creams, suntan lotions, toothpastes, and buffered aspirin contain aluminum. Additionally, aluminum is found in some medical vaccinations, intravenous solutions, wound and antacid irrigations, ulcer treatments, blood oxygenation, bone or joint replacement treatments, and burn treatments. Foods containing aluminum include baking powder, cake mixes, frozen dough, pancake mixes, self-rising flour, grains, and processed cheese. Aluminum cans, aluminum foil, disposable turkey roasting pans, and other containers are also sources of aluminum contamination.

## Studies of Aluminum Toxicity
### University of Western Ontario

*"Regardless of the host, the route of administration, or the speciation, aluminum is a potent neurotoxicant."*

—MJ Strong, Department of Clinical Neurological Sciences, University of Western Ontario, Canada

Seventh Edition | **Essential Oils Desk Reference** | **219**

## University of Stirling

*"Aluminum is acutely toxic to fish in acid waters. The gill is the principal target organ and death is due to a combination of ionoregulatory, osmoregulatory, and respiratory dysfunction. The mechanism of epithelial cell death is proposed as a general mechanism of aluminum-induced accelerated cell death."*

—C Exley, University of Stirling, Scotland

## Biofactors

*"Experimental evidence is summarized to support the hypothesis that chronic exposure to low levels of aluminum may lead to neurological disorders."*

—JG Joshi, Aluminum, a neurotoxin which affects diverse metabolic reactions. *Biofactors* (1990 Jul)

## Thomas Jefferson University

*"This data defines a new model in which aluminum kills liver cells by mechanisms distinct from previously recognized pathways of lethal cell injury. It is hypothesized that aluminum binds to cytoskeletal proteins intimately associated with the plasma membrane. This interaction eventually disrupts the permeability barrier function of the cell membrane, an event that heralds the death of the hepatocyte."*

—JW Snyder, et al. Department of Pathology, Thomas Jefferson University, Philadelphia, Pennsylvania (*Arch Biochem Biophys* 1995)

## State University at Ghent, Belgium

*"Epidemiological studies from Norway and England suggest a relation between the frequency of Alzheimer's disease and the concentration of aluminum in the drinking water. Estimates, made in this study, show that the role of aluminum from toothpastes may be even more important than that from the drinking water. For that reason we determined in samples of toothpastes taken from the Benelux market which brands contained aluminum. This appeared to be the case for about 22% of the brands which according to the manufacturers cover about 60% of the market."*

—RM Verbeeck, Laboratory for Analytical Chemistry, State University, Ghent, Belgium (*Acta Stomatol Belg* 1990 Jun)

## University of Virginia

*"Attention was first drawn to the potential role of aluminum as a toxic metal over 50 years ago. . . . the accumulation of aluminum is associated with the development of toxic phenomena; dialysis encephalopathy, osteomalacic dialysis, osteodystrophy, and an anemia. Aluminum has also been implicated as a toxic agent in the etiology of Alzheimer's disease, Guamiam amyotrophic lateral sclerosis, and parkinsonism-dementia."*

— CD Hewitt, et al., University of Virginia

## AromaGuard® Meadow Mist Deodorant

AromaGuard Meadow Mist Deodorant is aluminum-free, petrochemical-free, and made from edible ingredients and pure, therapeutic-grade essential oils. This deodorant contains coconut oil, beeswax, vitamin E, and essential oils like Lemon and Lavender for their skin care benefits.

**Ingredients:** coconut oil, white beeswax, pure ester 34, pure ester 40, zinc oxide, vitamin E (tocopheryl acetate)

**Essential Oils:** Lemon, Geranium, Rosemary, Coriander, Lavender, Bergamot, Tea Tree, Melaleuca Quinquenervia (Niaouli), Ylang Ylang, Clove

## AromaGuard® Mountain Mint Deodorant

AromaGuard Mountain Mint Deodorant is aluminum-free, petrochemical-free, and made from edible ingredients and pure, therapeutic-grade essential oils. Containing the natural, skin-soothing properties of coconut oil, beeswax, and vitamin E, this deodorant is infused with Lemon, Rosemary, and other pure essential oils.

**Ingredients:** coconut oil extract, white beeswax, pure ester 34, zinc oxide, pure ester 40, vitamin E (tocopheryl acetate)

**Essential Oils:** Clove, Lemon, Peppermint, Rosemary, Eucalyptus Radiata, White Fir

Personal Body Care | **Chapter 11**

# Hair Care

Many personal care products on the market today, including shampoos and conditioners, contain harmful chemicals. Unfortunately, too much of the public is unaware of the dangers and continue using these harmful products on themselves and their families, simply because they are uninformed and are bombarded with so much advertising touting the beauty and benefits of their synthetic products. Besides that, too many believe natural products do not work as effectively as their synthetic counterparts.

Recognizing that what you put on your body is as important as what you put in your body, the Young Living signature hair care line contains unique formulations of pure, therapeutic-grade essential oils and other plant-based ingredients to ensure not only a safe and toxin-free experience but also an effective one.

Benefits of the Young Living hair care products include sustainable plant-based products that are derived from actual botanicals, not synthesized in a lab, safe ingredients that have been shown by modern research to have no health risks, use recyclable packaging, and no animal testing. Our products are equally as good for the environment as they are for you.

## Copaiba Vanilla Moisturizing Conditioner

Plant-based, safe, and environmentally responsible, Copaiba Vanilla Moisturizing Conditioner is a rich, hydrating conditioner for dry or damaged hair.

Formulated with botanical extracts, vitamins, silk proteins, and the benefits of pure copaiba and vanilla essential oils, this gentle conditioner protects without over-drying for a soothing aromatherapy experience.

**Ingredients:** water, cetearyl alcohol, behenamidopropyl dimethylamine, glyceryl stearate, glycerin, levulinic acid, p-Anisic acid, lactic acid, inulin, hydrolyzed algin, chlorella vulgaris, orbignya speciosa kernel oil, astrocaryum murumuru seed butter, potassium sorbate, silk protein, panthenol, soybean seed extract, palm fruit extract, rice extract, undaria pinnatifida extract, phytic acid, Lycium barbarum (wolfberry) fruit extract, rosemary leaf extract, equisetum arvense extract, yucca root extract, vanilla absolute

**Essential Oils:** Lavender, Copaiba, Geranium, Lime

## Copaiba Vanilla Moisturizing Shampoo

Copaiba Vanilla Moisturizing Shampoo calms and moisturizes dry, irritated scalps and is a natural sealant that can help tame flyaways and lock in moisture. Plant-based, safe, and environmentally responsible, this shampoo is a rich, hydrating cleanser for dry or damaged hair.

**Ingredients:** water, decyl glucoside, coco betaine, lauryl glucoside, coco-glucoside, glyceryl oleate, sorbitan sesquicaprylate, glycerin, levulinic acid, p-Anisic acid, behenamidopropyl dimethylamine, lactic acid, inulin, xanthan gum, sodium phytate, Lycium barbarum (wolfberry) fruit extract, potassium sorbate, panthenol, silk protein, rosemary leaf extract, equisetum arvense extract, yucca (root) extract, hydrolyzed algin, chlorella vulgaris, soybean seed extract, palm fruit extract, rice extract, undaria pinnatifida extract, vanilla absolute

**Essential Oils:** Lavender, Copaiba, Geranium, Lime

## Lavender Mint Invigorating Conditioner

Plant-based, safe, and environmentally responsible, Lavender Mint Invigorating Conditioner is an invigorating moisturizing conditioner suitable for noncolor-treated hair. Containing botanical extracts, vitamins, silk protein, and the benefits of pure Lavender and mint essential oils, this conditioner provides an invigorating aromatherapy experience suitable for all hair types.

**Ingredients:** water, cetearyl alcohol, behenamidopropyl dimethylamine, glyceryl stearate, glycerin, levulic acid, p-Anisic acid, lactic acid, inulin, hydrolyzed algin, chlorella vulgaris, orbignya speciosa kernel oil, astrocaryum murumuru seed butter, potassium sorbate, silk protein, panthenol, soybean seed extract, palm fruit extract, rice extract, undaria pinnatifida extract, phytic acid, Lycium barbarum (wolfberry) fruit extract, rosemary leaf extract, equisetum arvense extract, yucca root extract

**Essential Oils:** Lavender, Peppermint, Spearmint

## Lavender Mint Invigorating Shampoo

Lavender Mint Invigorating Shampoo contains Lavender essential oil to soothe the scalp and calm unmanageable hair and Peppermint essential oil to stimulate the blood flow to the hair follicle—allowing hair to better absorb nutrients.

Plant-based, safe, and environmentally responsible, this shampoo is an invigorating cleansing blend suitable for noncolor-treated hair.

**Ingredients:** water, decyl glucoside, coco betaine, lauryl glucoside, coco-glucoside, glyceryl oleate, sorbitan sesquicaprylate, glycerin, levulinic acid, p-Anisic acid, behenamidopropyl dimethylamine, lactic acid, inulin, xanthan gum, sodium phytate, Lycium barbarum (wolfberry) fruit extract, potassium sorbate, panthenol, silk protein, rosemary leaf extract, equisetum arvense extract, yucca root extract, hydrolyzed algin, chlorella vulgaris, soybean seed extract, palm fruit extract, rice extract, undaria pinnatifida extract

**Essential Oils:** Lavender, Peppermint, Spearmint

## Lavender Conditioner

Lavender Conditioner moisturizes and conditions without weighing down the hair. It feeds the hair with MSM, amino acids, a multivitamin complex, and pure, therapeutic-grade essential oils.

**Ingredients:** natural vegetable fatty acid base, MSM (dimethyl sulfone), milk protein, phospholipids, quinoa extract, soybean protein, vitamin A (retinyl palmitate), vitamin C (ascorbic acid), rosemary leaf extract, amino acids, glycoproteins, sage extract, horsetail extract, coltsfoot extract, hydrolyzed wheat protein, vitamin E (tocopheryl), grape seed extract, vitamin B5 (panthenol), cetyl triethylmonium dimethicone copolyol phthalate, dimethicone copolyol meadowfoamate seed oil, acetamide MEA, dimethiconol panthenol, keratin, linoleic acid,

linolenic acid, sulfur, tocopheryl acetate, hyaluronic acid, sorbitol, wheat germ oil, dimethiconol cysteine, jojoba seed oil, guar gum

**Essential Oils:** Lavender, Clary Sage, Lemon, Jasmine

**Allergen Warning:** Contains wheat product.

## Lavender Shampoo

Lavender Shampoo contains all-natural ingredients for gently cleansing and moisturizing hair. It is fortified with a vitamin complex, including panthenol and vitamins A, C, and E. It also contains MSM, which provides sulfur to help build and strengthen hair, essential oils for healthy hair and scalp and a beautiful fragrance.

**Ingredients:** coconut oil, olive oil, decyl polyglucose, MSM (dimethyl sulfone), water, dimethicone copolyol meadowfoamate seed oil, soybean protein, wheat protein, oat kernel protein, lemon peel extract, sugar maple extract, orange fruit extract, aloe vera leaf gel, vitamin A (retinyl palmitate), vitamin C (ascorbic acid), vitamin B5 (panthenol), grape seed extract, vitamin B3 (niacin), vitamin E (tocopheryl acetate), keratin, dimethiconol panthenol, linoleic acid, linolenic acid, jojoba seed oil, tocopherol, hyaluronic acid, wheat germ oil, sorbitol, sweet almond oil, soap bark extract, soapwort extract, inositol, guar gum, sulfur, acetamide MEA, dimethyl lauramine oleate, dimethiconol cysteine, cetyl triethylmonium dimethicone copolyol phthalate, PG-hydroxyethycellulose cocodimonium chloride

**Essential Oils:** Lavender, Clary Sage, Jasmine, Lemon

**Allergen Warning:** Contains wheat product.

# Hand Purifier

## Thieves® Waterless Hand Purifier

This all-natural hand cleaner is designed to sanitize and refresh the hands. Thieves Waterless Hand Purifier conveniently promotes good hygiene whenever water or washing facilities are not available.

It contains Thieves blend essential oil, known for the powerful, antibacterial properties that penetrate the skin as the ethanol in this hand purifier evaporates. It also contains active skin-moisturizing ingredients to prevent dry skin.

**Ingredients:** alcohol (denatured with peppermint essential oil), water, aloe vera leaf powder, vegetable glycerin, hydroxylpropyl cellulose

**Essential Oils:** Peppermint, Thieves Blend: [Clove, Lemon, Cinnamon Bark, Eucalyptus Radiata, Rosemary]

**Directions:** Apply a nickel-size amount to the palm of the hand and rub until completely absorbed.

Personal Body Care | **Chapter 11**

# Hormone Balancing

## Prenolone® + Body Cream

Prenolone + Body Cream contains pregnenolone, DHEA, blue and black cohosh, and Ylang Ylang, Clary Sage, and other essential oils to nourish the skin and help maintain healthy estrogen levels.

**Ingredients:** water, dimethyl sulfone (MSM), caprylic/capric triglyceride, sorbitol, lecithin, pregnenolone, Lycium barbarum (wolfberry) seed oil, shea butter, glyceryl stearate, Roman Chamomile flower extract, rosebud flower extract, calendula flower extract, St. John's wort extract, gingko biloba leaf extract, grape seed extract, aloe vera leaf gel, green tea leaf extract, stearic acid, sodium PCA, algae extract, prasterone (DHEA), wild yam root extract, black cohosh root, blue cohosh root, eleuthero root extract, vitamin A (retinyl palmitate), kelp extract, flax seed oil, trace mineral complex, vitamin E (tocopheryl acetate), hydrolyzed wheat protein, vitamin E (tocopherol linoleate), wheat germ oil, allantoin, vitamin C (ascorbic acid), locust bean gum

**Essential Oils:** Ylang Ylang, Clary Sage, Geranium, Fennel, Sage, Blue Yarrow, Bergamot

**Directions:** Begin using one day after menstrual cycle ends. Apply ¼–½ teaspoon 2 times a day for 21 consecutive days. Discontinue for 7 days; then repeat. Massage thoroughly into soft tissue areas of the body until absorbed.

**Allergen Warning:** Contains wheat products.

## Progessence® Plus

As women age, progesterone levels drop, and staying hormonally balanced becomes increasingly challenging, causing everything from sleep and mood disorders to more serious health concerns. Progesterone deficiency is something that affects all women.

Progessence Plus increases hormonal balance the way nature intended. It is a balancing blend designed to enhance the natural effects of progesterone. Pure USP-grade, super-micronized progesterone from wild yam is purified into a pure, therapeutic-grade essential oil-infused serum.

The first-ever, pure progesterone serum on the market, Progessence Plus has a pleasant aroma, is easy to take with you, is easily absorbed into the skin, and does not require cycling the application sites like other progesterone supplements.

Progessence Plus contains Sacred Frankincense, Bergamot, and Peppermint essential oils, plus vitamin E for increased skin benefits.

**Ingredients:** caprylic/capric triglyceride, tocopherol, USP-grade progesterone (from wild yam extract)

**Essential Oils:** Copaiba, Sacred Frankincense, Cedarwood, Bergamot (Furocoumarin-free), Peppermint, Clove

**Directions:** Apply 2-4 drops 2 times daily on neck area. For added effect, apply 1-2 drops along forearms 2 times daily. Do not exceed 2 applications per day.

**Allergen Warning:** This product contains an ingredient known to the state of California to cause cancer.

## Protec™

Protec is a balancing blend of natural ingredients that supports health and hygiene for men and women. This formula is enhanced with Frankincense, Myrrh, Sage, and Cumin essential oils.

**Ingredients:** grape seed oil, wheat germ oil, sweet almond oil, olive oil

**Essential Oils:** Frankincense, Myrrh, Sage, Cumin

**Directions:** Use ½ to 1 fl. ounce rectally to support prostate health. It may also be balancing for women when used as a douche. Shake well before using.

**Allergen Warning:** Contains wheat product.

## Regenolone™ Moisturizing Cream

Regenolone is a natural moisturizer formulated to support proper estrogen levels in women. It contains wild yam, black and blue cohosh, Peppermint, and Wintergreen to invigorate the skin and enhance absorption.

**Ingredients:** water, dimethyl sulfone (MSM), fractionated coconut/palm oil, sorbitol, pregnenolone, lecithin, shea butter, wolfberry seed oil, glyceryl stearate, aloe vera leaf, sodium PCA, stearic acid, calendula flower extract, Roman chamomile flower extract, rosebud flower extract, green tea leaf extract, St. John's wort extract, ginkgo biloba leaf extract, grape seed extract, algae extract, vitamin E (tocopheryl acetate and linoleate), hydrolyzed wheat protein, locust bean gum, trace minerals, flaxseed oil, wheat germ oil, allantoin, wild

Seventh Edition | **Essential Oils Desk Reference** | 223

yam root extract, eleuthero root extract, kelp extract, vitamin A (retinyl palmitate), black cohosh root extract, blue cohosh extract, vitamin C (ascorbic acid)

**Essential Oils:** Wintergreen, Peppermint, Douglas Fir, Oregano

**Directions:** Apply a dime-sized amount directly onto dry skin as needed, not to exceed five applications per day.

**Allergen Warning:** Contains wheat products.

## Shutran™

Shutran is an empowering essential oil blend that is specifically designed for men to boost feelings of masculinity and confidence.

**Ingredients:** Idaho Blue Spruce, Ylang Ylang, Ocotea, Hinoki, Davana, Cedarwood, Lavender, Coriander, Lemon, Northern Lights Black Spruce

**Directions: Topical:** Apply 2-4 drops 2 times daily or as needed.

**Caution:** Possible sun sensitivity.

# Lip Balms

### Cinnamint™ Lip Balm

Moisturize and protect your lips with an all-natural lip balm. Featuring pure Cinnamon Bark and Peppermint essential oils, Cinnamint Lip Balm helps prevent skin dehydration for soft, smooth lips.

**Ingredients:** coconut oil, beeswax, sweet almond oil, jojoba seed oil, wolfberry seed oil, rosehip seed extract, tocopherol, vitamin E (tocopheryl acetate)

**Essential Oils:** Peppermint, Orange, Spearmint, Cinnamon Bark

### Grapefruit Lip Balm

This balm is infused with grapefruit essential oil, wolfberry seed oil, and antioxidants that seal in moisture to prevent dehydration for smooth, supple lips.

**Ingredients:** coconut oil, beeswax, jojoba seed oil, sweet almond oil, wolfberry seed oil, rosehip seed extract, tocopherol, vitamin E (tocopheryl acetate)

**Essential Oil:** Grapefruit

### Lavender Lip Balm

This balm soothes dry, chapped lips with gentle, protective Lavender essential oil and the moisturizing benefits of jojoba oil and vitamin E.

**Ingredients:** coconut oil, beeswax, jojoba seed oil, sweet almond oil, wolfberry seed oil, rosehip seed oil, tocopheryl, vitamin E (tocopheryl acetate)

**Essential Oil:** Lavender

# Lip Gloss/Essential Oil Duos

### ART L'Brianté – Neutral/Winter Scent

L'Brianté Neutral Lip Gloss and the sophisticated Winter Essential Oil Blend are perfect for revealing your natural beauty on the go.

**Lip Gloss Ingredients:** caprylic/capric triglyceride, castor seed oil, mica, candelilla wax, safflower seed oil, aloe leaf juice, iron oxide, spearmint leaf extract, carrot extract, maltodextrin (non-GMO)

**Lip Gloss Essential Oils:** Tangerine, Ocotea

**Essential Oil Blend Ingredients:** caprylic/capric triglyceride, Idaho Balsam Fir, White Fir, Royal Hawaiian Sandalwood, Vetiver, Ylang Ylang

### ART L'Brianté – Pink/Summer Scent

L'Brianté glowing Pink Lip Gloss and sweet Summer Essential Oil Blend helps you look and feel radiant.

**Lip Gloss Ingredients:** caprylic/capric triglyceride, castor seed oil, mica, candelilla wax, eclipta prostrata extract, melia azadirachta extract, moringa pterygosperma seed oil, purple carrot extract, maltodextrin (non-GMO), safflower seed oil, aloe leaf juice, spearmint leaf extract, citric acid

**Lip Gloss Essential Oils:** Tangerine, Ocotea

**Essential Oil Blend Ingredients:** caprylic/capric triglyceride, Tangerine, Mandarin, Lime, spearmint leaf extract, Vetiver, Patchouli, Idaho tansy extract

Personal Body Care | **Chapter 11**

## ART L'Brianté – Red/Amoressence Scent

L'Brianté rich Red Lip Gloss and romantic Amoressence Essential Oil Blend help you look and feel beautiful wherever you go.

**Lip Gloss Ingredients:** caprylic/capric triglyceride, castor seed oil, candelilla wax, eclipta prostrata extract, melia azadirachta extract, moringa pterygosperma seed oil, mica, carrot extract, maltodextrin (non-GMO), safflower seed oil, aloe leaf extract, iron oxides

**Lip Gloss Essential Oils:** Spearmint, Tangerine, Ocotea

**Essential Oil Blend Ingredients:** caprylic/capric triglyceride, Vetiver, Idaho Blue Spruce, Davana, Jasmine, Ocotea, Roman Chamomile, Ylang Ylang, Geranium, vanilla bean extract

# Massage Oils

Massage and therapeutic touch have long been part of both physical and emotional healing. Massage improves circulation and lymphatic drainage and aids in the elimination of tissue wastes. Massage also opens and increases the flow of energy, balancing the entire nervous system, and helping to release physical and emotional disharmony.

When essential oils are combined with massage, the benefits are numerous. The oils bring peace and tranquility as well as keen mental awareness.

The unrefined carrier vegetable oils are rich in fat-soluble nutrients and essential fatty acids

## Cel-Lite Magic™ Massage Oil

Cel-Lite Magic Massage Oil enhances circulation and provides nutrients that help reduce the appearance of fat and cellulite. This massage oil is formulated with pure vegetable oils, vitamin E, Grapefruit essential oil to improve skin texture, and Juniper essential oil to detoxify and cleanse.

**Ingredients:** caprylic/capric triglyceride, grape seed oil, wheat germ oil, sweet almond oil, olive oil

**Essential Oils:** Grapefruit, Cypress, Cedarwood, Juniper, Clary Sage,

**Directions:** Massage on locations where firming and toning are desired. Can be used in massage or added to bath water. Shake well before using.

**Allergen Warning:** Contains wheat product.

## Dragon Time™ Massage Oil

Dragon Time Massage Oil combines specially blended vegetable oils with pure Lavender, Ylang Ylang, and other essential oils that deliver natural phytoestrogens to balance and stabilize the body. Containing a blend of essential oils that have been researched in Europe for their

balancing effects on hormones, this massage oil is recommended for both young and mature women.

**Ingredients:** caprylic/capric triglyceride, grape seed oil, wheat germ oil, sweet almond oil, olive oil

**Essential Oils:** Lavender, Fennel, Clary Sage, Sage, Ylang Ylang, Yarrow, Jasmine

**Directions:** Shake well before using. Gently massage onto lower abdomen and lower back or add approximately ½ ounce to bath water.

## Ortho Ease® Massage Oil

Ortho Ease Massage Oil is a calming blend of vegetable oils and therapeutic-grade essential oils such as Wintergreen, Peppermint, Juniper, and Marjoram. This unique blend is anti-inflammatory and pain-killing, ideal for strained, swollen, or torn muscles and ligaments. It also combats insect bites, dermatitis, and itching.

**Ingredients:** caprylic/capric triglyceride, grape seed oil, wheat germ oil, sweet almond oil, olive oil

**Essential Oils:** Wintergreen, Peppermint, Juniper, Eucalyptus Globulus, Lemongrass, Marjoram, Thyme, Eucalyptus Radiata, Vetiver

**Directions:** Shake well before using. Gently massage into areas of body experiencing stress.

**Allergen Warning:** Contains wheat product.

## Ortho Sport® Massage Oil

Ortho Sport Massage Oil is an anti-inflammatory and pain-killing complex of vegetable and essential oils. Ideal for strained, swollen, or torn muscles and ligaments, it has higher phenol content than Ortho Ease and produces a greater warming sensation.

Seventh Edition | **Essential Oils Desk Reference** | 225

**Essential Oils Desk Reference** | Seventh Edition

**Ingredients:** caprylic/capric triglyceride, grape seed oil, wheat germ oil, sweet almond oil, olive oil

**Essential Oils:** Wintergreen, Peppermint, Oregano, Eucalyptus Globulus, Elemi, Vetiver, Lemongrass, Thyme

**Directions:** Shake well before using. Thoroughly massage into areas of the body feeling stress following exercise.

**Allergen Warning:** Contains wheat product.

## Relaxation™ Massage Oil

Relaxation Massage Oil promotes tranquility to the body, mind, and spirit and eases tension to restore vitality. This formula blends specially selected vegetable oils with soothing essential oils for maximum stress relief and relaxation.

**Ingredients:** caprylic/capric triglyceride, grape seed oil, wheat germ oil, sweet almond oil, olive oil

**Essential Oils:** Tangerine, Lavender, Spearmint, Ylang Ylang, Peppermint, Coriander, Bergamot (Furocoumarin-free), Geranium

**Directions:** Shake well before using. Gently massage onto skin as needed.

**Allergen Warning:** Contains wheat product.

## Sensation™ Massage Oil

Sensation Massage Oil inspires the senses and encourages feelings of passion, romance, and youthfulness. This special blend of vegetable oils and essential oils leaves skin feeling silky, smooth, and soft.

**Ingredients:** caprylic/capric triglyceride, grape seed oil, wheat germ oil, sweet almond oil, olive oil

**Essential Oils:** Ylang Ylang, Coriander, Bergamot (Furocoumarin-free), Jasmine, Geranium

**Directions:** Shake well before using. Massage liberally onto skin as desired.

**Allergen Warning:** Contains wheat product.

## V-6™ Vegetable Oil Complex

V-6 Vegetable Oil Complex is comprised of nourishing, antioxidant vegetable oils that are colorless and odorless. It is used to create custom massage oils or to dilute essential oils for sensitive skin. V-6 has a long shelf life, does not clog pores, and will not stain clothes.

**Ingredients:** caprylic/capric triglyceride, sesame seed oil, grape seed oil, sweet almond oil, wheat germ oil, sunflower seed oil, olive oil

**Directions: Direct application**: Mix 1 drop of chosen essential oil in 1-8 teaspoons of V-6 Vegetable Oil Complex and apply. May be applied to skin prior to the application of essential oils.

**Custom blend for topical applications**: Mix 15-30 drops of chosen essential oils in 1/8-1/4 cup V-6. Stronger oils such as Cinnamon Bark, Clove, Oregano, etc., require more dilution than gentler oils. Shake well before using.

**Allergen Warning:** Contains wheat product.

# Oral Health Care

### The Dirtiest Place on the Body

It is common medical knowledge that the dirtiest part of the body is not the colon or bowels—but the mouth. The back of the tongue is literally teeming with pathogenic microorganisms.

According to Dr. John Richter, founder of the Richter Center for the Diagnosis and Treatment of Breath Disorders, "more bacteria per square inch live on the back of the tongue than on any other part of the body."

The problem is that few people use a toothbrush to remove these bacteria, and even if the tongue were to receive a thorough scrubbing, many would remain and quickly repopulate the mouth.

### U.S. Surgeon General

Few people realize how important good oral hygiene is to wellness and reducing the risk of serious chronic diseases such as heart disease and cancer. According to the U.S. Surgeon General, "The terms oral health and general health should not be interpreted as separate entities. Oral health is integral to general health."

### The Heart Disease Link

At the 2001 annual session of the American College of Cardiology, researchers were stunned by new research that showed that gingivitis is actually linked to heart disease. "There is sufficient evidence to conclude that oral lesions, especially advanced periodontopathies, place certain patients at risk for cardiovascular disease and stroke," stated Louis F. Rose, DDS, MD, of the University of Pennsylvania.

The same oral pathogen *Porphyromonas gingivalis* that causes gum disease also contributes to the inflammation along arteries and arterial damage that leads to heart and vascular disease.

### The Cancer Link

Studies show a clear link between poor dental hygiene (i.e., gingivitis, cavities) and cancer.

A fascinating longitudinal study published in the *British Medical Journal* followed 1390 Swedish patients over the course of 25 years. Those with the most dental plaque (bacteria) were twice as likely to die of cancer as those who had low-to-normal levels.

"Poor oral hygiene, as reflected in the amount of dental plaque, was associated with increased cancer mortality," concluded researchers from the prestigious Karolinska Research Institute in Sweden.

### Oil Pulling

One of the oldest and most powerful ways of improving oral health is the ancient Ayurvedic practice of "oil pulling." Traditionally using sesame seed oil, this technique involves swishing vegetable oil in the mouth for between 5 and 15 minutes. It is important to push the oil under the tongue and between the teeth where most of the pathogenic microorganisms reside. The swishing action with the oil literally "pulls" or "extracts" inflammation-causing bacteria and fungi from the crevices in the mouth, which will then be spit out (**not** swallowed or gargled). A modern version of this practice replaces sesame seed oil with coconut oil. The coconut oil version has been reported to not only improve oral health but sinus function as well.

A new advancement in the practice of oil pulling is to combine coconut oil with an antiseptic essential oil such as clove. This can magnify the effectiveness of oil pulling to a huge degree, especially because the germ-killing clove oil will penetrate the nooks and crannies of the mouth along with the coconut oil to provide far reaching disinfecting benefits far exceeding that of the vegetable oil alone (which only mechanically removes microbes without actually killing them).

### Oral Hygiene: The Next Level

Combining oil pulling with a water-soluble antiseptic such as xylitol further improves oral hygiene. A five-carbon sugar derived from birch tree sap, xylitol is found in dental products such as chewing gum in order to reduce plaque and reduce dental decay.

Because xylitol is water soluble, it acts on a completely different level than oil-based solutions. Using a two-pronged approach in which both oil-soluble and water-soluble oral disinfectants are combined, xylitol takes oral health to an entirely new level and creates an unmatched oral treatment care system that is revolutionizing the way people approach general health.

### Brushing Teeth: Cosmetic Only

Most toothpastes work to prevent cavities by merely hardening the tooth enamel with fluoride or using abrasive salts to mechanically scrub away microorganisms from teeth and gums.

The problem is that brushing is not enough to reduce the persistent inflammation and the disease-causing bacteria, fungi, and viruses in the mouth. Such microorganisms typically hide between teeth and under the tongue. While brushing mechanically removes some of the plaque and pathogens, it still leaves countless microorganisms behind to later re-infest the mouth. Oral hygiene could be vastly improved by adding proven and potent antiseptics to the toothpaste matrix, rather than relying on either fluoride or scrubbing.

### Antibacterial and Antiseptic

Essential oils are ideal for use in oral care products because they are both antiseptic and nontoxic, a rare combination. Jean Valnet, MD, who used essential oils for decades in his clinical practice, emphasized this, "Essential oils are especially valuable as antiseptics because their aggression toward microbial germs is matched by their total harmlessness toward tissue."

Thieves AromaBright, Thieves Dentarome Plus, and Thieves Dentarome Ultra toothpastes; Thieves Fresh Essence Plus Mouthwash; and KidScents Slique Toothpaste use pure, therapeutic-grade essential oils at the heart of their formulas. These oils include Peppermint, Wintergreen, Eucalyptus Globulus, Thyme, and a proprietary blend of pure, therapeutic-grade essential oils called Thieves (includes Clove, Lemon, Cinnamon Bark, Eucalyptus Radiata, and Rosemary).

Thieves blend was tested at Weber State University in Ogden, Utah, and found to dramatically inhibit the growth of many types of bacteria (both gram negative and gram positive), including *Micrococcus luteus* and *Staphylococcus aureus*.

Even more remarkably, this blend exhibited a 99.96 percent kill rate against tough gram negative bacteria like *Pseudomonas aeruginosa*. These bacteria, because of their thicker cell walls, tend to be far more resistant to antiseptics.

**Essential Oils Desk Reference** | Seventh Edition

## Effectiveness of Chemical Constituents Against Strains of Bacteria

| Bacteria | Cinnam Aldehyde from cassia/cinnamon essential oil | Thymol from thyme essential oil | Carvacrol from oregano essential oil | Eugenol from clove essential oil |
|---|---|---|---|---|
| Streptococcus mutans | 250 | 250 | 250 | 500 |
| Streptococcus sanguis | 250 | 125 | 125 | 250 |
| Streptococcus milleri | 31 | 125 | 125 | 125 |
| Streptococcus mitis | 125 | 125 | 125 | 250 |
| Peptostreptococcus anaerobius | 500 | 500 | 500 | 1000 |
| Prevotella buccae | 125 | 250 | 250 | 500 |
| Prevotella oris | 63 | 250 | 250 | 500 |
| Prevotella intermedia | 125 | 125 | 125 | 250 |

Didry, et al., 1994

**MIC µg/ml (PPM or parts per million)**

### The Strength of Thyme Essential Oil

A comprehensive 2002 survey of medical literature has shown that Thyme essential oil is one of the strongest natural antiseptics known.

Researchers found that Thyme essential oil kills over 60 different strains of bacteria (both gram negative and gram positive) and 16 different strains of fungi.

A 1995 study by Nicole Didry at the College of Pharmaceutical and Biological Sciences in Lille, France, found that Thyme essential oil, even in very small concentrations (500 parts per million or less), killed the pathogenic organisms responsible for tooth decay, gingivitis, and bad breath—*Streptococcus mutans, Streptococcus sanguis, Streptococcus milleri, Streptococcus mitis, Peptostreptococcus anaerobius, Prevotella buccae, Prevotella oris*, and *Prevotella intermedia*.

### Clinical Research on Essential Oils in Dental Hygiene

Over 100 studies have documented how essential oils kill the microbes that cause tooth decay and gingivitis. According to Christine Charles and colleagues in a study published by the *Journal of the American Dental Association*, "The efficacy of an essential-oil-containing antiseptic mouth rinse has been demonstrated in numerous double-blind clinical studies."

Researchers at the University of Maryland have also stated in the *Journal of Clinical Periodontology* that "Antiseptic mouth rinses are well known for their antibacterial effectiveness and are widely used for the prevention and treatment of periodontitis and to prevent the formation of supragingival plaque."

*"The essential oils of thyme, clove, and cinnamon possess significant inhibitory effects against 23 different genera of bacteria."*

— International Journal of Food Microbiology

### Removing Plaque Naturally

Most toothpastes use questionable chemicals such as pentasodium triphosphate and tetrasodium pyrophosphate to control plaque, the scale that builds up on teeth and irritates gums, leading to gingivitis, tooth loss, and periodontal disease. Plaque is a bacterial community called a biofilm that is extremely difficult to eradicate.

However, studies published in the *American Journal of Dentistry* have documented the significant plaque-reducing effects of zinc citrate. Among these clinical studies was a randomized, double-blind, six-month trial that showed that zinc citrate-containing toothpaste could reduce plaque by 26 percent.

### Essential Oils as Effective Antiseptic Mouth Rinses

Essential oils have proven to be even more effective as antiseptic mouth rinses than even FDA-recognized, plaque-control, antiseptic drugs, such as stannous fluoride.

A 2015 study published in the journal *PLoS* found that an essential oil mouth rinse containing essential oil constituents thymol, menthol, methyl salicylate, and eucalyptol was as effective as a 0.2 percent solution of chlorhexidine against plaque biofilm without the gastrointestinal and tooth-staining effects of chlorhexidine.

**Personal Body Care** | **Chapter 11**

## Toothpaste Solutions (See chart on right)

The Thieves line of toothpastes represent a comprehensive, powerful, natural, and novel approach to dental health.

Thieves AromaBright contains key components of both the Dentarome Plus (sodium bicarbonate) and Dentarome Ultra (calcium carbonate). This combination is far more effective than each alone in promoting oral health and beauty. Sodium bicarbonate greatly enhances the antiseptic action of the essential oils, while calcium carbonate is essential for brightening teeth. In fact, these two carbonate salts are superior to enzymes in promoting tooth whiteness.

Thieves AromaBright also includes the powerful anti-inflammatory essential oil Ocotea for the first time, essential for reducing oral inflammation, gingivitis, and periodontitis. Ocotea is rich in alpha humulene and beta caryophyllene, which are some of the best-studied essential oil compounds to combat inflammation.

### Thieves® AromaBright™ Toothpaste

Thieves AromaBright Toothpaste gently removes stains while polishing and brightening the appearance of teeth for a sparkling smile. Significant attributes include:

- Anti-stain whitening enzymes
- Time-released essential oil mouthwash
- Therapeutic-grade essential oil blend of Thieves
- A low-abrasion formula
- Special plaque-control agents
- All food-grade, edible ingredients

**Ingredients:** water, calcium carbonate, coconut oil, sodium bicarbonate, vegetable glycerin, xylitol, xanthan gum, stevia leaf, lecithin

**Essential Oils:** Peppermint, Spearmint, Clove, Ocotea, Cinnamon Bark, Lemon, Eucalyptus Radiata, Rosemary

Contains NO fluoride, sodium lauryl sulfate, sugar, synthetic chemicals, or colors.

### Thieves® Dentarome® Plus Toothpaste

Thieves Dentarome Plus Toothpaste is formulated to provide long-lasting freshness by combining quality essential oils for natural, safe dental hygiene.

In addition, Dentarome Plus uses an exclusive formula of uniquely antiseptic, antimicrobial, therapeutic-grade essential oils to combat plaque-causing microorganisms.

The Thieves blend in Dentarome toothpaste was tested at Weber State University and found to have potent, antimicrobial properties against a wide range of oral microbes, including *Streptococcus oralis, Streptococcus pneumoniae,* and *Candida albicans.*

## Key Differences Between Thieves Toothpastes

| Oral Health Care Ingredient | AromaBright | Dentarome Ultra | Dentarome Plus |
|---|---|---|---|
| Calcium carbonate | ✔ | ✔ | |
| Sodium bicarbonate | ✔ | | ✔ |
| Virgin Coconut Oil | ✔ | | |
| Xylitol | ✔ | ✔ | |
| Thieves Essential Oil Blend | ✔ | ✔ | ✔ |
| Ocotea Essential Oil | ✔ | | |
| Peppermint Essential Oil | ✔ | ✔ | ✔ |
| Spearmint Essential Oil | ✔ | | |
| Wintergreen Essential Oil | | ✔ | ✔ |
| Lecithin | Sunflower | Soy | |

**Ingredients:** water, sodium bicarbonate, vegetable glycerin, xanthan gum, ionic trace minerals, stevia leaf

**Essential Oils:** Peppermint, Wintergreen, Thieves blend: [Clove, Lemon, Cinnamon Bark, Eucalyptus Radiata, Rosemary]

Contains NO fluoride, sodium lauryl sulfate, sugar, synthetic chemicals, or colors.

### Thieves® Dentarome® Ultra Toothpaste

Thieves Dentarome Ultra Toothpaste is a high-powered, essential oil toothpaste that provides long-lasting freshness. It is formulated with a special two-part essential oil system that has:

- Anti-stain whitening enzymes
- Time-released essential oil mouthwash
- Therapeutic-grade essential oil blend of Thieves
- A low-abrasion formula
- Special plaque-control agents
- All food-grade, edible ingredients
- Patented Liposome Technology
- Emulsifies and protects essential oils from oxidation
- Binds essential oils to the mucus membranes in the mouth for unmatched breath-freshening and oral hygiene

**Ingredients:** water, sodium bicarbonate, vegetable glycerin, xanthan gum, ionic trace minerals, stevia leaf

**Essential Oils:** Peppermint, Wintergreen, Thieves Blend: [Clove, Lemon, Cinnamon Bark, Eucalyptus Radiata, Rosemary]

Contains NO fluoride, sodium lauryl sulfate, sugar, synthetic chemicals, or colors.

Seventh Edition | **Essential Oils Desk Reference** | 229

# Excess Abrasion Destroys Tooth Enamel

The problem with many common brand toothpastes is that they contain very large-sized abrasive particles that can quickly wear away tooth enamel.

Because tooth enamel is not regenerated by the body, its loss is permanent. It is never replaced. As tooth enamel is lost, the softer dentin material underneath is exposed, thereby greatly enhancing the risk of dental decay and tooth loss.

To preserve dental enamel, toothpaste (dentifrice) should have extremely fine particles, which should be fine enough to not damage or wear away irreplaceable enamel but yet be sufficiently strong to remove the biofilm of dental plaque (caused by *Streptococcus mutans* bacteria) that can cause tooth decay, gingivitis, and dental disease.

Shown at 500 times magnification are scanning electron microscope photos of ultrafine particle zinc oxide **(image A)** and calcium carbonate **(image B)**, which form the base of the most advanced toothpastes in the world. These ultrafine particle sizes allow for gentle removal of dental plaque with minimal erosion of tooth enamel.

**Image C** shows a popular toothpaste that has article sizes so large that a single grain nearly fills up the entire image area. Such huge particles are extremely corrosive to teeth, cleaning teeth while at the same time accelerating the erosion of enamel.

**Image D** shows the large, angular structure of a leading whitening toothpaste, whose sharp, oversized structure whitens teeth by stripping away enamel with a sandpaper-like action.

**Image E** shows a popular household toothpaste with less angular but larger particle sizes with a rough, coarse, abrasive texture that can be highly damaging to dental structure. Long-term use of such dentifrices can hasten the loss of enamel and eventually increase the risk of tooth loss.

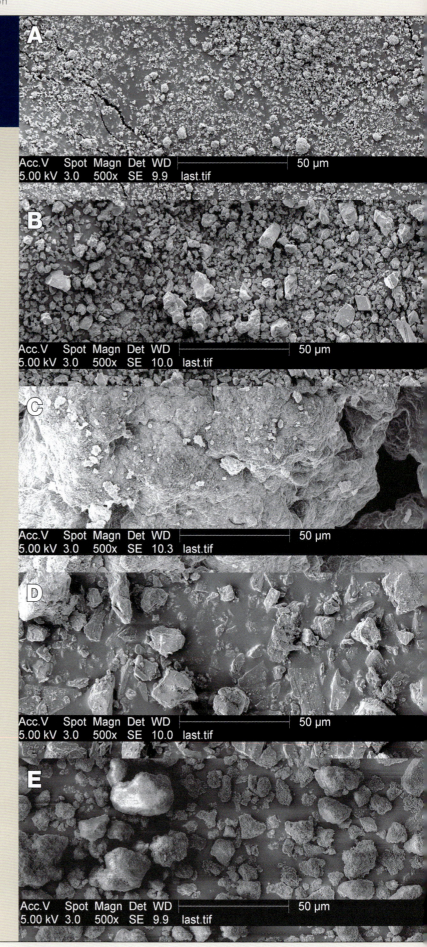

Personal Body Care | Chapter 11

# Comparing Toothpastes

| Oral Health Care Ingredient | Thieves AromaBright | Common Brand |
|---|---|---|
| **Primary Active Ingredient** | Thieves Essential Oil Blend* | Stannous Fluoride, Sodium Fluoride |
| **Germ-killing Ingredients** | Essential Oils of Clove, Cinnamon Bark, and Eucalyptus Radiata | None |
| **Antimicrobial Enhancer** | Lemon Essential Oil** | None |
| **Treats Tooth Sensitivity** | Clove Essential Oil | Potassium Nitrate |
| **Foaming Agent** | None | Poloxamer 407, PEG-12, Sodium Laurel Sulfate*** |
| **Plaque Control** | Sodium Bicarbonate | |
| **Tooth and Gum Health Agents** | Virgin Coconut Oil, Peppermint Essential Oil, Ocotea Essential Oil | Tetrasodium Pyrophosphate |
| **Moisturizer** | Vegetable Glycerin | Propylene Glycol, PEG-6, Glycerin |
| **Sweetener** | Xylitol, Pure Stevia Extract | Sorbitol, Sodium Saccharin |
| **Coloring** | None | Titanium Dioxide, FD&C Blue #1, Yellow #5 |
| **Cleansing Agent** | Nano-sized Calcium Carbonate | Abrasive Hydrated Silica, Mica, Sodium Hexametaphosphate |
| **Flavoring** | Spearmint Essential Oil | "Flavor" (Artifical and/or Natural Chemicals) |
| **Warnings on Usage** | None | Warning: When using this product, do not use for sensitivity for longer than four weeks, unless recommended by a dentist. |
| **Warnings on Ingestion** | None | Warning: Keep out of reach of children. If more than used for brushing is accidentally swallowed, get medical attention or contact a poison control center right away. |

\* A proprietary blend of Clove, Lemon, Cinnamon Bark, Eucalyptus Radiata, and Rosemary essential oils
\*\* Guerra FQ, et al. Increasing antibiotic activity against a multidrug-resistant Acinetobacter spp by essential oils of *Citrus limon* and *Cinnamomum zeylanicum*. Nat Prod Res. 2012;26(23):2235-8.
\*\*\* Also known as Sodium Laureth Sulfate

## KidScents® Slique® Toothpaste

KidScents Slique Toothpaste is a safe, natural alternative to commercial brands of toothpaste. The perfect choice for parents who want a safe, all-natural toothpaste for their kids.

Formulated with Slique Essence essential oil blend, this toothpaste gently cleans teeth and tastes great without synthetic dyes or flavors.

Thieves essential oil blend is used as a gum health agent with antibacterial properties.

KidScents Slique Toothpaste is perfect for children of all ages, and it makes a great training toothpaste for children during the crucial first years while they develop their primary teeth. Calcium carbonate, baking soda, and xylitol are used as tooth and gum health agents.

**Ingredients:** water, calcium carbonate, coconut oil, sodium bicarbonate, vegetable glycerin, xylitol, xanthan gum, stevia leaf, lecithin

**Essential Oils:** Slique Essence: [Grapefruit, Stevia, Tangerine, Spearmint, Lemon, Ocotea], Thieves: [Clove, Lemon, Cinnamon Bark, Eucalyptus Radiata, Rosemary]

Contains NO fluoride, sodium lauryl sulfate, sugar, synthetic chemicals, or colors

## Thieves® Dental Floss

Flossing is an essential part of the tooth-cleaning process because it removes plaque from between teeth and at the gum line, where periodontal disease often begins.

Thieves Dental Floss is made with strong fibers that resist fraying and easily glide between teeth for those

Seventh Edition | **Essential Oils Desk Reference** | 231

# Comparing Mouthwashes

| | **Thieves Fresh Essence Mouthwash** | **Common Brand** |
|---|---|---|
| Active Ingredients | Thieves*, Thyme oil, Eucalyptus oil, Wintergreen oil, Peppermint oil, Thymol, 1,8-cineole, Methyl Salicylate, Menthol | None |
| Base | Water | Alcohol, SD Alcohol |
| Sweetener | Stevioside, Sorbitol | Sodium Saccharin |
| Coloring | None | D&C Yellow #10, FD&C Green #3, FD&C Blue #1, FD&C Yellow #5 |
| Flavoring | Peppermint | Artificial Sources |
| Preservatives | None | Benzoic Acid, Polysorbate 80 |
| Dispersant | Natural Lecithin | Poloxamer 403, Sodium Hydroxide (Lye), Synthetic Glycerine |

\* A proprietary blend of Clove, Lemon, Cinnamon, Eucalyptus Radiata, Rosemary

hard-to-reach places. This floss combines the traditional benefits of regular dental floss with the antibacterial benefits of Thieves essential oil blend. The floss is infused with essential oils that help fight infection and cavities.

**Essential Oils:** Thieves: [Clove, Lemon, Cinnamon Bark, Eucalyptus Radiata, Rosemary], Peppermint

## Essential Oil Mouth Rinses Reduce Plaque and Fight Tooth Decay

A number of clinical studies over the past 20 years have documented the ability of essential oil mouth rinses to control plaque and fight gingivitis.

Typical of these is a 1999 study at Humboldt University in Berlin, Germany. Researchers using an observer-blind, randomized, cross-over design found that median plaque reductions generated by twice-daily essential oil mouth rinses were 23 percent greater than a placebo. The essential oils used were thyme, peppermint, wintergreen, and eucalyptus.

A six-month, double-blind, controlled clinical study at the University of Maryland similarly found that the essential oils of thyme, peppermint, wintergreen, and eucalyptus dramatically improved oral hygiene, killing the bacteria that cause plaque, tooth decay, and gingivitis.

In this case, 20 ml of mouth rinse used 2 times daily produced a 34 percent inhibition of both plaque and gingivitis compared with a control group.

## Slow Release Systems for Oral Soft Tissues

Liposomal systems that adhere to mucus membranes are designed to slowly release beneficial chemical compounds in the mucus membranes of the mouth and nose. This is useful in the slow release of flavors.

For example, a breath lozenge containing menthol that is contained in a mucin-binding system can provide extended oral freshness longer than a standard menthol lozenge (Figure 1).

In another experiment, two thymol-based mouthwashes were compared side by side. The first was a standard commercial product with no liposome-based delivery; the second used a liposomal delivery system. The results of the experiment are illustrated in Figure 2.

The level of thymol measured in saliva over a period of 5 minutes was measured. With the commercial product, thymol levels dropped off quickly, whereas with the liposome-based mouthwash, a significantly higher level of thymol was found in each saliva sample.

## Benefits of Liposomes in Thieves Fresh Essence Plus Mouthwash

Controlled-release liposomes are a key ingredient in Thieves Fresh Essence Plus Mouthwash. These liposomes adhere to either tooth enamel or mucus membranes in the mouth. The two primary benefits of using liposome technology are:

1. **Controlled release of active ingredients**
2. **Ingredient protection**

232 | **Chapter 11** | Personal Body Care

## Liposomal Binding to Teeth

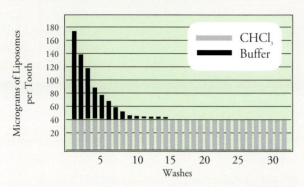

**Figure 1.** A saliva-coated human tooth was dipped in a solution of dental liposomes and rinsed repeatedly with 1.0 ml of water.

## Comparison of Coolness
Retention of menthol flavor in the mouth

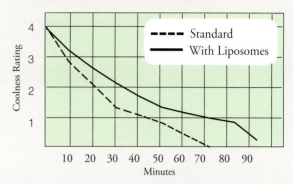

**Figure 2.** Lozenges made with mucin-binding system to release menthol flavor slowly are compared to control menthol lozenges. Timing began when the lozenge was completely dissolved in the mouth.

## Critical Kill Time Against Representative Oral Pathogens

| | TYPES of MOUTH RINSES | | |
|---|---|---|---|
| | Essential Oil | Stannous Fl | Sterile Water Control |
| Fusobacterium nucleatum | <0.5 min | <0.5 min | >5 min |
| Streptococcus mutans | <0.5 min | <1 min | >5 min |
| Prevotella intermedia | <0.5 min | <2 min | >5 min |
| Lactobacillus casei | <0.5 min | >2 min | >5 min |
| Candida albicans ATCC 28366 | <0.5 min | >5 min | >5 min |
| Candida albicans ATCC 18804 | <0.5 min | >5 min | >5 min |

Pan, et al., 1999

## Controlled Release
Retention of thymol in the mouth

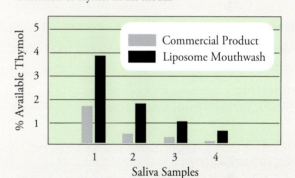

**Figure 3.** The retention of thymol was measured over a period of five minutes in various saliva samples. The level of thymol remaining in the saliva dropped off rapidly following usage of the commercial product. However, following usage of the liposome-based mouthwash, there was a significantly higher level of thymol in each saliva sample analyzed.

The controlled-release aspect of liposome technology is enhanced through the use of a patented "liposome anchoring" system. Liposomes that adhere to dental enamel can be used to improve dental health because they contain active materials to prevent plaque formation, treat periodontal disease, and prevent dental caries. These active materials can be released slowly, enhancing their benefits.

The ability of dental liposomes to slowly release their therapeutic cargo is demonstrated in Figure 3.

A saliva-coated tooth is dipped into a solution containing dental liposomes. The liposomes contain a test material. The tooth is sequentially washed with 1.0 ml of buffer 30 times. The test material is removed slowly with the washes. Even after 30 washes, some active material is retained on the tooth.

*"Essential oil constituents such as thymol, menthol, and eucalyptol have been used in mouth rinses for over 100 years [and] have been documented to be antibacterial in laboratory tests. With the association of microorganisms and plaque formation and [their] suspected involvement with carious lesions (tooth decay) and gingivitis, the effect of essential oils takes on new interest."*

—Journal of the Society of Cosmetic Chemists

## Thieves® Cough Drops

Thieves Cough Drops soothe sore throats, relieve coughs, and cool nasal passages. They are free from sugar, dyes, preservatives, and artificial flavors. With the Thieves blend, Lemon, and Peppermint essential oils, these sweet, spicy drops taste great and provide effective relief in combination with natural menthol.

**Ingredients:** menthol, isomalt, pectin, stevia leaf extract, water

**Essential Oils:** Cinnamon Bark, Clove, Eucalyptus Radiata, Lemon, Peppermint, Rosemary

**Directions:** Adults and children 5 years and over: dissolve 1 drop slowly in mouth and repeat every 2 hours as needed. Children under 5 years of age: ask a doctor.

## Thieves® Fresh Essence Plus™ Mouthwash

Thieves Fresh Essence Plus Mouthwash blends Thieves essential oil blend and Peppermint, Spearmint, and Vetiver essential oils for an extra clean mouth and fresh breath. It contains only natural ingredients and uses a patented, time-release technology for lasting freshness.

**Ingredients:** water, lecithin, quillaja saponaria wood extract, potassium sorbate, stevioside, vitamin E (alpha tocopheryl), colloidal silver, citric acid

**Essential Oils:** Peppermint, Clove, Spearmint, Lemon, Cinnamon Bark, Vetiver, Eucalyptus Radiata, Rosemary

**Directions:** Use 1 tablespoon or capful to gargle or swallow to ease a painful sore throat or upset stomach.

## Thieves® Hard Lozenges

Thieves Hard Lozenges deliver the cleansing power of Thieves essential oil blend with the sweet flavor of Peppermint, Lemon, and other natural ingredients for long-lasting relief. Both adults and children have found it to ease the pain of a sore throat and help with dryness. A convenient and portable way to enjoy this favorite dietary supplement.

Thieves is university tested for its ability to kill 99.6 percent of bacteria tested.

**Ingredients:** lemon rind, pectin, isomalt, stevia extract, water

**Essential Oils:** Lemon, Thieves: [Clove, Lemon, Cinnamon Bark, Eucalyptus Radiata, Rosemary], Peppermint

**Directions:** Dissolve 1 lozenge in mouth as needed.

## Thieves® Mints

Infused with the power of Thieves and Peppermint essential oils, Thieves Mints dissolve easily in the mouth and provide a healthy, sugar-free alternative to freshen your breath.

Thieves is university tested for its ability to kill 99.6 percent of bacteria tested.

**Ingredients:** sorbitol, calcium stearate, stevia rebaudiana extract

**Essential Oils:** Thieves blend: [Clove, Lemon, Cinnamon Bark, Eucalyptus Radiata, Rosemary], Peppermint

**Directions:** Dissolve 1 mint in mouth, as desired.

## Slique® Gum

This unique chewing gum promotes a healthy mouth and helps with appetite control. It is infused with frankincense resin, famous for its tooth and gum benefits. Natural sweeteners and the act of chewing alleviate snack cravings, making this gum a helpful tool in weight management. Peppermint and spearmint essential oils provide fresh breath.

**Ingredients:** frankincense gum resin, gum base, isomalt, sorbitol, natural flavors, calcium stearate, natural sweeteners, colors (red cabbage, turmeric), xylitol

**Essential Oils:** Peppermint, Spearmint

Personal Body Care | **Chapter 11**

# Pain Relief

## Cool Azul® Pain Relief Cream

Young Living's Cool Azul Pain Relief Cream provides penetrating and cooling relief from minor muscle and joint aches, simple backache, arthritis, strains, bruises, and sprains. This plant-based formula combines the power of Wintergreen essential oil and Cool Azul essential oil blend, while remaining free of synthetic ingredients. Get lasting comfort you can feel.

**Ingredients:** methyl salicylate, menthol, aloe vera leaf extract, safflower seed oil, glyceryl stearate, cetyl alcohol, stearyl alcohol, squalane, glycerin, rose hip seed oil, mango seed butter, water, alcohol, matricaria flower extract, green tea leaf extract, levulinic acid, benzyl alcohol, camphor, p-anisic acid, caraway seed oil, tocopheryl acetate

**Essential Oils:** Peppermint, Sage, Plectranthus Oregano, Balsam Copaiba, Melaleuca Quinquenervia (Niaouli), Lavender, Blue Cypress, Elemi, Vetiver, Dorado Azul, Matricaria (German Chamomile)

**Directions: Adults and children 12 years of age and older:** Apply to affected area not more than 3-4 times daily. **Children under 12 years of age:** Ask a doctor.

**Allergy alert:** If prone to allergic reaction from aspirin or salicylates, consult a doctor before use.

## Cool Azul™ Sports Gel

With 10 percent essential oils, Cool Azul Sports Gel is great to use before or after physical activity.

**Ingredients:** aloe extract, olive oil, glycerin, menthol, arnica extract, water, camphor, sodium hyaluronate, sunflower lecithin, xanthan gum, water, matricaria extract, willow bark extract, caraway seed oil, levulinic acid, p-Anisic acid

**Essential Oils:** Peppermint, Wintergreen, Sage, Copaiba, Plectranthus Oregano, Melaleuca Quinquenervia (Niaouli), Lavender, Blue Cypress, Elemi, Dorado Azul, Vetiver, German Chamomile (Matricaria)

**Directions:** Shake well before use. Rub and massage generously into skin.

**Caution:** Proceed with caution when applying to sensitive skin.

# Shaving

## Mirah™ Shave Oil

Mirah Shave Oil is formulated with a rich blend of essential oils, emollients, and botanical ingredients for a luxuriously close shave. Exotic baobab, meadowfoam, and avocado oils work together with our exclusive Mirah essential oil blend to reduce razor drag, bumps, and nicks.

**Ingredients:** fractionated coconut oil (caprylic/capric triglyceride), avocado fruit oils, meadowfoam seed oil, aloe vera leaf juice, baobab seed oil,

**Essential Oils:** Ylang Ylang, Idaho Blue Spruce, Ocotea, Hinoki, Coriander, Davana, Cedarwood, Lemon, Jasmine, Royal Hawaiian Sandalwood, Lavender, Rose

**Directions:** Pump shave oil into hands and rub a thin layer over skin. Shave.

## Shutran™ Aftershave Lotion

This aftershave lotion is light and soothing and moisturizes the skin with pure essential oils like Ylang Ylang, Lavender, and Northern Lights Black Spruce, as well as with other natural botanicals, including aloe and argan oil.

**Ingredients:** water, glycerin, caprylic/capric triglyceride, jojoba seed oil, coconut oil, polyglyceryl-10 pentastearate, sunflower seed wax, witch hazel, argan oil, lauryl laurate, sunflower seed oil, benzyl alcohol, aloe powder, sodium levulinate, behenyl alcohol, sodium stearoyl lactylate, xanthan gum, sodium anisate, citric acid, menthol, sodium hyaluronate, dandelion root extract, agar, sodium phytate

**Essential Oils:** Idaho Blue Spruce, Ylang Ylang, Ocotea, Hinoki, Davana, Cedarwood, Lemon, Coriander, Lavender, Northern Lights Black Spruce

**Directions:** Apply a small amount to face after shaving. Can also be applied in between shaves to keep skin moisturized.

Seventh Edition | **Essential Oils Desk Reference** | 235

**Essential Oils Desk Reference** | Seventh Edition

## Shutran™ Shave Cream

Made with pure essential oils and moisturizing botanicals, Shutran Shave Cream delivers an incredibly close, smooth shave. Combining hydrating palm, grape seed, and olive oils; naturally derived vitamin E complex; and mango and cocoa butter, this luxurious shave cream provides a frictionless glide to reduce razor burn and nicks.

**Ingredients:** aloe barbadensis leaf juice, caprylic/capric triglyceride, zinc oxide, palm oil, grape seed oil, olive oil, mango seed butter, glyceryl stearate, palm butter, cocoa seed butter, cera alba, xanthan gum, glycerin, cetearyl alcohol, menthol (natural source), organic sugar cane extract, mixed tocopherols (vitamin E), honey, sodium PCA, sodium stearoyl lactylate, water, bamboo extract, camellia oleifera leaf extract, levulinic acid, p-Anisic acid

**Essential Oils:** Tea Tree, Idaho Blue Spruce, Ocotea, Ylang Ylang, Hinoki, Cedarwood, Coriander, Davana, Lavender, Lemon, Northern Lights Black Spruce

**Directions:** Wet area with warm water. Apply a thin, even layer. Shave; rinse razor after each stroke. Rinse area with water.

# Skin Care

Human skin is like a large sponge and absorbs trace amounts of almost everything with which it comes in contact—both harmful and beneficial. The skin is especially vulnerable to solvents and petroleum-based chemicals. When some of these chemicals come in contact with the skin, they can be absorbed in far higher volumes than other types of substances.

This means that many questionable petrochemicals commonly found in personal care products such as sodium laurel sulphate (SLS), triethanolamine (TEA), polyethylene glycol (PEG), and quaterniums (ammonium salt) can be absorbed into the skin. Over time, some of these chemicals may accumulate in the organs and tissues and result in mounting brain, nerve, and liver damage.

### A Troubling Trend

The most troubling indication that showed that the synthetic chemicals in cosmetics and shampoos may be leaching into our bodies was provided by the government-funded Human Adipose Tissue Survey. According to this study, almost every person tested showed measurable levels of petroleum-based, carcinogenic chemicals, such as toluene, benzene, and styrene, in their fatty tissues.

This is why increasing numbers of health professionals are recommending personal care formulas that are completely natural and free of synthetic or petroleum-based ingredients.

"To stay healthy, people have to do more than just exercise and eat healthy," states Denver physician Terry Friedmann, MD. "Consumers should also avoid personal care products that contain toxic synthetic ingredients that can penetrate the skin and accumulate in their tissues. In some cases, these products can have a greater impact on health than either diet or exercise."

Many of the skin care products found here contain wolfberry seed oil, a costly, unusual ingredient that makes important contributions to healthy skin. Along with wolfberry seed oil, these unique products contain MSM, an essential nutrient that has an unsurpassed ability to strengthen the skin.

"MSM is absolutely dynamite for the skin," said international fashion model Teri Williams, who was a cover model for *Vogue Magazine*. She continued in an interview by saying, "In my experience, it is the single most important nutrient to support healthy skin and hair."

Ronald Lawrence, MD, PhD, agrees, "The importance of MSM for healthy skin and hair cannot be overemphasized. In my clinical practice, I have seen the difference that MSM makes. It is outstanding whether applied topically or taken as a dietary supplement."

In addition to wolfberry seed oil and MSM, these skin products also contain therapeutic-grade essential oils that have a long history of use in skin care. Pure Myrrh, Sandalwood, Geranium, Lavender, Ylang Ylang, Frankincense, and Roman Chamomile essential oils have been used to preserve the health of the skin throughout recorded history.

Also included in these personal care products is a proprietary blend of antioxidant herbal extracts such as ginkgo biloba, orange blossom, witch hazel, cucumber, horse chestnut, and aloe vera gel, as well as special blends of pure vegetable oils such as almond, jojoba, avocado, and rose hip seed oils.

"They feel fabulous on my skin," raved Kay Cansler, a former Director of Educational Diagnostics, in an interview. "Without question, these are products for the new millennium. I have been using them for six months, and I can feel and see a huge difference. I am very, very impressed."

**236** | **Chapter 11** | Personal Body Care

Personal Body Care | Chapter 11

## ART® Beauty Masque

The ART Beauty Masque features a concentrated formula designed to soothe skin and leave it feeling healthier and looking more radiant. This exotic blend of orchid petals and essential oils helps nourish stressed areas and promotes a more youthful appearance. It is suitable for all skin types.

**Ingredients:** water, aloe barbadensis extract, lactobacillus ferment, hyaluronic acid, astragalus membranaceus root extract, xanthan gum, morus alba leaf extract, torenia concolor whole plant extract, phalaenopsis orchid flower extract, *Boswellia carterii* resin extract, carthamus tinctorius flower extract, angelica polymorpha sinensis root extract, glycosphingolipids, vanilla absolute

**Essential Oils:** Stress Away blend: [Copaiba, Lime, Cedarwood, Ocotea, Lavender]

**Directions:** Wash and dry face. Remove masque from pouch and unfold with the plastic lining facing out. Place over entire face and remove the lining. Use hands to gently smooth masque for even coverage. Leave masque on for 20 minutes, then gently remove and discard. Use a damp cloth to remove any residue. For best results, use 3-4 times weekly in combination with ART Renewal Serum.

## ART® Chocolate Masque

Available at beauty school! The ART Chocolate Masque combines pure essential oils with exclusive Ecuadorian cacao to help nourish, soothe, and hydrate your skin.

**Ingredients:** raw cocoa mass

**Essential Oils:** Royal Hawaiian Sandalwood, Frankincense, Geranium, Amazonian Ylang Ylang

**Directions:** Place 1 piece of the ART Chocolate Masque in a double boiler pot. Allow chocolate to melt at a low temperature, not to exceed 113°F (about 45°C). Before applying, test the masque to ensure that it is not too hot. Apply using a facial brush, small spatula, or fingertips. Spread liberally over face and neck, avoiding the eyes and mouth. Leave masque on for 25-30 minutes and gently remove with lukewarm water. May also be used on hands.

**Caution:** For external use only.

## ART® Creme Masque

The ART Creme Masque is a blend of pure essential oils and spa-quality botanicals that help restore the look of youthfulness to the skin. We use hyaluronic acid and an exclusive blend of essential oils to moisturize and nourish skin, leaving it visibly more radiant. Other natural ingredients like cucumber extract, aloe vera, vitamin C, and green tea are added to soothe, protect, and tighten skin.

**Ingredients:** water, dicaprylyl carbonate, hydroxypropyl starch phosphate, maltodextrin, sorbitol, squalane, caprylic/capric triglyceride, cetearyl olivate, sorbitan olivate, aloe barbadensis leaf juice, pectin, oat kernel extract, panthenol, sodium hyaluronate, coconut alkanes, cetyl palmitate, sodium ascorbyl phosphate, sodium gluconate, lecithin, tocopheryl acetate, xanthan gum, sorbitan palmitate, glycerin, caprylyl glycol, phenoxyethanol, vanilla fruit extract, coco-caprylate/caprate, camellia oleifera leaf extract, cucumber fruit extract, hexylene glycol

**Essential Oils:** Vetiver, Davana, Ylang Ylang, Roman Chamomile, Jasmine, Ocotea, Geranium,

**Directions:** Wash and dry face. Apply evenly to face, avoiding eyes, and leave on for 20 minutes. Remove residue with moist towel. You may also use the masque overnight to help deepen the moisturizing effect.

## Chinese Secret to Youthful Skin

For centuries, the Chinese living in Inner Mongolia have been using a very unusual vegetable oil with exceptional benefits for the skin: Wolfberry seed oil. This rare and expensive oil from Inner Mongolia is painstakingly extracted from the seeds of the Ningxia variety of the Lycium berry. Not only is the oil rich in vitamin E, linoleic, and linolenic acids, but it also has an unusual chemistry that makes it ideal for nourishing and hydrating the skin. "The wolfberry seed oil is one of the best oils for the skin," according to researcher Sue Chao. "It is sought after throughout Asia and has some very unusual regenerative properties such as protecting aging skin and adding luster to skin."

Seventh Edition | **Essential Oils Desk Reference** | 237

# ART® Gentle Cleanser

This unique foaming cleanser was designed to cleanse the skin by gently removing oil, dirt, and makeup.

ART Gentle Cleanser is formulated from naturally occurring sugars and contains ingredients that penetrate the epidermis to remove unwanted oils and impurities. One quarter of this cleanser is composed of pure, therapeutic-grade essential oils that were specifically selected for their skin-enhancing benefits.

**Ingredients:** water, disodium cocoyl glutamate, coco-glucoside, decyl glucoside, glycerin, polyglyceryl-4 caprate, sodium cocoyl threoninate, sodium cocoyl glutamate, glyceryl oleate, honeysuckle flower extract (lonicera caprifolium), honeysuckle flower extract (lonicera japonica), sodium phytate, orchis mascula flower extract

**Essential Oils:** Frankincense, Royal Hawaiian Sandalwood, Melissa, Lemon, Lavender

**Directions:** Apply to wet hands and massage gently over face and neck with a circular motion. Rinse thoroughly. Use 2 times daily for a refreshing cleanse in the morning and a thorough cleanse at night. It is suitable for all skin types.

# ART® Intensive Moisturizer

ART Intensive Moisturizer is infused with exotic botanicals and essential oils, providing lasting hydration that produces the qualities of young-looking skin.

**Ingredients:** water, glycerin, coco-caprylate, cetearyl alcohol, glyceryl stearate, olive fruit unsaponifiables, apple fruit extract, murumuru seed butter, diheptyl succinate, capryloyl glycerin/sebacic acid copolymer, pentaclethra macroloba seed oil, benzyl alcohol, sodium stearoyl glutamate, physalis angulata extract, caprylic/capric triglyceride, sodium levulinate, alcohol denatured, sodium anisate, guar gum, hibiscus syriacus callus extract, terminalia ferdinandiana fruit extract, xanthan gum, sodium phytate, sodium hyaluronate, tocopherol, sunflower seed oil

**Essential Oils:** Hinoki, Royal Hawaiian Sandalwood, Cedarwood, Ylang Ylang, Frankincense

**Directions:** Apply on clean, dry face and neck with an upward, outward motion. Use morning, night, and throughout the day.

**Caution:** Patch test on small area of face before use.

# ART® Light Moisturizer

ART Light Moisturizer helps your skin retain proper hydration. With Young Living's essential oils and naturally derived ingredients, your face will feel soft and supple.

**Ingredients:** water, glycerin, coco-caprylate, coconut alkanes, polyglyceryl-6 distearate, cetearyl alcohol, microcrystalline cellulose, olive fruit unsaponifiables, cupuacu seed butter, benzyl alcohol (natural), jojoba esters, squalane, sodium levulinate, coco-caprylate/caprate, cellulose gum, cetyl alcohol, polyglyceryl-3 beeswax, xanthan gum, sodium anisate, senna alexandrina seed polysaccharide, dipotassium glycyrrhizate, prickly pear leaf cell extract, summer snowflake bulb extract, sodium phytate, asteriscus graveolens extract, purple orchid flower extract, aloe vera leaf juice, tocopherol, sunflower seed oil

**Essential Oils:** Royal Hawaiian Sandalwood, Frankincense

**Directions:** After cleansing and toning skin, apply moisturizer over dry face and neck. For best results, apply both morning and night and as needed throughout the day.

# ART® Refreshing Toner

A necessary step in any comprehensive skin care regimen, ART Purifying Toner helps support cleansing by removing unwanted oil, dirt, and impurities that can accumulate on the skin.

Designed to work in synergy with the other products in the ART Skin Care System, the Purifying Toner contains the essential oils of Frankincense and Sandalwood for their ability to replenish and revitalize skin, Lemon and Peppermint to cleanse and energize, and Melissa and Lavender to soothe and balance.

This mild formula absorbs quickly and leaves skin feeling clean, smooth, and soft. It minimizes oily shine and reduces the appearance of pores.

**Ingredients:** water, alcohol, heptyl glucoside, witch hazel water, glycerin, betaine, orchis mascula flower extract, aloe vera leaf juice, green tea leaf extract,

**Essential Oils:** Peppermint, Royal Hawaiian Sandalwood, Frankincense, Lavender, Lemon, Melissa

**Directions:** Shake well. After cleansing, sweep toner over face with a cotton ball. Use in the morning and evening as needed.

Personal Body Care | Chapter 11

## ART® Renewal Serum

ART Renewal Serum is an intricate blend of exotic botanicals chosen for their unique ability to soothe and protect the most delicate areas of the face. These premium ingredients work in harmony to deeply nourish, hydrate, and help restore youthfulness to skin.

**Ingredients:** water, glycerin, selaginella lepidophylla extract, lactobacillus ferment, condensed herbal extracts I: speranskia tuberculata whole plant extract, eucommia ulmoides extract, glycine tomentella root extract, polygonum cuspidatum root extract, vanilla extract, niacinamide, phalaenopsis orchid flower extract, condensed herbal extracts II: torenia concolor whole plant extract, *Commiphora myrrha* resin extract, *Boswellia carterii* resin extract, spatholobus suberectus stem extract, angelica polymorpa sinensis root extract, liquidambar formosana dried fruit extract, crocus sativus flower extract, Chamomilla recutita flower extract, sodium hyaluronate, ascorbyl glucoside

**Essential Oils:** Sensation blend: [Coriander, Ylang Ylang, Bergamot (Furocoumarin-free), Jasmine, Geranium]

**Directions:** Wash face. Apply to delicate areas of face 2 times daily and allow to absorb. For best results, follow with your choice of Young Living moisturizing creams.

**Cautions:** Avoid contact with eyes. Discontinue use if irritation occurs.

## ART® Sheerlumé™ Brightening Cream

This advanced formula combines a perfect blend of essential oils with skin-nourishing ingredients to visibly brighten and balance skin tone, unveiling a more radiant, youthful-looking glow.

**Ingredients:** water, glycerin, coconut alkanes, caprylic/capric tyriglyceride, glyceryl stearate SE, cetearyl alcohol, licorice root extract, sodium stearoyl lactate, centella asiatica extract, theobroma grandiflorum seed butter, physalis angulata extract, batyl alcohol, alcohol denatured, coco-caprylate/caprate, plumeria acutifolia flower extract, sodium PCA, meadowfoam seed oil, terminalia ferdinandiana fruit extract, lilium candidum leaf cell extract, sodium citrate, honeysuckle flower extract, citric acid, mallow extract, primula veris extract, alchemilla vulgaris extract, veronica officinalis extract, melissa officinalis extract, achillea millefolium extract, honeysuckle extract, sodium phytate, tocopherol

**Essential Oils:** Peppermint, Vetiver, Blue Cypress, Davana, Royal Hawaiian Sandalwood, Clove, Jasmine, Carrot, Spearmint, Geranium, Sacred Frankincense

**Directions:** Apply a thin layer of Sheerlumé on clean face, neck, or hands. For best results, use morning and night, either alone or under your favorite Young Living moisturizing cream.

## Boswellia Wrinkle Cream™

Boswellia Wrinkle Cream contains the pure essential oils of Frankincense, Sandalwood, Myrrh, Ylang Ylang, and Geranium that moisturize while minimizing shine, relaxing facial tension, and reducing the effects of sun damage. It tones, refines, and brightens the appearance of maturing skin.

This wrinkle cream may help build collagen and when used daily may help minimize and prevent wrinkles.

**Ingredients:** deionized water, glyceryl stearate, cetearyl alcohol, sodium stearoyl lactylate, caprylic/capric triglyceride, sweet almond oil, glycerin, levulinic acid, p-Anisic acid, olive oil, stearic acid, phellodendron amurense bark extract, barley extract, sorbic acid, shea butter, sodium hyaluronate, allantoin, xanthan gum, panthenol, sodium PCA, wolfberry seed oil, grapeseed extract, calendula extract, Roman chamomile flower extract, rose flower extract, orange flower extract, St. John's wort flower/leaf/stem extract, kelp extract, ginkgo biloba extract, sodium phytate, vitamin E (tocopheryl acetate), vitamin A (retinyl palmitate), aloe vera leaf juice, sodium hydroxide, citric acid

**Essential Oils:** Geranium, Ylang Ylang, Myrrh, Frankincense, Royal Hawaiian Sandalwood

**Directions:** After cleansing skin, apply gently over face and neck using upward strokes.

## ClaraDerm™

ClaraDerm spray soothes dry, chapped, or itchy skin. Its gentle blend is particularly helpful in relieving skin irritations, burning, and itching in sensitive female areas.

Its formula can assist in controlling rashes, candida, etc. It is especially suited for the vaginal area before and after childbirth. ClaraDerm is expertly formulated with a blend of Lavender, Frankincense, and other essential oils.

Seventh Edition | **Essential Oils Desk Reference** | 239

**Ingredients:** fractionated coconut oil

**Essential Oils:** Myrrh, Tea Tree, Lavender, Frankincense, Roman Chamomile, Helichrysum

**Directions:** Spray topically as needed.

## LavaDerm Cooling Mist™

Lavender essential oil has been highly regarded as a burn treatment since cosmetic chemist René Gattefossé used the oil to heal a severe burn he suffered in a laboratory explosion. Lavender oil has both antiseptic properties and an ability to reduce the formation of scar tissue.

LavaDerm Cooling Mist assists in the healing of most topical burns, ranging from sunburn to second-degree thermal burns. It also contains a highly purified concentrate of aloe vera gel, freshly processed from the leaves of *Aloe barbadensis*.

**Ingredients:** water, aloe vera leaf extract, vegetable glycerin, potassium sorbate, sodium levulinate, sodium anisate, ionic trace minerals, citric acid

**Essential Oils:** Lavender, Northern Lights Black Spruce, Helichrysum

**Directions:** Shake well before use. Spray topically onto desired area. Repeat every 10-15 minutes as needed to keep the skin cool and promote tissue regeneration.

## Orange Blossom Facial Wash™

This gentle, soap-free facial wash cleanses the skin without stripping natural oils. It contains MSM for softening, kelp to improve elasticity, and Lavender to soothe acne-prone skin and other problem areas.

**Ingredients:** deionized water, dimethyl sulfone (MSM), wolfberry seed oil, decyl polyglucose, mixed fruit acid complex, hydrolyzed wheat protein, citric acid, orange blossom extract, rosebud flower extract, calendula flower extract, aloe vera leaf juice, grape seed extract, St. John's wort extract, kelp extract, ginkgo biloba leaf extract, algae extract, demethyl lauramine oleate, citric acid

**Essential Oils:** Lavender, Patchouli, Lemon, German Chamomile, Rosemary

**Directions:** Gently lather over face and neck with warm water and rinse thoroughly. Use daily.

**Allergen Warning:** Contains wheat product.

## Rose Ointment™

Rose Ointment is a deeply soothing and nourishing blend for dry skin. Rose essential oil and vitamin A improve skin texture, while Tea Tree and Rose work to rejuvenate rough, irritated skin.

Use Rose Ointment over essential oils to lock in their benefits. Though not recommended for burns initially, this ointment can be very beneficial in maintaining, protecting, and keeping the scab soft.

**Ingredients:** mink oil, lecithin, beeswax, lanolin, sesame seed oil, wheat germ oil, rosehip seed oil

**Essential Oils:** Palmarosa, Patchouli, Coriander, Myrrh, Bergamot (Furocoumarin-free), Carrot Seed, Tea Tree, Ylang Ylang, Geranium, Rose

**Directions:** Apply to desired areas several times a day. Do not use on heat-stressed skin.

**Allergen Warning:** Contains wheat product.

## Sandalwood Moisture Cream™

Sandalwood Moisture Cream is an ultra-hydrating moisturizer infused with pure essential oils. MSM—a naturally occurring, plant-based chemical—softens skin and promotes elasticity. When used daily after cleansing and toning, this moisture cream promotes younger, healthier skin.

**Ingredients:** deionized water, glycerin, cetearyl alcohol, glyceryl stearate, caprylic/capric triglycerides, olive oil, stearic acid, pichia anomala extract, barley extract, sodium stearoyl lactylate, shea butter, sandalwood extract, phellondendron amurense bark extract, sodium levulinate, sorbic acid, sodium anisate, allantoin, xanthan gum, ascorbic acid, sodium PCA, hydrolyzed wheat protein, rose hip seed oil, wolfberry seed oil, calendula flower extract, chamomile flower extract, ginkgo biloba leaf extract, grape seed extract, kelp extract, orange flower extract, rosebud flower extract, St. John's wort extract, sodium phytate, vitamin E (tocopheryl acetate), vitamin A (retinyl palmitate), hydrolyzed wheat starch, aloe vera leaf juice, sodium hyaluronate, sodium hydroxide, citric acid

**Essential Oils:** Coriander, Royal Hawaiian Sandalwood, Lavender, Bergamot (Furocoumarin-free), Myrrh, Rosemary, Ylang Ylang, Geranium

**Directions:** Massage gently onto face, neck, and other desired areas. Use daily after cleaning and toning your skin.

**Allergen Warning:** Contains wheat products.

Personal Body Care | **Chapter 11**

## Satin Facial Scrub, Mint™

Satin Facial Scrub, Mint is a gentle, exfoliating scrub designed for normal skin. It contains jojoba oil, mango butter, MSM, aloe, and Peppermint essential oil to minimize the appearance of pores and rejuvenate dull skin.

This revolutionary formula gently eliminates layers of dead skin cells and can be used as a drying face mask to draw impurities from the skin.

**Ingredients:** water, glycerin, caprylic/capric triglyceride, jojoba seed oil, dimethyl sulfone (MSM), sorbitol, glyceryl stearate, aloe vera leaf gel, stearic acid, algae extract, vitamin E (tocopheryl acetate), vitamin A (retinyl palmitate), sodium PCA, shea butter, grape seed oil, zinc oxide, mango seed butter, vitamin C (ascorbic acid), sodium hyaluronate, tocopherol linoleate, allantoin, hydrolyzed wheat protein, hydrolyzed soy protein

**Essential Oils:** Peppermint, Rosemary, Roman Chamomile

**Directions:** Massage gently over face and neck with warm water and rinse thoroughly. Use as needed.

**Allergen Warning:** Contains wheat and soy products.

## Wolfberry Eye Cream™

Wolfberry Eye Cream is a natural, water-based moisturizer. Containing the antiaging properties of wolfberry seed oil, this cream soothes tired eyes and minimizes the appearance of bags, circles, and fine lines. Use in the evening. Repeat in the morning if desired.

**Ingredients:** deionized water, sorbitol, glycerin, cetearyl alcohol, glyceryl stearate, sodium stearoyl lactylate, oat kernel extract, stearic acid, caprylic/capric triglycerides, alfalfa seed extract, hydrolyzed lupine protein, levulinic acid, p-Anisic acid, sandalwood extract, phellodendron amurense bark extract, barley extract, olive fruit, wolfberry seed oil, avocado oil, kukui seed oil, rosehip seed oil, sweet almond oil, jojoba seed oil, mango seed butter, sorbic acid, witch hazel extract, allantoin, xanthan gum, shea butter, vitamin A (retinyl palmitate), sodium PCA, ascorbyl palmitate, cucumber fruit extract, hydrolyzed soy protein, hydrolyzed wheat protein, hydrolyzed wheat starch, horses chestnut seed extract, centella asiatica extract, sodium phytate, sodium hyaluronate, green tea leaf extract, ascorbic acid, sodium hydroxide, citric acid

**Essential oils:** Lavender, Coriander, Roman Chamomile, Frankincense, Geranium, Bergamot (Furocoumarin-free), Ylang Ylang

**Directions:** After cleansing and toning, massage gently onto soft skin under eyes. Use in the evening.

**Allergen Warning:** Contains wheat and soy products.

# Soaps, All Natural

### The Body's Largest Organ: The Skin

With skin covering approximately 22 square feet on the outside surface of the human body, it is the largest human organ and the first line of defense against harmful substances, infection, and dehydration. In adults, the skin is between 15 and 20 percent of total body weight.

Because of its large surface area, the skin can soak in many types of toxins and petrochemicals. This can result in cancer-causing compounds leaching into the body and accumulating in fat.

Many people complain that commercial soaps make their skin feel dry and itchy, or worse. Trapped "free alkali" is the most common irritant in soap, which is made from oils (acids) mixed with water and alkali (a base).

Acids and bases neutralize each other to form a salt, in this case soap, with glycerin as a byproduct.

Oils that do not combine with the alkali are "free," which creates a "superfatted" soap. These mild soaps are exceptionally good for the skin, even though they have a reduced lather and shelf life. Alkali that is not neutralized by essential oils is "free alkali," which makes soap harsh and drying.

The handcrafting process for natural soap removes the excess alkali that is left in commercial soaps.

### Benefits of Handmade, Natural Soaps

Handcrafted in small batches, natural bar soaps are not only pure, natural, and nontoxic, but they are also good for the skin.

Handmade soaps have a "hand-lotion-in-the-soap" effect, created by the natural vegetable oils and waxes in the soap, as well as an emulsion of water and glycerin that is formed when the soap was made. While the "hand-

Seventh Edition | **Essential Oils Desk Reference** | 241

lotion-in-the-soap" effect may reduce lathering, this is what makes handmade soap extraordinarily mild and moisturizing for dry and sensitive skin.

### Secret to Creating the Best Handmade Soap

The best handmade soaps are made exclusively with natural ingredients that are blended in small batches and poured into wooden block molds.

The soap is then wire cut into bars, dried on oak frames, and aged for over four weeks in a humidity- and temperature-controlled curing room. The extended curing process is usually time consuming and expensive, but it effectively eliminates most of the free alkali from the bar soap, a major cause of dryness and irritation.

Handmade, natural soap can be made from a number of vegetable ingredients such as saponified oils of palm, coconut, and olive and may include pure, therapeutic-grade essential oils. In addition, rosemary extract can be used as a natural preservative.

The result is a soap that does more than just cleanse the skin. It can also act as a therapeutic skin treatment with powerful antioxidant and skin-protecting properties that may be used to treat eczema, psoriasis, dermatitis, pigmentation, inflammation, and more.

### "Natural" Can be Unnatural

Unfortunately, the term "natural" can be used in very deceptive ways. If an ingredient is a five-generation derivative of coconut meat, some will claim it to be natural, even if you can't pronounce the name of the ingredient.

The main ingredients in many mass-produced bar soaps are substances known as "sodium tallowate" and "potassium tallowate." These are the fatty remains of slaughtered cows, sheep, and horses.

Brains, fatty tissues, and other unwanted parts of dead and sometimes diseased animals are collected into large vats and used to create "tallow." This tallow is shipped to commercial soap makers, where it is processed into bar soaps.

Unfortunately, the U.S. Food and Drug Administration does not regulate the ingredients in soap.

Some ingredients in mass-marketed soap, including isopropyl alcohol, fragrances, DEA, FD&C colors, propylene glycol, and triclosan, have been proven harmful to human health.

Isopropyl alcohol's drying effects can remove the skin's protective oils and cause irritation.

DEA (diethanolamine) is a hormone-disrupting chemical known to form cancer-causing nitrates and nitrosamines. Dr. Samuel Epstein of the University of Illinois has found that repeated skin applications of

DEA-based detergents resulted in a major increase in the incidence of liver and kidney cancers.

Regarding coal tar-derived FD&C colors, *A Consumer's Dictionary of Cosmetic Ingredients* states that "many pigments cause skin sensitivity and irritation . . ., and absorption (of certain colors) can cause depletion of oxygen in the body and death."

Instead of synthetic colors, German Chamomile may be used. Rich in chamazuline, an intense blue pigment, German Chamomile actually has anti-inflammatory properties that accelerate skin healing.

Moreover, other compounds in German Chamomile and other essential oils combine therapeutic action with delightful aromas.

Peppermint oil imparts a delightfully fresh fragrance to soap, while containing compounds such as menthol that act as pain relievers and anti-inflammatory agents.

Sadly, many of the compounds in the commercial fragrances used in bath and body products are carcinogenic or otherwise toxic.

The word "fragrance" on a soap label refers to over 4,000 ingredients, most of which are synthetic.

Not only are fragrances potentially carcinogenic, according to *Home Safe Home* author Debra Lynn Dadd, "Clinical observation by medical doctors has shown that exposure to synthetic fragrances can affect the central nervous system, causing depression, hyperactivity, irritability, inability to cope and other behavioral changes."

A surprising number of people experience a dry-skin reaction from many common synthetic fragrances.

# Moisturizing Bar Soaps

Moisturizing, all-natural bar soaps are created through a proprietary soap-making process derived from a 16th century Spanish recipe that was combined with modern technology and a proprietary blend of ultra-pure ingredients.

Hand poured and cured for almost a month, these bar soaps are unlike any other soaps on earth. Mild and long lasting, the soaps are made with pure, therapeutic-grade essential oils that are redefining natural skin therapy.

### Benefits

- Contain less than 1 percent free alkali; the proprietary soap-making process minimizes the presence of irritating, skin-drying, alkali salts

- Use a moisturizing, vegetable base that contains over 50 percent moisturizers

Personal Body Care | **Chapter 11**

- Include pure, therapeutic-grade essential oils, many of which have been studied for their antiseptic, anti-inflammatory, and antifungal properties and are added at the optimum moment of the soap-making process to preserve their beneficial compounds
- Contain only the finest organic ingredients, including:
  - Saponified oils of palm, coconut, jojoba, and olive
  - Organic oatmeal
  - Pure, therapeutic-grade essential oils
  - Ningxia wolfberry seed oil
  - Liquid aloe vera extract
  - Rosemary extract (as an antioxidant)
  - Glycerin

## Háloa Áina™ Royal Hawaiian Sandalwood™* Soap Collection

Royal Hawaiian Sandalwood comes from Háloa Áina, a family-owned business dedicated to restoring the native dryland forest of the big island of Hawaii. Found nowhere else in the world, this species of Sandalwood grows at an elevation of 5,000 feet on the slopes of Mauna Loa and is known for its rich, sweet, warm, and woodsy aroma. Each of these soaps pairs Royal Hawaiian Sandalwood essential oil with a complementary oil so that you can experience its soothing aroma in three distinct ways.

**Ingredients:** Royal Hawaiian Sandalwood wood distillate, sodium cocoate, sodium palmitate, sodium olivate, sodium castorate, oat kernel flour, kukui seed oil, iron oxides

## Royal Hawaiian Sandalwood™ Soap with Frankincense Oil

**Essential Oils:** Frankincense, Royal Hawaiian Sandalwood

## Royal Hawaiian Sandalwood™ Soap with Lavender Oil

**Essential Oils:** Lavender, Royal Hawaiian Sandalwood

## Royal Hawaiian Sandalwood™ Soap with Ylang Ylang Oil

**Additional Ingredient:** Royal Hawaiian Sandalwood wood powder

**Essential Oils:** Ylang Ylang, Royal Hawaiian Sandalwood

## Lavender-Oatmeal Bar Soap

Lavender-Oatmeal Bar Soap is a gentle formula that creates a creamy lather, relaxing and calming scent, and natural cleansing that is suitable for all skin types that the whole family can enjoy. It is formulated with 100 percent vegetable base and naturally derived ingredients, which includes oats that gently exfoliate and remove flaky, dull skin and excess oil. Infused with five therapeutic-grade essential oils, it moisturizes and soothes skin for a more radiant appearance and soft, supple feeling.

**Ingredients:** sodium palmate, sodium cocoate, water, glycerin, oat kernel flour, olive oil, sodium citrate, fractionated coconut oil (caprylic/capric triglyceride), oat bran, jojoba seed oil, wolfberry seed oil, oat kernel meal, aloe vera leaf extract, rosemary leaf extract

**Essential Oils:** Lavender, Coriander, Bergamot (Furocoumarin-free), Ylang Ylang, Geranium

## Lemon-Sandalwood Cleansing Soap

Lemon-Sandalwood Cleansing Soap is cleansing and purifying to the skin. Lemon oil is highly antifungal, so this soap can be effective at combating ringworm, athlete's foot, and other fungal infections. Sandalwood has been shown to protect the skin against viruses such as the human papilloma virus, which is related to herpes.

**Ingredients:** sodium palmate, sodium cocoate, water, glycerin, olive oil, sodium citrate, jojoba seed oil, aloe vera leaf extract, rosemary leaf extract, wolfberry seed oil, oat bran

**Essential Oils:** Lemon, Royal Hawaiian Sandalwood

## Melaleuca-Geranium Moisturizing Soap

Melaleuca-Geranium Moisturizing Soap is designed specifically to combat acne, while soothing and moisturizing the skin. Creating healthy skin naturally, this soap contains highly antiseptic essential oils to disinfect the skin.

**Ingredients:** sodium palmate, sodium cocoate, water, glycerin, olive oil, sodium citrate, jojoba seed oil, aloe vera leaf extract, rosemary leaf extract, wolfberry seed oil, oat bran

**Essential Oils:** Tea Tree, Geranium, Melaleuca Ericifolia, Vetiver

---

*Háloa Áina™ and Royal Hawaiian Sandalwood™ are trademarks of Jawmin, LLC.

Seventh Edition | **Essential Oils Desk Reference** | 243

## Morning Start® Moisturizing Soap

Morning Start Moisturizing Soap contains Lemongrass, Peppermint, Rosemary, and Juniper oils that revitalize the mind and awaken the skin each morning. Lemongrass has been documented as a powerful antifungal agent in clinical studies, ideal for combating ringworm, athlete's foot, and other fungal skin conditions.

**Ingredients:** sodium palmate, sodium cocoate, water, glycerin, olive oil, sodium citrate, jojoba seed oil, aloe vera leaf extract, rosemary leaf extract, wolfberry seed oil, oat bran

**Essential Oils:** Lemongrass, Rosemary, Juniper, Peppermint

## Peppermint-Cedarwood Moisturizing Soap

Peppermint-Cedarwood Moisturizing Soap offers ultra-cleansing benefits to cleanse and invigorate the skin. It also contains a blend of essential oils designed to combat pain and itching. Analgesic and pain-relieving, Peppermint-Cedarwood Moisturizing Soap combats tendon, ligament, bone, and muscle pain.

**Ingredients:** sodium palmate, sodium cocoate, water, glycerin, olive oil, sodium citrate, jojoba seed oil, aloe vera leaf extract, rosemary leaf extract, wolfberry seed oil, oat bran

**Essential Oils:** Peppermint, Cedarwood

## Sacred Mountain™ Moisturizing Soap

Sacred Mountain Moisturizing Soap soothes dehydrated skin, and the essential oil blend of Sacred Mountain promotes feelings of protection and empowerment. Designed for oily skin, this soap dissolves away excess sebum and gently exfoliates.

**Ingredients:** sodium palmate, sodium cocoate, water, glycerin, olive oil, sodium citrate, jojoba seed oil, aloe vera leaf extract, rosemary leaf extract, wolfberry seed oil, oat bran

**Essential Oils:** Black Spruce, Ylang Ylang, Idaho Balsam Fir, Cedarwood

## Shutran™ Bar Soap

Enriched with aloe, wolfberry seed oil, and Shutran essential oil blend, this vegan-friendly bar soap's creamy lather leaves skin feeling smooth, clean, and refreshed.

**Ingredients:** sodium palmate, sodium palm kernelate, water, glycerin, olive oil, shea butter, sodium gluconate, wolfberry seed oil, jojoba seed oil, carbon, aloe leaf extract

**Essential Oils:** Idaho Blue Spruce, Ylang Ylang, Ocotea, Hinoki, Davana, Cedarwood, Lavender, Coriander, Lemon, Northern Lights Black Spruce, Rosemary

## Thieves® Cleansing Soap

Thieves Cleansing Soap is enriched with the powerful Thieves essential oil blend, moisturizing plant oils, and botanical extracts to help cleanse, purify, and promote soft, healthy skin. Thieves is known for its antibacterial and antiseptic properties, making this soap ideal for purifying the skin.

**Ingredients:** sodium palmate, sodium cocoate, water, glycerin, olive oil, sodium citrate, jojoba seed oil, aloe vera leaf extract, rosemary leaf extract, wolfberry seed oil, oat bran

**Essential Oils:** Thieves Blend: [Clove, Lemon, Cinnamon Bark, Eucalyptus Radiata, Rosemary]

## Valor® Moisturizing Soap

Valor Moisturizing Soap is made with the empowering scent of Valor essential oil blend. Its all-natural ingredients help moisturize, cleanse, and rejuvenate the skin.

**Ingredients:** sodium palmate, sodium cocoate, water, glycerin, olive oil, sodium citrate, jojoba seed oil, aloe vera leaf extract, rosemary leaf extract, wolfberry seed oil, oat bran

**Essential Oils:** Valor Blend: [Black Spruce, Rosewood, Blue Tansy, Frankincense]

Personal Body Care | **Chapter 11**

# Foaming Hand Soaps

## Lavender Foaming Hand Soap

Lavender Foaming Hand Soap cleanses and conditions your hands without leaving them dry or irritated. Infused with Lavender essential oil, vitamin E, and aloe, this soap is effective yet gentle enough for the most sensitive skin.

**Ingredients:** water, decyl glucoside, cocamidopropyl hydroxysultaine, green tea leaf extract, vitamin A (retinyl palmitate), aloe vera leaf juice, p-Anisic acid, vitamin E (tocopheryl acetate), ginkgo biloba leaf extract, glycerin, citric acid, levulinic acid, phytic acid, cetyl hydroxyethylcellulose, sodium hydroxide, potassium sorbate

**Essential Oils:** Lavender, Myrrh, Lemon

**Caution:** Avoid contact with eyes. Not for internal use.

## Thieves® Foaming Hand Soap

Thieves Foaming Hand Soap is a natural hand-cleansing formula that contains Thieves essential oil blend, known for its powerful antibacterial properties. Thieves essential oil blend penetrates beneath the skin's surface, providing a long-lasting barrier of protection. This gentle, foaming soap also contains ingredients such as vitamin E, aloe vera, and ginkgo biloba to moisturize and soften the skin and provide a balanced pH to support the skin's natural moisture complex.

**Ingredients:** water, decyl glucoside, cocamidopropyl hydroxysultaine, alcohol denatured, aloe vera leaf juice, vitamin E (tocopheryl acetate), ginkgo biloba leaf extract, vitamin A (retinyl palmitate), camellia sinensis leaf extract, cetyl hydroxyethylcellulose, sodium hydroxide, citric acid

**Essential Oils:** Thieves: [Clove, Lemon, Cinnamon Bark, Eucalyptus Radiata, Rosemary], Orange

**Caution:** Avoid contact with eyes. Not for internal use.

# Safe, Natural Products
## (Do-It-Yourself)

## First-aid Spray

### Ingredients

- 2 drops Lavender
- 3 drops Tea Tree
- 2 drops Cypress
- 3 droppers (for dropping each oil on gauze)
- 8 oz. distilled water
- 1 spray bottle
- 1 sterile gauze pad with 3 drops of Lavender oil

### Directions

This first-aid spray is for minor cuts and abrasions. If you have a serious cut or wound, consult your physician.

Mix the three essential oils with the distilled water and put into a spray bottle. Clean all cuts and abrasions thoroughly and then spray the area with the first-aid spray.

You may want to cover the area with the sterile gauze to which you have applied 3 drops of Lavender.

This application should be repeated 2 times daily as necessary. After 3 days, you should allow the cut or abrasion to be exposed to the air, if possible.

## Spa Foot Scrub

### Ingredients

- ¼ cup sea salt or Epson salts
- Almond, coconut, avocado, or grape seed oil
- 10 to 15 drops of Lavender

### Directions

Treat your feet to a luxurious spa experience to exfoliate and pamper your feet. Mix ingredients and massage your feet with this mixture, which will soothe and soften your feet. Be sure to rinse and dry your feet when finished.

Seventh Edition | **Essential Oils Desk Reference** | 245

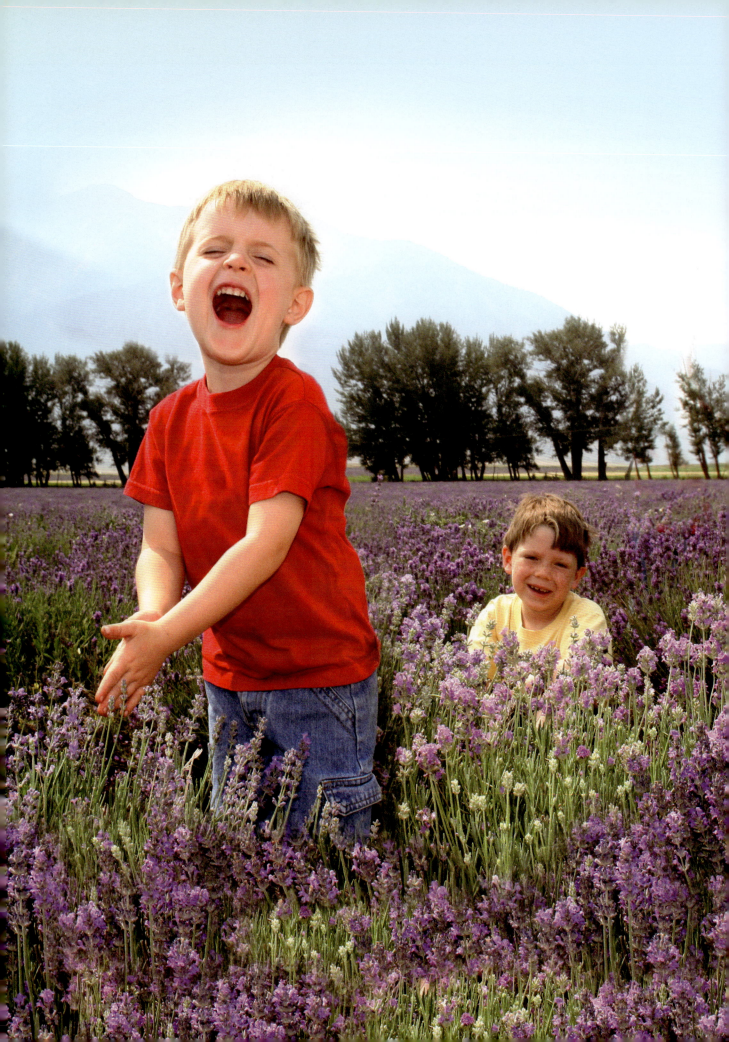

# Chapter 12
## Healthy Choices for Children

## KidScents® Body Care for Children

Our KidScents proprietary blends and other products are safe alternatives to products for children commonly found in the market today. You'll love our kid-focused essential oil blends and other products.

### KidScents Bath Gel

KidScents Bath Gel is a safe and gentle formula with a neutral pH balance perfect for young skin. It contains no mineral oils, synthetic perfumes, artificial colorings, or toxic ingredients.

**Ingredients:** water, decyl glucoside, glycerin, sorbitol, dimethyl sulfone (MSM), Roman chamomile flower extract, aloe vera leaf juice, panthenol, tocopheryl acetate (vitamin E), PG-hydroxyethylcellulose cocodimonium chloride, coneflower extract, grape seed extract, soap bark extract, soapwort extract, kiwi seed oil, jojoba seed oil, grapefruit seed extract, babassu seed oil, dimethicone PEG-8 meadowfoamate, hyaluronic acid, wheat germ oil, keratin, linoleic acid, linolenic acid

**Essential Oils:** Cedarwood, Geranium

**Directions:** Apply a small amount of KidScents Bath Gel to washcloth or directly to the skin. Rub gently, then rinse.

### KidScents Lotion

KidScents Lotion is safe, gentle, and pH neutral, ideal for young skin. It contains no mineral oils, synthetic perfumes, artificial colorings, or toxic ingredients.

**Ingredients:** water, dimethyl sulfone (MSM), glyceryl stearate, stearic acid, glycerin, grape seed extract, sodium hyaluronate, sorbitol, rose hip seed oil, shea butter, mango seed butter, wheat germ oil, kukui seed oil, lecithin, safflower seed oil, apricot kernel oil, sweet almond oil, vitamin E (tocopheryl acetate), vitamin A (retinyl palmitate), jojoba seed oil, sesame seed oil, marigold flower extract, matricaria (Roman chamomile) flower extract, green tea leaf extract, St. John's wort extract, algae extract, aloe vera leaf juice, ascorbic acid, ginkgo biloba leaf extract

**Essential Oils:** Cedarwood, Coriander, Geranium, Western Red Cedar, Bergamot (Furocoumarin-free), Ylang Ylang

**Directions:** Apply liberally to skin as needed.

### KidScents Shampoo

KidScents Shampoo contains the finest natural ingredients for gently cleansing children's delicate hair. A mild formula designed to provide the perfect pH balance for children's hair, it contains no mineral oils, synthetic perfumes, artificial colorings, or toxic ingredients.

**Ingredients:** water, decyl glucoside, dimethyl sulfone (MSM), Roman chamomile flower extract, aloe vera leaf juice, vitamin B5 (panthenol), vitamin E (tocopheryl acetate), babassu seed oil, coneflower extract, kiwi seed oil, jojoba seed oil, grape seed extract, dimethicone PEG-8 meadowfoamate, glycerin, hyaluronic acid, wheat germ extract, grapefruit seed extract, keratin, linoleic acid, linolenic acid

**Essential Oils:** Tangerine, Lemon

**Directions:** Apply a small amount to hair. Lather, then rinse.

### KidScents Slique® Toothpaste

KidScents Slique Toothpaste is a safe, natural alternative to commercial brands of toothpaste. Formulated with Slique Essence and Thieves essential oil blends, this toothpaste gently cleans teeth and tastes great without synthetic dyes or flavors. Slique Essence is antibacterial, antifungal, a lipid regulator, and a glucose regulator. Thieves is antiseptic and antimicrobial and combats plaque-causing microorganisms.

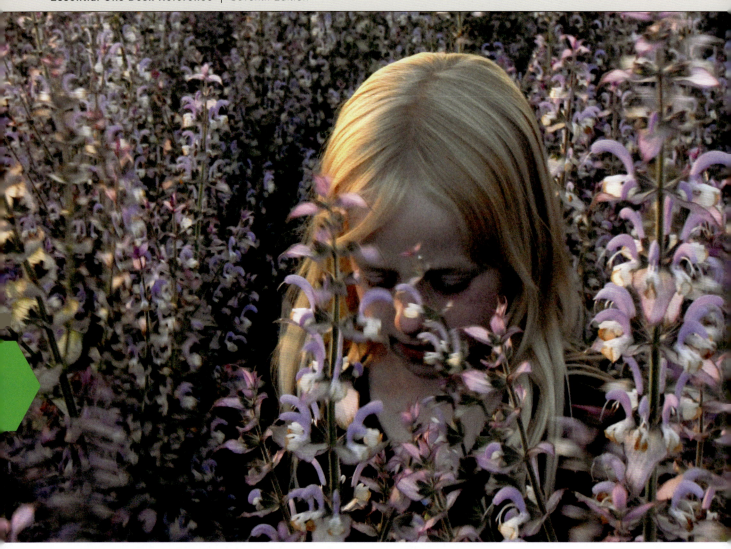

KidScents Slique Toothpaste is perfect for children of all ages, and it makes a great training toothpaste for children during the crucial first years while they develop their primary teeth. Calcium carbonate, baking soda, and xylitol are used as tooth and gum health agents. It includes an amazing blend of highly antiviral, antiseptic, antibacterial, and anti-infectious essential oils.

**Ingredients:** water, calcium carbonate, coconut oil, baking soda (sodium bicarbonate), vegetable glycerin, xylitol, xanthan gum, stevia leaf extract, lecithin

**Essential Oils:** Grapefruit, Tangerine, Spearmint, Lemon, Ocotea, Clove, Cinnamon Bark, Eucalyptus Radiata, Rosemary

**Directions:** Brush teeth thoroughly after meals or at least 2 times daily.

**Caution:** Use caution to keep KidScents Slique Toothpaste out of children's eyes.

## KidScents Tender Tush

KidScents Tender Tush is a gentle ointment designed to protect and nourish young skin and promote healing. This ointment soothes dry, chapped skin and offers protection for delicate skin. It is also great for expectant mothers who are concerned about having stretch marks.

**Ingredients:** coconut oil, cocoa seed butter, olive fruit oil, sweet almond oil, beeswax, wheat germ oil

**Essential Oils:** Royal Hawaiian Sandalwood, Coriander, Roman Chamomile, Lavender, Frankincense, Bergamot (furocoumarin-free), Cistus, Ylang Ylang, Geranium

**Directions:** Apply liberally to diaper area as often as needed to help soothe diaper rash, redness, or irritation.

Healthy Choices for Children | **Chapter 12**

# KidScents Nutritional Support for Children

## KidScents MightyVites™

KidScents MightyVites are great-tasting, chewable multivitamin tablets, perfect for children's developing bodies, including increased immune function, brain development, and bone and joint health. Made with Ningxia wolfberry (*Lycium barbarum*), KidScents MightyVites contain superfruits, plants, and vegetables that deliver the full spectrum of vitamins, minerals, antioxidants, and phytonutrients in their whole, synergistic, and easily-absorbable form. KidScents MightyVites come in two flavors, orange cream and mixed berry.

**Ingredients:** vitamin A (alpha and beta carotene), vitamin C (ascorbic acid) from oranges, vitamin D (as cholecalciferol), vitamin E (as d-α tocopheryl acid succinate), vitamin K (as phytonadione), thiamin (vitamin B1 as thiamine mononitrate), riboflavin (vitamin B2), niacin (as niacinamide), vitamin B6 (as pyridoxine HCl), vitamin B6 (as pyridoxal-5-phosphate), folate (folic acid), vitamin B12 (as methylcobalamin), biotin (vitamin H), pantothenic acid (as d-calcium pantothenate), iodine (as potassium iodide), magnesium (as magnesium oxide), zinc (from zinc yeast complex), selenium (from selenium yeast complex), copper (from copper yeast complex), chromium (from chromium yeast complex), sorbitol, fructose, natural flavors, lecithin (soy), citric acid, silica, magnesium stearate, dicalcium phosphate

**Directions:** Children ages 6-12 years old, take 3 chewable tablets daily prior to or with meals.

**Allergen Warning:** Contains an ingredient derived from soy

## KidScents MightyVites™
## Orange Cream Flavor

**Additional Ingredients:** Proprietary Blend: orange juice powder, Ningxia wolfberry fruit, malic acid, broccoli floret, methylsulfonylmethane (MSM), barley grass, curcumins, citrus flavonoids (from tangerine), spirulina algae, grape skin powder, tocotrienols (from natural palm oil), olive leaf extract, boron (as boron AAC), lutein (from marigold flowers)

## KidScents MightyVites™
## Wild Berry Flavor

**Additional Ingredients:** Proprietary Blend: grape skin powder, Ningxia wolfberry fruit, cherry juice powder, strawberry juice powder, malic acid, broccoli floret, methylsulfonylmethane (MSM), barley grass, curcumins, citrus flavonoids (from tangerine), spirulina algae, tocotrienols (from natural palm oil), olive leaf extract, boron (as boron AAC), lutein (from marigold flowers)

## KidScents MightyZyme™

KidScents Mightyzyme is a special formulation containing nine different digestive enzymes and other nutrients designed to support healthy digestion in children. It also aids in the relief of occasional symptoms, including fullness, pressure, bloating, gas, pain, or minor cramping that may occur after eating.

**Ingredients:** folate (as folic acid), calcium (from calcium carbonate), Proprietary Mightyzyme Blend: protease 3.0, protease 4.5, protease 6.0 amylase, peptidase, bromelain, cellulase, lipase, alfalfa leaf, carrot root, carnauba wax, fructose, maltodextrin, apple juice concentrate, coconut oil, silica

**Essential Oils:** Peppermint

**Directions:** For children age 6 or older: Chew 1 tablet 3 times daily prior to or with meals. For children under 6 years of age: Chew 1/2 to 1 tablet (crushed if needed and mixed with yogurt or applesauce).

Seventh Edition | **Essential Oils Desk Reference** | 249

# KidScents Oil Collection

The KidScents Oil Collection includes six oil blends formulated especially for kids to help them through the common ups and downs of childhood. See below.

## Bite Buster™

Bite Buster is an excellent insect repellant formulated especially for kids.

**Ingredients:** caprylic/capric glycerides, Idaho Tansy, Citronella, Palo Santo

**Directions: Aromatic:** Diffuse up to 1 hour 3 times daily. **Topical:** Recommended application is for children ages 2-12. To be applied only by a trusted adult or under adult supervision. Apply 2-4 drops directly to desired area. Dilution not required, except for the most sensitive skin. Use as needed.

## GeneYus™

Diffuse GeneYus to help young minds focus and concentrate on projects.

**Ingredients:** fractionated coconut oil, Sacred Frankincense, Blue Cypress, Cedarwood, Idaho Blue Spruce, Palo Santo, Melissa, Northern Lights Black Spruce, almond oil, Bergamot, Myrrh, Vetiver, Geranium, Royal Hawaiian Sandalwood, Ylang Ylang, Hyssop, Rose

**Directions: Aromatic:** Diffuse up to 1 hour 3 times daily. **Topical:** Recommended application is for children ages 2-12. To be applied only by a trusted adult or under adult supervision. Apply 2-4 drops directly to desired area. Dilution not required, except for the most sensitive skin. Use as needed.

**Caution:** Avoid direct sunlight and UV rays for up to 12 hours after applying product.

## Owie™

Apply Owie topically to improve the appearance of your child's skin and to help heal a wound.

**Ingredients:** caprylic/capric glycerides, Idaho Balsam Fir, Tea Tree, Helichrysum, Elemi, Cistus, Hinoki, Clove

**Directions: Aromatic:** Diffuse up to 1 hour 3 times daily. **Topical:** Recommended application is for children ages 2-12. To be applied only by a trusted adult or under adult supervision. Apply to desired area as needed. Dilution not required, except for the most sensitive skin. Use as needed.

## SleepyIze™

SleepyIze calms and relaxes the mind and body prior to bedtime for kids.

**Ingredients:** caprylic/capric glycerides, Lavender, Geranium, Roman Chamomile, Tangerine, Bergamot, Sacred Frankincense, Valerian, Ruta (Rue)

**Directions: Aromatic:** Diffuse up to 1 hour 3 times daily. **Topical:** Recommended application is for children ages 2-12. To be applied only by a trusted adult or under adult supervision. Apply 2-4 drops directly to desired area. Dilution not required, except for the most sensitive skin. Use as needed.

**Caution:** Avoid direct sunlight or UV rays for up to 12 hours after applying product.

## SniffleEase™

SniffleEase is a refreshing, rejuvenating blend formulated just for kids for when they have congestion.

**Ingredients:** caprylic/capric glycerides, Eucalyptus Blue, Palo Santo, Lavender, Dorado Azul, Ravintsara, Myrtle, Eucalyptus Globulus, Marjoram, Pine, Eucalyptus Citriodora, Cypress, Eucalyptus Radiata, Black Spruce, Peppermint

**Directions: Aromatic:** Diffuse up to 1 hour 3 times daily. **Topical:** Recommended application is for children ages 2-12. To be applied only by a trusted adult or under adult supervision. Apply 2-4 drops directly to desired area. Dilution not required, except for the most sensitive skin. Use as needed.

## TummyGize™

TummyGize™ is a quieting, relaxing blend that can be applied to little tummies that are upset. It also supports proper digestion.

**Ingredients:** caprylic/capric glycerides, Spearmint, Peppermint, Tangerine, Fennel, Anise, Ginger, Cardamom

**Directions: Aromatic:** Diffuse up to 1 hour 3 times daily. **Topical:** Recommended application is for children ages 2-12. To be applied only by a trusted adult or under adult supervision. Apply 2-4 drops directly to desired area. Dilution not required, except for the most sensitive skin. Use as needed.

**Caution:** Avoid direct sunlight and UV rays for up to 12 hours after applying product.

# Chapter 13
## Fortifying Your Home with Essential Oils

## Protecting Your Home

Essential oils have been used since the beginning of time for a vast array of applications. They were most noticeably used for religious ceremonies, healing, perfumery, cosmetics, beautifying the body, etc.

Over the last three or four decades, the perfume and food-flavoring industries have used the majority of the essential oil production in the world for their purposes. However, in the last few years, since essential oils have made their re-entrance into our modern world on a more dramatic scale, they are being used for many things.

If you start reading labels, you will be astounded at how many products contain essential oils. It is easy to understand why they would be used in toothpastes, mouthwashes, deodorants, perfumes, sprays, sauces, preservatives, liquors, air fresheners, and pharmaceuticals.

But could you imagine that they would be used for glue, tape, cement, paint, paint removers, upholstery materials, finishing materials, carbon paper, crayons, ink, ribbons, writing paper, labels, wrappers, polishes, cleaners, solvent lubricating oils and waxes, grease, rubber toys, waterproofing compounds, and plastics?

What you will read in this chapter are but a few of the many ways you can use essential oils to deodorize and protect your home. It is for you to make those discoveries and share them with your family and friends.

## Thieves® Products

Protect yourself from harmful bacteria, naturally. Thieves products provide a natural, safe, and highly effective defense against germs that can make us sick. Every day we touch door handles, tabletops, and other surfaces covered with bacteria. Chemical-filled antibacterial soaps and hand sanitizers may or may not be effective but are filled with synthetic ingredients that can be highly toxic.

All-natural Thieves household products contain the proven antibacterial properties of Thieves essential oil blend, other complementary essential oils, and plant-based ingredients. With their eco-friendly packaging and effective results, Thieves natural household products should be in every home.

### Thieves Automatic Dishwasher Powder

This gentle yet effective formula uses Thieves, Lemongrass, and Orange essential oils combined with other naturally derived ingredients to safely tackle even stuck-on food, and it dries without hard water spots for sparkling dishes.

**Ingredients:** sodium carbonate, sodium citrate dihydrate, sodium percarbonate, sodium silicate, sapindus mukorossi fruit extract, rice oligodextrin, silica, protease, sunflower seed oil, amylase

**Essential Oils:** Orange, Lemongrass, Clove, Lemon, Cinnamon Bark, Rosemary, Eucalyptus Radiata

**Directions:** Place 1 scoop in the dishwasher dispensers. Use 2 scoops for heavy loads or with hard water.

**Caution:** Keep out of reach of children. In case of eye contact, immediately flush thoroughly with water. If swallowed or inhaled, drink plenty of water and seek medical help. Flush immediately if product comes in contact with skin.

Essential Oils Desk Reference | Seventh Edition

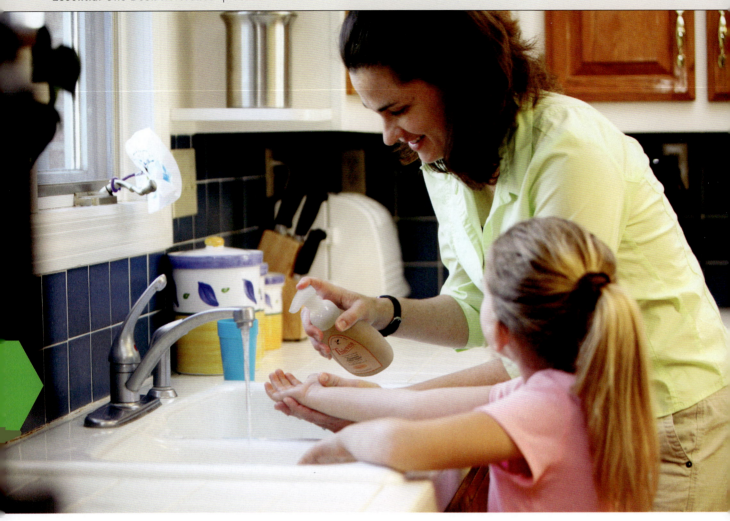

## Thieves Dish Soap

Thieves Dish Soap naturally and effectively cleans your dishes without chemicals, dyes, or synthetics. Featuring Thieves, Jade Lemon, Bergamot, and other plant-based ingredients, this dish soap leaves dishes sparkling clean.

**Ingredients:** water, decyl glucoside, sodium lauroyl lactylate, lauryl glucoside, sodium oleate, caprylyl glucoside, sodium sesquicarbonate

**Essential Oils:** Jade Lemon, Bergamot (furocoumarin-free), Thieves essential oil blend: [Clove, Lemon, Cinnamon Bark, Eucalyptus Radiata, Rosemary]

**Directions:** Dispense a small amount of soap with warm running water. Add additional soap as needed.

## Thieves Foaming Hand Soap

A natural alternative to chemical soaps, Thieves Foaming Hand Soap contains the essential oil blend Thieves, known for its powerful cleansing and antibacterial properties. Thieves essential oil blend penetrates beneath the skin's surface, providing a long-lasting barrier of protection. This gentle, foaming soap also contains ingredients such as vitamin E, aloe vera, and *Ginkgo biloba* to moisturize and soften the skin and provide a balanced pH to support the skin's natural moisture complex.

**Ingredients:** water, decyl glucoside, cocamidopropyl hydroxysultaine, alcohol denatured, aloe vera leaf juice, tocopheryl acetate, *Ginkgo biloba* leaf extract, retinyl palmitate, *Camellia sinensis* leaf extract, cetyl hydroxyethylcellulose, sodium hydroxide, citric acid

**Essential Oils:** Thieves essential oil blend: [Clove, Lemon, Cinnamon Bark, Eucalyptus Radiata, Rosemary], Orange

**Directions:** Pump foam onto hands, lather, and then rinse thoroughly.

Fortifying Your Home with Essential Oils | Chapter 13

## Thieves Fruit & Veggie Soak

Formulated with DiGize, Purification, and Thieves essential oil blends, the Thieves Fruit & Veggie Soak safely and efficiently cleans large amounts of produce at one time.

**Ingredients:** water, decyl glucoside, glycerin, citric acid, sodium citrate

**Essential Oils:** Tarragon, Ginger, Peppermint, Juniper, Fennel, Lemongrass, Clove, Rosemary, Citronella, Anise, Lemon, Patchouli, Cinnamon Bark, Tea Tree, Lavandin, Eucalyptus Radiata, Tunisian Myrtle, Moroccan Myrtle

**Directions:** Pour 1 fl. oz. (2 tablespoons) for every gallon of water. Make enough solution to completely cover produce. Soak produce in solution for 1-2 minutes. Rinse under running water.

## Thieves Fruit & Veggie Spray

Powered by five essential oils, the Thieves Fruit & Veggie Spray is formulated to quickly and naturally clean fruits and vegetables.

**Ingredients:** water, citric acid, decyl glucoside, glycerin, sodium citrate

**Essential Oils:** Lime, Thieves essential oil blend: [Clove, Lemon, Cinnamon Bark, Eucalyptus Radiata, Rosemary]

**Directions:** Spray to cover produce. Rub for 30 seconds. Rinse under running water.

## Thieves Household Cleaner

Thieves Household Cleaner offers a nontoxic, biodegradable, all-purpose cleaning solution using therapeutic-grade essential oils as emulsifiers and germ killers. Containing Thieves essential oil blend, proven in a 1997 Weber State University (Ogden, Utah) study to kill over 99.96 percent of bacteria like *Pseudonomas aeroginosa*, this cleaner is fully biodegradable and complies with EPA standards.

**Ingredients:** water, alkyl polyglucoside, sodium methyl 2-sulfolaurate, disodium 2-sulfolaurate, tetrasodium glutamate diacetate

**Essential Oils:** Thieves essential oil blend: [Clove, Lemon, Cinnamon Bark, Eucalyptus Radiata, Rosemary], Lemon

**Directions:** Use for household cleaning purposes as needed. Dilute or use straight for extra strength. Dilution ratios are listed on the label.

## Thieves Laundry Soap

With a plant-based formula, Thieves Laundry Soap gently and naturally washes clothes without using chemicals or synthetics. Natural enzymes and powerful essential oils enhance the formula's strength and give a pleasant light citrus scent.

**Ingredients:** water, decyl glucoside, sodium oleate, glycerin, caprylyl glucoside, lauryl glucoside, sodium chloride, sodium gluconate, carboxymethyl cellulose, alpha-amylase, protease, lipase

**Essential Oils:** Jade Lemon, Bergamot (furocoumarin-free), Thieves essential oil blend: [Clove, Lemon, Cinnamon Bark, Eucalyptus Radiata, Rosemary]

**Directions:** Follow garment-care label instructions. Add clothes. Start machine and add the proper amount of soap for load size. Standard: ½ cap for conventional washers; ¼ cap for High Efficiency (HE) washers. Adjust for smaller, larger, and heavily soiled loads. PRETREAT: Pour onto stained fabric, gently rub, and soak. This natural formula is safe to add directly to clothes.

## Thieves Spray

Thieves Spray is an all-natural, petrochemical-free antiseptic spray ideal for purifying small surfaces like doorknobs, handles, toilet seats, and more. Containing Thieves essential oil blend, proven in a 1997 Weber State University (Ogden, Utah) study to kill bacteria like *Pseudonomas aeroginosa,* this antiseptic spray may be used to spray any surface that needs cleaning and protection from dust, mold, and other undesirable microorganisms.

**Ingredients:** alcohol denatured, water, caprylic/capric triglyceride, lecithin, polysorbate 80

**Essential Oils:** Thieves essential oil blend: [Clove, Lemon, Cinnamon Bark, Eucalyptus Radiata, Rosemary]

**Directions:** Spray on surfaces such as kitchen and bathroom counters, public seating, and anywhere germs may be present. Clean as needed.

## Thieves Waterless Hand Purifier

An all-natural hand cleaner, Thieves Waterless Hand Purifier conveniently promotes good hygiene whenever water or washing facilities are not available. This purifier contains the essential oil blend of Thieves, known for its powerful antibacterial properties, which penetrates the skin as the ethanol evaporates. It also contains active moisturizing ingredients to prevent dry skin.

Seventh Edition | **Essential Oils Desk Reference** | 253

**Ingredients:** denatured ethanol SD-38B (denatured with Peppermint essential oil), water, aloe vera leaf powder, vegetable glycerin, hydroxypropyl cellulose

**Essential Oils:** Thieves essential oil blend: [Clove, Lemon, Cinnamon Bark, Eucalyptus Radiata, and Rosemary]

**Directions:** Use daily as often as necessary to purify hands. Apply a nickel-size amount to the palm of the hand and rub in until completely absorbed

## Thieves Wipes

Thieves Wipes are antiseptic cleaners infused with Thieves essential oil blend, proven in a 1997 Weber State University (Ogden, Utah) study to kill bacteria like *Pseudonomas*

*aeroginosa* and are ideal for use on door handles, toilet seats, and any surface in need of cleaning and protection from dust, mold, and undesirable microorganisms.

**Ingredients:** pure grain alcohol, deionized water, soy lecithin, and polysorbate 80

**Essential Oils:** Thieves essential oil blend: [Clove, Lemon, Cinnamon Bark, Eucalyptus Radiata, Rosemary]

**Directions:** Wipe surfaces to clean as needed. Ideal for use on door handles, toilet seats, and anywhere undesirable organisms may be present.

# Personal Uses for Essential Oils

There are far too many uses of essential oils to list here; nevertheless, they have really taken their place in our world. You will have fun and many amazing experiences as you use them in your daily household activities. How nice to open the dryer door and take a breath of the fresh smell of Lemon as you take out your clothes.

## Laundry Freshener
**Ingredients:**
- 2 drops Lavender (or Lemon)
- 2 drops Tea Tree

**Directions:**

There is nothing new about the idea of scented laundry. Our ancestors used to dry their clothes on rosemary or lavender bushes to scent them. It was also popular to lay sprigs of lavender between the clean linens in cupboards to keep them smelling fresh.

Today you may add Lavender, known for its fresh scent; Tea Tree, known for its disinfecting power; or any other oil of your choice to a washcloth and put this into your washer with the rest of your laundry. You may also add a washcloth with Lavender, Lemon, or other essential oil to your dryer for fresh smelling linens and towels.

## Kitchen Deodorizing Spray
**Ingredients:**

- 2 drops Rosemary
- 4 drops Lemon
- 2 drops Eucalyptus Globulus
- 4 drops Lavender
- 1 quart distilled water

**Directions:**

The kitchen and bathroom are often sources of odors and bacteria. This spray deodorizes and cleans the air instead of merely covering up odors.

Fill a 1-quart spray bottle with the distilled water, add the essential oils, and mix by shaking. You may use this to deodorize and freshen the air after cooking or to wipe work areas, cupboards, sinks, tiles, or woodwork. It will deodorize and help keep the areas disinfected.

Use as directed. Kitchen deodorizing spray is safe for your family and the environment.

Fortifying Your Home with Essential Oils | **Chapter 13**

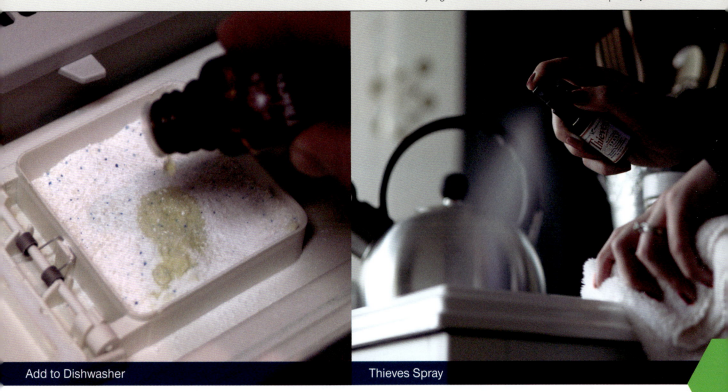

Add to Dishwasher

Thieves Spray

### Essential Oils for Cooking

Many essential oils and some essential oil blends may be used as ingredients for cooking and baking, in addition to their being used as supplements. Please see the Vitality essential oils and blends and their usage directions in Chapter 6 (Single Oils) and Chapter 7 (Essential Oil Blends).

### Directions:

When using essential oils for cooking and baking, keep in mind that they are very concentrated and that you will need only 1 or 2 drops per recipe that serves at least 4 people if the oils are added after cooking and baking. However, you may find that you will need more drops of oils if they are added before cooking and baking.

### Examples

Here are some examples of uses. Be creative; see what your family likes. You may find that you can include the oils in many of your own favorite recipes. The essential oils are better added at the end of cooking or boiling to keep the flavor strong.

- Season salad dressings with Lemon Vitality, Rosemary Vitality, Clove Vitality, Orange Vitality, Cinnamon Bark Vitality, Tangerine Vitality, Peppermint Vitality, or any other oil or blend of your choice.
- Season cakes, frostings, puddings, fruit pies, and salads with Lemon Vitality, Orange Vitality, Cinnamon Bark Vitality, Lavender Vitality, Clove Vitality, Spearmint Vitality, Nutmeg Vitality, Peppermint Vitality, or any other oil or blend of your choice.
- Flavor homemade ice cream with Lavender Vitality, Lemon Vitality, Orange Vitality, Peppermint Vitality, Slique Essence, or any other oil or blend of your choice.
- Season meat with Oregano Vitality, Basil Vitality, Clove Vitality, Rosemary Vitality, Nutmeg Vitality, Thyme Vitality, or any other oil or blend of your choice.
- Add Lavender Vitality, Lemon Vitality, Orange Vitality, Tangerine Vitality, Clove Vitality, Spearmint Vitality, Cinnamon Bark Vitality, Peppermint Vitality, Slique Essence, or any other oil or blend of your choice to your favorite herbal tea after brewing.
- For a cold drink that even children will love, add Lemon Vitality, Orange Vitality, Spearmint Vitality, Peppermint Vitality, Citrus Fresh Vitality, Slique Essence, or any other oil or blend of your choice to a pitcher of iced, distilled water as an alternative to sweetened sodas.
- Flavor honey by stirring in an essential oil or blend of your choice. If the honey is too solid to stir, cook it on low heat until it becomes liquid and then stir in the essential oil.

Have fun cooking and baking with the essential oils and blends of your choice.

Seventh Edition | **Essential Oils Desk Reference** | 255

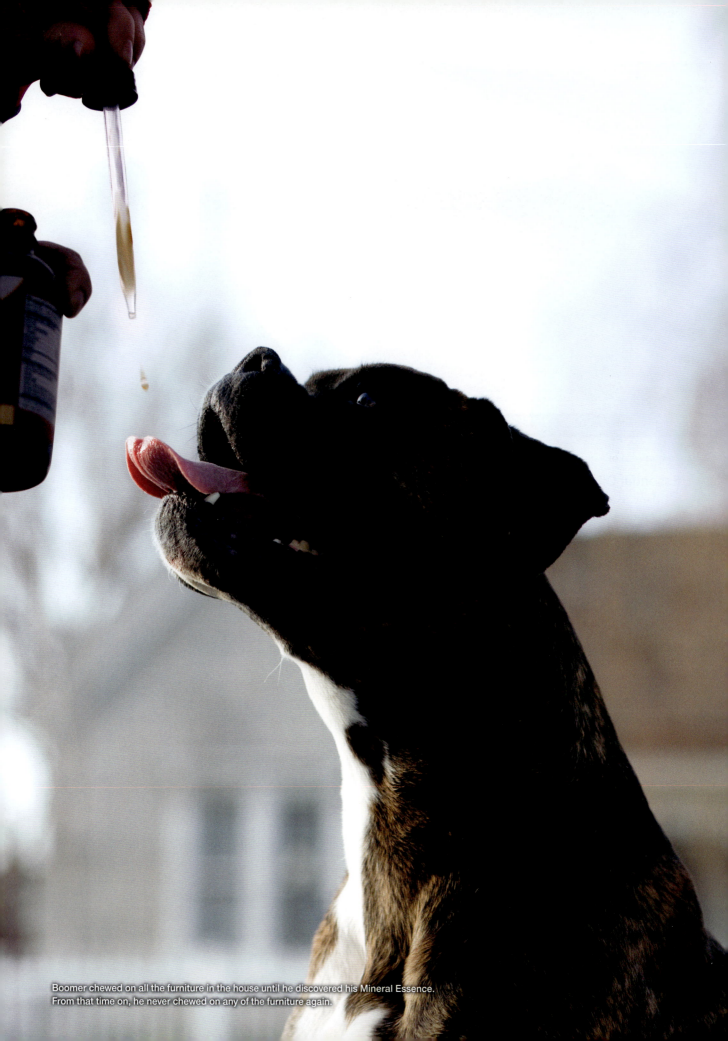

Boomer chewed on all the furniture in the house until he discovered his Mineral Essence.
From that time on, he never chewed on any of the furniture again.

# Chapter 14
## Animal Care

# Veterinary Medicine

Essential oils have been used very successfully on many different kinds of animals, and veterinarians have now witnessed the use of essential oils with almost every form of the animal kingdom. The amazing realization that every animal in nature would be exposed to nature's powerful medicine has propelled the use of essential oils to include everything from honey bees to elephants. In general, animals respond to essential oils in much the same way as humans.

## How Much Should I Use?

Most animals are more sensitive to the effects of essential oils than humans. They often seem to have a natural affinity to the healing influence of the oils. Hair follicles may enhance the absorption of essential oils. As animals clearly have more hair follicles than humans, we can see the potential for animals to effectively absorb essential oils, even from exposure to basic diffusion.

The sensitivity to essential oils, which was once thought to be purely an animal trait, may have a great deal to do with the density, or number, of hair follicles on a particular animal. The more follicles per square inch of skin, the more enhanced the absorption of essential oils. Therefore, cats can absorb more essential oils through their skin more efficiently than a horse or a dog with a coarser hair coat. When we consider which animal species seem most sensitive to exposure to essential oils, it often has a strong correlation with density of hair follicles.

While adjusting the dosage proportionately based on the animal's body weight is a sound first start, one must consider this enhanced ability for absorption as well. It would seem logical that if the protocol for a human being weighing 160 pounds calls for 3-5 drops, then a horse at 1,600 pounds or more could use as much as 10 times that amount, and a dog weighing 16 pounds would need as little as one tenth of that amount. Although this increase for the horse is likely accurate for oral use, topical applications may actually require less, considering hair follicle interactions.

In animals smaller than humans, it has remained mostly accurate to adjust the protocols based on body weight. If one drop of an essential oil can aid a headache in a 160-pound human, a bird weighing less than 1 pound may require only the minute amounts reached by diffusion to attain therapeutic levels. Thankfully, veterinarians have documented wide ranges of safety within the animal kingdom when truly therapeutic-grade oils are used, and even small birds can use essential oils in wondrous ways.

Start with protocols that are known to be used for your particular species, using small amounts initially and then gradually increasing in concentration and frequency. It is easy to reapply essential oils in an hour or more if additional oil is needed, but it's impossible to take back drops that were applied to the skin.

While applying oils to the feet has long been considered the safest location for humans, evidence suggests that animals carry many more toxins within their foot pads. Applying essential oils (especially neat) to the pads and feet of dogs and cats may create an uncomfortable detoxification of every-day exposures to toxins such as fabric softeners, floor cleaners, lawn and ice melting chemicals, outdoor pollutants, topical medications, air fresheners, odor eliminators, and more. For large animals such as horses and cows, applying to the hooves and along the frog or coronet band region remains a well-tolerated site.

In the case of small dogs, cats, and exotic pets, essential oils should generally be diluted before applying. Many factors play a role in why animals are more sensitive to essential oils than humans, and understanding each species' unique needs for dilution, oil selection, and applications of oils is mandatory.

Some species are truly more sensitive to the biochemicals in the oils than humans. Cats are notoriously deficient in the Cytochrome P450 liver metabolism pathway. This pathway is used for the metabolism and excretion of all sorts of chemicals from their body, including traditional

Seventh Edition | **Essential Oils Desk Reference** | 257

medications. This fact has made cats unique in veterinary medicine, no matter what the substance may be to which they are exposed.

It is wise to use caution when choosing oils high in phenols and eugenols (such as Oregano, Thyme, Clove, and Cinnamon) with cats because they can be extremely sensitive to these stronger oils. These oils should be used in only high rates of dilution; for example, the Kitty Raindrop® Technique contains 4 drops each of Oregano (or Plectranthus Oregano), Thyme, Basil, Cypress, Wintergreen, Marjoram, and Peppermint in 30 ml (1 ounce) of V-6 Vegetable Oil Complex, resulting in an approximate 95% dilution.

## Percentages

Understanding percentages of dilution can be difficult for even the most experienced aromatherapist. Clear communication about how to dilute essential oils is critical for proper use, especially for animals. Describing dilution in multiple ways can be helpful for those of us without a mathematical strong suit. Confusion can ensue when someone is uncertain if the oil should be used at 90% "strong" or 90% "diluted." In most situations, it may be best to clearly describe the dilution of essential oils in terms of how many drops of essential oils are added to a certain quantity of carrier oil.

A solution referred to as 90% can be thought of as 1 drop of essential oil in 9 drops of carrier oil. An 80% solution will be 2 drops of essential oil in 8 drops of carrier oil. Below is a quick reference for the percent of dilution in terms of drops of essential oil per carrier oil.

90% = 1 drop essential oil + 9 drops carrier oil
80% = 2 drops essential oil + 8 drops carrier oil
70% = 3 drops essential oil + 7 drops carrier oil
60% = 4 drops essential oil + 6 drops carrier oil
50% = 5 drops essential oil + 5 drops carrier oil
*(also called 50:50=1 drop essential oil + 1 drop carrier oil)*
40% = 6 drops essential oil + 4 drops carrier oil
30% = 7 drops essential oil + 3 drops carrier oil
20% = 8 drops essential oil + 2 drops carrier oil
10% = 9 drops essential oil + 1 drop carrier oil

## General Guidelines
• For small animals (cats, small dogs, and exotics): Apply 3-5 drops of diluted (80-90%) oil mixture per application.
• For larger animals (large dogs, goats, and pigs): Apply 3-5 drops neat (dilute if using oils high in phenol) per application.

• For large animals (cattle, horses, and elephants): Apply 10-15 drops neat (dilute if using oils high in phenol) per application.

## Aversions to Essential Oils

For those new to essential oils, start with very light, "species specific" applications. When animals appear to "dislike" essential oils, it is often because they have been exposed to an inappropriate use of the essential oil. Aversion to a negative event is strongly ingrained in an animal's memory, according to a lecture presented by Dr. Temple Grandin (PhD and professor of animal science at Colorado State University.) Therefore, if a situation resulted in essential oils accidently coming into contact with sensitive tissues (eyes), the use and smell of essential oils in the future, may "remind" an animal of that past occurrence, and an aversion is born.

Animals truly do have a more acute sense of smell, and often this is interpreted as an aversion to essential oils. In actuality, it is purely that the animal has much less need to be in close proximity to an essential oil to smell it. Surely, we can recognize how strong an essential oil smells when the bottle is directly under our nose. Imagine that intensity of smell being appreciated from across the room, and you will start to understand how animals may perceive an essential oil as too intense when we bring a bottle close to them. We do not need to avoid using essential oils around our animals, but we do need to understand and be respectful that some animals can smell the essential oil from across the room—with the bottle still closed!

## Detoxifications to Essential Oils

Many veterinarians are currently documenting the use of Young Living Essential Oils in veterinary practices around the world.

Many cases concerning essential oil safety and use have been wrongly interpreted due to the lack of pre-exposure blood work. When oils are applied to an animal, it is often because it is already ill. It is important to note that true toxicity to nontherapeutic-grade oils does exist, as well it should. Adulterated, synthetic, and contaminated oils are just not tolerated by sensitive animals with highly intelligent bodies.

Consulting with a veterinarian and having blood and urine evaluations prior to starting the use of essential oils is always recommended. Then, working with your veterinarian, the frequency of follow up examinations and laboratory testing can be determined.

Animal Care | Chapter 14

# Techniques for Different Animal Species

The use of essential oils has been documented in almost every species; however, each species has a slightly different set of techniques and methods used to safely and easily expose them to essential oils.

## Fish

Fish are exposed to plant matter decomposing in their water environment. Peppermint and Lemon essential oils and the oil blend Purification have been used frequently and with great results for a multitude of concerns from fungal infections, parasites, and bacterial concerns.

Start by introducing very small amounts of oil into a glass aquarium or pond by dipping a toothpick into the oil and then putting it into the water. After several days, amounts can be increased according to the volume of water in the enclosure. Often when drops of essential oil are placed on the water's surface, fish will orally ingest the oil droplets. This is truly an amazing sight to see.

## Insects

Likewise, insects can be affected by essential oils. For example, honey bees are suffering from mysterious conditions. Dripping essential oils like Frankincense onto cotton balls and placing them in or around the beehive is currently being used to boost honey bee health.

Essential oils are also used as pest control to repel insects.

## Birds

Birds (especially parrots) are a more recent addition to the world of veterinary aromatherapy. Pet birds are extremely sensitive to household toxins, and even the spray of an air freshener or the burning of a candle can be dangerous to a bird. Since many household fragrances are created with poor grade, adulterated, or synthetic essential oils, it was commonly thought that all essential oils were toxic to birds. This has been found to be untrue. While birds have a distinct way in which they should be exposed to essential oils, they not only benefit from but also thrive with the addition of essential oils into their lives.

A favorite technique that is being used currently with thousands of birds is the Feather Spray Recipe. This amazing spray was created by Leigh Foster and carries benefits for everything from bacterial, viral, and fungal conditions to cancer prevention and immune system support.

### Feather Spray Recipe

Place 20 drops of Lavender, 20 drops of Lemon, and 20 drops of Orange essential oils into a 4-ounce glass spray bottle. Add distilled water to fill the bottle. Shake well before each application and then mist the bird directly with the spray up to 2 times a day. Birds love this spray, including those who routinely dislike a shower from a traditional spray bottle.

### Diffusing

Diffusing from one of the water-based diffusers is recommended for use with birds. Air diffusers may be used; however, they require being farther away from the bird or used in a much larger room (such as a barn or large aviary). Almost all essential oil singles and blends have been diffused around birds from water-based diffusers such as the Aria or Home Diffuser.

In general, start with 3 drops of oil added to the water of the diffuser. Monitor the bird(s) closely for the first 5-10 minutes of diffusing and gradually increase the length of time and frequency. Often, you can diffuse on an almost continual basis—bringing amazing benefits and health to your birds.

## Exotic Pets

You can use essential oils for ferrets in the same way as for cats. For other exotic animals, start with water-based diffusing, as outlined for birds. For animals that may soak in water, such as turtles or lizards, the recommendations made for fish can easily be used. Many exotic pets enjoy small amounts of Citrus Fresh or other citrus oils added to their drinking water. Use approximately 1 drop per liter of water. Make sure that the animal drinks adequately and that plastic dishes are not used to hold the water. Glass, ceramic, and stainless steel water containers are recommended for use with essential oils.

## Cats

Cats present their own unique controversies and requirements for essential oil use. Most cat owners would agree that cats have distinct opinions of the world, and this certainly holds true for aromatherapy. Diffusing is usually a method that is well tolerated by all cats, especially from water-based ultrasonic diffusers.

Many misconceptions have been made about what cats like or don't like. Apparently, these generalizations may have been made based on individual reports and not from cats as a species. For example, one cat may dislike citrus

Seventh Edition | **Essential Oils Desk Reference** | 259

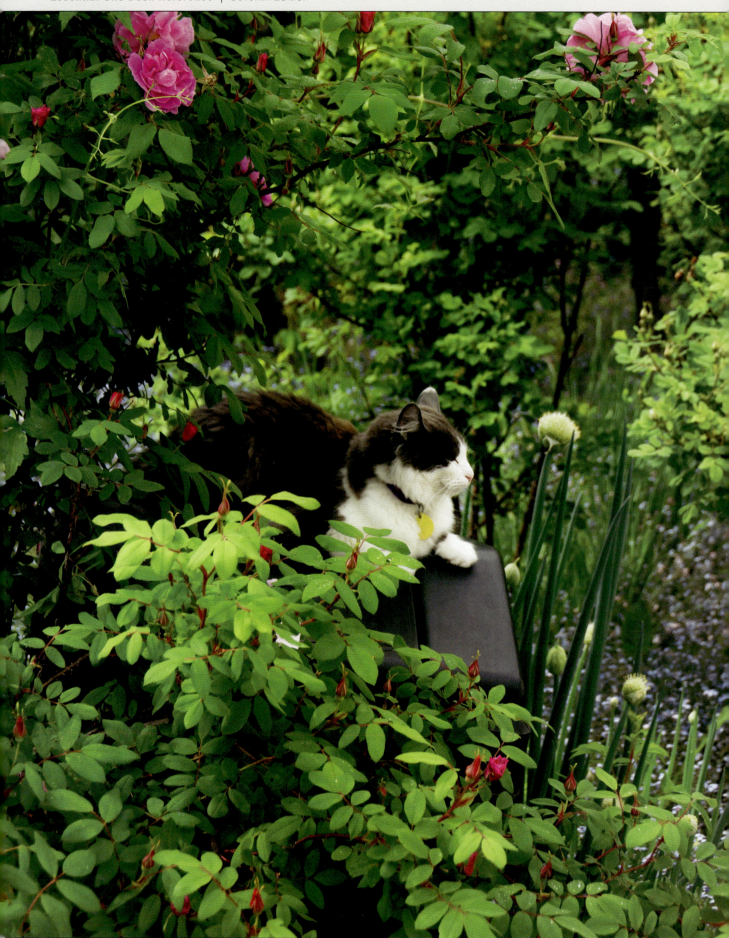

Animal Care | **Chapter 14**

oils, but then another cat is found to be attracted to them. Allowing cats to show you their individual preferences is a good idea. If a cat leaves or enters the room when you diffuse a certain essential oil, you will quickly find out its preferences every time that particular oil is diffused.

The wisest choice is to use oils that are used often or have been used with many cats and to use them with techniques that cats enjoy. The best choice is to first select an oil that is known to be very safe and well tolerated by cats.

Presented here are the application methods most commonly used on cats. Start with techniques that are widely used and shown to be safe. Animals are individuals so there could be a specific cat that will not respond well to an application method or that may prove to be more sensitive than another cat. Common sense and a tailored approach for each cat are important. A good policy is to consult with a veterinarian and have blood and urine evaluations prior to starting the use of essential oils.

### *Diffusing*

Diffusing by a water-based ultrasonic diffuser is the most tolerated by cats. Start by adding 3-5 drops of essential oil to the diffuser. If cats tolerate and like particular essential oils, concentrations and times may be increased.

### *Kitty Raindrop Technique*

This technique was also created by Leigh Foster and had been used on many of her own rescued cats prior to its now mainstream use. Although this technique includes oils that are typically contraindicated for cats, veterinarians and cat owners alike have witnessed amazing health benefits with this technique. The formula and technique were designed specifically for cats, and it is remarkable to watch them enjoy this application.

### *Kitty Raindrop Solution*

Add 4 drops each of Oregano (or Plectranthus Oregano), Thyme, Basil, Cypress, Wintergreen, Marjoram, and Peppermint to a 30-ml (1-ounce) glass essential oil bottle. Add V-6 Vegetable Oil Complex to fill the remainder of the bottle.

Mix by rocking the bottle; then apply approximately 6 drops of the solution up the spine of the cat, from tail to head. Next, gently stroke or feather the essential oil solution up the back of the cat, similar to the methods used with the human Raindrop Technique. Amazingly, cats often enjoy this backward stroke! If you encounter one that does not, just pet the cat "normally" from head to tail or omit the strokes all together.

Balancing the cat with Valor or Valor II (neat or diluted) can be performed prior to the KRDT. Place Valor or Valor II in the palms of your hands; then rub your hands together, allowing the Valor or Valor II to almost completely absorb into your palms. Place your hands over the shoulder and rump area, and the balancing procedure is completed much like that described for humans. In some situations, this step is omitted, mainly in cats who are unable to be handled easily.

### *Petting the Cat*

This method is well tolerated by cats and seems to be far superior to dripping oils directly onto their skin. Since hair follicles may enhance absorption, spreading the essential oils over a larger area of the cat may indeed prove more effective. This method involves placing a neat or diluted oil into your hand. Circling your hands together, the essential oils are allowed to absorb in varying degrees into your skin. Once you have the amount of oil on your hands that you desire—which can vary from completely absorbed to a thin coating— you simply pet your cat. Even with oils completely absorbed into your hand, if you smell your cat after petting, you will find that it smells like essential oils. Since cats groom themselves, oral ingestion of the essential oil is also likely to occur.

### *Kitty Litter*

Kitty litter is possibly one of the easiest methods by which to expose cats to the health benefits of essential oils. It not only replaces the toxic fragrances found in commercial kitty litter, but it also offers a way to provide preventive and continued health benefits from essential oils on a regular basis.

Start with unscented kitty litter. Staying with the same brand that you currently use is often advisable. Add 1-3 drops of your chosen essential oil to 1 cup of baking soda. Store this mixture in a glass jar and allow it to "marinade" for several hours, shaking the mixture several times. Later, you may find you can add more essential oil drops to this recipe.

Sprinkle a small amount of the baking soda mixture onto your kitty litter. Mix well. Provide a separate litter box that does not contain essential oils to make sure that your cat does not have an aversion to the essential oil that was selected. Once you are sure your cat is using the litter box with your oil selection and concentration, you can then omit the use of the plain litter box.

Selecting and rotating various oils can bring big benefits to your cat. Copaiba can aid with arthritis pains, DiGize or DiGize Vitality can aid in intestinal upset, and Frankincense or Frankincense Vitality may bring anticancer benefits. The choices are endless and can provide powerful preventive measures to your feline friends.

Seventh Edition | **Essential Oils Desk Reference** | 261

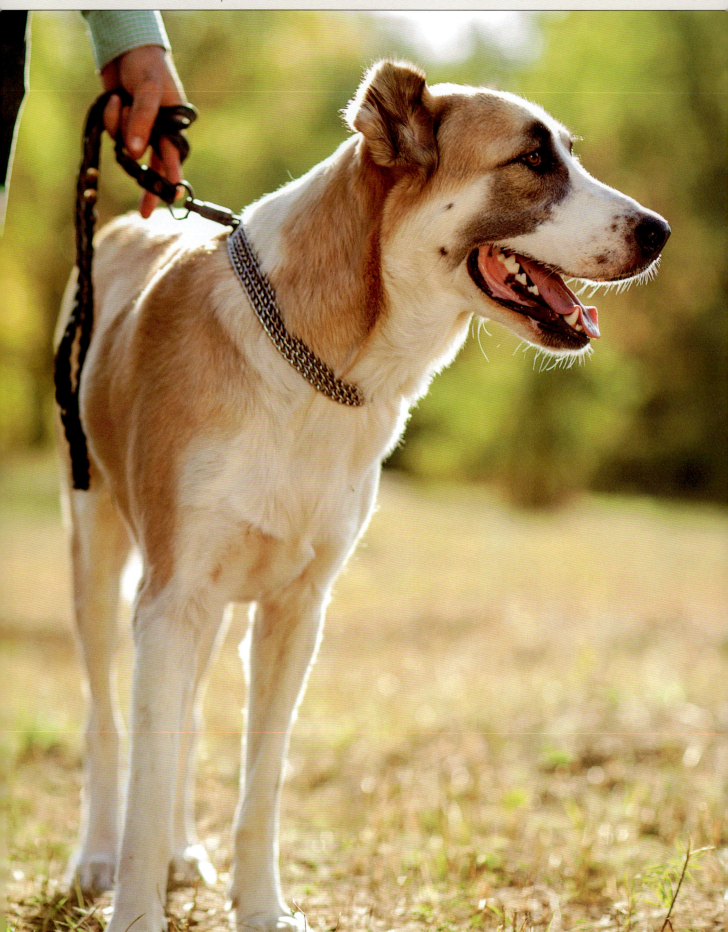

Animal Care | **Chapter 14**

## Dogs

Dogs come in various sizes, so techniques will often need to be modified accordingly. Dogs the size of cats and smaller may initially do best when exposed to essential oils with the recommendations made for cats. Larger concentrations of oils may then be used as needed. On average, dogs can use oils more freely and easily than cats and smaller-sized animals, much like we would use oils for young children.

### Raindrop Technique

Raindrop Technique has become a very common and regular treatment course for animals. This powerful technique is indicated for almost any concern; however, streamlining this application into approximately 15-20 minutes is mandatory to be able to provide the procedure to every patient who is in need. When possible, a full Raindrop Technique, similar to that described and used for humans, is recommended.

However, when multiple animals in a hospital, farm, or household would benefit from a Raindrop Technique, the oils are far more important than the actual procedure. Learning the very simple and basic procedure allows for a level of comfort to be established, and future skills may be incorporated when the facilitator is ready.

Balancing with Valor can occur as an optional step for dogs as well. Several drops are placed into the palms of your hand, generally neat, and are usually left "wet" in the palm. The hands are placed over the shoulder and rump, and balancing is performed, much as it is described for humans.

Next, the Raindrop Technique oils are applied one at a time up the spine, dripping from approximately 6 inches above the dog. The oils are not mixed together for dogs as they are for cats. Some dogs may require oils to be diluted prior to application, and in that case we generally dilute each oil individually.

Very small or sensitive dogs can use the Kitty Raindrop Technique as well. For very small dogs, generally under 20 pounds (9 kg), approximately 3 drops of each oil are applied. For dogs 20-50 pounds (9-23 kg), approximately 3-6 drops of each oil are applied. Dogs over 50 pounds (23 kg) can generally receive approximately 6-9 drops of each Raindrop oil.

The sequence of oil application is generally Oregano (or Plectranthus Oregano), Thyme, V-6, Basil, Cypress, Wintergreen, Marjoram, and Peppermint.

After each oil is dripped up the spine, the oils are stroked up the back from tail to head. For this abbreviated version of the Raindrop Technique, don't be concerned with the length of the strokes or how many times you perform them. Stimulating the spinal area in which the oils are dripped is the main goal, and even normal petting can accomplish this when needed.

After Oregano and Thyme, you will notice that V-6 is listed. There are a variety of ways to provide a calming or diluting of the essential oils that are applied during the Raindrop Technique. However, no technique is incorrect and the one that works for you is the best one.

So, after Oregano and Thyme are applied and stroked in, a fairly generous strip of V-6 is applied along the spine. Fur does not need to be parted for any part of the application, except with extremely long-haired dogs whose hair naturally parts.

The V-6 is massaged in, and then the rest of the essential oils are dripped on in sequence and stroked in, right on top of the V-6. It has a much better handling quality and does not leave as much of a greasy residue behind (for fur or furniture.)

After all of the essential oils are applied and stroked in, Vita Flex may also be performed up the spine in a final closing procedure.

If irritation to the skin or animal occurs at any stage of the Raindrop Technique, it is suggested that you stop the procedure and not apply any more oils. Apply more V-6 to the area of detoxification and irritation and allow approximately 10-15 minutes for full calming effects to be seen. Generally, do not try to "fix" any skin irritation by applying another calming or skin-soothing essential oil to the site.

Many dogs have been exposed to toxic chemicals, repeat vaccinations, or chronic medications and are in great need of detoxification. Since essential oils are so powerful in evoking this detoxification, sometimes more is not better. For dogs that do have a larger need for detoxification, using diluted or milder oils will gradually detoxify them in a more comfortable manner. After a time, their body will grow healthier, and they will be able to enjoy a full-fledged Raindrop Technique.

### Petting the Dog

Just as described for cats, petting dogs is a wonderful application method. You can usually have much more essential oil left on the palms of your hands prior to petting dogs, and dilution is not commonly needed.

### Diffusing

Dogs benefit greatly from regular daily diffusion and tolerate well both air-style and water-based diffusing. The previous directions regarding diffusing may be followed for dogs as well.

Seventh Edition | **Essential Oils Desk Reference** | 263

# Other Helpful Tips

- When treating large animals for viral or bacterial infection, arthritis, or bone injury, generally use the same oils and protocols recommended for humans.

- For applying to large, open wounds or hard-to-reach areas, it helps to put the oils in a spray bottle; dilute the oils with V-6 Vegetable Oil Complex, other vegetable oil, or olive oil; and spray the mixture directly on the location.

- After applying oil to an open wound, cover the wound with Animal Scents Ointment to seal and protect it from further infection. The ointment will also prevent the essential oils from evaporating.

- There is no right or wrong way to apply essential oils. Every animal is a little different. Use common sense and good judgment as you experiment with different methods. Observe carefully how the animal responds to the treatment.

- Take special care not to get essential oils in the animal's eyes.

- Make sure the animal is drinking pure water. **Chlorinated water will suppress thyroid and immune function** in animals even quicker than in humans. When that happens, you will suppress the healing process of that animal, whether it is a dog, horse, or cat.

- Quality protein is vitally important to promote healing, which makes the use of organic feed essential. Unfortunately, many commercial feeds contain bovine byproducts that have high risk for BSE disease (Bovine Spongiform Encephalopathy or "Mad Cow Disease") and make them unfit for animal care. Avoid these at all costs. Enzymes are also essential to maximize digestion and protein assimilation.

## Small Ruminants, Pigs

These animals can often be exposed to oils in similar ways as dogs. Raindrop Technique is often used. Diffusing for these animals is best with an "air-style" diffuser such as the TheraPro or Essential Oil Diffuser, as they are often in barns or larger areas. Oral essential oils are commonly used and are easily added to feed.

## Horses

Favorite methods of oil use for horses include Raindrop Technique, oral oils, topical applications (neat or diluted), massage, and petting. Oils can also be added to the water trough.

## Cattle and Livestock

Oils are used similarly to horses for these animals. Regular use of oils in feeds, water, udder washes, and post-milking teat dips are wonderful ways to gain health benefits on a routine basis.

## How to Administer Essential Oils Internally

For ingestion, the essential oils can be put into a capsule or mixed with the animal's food. A few drops can be added to soft, moist foods or to gravy on food when giving to dogs or cats. Mixing an essential oil with NingXia Red juice and giving it by syringe is also a common technique. Many animals will also ingest essential oils added to their drinking water.

For large animals, the animal's bottom lip can be pulled out, and as in the case of a horse, 10 or 15 drops of oil put in. The animal will feel the effect quickly because capillaries in the lip will carry the oil into the bloodstream immediately. For a large dog, 1 to 3 drops are sufficient. When cats have received essential oils orally, they often display a very typical salivation response. This response is not specific to essential oil use; many cats salivate profusely when traditional medications have been given by mouth.

When treating animals with essential oils internally, it is critical to make certain the oils used are pure and free of chemicals, solvents, and adulterants.

## Applying Essential Oils on a Jittery, Resistant Animal

If you have a high-spirited, jittery animal that will not be still to receive the application, apply Peace & Calming and/or Valor or Valor II on yourself first. As you approach the animal, it should react calmer as it smells the aroma.

Kneel down or squat beside the animal and remain still for several minutes so that it can become accustomed to the smell. As the animal breathes in the fragrances, it will become calmer and easier to manage.

Animal Care | Chapter 14

# Animal Scents® Products

## Animal Scents Dental Pet Chews

Animal Scents Dental Pet Chews are a fast and easy way to clean your pet's teeth without having to use a toothbrush. Their naturally derived ingredients help to freshen your pet's breath; your pet will love it and so will you.

**Ingredients:** potato starch, pea fiber, gelatin, beet pulp, tapioca syrup, glycerin, calcium carbonate, coconut oil, natural poultry flavor, safflower oil, salt, kelp powder, dill, blueberry juice, gum arabic, mixed tocopherols (preservative), green tea extract, parsley, rosemary extract

**Essential Oils:** Spearmint, Tarragon, Ginger, Peppermint, Juniper, Fennel, Anise, Patchouli, Lemongrass, Cumin

**Directions:** For 20+ lb. pets: give 2 chews per week. For 5-19 lb. pets: give ½ a chew 2 times a week. This product is intended for intermittent or supplemental feeding only. Adjust diet as needed to accommodate this chew. Consult a veterinarian for pets that are pregnant or under 5 lbs. before use.

**Caution:** Always offer sufficient water when giving your pet treats or food. Make sure your pet chews the treat completely, as gulping any item can be harmful. This product is not recommended for pets with a history of gulping, choking, or poor chewing capability.

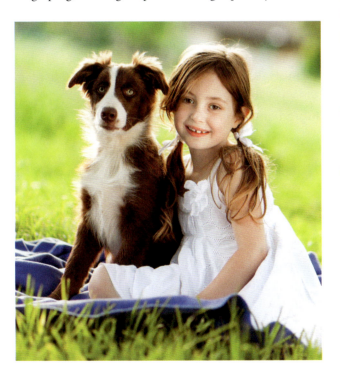

## Animal Scents Ointment

Animal Scents Ointment is blended with Tea Tree and Myrrh, two of nature's most powerful essential oils. It is a protective and soothing salve formulated for external use on animals. Tested in the field for many years, this ointment is typically used for minor skin irritations, cuts, and abrasions. It is designed to cover infected wounds and seal in the essential oils.

Animal Scents Ointment offers an effective yet gentle and safe approach to soothing your pets without using harmful chemicals or synthetic products.

**Ingredients:** mink oil, lecithin, beeswax, lanolin, sesame seed oil, wheat germ oil, rose hip seed oil

**Essential Oils:** Palmarosa, Carrot Seed, Geranium, Patchouli, Coriander, Idaho Balsam Fir, Myrrh, Tea Tree, Bergamot (furocoumarin-free), Ylang Ylang

**Directions:** Clean area and apply as needed. If using Young Living's essential oils, apply oil(s) prior to application of Animal Scents Ointment.

## Animal Scents Shampoo

Animal Scents Shampoo is formulated to clean all types of animal fur and hair. It has insect-repelling and killing properties and is designed to rid hair of lice, ticks, and other insects. This all-natural shampoo contains five powerful essential oils that are blended to gently cleanse, increase luster, and enhance grooming without the harmful ingredients often found in pet care products.

**Ingredients:** water, decyl glucoside, coco betaine, lauryl glucoside, coco-glucoside, glycerin, glyceryl oleate, citric acid, xanthan gum, inulin, sodium levulinate, sodium anisate, sodium phytate

**Essential Oils:** Lavandin, Lemon, Geranium, Citronella *(C. Nardus)*, Citronella Java Type *(C. winterianus)*, Northern Lights Black Spruce, Vetiver

**Directions:** Pour a small amount of shampoo into your palm and rub gently between your hands. Massage thoroughly into your pet's wet coat. Lather. Rinse thoroughly. Repeat if necessary.

Seventh Edition | Essential Oils Desk Reference | 265

# Animal Scents Essential Oil Blends

## Infect Away™

Infect Away utilizes six essential oils for a gentle cleansing effect on your animal. For best results, use as the second part to a three-part system, with PuriClean being used first, then Infect Away, followed by Mendwell. It supports a healthy skin barrier.

**Ingredients:** caprylic/capric glycerides

**Essential Oils:** Myrrh, Patchouli, Dorado Azul, Palo Santo, Ecuador Plectranthus Oregano, Ocotea

**Directions:** Carefully apply according to the size and species of the animal. Additional dilution is recommended for smaller species.

## Mendwell™

Mendwell is a blend of oils that supports healthy skin repair and is specifically formulated for animals. For best results, use as the last step in a three-part system, with PuriClean and Infect Away being used first.

**Ingredients:** caprylic/capric glycerides

**Essential Oils:** Geranium, Lavender, Hyssop, Myrrh, Frankincense, Hinoki

**Directions:** Carefully apply according to the size and species of the animal. Additional dilution is recommended for smaller species.

## ParaGize™

Created with animals in mind, ParaGize is a proprietary blend of essential oils that promotes healthy digestion and helps expel worms and parasites.

**Ingredients:** caprylic/capric glycerides

**Essential Oils:** Tarragon, Ginger, Peppermint, Juniper, Fennel, Anise, Patchouli, Lemongrass, Cumin, Spearmint, Rosemary

**Directions:** Carefully apply according to the size and species of the animal. Additional dilution is recommended for smaller species.

## PuriClean™

PuriClean is a unique blend of eleven essential oils that is specifically formulated for animals that cleanses and refreshes the skin. For best results, use as the first step in a three-part application, with Infect Away and Mendwell being used after PuriClean.

**Ingredients:** caprylic/capric glycerides

**Essential Oils:** Citronella, Lemongrass, Rosemary, Tea Tree, Lavandin, Myrtle, Patchouli, Lavender, Mountain Savory, Palo Santo, Cistus

**Directions:** Carefully apply according to the size and species of the animal. Additional dilution is recommended for smaller species.

## RepelAroma™

A natural insect repellant for animals, RepelAroma™ is a unique combination of essential oils that helps animals enjoy the outdoors without annoyance.

**Ingredients:** caprylic/capric glycerides

**Essential Oils:** Citronella, Idaho Tansy, Palo Santo, Tea Tree

**Directions:** Carefully apply according to the size and species of the animal. Additional dilution is recommended for smaller species.

## T-Away™

T-Away™ is formulated with a powerful combination of essential oils to promote new levels of emotional freedom and joyful feelings.

**Ingredients:** caprylic/capric glycerides

**Essential Oils:** Tangerine, Lavender, Royal Hawaiian Sandalwood, German Chamomile, Frankincense, Valerian, Ylang Ylang, Black Spruce, Geranium, Davana, Orange, Angelica, Ruta (Rue), Helichrysum, Hyssop, Spanish Sage, Citrus Hystrix, Patchouli, Coriander, Blue Tansy, Bergamot (furocoumarin-free), Rose, Lemon, Jasmine, Roman Chamomile, Palmarosa

**Directions:** Carefully apply according to the size and species of the animal. Additional dilution is recommended for smaller species.

Animal Care | **Chapter 14**

# Products for First Aid for Animals

**Animal Scents Ointment** to seal and disinfect open wounds

**Copaiba** for bruising and soreness on small animals; used as a replacement for traditional Non-Steroidal Anti-Inflammatory Drugs (NSAIDs)*

**Exodus II** for infection and inflammation and to promote tissue regeneration

**Helichrysum** as a topical anesthetic and for neurologic conditions

**Idaho Tansy** is one of the most versatile oils for animals. It is purifying, cleansing, tissue-regenerating, anti-inflammatory, anesthetic, and is used for bruised bones, cuts, wounds, and colic. It also repels flies. Palo Santo may be used in place of Idaho Tansy.

**Lavender** for tissue regeneration and desensitizing the wound; effective against ringworm

**Melrose** for disinfecting and cleaning wounds; accelerates healing of wounds

**Mountain Savory** for reducing inflammation

**Myrrh** for infection, inflammation, and promoting tissue regeneration

**Ocotea** for bruising and soreness on large animals; oil of choice for diabetes

**Ortho Ease** to dilute essential oils and act as a pain reliever and anti-inflammatory; also has insect-repelling actions

**PanAway** as a pain killer if the pain originates from a broken bone rather than an open wound; make sure there is no visible, open, raw tissue.

***Note:*** Do not apply PanAway to open wounds because it will sting and traumatize the animal. Instead, use Helichrysum and Idaho Balsam Fir to reduce bleeding and pain.

**Purification** is more effective than using iodine or hydrogen peroxide for washing and cleansing wounds. It also repels ticks and mites.

**Roman Chamomile** for tissue regeneration and desensitizing wounds

**Thieves** for inflammation, infection, bacteria, proud flesh (a condition where new tissue continues to rebuild itself, causing excessive granulation), and promoting tissue regeneration

**Valerian** can be used internally and externally for controlling pain

**Vetiver** can be used internally and externally for controlling pain

# Animal Treatment

**Arthritis** (common in older animals and purebreds)

Ortho Ease or PanAway: Massage on location or put several drops in animal feed.

Use Raindrop-like application of PanAway, Wintergreen, Pine, or Spruce and massage the location. For larger animals, use at least 2 times more oil than a normal Raindrop Technique would call for on humans.

Copaiba can be given orally as a replacement for traditional NSAID's.

For prevention: Put Power Meal or Pure Protein Complete and Sulfurzyme in feed or fodder. Small animals need 1/8 to 1/4 serving per day. Large animals need 2 to 4 servings per day.

**Birthing**

Gentle Baby

**Bleeding**

Geranium, Helichrysum, and Cistus: Shave the hair over the area being treated. For internal hemorrhage, the use of Cistus orally is recommended.

**Bones** (pain and spurs on all animals)

R.C., PanAway, Wintergreen, Lemongrass, and Spruce. All conifers are very powerful in the action for bones and in promoting bone health. For more effective absorption, it is helpful to shave the fur/hair away from the area being treated. AgilEase is an excellent supplement for building animal bones.

**Bones** (fractured or broken)

Mix PanAway with 15-25 drops of Wintergreen and Spruce. Cover the area. After 15 minutes rub in 10-15 more drops of Wintergreen and Spruce and cover with Ortho Sport Massage Oil. AgilEase can be used as a supplement to help speed bone healing.

**Calming**

Peace & Calming, T-Away, Trauma Life, and Lavender; domestic animals respond very quickly to the smell.

Seventh Edition | **Essential Oils Desk Reference** | **267**

**Essential Oils Desk Reference** | Seventh Edition

## Colds and Flu

For small animals, put 1-3 drops of Exodus II, Immu-Power, DiGize, or DiGize Vitality in feed or fodder. For large animals, use 10-20 drops.

## Colic

For large animals like cows, put 10-20 drops of DiGize or DiGize Vitality in feed or fodder. For small animals, use 1-3 drops.

Horse Colic Protocol: Administer 20 drops of Peppermint or Peppermint Vitality and 20 drops of DiGize or DiGize Vitality orally, as well as apply to the umbilical area of the abdomen. Repeat every 20 minutes, as needed.

## Fleas and Other Parasites

**Singles:** Lemongrass, Tea Tree, Eucalyptus (all types), Peppermint

**Blends:** RepelAroma, ParaGize, DiGize; also add 1-2 drops of Lemongrass to Animal Scents Shampoo.

Oils repel fleas and other external parasites. Wash blankets with oils added to the wash during the rinse cycle. Also, place 1-2 drops of Lemongrass on the collar to help eliminate fleas.

For internal parasites, rub ParaGize and/or DiGize on the pads (bottoms) of the feet daily. Many people have reported that they have seen the parasites eliminated from the animal within days after starting this procedure.

## Inflammation

Apply Ortho Ease, PanAway, Pine, Wintergreen, or Spruce on location. Put Sulfurzyme in feed. Mineral Essence may also be helpful.

## Insect Repellent

Use RepelAroma. Put 10 drops each of Palo Santo, Idaho Tansy, Eucalyptus Globulus, and Peppermint in an 8-ounce spray bottle with water.

Alternate formula: Put 2 drops Pine, 2 drops Eucalyptus Globulus, and 5-10 drops Purification in a spray bottle of water. Shake vigorously and spray over area.

## Ligaments/Tendons (torn or sprained)

Apply Lemongrass and Lavender (equal parts) on location and cover area. For small animals or birds, dilute essential oils with V-6 Vegetable Oil Complex (2 parts mixing oil to 1 part essential oil). Palo Santo is an excellent oil for use on smaller animals and is generally milder than Lemongrass.

## Mineral Deficiencies

Mineral Essence. In one case, an animal stopped chewing on furniture once his mineral deficiency was met.

Mineral deficiency is also an important aspect of anxiety in animals, so supplementing with Mineral Essence can show beneficial calming effects.

## Mites (ear mites)

Apply Purification and/or Peppermint to a cotton swab and swab just the inside of the ear.

## Nervous Anxiety

Valor, T-Away, Trauma Life, Roman Chamomile, Geranium, Lavender, Valerian

## Pain

Helichrysum, PanAway, Relieve It, Cool Azul Pain Relief Cream, Deep Relief, Cool Azul, Cool Azul Sports Gel, Clove, or Peppermint diluted 50/50 with V-6 Vegetable Oil Complex

## Shiny Coats

Tail & Mane Sheen, Shampoo, PuriClean, Rosemary, Sandalwood, Sulfurzyme

## Sinus Problems

Diffuse Raven, R.C., Pine, Myrtle, and Eucalyptus Radiata in the animal's sleeping quarters or sprinkle on the bedding. Thieves, Super C, Exodus II, and ImmuPro have been reported as being extremely beneficial for sinus and lung congestion.

## Skin Cancer

Frankincense, Lavender, Clove, Myrrh; apply neat.

## Ticks

To remove ticks, apply one drop of Cinnamon Bark or Peppermint on a cotton swab and apply directly to the tick. Then wait for it to release its head before removing from the animal's skin.

## Trauma

T-Away, Trauma Life, Valor, Peace & Calming, Melissa, Gentle Baby, Lavender, Valerian, Roman Chamomile

## Tumors or Cancers

Mix Frankincense with Ledum, Lavender, or Clove and apply on the area of tumor.

## Worms and Parasites

ParaGize, ParaFree, DiGize

## Wounds (open or abrasions)

PuriClean, Infect Away, Mendwell, Melrose, Helichrysum, Animal Scents Ointment

268 | Chapter 14 | Animal Care

Animal Care | **Chapter 14**

# Specific Care for Horses

**Bruised Ankle** (e.g., from hobble injury)

Melrose, Mountain Savory, Ocotea, Cool Azul, Cool Azul Pain Relief Cream, Cool Azul Sports Gel, and Deep Relief to reduce tenderness, bruising, and inflammation

## Cancer

Shave area near the tumor and inject Sacred Frankincense or Frankincense with a hypodermic syringe. Alternate with Clove oil every four days. Keep saturated with Sacred Frankincense or Frankincense. If the area is open, put a plug in the opening to hold the oil in the tumor cavity. Continue for six months.

## Colic (The leading cause of death in horses)

**Symptoms**
- Pawing the ground with head down
- Trotting in circles
- Lying down and looking bloated
- No churning or rumbling in the stomach
- Being quiet

**Causes**
- Eating off the ground and a mineral imbalance (getting too much dirt in the gut). The accumulated dirt can cause the gut to twist, abscess, and spasm.
- Parasites
- Eating too much alfalfa and not enough feed. Alfalfa can stress the kidneys and liver in horses. In general, grass hay is best for horses of all kinds. As a rule of thumb, the more a horse works, the more alfalfa it needs and can tolerate.
- Getting too hot

**Treatment Protocol**

Keep the horse standing or walking. If the horse lies down, keep the animal's head tied up to prevent him from rolling.

**1st hour**

*Internal Use*
- 8 to 10 Detoxzyme capsules
- 15 drops of DiGize Vitality
- Put into animal's feed grain or drop inside lip. You can open the capsules and make an enzyme and oil paste to put inside the horse's lip.

*Massage*
- Rub 10 drops DiGize up each flank and massage out toward umbilical area.
- Rub 10 drops DiGize around the coronet band.
- Rub DiGize on auricular points of ears.

*Enema*
- Mix 30 drops of DiGize in 6 oz. V-6 Vegetable Oil Complex or olive oil and insert in the horse's rectum as an enema. Do not use castor oil as it dehydrates the colon.

**2nd hour**
- Put 10-20 drops DiGize Vitality in the mouth and on the flanks and coronet band.

**4th hour**
- Repeat 1st-hour protocol except for enema.

**6th hour**
- Repeat 1st-hour protocol, adding 5 drops of Peppermint to the 10-20 drops of DiGize Vitality.

**8th hour**
- Repeat 1st-hour protocol, except for enema, and add one scoop of Power Meal or Pure Protein Complete (add to water if the animal is drinking).

**10th hour**
- Continue administering 6-8 Detoxzyme capsules every 2 hours until the horse's bowels are moving well.

## Distemper, Whooping Cough, or Asthma

**Daily Regimen**
- Mix 30 drops each of R.C. and Raven in 4 oz. of V-6 Vegetable Oil Complex and insert into the rectum.
- Put 15 drops each of R.C. and Raven in the bottom lip.
- Massage oils on the chest between the front legs and auricular points of ears.
- Apply Raindrop Technique down the spine and neck hair.
- Administer 4 Longevity Softgels.

## Fractures/Bone Chips

Shave area around affected bone. Apply mixture of:
- 5 drops Wintergreen
- 5 drops Idaho Balsam Fir
- 2 drops Oregano (or Plectranthus Oregano)
- Add 2 tablespoons Sulfurzyme to feed.
- Continue the above regimen daily for 3 months.

**Case History**

In 1997 a horse's back hock was fractured with two 50-cent-sized pieces splintered off. The animal was diagnosed at stage five lameness, and the vet urged to have the animal euthanized.

After Wintergreen essential oil was applied for several months, the bone regenerated and the break healed.

Seventh Edition | **Essential Oils Desk Reference** | 269

## Gary's Equine Essentials *(Products specially formulated for equine use.)*

### Massage Oil

This blend is diluted specifically for equine use to give your horse a well-deserved cool-down before, during, or after physical activity.

**Ingredients:** coconut oil (caprylic/capric triglyceride)

**Essential Oils:** Wintergreen, Peppermint, Sage, Plectranthus Oregano, Copaiba (Balsam Copaiba), Melaleuca Quinquenervia (Niaouli), Lavender, Blue Cypress, Elemi, Vetiver, Caraway, Dorado Azul, Matricaria (German Chamomile)

**Directions:** Apply to desired area and massage as needed. Dilute with V-6 or other pure carrier oil as needed.

### Shampoo

Equine Essentials Shampoo provides safe and effective cleansing and conditioning to leave the coat smooth, lustrous, and looking its best.

**Ingredients:** water, decyl glucoside, alkyl polyglucoside, coco betaine, sodium methyl 2-sulfolaurate, lauryl glucoside, tetrasodium glutamate diacetate, coc-glucoside, glycerin, glyceryl oleate, citric acid, xanthan gum, inulin, sodium levulinate, disodium 2-sulfolaurate, sodium anisate, sodium phytate

**Essential Oils:** Clove, Lemon, Cinnamon Bark, Rosemary, Lavandin, Geranium, Citronella *(C. Nardus)*, Cintronella Java Type *(C. winterianus)*, Northern Lights Black Spruce, Vetiver

**Directions:** Mix a generous amount of Equine Shampoo in a bucket of warm water. Lather into a wet coat and massage. Rinse thoroughly and repeat if necessary.

### Tail & Mane Sheen™

Gary's Tail & Mane Sheen smooths hair, can be used as a detangler, and brings out the hair's natural, healthy shine. Monoi oil is a fragrant oil consisting of gardenias soaked in coconut oil and is widely used among French Polynesians as a skin and hair softener.

**Ingredients:** coconut oil (caprylic/capric triglyceride), wheat germ oil, mink oil, monoi extract

**Essential Oils:** Hinoki, Northern Lights Black Spruce, Lemon, Lavender, Geranium, Royal Hawaiian Sandalwood

**Directions:** For best results, wash and groom before application. Spray on tail and mane and comb through to achieve a glossy appearance.

---

The horse returned to the jousting arena stronger and more powerful than ever and spent several more years entertaining the crowds.

**Note:** Other oils that may be effective for this condition include Helichrysum, Northern Lights Black Spruce, and Idaho Balsam Fir. Sulfurzyme may be used internally.

### Hide Injuries

**Case History**

A 4-month-old colt had the hide on one side of its body stripped off. The wound was sprayed with Melrose to disinfect and Helichrysum to control the pain. The wound was then sealed with the formula now known as Animal Scents Ointment. Within several months, the hair and skin had completely grown in, and the animal had made a full recovery.

### Hoof Infections

**Case History**

In 2000 a show horse received some kind of severe bite on the pastern. Although the vet diagnosed a rattlesnake bite, it may have been caused by something else.

Two weeks later, the entire pastern and coronet band were inflamed (the size of a cantaloupe), and the rotting, decaying flesh revealed a large hole where the bone was visible and had separated from the hoof.

The vet suggested amputating the foot. Instead, the following protocol was initiated:

- **Day 1:** The wound was cleaned and disinfected with Thieves and Helichrysum, and the foot was bandaged. This treatment decreased pain enough to allow the mare to put weight on the foot.
- **Day 2:** The swelling had dropped by 50 percent. The wound was again cleaned with Thieves and Helichrysum and then packed with Animal Scents Ointment.

Animal Care | Chapter 14

- **Days 3 to 14:** The wound was washed morning and night with Thieves, Melrose, and Helichrysum and packed with Animal Scents Ointment.
- **Result:** Today the animal walks with no discomfort. A brand new hoof has appeared with only a small scar on the wound site. Although there was minor swelling in the pastern for a while, it had faded eight months later.

## Imprinting on New Foals

**Recommended Essential Oils:** Valor, Highest Potential, Sacred Mountain, Joy, Surrender, Acceptance

As soon as a colt is born, pick up the foal and hold it in your arms. Massage 5-6 drops of oil along the spine and place a drop on each ear. Then rub oils all over the colt's body a few drops at a time. Lay the colt in your lap and position it with its head back, stroke its neck, and pass all the way over its nose (avoid putting any oils on the nose as it is very sensitive). Repeat every day for 21 days.

## Jitteriness

To calm a horse, apply a few drops of oil on your hands and put one hand on the base of the tail and the other on the withers. The animal should relax. Relaxation is the first step to healing.

Put several drops of T-Away, Trauma Life, Surrender, Peace & Calming, or Peace & Calming II in your hand and briefly hold it up to the animal's muzzle or nostrils. If the horse pulls away and returns to it several times, perhaps out of curiosity or perhaps thinking that food may appear, feed him some grain as a reward and then put your hand with oil on his muzzle and gently rub it in.

As he relaxes, work your hand around the side of his jaw and up along the neckline to the ears. Then rub his ears and the top of his head and crop. As he relaxes further, you can add more oil to the palm of your hand (Peace & Calming, Peace & Calming II, or Valerian) and continue rubbing his ears, head, and crop.

## Kidney Failure

- Administer 10 drops (about 1/2 of a dropper) of K&B tincture morning and night.
- Using a Raindrop application on the spine, apply 5 drops each of Cypress and Juniper daily for 10 days.

## Laxative for Foals

Put 4 drops of DiGize Vitality in bottom lip daily until bowels are moving.

## Open Wounds

### Case History

A large thoroughbred gelding was attacked by a cougar that clawed a chunk of flesh half the size of a soccer ball out of the horse's buttocks. The horse bled terribly, blood squirting from ruptured blood vessels.

The vet said the prognosis was grim because there was too much torn, damaged, and removed tissue. Even if the horse didn't die, the wound would leave a sizeable scar and indentation.

### Treatment Protocol

**Day 1**

To reduce the pain and stop the bleeding, a 5 cc hypodermic syringe was filled with Helichrysum and sprayed into the wound. The horse became less jittery, and the bleeding stopped. Several minutes later a larger 10 cc syringe of Purification was sprayed into the open wound. It took over 15 ml of Purification to spray down and cover the entire wound.

After several hours, the wound was sprayed with Melrose to disinfect it and was packed with Animal Scents Ointment. To keep hair out of the wound and reduce the possibility of infection, the tail was wrapped and tied up. Because there was no way to cover or close the wound, the horse was kept in the stable to prevent him from moving around. The animal was closely monitored to reduce the possibility of reinfection caused by the animal lying down, rolling around, and scratching the wound.

**Days 2-7**

The horse's grain was supplemented with crushed up Essentialzyme, the yellow capsule in Essentialzymes-4, and four scoops of Power Meal, which is dense in the nutrients required for healing and tissue rebuilding.

Three times a day, the open wound was irrigated with Purification and Helichrysum. The vet came regularly to monitor the horse's progress. He remarked that he had never seen muscle tissue regenerate to such a degree.

**Weeks 2 to 4**

Two times a day, the open wound was irrigated with Purification and Helichrysum.

**Weeks 4 to 8**

Once a week, the wound was irrigated with Purification and Helichrysum until it was closed.

### Results

Today, no indentation or concavity is visible, only a small, circular 2-inch scar.

Seventh Edition | **Essential Oils Desk Reference** | 271

## Puncture Wounds

Put 1 cc of Thieves in a hypodermic syringe, insert the needle deeply into the wound, and irrigate thoroughly. Repeat 1 to 2 times a day for 2 to 3 days if still infected or swollen. Continue this process for up to 10 days.

## Saddle Sores and Raw Spots

(i.e., where packs rub against flesh)

Use PuriClean, Infect Away, and Mendwell as a three-part system; may also use Melrose and Animal Scents Ointment for at least 3 days.

## Scours (diarrhea caused by bacteria)

- Put 5 drops ParaGize or DiGize Vitality in the horse's lower lip and rub 5-8 drops in the flank.
- Place ICP in water and pour it down the throat. Continue for four days.

## Screw Worm

There is a round worm called a bore or screw worm that bores into the spine of a horse (especially wild horses). It will cause a huge boil-like abscess on the spine. When lanced, a larva worm will come out of that abscess. Sometimes the abscess will actually break open and ooze.

Pour Thieves into the hole to flush out the larva worm and then fill the hole with a mixture of 12 drops of Melrose and 5 drops of Mountain Savory.

## Strangles (*Streptococcus equi* infection)

- Perform the Raindrop Technique with Thieves.
- Apply 4 drops of Thieves Vitality on the inside of the bottom lip (for a large horse, 8 drops).
- After 2 hours repeat Raindrop Technique with Oregano Vitality (or Plectranthus Oregano) and Thyme Vitality. Put 2 drops of Oregano Vitality and 2 drops of Thyme Vitality on the inside of the bottom lip (for a large horse, 4 drops each).
- Repeat the last two steps every 2 hours until the horse begins to improve. As the horse continues to improve, alternate treatments every 4 hours, every 6 hours, and then morning and night.

## Swollen Sheath

Geldings and stallions occasionally suffer from swollen sheath with an abscess and infection. It can be caused by:

- Eating hay too rich in protein. Ideal levels of protein should be 12 to 15 percent, and alfalfa hay can have protein as high as 26 percent.
- Not extracting the penis and letting it clean off.

**Treatment**

- Put on rubber gloves.
- Clean inside the sheath and remove debris with soap and water. Use a half cap of Thieves Household Cleaner diluted in a half gallon of water.
- Clean outside the sheath by applying Myrrh oil and Rosemary with Tea Tree. The ratio is 15 drops of Myrrh, 15 drops of Rosemary, and 10 drops of Tea Tree.
- Clean and disinfect morning and night until infection and swelling subside.
- Maintenance: The sheath should be cleaned out once a month. Make sure the horse is fed adequate water and grass hay and gets sufficient exercise to increase circulation.
- Perform a Raindrop Technique with Oregano (or Plectranthus Oregano), Thyme, and Mountain savory every 3 to 6 months.

## Umbilical Cords of Newborn Foals

Instead of iodine, put Myrrh oil on the umbilical cord of newborn foals. Myrrh will dry the umbilical cord and facilitate a good separation. Exodus II can also be used to treat infections in a foal's umbilical cord.

Animal Care | Chapter 14

# Raindrop Technique® for Horses

Although many veterinarians have developed their own variations of this technique, the simplicity of this procedure is what makes it effective.

Raindrop Technique for horses is similar to that for humans, except that there must be practical modifications because of the difference in size and shape of the patient. Trying to exactly duplicate the human version of the Raindrop Technique on animals is not advised.

## Starting Point

Apply 6 drops of Valor to the tailbone (the base of the tail where it connects with the spine). Next, place one hand on the withers and the other on the tailbone and hold for 5 minutes. There is no difference energetically whether you use your right or left hand in these spots. Once the horse relaxes (i.e., drops its head and eyelids droop), the procedure can start.

## Don'ts

- Do not spend too much time stroking the horse's spine. Usually, three repetitions are sufficient.
- Avoid dripping oils on the hair of the horse's spine and stroking them in. You will be stroking against the grain of the hair, and oil will be flicked off the spine rather than rubbed in. This is not as important for animals with fine hair.
- Once you make contact with the animal on which you are applying oils, never break it.
- Do not work on the animal with multiple partners. Raindrop Technique is more effective when only one pair of hands makes continuous contact with the animal because the energy stays the same, and animals get skittish when two or more people touch them at the same time.

## How to Apply Oils

- Where feasible, shave the spine area for direct application of the oil (you will use less oil).
- If shaving is not feasible, stand the hair up and part it, then drip the oil down through the hair so that the oil contacts the spine. Hold the oil 6 inches above the spine as you drop it in.
- For coarse-haired animals, stroke in the oils using small, circular motions, working from the base of the tail to the shoulders of the spine.
- For fine-haired animals, stroke in the oils using regular Raindrop Technique straight strokes.
- Spend enough time massaging to get the oils down into the skin and not sitting on top of the hair.

- When dripping the oils on the spine, use 12 drops on a draft horse, 6 drops on a saddle horse, or 3-4 drops on a miniature horse, Shetland, or Welch pony.

## Additional Tips

- Carefully use your fingertips and thumb tips to perform Vita Flex along the auricular points of the ear. Be gentle. If you inflict even a little discomfort, the horse will distrust you and pull away.
- Stretching the spine is problematic in horses, so instead, place one hand over the tail, the other hand on the withers, and focus moving the energy along the spine.
- Rubbing oils around the coronet band will allow the oils to reach the bloodstream and travel through the nerves in the legs to the spine.
- Drip Marjoram and Aroma Siez into the hair of the outside muscles away from the spine and rub in with a larger circular motion massage. Idaho Tansy, Palo Santo, or Melrose—which are anti-inflammatory, anesthetic, insect-repelling, relaxing, and healing—can also be used. This is important because horses used for packing, riding, or working have extra stress placed on the spine and muscles in the back.
- Avoid having two people working on opposite sides of the horse at the same time. No two people's energy is the same, and this produces an energetic imbalance.
- Use a stool (mounting block) to reach both sides of the spine without having to break contact, potentially creating tension in the animal.
- Some people mistakenly believe that if they don't have all the oils in the Raindrop Kit, they can't do a Raindrop. You do not need to apply every oil to have an effective treatment.
- You can perform an excellent, beneficial Raindrop procedure with one oil, if that's all you have. Using just Oregano (or Plectranthus Oregano) and Thyme, Palo Santo, or even Idaho Tansy can produce excellent results. Similarly, Melrose, Tea Tree, or Mountain Savory can also be used.
- It is okay to stroke oils down off the hips and down the legs.
- It is okay to put a hot towel on the spine. In fact, it is recommended.
- Following a Raindrop Technique, you can apply a saddle blanket and then a horse blanket and leave the animal standing in the stall. Usually after about 10 minutes, it will lie down and go to sleep.

Seventh Edition | **Essential Oils Desk Reference** | 273

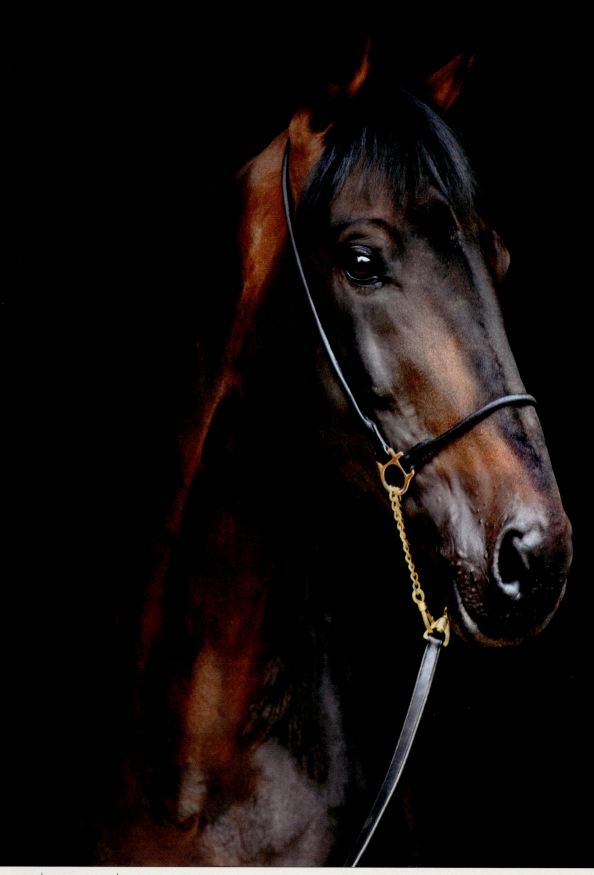

Animal Care | **Chapter 14**

# Essential Oil Testimonials About Animals
## The following is a small selection of the dozens of testimonials received from animal owners

"Since 1997 I have had phone consultations with Young Living Essential Oil enthusiasts and have found that many issues have been solved in many animals with the simple introduction of NingXia Red and Power Meal. Often nothing else was done except to add these powerful, nutrient-rich supplements to the pet's diet. The symptoms have then disappeared, and the pets have returned to being normal, vibrant animals.

"I have many success stories in returning pets to their normal, vibrant, healthy state. For example, animals having osteosarcoma (bone cancer) and mast cell tumors have outlived their expectancy by a year with the introduction of oils and supplements from Young Living.

"In addition, many times I have used Frankincense to lower the mitotic (aggressiveness) index of cancer cells, documenting these with before and after cytology. I highly recommend applying Frankincense topically on tumors to decrease their rate of growth."

"I have also developed a technique using Young Living essential oils to decrease the inflammation of the anal gland sac and the scarring due to chronic infection.

"Currently, there is an ongoing case study at my practice and a paper to be published soon regarding using these oils for specific diseases.

"I believe in numbers when it comes to knowing if a product will benefit animals and have had the amazing privilege of collecting thousands of case studies of using Young Living essential oils and products on animals. Many veterinarians can benefit from these case studies.

— *Nancy Brandt, DVM, CVA, CVC,*
*Las Vegas, Nevada*

"I have been using essential oils in my home for many years and had never thought that I could use them around my parrots. Not only can I use them, but my birds' health has only gotten better. I have been able to replace prescription drugs and helped problems that traditional vets have no answers to. My birds get sprayed everyday with the Feather Spray, drink essential oils in their water, and even eat them in their foods. I can't imagine life without these oils!"

— *Norma Ameling*
*South Haven, Minnesota*

"My cat developed a pink bald spot near his tail, which was losing hair by the day. The veterinarian did not know what it was, so she tested for a virus and sold me antibiotics to give him just in case. She mentioned that the spot had the appearance of a burn.

"When I got home, I decided to re-think the antibiotic idea: 'If it might be a burn, why not simply put Lavender on it?' I asked myself. So I applied less than a drop on that spot by just barely touching it. In the morning it was clearly improved. I applied Lavender again the same way, a second time only. His fur grew back in so fast that I didn't worry about it again.

"Later I learned that this is a common spot where a cat will scratch another when it runs away from a standoff. In hindsight, I believe the bald spot was just that: a cat scratch infection."

— *Barbara J. Ullrich, Tacoma, WA*

Seventh Edition | **Essential Oils Desk Reference** | **275**

"Purification is our favorite oil to diffuse in our house. We have high ceilings over Izzie's cage (she is an Orange Bearded Dragon about a foot long, nose to tail). We often leave the cool-mist diffuser on for much of the day due to high winds and dust here in Las Vegas. If we keep our fish in the same area, then we don't add any extra oil to their bowls. The Purification sanitizes the air around the cage and keeps Izzie parasite free and healthy.

"We use Thieves Household Cleaner to clean her tank and wash her bowls, toys, etc. We dilute a cap full in a cup of water in a glass spray bottle and wipe her tank down while she gets a bath and sunshine outside. Once everyone and everything dries, we put them all back together, and she sleeps like a baby.

"Worth noting: We have children with food and environmental allergies, and diffusing Purification helps keep all the critter odors and danders from irritating the allergy sufferers in the house."

Tara also comments on the use of essential oils for her fish:

"Only add essential oils to their water if they are in glass bowls. Essential oils leach toxins from plastic, and you wouldn't want your fish swimming in toxins. For small glass Betta bowls under a gallon: Start with dipping a toothpick in Purification oil and dip it into the bowl. If all is well with the fish and you are comfortable, put in one drop of Purification. You can use a toothpick to mix it around so that your fish don't take one big gulp. Although, don't be surprised if they do! For larger tanks: Still start off small with a toothpick or 1 drop and work your way up to 2 or 3 drops. Purification is a great antiseptic for the fish and the tank."

— *Tara Rayburn, Las Vegas, Nevada*

"Three years ago, my corgi, Dickens, ruptured a disc in his back. As a result, his back legs were paralyzed. He was five years old at the time. He underwent surgery and recovered very well, but he was left with an odd gait with swinging hips. He was able to run and play, go on long walks, and, most importantly, was pain free.

"But a year and a half ago, while lying on the sofa, he rolled over on his back and immediately began yelping in pain. We had no idea what was wrong.

"Since it was 8 p.m. on a Friday night, we took him to an emergency animal clinic. He was examined and x-rayed. Nothing showed up on the x-ray, but Dickens continued to howl and shake, so the vet thought that maybe he had a pinched nerve in his neck. She gave him a shot for pain as well as a cortisone shot and prescribed both pain and cortisone pills.

"We took him to our regular vet the following Monday, who agreed that the problem was most likely a pinched nerve and gave us enough pills to last two weeks. Dickens did fine for two weeks, and after a final checkup, the vet released him. He recommended that we use a harness, not a leash, to relieve any neck stress.

"Things went along well for about ten days. Then all at once, Dickens started howling in pain. This time I decided to try my own therapy. I got out a 15-ml bottle and made up a "Raindrop concoction" consisting of 5 ml of Valor, 2 ml of Aroma Siez, and 1 ml each of Oregano, Thyme, Basil, Wintergreen, Cypress, Marjoram, and Peppermint.

"I applied 5-7 drops of this mixture along his spine, starting at the atlas and moving down to his tail bone. I massaged it in and then applied a little V-6 Vegetable Oil Complex to "seal" it. I repeated this treatment 3-4 times daily. On the second day, Dickens was running and playing again.

"I continued the treatment for about three weeks. Several times since then, Dickens has come over to me and stared expectantly until I got out the "Raindrop concoction" and applied it to his back.

"Now over eight years old, he has remained healthy and happy, and I know what to do if the condition flares up again."

— *Linda Chandler, Carmel, CA*

Animal Care | Chapter 14

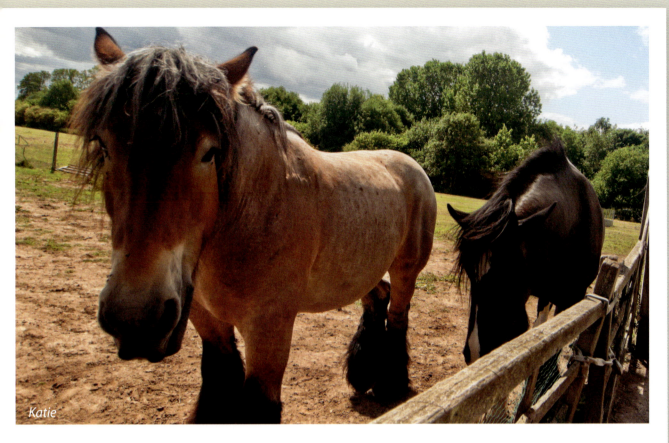

Katie

"My horse, Katie, is a beautiful Shire draft horse, the type used in jousting. Katie had a serious abscess on the bottom of her foot. Fixing this involves digging a huge hole into the foot to get the abscess out and is painful for the horse—which is very rarely anaesthetized.

"My vet was trying to get to the abscess; and, of course, Katie was skittish. The farrier was helping the vet, but Katie weighs a ton (yes, a ton—as I said, she is a jousting-type horse) and it was very slow going.

"Katie was upset and scared, and I knew she was in pain. It's hard because you can't tell an animal "it's going to be all right" when the doctor is done. I didn't know what to do.

"So I had my friend go to my car to get some Peace & Calming, as I figured anything could help. She mistakenly brought back PanAway; and before realizing it was a different blend, I put it up to Katie's nose. At that moment, I realized it was not the oil I had intended to use and had my friend go back to the car to get the Peace & Calming.

"However, as soon as I had put the PanAway to Katie's face, she had gotten "interested" in the smell, her ears had pricked forward, and she had stopped moving around as much. Then when I put the Peace & Calming up to her nostrils, it calmed her down *immediately.* The vet was able to 'doctor her up,' and an unpleasant task became manageable. In fact, the farrier didn't even have to continue to help the vet.

"Katie relaxed so much that we could see her shoulder go down, and she stopped trying to pull her foot away from the vet, even though there was blood all over her hoof from the vet trying to dig out that abscess! My friend and I were honestly amazed that suddenly she just relaxed and even dropped her head down.

Now, mind you, I used almost the entire bottle of Peace & Calming because the work on the abscess took a long time. But from the moment I put it up to her nostrils until the vet packed her foot and wrapped it with an enormous bandage, her shoulders were relaxed and her head was down, a good sign that a horse is not stressed. The vet didn't even give her a 'butte' (horse painkiller); he just said, "Whatever you were doing, keep doing that."

— *Sandra Shepard, CMT, JD, Petaluma, CA*

Seventh Edition | Essential Oils Desk Reference | 277

"Early one morning I received a call from Marie, one of my massage clients I had seen the day before. Her 14-year-old dog, Precious, had been to the groomer—whom she doesn't like—and fell off the table while the groomer wasn't watching. The dog could not walk or squat.

"Marie took her dog to the vet, who examined and x-rayed Precious but found no broken bones. Precious received a shot and an anti-inflammatory, but she still could not walk.

"Marie wanted me to help with her dog. Although Marie had complete faith in my abilities, I was hesitant to go. I suggested other things that might help, but Marie was insistent so I told her I would be there within the hour.

"On the way I was sorting out what I could do for the dog. I had the essential oil blend PanAway with me, but I wasn't sure the dog would like the aroma and wondered if an animal in pain would allow me to work on it.

"I know Precious so that was a help, and she was glad to see me. She was on Marie's bed, which was a good place to work.

"I tried gentle massage to the back and spinal area, and it was soon evident that she liked what I was doing and seemed to know I was trying to help her.

"After about 10 or 15 minutes, we encouraged her to get up. She stood, but her hind legs were rubbery, and she could not walk. As she lay down, I noticed her left back leg was stuck out straight. I massaged the left leg, hip, and knee with PanAway, especially the tendons in the knee, and then we took her outside. She emptied her bladder, came inside under her own power, drank a whole bowl of water, and ate a little food, even though she had not previously been drinking or eating.

"Marie called me the next day to say Precious was walking and feeling fine. 'It's a miracle!' she joyfully exclaimed."

— *Kathy Smith, CMS, NMT, Atlanta, GA*

"I recently used the oils in a case with a mare that had colic, and they seemed to work just like the drug, Banamine. I had on hand three oils that were suggested in the *Desk Reference* for use on smooth muscles (intestines)—Marjoram, Clary Sage, and Lavender.

For each application, I used 5 drops of the same oils on each flank with a warm compress. Each application took effect in about 30 minutes and kept the mare calm and comfortable for 2½–3 hours. I alternated oils throughout the night with each application. Marjoram and Clary Sage seemed to work better than Lavender. By 7:30 the next morning, the mare showed marked improvement and went for water."

— *Janis Early, Tallahassee, FL*

"My cat, Nigel, had to be rushed to three different animal hospitals one night due to a ruptured urethra. He was in severe pain and had been anesthetized twice over the course of about six hours.

"By 11 p.m. we were wearily on our way to the third hospital, which was over an hour away, when I thankfully found my Young Living Lavender oil in my coat pocket. After applying several drops to my forehead, temples, and neck to help calm me down, I simply held the open bottle next to Nigel's carrier, where he was loudly despairing and restlessly trying to stand, despite his dizziness from the anesthesia.

"Within seconds of introducing the oil to him, he became silent. I was so amazed that I had to check to make sure he was still alive! I left the bottle open for the duration of the trip. He remained calm for the remainder of the drive, meowing only occasionally, and made it through his final surgery beautifully.

"Thanks to the Lavender oil, Nigel and I got through the final hours of that very long, traumatic night with comfort and ease."

— *Sarah George, Newburyport, MA*

# Section 3
## Application

**CHAPTER 15**

Techniques for Essential Oil Application. . . . . . . . . . . . . . . . . . . . . . . . . .281

Neuro Auricular Technique. . . . . . . . . . . . . . . . . . . . . . . . . . . . . . . . . . . . .282

Lymphatic Pump . . . . . . . . . . . . . . . . . . . . . . . . . . . . . . . . . . . . . . . . . . . .284

Vita Flex . . . . . . . . . . . . . . . . . . . . . . . . . . . . . . . . . . . . . . . . . . . . . . . . . . .285

Raindrop Technique . . . . . . . . . . . . . . . . . . . . . . . . . . . . . . . . . . . . . . . . . .290

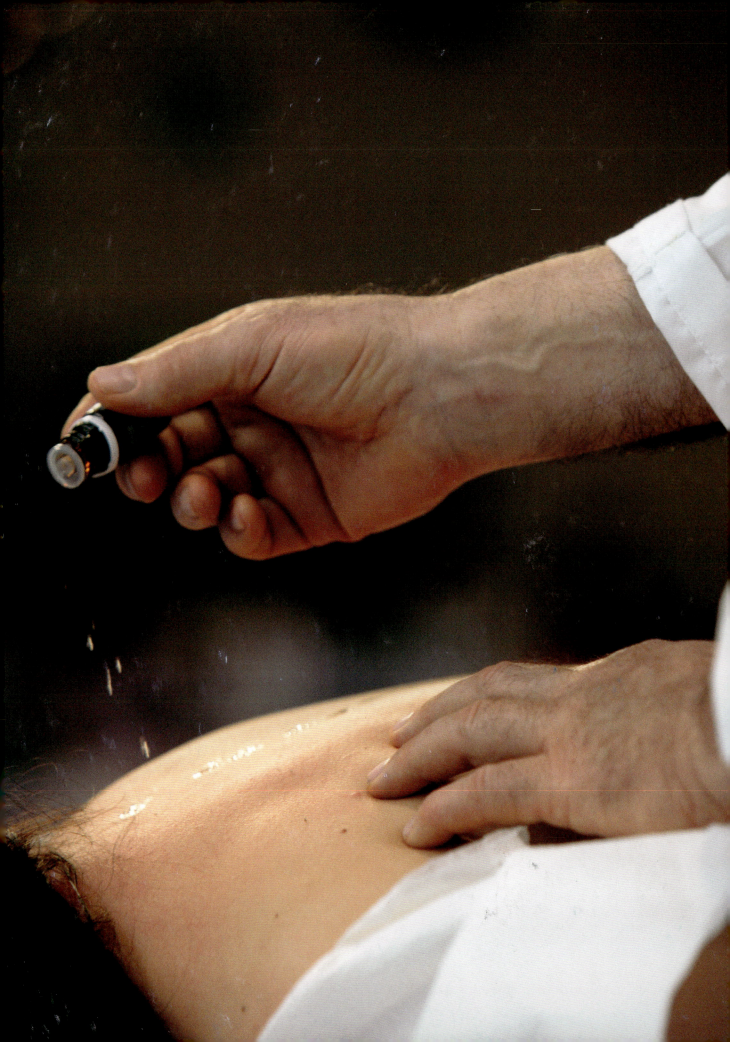

# Chapter 15
## Techniques for Essential Oil Application

## The Use of Different Techniques

People use essential oils in many creative ways for healing and supporting the human body that open a world of great discovery and untapped potential. It does not seem to matter how the essential oils are used, as long as their energy penetrates the body through direct application, inhalation, or ingestion.

The possibilities become very exciting as the essential oils are used by individuals new and/or inexperienced, and they begin to discover unexpected and fascinating benefits. However, as with any natural substance, essential oils should be used carefully, intelligently, and most importantly, with common sense. Keeping this in mind, common sense will enable you to enjoy the benefits and immense pleasure in using the essential oils as you learn to apply them through these techniques that have brought Peace & Calming, Joy, Harmony, and Abundance to thousands of people throughout the world.

The five specific techniques explained in this chapter have been studied and used in research as the development of their application has been refined and documented. Numerous doctors and health professionals are now acknowledging the benefits of these natural techniques, and thousands of individuals throughout the world have had tremendous benefits.

This knowledge is available to those who are interested in learning about essential oils, God's gifts that Mother Nature eagerly provides, and how to use these brilliant but simple techniques in order to help themselves, their families, friends, and those in their world of influence.

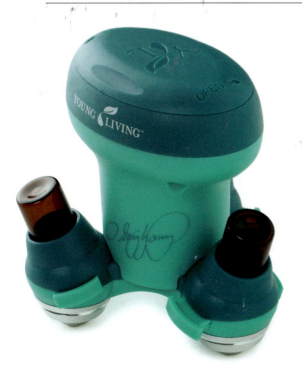

### Vitassage™ Essential Oil Dispensing Massager

The Vitassage is a one-of-a-kind creation by D. Gary Young that incorporates Young Living essential oils into the massage experience.* Three stainless-steel roller balls simultaneously disperse up to three different oils onto the skin, while the powerful vibration technology allows the oils to penetrate deep into stressed tissue.

The Vitassage offers the power of Young Living's pure, therapeutic-grade essential oils and massage to both professionals and casual users alike.

- The ultimate aromatherapeutic massage experience
- Profound vitality using YL patent-pending* aroma vibration
- Sliding mechanism for independent oil dispersion
- Unique 2-ml bottle replacement system that allows for customizable oil combinations

* Patents Pending

# Neuro Auricular Technique

D. Gary Young developed the Neuro Auricular Technique, NAT, which integrates the use of pure, therapeutic-grade essential oils with acupressure by using a small, pen-shaped instrument with a rounded end to apply the oils to the acupressure meridians or Vita Flex points on the ears.

He discovered that using essential oils in conjunction with acupressure was extremely beneficial. Interestingly, he found that acupressure stimulation on specific neurological points with the essential oils evoked a quicker response to specific conditions. The combination of acupressure with essential oils seemed to substantially increase benefits in targeted areas.

The Neuro Auricular Technique has shown remarkable benefits in both the emotional and physical realm. When working on a physical need, an emotional release is often experienced that can bring about a positive attitude of hope and renewed vitality.

In relationship to the spine and dealing with neurological problems that exist because of spinal cord injury, the Neuro Auricular Technique has been extremely beneficial in delivering the oils to the exact location of the neurological damage.

The Neuro Auricular Technique is a program that Gary continues to research, develop, and teach worldwide to doctors and other health practitioners. It has proven to have tremendous results and has the potential to be a well-known modality in the future.

## Emotional Ear Chart

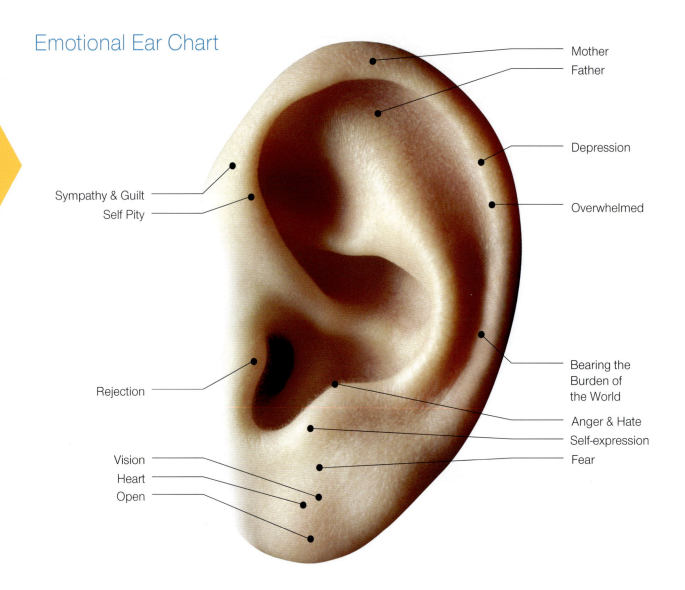

Techniques for Essential Oil Application | **Chapter 15**

# Physical Ear Chart

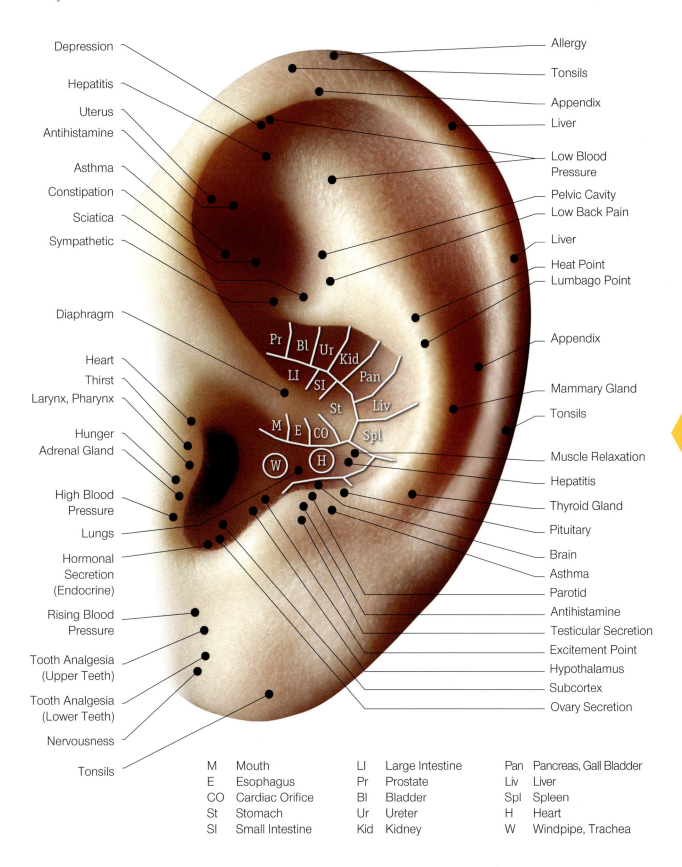

| | | | | | | | |
|---|---|---|---|---|---|---|---|
| M | Mouth | LI | Large Intestine | Pan | Pancreas, Gall Bladder |
| E | Esophagus | Pr | Prostate | Liv | Liver |
| CO | Cardiac Orifice | Bl | Bladder | Spl | Spleen |
| St | Stomach | Ur | Ureter | H | Heart |
| SI | Small Intestine | Kid | Kidney | W | Windpipe, Trachea |

Seventh Edition | **Essential Oils Desk Reference** | 283

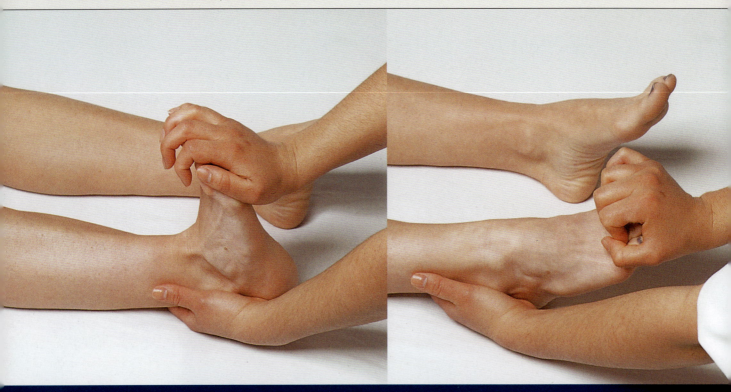

Figure A — Pushing the foot

Figure B — Pulling the foot

## Lymphatic Pump

Maintaining lymph circulation is one of the keys to keeping the immune system adequately functioning. This technique is designed to promote lymph circulation. It is an excellent tool for those who are sedentary or bedridden.

1. With the recipient lying on his or her back, hold one leg with one hand just above the ankle with your palm on the underside of the leg (covering the Achilles tendon).
2. Place the other hand on the bottom of the recipient's foot with your palm over the ball of the foot and your fingers curled around the toes.
3. Push the top of the foot away from you (See Figure A).
4. Then pull the foot toward you by the toes until the ball of the foot is as close to the table as possible (See Figure B).
5. Check with the recipient during the pump to verify that the muscles in the foot are not being overextended. This should be an active process, but not a painful one.
6. Pull and push the foot using this "pumping motion" at least 10 times on each leg for maximum benefit. Note that the recipient's entire body should move during each step of the Lymphatic Pump.

# Vita Flex Technique

Vita Flex means "vitality through the reflexes" and is an easy way to apply essential oils through the bottoms of the feet. It is a very important technique that can facilitate the relief of pain and suffering quickly, as well as improve physical and emotional well-being.

It helps identify different structural and health needs of the body and together with the Raindrop Technique increases the opportunity for healing and rejuvenation. Vita Flex is a specialized form of hand and foot massage that is exceptionally effective in delivering the benefits of essential oils throughout the body.

It is said to have originated in Tibet thousands of years ago and was perfected in the 1960s by Stanley Burroughs long before acupuncture was popular in Western medicine.

Vita Flex is based on a complete network of reflex points that stimulate all the internal body systems. When the fingertips connect to specific reflex points with essential oils using the special Vita Flex application, an electrical charge is released that sends energy through the neuroelectrical pathways.

This electrical charge follows the pathways of the nervous system to where there is a break in the electrical circuit, usually related to an energy block caused by toxins, damaged tissues, or loss of oxygen.

More than 1,500 Vita Flex points are located throughout the body in comparison to only 365 acupuncture points used in reflexology. Vita Flex is similar to but different from reflexology. As it is used today, reflexology has a tendency to ground out the electrical charge from constant compression and rotation pressure, which causes cell separation and loss of oxygen to subdermal tissues, causing further injury.

In contrast to the steady stimulation of reflexology, Vita Flex uses a rolling and releasing motion that involves placing the fingers flat on the skin, rolling up onto the fingertips, and continuing over onto the fingernails, using medium pressure, and then sliding the hand forward about ½ inch, continually repeating this rolling and releasing technique until the specific Vita Flex area is covered. This rolling motion is repeated over the area three times.

Vita Flex corrects weakened or injured areas through the electrical reflex points, preventing further injury and less stress and allowing for quicker, more efficient healing. Combining the electrical frequency of the oils and that of the person receiving the application creates rapid and phenomenal results.

This ancient technique has brought healing of a greater dimension to our modern world with its complete, scientific, workable system of controls that releases the unlimited healing power within the human body.

The diagram of the nervous system shows the points on the spine and their electrical connection to specific areas throughout the entire body.

## Vita Flex on the Hands

The hands also have specific reflex points that correspond to different organs and systems of the body. Although the hands are smaller and perhaps not as comfortable to work on, if you are in a hurry or are unable to get to the feet, there are still definite benefits in using the Vita Flex technique on the hands.

**Essential Oils Desk Reference** | Seventh Edition

# Vita Flex Foot Chart

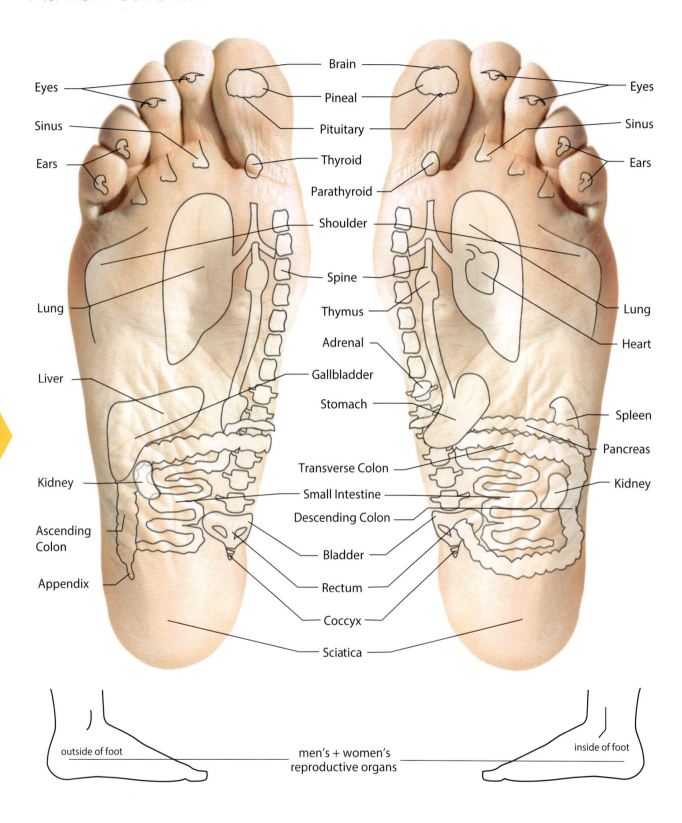

Chapter 15 | Techniques for Essential Oil Application

Techniques for Essential Oil Application | Chapter 15

## Nervous System Connection Points

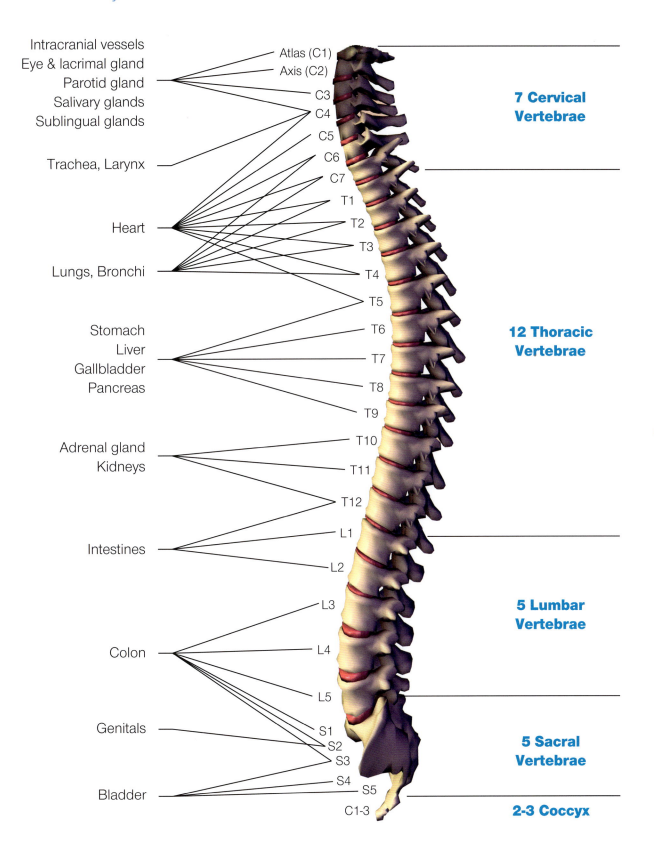

**Essential Oils Desk Reference** | Seventh Edition

# Palm of Left Hand

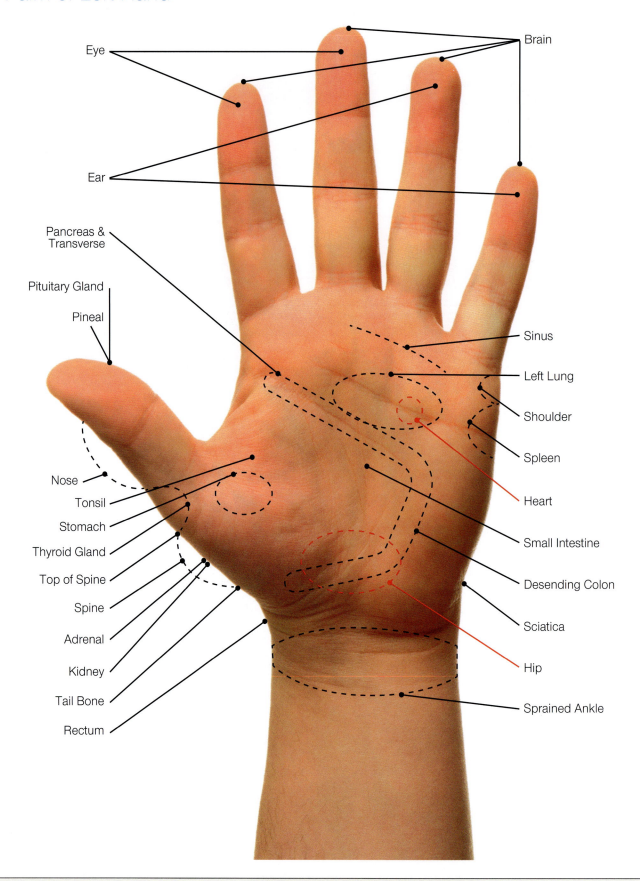

288 | Chapter 15 | Techniques for Essential Oil Application

## Techniques for Essential Oil Application | Chapter 15

# Palm of Right Hand

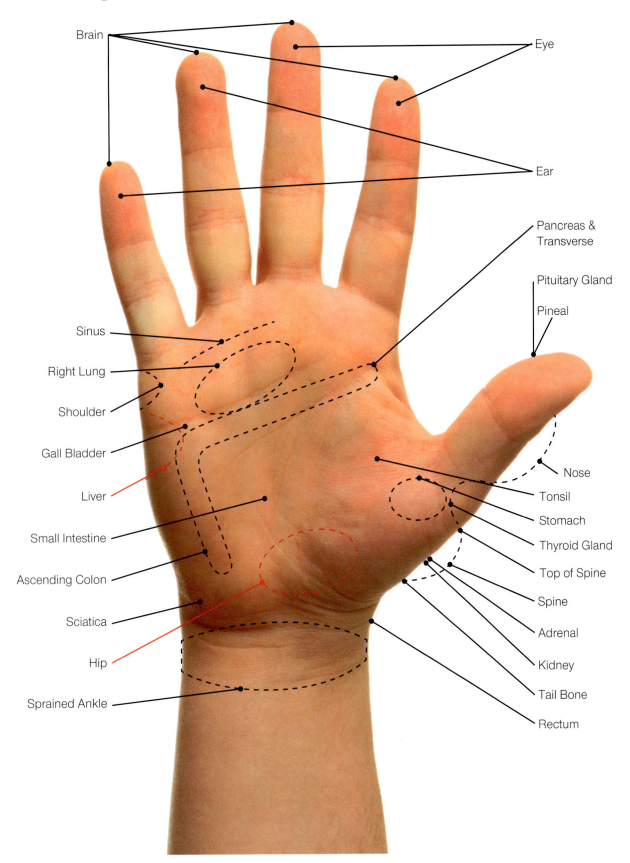

# Raindrop Technique®

Most people would agree that massage is soothing, relaxing, and pleasurable. But Raindrop Technique is unquestionably far superior as it combines essential oils with special massage techniques to add greater therapeutic benefits to a pleasurable massage.

Anyone who has experienced Raindrop Technique is very quick to get on the massage table again to enjoy and discover new benefits of this most remarkable application of essential oils.

Raindrop Technique is one of the safest, noninvasive regimens available for spinal health. It is also an invaluable method to promote healing from within using topically applied essential oils.

## The Development of the Raindrop Technique

D. Gary Young developed the Raindrop Technique based on his research of essential oils and their antimicrobial properties, his knowledge of the Vita Flex technique and its reflex points on the feet, and fascinating information on the light stroking called "effleurage" and its effect on the muscles and the nervous system.

## Lakota Indians

While visiting with the Lakota people, Gary learned that for several generations before the U.S./Canadian border was established, the Lakota Indians migrated across the Canadian border into the northern regions of Saskatchewan and Manitoba. There, they often witnessed the Northern Lights, or Aurora Borealis.

Those who were ill or had complicated health problems would stand facing the Aurora Borealis, hold their hands toward the lights, and inhale deeply.

The Lakota believed that when the Aurora Borealis was visible, the air was charged with healing energy. They would mentally "inhale" this energy, allowing it to pass through their spine and on to other afflicted areas of the body through neurological pathways. Many experienced dramatic healing effects through this practice.

Eventually, after the border divided the U.S. from Canada, making migrations to the north impossible, the Lakota began practicing this energy process mentally, coupled with light stroking to facilitate the spreading of energy through the body.

## Effleurage

Gary has said that he does not know if this is where the effleurage he teaches (feathered finger-stroking) first originated, but it has become associated with this healing technique. It is believed that the Lakota people continued their practice of mentally processing energy, coupled with effleurage, to distribute healing energy throughout the body.

Gary found that when this practice of effleurage was coupled with the therapeutic power of essential oils and the stimulation of Vita Flex, its effects were greatly heightened. Since this therapeutic practice was adopted in 1989, Raindrop Technique has been embraced by massage therapists, chiropractors, and other medical professionals around the world for its help with relaxation, correcting spinal misalignments, and antiviral effects.

## Statistical Validation

In 2001 David Stewart, PhD, circulated a questionnaire to over 2,000 health practitioners, massage therapists, aromatherapists, and their clients to gain insight on the results that were accruing from Raindrop Technique.

He received 422 responses summarizing the experiences of some 14,000 Raindrop sessions. His findings are summarized in his booklet *A Statistical Validation of Raindrop Technique* (available through Life Science Publishing; order online at discoverlsp.com or by calling toll-free 1.800.336.6308).

Overall, the 416 respondents who had received a Raindrop Technique rated it positive (97 percent), pleasant (98 percent), resulted in improved health (89 percent), resulted in an improved emotional state (86 percent), and would choose to receive Raindrop Technique again (99.9 percent).

## Consistent with the French Model

The use of undiluted essential oils in Raindrop Technique is consistent with the French model for aromatherapy—which is the most extensively practiced and studied model in the world. Having used essential oils clinically since the 1920s, the French have consistently recommended neat (undiluted) use of essential oils.

An illustrious roster of 20th century French physicians provides convincing evidence that undiluted essential oils have a valuable place in the therapeutic arsenal of clinical professionals. René Gattefossé, PhD; Jean Valnet, MD; Jean-Claude Lapraz, MD; Daniel Pénoël, MD; and many others have long attested to the safe and effective use of undiluted essential oils and the dramatic and powerful benefits they can impart.

Techniques for Essential Oil Application | **Chapter 15**

## Skin Warming or Reddening

In the case of Raindrop Technique, the use of certain undiluted essential oils typically causes minor reddening and "heat" in the tissues. Normally, this is perfectly safe and not something to be overly concerned about. Individuals who have fair skin such as blondes and redheads or those persons whose systems are toxic are more susceptible to this temporary reddening.

If the reddening or heat becomes excessive, it can be remedied within a minute or two by immediately applying several drops of V-6™ Vegetable Oil Complex or a pure, high quality vegetable oil like jojoba, almond, avocado, olive, or coconut oil on the affected area. This effectively dilutes the oils and the warming effect.

Temporary, mild warming is normal for Raindrop Technique. Typically, it is even milder than that of many capsicum creams or sports ointments. Indeed, rather than being a cause for concern, this warming indicates that positive benefits are being received.

In cases where the warmth or heat exceeds the comfort zone of the recipient, as mentioned before, the facilitator can apply any pure vegetable oil to the area until the comfort level is regained and reddening dissipates (usually within 2-5 minutes).

**Note:** If a rash should appear, it is an indication of a chemical reaction between the oils and synthetic compounds in the skin cells and the interstitial fluid of the body (usually from conventional personal care products).

Some misconstrue this as an allergic reaction; when in fact, the problem is not caused by an allergy but rather by foreign chemicals already imbedded in the tissues. Essential oils are known to digest toxic waste, chemicals, and other unwanted toxins in the body; and sometimes that process starts to work very quickly.

## Medical Professionals

A number of medical professionals throughout the United States have adopted Raindrop Technique in their clinical practice and have found it to be an outstanding method to relieve the problems associated with sciatica, scoliosis, kyphosis, and chronic back pain.

Ken Krieger, DC, a chiropractor practicing in Scottsdale, Arizona, states, "As a chiropractor, I believe that the dramatic results of Raindrop Technique are enough for me to rewrite the books on scoliosis."

Similarly, Terry Friedmann, MD, of Westminster, Colorado, stated that ". . . these essential oils truly represent a new frontier of medicine; they have resolved cases that many professionals had regarded as hopeless."

## Microorganisms May Cause Scoliosis and Sciatica

A growing amount of scientific research shows that certain microorganisms lodge near the spinal cord and contribute to deformities. These pathogens create inflammation, which, in turn, contorts and disfigures the spinal column.

Raindrop Technique uses a sequence of highly antimicrobial essential oils dropped on the back as a noninvasive therapy for fighting against pathogens lying dormant against the spine, which alleviates symptoms of scoliosis, kyphosis, and other back ailments while strengthening the immune system.

Studies at Western General Hospital in Edinburgh, Scotland, linked virus-like particles to idiopathic scoliosis.[1,2]

Researchers at the University of Bonn have also found that the varicella zoster virus can lodge in the spinal ganglia throughout life.[3]

Research in 2001 further corroborated the existence of infectious microorganisms as a cause of spine pain and inflammation. Alistair Stirling and his colleagues at the Royal Orthopedic Hospital in Birmingham, England, found that 53 percent of patients with severe sciatica tested positive for chronic, low-grade infection by gram-negative bacteria (particularly *Propionibacterium acnes*), which triggered inflammation near the spine. Stirling suggested that the reason these bacteria had not been identified earlier was because of the extended time required to incubate disc material (7 days).[4]

The tuberculosis mycobacterium has also been shown to contribute to spinal disease and possibly deformations. Research at the Pasteur Institute in France, published in *The New England Journal of Medicine*, documented increasing numbers of patients showing evidence of spinal disease (Pott's disease) caused by tuberculosis.[5, 6, 7, 8]

In addition, vaccines made from live viruses have been linked to spinal problems. A 1982 study by Pincott and Taff found a connection between oral poliomyelitis vaccines and scoliosis.[9]

Raindrop Technique is a powerful, noninvasive technique utilizing the antiviral, antibacterial, and anti-inflammatory action of several key essential oils to assist the body in maintaining or retraining the spinal column's natural curvature.

During the past 18 years, this technique has helped alleviate or resolve many cases of scoliosis, kyphosis, and chronic back pain and has eliminated the need for back surgery for hundreds of people.

Seventh Edition | **Essential Oils Desk Reference** | 291

## Powerful Antibacterial Agents

Essential oils are some of the most powerful inhibitors of microbes known and as such are an important, new weapon in combating many types of tissue infections. A 2015 study tested a number of essential oils against several gram positive and gram negative bacteria like *Klebsiella pneumoniae, Pseudomonas aeruginosa, Staphylococcus aureus,* and *E. coli.* The study authors concluded that the "components of essential oil of thyme and pine are highly active against food borne pathogens, generating the largest zones of inhibition."[10]

Similarly, basil essential oil also demonstrated strong bactericidal action against microorganisms *Aeromonas hydrophila* and *Pseudomonas fluorescens.*[11]

A study at the Central Food Technological Institute in Mysore, India, found that a large number of essential oil components had tremendous germ-killing effects, inhibiting the growth of Staphylococcus, Micrococcus, Bacillus, and Enterobacter strains of bacteria.

These germ-killing compounds included menthol (found in Peppermint), eucalyptol (found in Rosemary, Eucalyptus Radiata, and Geranium), linalool (found in Marjoram), and citral (found in Lemongrass).[12]

A 2001 study conducted by D. Gary Young, Diane Horne, Sue Chao, and colleagues at Weber State University in Ogden, Utah, found that Oregano, Thyme, Peppermint, and Basil exhibited very strong antimicrobial effects against pathogens such as *Streptococcus pneumoniae,* a major cause of illness in young children and death in elderly and immune-weakened patients.[13] Many other studies confirm these findings.[14]

The ability of essential oils to penetrate the skin quickly and pass into body tissues to produce therapeutic effects has also been studied. Hoshi University researchers in Japan found that cyclic monoterpenes (including menthol, which is found in Peppermint) are so effective in penetrating the skin that they can actually enhance the absorption of water-soluble drugs.[15] North Dakota State University researchers have similarly found that cyclic monoterpenes such as limonene and other terpenoids such as menthone and eugenol easily pass through the dermis, magnifying the penetration of pharmaceutical drugs such as tamoxifen.[16]

## Ingesting Essential Oils

It is interesting to note that many essential oils used in Raindrop Technique—in addition to being highly antimicrobial—are also among those classified as GRAS (Generally Regarded As Safe) for internal use by the U.S. Food and Drug Administration. These include Basil, Marjoram, Peppermint, Oregano, and Thyme. These and many other essential oils on the GRAS list have had a long history for decades as foods or flavorings, with virtually no adverse reactions. It is interesting how the people of the world were ingesting essential oils long before the FDA determined they were safe.

In sum, Raindrop Technique is a safe, noninvasive way to achieve spinal health. It is an invaluable method to promote healing from within using topically applied essential oils.

## The Raindrop Technique Experience

Most people would agree that massage is soothing, relaxing, and pleasurable. But Raindrop Technique is unquestionably far superior as it combines essential oils with special massage techniques to add greater therapeutic benefits to a pleasurable massage.

Anyone who has experienced Raindrop Technique is very quick to get on the massage table again to enjoy and discover new benefits of this most remarkable application of essential oils.

## Physical Relief and Emotional Release

When D. Gary Young developed Raindrop Technique in 1991, he first chose nine pure, therapeutic-grade essential oils that would synergistically combine to kill viral and bacterial pathogens, reduce inflammation, support the immune system, ease respiratory discomfort, relax stressed muscles, and relieve the body of bone and joint discomfort.

He felt this combination of oils would also balance the energy, lift the spirit by reducing stress, and calm a troubled and confused mind. This began a new realm of healing that emerged from within the confines of emotional bondage.

In the cerebral cortex is a structure called the amygdala that is affected only by scent. It is here that the emotions and memories of life are stored. Since essential oils have the ability to cross the blood-brain barrier and stimulate the amygdala, buried feelings of past trauma, emotional upset, and unhappy memories are often released to the cognizant mind, bringing those feelings and consequences to the surface of awareness.

Many physical and emotional problems become dim or completely disappear as the foundation of the emotion is discovered and released. Raindrop Technique has vast benefits only to be realized by the individual receiving the application. It is different for each individual, unlike anyone else, and is very personal and specific to each person's needs.

Children tend to respond even faster than adults because they do not have any preconceived ideas about what they want to have happen or experience. They just love it and often fall asleep, while the essential oils and the touch of massage fill them with peace and contentment as body systems harmonize together.

Raindrop Technique is an experience for everyone at any age for whatever the need or desire may be, and perhaps it is just a time of quiet relaxation and enjoyment.

## Raindrop Technique and Essential Oils

Raindrop Technique is one of the safest, most noninvasive regimens available for spinal health. It is also an invaluable method for promoting healing from within using topically applied essential oils.

### Single Oils
- **Oregano** (or **Plectranthus Oregano**): Awakens receptors, kills pathogens, and helps digest toxic substances on the receptor sites
- **Thyme**: Kills pathogens and digests waste and toxic substances on the receptor sites
- **Basil**: Releases muscle tension
- **Cypress**: Improves circulation and is oil for the pituitary gland
- **Wintergreen**: Reduces pain
- **Marjoram**: Strengthens muscles
- **Peppermint**: Promotes greater oil penetration

### Essential Oil Blends
- **Valor** (or **Valor II**): Structural balancing and alignment
- **Aroma Siez:** Muscle relaxation and pain reduction
- **White Angelica:** Protection for adversarial energies

### Simple Explanation

The oils are dispensed like drops of rain from a height of about 6 inches above the back. Starting from the low back, the oils are feathered with the back of the fingers up along the vertebrae, out over the back muscles, and over the shoulders to the neck. Although the entire technique takes from 30-45 minutes to complete, the oils continue to work for several days as the healing and realignment processes take place.

Many recipients feel the benefits of the oils for several days afterward, as they recognize that the pain has decreased or is completely gone, there is no fever, they have more mobility, and they have an overall feeling of peace and a renewed zest for life.

Experiencing the wonderful results of a first-time Raindrop application does not mean that all the desired benefits will be realized. One Raindrop session might be just a time to balance and relax the body. Some individuals may feel they want to have Raindrop once a week, once a month, or every three or four months. Other individuals working on structural realignment or needing emotional support may choose to have Raindrop done on a weekly basis to continue with their progress.

It is important to recognize that a healthy body is not attained by doing just one thing. It is a result of a well-rounded program of exercise, proper diet, and sufficient sleep. Health is everything we do, say, see, eat, and think, along with drinking plenty of water and getting enough sleep.

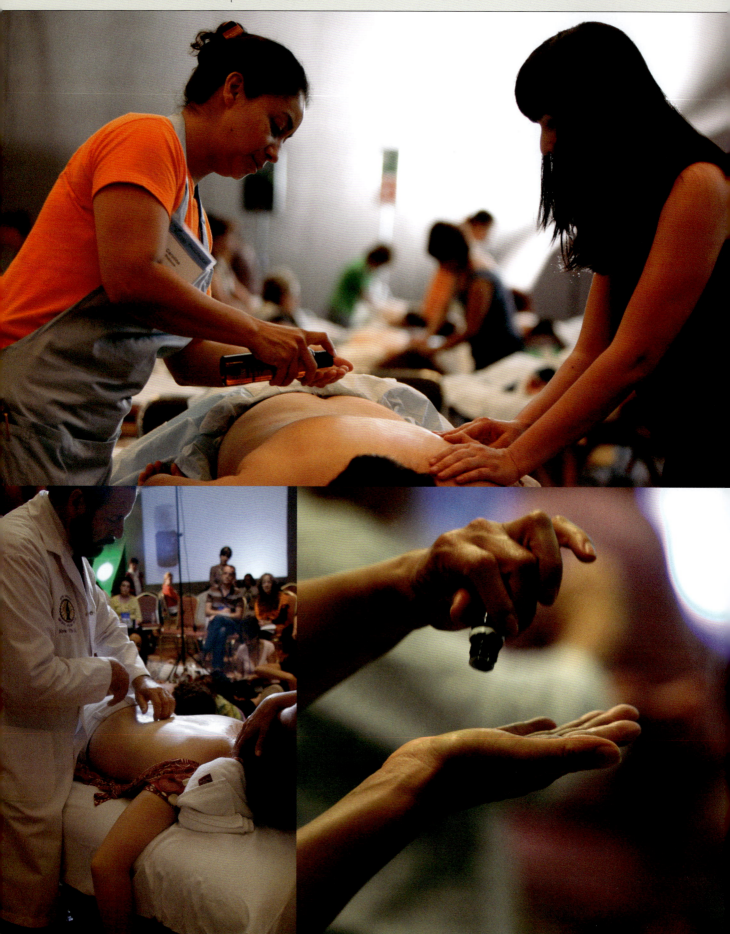

Techniques for Essential Oil Application | **Chapter 15**

# Preparation

To properly perform the Raindrop Technique, the following items and guidelines are necessary:

1. **A massage table or comfortable, flat surface.**
   The surface should be high enough that the facilitator can perform the technique without back strain. Use sheets or towels as a barrier, being sensitive to the fact that essential oils may damage or stain vinyl and other fabrics.

2. **Respect the receiver's modesty at all times.** The use of a blanket or sheet provides the best protection. Make sure the environment and your actions promote a sense of security and protection for the receiver.

3. **Raindrop Technique Kit:**
   - Valor (or Valor II)
   - Oregano (or Plectranthus Oregano)
   - Thyme
   - Basil
   - Cypress
   - Wintergreen
   - Marjoram
   - Aroma Siez
   - Peppermint
   - White Angelica*
   - V-6 Vegetable Oil Complex
   - Ortho Ease Massage Oil

   *White Angelica is needed but is not included in the kit.*

# Be sure to remember the following:

1. The Raindrop Technique should be performed only if the facilitator is feeling balanced and focused. Time should be spent developing clarity and energy for transfer to the receiver during the technique.

2. Both facilitator and receiver should be relaxed and comfortable. Appropriate clothing should be worn.

3. An environment should be created that is warm, quiet, relaxing, and comfortable. Soft music and lighting generally prove to be beneficial to the receiver.

4. Both the facilitator and the receiver should remove all jewelry. This includes watches, pendants, chains, rings, bracelets, belts, earrings, etc. These items produce an electrical energy that may interfere with the technique. Metal eyeglasses are acceptable.

5. Facilitators should make sure their fingernails are clipped and filed to prevent scratching the receiver's skin, particularly when performing Vita Flex. Nails should also be free of polish, since essential oils can remove polishes and lacquers.

6. Inquire as to whether the receiver has been exposed to chemicals or has worked in a toxic environment.

7. Ask the receiver if he or she needs to use the restroom prior to beginning.

8. Request permission to begin the Raindrop Technique.

9. It is necessary to access the receiver's back for application of the oils. The use of clothing that fully exposes the spine works best. If modesty can be preserved, remove all clothing from the waist up for easier application.

10. To begin, the receiver should lie as straight as possible on his or her back, face up, on the massage table. Arms should rest alongside the body with the palms touching the sides of the thighs. This will help direct the flow of energy and keep it connected to the receiver.

11. Once contact is made with the receiver, the facilitator should maintain a constant physical connection. This promotes feelings of calmness and security while developing a sense of trust with the facilitator.

12. While applying the Raindrop Technique, use caution when working near the spine or applying direct pressure.

13. Offer assistance to the receiver when dismounting the table.

14. Have plenty of water available for the receiver after the Raindrop Technique is complete.

15. Provide detailed instructions to the receiver for post-Raindrop Technique care.

*Caution: Some of the oils may feel hot to the receiver. You may apply V-6 at any time. This will create a cooling effect on any area of discomfort.*

Seventh Edition | **Essential Oils Desk Reference** | 295

**Essential Oils Desk Reference** | Seventh Edition

# Overview of Application

**Step 1:** Balance energy. Apply **Valor** (or **Valor II**) on the soles of the feet. If a second person is assisting, then that person can put the oils on the shoulders.

**Step 2:** Vita Flex Technique. Work the same Raindrop Technique oils into the spinal reflex areas of the feet.

Vita Flex facilitates quick absorption of the oils through the bottoms of the feet and prepares the body for Raindrop on the back. It is also highly relaxing.

**Step 3:** The 5-step Feathering Technique. Use with each of the oils as they are applied on the back, starting at the base of the spine and working upwards to stimulate the cell receptors and activate energy centers along the spine, as well as to distribute the oil drops over the back for rapid penetration.

**Step 4:** Feather 3-5 drops of **Oregano** (or **Plectranthus Oregano**)—from the spine outwards.

**Step 5:** Feather 3-5 drops of **Thyme**—from the spine outwards.

**Step 6:** Stretch and release. Feather 4-6 drops of **Basil** along both sides of the spine and feather out and upwards. Then take hold of the feet and gently pull to stretch the spine, releasing tension from the vertebra, back muscles, and tissue.

**Step 7:** Finger Straddle Massage. Apply 5-8 drops of **Cypress** on the spine and feather; then perform the Spinal Finger Straddle.

**Step 8:** Vita Flex Thumb Roll. Apply 5-8 drops of **Wintergreen** on the spine and feather; then perform the Vita Flex Thumb Roll.

**Step 9:** Circular Hand Massage. Apply 8-10 drops of **Marjoram** on the back and feather; then perform the Circular Hand Massage.

**Step 10:** Palm Slide. Apply 8-10 drops of **Aroma Siez** over the entire back and feather; then perform the Palm Slide.

**Step 11:** Feathering Technique. Apply 3-5 drops of **Peppermint** on the spine and feather.

**Step 12:** Feathering Technique. Apply 8-10 drops of **Valor (or Valor II)** over the back and feather.

# Explanation of Terms

**Facilitator:** The person conducting the Raindrop Technique; if there are two facilitators, one will work at the feet, and the other will work at the shoulders.

**Receiver:** The person receiving the Raindrop Technique

**Malleolus:** Hammer-shaped protuberance at each side of the ankle joint

**Sacrum:** Base of the spine

**Atlas:** Hairline or top of the neck

**Lumbar:** Part of the back between the lowest ribs and the pelvis

**Cervical:** Upper part of the spine/neck

**Thoraces:** Middle of the spine

**Feather:** Alternating the use of the hands to brush the backs of your fingertips along the spine from sacrum to atlas

**Spinal Tissue Pull:** Using circular, clockwise motions with fingertips to gently pull the muscle tissue away from the spine

**Finger Straddle:** Straddling the spine with the index and middle fingers and using the bottom edge of the right hand to create a sawing motion over the straddled fingers, while at the same time slowly pulling hands toward the atlas

**Thumb Roll:** Rolling thumbs along either side of the spine, moving toward the atlas

**Circular Hand Massage:** Rotating hands, palms down, along the spine in a clockwise motion

**Palm Slide:** Sliding palms in opposite directions along the spine

**Fan:** Using long strokes with the hands to fan up the spine and to the sides

**296** | **Chapter 15** | Techniques for Essential Oil Application

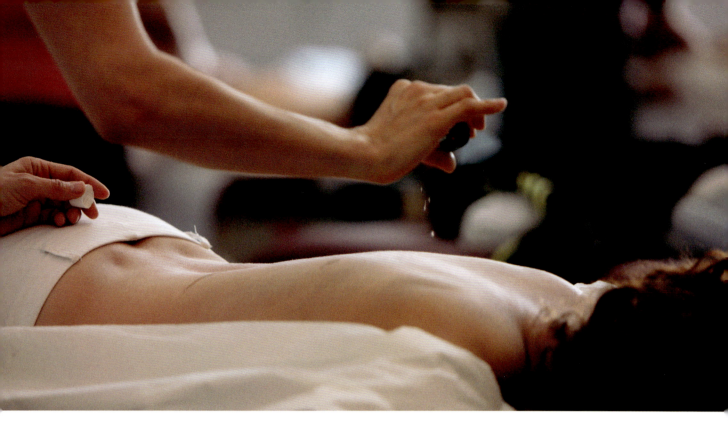

## 1. BALANCING BODY ENERGY

### Application of Valor (or Valor II)

Valor (or Valor II) serves as the foundation for all work performed during the Raindrop Technique. This essential oil blend helps regulate the electromagnetic energy that flows through the body and balances the receiver's emotional, spiritual, and physical energy. By balancing these energies, the receiver's connections are dramatically improved.

It is only necessary for one facilitator to perform this process by using the foot application. If two facilitators are present, work in unison: one at the shoulders and one at the feet. Both will apply Valor (or Valor II) and remain in contact until the energy is balanced.

### Shoulder Application

1. The facilitator should put White Angelica essential oil blend on his or her shoulders, back of the neck, and thymus area before starting the Raindrop Technique.
2. The facilitator places 3 drops of Valor (or Valor II) in each hand.
3. With both palms up, cup under the receiver's right shoulder with the right hand and cup under the left shoulder with the left hand.
4. Hold this position until the facilitator at the feet completes the same technique.
5. Continue with the foot application as described.

**BALANCING BODY ENERGY**

*Placing hands on the recipient's feet*

### Foot Application

1. Facing the receiver, place 6 drops of Valor (or Valor II) in each hand.
2. Make contact with the receiver's feet, with the palm of the right hand to the right foot and the palm of the left hand to the left foot. The feet should be held snug with the palms of the hands against the soles of the feet. The facilitator should have firm, but comfortable, contact with the receiver.

Seventh Edition | Essential Oils Desk Reference | 297

## VITA FLEX ON THE SOLES OF THE FEET

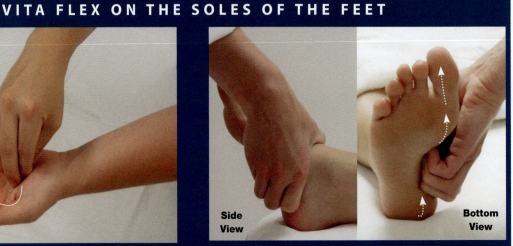

Dipping fingertips into essential oil

Vita Flex along the spinal reflex point, step 2

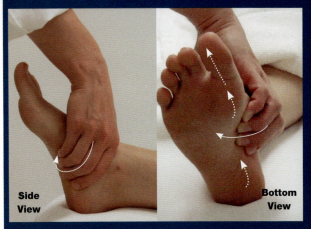

Vita Flex along the spinal reflex point, step 1

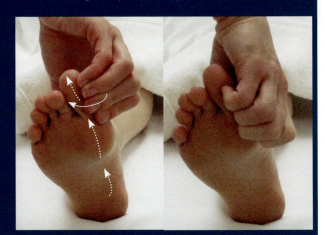

Vita Flex at the big toe, step 1    Vita Flex at the big toe, step 2

### 2. VITA FLEX

To use this technique, nine essential oils are applied to the spinal Vita Flex area on the soles of the feet. These nine oils and blends, in application sequence, are:

1. Oregano (or Plectranthus Oregano)
2. Thyme
3. Basil
4. Cypress
5. Wintergreen
6. Marjoram
7. Peppermint
8. Aroma Siez
9. White Angelica

**Things to Remember**

1. Always begin with the right foot for consistency purposes.
2. Use firm, but not painful, pressure; roll and press to the first knuckle.
3. Move slowly and evenly, one finger width at a time.
4. Repeat everything in three's.

**Procedure**

The following procedure is to be repeated for each of the seven oils, using the appropriate sequence (see the *10 Steps for Vita Flex* worksheet for more detailed instructions).

1. Place 2–3 drops of essential oil (1–2 drops for smaller feet) in the palm of the left hand. Dip the fingertips of the right hand in the oil and stir clockwise three times to energize the oil. Apply along the spine Vita Flex points (bottom inside edge of the foot from heel to the tip of the big toe).

2. Cup the hand so that the fingertips rest on the Vita Flex points at the heel while the thumb rests on the top of the foot.

3. Rock the hand forward so the nail ends up flat against the bottom of the foot (about half a finger length). Then rock backward to the original position.

4. Continue this technique all the way up the foot to the tip of the big toe. End with several Vita Flexes on the neck and center pad of the big toe. Repeat two times before moving to the other foot.

5. Continue this process with the remaining oils.

**Remember:** Right hand to right foot and left hand to left foot. Do both right and left feet before moving to the next oil in the sequence.

### 3. SPINAL APPLICATION OF ESSENTIAL OILS

After Vita Flex is complete, have the receiver turn over and lie on his or her stomach. Be sure that the receiver is comfortable and that modesty is respected. The receiver should place his or her arms comfortably along the sides of the body. The entire back needs to be exposed for application of the Raindrop oils. The oils will be applied from the sacrum to the atlas.

Feather strokes are used in addition to stretching, Vita Flex, and rubbing techniques. For both Vita Flex and other procedures within the Raindrop, specific steps are performed three complete times.

The oils used here mirror those that were used in the Vita Flex application and should be used in the same sequential order.

#### A. OREGANO (or Plectranthus Oregano)
1. Hold the bottle 6 inches above the skin and evenly place 2–4 drops of Oregano (or Plectranthus Oregano) along the spine, extending from the sacrum to the atlas.

**Feather**
2. Use 6-inch brush strokes to "feather" up the spine. To feather, gently brush the back of the fingertips up the spine while alternating hands.
3. Use 12-inch brush strokes to feather up the length of the spine.
4. Feather the entire length of the spine using three long brush strokes.
5. Repeat this process two or three more times.

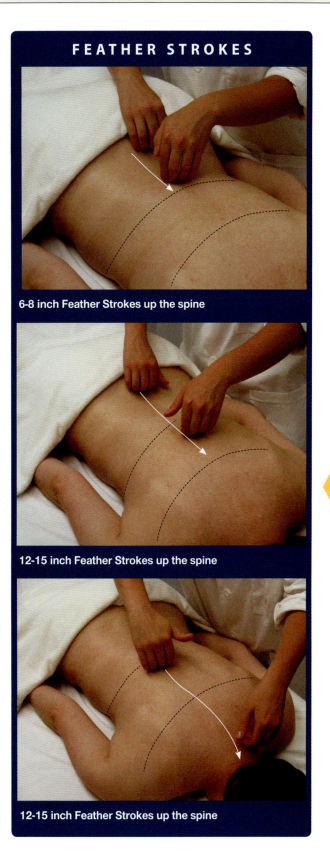

**FEATHER STROKES**

6-8 inch Feather Strokes up the spine

12-15 inch Feather Strokes up the spine

12-15 inch Feather Strokes up the spine

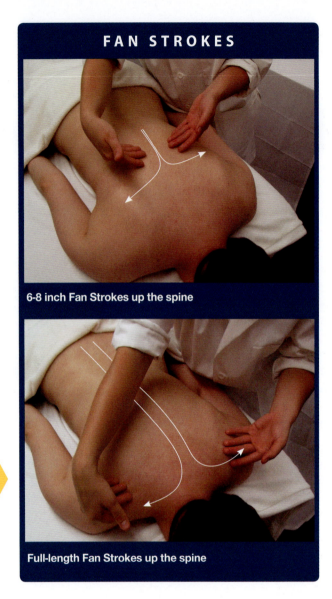

6-8 inch Fan Strokes up the spine

Full-length Fan Strokes up the spine

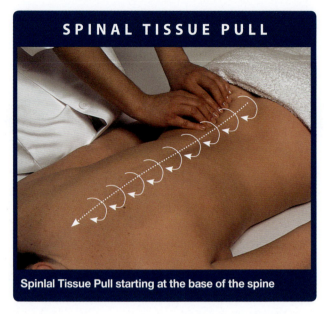

Spinlal Tissue Pull starting at the base of the spine

### C. BASIL

1. Apply 3–4 drops of Basil evenly along both sides of the spine.
2. Immediately feather up the spine according to the technique previously described.

*Spinal Tissue Pull*

3. Alongside the spine, place hands side by side with fingers curved and the heels of the hands resting on the back. Complete three rotations using the pads of the fingertips to create small, circular, clockwise motions to gently pull the muscle tissue away from the spine.
4. After finishing one side of the spine, move to the other side of the receiver and repeat the procedure on the opposite side. Do not apply direct pressure to the spinal vertebrae.
5. Repeat this step two more times.

*Fan*

6. Use 6-inch fanning strokes to fan up the spine and to the sides of the receiver. To fan, gently brush the back of the fingertips up and away from the spine.
7. Fan the entire length of the spine using three long fanning strokes.

**Note:** Do not repeat this process.

### B. THYME

1. Hold the bottle 6 inches above the skin and evenly place 2–4 drops of Thyme along the spine, extending from the sacrum to the atlas.
2. Immediately feather up the spine according to the technique previously described.

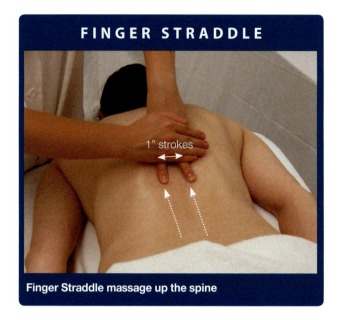

**FINGER STRADDLE**

Finger Straddle massage up the spine

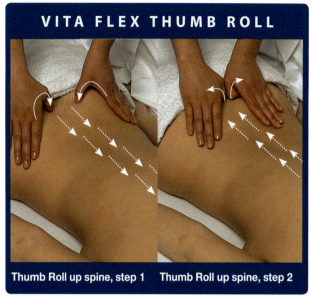

**VITA FLEX THUMB ROLL**

Thumb Roll up spine, step 1    Thumb Roll up spine, step 2

### D. CYPRESS

1. Hold the bottle 6 inches above the skin and evenly place 4–6 drops of Cypress along both sides of the spine, extending from the sacrum to the atlas.
2. Immediately feather up the spine according to the technique previously described.

*Finger Straddle*

3. Stand on the receiver's left side, near the shoulder area, facing the receiver's feet.
4. With the index and middle fingers of the left hand, straddle the spine at the sacrum. Place the bottom edge of the right hand ulna or pinky-side down, just below the middle joints of the two straddling fingers.
5. Apply moderate, downward pressure with the straddling fingers while pulling them slowly to the atlas of the spine. At the same time, saw with the right hand using short, rapid, back-and-forth motions.
6. Once at the atlas, use the straddled fingers to gently pull toward the head three times.
7. Repeat this process two more times.

### E. WINTERGREEN

1. Hold the bottle 6 inches above the skin and evenly space 6–10 drops of Wintergreen along both sides of the spine, extending from the sacrum to the atlas.
2. Immediately feather up the spine according to the technique previously described.

*Vita Flex Thumb Roll*

3. At the sacrum, place both thumbs 1 inch apart on either side of the spine with the tip of the thumbs down, one slightly higher on the back than the other.
4. Begin rolling thumbs from the tip to the nail, back and forth, working up the spine in small increments from the sacrum to the atlas, applying mild pressure the entire time.
5. Continue to roll your thumbs lightly over onto the knuckles and then back to their stand-up position. When doing this process, the knuckles should make contact with the spine. Work up the spine 1 inch at a time.
6. Repeat this step two more times.

**Note:** For clients who have neurological conditions, it is important to work down from the atlas to the sacrum instead of working up the spine.

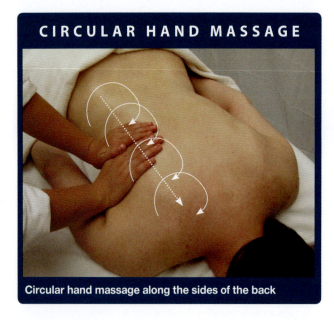

Circular hand massage along the sides of the back

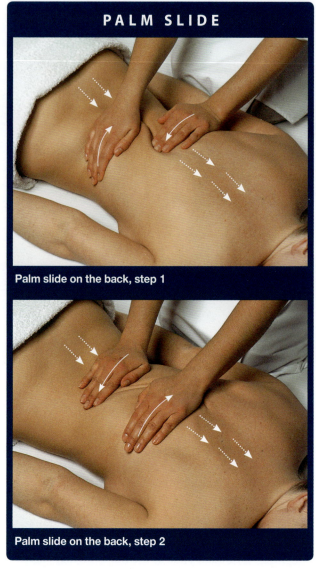

Palm slide on the back, step 1

Palm slide on the back, step 2

### F. MARJORAM

1. Hold the bottle 6 inches above the skin and evenly space 10–15 drops of Marjoram over the entire back, extending from the sacrum to the atlas.
2. Immediately feather as needed to evenly distribute the oil.

*Circular Hand Massage*

3. Place your hands palms down on the lower right side of the back. Rotate hands in a firm, clockwise motion up the right side of the spine.
4. Walk to the left side of the receiver and place your hands palms down on the lower left side of the back. Rotate hands in a firm, clockwise motion up the left side of the spine. Walk back to the right side of the receiver.
5. Repeat steps 3 and 4 two more times.

### G. AROMA SIEZ

1. Hold the bottle 6 inches above the skin and evenly place 10 drops of Aroma Siez all over the back, extending from the sacrum to the atlas.
2. Immediately feather as needed to evenly distribute the oil.

*Palm Slide*

3. Place both hands palm down on the receiver's back on each side of the spine near the sacrum. One hand should be slightly higher than the other.
4. Slide palms, with mild downward pressure, in opposite directions, working slowly up the spine using a back and forth motion up to the nape of the neck.
5. Slide back to the base using the same movements.
6. Repeat this process two more times.

Techniques for Essential Oil Application | Chapter 15

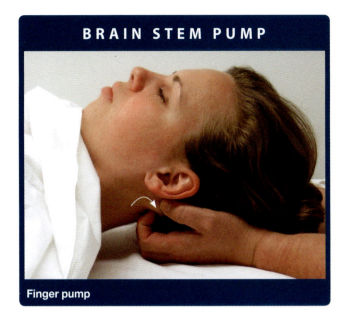

**BRAIN STEM PUMP**

Finger pump

### H. PEPPERMINT
1. Hold the bottle 6 inches above the skin and evenly space 3–5 drops of Peppermint along the spine, extending from the sacrum to the atlas.
2. Immediately feather up the spine according to the technique previously described.

### I. VALOR (or Valor II)
1. Hold the bottle 6 inches above the skin and evenly space 10–12 drops of Valor (or Valor II) along the spine, extending from the sacrum to the atlas.
2. Immediately feather up the spine according to the technique previously described.

### 4. LYMPHATIC PUMP *(Brain Stem Pump Technique)*
1. Have the receiver lie facing up.
2. Place both hands under the back of the head with fingertips resting at the base of the skull.
3. Gently pull the head toward you in a soft, rocking motion, so the entire body moves. Sustain motion for one minute, then rest for one minute.
4. Repeat this process one more time. This movement provides an excellent lymphatic pump effect.

### 5. STRETCH AND RELAX PULL
1. Sit so that your shoulders are parallel to the receiver's shoulders.
2. Hold the receiver's head, using the cranial hold, with your less dominant hand under the base of the receiver's head and the dominant hand cradling the chin.
3. Next, place together your pointer finger and your middle finger and place them under the receiver's chin, just above the Adam's apple, keeping your ring and pinky fingers from touching the receiver's throat.
4. Pull straight back, gently toward you, with the hand under the base of the skull and gently pull with the fingers on the chin. Hold for three to five seconds and gently release.
5. Repeat this movement two more times.

**Note:** If there is another facilitator to assist with this process, he or she should stand at the feet of the receiver and hold the ankles. When the gentle pull is being done at the head, the facilitator at the feet holds the ankles and gently pulls and then releases at the same time as the facilitator at the head.

### FINAL NOTES
- Finish by having the receiver place White Angelica on his or her shoulders, back of the neck, and thymus.
- It is possible that the receiver may have some emotions surface during the application of the Raindrop Technique. Be sure to have the emotional oils ready to assist him or her through the process of releasing those emotions.
- It is important that BOTH the receiver and facilitator drink plenty of water when giving and receiving the Raindrop Technique.

Seventh Edition | Essential Oils Desk Reference

## Customizing Raindrop Technique

Raindrop Technique may be customized to address different health issues that are not directly related to back problems. Lung infections, digestive complaints, hormonal problems, liver insufficiencies, and other problems can all be dealt with by substituting standard Raindrop Technique essential oils with other oils that are specifically targeted for that body system.

As a rule, when customizing, start with Valor (or Valor II), Oregano (or Plectranthus Oregano), and Thyme. For extra antiviral effect, add Mountain Savory. The other essential oils such as Basil, Wintergreen, Marjoram, Thyme, or Cypress can be omitted or replaced by essential oils specific for the condition being targeted.

For example, if targeting a lung infection, replace Basil and Wintergreen with Ravintsara. Cypress is replaced with Eucalyptus Radiata, and Marjoram is replaced with R.C.

Use "The Personal Usage Guide" to see other essential oils that would be applicable for what the individual needs are.

The basic Raindrop Technique has several variations, but these variations are not easy to explain and require class instruction and demonstration.

It would be informative to attend a Raindrop Technique Training with D. Gary Young or one of his trainers and learn the Raindrop Technique from someone who has the knowledge of essential oils and their application.

Raindrop Technique has assisted both professionals and lay people to achieve true balance in the body. Out of the thousands of Raindrop Technique sessions that have been performed, hundreds of instances have been reported where the results were amazingly profound and immediate. Here are just a few examples:

A young man from Denver, Colorado, who suffered from chronic scoliosis, was able—for the first time in eight years—to fully bend over after the application of Raindrop Technique. With an overhead camera televising an image of his spine as he bent over, an audience of over 400 watched the vertebrae in his spine literally move into place. When he stood up, he was measured and had gained an inch in height.

Another instance involved a professional model in her early 40s who had developed early adult-onset scoliosis. She had to alter clothing so that it would fit properly for modeling sessions. She was not able to sit still for any length of time. After a Raindrop session, her spine straightened to such a degree that she, too, had gained an inch in height. She followed up with more sessions, and in the next few months reported that all discomfort was gone. She now dances and rides horses, pain free.

It is quite common for individuals with scoliosis who receive Raindrop Technique to gain ½ inch or more in stature from a single application.

Many others have reported pain relief, congestion relief, and cold and flu relief as a result of Raindrop Technique, which is why it has captured so much interest among those involved in the healing arts.

---

ENDNOTES

1. Green RJ, Webb JN, Maxwell MH. The nature of virus-like particles in the paraxial muscles of idiopathic scoliosis. *J Pathol.* 1979 Sep;129(1):9-12.

2. Webb JN, Gillespie WJ. Virus-like particles in paraspinal muscle in scoliosis. *Br Med J.* 1976 Oct 16;2(6041):912-3.

3. Wolff MH, Buchel F, Gullotta F, Helpap B, Schneeweiss KE. Investigations to demonstrate latent viral infection of varicella-Zoster virus in human spine ganglia. *Verh Dtsch Ges Pathol.* 1981;65:203-7.

4. Stirling A, et al. Association between sciatica and *Propionibacterium acnes. Lancet* 2001 Jun 23:357(9273):2024-5.

5. Nagrath SP, Hazra DK, Pant PC, Seth HC. Tuberculosis spine—a diagnostic conundrum. Case report. *J Assoc Physicians India.* 1974 May;22(5):405-7.

6. Jenks PJ, Stewart B. Images in clinical medicine. Vertebral tuberculosis. *N Engl J Med.* 1998 June 4;338(23):1677.

7. Monaghan D, Gupta A, Barrington NA. Case report: Tuberculosis of the spine—an unusual presentation. *Clin Radiol.* 1991 May;43(5):360-2.

8. Petersen CK, Craw M, Radiological differentiation of tuberculosis and pyogenic osteomyelitis: a case report. *J Manipulative Physiol Ther.* 1986 Mar;9(1):39-42.

9. Pinott JR, Taffs LF. Experimental scoliosis in primates: a neurological cause. *J Bone Joint Surg Br.* 1982;64(4):503-7.

10. Ozogul Y, et al. Antimicrobial Impacts of Essential Oils on Food Borne-Pathogens. *Recent Pat Food Nutr Agric.* 2015;7(1):53-61

11. Wan J, Wilcock A, Coventry MJ. The effect of essential oils of basil on the growth of Aeromonas fluorescens. *Journal of Applied Microbiology,* 1998, 84: 152-158.

12. Beuchat LR. Antimicrobial properties of spices and their essential oils. Center for Food Safety and Quality Enhancement, Department of Food Science and Technology, University of Georgia, Griffin, Georgia.

13. Horne D, et al. Antimicrobial effects of essential oils on Streptococcus pneumoniae. *Journal of Essential Oil Research,* (September/October 2001), 13: 387-392.

14. Moleyar V, Narasimham P. Antibacterial activity of essential oil components. *International Journal of Food Microbiology,* Vol. 16 (1992): 337-32.

15. Obata Y, et al. Effect of pretreatment of skin with cyclic monoterpenes on permeation of diclofenac in hairless rat. *Biol Pharm Bull.* 1993 Mar;16(3):312-4.

16. Zhao K, Singh J. Mechanisms of percutaneous absorption of tamoxifen by terpenes: eugenol, d-limonene and menthone. *Control Release.* 1998. Nov 13;55(2-3):253-60.

# Section 4
## Special Issues

**CHAPTER 16** Essential Oils: Spiritual, Mental, and Emotional. . . . 307

**CHAPTER 17** Cleansing and Diet . . . . . . . . . . . . . . . . . . . . . . . . 317

**CHAPTER 18** Building Blocks of Health . . . . . . . . . . . . . . . . . . . . 343

**CHAPTER 19** Longevity and Vitality—Special Features . . . . . . . . . 361

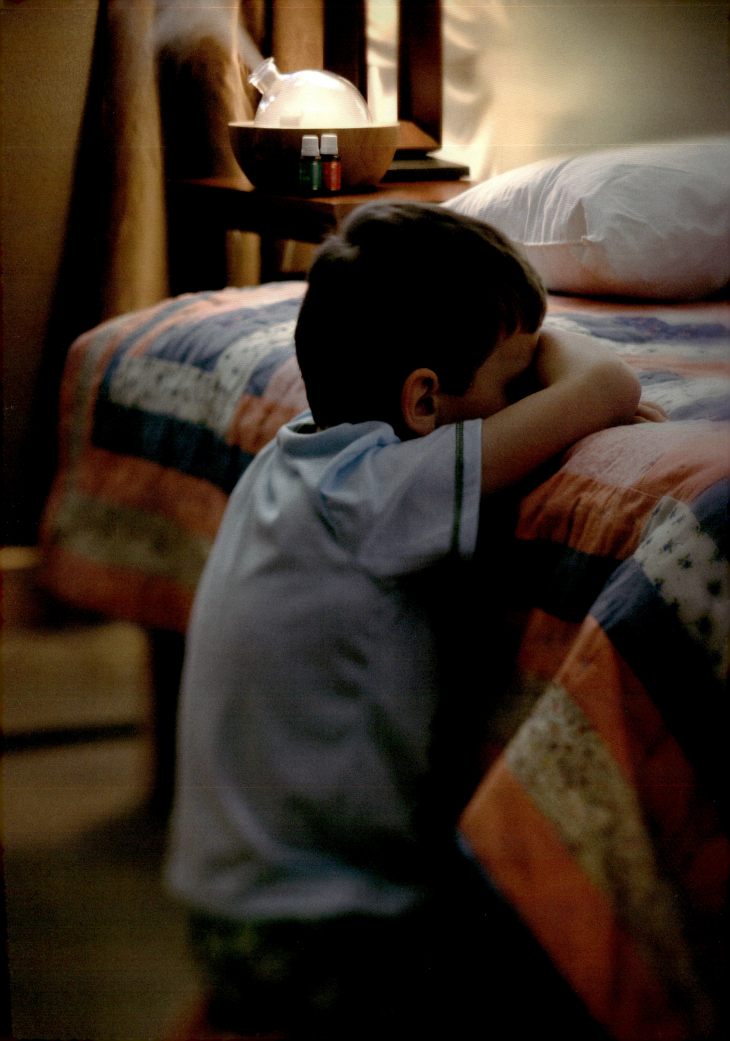

# Chapter 16
## Essential Oils: Spiritual, Mental, and Emotional

## Support with Essential Oils

For literally thousands of years, the sacred smoke of frankincense rose in fragrant columns from temples across the ancient world. Why was it given so much importance in worship and as an offering to the gods? Why do some churches even today still burn frankincense for incense as a major procedure in their worship services?

### The Appeal of Frankincense

The appeal of frankincense has not lessened as ancient days have rolled into the 21st century. As essential oils have gained prominence in our world, people are drawn to the rich aromas of frankincense and myrrh. Fittingly, it is only in our time, as recent as 2008, that scientists have discovered that we are apparently "hardwired" to have feelings of peace, awe, and reverence when using frankincense.

A young Israeli researcher named Arieh Moussaieff joined others from the Hebrew University in studying the Jerusalem Balsam, an herbal remedy that was formulated in 1719 in the Saint Savior monastery pharmacy in the old city of Jerusalem. Of the five different formula variations, the researchers chose to focus on one found in manuscript form in the monastery's archives. It contained four plants: olibanum (*Boswellia* species), myrrh (*Commiphora* species), aloe (*Aloe* species), and mastic (*Pistacia lentiscus L.*). The study that was published in 2005 showed the formula to have anti-inflammatory, antioxidative, and antiseptic properties.

In further frankincense studies, Dr. Moussaieff discovered that a compound of frankincense resin provides protection for the nervous system. Continuing his research, he was the lead researcher on a study that made news around the world.

As the Weizmann Institute of Science wrote in its science newsletter *Interface*, Dr. Moussaieff noticed " . . . the resin's antidepression and antianxiety properties and, investigating further, found that they act on a previ-

ously unknown pathway in the brain that regulates emotion. These findings not only help explain the ubiquity of frankincense in religion, they also hint that the active compounds may be used in the future to treat any number of neurological diseases, from Parkinson's to depression."[1]

Dr. Moussaieff's study was published in 2008 and documented for the first time that an ion channel in the brain (TRPV3) that was previously known only to be implicated in the perception of warmth in the skin had the much more important effect of causing antidepressive and antianxiety behavioral changes when triggered by a component of frankincense, incensole acetate. Dr. Moussaieff's study concluded that "TRPV3 channels in the brain may provide a biological basis for deeply rooted cultural and religious traditions."[2]

Truly, can one come to any other conclusion than we are hard-wired to experience calming and mood-enhancing effects when inhaling the scent of *Boswellia carterii* or *Boswellia sacra*, the two frankincense species known and loved for thousands of years?

You may wonder if being uplifted in mood and having your anxiety quelled by Sacred Frankincense or Frankincense is really a requisite for worship or meditation. The ancient Egyptians apparently thought so, even though they had no idea how frankincense actually accomplished this. The late Professor Gonzague Ryckmans wrote that the Egyptian word for frankincense is SNTR, and it can be translated as "scent of the deity" or "what qualifies man to communicate with the deity."[3]

Religion scholar Scott Hahn, PhD, wrote a chapter on incense in his book, *Signs of Life: 40 Catholic Customs and Their Biblical Roots.* He wrote: "Incense became the most emblematic form of worship. Grains of incense, once dropped into a thurible with hot coals, rise heavenward as fragrant smoke. It's meant to be an outward sign of the inner mystery that is true prayer."[4]

Seventh Edition | **Essential Oils Desk Reference** | 307

## Energy Centers (Chakras) and Associated Glands

**CROWN—Thought—Violet**
Pineal: Controls cerebrum, right brain hemisphere, central nervous system, and right eye

**3RD EYE—Light—Indigo**
Pituitary: Controls endocrine system, left brain hemisphere, left eye, nose, ears, sinuses, and parts of nervous system

**THROAT—Ether/Sound—Blue**
Thyroid: Controls jaw, neck, throat, voice, airways, upper lungs, nape of neck, and arms

**HEART—Air/Touch—Green**
Thymus: Controls heart, blood circulation, immune system, lower lungs, rib cage, skin, upper back, and hands

**SOLAR PLEXUS—Fire/Sight—Yellow**
Pancreas: Controls liver, digestive system, stomach, spleen, gall bladder, muscles, autonomic nervous system, and lower back

**SACRAL—Water/Taste—Orange**
Adrenal: Controls all solid parts—spinal column, bones, teeth, nails; also controls blood and building of cells, kidneys, and bladder

**BASE/ROOT—Earth/Smell—Red**
Reproductive: Controls pelvic area, sex organs, potency, and fluid functions

Hahn mentioned that from Psalm 141:2 in the Old Testament ("Let my prayer be counted as incense before you,") to Philippians 4:18 in the New Testament ("an odour of a sweet smell, a sacrifice acceptable, wellpleasing to God."), incense permeates the Bible. The last book of the New Testament, Revelation, also connects incense with prayer: ". . . and there was given unto him much incense, that he should offer it with the prayers of all saints upon the golden altar which was before the throne. And the smoke of the incense which came with the prayers of the saints, ascended up before God out of the angel's hand" (Rev. 8:3-4).

Hahn also observed that some biblical people used incense and prayer merely as a rote ritual or offered it to strange gods, causing Isaiah to declare these words of the Lord: "Bring no more vain offerings; incense is an abomination to me" (Isaiah 13:1).

True worship is always within a sincere heart. Hahn notes that, "In fact, through the prophet Malachi, he [God] foretold a day when 'from the rising of the sun to its setting . . . in every place incense is offered unto my name, and a pure offering' (Malachi 1:11)."[5]

### How to Enhance Worship and Meditation with Essential Oils

When you want to be "centered" and to quiet a busy mind during meditation so you can focus on worshipful prayer, Frankincense brings peace and a sense of calming to your heart. You need not burn the precious resin to achieve this calmness. Simply breathe in deeply the aroma of Sacred Frankincense or Frankincense.

You may wish to apply (anoint) a few drops of these precious oils on your crown chakra and over your heart. Imagine being away from the busyness of life and perhaps resting on a solitary hill in Oman that overlooks the blue waters of the Arabian Sea, looking in the other direction and feeling the quietness of the immense desert with mystifying sand dunes that seem to shimmer in the sun, or taking refuge under a large frankincense tree that offers a little shade and a place of rest.

Prayer and meditation are ways of preparing that many energy workers and healers use before they begin their day.

The negative energy that also inhabits this world can have no influence while you become quiet and communicate with God. Simply apply a few drops of White Angelica on

308 | Chapter 16 | Spiritual, Mental, and Emotional Support with Essential Oils

your shoulders to wrap yourself in its energetic protection. A drop of rose oil over your heart or on the crown chakra can also help you rise up to a meditative state above the worries of the world.

It is a scientific fact that meditating is healthful and prayer is calming to the soul. You may find singing a quiet hymn a joyful experience. Poet Paul Gerhardt (1607-1676) wrote that hymns can be offerings to God: "Hymns of praise are incense and rams."

## Mental and Emotional Support

Today we live in a society of emotional turmoil. More and more the evidence is accumulating that our emotional health can have a profound effect on our physical health. More than ever before, researchers are probing the impact that emotional states have on the physical condition of the body.

Many doctors are recognizing the possibility that a number of diseases are caused by emotional problems that link back to infancy and childhood—and perhaps even to the womb. These emotional problems can compromise body systems and even genetic structuring through a process that creates the equivalent of a molecular "memory" in key organs and structures of the body.

The idea that memories and traumas can be embedded in the brain is not new, but scientists are now saying that these brain imprints may extend throughout the body. Well-known author and Georgetown University research professor Candace Pert states, "Repressed traumas caused by overwhelming emotion can be stored in a body part, thereafter affecting our ability to feel that part or even move it."

"To some degree, all of the organ systems in the human body have 'memory,'" agrees Bruce D. Perry, MD, PhD. "All nerve cells 'store' information in a fashion that is contingent upon previous patterns of activity," he noted. Dr. Perry is with the Child Trauma Program sponsored jointly by Baylor College of Medicine and Texas Children's Hospital. Perry says further that the ability to "carry elements of previous experience forward in time is the basis of the immune, the neuromuscular, and the neuroendocrine systems."

## Sense of Smell Links Emotion and Memory

As scientists have studied to understand the neural basis of emotion, they have discovered that the limbic system of the brain plays a vital role in interpreting and channeling intense experiences, particularly memories of fear or trauma. Interestingly, the two parts of the limbic system that play a major role in emotional processing—the amygdala and the hippocampus—are located within less than an inch of the olfactory nerve (See diagram above).

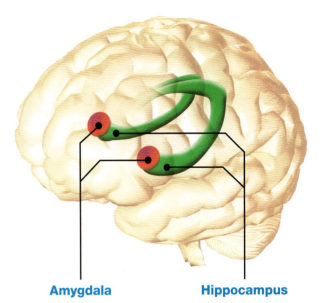

**Amygdala**
Influences behaviors and activities. It is also concerned with emotions such as anger and jealousy, as well as drives such as hunger, thirst, and sexual desire.

**Hippocampus**
Involved with recognizing new experiences, learning, and memory—especially sort-term memory.

Olfaction or smell is the sense that is physically the closest to the limbic system structures of the amygdala, which is involved in experiencing emotion and also in emotional memory, and the hippocampus, which encompasses memory: working memory and short-term memory. This gives you an idea of how closely linked the sense of smell is to emotion and memory.

In 1989 researchers agreed that the amygdala—one of several structures in the cerebral cortex—plays a major role in storing and releasing emotional trauma and that aromas have a profound effect in triggering those responses.

Joseph Ledoux, MD, of the New York Medical University, was one of the first to suggest that the use of aroma could be a major breakthrough in helping to release hidden and suppressed feelings and memories of emotional bondage.

Fear and trauma can produce conditioned emotional responses that—unless released—will not only hamper our ability to live and enjoy life fully but can also limit the ability of some body systems to function properly, particularly the immune system. This can result in unexplained pain and illness as well as depression and other psychological "issues."

Many of the biochemicals in essential oils—particularly sesquiterpenes—can increase blood oxygen levels in the brain. The stimulation of both aroma and oxygenation seems to affect the amygdala in ways that

**Essential Oils Desk Reference** | Seventh Edition

facilitate the release of stored emotional blocks, both in the subconscious and in various body systems.

Combining the aroma of essential oils and oxygenation regularly over time—accompanied by mental focus and intent—has proven to be effective in many cases for resolving unexplained physical problems that were rooted in past emotional trauma.

### Relaxing with Essential Oils

Another way in which essential oils can assist in helping people to move beyond emotional blocks is through their relaxing effect. The aldehydes and esters of certain essential oils such as Lavender, Ruta (Rue), Frankincense, etc., are very calming and sedating to the nervous system (including both the sympathetic and parasympathetic systems). These substances allow us to relax instead of getting caught in an anxiety spiral.

Anxiety creates an acidic condition that activates the transcript enzyme, which then transcribes that anxiety on the RNA template and stores it in the DNA. That emotion then becomes a predominant factor in our lives from that moment on.

### Releasing with Essential Oils

The process of emotional release using essential oils should not be dramatic, but gentle, occurring step-by-step over a period of time. Application of the oils accompanied by mental focus and relaxation should occur multiple times per day. Some emotional blocks will require only a day or two to begin releasing; others may require weeks.

Many essential oil blends have been created precisely for the purpose of helping to release emotional patterns. The protocol outlined below is one that can be used very

flexibly. One can use just the first step or two, a selection of steps, or use all the steps, depending on inclination and need. Each succeeding step involves another essential oil, which may further stimulate the release process.

It is important to remember that this process should not be uncomfortable. As you reach a step during which you begin to feel uncomfortable, there is no need to go further. It is better to wait for a future application when you feel confident before going to that next step. The applications should be accompanied by mental effort focusing on reprogramming negative emotions with positive emotions and images.

**Note:** Some people may find the idea that essential oil scents can be healing and therapeutic just a bit strange or somewhat "woo-woo." Perhaps a testimonial will be instructive.

A lady in her early forties tells of her experience. She had the opportunity to smell several essential oil blends and was drawn to the blend of Release. Her friend gave it to her so that she could experiment to see if she noticed anything. Day after day she opened the bottle, inhaled deeply, and put it on her wrist so that she could smell it throughout the day.

A few months later she had a marvelous dream that went back to a long-repressed memory. A new experience occurred in the dream that gave balance and perspective to the traumatic memory. She was able to heal her feelings as though they just "wafted away in a gentle breeze."

It was many months later that she realized that it was the power of the oil blend Release that allowed this healing to take place. You would have a difficult time telling this lady that oils cannot possibly be healing!

# "Letting Go" with Essential Oils

This is a very simple guideline for "letting go" of some old emotional baggage, releasing, allowing the up-lifting feeling of peace and emotional freedom to take root.

Emotional health is a precious gift to our physical health and well-being.

It is important to be in a quiet place and setting with no cell phone, no TV, and no noisy environment.

**STEP 1. Valor or Valor II** should be the first blend used when preparing for an emotional release. It helps balance the energies within the body and helps to give courage, confidence, and self-esteem. Apply 3-6 drops on each foot and top of shoulders, cup hands,

and breathe in the beautiful strength-giving aroma as it balances the body.

**STEP 2. Harmony** is an exquisite blend of 12 essential oils and promotes physical and emotional healing through harmonic balance of the energy centers of the body, enabling energy to flow more efficiently. It helps reduce stress and creates an overall sense of well-being. Apply a drop on each of the chakra points.

**STEP 3. Sacred Frankincense** helps to regulate emotions, reduces the feelings of stress, and is very calming. It eases the depression around the traumatic experiences of life, whether in times of bereavement, divorce, or

**310** | **Chapter 16** | Spiritual, Mental, and Emotional Support with Essential Oils other emotional losses. It promotes confidence and purpose as the feelings of negativity disappear and stimulates the body's immune system.

When used during yoga, meditation, or prayer, the fullness and capacity of this oil brings support physically, emotionally, and spiritually, offering healing to those who use it. Placing this oil on the temples, back of neck, top of head, and over the heart allows the opportunity for deeper spiritual connection.

**STEP 4.** The **3 Wise Men** blend was formulated to open the subconscious mind through pineal stimulation to release deep-seated trauma encoded in the DNA. This blend opens the crown chakra and stimulates the limbic system, bringing a sense of grounding and uplifting through positive memory recall. Place 2-3 drops on the crown of the head.

**STEP 5. Release** or **Divine Release** helps a person let go of the energy that comes from anger and hate held within the cells of the liver in order to create emotional peace and well-being. Freedom comes from being at peace rather than from harboring negative emotions. Rub 1-2 drops over the front and back of the liver area in a circular motion.

**STEP 6: Idaho Balsam Fir** is a wonderful aroma that is very grounding and relaxing to the body. It helps with the effects of seasonal affective disorder, lifting depression. This strengthening oil stimulates the immune system, creating an increase of energy and sense of well-being. Rub a drop on the brain stem and under the nose. Breathe in the fortifying and balancing fragrance, bringing in the feeling of security.

**STEP 7. Inner Child** is a blend that may stimulate childhood memory. When children experience abuse or trauma, they can become "disconnected" from their inner child or identity. This disconnection may not be apparent until many years later, manifesting itself as a "midlife crisis." The Inner Child fragrance may stimulate memory response, helping one reconnect with his or her fundamental identity. This is an essential step or condition to achieving emotional balance. Apply 1 drop under the nose and 1 drop around the navel.

**STEP 8. Forgiveness** has high electrical frequencies that can help release negative memories to facilitate forgiveness, letting go, and moving on. Apply 1-2 drops around the navel and massage in a clockwise motion.

**STEP 9. Grounding** may be helpful in situations where one is overexcited about new ideas or wants to escape into a protective fantasy. In this kind of mental state, it is easy to make choices that lead to bad relationships, bad business decisions, and other unfortunate circumstances. We seek for an escape because we have no anchor to know how to deal with negative emotions.

The aroma of Grounding helps restore confidence and peace, enabling us to deal logically and peacefully with life's decisions. Apply 1-2 drops to the back of the neck and on the sternum.

**STEP 10. Hope** is formulated to reconnect with a feeling of strength and optimism for the future. Hope must be in place in order to move forward in life. Hopelessness can cause a loss of vision of goals and dreams, making it impossible to release emotional blocks. This aroma may also help in overcoming tendencies toward depression. Massage 1 drop on the outer edge of each ear.

**STEP 11. Joy** is an exotic blend of Ylang Ylang, Bergamot, and pure Bulgarian Rose oil and produces a magnetic energy to attract love and enhance self-love, bringing joy to the heart. Apply 1-2 drops over the heart area and massage in a clockwise motion.

**STEP 12. Present Time** has an empowering fragrance that gives a feeling of being "in the moment." One can only progress through emotional release when in the present time. Apply 1-2 drops on the thymus (top of the sternum) in a circular motion.

**STEP 13. SARA** is an essential oil blend formulated specifically for opening the limbic system to release the memories of serious trauma connected with **S**exual **A**nd/or **R**itual **A**buse. Apply 1 drop over the energy centers (chakras), navel, and chest.

**STEP 14. White Angelica** is an amazing blend of 18 different oils, some of which were used during ancient times to increase the aura around the body, bringing a delicate sense of strength and protection. Its frequency protects against negative energies and helps to create a feeling of wholeness and oneness with the Creator. Apply 1-2 drops on the crown and on the shoulders.

**STEP 15: Take time** while still in the quiet, meditative space and select an oil or oil blend of your choice to enhance this process, reflect on your goals, your dreams, and on the positive things in your life, along with the things that you are choosing to change in your life.

Place a couple of drops of your oil or blend of choice over your heart, back of neck, and then cupping your hands together, breathe in the life-giving, minute, fragrant molecules.

This can be a fortifying process, so take time to write some notes about your experience.

You can choose many oils and blends for this quiet time such as Rose, Ylang Ylang, Sacred Frankincense, Frankincense, Northern Lights Black Spruce, Highest Potential, Gathering, The Gift, Envision, Motivation, Into The Future, Magnify Your Purpose, Joy, Gratitude, Believe, Build Your Dream, Light the Fire, Live Your Passion, Transformation, Oola Balance, Oola Grow, etc. They are all wonderful oils and oil blends to anchor emotional balance and stability.

When you are finished with your quiet time or meditation, do not distract your focus by immediately watching TV or going out to a social event. Remember that the oils may continue to work on an emotional level for several days.

Several oils that you can carry with you that are easily available are the roll-on oils of Valor, Tranquil, RutaVaLa, and Stress Away, for those times when you need some emotional support immediately. Use them on a regular basis, especially at nighttime before you go to sleep. Roll the oils on behind your neck and along the rims of your ears; rub some on your hands until dry and then rub inside the pillow cover; or rub some on the pillow for a wonderful, aromatic, wafting fragrance to lull you off to sleep.

For a much more thorough explanation of emotional release and for specific emotional issues, consult the two books by Karol K. Truman entitled *Feelings Buried Alive Never Die* and *Healing Feelings from Your Heart* and the book by Dr. Carolyn L. Mein entitled *Releasing Emotional Patterns with Essential Oils*. These books are available through Life Science Publishing.

# Oils for Specific Emotional Challenges

## Abuse
**Singles:** Geranium, Ylang Ylang, Palo Santo, Ocotea, Frankincense, Sacred Frankincense

**Blends:** SARA, Hope, Freedom, Joy, Peace & Calming, Inner Child, AromaSleep, SleepyIze, Grounding, Trauma Life, Divine Release, Release, Valor, Valor Roll-On, Valor II, Forgiveness, White Angelica, Inner Harmony, T.R. Care, Oola Faith, Oola Family, Oola Friends

## Agitation
**Singles:** Idaho Blue Spruce, Bergamot, Cedarwood, Idaho Balsam Fir, Jade Lemon, Clary Sage, Frankincense, Sacred Frankincense, Geranium, Juniper, Dalmatia Juniper, Lavender, Myrrh, Marjoram, Rose, Ylang Ylang, Laurus Nobilis, Cistus, Hinoki

**Blends:** Peace & Calming, Peace & Calming II, Freedom, Joy, InTouch, Valor, Valor Roll-On, Valor II, AromaEase, Tranquil Roll-On, Harmony, AromaSleep, Inner Harmony, Forgiveness, T.R. Care, Oola Faith, Oola Family, Oola Fun, RutaVaLa, RutaVaLa Roll-On, Abundance, Australian Blue, White Light

## Anger
**Singles:** Idaho Blue Spruce, Bergamot, Cedarwood, Frankincense, Sacred Frankincense, Lavender, Myrrh, Orange, Rose, Roman Chamomile, Ylang Ylang, Laurus Nobilis, Jade Lemon, Pine, Ponderosa Pine

**Blends:** Release, Divine Release, InTouch, Valor, Valor Roll-On, Valor II, Sacred Mountain, AromaEase, Harmony, Hope, Forgiveness, Freedom, Oola Family, AromaSleep, SleepyIze, Inner Harmony, Transformation, Present Time, T.R. Care, Trauma Life, Joy, Oola Faith, Tranquil Roll-On, Surrender, Christmas Spirit, White Angelic, White Light

## Anxiety
**Singles:** Idaho Blue Spruce, Orange, Roman Chamomile, Ylang Ylang, Lavender, Sacred Frankincense, Frankincense, Clary Sage, Jade Lemon, Angelica, Laurus Nobilis, Hinoki, Cistus, Palmarosa, Pine, Idaho Ponderosa Pine

**Blends:** Freedom, InTouch, Valor, Valor Roll-On, Valor II, AromaSleep, SleepyIze, Hope, Peace & Calming, AromaEase, T.R. Care, Tranquil Roll-On, Joy, Present Time, Divine Release, The Gift, Oola Faith, Oola Family, Oola Finance, Oola Fun, Reconnect, Inner Harmony, Abundance, Surrender, Believe, Shutran, White Angelica, White Light, Oola Balance, Oola Grow, Australian Blue

## Apathy
**Singles:** Frankincense, Sacred Frankincense, Geranium, Marjoram, Jasmine, Orange, Peppermint, Rose, Sandalwood, Jade Lemon, Thyme, Ylang Ylang, Lime

**Blends:** Joy, Harmony, Valor, Valor Roll-On, Valor II, T.R. Care, 3 Wise Men, Hope, Believe, White Angelica, Motivation, Live with Passion, Live Your Passion, Highest Potential, Build Your Dream, Shutran, Inner Harmony, GeneYus, Iron Will, Peak Performance, Oola Fun, Oola Balance, Oola Grow

Spiritual, Mental, and Emotional Support with Essential Oils | **Chapter 16**

## Argumentative

**Singles:** Idaho Blue Spruce, Cedarwood, Palo Santo, Idaho Balsam Fir, Roman Chamomile, Frankincense, Sacred Frankincense, Jade Lemon, Jasmine, Orange, Ylang Ylang, Cistus, Palmarosa, Pine, Idaho Ponderosa Pine

**Blends:** Peace & Calming, Peace & Calming II, Freedom, InTouch, Egyptian Gold, Joy, Harmony, Hope, Valor, Valor Roll-On, Valor II, AromaSleep, SleepyIze, Acceptance, AromaEase, Oola Faith, Oola Family, Humility, Surrender, Divine Release, Release, T.R. Care, Inner Harmony, RutaVaLa, RutaVaLa Roll-On

## Boredom

**Singles:** Cedarwood, Northern Lights Black Spruce, Black Spruce, Black Pepper, Roman Chamomile, Sacred Frankincense, Frankincense, Juniper, Dalmatia Juniper, Lavender, Rosemary, Jade Lemon, Thyme, Ylang Ylang

**Blends:** Build Your Dream, Dream Catcher, Light the Fire, Reconnect, InTouch, T.R. Care, Citrus Fresh, Motivation, Transformation, Inner Child, Valor, Valor Roll-On, Valor II, GeneYus, Awaken, Live with Passion, Live Your Passion, Oola Fun, Gathering, En-R-Gee

## Concentration

**Singles:** Cedarwood, Cypress, Juniper, Dalmatia Juniper, Lavender, Lemon, Jade Lemon, Lemon Myrtle, Basil, Helichrysum, Myrrh, Orange, Peppermint, Rosemary, Sandalwood, Ylang Ylang

**Blends:** Brain Power, Clarity, Reconnect, GeneYus, Highest Potential, Oola Faith, InTouch, T.R. Care, Common Sense, Awaken, Gathering, Dream Catcher, Build Your Dream, Light the Fire, Citrus Fresh, Magnify Your Purpose, Brain Power, Freedom, Oola Finance, Oola Balance, Oola Grow

## Confusion

**Singles:** Cedarwood, Northern Lights Black Spruce, Black Spruce, Peppermint, Sacred Frankincense, Frankincense, Jade Lemon, Ginger, Juniper, Dalmatia Juniper, Copaiba, Lemon Myrtle, Rosemary, Basil, Thyme, Ylang Ylang

**Blends:** Clarity, Light the Fire, Reconnect, GeneYus, Citrus Fresh, Common Sense, Harmony, Valor, Valor Roll-On, Valor II, AromaEase, Freedom, Present Time, Awaken, Brain Power, T.R. Care, Oola Faith, Gathering, Inner Harmony, InTouch, Grounding, Abundance, AromaSleep, SleepyIze, Oola Balance, Oola Grow, Oola Finance, Divine Release, Shutran, Oola Fun, Build Your Dream, Iron Will, Peak Performance, White Light

## Day-Dreaming

**Singles:** Ginger, Cedarwood, Ocotea, Northern Lights Black Spruce, Black Spruce, Lemon, Peppermint, Rose, Rosemary, Tangerine, Jade Lemon, Lemon Myrtle, Spearmint

**Blends:** Reconnect, GeneYus, Sacred Mountain, Gathering, Common Sense, InTouch, Harmony, Present Time, Dream Catcher, Build Your Dream, 3 Wise Men, Magnify Your Purpose, Envision, Light the Fire, Live with Passion, Live Your Passion, Oola Faith, Brain Power, Highest Potential

## Depression

**Singles:** Sacred Frankincense, Idaho Blue Spruce, Frankincense, Copaiba, Palo Santo, Jade Lemon, Lemon, Sandalwood, Geranium, Lavender, Angelica, Orange, Grapefruit, Cistus, Ylang Ylang, Hinoki, Melissa, Lime, Palmarosa, Pine, Idaho Ponderosa Pine, Tsuga, Western Red Cedar, Mastrante

**Blends:** Valor, Valor Roll-On, Valor II, AromaEase, Divine Release, Freedom, T.R. Care, Oola Friends, Motivation, Live with Passion, Live Your Passion, Hope, Believe, Christmas Spirit, Reconnect, InTouch, Inner Harmony, Shutran, Citrus Fresh, Brain Power, Present Time, Oola Balance, Envision, Sacred Mountain, Harmony, Oola Field, Highest Potential, Build Your Dream, Light the Fire, Oola Faith, Oola Finance, Oola Fitness, Joy, Australian Blue, AromaSleep, Oola Fun, White Light, Dragon Time, En-R-Gee, Gentle Baby, SARA

## Despair

**Singles:** Cedarwood, Northern Lights Black Spruce, Black Spruce, Sacred Frankincense, Idaho Blue Spruce, Frankincense, Lavender, Geranium, Jade Lemon, Lemon, Orange, Peppermint, Rosemary, Thyme, Cistus, Ylang Ylang, Hinoki, Melissa, Lime, Palmarosa, Pine, Idaho Ponderosa Pine, Tangerine, Tsuga, Western Red Cedar, Mastrante

**Blends:** Joy, Believe, Christmas Spirit, Freedom, Reconnect, T.R. Care, InTouch, AromaEase, Valor, Valor Roll-On, Valor II, AromaSleep, SleepyIze, Inner Harmony, Harmony, Gathering, Grounding, Inner Child, Forgiveness, Oola Field, Oola Finance, Oola Friends, Motivation, Divine Release, Oola Faith, Hope, Oola Balance, RutaVaLa, RutaVaLa Roll-On, Citrus Fresh, Abundance, Australian Blue, En-R-Gee, Gentle Baby, SARA, Oola Fitness, Oola Fun, Build Your Dream, Light the Fire, White Light

Seventh Edition | **Essential Oils Desk Reference** | 313

## Despondency

**Singles:** Idaho Blue Spruce, Geranium, Sacred Frankincense, Frankincense, Jade Lemon, Ginger, Orange, Rose, Ylang Ylang, Idaho Balsam Fir, Hinoki, Melissa, Lime, Cistus, Nutmeg, Palmarosa, Pine, Idaho Ponderosa Pine, Tangerine, Tsuga, Western Red Cedar, Mastrante

**Blends:** Oola Faith, Inspiration, Reconnect, Common Sense, Shutran, InTouch, Inner Harmony, Harmony, Christmas Spirit, Valor, Valor Roll-On, Valor II, Hope, Freedom, T.R. Care, Oola Field, Joy, Build Your Dream, Light the Fire, Present Time, Gathering, Inner Child, Trauma Life, Australian Blue, AromaEase, Envision, AromaSleep, SleepyIze, Oola Balance, Oola Finance, Oola Fitness, Oola Friends, Oola Fun, White Light, Citrus Fresh, En-R-Gee, Gentle Baby

## Disappointment

**Singles:** Copaiba, Sacred Frankincense, Frankincense, Palo Santo, Geranium, Ginger, Juniper, Dalmatia Juniper, Lavender, Jade Lemon, Northern Lights Black Spruce, Black Spruce, Orange, Thyme, Ylang Ylang, Hinoki, Laurus Nobilis, Melissa, Cistus, Tangerine, Tsuga, Western Red Cedar, Mastrante

**Blends:** Oola Faith, Hope, Joy, Christmas Spirit, Valor, Valor Roll-On, Valor II, Reconnect, T.R. Care, AromaSleep, SleepyIze, Present Time, Inner Harmony, Harmony, Build Your Dream, Dream Catcher, Light the Fire, Abundance, Divine Release, Release, Freedom, Gathering, Magnify Your Purpose, Live with Passion, Live Your Passion, Believe, Shutran, InTouch, AromaEase, Oola Finance, Oola Friends, Oola Balance, Oola Fitness, Oola Fun, Motivation, White Light, Australian Blue

## Discouragement

**Singles:** Idaho Blue Spruce, Bergamot, Idaho Balsam Fir, Cedarwood, Sacred Frankincense, Frankincense, Geranium, Juniper, Dalmatia Juniper, Lavender, Jade Lemon, Lemon, Orange, Northern Lights Black Spruce, Black Spruce, Hinoki, Melissa, Cistus, Laurus Nobilis, Lime, Cardamom, Nutmeg, Palmarosa, Pine, Idaho Ponderosa Pine, Tangerine, Tsuga, Western Red Cedar, Mastrante

**Blends:** Oola Faith, Valor, Valor Roll-On, Valor II, Shutran, AromaSleep, SleepyIze, Light the Fire, Oola Friends, The Gift, Sacred Mountain, Freedom, Common Sense, InTouch, Hope, Joy, Build Your Dream, Dream Catcher, Divine Release, Release, Inner Harmony, Reconnect, Abundance, Into the Future, Magnify Your Purpose, Envision, Believe, AromaEase, Iron Will, Peak Performance, Oola Family, Oola Field, Oola Finance, Oola Fitness, Oola Fun, Gathering, Christmas Spirit, Australian Blue, Oola Balance, White Light, Citrus Fresh, En-R-Gee

## Fear

**Singles:** Idaho Blue Spruce, Palo Santo, Cypress, Roman Chamomile, Geranium, Juniper, Dalmatia Juniper, Myrrh, Northern Lights Black Spruce, Black Spruce, Orange, Sacred Frankincense, Hinoki, Jade Lemon, Cistus, Pine, Idaho Ponderosa Pine, Tangerine, Tsuga, Western Red Cedar

**Blends:** Oola Faith, Valor, Valor Roll-On, Valor II, T.R. Care, AromaEase, AromaSleep, SleepyIze, Freedom, InTouch, Present Time, The Gift, Tranquil Roll-On, Divine Release, Release, Hope, Inner Harmony, White Angelica, Trauma Life, Oola Friends, Gratitude, Gathering, Abundance, Highest Potential, Shutran, Australian Blue, Light the Fire, Christmas Spirit, Oola Field, Oola Finance, Oola Fun, Oola Balance, White Light

## Forgetfulness

**Singles:** Cedarwood, Roman Chamomile, Sacred Frankincense, Frankincense, Rosemary, Copaiba, Idaho Balsam Fir, Peppermint, Thyme, Jade Lemon, Lemon Myrtle, Ylang Ylang

**Blends:** Reconnect, GeneYus, Clarity, Valor, Valor Roll-On, Valor II, Present Time, Gathering, 3 Wise Men, Dream Catcher, Citrus Fresh, Acceptance, Brain Power, Highest Potential, Inner Harmony, Oola Grow, Egyptian Gold, Gathering

## Frustration

**Singles:** Idaho Blue Spruce, Roman Chamomile, Palo Santo, Ocotea, Ginger, Juniper, Dalmatia Juniper, Lavender, Jade Lemon, Lemon, Orange, Peppermint, Thyme, Ylang Ylang, Northern Lights Black Spruce, Black Spruce, Hinoki, Melissa, Cistus, Angelica, Palmarosa, Tangerine

**Blends:** Valor, Valor Roll-On, Valor II, T.R. Care, Light the Fire, Hope, AromaEase, Present Time, Oola Faith, Sacred Mountain, 3 Wise Men, Inner Harmony, Humility, Peace & Calming, Peace & Calming II, Oola Friends, AromaSleep, SleepyIze, Hope, Freedom, Iron Will, Peak Performance, Oola Field, Oola Fun, Reconnect, GeneYus, InTouch, Tranquil Roll-On, Divine Release, Release, Surrender, Gratitude, Gathering, Abundance, Oola Balance, Oola Family, Oola Finance, Oola Fitness, Shutran, White Light, Australian Blue

Spiritual, Mental, and Emotional Support with Essential Oils | **Chapter 16**

## Grief/Sorrow

**Singles:** Bergamot, Palo Santo, Roman Chamomile, Clary Sage, Eucalyptus Globulus, Juniper, Dalmatia Juniper, Lavender, Hinoki, Laurus Nobilis, Melissa, Cistus, Tsuga, Jade Lemon, Western Red Cedar, Mastrante

**Blends:** Oola Faith, Valor, Valor Roll-On, Valor II, T.R. Care, AromaEase, AromaSleep, SleepyIze, Release, Divine Release, Freedom, Inspiration, Inner Child, Gathering, Inner Harmony, Harmony, Present Time, Magnify Your Purpose, Abundance, Australian Blue, Christmas Spirit, Oola Balance, Oola Finance, Egyptian Gold, Oola Field, White Light, InTouch, SARA

## Guilt

**Singles:** Roman Chamomile, Cypress, Juniper, Dalmatia Juniper, Geranium, Sacred Frankincense, Frankincense, Northern Lights Black Spruce, Black Spruce, Rose, Jade Lemon, Thyme

**Blends:** Oola Faith, Oola Field, Valor, Valor Roll-On, Valor II, T.R. Care, AromaEase, Divine Release, Release, Freedom, AromaSleep, SleepyIze, Inspiration, Common Sense, Inner Child, Gathering, Inner Harmony, Harmony, Present Time, Oola Friends, Oola Finance, Magnify Your Purpose, Gratitude, Egyptian Gold, SARA

## Irritability

**Singles:** Idaho Blue Spruce, Idaho Balsam Fir, Lavender, Ocotea, Melissa, Palo Santo, Copaiba, Dorado Azul, Valerian, Western Red Cedar, Ylang Ylang, Angelica, Jade Lemon, Tangerine, Cistus, Tsuga, Palmarosa

**Blends:** Valor, Valor Roll-On, Valor II, Freedom, T.R. Care, Oola Faith, Hope, AromaEase, Peace & Calming, Peace & Calming II, AromaSleep, SleepyIze, Divine Release, Release, Surrender, Transformation, Oola Family, Forgiveness, Inner Harmony, Oola Field, InTouch, Present Time, Inspiration, White Angelica, White Light, Abundance, Oola Fitness, Dragon Time, Lady Sclareol

## Jealousy

**Singles:** Ocotea, Palo Santo, Idaho Balsam Fir, Dorado Azul, Sacred Frankincense, Frankincense, Lemon, Orange, Rose, Rosemary, Thyme

**Blends:** The Gift, Chivalry, Sacred Mountain, Valor, Valor Roll-On, Valor II, White Angelica, Joy, Inner Harmony, Harmony, AromaSleep, SleepyIze, Humility, Forgiveness, Oola Family, Oola Field, Oola Fitness, Surrender, Release, Gratitude

## Mood Swings

**Singles:** Idaho Blue Spruce, Idaho Balsam Fir, Clary Sage, Sage, Dalmatia Sage, Geranium, Juniper, Dalmatia Juniper, Fennel, Lavender, Peppermint, Rose, Jasmine, Rosemary, Jade Lemon, Lemon, Northern Lights Black Spruce, Black Spruce, Angelica, Yarrow, Hinoki, Laurus Nobilis, Melissa, Cistus, Lime, Ylang Ylang, Nutmeg, Vetiver

**Blends:** Peace & Calming, Peace & Calming II, Reconnect, GeneYus, AromaEase, RutaVaLa, RutaVaLa Roll-On, Gathering, Valor, Valor Roll-On, Valor II, AromaSleep, SleepyIze, Dragon Time, Mister, Oola Faith, Inner Harmony, Harmony, Joy, Present Time, Freedom, Envision, Magnify Your Purpose, Abundance, White Angelica, InTouch, Brain Power, Australian Blue, Christmas Spirit, Oola Field, Oola Fun, Tranquil Roll-On, T.R. Care, Oola Balance, Oola Family, Oola Finance, Oola Fitness, Oola Friends, Egyptian Gold, En-R-Gee, Shutran, Lady Sclareol, White Light

## Obsessiveness

**Singles:** Clary Sage, Ocotea, Palo Santo, Cypress, Geranium, Lavender, Ylang Ylang, Jade Lemon, Patchouli

**Blends:** Sacred Mountain, The Gift, Valor, Valor Roll-On, Valor II, Forgiveness, Acceptance, Humility, Inner Child, Present Time, Awaken, Motivation, Surrender, Transformation, Inner Harmony, AromaEase, Divine Release, Release, Common Sense, Joy, Gratitude

## Panic

**Singles:** Idaho Blue Spruce, Bergamot, Idaho Balsam Fir, Roman Chamomile, Myrrh, Sacred Frankincense, Frankincense, Lavender, Marjoram, Rosemary, Jade Lemon, Thyme, Ylang Ylang, Northern Lights Black Spruce, Black Spruce, Angelica, Cistus, Palmarosa, Pine, Idaho Ponderosa Pine

**Blends:** Harmony, Valor, Valor Roll-On, Valor II, InTouch, T.R. Care, AromaEase, AromaSleep, SleepyIze, Oola Faith, Freedom, RutaVaLa, RutaVaLa Roll-On, The Gift, Gathering, White Angelica, Peace & Calming, Peace & Calming II, Trauma Life, Tranquil Roll-On, Inner Harmony, Awaken, Grounding, Abundance, Believe, Reconnect, Oola Balance, Oola Finance, Shutran, Australian Blue

Seventh Edition | **Essential Oils Desk Reference** | 315

## Resentment

**Singles:** Jasmine, Rose, Idaho Tansy, Ocotea, Jade Lemon, Palo Santo

**Blends:** Forgiveness, RutaVaLa, RutaVaLa Roll-On, Inner Harmony, Harmony, T.R. Care, Believe, Common Sense, Humility, White Angelica, Surrender, Joy, Oola Faith, Oola Finance, Divine Release, Release, Oola Field, Oola Family, AromaEase, AromaSleep, SleepyIze, Oola Balance

## Restlessness

**Singles:** Idaho Blue Spruce, Bergamot, Ocotea, Idaho Balsam Fir, Dorado Azul, Sacred Frankincense, Frankincense, Geranium, Lavender, Jade Lemon, Orange, Ylang Ylang, Northern Lights Black Spruce, Black Spruce, Angelica, Valerian, Cistus, Cardamom, Palmarosa

**Blends:** Reconnect, GeneYus, InTouch, T.R. Care, RutaVaLa, RutaVaLa Roll-On, AromaEase, Common Sense, Peace & Calming, Peace & Calming II, Freedom, Inner Harmony, Oola Faith, Tranquil Roll-On, Build Your Dream, The Gift, Sacred Mountain, Gathering, Valor, Valor Roll-On, Valor II, Inspiration, Acceptance, Surrender, Light the Fire, Live with Passion, Live Your Passion, White Angelica, Oola Field, Oola Finance, Oola Fitness, Oola Grow, Oola Balance, Oola Friends, Oola Fun, Shutran, AromaSleep, SleepyIze, Abundance, Iron Will, Peak Performance

## Shock

**Singles:** Idaho Blue Spruce, Helichrysum, Basil, Dorado Azul, Copaiba, Roman Chamomile, Ylang Ylang, Rosemary, Cardamom

**Blends:** Clarity, Common Sense, Reconnect, AromaEase, Chivalry, Valor, Valor Roll-On, Valor II, Inspiration, Joy, AromaSleep, SleepyIze, Tranquil Roll-On, Grounding, Trauma Life, T.R. Care, Freedom, White Light, Brain Power, Australian Blue, Abundance

## Stress

**Singles:** Idaho Blue Spruce, Roman Chamomile, Ylang Ylang, Angelica, Frankincense, Sacred Frankincense, Cistus, Cardamom, Cedarwood, Hinoki, Laurus Nobilis, Melissa, Lime, Jade Lemon, Clove, Dill, Palmarosa

**Blends:** Stress Away, Stress Away Roll-On, AromaEase, AromaSleep, SleepyIze, Freedom, Reconnect, GeneYus, Tranquil Roll-On, Oola Faith, T.R. Care, Divine Release, Release, Hope, Magnify Your Purpose, Christmas Spirit, Live with Passion, Live Your Passion, Light the Fire, Iron Will, Peak Performance, Citrus Fresh, En-R-Gee, Into the Future, Highest Potential, Gathering, Mister, RutaVaLa, RutaVaLa Roll-On, Transformation, Oola Finance, Oola Balance, Oola Grow, Oola Family, Oola Friends, InTouch, Oola Field, Oola Fitness, Oola Fun, Shutran, White Light, Inner Harmony, White Angelica

---

ENDNOTES:

1. http://wis-ks.gsites.co.il/site/en/weizman.asp?pi=421&doc_id=6120&interID=6107.
2. Moussaieff A, Friede E, Amar Z, Lev E, Steinberg D, Gallily R, Mechoulam R. The Jerusalem Balsam: from the Franciscan Monastery in the old city of Jerusalem to Martindale 33, *J Ethnopharmacol.* 2005 Oct 3;101-(1-3):16-26.
3. Der Weihrauch: Geschichte, Bedeutung, Vervendung, Regensburg, 1977:17.
4. Hahn S. *Signs of Life: 40 Catholic Customs and their Biblical Roots*, Doubleday, 2009:159.
5. Ibid:158.

# Chapter 17
## Cleansing and Diet

## The Importance of Cleansing

As the human body ages, there is a greater buildup of chemical contamination in our tissues. As toxins accumulate, the body is more likely to suffer the energy-robbing effects of poor health and degenerative diseases.

This is why cleansing the body is so important. When the body is purging itself of heavy metal contamination, undigested foods, and internal pollution, it relieves enormous stress on the organs and tissues, immune function is enhanced, and the stress on the liver is reduced.

Cleansing helps with weight reduction and brings back the creative energy, motivation, and vitality that are especially healing when suffering from degenerative diseases.

### Everyone Needs Cleansing

Babies, who are at the beginning of their lives, and the elderly, who have lived long lives, all need cleansing.

All of us are stressed, to a lesser or greater degree, by an ever-mounting buildup of toxins, chemicals, bacteria, parasites, industrial wastes, herbicides, pesticides, additives, and heavy metals we unknowingly absorb from our food, cosmetics, air, water, and even from the mercury fillings in our teeth.

Moreover, humans are subjected to concentrated doses of potentially harmful chemicals from the meats and dairy products consumed.

According to a 1990 survey taken by the Environmental Protection Agency (EPA), every single person tested showed some evidence of petrochemical pollution in their body tissues and fat. Some of the chemicals found included styrene (used in plastics), xylene (a solvent in paint and gasoline), benzene (a chemical found in gasoline), and toluene (another carcinogenic solvent).

If that survey were taken today, how many more chemicals and pollutants would be found? How much radiation contamination is our world experiencing from just the atomic energy disaster in Japan? It all adds up to a world of disease and suffering.

Inflammation is one of the main factors contributing to disease in the human body today, heart disease being a prime example. Many people do not understand how someone relatively healthy, with low cholesterol levels, normal arterial function, and healthy arterial walls, can unexpectedly suffer a heart attack; yet it happens all too often. The explanation is inflammation.

What causes this inflammation and how does it occur in the body? Inflammation has various causes: bacterial infection (such as *Chlamydia pneumoniae*), poor diet, chemicals, hormonal imbalance, or physical injury.

Inflammation can come just from an organ or a body system not functioning properly—a system plugged with a vast number of toxins and waste debris, unable to absorb all the necessary life-giving nutrients.

A protein called "C-reactive" is released by the liver when inflammation is present. The level of this protein indicates the degree of inflammation in places like the linings of the arteries of the heart.

Accumulation of C-reactive protein and an excess of blood protein plasma can change pH in the blood and cellular function and hasten the onset of tumors and a predisposition for heart disease. In fact, C-reactive protein testing may help doctors predict heart attack or stroke risk.

Cleansing gives the body the strength to fight off the disease and not be encumbered or overloaded with the accumulation of toxins, mucous, and parasites that have built up over the years.

Seventh Edition | **Essential Oils Desk Reference** | 317

**Essential Oils Desk Reference** | Seventh Edition

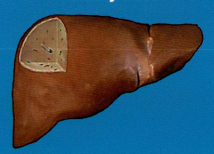

**Healthy Liver**

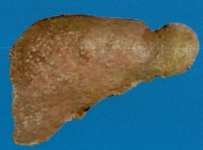

**Cirrhotic Liver**

This type of degeneration is created whenever functioning liver cells are replaced by non-functioning, scar tissue cells. Eventually, the liver ceases to function, leading to death. Cirrhosis is usually the end-result of cumulative liver overload, toxicity, and hepatitis infection.

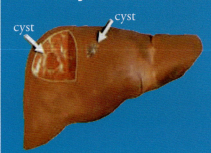

**Cystic Liver**

Cumulative DNA damage results in this condition, which is usually caused from excess lipid peroxidation and lack of dietary antioxidants.

# Liver Health

**The Importance of Liver Health**

"The liver is one of the most important organs in the body, playing a major role in detoxifying the body. When the liver is damaged due to excess alcohol consumption, viral hepatitis, or poor diet, an excess of toxins can build up in the blood and tissues that can result in degenerative disease and health."

—D. Gary Young, ND
*Essential Oils Integrative Medical Guide*

The quality of virtually every body function depends on the liver, which is essential for life. The liver is responsible for removing and neutralizing toxins and germs from the blood, promoting digestion, maintaining hormone balance, regulating blood sugar levels, and making proteins that regulate blood clotting.

Cumulative liver stress caused by toxins, poor diet, or disease inevitably leads to irreversible liver damage and death. The first stage is a condition known as fatty liver in which fat deposits accumulate and poison the liver. It has been estimated that 5 percent of the general population and 25 percent of patients with obesity and diabetes suffer from fatty liver.

With time, fatty liver eventually progresses to cirrhosis, a condition in which nonfunctioning scar tissue replaces working tissue; it is the eighth leading cause of death by disease, killing over 22,000 people a year.

The liver is one of the most important organs in the body. It is pivotal for purifying the blood and plays a key role in converting carbohydrates to energy, as well as storing energy in the form of glycogen and fats.
It is responsible for these vital functions:

- Filtering and processing all food, nutrients, alcohol, drugs, and other materials that enter the bloodstream and letting them pass, breaking them down or storing them
- Manufacturing bile needed to emulsify fats for digestion
- Making and breaking down many hormones, including cholesterol, testosterone, and estrogens
- Regulating blood sugar levels

Virtually every function of the human body depends on the liver. Beyond the physiological importance of the liver, it is the anchor of all emotions, meaning that the negative emotions we experience are stored in the liver.

With the health challenges we all face in our modern world, it has never been more important to maintain a fully functioning, healthy liver. An overburdened liver can

Cleansing and Diet | **Chapter 17**

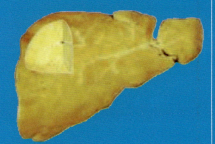

**Extreme Fatty Liver**

This becomes more common later in life or because of severe liver stress. A liver that displays this level of fatty degeneration would eventually become scarred and contribute to cirrhosis. Overcooked and refined foods can also contribute to the progression of severe fatty liver.

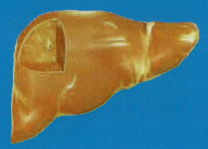

**Fatty Liver**

This disease is found in 5 percent of the general population and over 25 percent of patients with obesity and type II diabetes. The condition usually comes from cumulative liver stress caused by excess sugars in the diet, deficiency in choline, chemical stress and toxicity, lipid peroxidation (fats becoming rancid in the liver), and/or alcohol

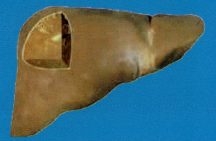

**Haemo-type Liver**

Excessive iron in the diet can lead to cumulative liver damage and cirrhosis.

negatively affect our energy, digestion, skin, and blood. That is why cleansing and detoxifying the liver is so fundamental for good health.

### Facts About the Liver
- About one fourth of your total blood volume passes through your liver **every minute**.
- It is the largest organ in the body, essential for life.
- It produces bile to help absorb fats and fat-soluble vitamins.
- It removes or neutralizes poisons from the blood.
- It removes germs and bacteria from the blood.
- It makes proteins that regulate blood clotting.

### Things that Stress the Liver
- **Blocked bile ducts**—When the ducts that carry bile out of the liver are blocked, bile backs up and damages liver tissue (biliary cirrhosis).
- **Chronic hepatitis B and C**—The hepatitis virus is a major cause of chronic liver disease and cirrhosis in the United States. Hepatitis viral infections cause inflammations and low-grade damage to the liver, which eventually leads to cirrhosis and death.
- **Diabetes, protein malnutrition, obesity, and corticosteroid use**—Any of these can cause nonalcoholic steatohepatitis (NASH). NASH results in deadly fat buildup and eventual cirrhosis in the liver.
- **Exposure to chemicals and parasites**—Toxins, pharmaceutical drugs, and parasites contribute to liver problems. Many pesticides, petrochemicals, and environmental toxins are potent liver stressors. Parasitic infection (schistosomiasis) can also contribute to cirrhosis.

  Acetaminophen can also stress the liver, as can reactions to prescription drugs. Acetaminophen is found in both over-the-counter and prescription drugs; and accidental overdoses each year result in 56,000 emergency room visits, 1,600 cases of acute liver failure, and 458 deaths.

  On January 13, 2011, the FDA announced that products containing acetaminophen cannot contain more than 325 milligrams of acetaminophen, and the labels must warn of the potential risk of severe liver injury.

- **Inherited diseases**—Alpha-1 antitrypsin deficiency, Wilson's disease, galactosemia, and glycogen storage diseases are inherited disorders that result in malproduction, malprocessing, and malstorage by the liver of enzymes, proteins, and metals.
- **Iron overload**—Excess iron in the diet can stress the liver, especially in individuals who are genetically unable to dispose of or sequester dietary iron (hemochromatosis). It creates a haemo-type liver pathology.

Seventh Edition | **Essential Oils Desk Reference** | 319

**Essential Oils Desk Reference** | Seventh Edition

# Signs of an Overloaded and/or Toxic Liver

Here are some clues that could mean your liver is in trouble:

- Overweight
- Inability to lose weight
- Weight loss
- Loss of appetite
- Abdominal bloating after eating
- Excessive gas
- Poor and inadequate digestion
- Nausea
- Bad breath
- Coated tongue when going without food for a half or full day
- Sluggish metabolism
- High cholesterol
- Sugar cravings
- Excessive alcohol intake
- Sensitivity to medication—*Because of the liver's inability to remove drugs from the blood at the usual rate, drugs act longer than expected.*
- Irritable bowel syndrome
- Frequent or continued fatigue
- Weakness
- Frequent headaches or migraines

- Mood and behavior swings
- Unpleasant moods
- Forgetfulness, poor concentration, or disturbed sleep
- Lowered immunity—*A liver not able to work at the optimum level will result in immune system dysfunction, which leads to infection and many other problems.*
- Over-burdened immune system
- Recurring colds, fevers, and mucus
- Excessive body heat
- Gallbladder problems
- Gallstones
- Fatty liver
- Allergies
- High blood pressure
- Hormonal imbalance
- Rashes
- Chemical intolerance
- Bruising and bleeding—*This is caused when the liver is unable to produce sufficient clotting proteins.*

- Portal hypertension—*When the flow of blood through the portal vein is slowed, pressure increases inside.*
- Varices (distended veins)—*When blood from the intestines and spleen backs up into blood vessels in the stomach and esophagus, the varices swell and are more likely to burst.*
- Jaundice—*The liver's inability to cleanse the blood may result in yellowing of the skin and eyes.*
- Itching—*Intense itching may be a result of bile waste residue deposited in the skin.*
- Oily skin
- Skin blemishes
- Edema and ascites—*Excessive fluid in the abdomen between the lining and the abdominal organs is caused when the liver stops making the protein albumin, holding water in the leg (edema) and abdomen (ascites), often referred to as fluid retention.*

- **Nonalcoholic steatohepatitis (NASH)**—This condition causes fat buildup and eventual cirrhosis of the liver. This type of hepatitis appears to be associated with diabetes, protein malnutrition, obesity, coronary artery disease, and corticosteroid treatment.

- **Poor diet**—Excess intake of refined carbohydrates and sugars can cause fatty liver or liver degeneration over time. Diabetes, protein malnutrition, obesity, and corticosteroid treatment can also cause fatty liver.

- **Coffee and colas**—Because the liver is the cleansing organ of the body, it has to cleanse and filter the toxins and waste out of the blood. If the liver is too overloaded and cannot function optimally, then other systems begin to break down, and the liver starts to deteriorate.

  Coffee is a drink loved by millions of people all over the world, but that does not change the fact that

it has damaging effects on the liver and other organs of the body.

- Coffee promotes aging because of high amounts of cadmium.

- Cadmium, a toxic heavy metal, interferes with immune function, nerve conduction, and hundreds of other physiological systems.

- High quantities of cadmium in the diet have been correlated with shortened life span.

- Cadmium stays locked in the body for decades. Researchers estimate that its biologic half-life is up to 38 years, according to the Agency for Toxic Substances & Disease Registry.

- Coffee blocks the absorption of zinc, which is one of the few minerals that can counteract and neutralize cadmium.

320 | **Chapter 17** | Cleansing and Diet

Cleansing and Diet | **Chapter 17**

- The caffeine in coffee and colas acts as both a stimulant and a diuretic and is related to lower calcium and trace mineral levels in the body.

- Caffeine increases the stress hormone cortisol in the body, which, if produced in excess, can result in high blood pressure, adrenal exhaustion, and diabetes.

Colas containing phosphoric acid can leach magnesium from the body. Magnesium-deficiency is directly linked to degenerative diseases like heart disease and diabetes.

- **Viruses**—The hepatitis B and C viruses are major causes of chronic liver disease and cirrhosis in the United States. Hepatitis viral infections cause inflammation and low-grade damage to the liver that eventually leads to cirrhosis and death.

  A 2003 study conducted by Roger Lewis, MD, at the Young Life Research Clinic in Springville, Utah, evaluated the efficacy of Helichrysum, Ledum, and Celery Seed, essential oils in the JuvaCleanse blend, in treating cases of advanced hepatitis C.

In one case, a male, age 20, was diagnosed with a hepatitis C viral count of 13,200. After taking two capsules (approximately 750 mg each) of JuvaCleanse per day for a month with no other intervention, the patient's viral count dropped to 2,580, an over 80 percent reduction.

### Nonalcoholic Fatty Liver Disease

Nonalcoholic fatty liver disease is caused not by alcohol but by excess fat accumulation in the liver that affects up to 25 percent of the people in the United States, according to the American Liver Foundation. It has been reported that this condition is even appearing in children. Medscape reported that choline deficiency has been suggested as a possible cause of NAFLD, although further evaluation is needed.

# Alkalinity

### The Importance of Alkalinity to Health

The pH of the blood is very tightly controlled by the body. When serum pH becomes too acidic, then calcium is robbed from the bones, and biochemical changes begin to slowly tax and stress liver tissues.

As the liver's ability to filter becomes impaired, the blood becomes increasingly acidic. Unfriendly bacteria and fungi that populate our intestinal tracts thrive in an acid environment and are responsible for secreting mycotoxins, which are the root cause of many debilitating human conditions.

In fact, many researchers believe that most diseases can be linked to blood and intestinal acidity, which contributes to an acid-based yeast and fungus dominance.

### The symptoms of excess internal acidity include:

- Fatigue/low energy
- Unexplained aches and pains
- Overweight conditions
- Low resistance to illness
- Unbalanced blood sugar
- Allergies
- Headaches
- Irritability/mood swings
- Indigestion
- Colitis/ulcers
- Diarrhea/constipation
- Urinary tract infections
- Rectal itch/vaginal itch

The ideal pH for human blood is between 7.4 and 7.6. Preserving this alkalinity (pH balance) is the bedrock on which sound health and strong bodies are built. When the blood loses its alkalinity and starts to become more acidic, the foundation of health is undermined. This creates an environment where we become vulnerable to disease, runaway yeast, and fungus overgrowth.

The naturally occurring yeast and fungi in the body thrive in an acidic environment. These same yeast and fungi are responsible for secreting a large number of poisons called mycotoxins, which are believed to be one of the root causes of many diseases and debilitating conditions.

When yeast and fungus decline in the body, so do their production of mycotoxins, the poisonous waste products and byproducts of their life cycles.

There are numerous varieties of these mycotoxins, many of which are harmful to the body and must be neutralized by our immune systems. When our bodies are overwhelmed by large quantities of these toxins, our health becomes impaired, and we become susceptible to disease and illness.

Many cancers have been linked to mycotoxins. For example, the fungus *Aspergillus flavus*, which infests stored peanuts, not only generates cancer in laboratory animals but has been documented as the prime culprit in many liver cancers in humans.

By balancing the body's pH and creating a more alkaline environment, you can rein in the microbial overgrowth and choke off the production of disease-producing mycotoxins. With pH balance restored, the body can regain newfound vigor and health.

Seventh Edition | **Essential Oils Desk Reference** | 321

## How to Restore Alkalinity

An alkaline environment is hostile to fungi, which require acidity to survive and thrive. Lowered yeast and fungus populations translate into lower levels of body-damaging, disease-inducing mycotoxins.

Some of the most common varieties of pathogenic bacteria, yeast, and fungi that live in the intestines are inactive. However, when the body is weakened by illness, stress, and excess acidity caused by stress, these bacteria become harmful and active, changing into an invasive mycolic form. Here are six suggestions to help you achieve and maintain an alkaline pH blood environment.

1. **Carefully monitor your diet.** Avoiding yeast- and fungus-promoting foods is a crucial factor in combating excess acidity and fungus over-growth. Meats, sugars, dairy products, pickled foods, and malted products can be especially acidic. On the other hand, garlic is excellent for controlling fungi and yeast. Other high-alkaline, fungus-inhibiting foods include green and yellow vegetables, beans, and whole nuts.

   The natural ratio between alkaline and acidic foods in the diet should be 4:1—four parts alkaline foods to one part acidic. JuvaPower and JuvaSpice are mixtures of extremely alkaline and high-antioxidant foods that nourish the liver and combat toxic acidity.

   The pH of a raw food does not always determine its acidity or alkalinity in the digestive system. Some foods, like lemons, might be acidic in their natural state but when consumed and digested are converted into alkaline residues.

   Thus, the true determinant of a food's pH is whether it is an alkaline-ash or acidic-ash food. In this case, lemons are an alkaline-ash food.

2. **Avoid the use of antibiotics.** The overuse of antibiotics for incidental, minor, or cosmetic conditions not only increases the resistance of pathogenic microorganisms, but it kills the beneficial bacteria in your body, leaving the mycotoxin-generating yeast and fungi intact. This is why many women suffer outbreaks of yeast infections after antibiotic use.

3. **Essential oils.** Many essential oils possess important antimicrobial, antibacterial, and antifungal properties. Clove and Thyme essential oils have been documented to kill over 15 different strains of fungi.

   Essential oils work best when blood and tissues are alkaline. When our systems become acidic—due to poor diet, illness, or emotional stress—essential oils lose some of their effects. So the best way to enhance the action of essential oils is to alkalize your body.

4. **Alkaline minerals.** Increasing the intake of calcium can dramatically boost blood and intestinal alkalinity.

   - Calcium and magnesium-rich supplements such as MegaCal and SuperCal can help alkalinize both blood and body tissues.

   - AlkaLime is an outstanding source of alkaline salts that can help reduce internal acidity.

   - Mineral Essence supplies the body with more than 60 of the most efficiently absorbed ionic minerals available.

   - JuvaPower and JuvaSpice (for salads and cooking) are also rich in minerals and yeast-fighting phytonutrients.

5. **Lower stress.** Emotional and psychological tension can be especially damaging to body systems and act as a prime promoter of acid formation in the body. To properly appreciate how acidic stress can be, just think back to the last time you were seriously stressed out and had to reach for an antacid tablet to soothe your heartburn or stomach discomfort.

   Blends of essential oils high in sesquiterpenes such as Myrrh, Sandalwood, and Cedarwood can produce profound balancing and calming effects on emotions. They work by affecting the limbic system of our brain, the seat of our emotions.

6. **Boost friendly flora.** From 3 to 4 pounds of beneficial bacteria permanently reside in the intestines of the average adult. Not only are they the first line of defense against foreign invaders, but they are also absolutely essential for health, energy, and optimum digestive efficiency. These intestinal houseguests not only control mucus and debris, but they also produce B vitamins and vitamin K and maintain the all-important pH balance of the body.

   These friendly floras are also important in counteracting and opposing yeast and fungus overgrowth. When our natural cultures are compromised or disrupted by taking antibiotics or by poor dietary practices, yeast and fungus start growing unopposed and begin colonizing and invading larger swaths of our internal terrain, secreting ever-increasing volumes of poisonous mycotoxins.

   Using an acidophilus and bifidus supplement (such as Life 9) may be especially valuable in boosting levels of naturally occurring beneficial bacteria in the body and preventing fungal and yeast overgrowth. They also help the body maintain proper pH balance for nutrient digestion and absorption.

Cleansing and Diet | **Chapter 17**

Ideally, the lactobacillus acidophilus and bifido-bacterium cultures must be combined with plantain to promote implantation on the intestinal wall. Life 9 capsules are most beneficial at night while the body is busy cleansing and repairing while you sleep.

Research indicates a significant proportion of bacteria from many acidophilus supplements do not reach the lower intestine alive, or they arrive in such a weakened state that they are not of much benefit. Combining the acidophilus and bifidus cultures is stronger in helping these cultures adhere to the intestinal walls.

An even more effective means of fortifying the friendly flora in our intestines is by consuming fructooligosaccharides (also known as FOS).

FOS is one of the most powerful natural agents for feeding our friendly flora and is made up of medium-chain sugars that cannot be used by pathogenic yeast and fungi. The end result is that FOS starves fungi while feeding the acidophilus and bifidus cultures that are our main defense against disease.

But FOS is far more than just an outstanding means of rebuilding and protecting the beneficial bacteria inside the body. Over a dozen clinical studies have documented the ability of fructooligosaccharides to prevent constipation,[1,2] lower blood sugar,[3] reduce cholesterol levels,[4] and even prevent cancer.[5,6]

### Testing Your pH

You can easily test your pH at home by purchasing small litmus-paper strips at your drug store or pharmacy. To get the most accurate reading, expose the strip to a sample of your saliva immediately after awakening in the morning and before eating breakfast. Color changes on the litmus paper will determine pH; check the instructions in your kit for specific details on how to read the litmus paper.

# Cleansing Programs

Cleansing and the commitment you make to it is a personal choice. You have to decide what program you want to follow and then discipline yourself to accomplish what you desire. Even drinking enough water takes discipline.

However, the reward is worth the denial of food and the pleasure of eating. You cannot put a price on health, because the price of not having good health is too high. You simply have to plan your protocol, get started, and stay with it. Those are the only requirements.

### The Ideal Program

The ideal cleansing program requires a high consumption of water, and that means distilled or purified water, never chlorinated tap water. You should work up to a gallon of water each day. Then with strong digestive enzymes, minerals, high-potency herbs, and therapeutic-grade essential oils, the body is ready to go to work.

Essential oils have a special, lipid-soluble makeup, which gives them a remarkable ability to penetrate cell membranes, break up undigested food, and digest toxins. Essential oils deliver oxygen that inhibits the growth of many types of microbes. In fact, many essential oils have been studied and documented for their unique antimicrobial, antifungal, and antiparasitic properties. Some oils, like Rosemary, have demonstrated significant antiseptic activity, with documented research appearing in many scientific journals.

### Cleanse Often

Cleansing should be done two to three times a year, but eating healthy cleansing foods and supplements should be a daily part of your life throughout the year. It is important to have this kind of awareness at a young age to be able to enjoy the "older" years without health problems. Just because an individual is 40 years old does not mean that the body has to start breaking down and taking on disease.

Naturally, with age comes a greater buildup of debris in our bodies caused by the food we eat and the pollutants in our environment, as well as less production of stomach acids and enzymes.

Without proper enzyme production, the body is not able to properly break down undigested proteins and other fermenting debris that obstruct our digestive system and impede the assimilation of nutrients.

### Cleanse Completely

It is difficult to control internal pollution with a simple one-time fix or a single magic bullet. Complete cleansing requires many different solutions targeted at specific systems of the body. Cleansing the liver requires a different combination of herbs, oils, and minerals than those required for the colon.

A complete cleansing requires a broad array of products that are effective against a wide variety of contaminants and microorganisms, not just one or two. Contaminants,

Seventh Edition | **Essential Oils Desk Reference** | **323**

like heavy metals, need a different set of tools to deactivate and purge them from the body than parasites do.

Essential oils are an important part of a complete cleansing program. Essential oils are highly antibacterial, antifungal, antiviral, and anti-inflammatory. They digest and chelate toxic chemicals and poisons in the body. Essential oils promote the body's production of enzymes, which improve colon peristalsis, the key to waste elimination.

## Fasting

Fasting is the avoidance of solid food, with liquid intake varying from no liquids (1–2 days) to just water or water and fresh juices. A fast can last 24 hours or several weeks.

Fasting has long been a tradition in Judaism, Christianity, and the Eastern religions. Religious fasting can involve purification, penitence, or preparation for approaching God.

Fasting has been called "nature's single-greatest healing therapy."

An increasing number of doctors are recognizing that fasting can be physically healing while allowing us to focus our energy inward, bringing clarity and change.

Fasting is generally safe, but those with medical conditions should check with their health care professional.

An extremely important benefit of fasting is the elimination of toxins. By minimizing the work our digestive system must do, we allow it to repair itself and expel stored toxins.

In the beginning of a fast, the liver will convert stored glycogen to energy. As the fast continues, some proteins will break down unless calories are provided through juices and sweeteners such as maple syrup.

The first 2 to 4 days of the fast are often the most difficult, since you will be overcoming the powerful psychological need to eat. As the body begins to cleanse itself of parasites and putrefying toxins, a person may experience a sudden surge in energy and well-being.

Tapeworms, pinworms, roundworms, etc., may be seen in the stools after 4 to 6 days. As the cleansing progresses, the mind will become sharper, the memory will improve, and the spirit will become more buoyant.

**Pregnant or lactating women should not fast.**

## Cleansing Through Fasting

This is the most disciplined, comprehensive way to cleanse the body. It is a time when the body can work on revitalizing cells and stopping degeneration that has already started. It enables the body to cleanse and rebuild an overworked liver. This is when longevity is put in motion.

---

### Consult Your Physician

Anyone cleansing or fasting for more than three days should do so under the supervision of a health care professional.

Never begin a shut-down fast unless you have been fasting regularly for at least two years. This type of fast should always be done under supervision.

---

A true fast consists of only water, but very few people are able to sustain this type of a fast.

### The Master Cleanse—Stanley Burroughs (Lemonade Diet)

The Master Cleanse, as it is called, was developed by Stanley Burroughs and has been used successfully by thousands of people. It takes time, but although it is still a liquid diet, it provides certain nutrients to sustain the body and help with cleansing. Stay focused and determined and you will have success, too.

The Master Cleanse is a mixture of lemon juice, Grade B maple syrup, and cayenne pepper that is consumed throughout the day and is the source of calories, vitamins, and minerals for the body.

The Master Cleanse is for almost anyone, except young children, diabetics, and those who are very weak and cannot stay with their own commitment of cleansing or who need supervised help.

Most people can safely cleanse for at least 7–10 days. As with any program of caloric restriction, however, it is strongly recommended that you consult with your health care professional before undertaking any extended fast or cleanse.

### The Master Cleanse Protocol

- Squeeze the juice from ½ fresh organic lemon.
- Mix juice into 8 oz. distilled water.
- Add 1–2 tablespoons Grade B maple syrup or Yacon Syrup. Both are available at the health food store.
- Add up to 1/10 teaspoon cayenne (red) pepper (capsicum).

Start with a pinch or two of cayenne pepper and gradually increase to 1/10 teaspoon. Do not put it in capsules and swallow separately. The cayenne pepper is specific to the formula, and with it the action of the formula changes. If sent directly to the stomach, it can cause inflammation and excessive mucous that may lead to sinusitis or too much bowel mucus and can even contribute to inflammatory bowel syndrome.

Drink 6 to 12 10-ounce glasses of lemonade daily. Every time you begin to feel hunger, have another glass of the lemonade. Remember, it is extremely important to also drink water to help flush out toxins.

Grade B maple syrup contains minerals and nutrients that support the body nutritionally during the cleansing period. Diabetics should substitute molasses for maple syrup. Available at most health food stores, about ¼ to ½ tablespoon is usually sufficient for sweetening.

Contrary to popular belief, lemon is not acidic in the body. As the lemon juice mixes with the salvia, it gradually starts to change its pH, and then in the stomach it turns completely alkaline as it mixes with the hydrochloric acid.

If an acid-like reaction is observed when using lemon with water, it is because of the minerals in the water. Distilled water will not react in this manner.

Cayenne pepper is a blood vessel dilator, a thermal warmer, and provides vitamin A. People who have Type O blood tend to have poor circulation and will need to drink the lemonade every ½ hour to maintain proper blood sugar levels, or else the body temperature may drop during the cleanse.

Cayenne is a thermogenic herb known for its ability to warm and improve circulation. When used in a dietary program, it can promote greater fat burning. Moderate exercise enhances the cleansing action of the program.

During the middle and later phases of the lemon cleanse, typically between day 3 and day 7, the body chemistry changes, and energy levels usually begin to rise. You may experience minor discomfort such as headaches, upset stomach, or low energy, while toxins and parasites are released from the body.

If your energy decreases, then drink another glass of the juice. Sometimes when on this type of cleanse, if you are not watching the clock to make sure you are drinking the juice on a regular schedule, you may feel weak and develop a headache.

A Type O person will need to drink it more often than a Type A person. Remember—drinking plenty of water is also very important.

These symptoms should pass. If not, ask your health practitioner to monitor the situation, gently come off the lemon cleanse, or begin to add foods that are cleansing such as salads, fruits, etc. Grapefruit makes a good cleansing juice. Follow the recipe and sweeten to taste.

You can also experiment with adding different essential oils like Lemon, Orange, or Grapefruit, which will provide additional benefit. Add only 1 drop of oil per glass as the oils are very concentrated.

## Wanting to Eat

If you feel that you need or want to eat, add only foods that are compatible with your cleansing program. Salads, vegetables, fruit, Pure Protein Complete, ICP, and JuvaPower are immensely supportive to the elimination process.

Take different enzymes at varied times for their particular benefits: Allerzyme, Detoxzyme, Essentialzyme, Esssentialzymes-4, and MightyZyme increase the enzymatic action for better detoxification.

See the recipes at the end of this section for healthy eating choices with or without your cleansing program. Use them as examples and modify them for your taste.

## A Positive Mental Attitude Is Important

Having a positive attitude during cleansing or fasting is important. If you are learning how to fast, start by fasting one day a week. Start on a Sunday or a day that is more restful and not filled with normal, everyday stress. The biggest obstacle to successful cleansing is fear of failure and not knowing what to expect.

To fast for 24 hours, it is easiest to begin at noon and finish at noon on the following day or fast from one dinner to the next.

Again, drink plenty of water, as water is the catalyst to all cleansing. At the beginning of the fast, you might experience some unpleasant side effects such as headache, nausea, bloating, or irritability. These symptoms are part of the cleansing response and are often a result of toxins and waste matter being purged from the body, which usually begins to take place within 12 to 36 hours.

If you experience these symptoms, simply cut back on fluid intake and drink vegetable juices such as carrot and celery. Try mixing carrot, celery, spinach, and broccoli together and see how your body feels.

Carrot juice with a little apple juice or carrot, apple, and a little lemon juice promote continuous cleansing. A mixture of 6 ounces of carrot juice, 1 ounce of apple juice, and ½ ounce of lemon juice will help keep the pH balanced, slow down any diarrhea, and keep the cleansing action going.

Nausea and bloating are an indication that the poisons are being released at a very rapid rate and may be backing up into the liver. Keeping the liver cleansed and flushed is extremely important.

The essential oil of Ledum works well as a diuretic and dilates the bile duct between the liver and kidneys. One or two capsules morning or night is probably sufficient. Other essential oil blends such as GLF, JuvaCleanse, and JuvaFlex all aid in the cleansing process.

Peristalsis is a wave-like motion of the intestines as it moves waste matter out of the body. A spastic or prolapsed colon from loss of peristalsis or restrictions from kinks, loops, or twists in the colon make proper elimination difficult and often painful.

## Colon Hydrotherapy Cleanse

Colon hydrotherapy is a powerful treatment for cleansing the colon and helps restore peristalsis. Make an appointment with a colon hydrotherapist to have a colonic treatment or buy a colima board to give yourself a colonic at home. Portable colon hydrotherapy units are also available for home use. The Colonet JR-4 is an advanced, free-gravity-flow, in-home enema unit that is lightweight, portable, and specifically designed for easy use in a private bathroom.

### Colon Cleanse Recipe #1

- 5 drops Rosemary
- 5 drops Basil
- 5 drops ParaFree
- 4 drops Fennel

### Colon Cleanse Recipe #2

- 15–20 drops of ParaFree alone in water
  Add to colonic water and mix well.

During cleansing, you might have an unexpected emotional clearing. Various essential oils have a direct effect on the emotional centers of the brain. They can help control, calm, release, and facilitate the emotional response.

Essential oil blends such as Release, Inner Child, Valor, Valor II, Grounding, Peace & Calming, and Peace & Calming II offer good emotional support during such times. Roll-on blends such as Stress Away Roll-On, Tranquil Roll-On, Breathe Again Roll-On, and RutaVaLa Roll-On are easy to carry in your pocket and can offer immediate relief.

The essential oils of Valerian, Roman Chamomile, Idaho Balsam Fir, and Lavender are very calming and relaxing. In addition, Peace & Calming, Peace & Calming II, Release, and JuvaFlex oil blends, used topically or diffused, promote a calming environment. Most citrus oils contain aldehydes that are very calming as well. Vitamin B12 (Super B) and folic acid are also important for emotional stability.

## Liquid Cleansing Recipes

There are many other liquid recipes and protocols for easier and simpler cleansing. Some of the recipes are used as daily maintenance with or without food, and some are used for one or two weeks with or without food. Some are specific for a particular need, some are used once a year, some are used once a month, and some are used just for the experience. Whatever the reason, your body will benefit with improved health and vitality.

## Vital Life Juice Recipe

D. Gary Young first created this recipe over 35 years ago for detoxification for patients with degenerative disease. Since that time, it has been very successful in providing the needed benefits to those with greater health challenges. It has become a very popular juice for many who just want the concentrated nutrients and a simple cleansing.

Use a juicer (not a blender):
- 3 oz. beet juice
- 1 oz. celery juice
- 1 oz. carrot juice
- 1/3 oz. white radish juice
- 1/3 oz. red potato juice (optional)
- 1/8 oz. ginger (Whole ginger may be juiced while juicing other vegetables.)

Directions:
- Drink ¼–½ cup every 2–3 hours.
- The potato is optional except when fighting liver cancer.
- The Vital Life Juice is good to drink while on the Master Cleanse.

## Grapefruit Juice Recipe

This fruit has a history of cleansing and promoting fat burning. It is simple to make and enjoyable to drink throughout the day.
- About ½ cup freshly pressed grapefruit juice
- 1 quart distilled or purified water
- 3 drops of Spearmint
- 3 drops of Tangerine
- Blue Agave or Yacon Syrup to taste

The more frequent the elimination, the better. There may be some discomfort or bloating if the body is not eliminating several times a day. There should be at least 2–3 or more bowel movements every day to constantly be moving the waste out of the body that is being loosened from the various organs and intestines.

If there is some discomfort and elimination is slow, add ComforTone, one of the first herbal supplements formulated with essential oils to help relieve constipation, enhance colon and digestive functions, and dispel parasites and toxins. Increase the number of enzyme capsules as well.

## Cleansing with Supplements

### Blood Cleanse

The tincture Rehemogen contains herbs that were traditionally used by Native Americans for cleansing and purifying the blood. It builds red blood cells and is recommended for any blood disorder.

- Put 2–3 droppers of Rehemogen (50–75 drops) in distilled water and drink every 2–3 hours.
- Rehemogen and JuvaTone together work well to assist in cleansing the blood and the liver.

## Enzymes and Daily Maintenance
- Take 2–3 enzyme capsules of your choice 3 times daily before meals.
- Always carry enzymes with you when eating out or remember to take them when you return home. If you have eaten a heavy meal at night, be sure to take your enzymes before going to bed to keep the food digesting and prevent fermenting.
- A, B, and AB blood types: 2–4 capsules
- O blood types: 3–6 or more capsules, if necessary

## Enzyme Cleanse

Enzymes break down foods and proteins that might otherwise ferment and putrefy in the gastrointestinal tract. Undigested foods tax our bodies, sap our energy, and spur the overgrowth of yeast, fungi, parasites, bacteria, and microorganisms that contribute to viral conditions, gastritis, Crohn's disease, diverticulitis, and other inflammatory conditions.

Inadequate digestive enzyme activity has also been linked to chronic inflammation elsewhere in the body such as fibromyalgia, inability to gain or lose weight, bad breath, body odor, skin rashes, and migraines.

Enzymes like pancreatin, pancrelipase, chymotrypsin, and trypsin are very efficient in breaking down proteins.

However, if the body is acidic, chymotrypsin, trypsin, and other enzymes will not effectively activate in the body.

Vegetable enzymes from the unripe papaya and pineapple (papain and bromelain) provide enzyme support.

Digestive enzymes promote complete digestion and help those who have difficulty digesting and assimilating food. As we age, we need more enzymes for complete digestion. Enzymes are essential in unlocking and metabolizing the vitamins, minerals, and amino acids in food.

Detoxzyme, Allerzyme, Essentialzyme, Essential-zymes-4, and MightyZyme all help digest cooked and processed foods that lack the natural enzymes of fresh foods.

## Enzyme Ramping Protocol

Essentialzyme was formulated in 1984 with this protocol for someone suffering from a degenerative disease such as cancer.

Most people would not need to follow this protocol, but it will help you to understand the commitment it takes to fight disease.

**Phase 1:** Take 3 caplets 3 times daily. Increase by 1 caplet every day until you become nauseated. Then discontinue Essentialzyme for 24 to 36 hours.

**Phase 2:** Take 4 caplets 3 times daily. Increase daily by 1 caplet until you become nauseated. Rest (discontinue) again for 24–36 hours.

**Phase 3:** Take 5 caplets 3 times daily. Increase daily by 1 caplet until you become nauseated. Rest again for 24–36 hours.

**Phase 4:** Start again with the amount that you were taking before the nausea occurred the third time. For example: If you were taking 18 caplets, you would have been taking 6 caplets 3 times a day when you became nauseated. Therefore, start Phase 4 again with 6 caplets 3 times daily and continue with this amount for 6 weeks.

**Phase 5:** In the 7th week, start the enzyme-ramping program all over again. This means to begin Phase 1 again and increase the amount by 1 each day until nausea or vomiting starts again. Repeat and continue for 6 weeks as previously described.

If your doctor determines that you are in remission, you can maintain with 5–10 caplets daily for one year, 6 days a week.

**Maintenance:** Take 5–10 Essentialzyme caplets 3 times daily.

**Caution:** This is a very rigorous program, so you should consult with your doctor or health care professional before starting and have your doctor monitor your progress during the program.

## Heavy Metals Cleanse

Heavy metals are some of the most toxic poisons on earth and can slowly accumulate in human tissues and cause neurological diseases, cardiovascular problems, and some types of cancers.

The problem is that heavy metals such as mercury and lead form insoluble metallic salts that become trapped in the fat and in the kidneys and cannot be easily excreted from the liver. Because the liver plays a major role in trapping and stabilizing mercury, liver cleansing using essential oils can be an outstanding treatment in purging the body of heavy metal contamination that contributes to many chronic neurological diseases.

Mercury is present in harmful amounts in almost every person in the United States, due to the consumption of seafood (methyl mercury levels in canned tuna are especially problematic) and amalgam dental fillings (which are about 50 percent mercury).

**Essential Oils Desk Reference** | Seventh Edition

# Food "Ash" pH

pH measures **below** +7.0 are considered acidic; those **above** +7.0 are considered alkaline. The determination of whether a food is acid or alkaline is not gauged by its pH but by the pH of its residues or metabolites.

| | |
|---|---|
| Alfalfa Grass | +29.3 |
| Almond | +3.6 |
| Apricot | -9.5 |
| Artichokes | +1.3 |
| Asparagus | +1.1 |
| Avocado (Protein) | +15.6 |
| Banana, Ripe | -10.1 |
| Banana, Unripe | +4.8 |
| Barley Grass | +28.7 |
| Barley Malt Syrup | -9.3 |
| Beans, French Cut | +11.2 |
| Beans, Lima | +12.0 |
| Beans, White | +12.1 |
| Beef | -34.5 |
| Beer | -26.8 |
| Beet Sugar | -15.1 |
| Beet, Fresh Red | +11.3 |
| Biscuit, White | -6.5 |
| Blueberry | -5.3 |
| Borage | +3.2 |
| Brazil Nuts | -0.5 |
| Bread, Rye | -2.5 |
| Bread, White | -10.0 |

| | |
|---|---|
| Bread, Whole-grain | -4.5 |
| Bread, Whole-meal | -6.5 |
| Brussels Sprouts | -1.5 |
| Buckwheat Groats | +0.5 |
| Butter | -3.9 |
| Buttermilk | +1.3 |
| Cabbage, Green December Harvest | +4.0 |
| Cabbage, Green March Harvest | +2.0 |
| Cabbage, Red | +6.3 |
| Cabbage, Savoy | +4.5 |
| Cabbage, White | +3.3 |
| Cantaloupe | -2.5 |
| Caraway | +2.3 |
| Carrot | +9.5 |
| Cashews | -9.3 |
| Cauliflower | +3.1 |
| Cayenne Pepper | +18.8 |
| Celery | +13.3 |
| Cheese, Hard | -18.1 |
| Cherry, Sour | +3.5 |
| Cherry, Sweet | -3.6 |
| Chia, Sprouted | +28.5 |
| Chicken | -18.0 to -22.0 |
| Chives | +8.3 |
| Coconut, Fresh | +0.5 |
| Coffee | -25.1 |
| Comfrey | +1.5 |
| Corn oil | -6.5 |
| Cranberry | -7.0 |

| | |
|---|---|
| Cream | -3.9 |
| Cucumber, Fresh | +31.5 |
| Cumin | +1.1 |
| Currant | -8.2 |
| Currant, Black | -6.1 |
| Currant, Red | -2.4 |
| Dandelion | +22.7 |
| Date | -4.7 |
| Dog Grass | +22.6 |
| Eggs | -18.0 to -22.0 |
| Endive, Fresh | +14.5 |
| Fennel | +1.3 |
| Fig Juice Powder | -2.4 |
| Filbert | -2.0 |
| Fish, Fresh Water | -11.8 |
| Fish, Ocean | -20.0 |
| Flax Seed Oil | -1.3 |
| Flax Seed | +3.5 |
| Fructose | -9.5 |
| Garlic | +13.2 |
| Gooseberry, Ripe | -7.7 |
| Grapefruit | -1.7 |
| Grapes, Ripe | -7.6 |
| Hazelnut | -2.0 |
| Honey | -7.6 |
| Horseradish | +6.8 |
| Juice, Natural Fruit | -8.7 |
| Juice, White Sugar Sweetened Fruit | -33.4 |
| Kamut Grass | +27.6 |
| Ketchup | -12.4 |

*Source: Young, Robert O. Sick and Tired. Alpine, UT, 1977.*

According to the Mercury Policy Project, dental amalgam is the largest source of mercury pollution to reach waste water treatment plants.

Mercury discharges [in wastewater] from dental offices far exceeded all other commercial and residential sources. EPA cited an estimate in 2007 that 36 percent of the mercury reaching municipal sewage treatment plants is released by dental offices. Other investigations have put the figure closer to 50 percent.[7]

According to Mercola.com, a 44-pound child consuming 6 ounces of tuna a week would be exposed to 4 times the EPA reference dose for mercury, and a 120-pound woman consuming the same amount would be exposed to 1½ times the EPA reference dose.

Women of childbearing age in the United States suffer from tissue levels of mercury that can be dangerous to a developing fetus.

## Clinical Studies with Heavy Metals

Clinical studies show that the essential oil blends of JuvaCleanse, JuvaFlex, and GLF, which contain the essential oils of Helichrysum, Ledum, and Celery Seed, dramatically amplified the elimination of heavy metals from the body, especially mercury, one of the most toxic of all nonradioactive metals.

Cleansing and Diet | **Chapter 17**

## Food "Ash" pH *(continued)*

| | | |
|---|---|---|
| Kohlrabi . . . . . . . . . . . . . . . . . +5.1 | Pear . . . . . . . . . . . . . . . . . . . . .-9.9 | Spinach, March Harvest . . . . . +8.0 |
| Lecithin, Pure (Soy) . . . . . . . +38.0 | Peas, Fresh . . . . . . . . . . . . . . +5.1 | Straw Grass . . . . . . . . . . . . . +21.4 |
| Leeks (Bulbs) . . . . . . . . . . . . . +7.2 | Peas, Ripe . . . . . . . . . . . . . . . +0.5 | Strawberry . . . . . . . . . . . . . . .-5.4 |
| Lemon, Fresh . . . . . . . . . . . . . +9.9 | Pineapple . . . . . . . . . . . . . . .-12.6 | Sugar Cane Juice |
| Lentils . . . . . . . . . . . . . . . . . . +0.6 | Pistachios . . . . . . . . . . . . . . .-16.6 | Dried (Sucanat). . . . . . . . . .-9.6 |
| Lettuce . . . . . . . . . . . . . . . . . . +2.2 | Plum, Italian . . . . . . . . . . . . .-4.9 | Sugar Cane, Refined (White). .-17.6 |
| Lettuce, Fresh Cabbage . . . . +14.1 | Plum, Yellow . . . . . . . . . . . . .-4.9 | Sunflower Oil. . . . . . . . . . . . . .-6.7 |
| Lettuce, Lamb's . . . . . . . . . . . +4.8 | Pork . . . . . . . . . . . . . . . . . . . .-38.0 | Sunflower Seeds . . . . . . . . . . . .-5.4 |
| Limes . . . . . . . . . . . . . . . . . . . +8.2 | Potatoes, Stored . . . . . . . . . . +2.0 | Sweeteners, Artificial . . . . . . .-26.5 |
| Liquor . . . . . . . . . . .-28.6 to -38.7 | Primrose. . . . . . . . . . . . . . . . +4.1 | Tangerine . . . . . . . . . . . . . . . .-8.5 |
| Liver. . . . . . . . . . . . . . . . . . . . .-3.0 | Pumpkin . . . . . . . . . . . . . . . .-5.6 | Tea (Black) . . . . . . . . . . . . . .-27.1 |
| Macadamia Nuts . . . . . . . . . .-11.7 | Quark . . . . . . . . . . . . . . . . . .-17.3 | Tofu . . . . . . . . . . . . . . . . . . . . +3.2 |
| Mandarin Orange. . . . . . . . .-11.5 | Radish, Sprouted . . . . . . . . . +28.4 | Tomato . . . . . . . . . . . . . . . . +13.6 |
| Mango . . . . . . . . . . . . . . . . . . .-8.7 | Radish, Black (Summer). . . . +39.4 | Turbinado . . . . . . . . . . . . . . . .-9.5 |
| Margarine. . . . . . . . . . . . . . . .-7.5 | Radish, White (Spring). . . . . . +3.1 | Turnip . . . . . . . . . . . . . . . . . +8.0 |
| Marine Lipids. . . . . . . . . . . . . +4.7 | Raspberry. . . . . . . . . . . . . . . . .-5.1 | Veal . . . . . . . . . . . . . . . . . . . .-35.0 |
| Mayonnaise . . . . . . . . . . . . . .-12.5 | Red Radish. . . . . . . . . . . . . . +16.7 | Walnuts . . . . . . . . . . . . . . . . .-8.0 |
| Meats, Organ . . . . . . . . . . . . .-3.0 | Rhubarb Stalks. . . . . . . . . . . . +6.3 | Watercress . . . . . . . . . . . . . . . +7.7 |
| Milk Sugar . . . . . . . . . . . . . . .-9.4 | Rice Syrup, Brown . . . . . . . . .-8.7 | Watermelon . . . . . . . . . . . . . . .-1.0 |
| Milk, Homogenized . . . . . . . .-1.0 | Rice, Brown . . . . . . . . . . . . .-12.5 | Wheat Germ . . . . . . . . . . . . .-11.4 |
| Millet. . . . . . . . . . . . . . . . . . . +0.5 | Rose Hips. . . . . . . . . . . . . . .-15.5 | Wheat Grass. . . . . . . . . . . . . +33.8 |
| Molasses. . . . . . . . . . . . . . . . .-14.6 | Rutabaga . . . . . . . . . . . . . . . +3.1 | Wheat . . . . . . . . . . . . . . . . . .-10.1 |
| Mustard . . . . . . . . . . . . . . . .-19.2 | Sesame Seeds . . . . . . . . . . . . +.5 | Wine . . . . . . . . . . . . . . . . . . .-16.4 |
| Nut, Soy (Soaked, | Shave Grass . . . . . . . . . . . . +21.7 | Zucchini. . . . . . . . . . . . . . . . . +5.7 |
| then Air Dried) . . . . . . . . +26.5 | Sorrel . . . . . . . . . . . . . . . . . +11.5 | |
| Olive Oil . . . . . . . . . . . . . . . . +1.0 | Soy Beans, (Cooked, | |
| Onion . . . . . . . . . . . . . . . . . . +3.0 | then Ground) . . . . . . . . . +12.8 | |
| Orange. . . . . . . . . . . . . . . . . .-9.2 | Soy Flour . . . . . . . . . . . . . . . +2.5 | |
| Oysters. . . . . . . . . . . . . . . . . .-5.0 | Soy Sprouts . . . . . . . . . . . . . +29.5 | |
| Papaya . . . . . . . . . . . . . . . . . .-9.4 | Soybeans, Fresh . . . . . . . . . . +12.0 | |
| Peach . . . . . . . . . . . . . . . . . . .-9.7 | Spelt. . . . . . . . . . . . . . . . . . . +0.5 | |
| Peanuts. . . . . . . . . . . . . . . . .-12.8 | Spinach (other than March) . +13.1 | |

Mercury is particularly damaging to the brain and nervous system because it passes through the blood-brain barrier, accumulates indefinitely in motor neurons, and destroys healthy growth of the dendrites.

JuvaCleanse may be applied over the liver and also taken as a dietary supplement. Put 10–20 drops into one 00 capsule and take it in the morning and evening.

One of the most difficult aspects of cleansing is refraining from food or reducing our food intake, and besides, most of the food we eat is not very complimentary to our cleansing. If you eat in a healthy manner that will not compromise your cleansing program, you will not defeat your purpose. Too many people feel confused and do not know what foods are basically supporting to the cleansing process.

### ComforTone®—Herbal Colon Cleanse

ComforTone is formulated with cascara sagrada, diatomaceous earth, licorice root, apple pectin, bentonite, licorice, psyllium, cayenne pepper, and garlic. These herbs are particularly effective in purging the colon of toxins and impurities, which is just as important as cleansing the small intestine.

Waste products and gases held in the colon have a much higher concentration of toxic byproducts than those in the small intestine. When these leach into the

Seventh Edition | **Essential Oils Desk Reference** | 329

organs and tissues, they can wreak havoc in our bodies.

The essential oil blends of DiGize and JuvaFlex, formulated with the single oils of Peppermint, Rosemary, Tarragon, Ginger, Anise, and Fennel, promote peristalsis and increase digestive secretions for better digestion.

## ComforTone Protocol

- Two capsules every morning and night for two days should increase bowel movements to 3–4 daily.
- If elimination does not improve, then increase capsules to 3 each night and morning.
- Do not exceed 10 capsules per day without advice from a health care practitioner.
- If you start to have cramps, you may be dehydrated and may have a spastic or prolapsed colon, causing loss of peristalsis. This is when colon hydrotherapy may be helpful.
- Aloe vera juice and/or prune juice work as natural laxatives. Drink 8 ounces a day and take 5–6 capsules of ComforTone and 1–2 tablespoons of JuvaPower in water morning and night.
- Drink half your body weight of water in fluid ounces daily, and when cleansing, drink 20 percent more water. It softens clay-like, hard waste matter trapped in tissue pockets in the intestinal tract, caused from not drinking enough fluids.
- When bowel movements increase up to 3 to 4 times per day, you know ComforTone is working. If when you stop taking ComforTone, your bowel movements slow down or become sluggish, then begin again until ComforTone is again working.
- If diarrhea occurs for more than 1 or 2 days, stop the ComforTone, rest for 1–2 days, and then start again with a smaller amount. ComforTone is safe and can be very helpful during an entire pregnancy, if necessary. A little diarrhea is easier to take care of than the misery of being constipated. The object is to eliminate easily and often.
- ComforTone and JuvaPower work very well together for synergistic cleansing through the digestive system.

## ICP™—Intestinal Fiber Cleanse

Coarsely ground grains rich in soluble and semisoluble fiber are some of the best intestinal cleansers known. ICP's psyllium powder and husks, rice bran, oat bran, flax seed, and fennel seed help loosen and expel undigested and fermenting materials from the intestines that block nutrient absorption and cause poison to be reabsorbed into the body.

Fibers act as a biochemical sponge for the body, absorbing impurities, gases, and toxins and increasing the flow of waste matter through the intestines, helping to minimize the exposure to harmful substances. The slower the "transit time" of waste matter through the intestinal tract, the higher the incidence of disease.

Fiber satisfies the appetite by giving people a feeling of fullness without adding excessive calories. Fiber may also help balance blood sugar levels. It also helps maintain regularity as we age, preventing and overcoming constipation, diarrhea, and gas.

The essential oil blend DiGize and the supplement Digest & Cleanse are formulated with the single oils of Fennel, Tarragon, Ginger, Lemongrass, Rosemary, Basil, Bergamot, and Melissa that not only help dissolve and chelate toxins but also combat pathological microorganisms that reside in the intestines.

## ICP Protocol
### When the bowels are moving regularly:

- Take 1 tablespoon ICP mixed in a glass of water morning and night for 2–3 days.
- After 2–3 days, increase dosage to 2 tablespoons morning and night while you cleanse; drink plenty of water.
- Maintenance dosage: Take 2 tablespoons 3–4 times per week.
- Beta-carotene, found in carrot juice and beet juice, also helps with elimination.
- Carrot Seed oil detoxifies the liver and in combination with the essential oils of Geranium and Lemongrass may help in eliminating gallstones, cleansing the bowel, and relieving flatulence.
- Lemon, Frankincense, and Idaho Balsam Fir help dissolve, eliminate, and decrease the pain of kidney stones.
- Ledum, Juniper, and Geranium also work well together for an intestinal cleanse.
- DiGize, Fennel, Tarragon, and Peppermint help relieve flatulence.

To maintain a healthy colon, it is best to stay away from processed and pasteurized dairy products, including all cheeses except goat cheese. Avoid refined white sugar, white flour, processed salt, starchy processed foods, and fried foods. These are deadly to the intestinal tract.

Breads made from hybrid wheat and other grains are also damaging to the digestive tract. Both whole wheat and white bread are converted into sugar by the body, and the sugar turns to fat.

If you have heartburn while taking ComforTone or ICP, your digestive system is obviously not working

Cleansing and Diet | **Chapter 17**

properly. If the cleansing process reduces the intestinal flora, begin adding the following to the program:

- Essentialzyme: Take 1–3 caplets per meal and up to 6 with heavy meat meals late in the day or at night. Oils that can accelerate digestion are Tarragon, Fennel, Anise, and the essential oil blend of DiGize. Take 3 or 4 drops of each essential oil mentioned above in a double 00 capsule before or after a meal to enhance digestion.
- Take 5 capsules of Life 9 at nighttime to help build up the intestinal flora. Consume organic yogurt or kefir without sugar or artificial sweeteners ½ hour before meals on an empty stomach.

These supplements provide the stomach with the friendly bacteria and enzymes necessary for good digestion, conversion, and assimilation. Master Formula, MultiGreens, and Mineral Essence provide trace minerals that the body requires to produce enzymes.

When taken together, ComforTone and Essentialzyme have synergistic effects, so less of each is required to achieve similar benefits.

## Liver Cleansing Supplements

The Juva products will bring restoration and support for optimal liver function.

- **JuvaCleanse®**
  This oil blend was formulated with Celery Seed, Helichrysum, and Ledum essential oils to help detoxify while enhancing liver function. It offers both hepatoprotective activity and antioxidant protection. Antioxidants neutralize the effects of free radicals, the oxidizing agents that cause aging and degenerative conditions.

- **JuvaFlex™**
  With the essential oils of Fennel, Rosemary, Blue Tansy, Geranium, Roman Chamomile, and Helichrysum, this blend provides liver and digestive system support.

- **JuvaPower® and JuvaSpice®**
  These dietary supplements are delicious and convenient additions to a healthy diet with advanced phytonutrient fibers to cleanse the liver and intestines simultaneously. Both products contain the highest acid-binding foods for superior results.

- **JuvaTone®**
  This dietary supplement provides choline, a nutrient that is known for supporting optimal liver health, along with healing herbs and essential oils, including Lemon, German Chamomile, Geranium, and Blue Tansy.

## Liver Cleanse Recipes

This liver cleanse designed by D. Gary Young will help detoxify the liver and help maximize normal liver function in a natural, effective way.

This program combines the Master Cleanse, Vital Life Juice (recipe below), salads, and the nutritional supplements for a minimum of five days.

**Immediately after you awaken (6 a.m.):**
Drink a 10-oz. glass of Master Cleanse:
- 10 oz. purified water
- ½ lemon (squeezed)
- Pinch of cayenne pepper
- 2 teaspoons Blue Agave, maple syrup, or Yacon Syrup

**Then take the following supplements:**
- 2 JuvaTone
- 2 Detoxzyme
- 1 Essentialzymes-4 (white capsule)
- 20 drops JuvaCleanse in one 00 capsule

  Wait for 30–60 minutes and then drink ¼ cup Vital Life Juice

## Vital Life Juice Recipe:

Mix in a juicer (not a blender):
- 3 oz. beet juice
- 1 oz. carrot juice
- 1 oz. celery juice
- 1/3 oz. white radish juice
- 1/8 oz. ginger (Whole ginger may be juiced while juicing other vegetables.)
- 1/3 oz. red potato juice (optional)

**7 a.m.:** Drink 10 oz. of the Master Cleanse drink.

**8 a.m.:** Eat quinoa and oatmeal with coconut or other alternative milk.

**9 a.m.–10 a.m.:** Drink Vital Life Juice followed by 1 package of Slique Shake and 1 tablespoon JuvaPower in liquid of choice.

**11 a.m.:** Drink 10 oz. of the Master Cleanse drink.

**12 noon–Lunch:** Lunch may include any of the salad recipes that follow. Eat lunch along with drinking the Master Cleanse drink. One tablespoon of JuvaPower may be added to the salad.

**1 p.m.:** Drink 10 oz. of the Master Cleanse drink.

**2 p.m.:** Drink Vital Life Juice.

**3 p.m.:** Drink Slique Shake and NingXia Red.

**4 p.m.:** Drink Vital Life Juice.

**6 p.m.:** Eat a salad of your choice, white basmati rice with coconut or other alternative milk, or one of the dinner recipes listed below. If you have not used JuvaPower before, take 1 tablespoon of JuvaPower at

Seventh Edition | **Essential Oils Desk Reference** | 331

dinnertime along with two Allerzyme capsules.

**7 p.m.:** Drink Master Cleanse drink.

**8 p.m.:** Drink Vital Life Juice.

**9 p.m.:** Take 2 JuvaTone, 2 Detoxzyme, 1 Essential-zymes-4 (white capsule), and 1 Essentialzymes-4 (yellow capsule), followed by 1 capsule of JuvaCleanse and the Master Cleanse drink.

Drink 2–4 oz. of NingXia Red during the day as desired.

If there are any problems with bowel function or movement, incorporate ComforTone and ICP into one of your drinks. This will enhance the cleansing action of the liver.

You may want to check with your health care professional before beginning any dietary change, especially if serious degenerative disease is a condition.

## ParaFree™ and Parasites

Almost everyone has parasites in one form or another. For the most part, they go entirely unnoticed until the person begins to feel "achy" and fatigued.

Pure essential oils have some of the strongest antiparasitic properties known, including Thyme, Clove, Anise, Nutmeg, Fennel, Vetiver, Idaho Tansy, Cumin, Tea Tree, Ledum, Melissa, and Bergamot. ParaFree, DiGize, Digest & Cleanse, and Inner Defense are supplements that aid the body in killing and ridding itself of parasites.

### ParaFree Protocol

- Take 3–6 ParaFree softgels 2–3 times daily for one week. Rest for one week to allow the parasite eggs to hatch.
- Start again and continue for 3 weeks and then rest for 3 weeks. Repeat this cycle three times.

# Establishing and Maintaining Good Health

## Babies and Children

Babies and children respond very well to essential oils and nutritional supplements. The only difference is the amount. KidScents MightyZyme and MightyVites and NingXia Red are products specific to children. The Super C Chewables are a good companion to MightyVites and MightyZyme.

Children have an innate sense about essential oils. Most children are very drawn to the aromas. They love to have them massaged on their feet and backs as much as they love to feel them in their own hands and massage them on someone else. They just want to put them on without questions and concerns.

- **Babies:** Put 1–2 drops of oil in your hand and rub your hands together until they are practically dry. Then hold them over any area of the baby. This works very well without direct application.
- **Direct application:** Mix 1–2 drops of an essential oil in V-6 Vegetable Oil Complex and apply to the bottoms of feet.
- **Children:** Put 1–2 drops on bottoms of feet or anywhere else on the body as long as the oil is diluted in V-6 Vegetable Oil Complex or in any vegetable oil. Although dilution is recommended, it is not always necessary. The essential oil roll-ons are perfect for babies and children of all ages as well as for adults.

## Balancing Body Frequency

When the body is overloaded with toxins and is not able to cleanse properly, the endocrine system is not able to maintain good electrical balance throughout the physical body. The first solution is to begin a cleanse, as has been written about in this chapter.

- Where the imbalance is due to allergies in the sinuses, throat, or pituitary, apply 1–3 drops of The Gift, Valor, Sacred Mountain, etc., to the crown of the head, the forehead, and the thymus.
- The essential oil blends Release, Divine Release, Freedom, Inner Harmony, Reconnect, T.R. Care, etc., stimulate harmony and balance by releasing memory trauma from liver cells, where the emotions of anger, hate, and frustration are stored. Apply neat or diluted with V-6 or other massage oil over liver, apply compress over liver, or massage Vita Flex points on feet and hands.
- Sandalwood oxygenates the pineal/pituitary gland, thus improving attitude and body balance. Rose has a frequency of 320 MHz, the highest of all oils. Its beautiful fragrance is aphrodisiac-like and almost intoxicating. The frequency of every cell is enhanced, bringing balance and harmony to the body. Rose is stimulating and elevating to the mind, creating a sense of well-being.
- A blend of 5 drops each of Frankincense, Myrrh, and Idaho Balsam Fir with 1 drop of Rose oil is very helpful for depression. Put a drop of the blend on the thumb and press the thumb against the roof of the mouth. This opens the cranial sutures and is a powerful way to amplify the benefits and change the feelings of depression, sadness, despair, etc.
- Idaho Balsam Fir rubbed under the nose and even up the nostrils is very uplifting and mood enhancing. There is usually a noticeable change of emotion immediately.

Cleansing and Diet | **Chapter 17**

- Lavender, Aroma Ease, Inner Harmony, Peace and Calming, Peace & Calming II, etc., are excellent for calming a troubled mind and creating a peaceful environment.
- Harmony and Inner Harmony will probably work in most situations because they bring harmonic balance to the energy centers of the body.
- Inner Child, Reconnect, T.R. Care, SARA, Divine Release, InTouch, etc., stimulate memory response, enabling a person to get in touch with the feelings connected to trauma and negative memories and to let them go, thus allowing the person to create positive attitudes and intentions for the future.
- For overall body electrical imbalance, put 1–2 drops of Sacred Frankincense, 3 Wise Men, Reconnect, Gathering, Inspiration, etc., in each palm. Rub the hands together and then hold the right palm over the navel and the left palm over the thymus and take three slow, deep breaths.

Next, place the dominant hand over the navel, the other hand over the thymus, and rub clockwise three times. This works through the body's electrical field by pulling the frequency in through the umbilicus, the thymus, the olfactory, and then to the limbic system in the brain to create electrical balance.

The same procedure may be repeated with any of the different oils. Grounding is good for balancing frequencies when disrupted by disease.

- Harmony and Inner Harmony on the energy centers (or chakras) help to balance the body, thus improving the healing process and facilitating the release of stored emotions.
- Massage 3–4 drops of Thieves on the bottoms of the feet.

The energy points corresponding to the endocrine glands are:

- The crown (top) of the head (pineal)
- Forehead (pituitary)
- Neck (thyroid)
- Thymus
- Solar plexus (adrenal)
- Navel (pancreas)
- Groin (ovaries/gonads)

Other oils and oil blends that can be used to balance frequency are Frankincense, Sacred Frankincense, The Gift, Common Sense, Idaho Balsam Fir, Valor, Valor II, 3 Wise Men, Gathering, Northern Lights Black Spruce, Highest Potential, Transformation, Joy, White Angelica, and many others.

Any of the roll-ons really work well in applying oils to the energy points of the body: RutaVaLa, Tranquil, Stress Away, Valor, and Breathe Again. You can also transform your favorite Young Living oils and blends into easy-to-use roll-on bottles by inserting an AromaGlide™ advanced roller fitment into any 5-ml or 15-ml bottle with an "Sb" marking on the bottom.

## Fortifying the Immune System

The immune system must be strong and responsive in order to combat all types of disease brought on by pollution and undigested toxins that can lower the immune system response. Dietary supplements containing essential oils can boost and strengthen the immune system.

**ImmuPro**™—combines complex polysaccharides, beta glucans, minerals, essential oils, and melatonin, one of the most powerful immune stimulants known.

- Take 1 or more chewable tablets at night before retiring. Some people enjoy the taste as well as the added benefits of 3–4 tablets. If you take them during the day, you will probably feel like you would like to take a nap.
- Children love them and so do parents who have a hard time getting their children to sleep. Try ½ tablet to begin with, as that may be sufficient. However, 1–2 tablets are not harmful and may even be "helpful."

**Exodus II**™ and **Thieves**®—are essential oil blends that contain immune-stimulating and antimicrobial-compounds. Because essential oils have such complex chemistry, viruses and bacteria have difficulty living in an essential oil solution.

- Massage: 3–6 drops on thymus, throat, bottoms of feet, or wherever desired
- Maintenance: 2–4 capsules daily
- Health challenges: 6–10 capsules 3 times daily for 10 days and then reduce

**Sulfurzyme**®—contains MSM and Ningxia wolfberry for powerful nutritional support.

- Maintenance: 1–2 teaspoons daily in water or juice or as needed
- Additional health support: Begin with 1–2 teaspoons daily and work up to 3–4 tablespoons daily or more if desired

**ImmuPower**™—is an essential oil blend used to strengthen, build, and protect the body.

- Maintenance: 1 capsule 3–4 times weekly
- Pneumonia, flu, or colds: 4 capsules daily for 10 days, rest 4 days, and then 1 capsule daily for another 10 days

**Inner Defense**®—Take 2–4 capsules daily

**OmegaGize³**®—Take 1–2 capsules daily

**Super B**™—Take 1 tablet daily after eating

**Thyromin**™—is a very unique blend of glandular extracts, herbs, amino acids, minerals, and essential oils to support the thyroid. This gland regulates body metabolism and temperature and is important for immune function.

- Maintenance: Take 1 capsule immediately before going to bed.

Seventh Edition | **Essential Oils Desk Reference** | 333

- Additional health support: Take 3 capsules immediately before going to bed and 2 in the morning.

**Mineral Essence™**—is a precisely balanced complex of essential oils and more than 60 trace minerals that are essential to a healthy immune system. It includes well-known antioxidants and immune-supporters such as zinc, selenium, and magnesium.

- Maintenance: Take 1–2 droppers 1–3 times daily in water or NingXia Red.
- Additional health support: Take 2–5 droppers 2 times daily.

**Singles:** Sacred Frankincense, Palo Santo, Eucalyptus Blue, Ocotea, Ravintsara, Thyme, Oregano, Rosemary, Idaho Tansy, Mountain Savory, Melissa, Lemon, Cinnamon, Clove, Cistus, Tea Tree, Myrrh, Myrtle

**Blends:** The Gift, Thieves, Melrose, Purification, ImmuPower, Exodus II, DiGize, GLF, JuvaCleanse, JuvaFlex, Longevity Softgels

**Supplements:** Super B, MultiGreens, Slique Shake, Pure Protein Complete, Rehemogen, AlkaLime, Life 9, NingXia Red, JuvaTone, Super C, and Inner Defense

**NingXia Red® Juice** is the highest-ranked antioxidant liquid dietary supplement that combines the wolfberry fruit (*Lycium barbarum*), pomegranates, blueberries, raspberries, and other fruit juices with essential oils. It is delicious and provides a great many nutrients that promote strength, vitality, and longevity.

# Daily Maintenance

## Strength-building Protocol

Nutritional supplements enhanced with essential oils can help support and balance body systems. The following products will nourish, strengthen, and build your body.

**Slique Shake™**—Vegan protein drink with Chinese wolfberries

- Mix 1 package in water or milk of choice and drink 2–3 times daily. It can be mixed in orange or apple juice, but this may make it too sweet and lower the pH. It also may be mixed with cereal, fruits, desserts, and other foods.
- Combine equal parts Slique Shake and Pure Protein Complete for a high-powered protein blend.
- Drink as needed or as a meal replacement.

**Essentialzyme™**—Enzyme-rich ingredients for better digestion and nutrient absorption for improved mental clarity and physical activity

- O Blood Type: 3–5 caplets daily (depending on type of food eaten and time of day)
- B Blood Type: 4–6 caplets daily
- A Blood Type: 5–7 caplets daily (A types tend to have more digestive needs)
  **Note:** When eating heavy protein foods after 3 p.m., take Essentialzymes-4 (yellow capsule), which will help with evening and nighttime digestion.

**MultiGreens™**—Protein-rich chlorophyll to facilitate balanced pH

- O Blood Type: 8–10 capsules daily
- B Blood Type: 6–8 capsules daily
- A Blood Type: 4–6 capsules daily

**Super C™ Chewable Tablets**—The only vitamin C chewable vitamin in the world that combines citrus essential oils; citrus bioflavonoids; and whole-food, natural vitamin C in one tablet.

It is a powerful antioxidant vitamin with minerals, bioflavonoids, and trace minerals to balance electrolytes and assist in the absorption of vitamin C.

Pure essential oils of Orange, Grapefruit, Tangerine, Lemon, and Lemongrass help increase digestion and nutrient absorption and are enjoyed by both adults and children.

**Super C™ Tablets**—Properly balanced with rutin, biotin, bioflavonoids, and trace minerals, Super C works synergistically in balancing the electrolytes and increasing the absorption rate of vitamin C.

Without bioflavonoids, vitamin C has a hard time getting inside cells; and without proper electrolyte balance and trace minerals, it will not stay there long.

**SuperCal™** or **MegaCal™**—Contain minerals, calcium, magnesium, potassium, and zinc combined with essential oils to maintain proper health. Take 2–6 capsules or 1-2 scoops daily or as needed.

**Sulfurzyme®**—A natural form of dietary sulfur to support normal metabolic functions, circulation, and help strengthen the body's natural defense system. It builds strong hair and nails.

- Start: 1–2 teaspoons daily for 1–2 days
- Increase: 1–2 tablespoons 2 times daily for maximum results

Cleansing and Diet | **Chapter 17**

## Maintenance Protocol

Our lifestyles should incorporate cleansing at all times. The intensity of cleansing depends on the individual. ComforTone, Essentialzyme, Detoxzyme, JuvaPower, and ICP taken at the same time provide a powerful, synergistic cleansing force.

- **ComforTone®:** 3–5 capsules morning and night
- **Essentialzyme™:** 3 caplets 3 times daily to digest toxic waste from everyday metabolism
- **Detoxzyme®:** 2 capsules morning and noon, 4 capsules at night
- **ICP™:** 1 teaspoon of powder in water, carrot juice, or apple juice morning and night
- **JuvaPower®:** 1–2 tablespoons of powder in water 2 times daily
- **JuvaSpice®** is made to sprinkle on salads and to use in cooking

| A Simple Guide for Daily Maintenance | |
|---|---|
| Longevity (oil blend) | Children over age 8: 6 drops per capsule 2 times daily or in yogurt; Adults: 20 drops per capsule, 1–2 capsules, 2 times daily or in yogurt |
| Longevity Softgels | Children and teens ages 10–18: 1–2 capsules daily. Adults: 2–4 capsules daily |
| Melrose | Children over age 8: 6 drops per capsule 2 times daily or in yogurt; Adults: 20 drops per capsule, 1–2 capsules, 2 times daily or in yogurt |
| Super C | 4–6 tablets daily |
| Super C Chewable | 4–6 tablets or as desired |
| Thyromin | 1 capsule 3 times daily |
| Citrus Fresh | Children over age 8: 6 drops per capsule 2 times daily or in yogurt; Adults: 20 drops per capsule, 1–2 capsules, 2 times daily or in yogurt |
| EndoFlex | 1–2 capsules daily |
| Allerzyme | 2–4 capsules 3 times daily |
| Detoxzyme | 5–10 capsules at night |
| DiGize | 1–2 capsules daily |
| Essentialzyme | 2 tablets 3 times daily |
| ICP | 1–2 tablespoons in the morning |
| JuvaPower | 1–2 tablespoons at night |
| NingXia Red | 4–6 oz. daily |
| Water | Drink 3 liters daily |

## Good Eating Habits

Breakfast is the most important meal of the day. Some people work for an hour or two prior to having breakfast to promote appetite and prime the digestive system.

Generally, eat breakfast between 6 and 7 a.m. Protein and complex carbohydrate foods are best for energy conversion in the morning. Strawberries or raspberries are the only fruits recommended to eat with cereal.

Plain yogurt or Kefir without sweeteners are good sources of acidophilus and bifida bacteria cultures essential for proper intestinal flora. Sugar, synthetic sweeteners, and other foods high on the glycemic index should be avoided.

Sometimes people who have health challenges and have digestive systems that do not function properly feel better eating fruit like papaya, mango, pineapple, and watermelon, which are easier to digest.

Cereals can include oatmeal, millet, barley, quinoa, or a mixture of these, with your choice of milk.

However, it is best not to tax the body with too many grains, which make digestion more difficult.

Bread is better toasted to change it from a wet food to a dry food, making it more digestible. However, bread made with today's modern hybrid wheat is not healthy for the body. A and B blood types gain weight more easily than O types because of the difference in digestive systems.

Breakfast is the best time to eat proteins such as beans, rice, eggs, fish, etc., providing more energy and stamina throughout the day. Be sure to take 1–3 Essentialzymes-4 (yellow capsule) with high-protein meals.

Lunch should consist of carbohydrates such as mixed vegetables or salads (particularly greens) along with free-range chicken or turkey or freshwater fish (not farm raised). Drink plenty of water with every meal.

A simple meal of organic, white basmati rice with cinnamon, Blue Agave, maple syrup, or Yacon Syrup with your choice of milk is a perfect acid-binding food for an evening meal. White basmati rice is an alkaline food that is easier for the body to digest at night. A Slique Shake drink is also a simple replacement meal in the evening.

Dinner should be eaten in the late afternoon or early evening, if possible. It is much better to eat a bigger meal midday and not as heavy in the evening. Both fruit and solid vegetables are suitable for evening meals. If an individual must eat a large, heavy meal late in the day or evening, Essentialzyme or Essentialzymes-4 (yellow capsule) is needed to promote proper digestion, reduce gas, and prevent putrefaction and fungal growth in the intestines.

Seventh Edition | **Essential Oils Desk Reference** | **335**

## Environmental Protection
*(See also Chapter 19)*

Daily radiation bombardment from our highly technical, electrical world does not make the body healthier. If you know you have been exposed to radiation, feeling fatigued from it, or are flying on commercial airlines, because of the greater exposure to radiation due to the high altitude, an increased daily number of antioxidant supplements is needed.

An important supplement to take when flying is Thyromin, which supports the thyroid. Increase the number of antioxidant supplements you take 10 days before flying and increase the number for 10 days after traveling.

**Suggestions:** Inner Defense, Super C (or Chewable), Detoxzyme, Essentialzyme, Essentialzymes-4, NingXia Red, and many others.

The Environmental Protection Kits, QuadShield and EndoShield, are convenient, easy ways to help you maintain your protection against the dangers of daily radiation bombardment and in the case of a more serious threat—radioactive poisoning. Refer to the chart titled Environmental Protection Kits for products and details about how these products can protect you, your family, your friends, and those around you from the dangers of environmental pollution and potential daily radiation exposure.

### Restoring Proper Bowel Flora

Antibiotics, chemotherapy, or radiation destroy the good bacteria in the body. A good probiotic (acidophilus and bifidus) such as Life 9 probiotic will help restore proper flora in the digestive system.

Take 5 at night daily for one week after finishing with antibiotics or other medicines. Plain, unflavored yogurt taken before lighter meals also helps provide friendly bacteria.

For patients undergoing radiation, saturate the site 10 days prior to treatment with Tea Tree and Melaleuca Ericifolia. Take 4 double 00 capsules per day before, during, and for 30 to 60 days following radiation treatment.

## Environmental Protection Kits

The QuadShield and EndoShield kits each combine four powerful products to help people protect themselves against daily radiation bombardment of cell phones, computers, electrical appliances, and other potential dangers.

The QuadShield kit contains Longevity Softgels, the essential oil blend Melrose, and the nutritional supplements Super C (or Chewable), and Thyromin. The EndoShield kit contains Longevity Softgels and the essential oil blends Melrose, EndoFlex, and Citrus Fresh.

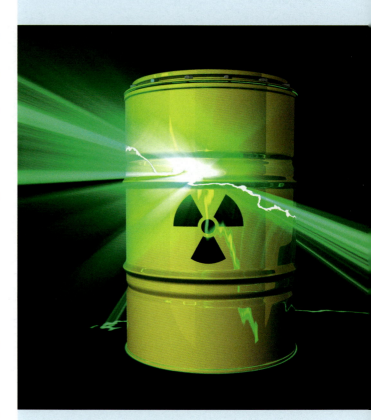

The Japanese earthquake of March 11, 2011, has taught the world that nuclear power plants are vulnerable to natural disasters, as well as from years of use that have caused deterioration and weakness.

Of the 104 nuclear power plants in the United States, six are identical to the damaged Fukushima plant, 17 others are very similar, and several are close to major earthquake faults.

The "giant" that has been sleeping since the days of the Three Mile Island and Chernobyl disasters has awakened.

Cleansing and Diet | **Chapter 17**

# Environmental Protection Kits

## QuadShield™

**Longevity Softgel**—The essential oils in Longevity Softgels increase the oxygen and ATP (adenosine triphosphate) cellular fuel for increasing cell life and immunity for stronger resistance against damage from environmental pollution.
- **Children and teens ages 10–18:** 1-2 capsules daily
- **Adults:** 2–4 capsules daily

**Melrose**—This blend is formulated with two species of Melaleuca oil: *M. alternifolia* and *M. quinquenervia*, also known as Niaouli, which were found through research by Daniel Pénoël, MD, and Pierre Franchomme, PhD, to prevent cellular damage from environmental pollution and potential daily radiation exposure.
- **Children ages 1–3:** 1 drop in yogurt or other liquid
- **Children ages 4–7:** 2 drops in yogurt or other liquid
- **Children 8 and older:** 6 drops per capsule 1–3 times daily or in yogurt or other liquid
- **Adults:** 20 drops per capsule, 1–2 capsules, 1–3 times daily or in yogurt or other liquid

**Super C (or Chewable)** —Super C provides the body with 2,166 percent of the recommended dietary intake of the powerful antioxidant vitamin C and is enhanced with minerals, bioflavonoids, and pure Orange, Lemon, and other essential oils. It is a natural antioxidant and free radical scavenger that supports the immune system and protects healthy cells from becoming damaged by the effects of environmental pollution.
- **Children ages 1–3:** 1–2 MightyVites daily
- **Children ages 4–7:** 2–3 MightyVites or Super C Chewables daily
- **Children 8 and older:** 3–4 MightyVites or Super C Chewables daily
- **Adults:** 4–6 tablets daily

**Thyromin**—Thyromin contains ingredients that give support and nutrition to both the thyroid and adrenal glands for a healthier glandular system.
- **Children:** continue to use MightyVites 2–4 daily
- **Adults:** only 1 capsule, 3 times daily

**NingXia Red**—Drink 4–6 oz. of NingXia Red for a delicious and healthy addition to your diet.

## EndoShield™

**Longevity Softgel**—The essential oils in Longevity Softgels increase the oxygen and ATP (adenosine triphosphate) cellular fuel for increasing cell life and immunity for stronger resistance against damage from environmental pollution.
- **Children and teens ages 10–18:** 1–2 capsules daily
- **Adults:** 2–4 capsules daily

**Melrose**—This blend is formulated with two species of Melaleuca oil: *M. alternifolia* and *M. quinquenervia*, also known as Niaouli, which were found through research by Daniel Pénoël, MD, and Pierre Franchomme, PhD, to prevent cellular damage from environmental pollution and potential daily radiation exposure.
- **Children ages 1–3:** 1 drop in yogurt or other liquid
- **Children ages 4–7:** 2 drops in yogurt or other liquid
- **Children 8 and older:** 6 drops per capsule 1–3 times daily or in yogurt or other liquid
- **Adults:** 20 drops per capsule, 1–2 capsules, 1–3 times daily or in yogurt or other liquid

**EndoFlex** —This blend contains oils very specific to the thyroid while at the same time addressing the entire endocrine system. Myrtle oil stimulates and promotes good thyroid health when combined with Spearmint, encouraging better circulation, stronger metabolism, and production of digestive enzymes. Geranium contains esters that protect the thyroid, which may explain why it is so heralded in French publications as a general tonic for the body. It supports the thyroid in being able to uptake iodine from food.
- **Children ages 1–3:** 1 drop in yogurt or other liquid
- **Children ages 4–7:** 2 drops in yogurt or other liquid
- **Children 8 and older:** 6 drops per capsule 2 times daily or in yogurt or other liquid
- **Adults:** 20 drops per capsule, 1–2 capsules, 1–3 times daily or in yogurt or other liquid

**Citrus Fresh**—This blend combines six citrus oils that are naturally antioxidant, antibacterial, and increase the uptake of vitamin C.
- **Children ages 1–3:** 1 drop in yogurt or other liquid
- **Children ages 4–7:** 2 drops in yogurt or other liquid
- **Children 8 and older:** 6 drops per capsule 2 times daily or in yogurt or other liquid
- **Adults:** 20 drops per capsule, 1–2 capsules, 1–3 times daily or in yogurt or other liquid

**NingXia Red**—Drink 4–6 oz. of NingXia Red for a delicious and healthy addition to your diet.

Seventh Edition | **Essential Oils Desk Reference** | **337**

# Recipes—Delicious and Nutritious

These recipes for salads and smoothies are very tasty and give you an idea for nutritious eating while on a cleansing program. Everyone loves the smoothies as a treat anytime, especially the children.

## Smoothie and Popsicle Recipes
*Created by Vallorie Judd*

### Protein Power
**(A nutritional protein drink for all ages!)**
- 1–2 scoops Balance Complete
- ½ cup carrot juice
- ½ cup fresh coconut milk
- 1 drop Orange essential oil
- ¼–½ cup water or an equivalent amount of ice

**Directions**
- Blend and enjoy nutrition at its best! It tastes like a "Creamsicle" but even better.
- This can be enjoyed fresh or frozen in little containers for a frozen "Proteinsicle."
- The carrot juice provides enzymes, and the coconut milk is full of essential omegas.
- It also makes a great replacement meal and is very satisfying to children who want to eat all the time.

**Variations**
- Use 1 scoop Pure Protein Complete and 1 scoop Balance Complete.
- Mangos are another wonderful fruit to blend into the protein drinks.
- Another healthful drink can be made using kefir (probiotics) and pineapple (bromelain).

### Pina Colada Delight
- 1 cup kefir milk
- 1 cup coconut milk
- 1–2 scoops Balance Complete or Pure Protein Complete
- ½ cup fresh chopped pineapple
- 1 frozen banana (or fresh banana with ice cubes)
- ½ cup ice cubes or water

**Directions**
- Blend and enjoy as a nutritious drink or freeze for a frozen treat.
- If you do not have kefir, then use coconut milk in its place.

### Frozen NingXia Popsicles
- 1 cup NingXia Red
- ¼–½ cup water
- ½ cup blueberries
- ½ cup strawberries
- 1 drop Orange or Lemon oil (optional)

**Directions**
Blend and pour into Popsicle trays and freeze.
*Also, the next recipe is very delicious!*

### NingXia Red Watermelon Juice or Popsicles
- ¼–½ cup NingXia Red
- 1 cup watermelon juice

**Directions**
- Mix together.
- Drink fresh or freeze for popsicles.

## Recipes for Healthful Eating
*Created by D. Gary Young*

The following recipes, created by D. Gary Young, are compatible meals with any cleansing program and are examples of healthful eating anytime.

**Note:** Basmati white rice is acid binding; brown rice is acid forming.

### Beet Salad with Apples and Carrots
- 3 medium cooked beets, diced
- 1 large apple, diced (Golden Delicious or Gala)
- 3 carrots, diced
- 2 fresh limes
- 2 tablespoons coconut, avocado, or olive oil
- 1 dash of JuvaSpice
- 1 dash of cayenne pepper
- 2 teaspoons Blue Agave or Yacon Syrup
- 1 head romaine lettuce
- 1 head red leaf lettuce

**Directions**
- Grate or dice the carrots and apples.
- Steam the beets for 1 minute and then run under icy water for 3 minutes to prevent overcooking.
- Slice, dice, and mix together. Squeeze limes for juice.

Cleansing and Diet | **Chapter 17**

## Spinach Delight

- 2 bunches spinach leaves (torn)
- 4 tablespoons sesame seeds
- 2 cups coconut, avocado, or olive oil
- 2 squeezed lemons
- 1 tablespoon JuvaSpice
- 1 dash Tabasco sauce
- 1 can diced water chestnuts
- 6 button mushrooms
- 2 beets, steamed, chilled, and diced
- 4 figs, diced

**Directions**
- Mix together and add a dressing of your choice.

## Mandarin Avocado Salad

- 4 heads romaine lettuce (chilled and torn)
- 1 avocado (peeled and chopped)
- 3 fresh mangos (chilled and diced)
- 1 small red pepper (finely chopped)
- 1 small green pepper (finely chopped)
- 8 green onions (finely chopped)
- 1 tablespoon fresh chives (finely chopped)

**Directions**
- Mix together; then add dressing.

## Tuna Mandarin Salad

- Use the same recipe as above but add fresh albacore tuna.

## Essential Rice Salad

- 3 cups cooked basmati rice (chilled)
- 1 cup cooked corn kernels
- 1 cup chopped celery
- 1 cup chopped almonds
- 1 cup grated carrots
- 3 green onions (finely sliced)
- 2 tablespoons sesame seeds (toasted)
- 4 cups raisins

**Directions**
- After cooking rice, place it in the refrigerator.
- When rice is chilled, toss all ingredients in a salad bowl along with the dressing of your choice.

## Bean Salad

- 1 cup chickpeas (garbanzo beans)
- 1 cup kidney beans
- 2 cups butter beans
- 1 cup black eyed beans
- 1 cup pinto beans
- 2 cups diced green beans

**Directions**
- Soak all beans for 12 hours, except the green beans.
- Next, boil for approximately 30 minutes and let simmer for 40 minutes or until beans are tender.
- Rinse, dry, and chill in the refrigerator.
- Add a dressing of your choice and serve.

## Garden Salad

- 2 heads romaine lettuce, torn
- 1 head red leaf lettuce, torn
- 1 bunch spinach leaves, torn
- 2 cups snow pea sprouts or pea sprouts
- 3 cups alfalfa, chopped
- 1 cup watercress, chopped
- 4 cups fresh dill, finely chopped
- 8 basil sprigs, chopped
- 4 fennel sprigs, chopped

**Directions**
- Mix together and add the dressing of your choice.

## Potato/Vegetable Salad

- 1 dozen small red potatoes
- 4 teaspoons paprika
- 2 tablespoons organic coconut, avocado, or olive oil
- 2 cups broccoli
- 6 cups romaine lettuce, torn
- 2 cups green beans or spinach, chopped
- 2 cups alfalfa sprouts
- 2 cups bean sprouts
- 1 cup finely sliced red cabbage

**Directions**
- Cook the potatoes for 20 minutes— with or without skins.
- Preheat oven to 400°F and place potato mixture in a glass casserole dish; bake for 5–10 minutes on the top rack of the oven.
- Steam the broccoli; then wait for 5 minutes and remove from heat.
- Run under cold water for 30 seconds; drain well.
- Mix lettuce and spinach.
- Cut the broccoli lengthwise and dice. Add the greens and dressing of your choice.
- Use JuvaSpice with an additional pinch of cayenne pepper for extra flavor.

## Minestrone Soup

- 1 cup basmati rice, cooked
- 2 cups navy beans, cooked
- 2 cups green beans, diced
- 2 teaspoons oregano, chopped
- 2 teaspoons basil, chopped
- 2 drops coconut oil
- 2 large potatoes, diced
- 3 average-size zucchini, chopped
- 2 large leeks (use whole)
- 4 celery stocks, diced
- 2 large carrots, diced
- 10 cups vegetable or chicken stock
- 2 garlic cloves, minced
- 1 large onion, chopped
- 2 cups mushrooms, sliced
- 4 large tomatoes, diced
- 1 tablespoon JuvaSpice

### Directions

- Cook beans and rice separately.
- Mix all the rest of the ingredients and let simmer in the chicken stock for 15 minutes.
- When beans appear to be tender (but not mushy) and the rice is done, add beans and rice to the vegetable mixture.
- Add 1 tablespoon of JuvaSpice and let simmer for 15 minutes.
- It will take approximately 45 minutes to cook the beans and 20-30 minutes to cook the rice.

## Pumpkin Pinch

- 3 butternut squash, diced
- 2 cups winter squash, diced
- 1 cup acorn squash, diced
- 2 onions, diced
- 1 garlic clove, minced
- 6 cups vegetable stock
- 4 bunches of fresh basil, chopped
- Coriander (to taste)
- 2 tablespoons soy sauce
- 1 dash cayenne pepper
- 1 tablespoon JuvaSpice
- 4 bunches flat leaf parsley, chopped and minced
- 1 cup milk of choice
- 2 bay leaves (remove after cooking)

### Directions

- Place all vegetables in a large pot and simmer slowly (approximately 45 minutes to 1 hour).
- Add seasoning about halfway through.
- Blend soup in a food processor until smooth—then add milk.
- Tastes great over basmati rice.

## Dinner Delight

- 1 cup basmati rice
- Shrimp and red snapper
- 1 onion, chopped
- 1 stalk celery, chopped
- 1 carrot, chopped
- Ginger root, minced
- Garlic clove, minced
- 1 bunch Brussels sprouts, chopped
- 1 medium-size zucchini, chopped or sliced
- 1 large winter squash or butternut squash

### Directions

- Cover squash with coconut or avocado oil and sesame seeds and bake at 350°F for 45–60 minutes until completely done.
- Cook basmati rice.
- Cook all the vegetables and spices together in a frying pan for about 20 minutes or until they start to become soft. Then add shrimp or fish and cook together on low heat for 15 to 20 minutes or until done.
- Take squash out of the oven and serve with vegetables, shrimp, or fish.

## Stir Fry

- 2 teaspoons coconut or avocado oil
- 10 scallions, minced
- 2 garlic cloves, minced
- 2 tablespoons ginger
- 2 lbs. red chili peppers, minced
- 1 teaspoon sesame oil
- 1 tablespoon mild chili powder

### Directions

- Cook 1 lb. Brussels sprouts for 10 min., let cool, and dice.
- Then mix the Brussels sprouts with the rest of the ingredients.
- Stir in hot frying pan or wok until tender.
- Eat with rice or potatoes.

Cleansing and Diet | **Chapter 17**

## Chicken with Onion Pineapple Sauce

- 6 chicken breasts
- 1 pineapple, cubed
- 2 cloves of garlic, minced
- 1 onion, chopped
- 1 red pepper, chopped
- ½ cup water
- JuvaSpice
- Mixed herbs/seasonings for chicken
- Basmati white rice (optional)

### Directions

- Sauté garlic and onions in a small amount of coconut or avocado oil; you also can use a small amount of water in a frying pan until lightly cooked.
- Add chicken and red pepper; brown with the onion and garlic.
- Add spices, water, and ½ of the pineapple that is cut in cubes.
- Put a lid on the pan and let cook for about ½ hour until the chicken is cooked.
- Take the other half of the pineapple and process in a blender; pour over chicken and stir.
- Sprinkle a liberal amount of JuvaSpice into the sauce. Let simmer for about 5 minutes.
- This becomes like gravy. You can add a mixture of flour, guar gum, or natural thickener for a more gravy-like texture.
- This is great served over basmati white rice and served with baked yams and salad.

## Gary's Chocomolie

- 1 cup avocado
- 4 tablespoons carob
- 16 dates
- 2 teaspoons vanilla extract
- 2 tablespoons maple syrup
- 34 ounces water

## Healthy Snacks

Everyone loves to snack, so why not snack in a healthy way? Slique Shake, Wolfberry Crisp Bars (Chocolate Coated), Slique Bars, Slique Bars (Chocolate-Coated), and Ecuadorian Dark Chocolessence bars are always a treat. They add protein, good fiber, and are packed with nutrients and essential oils that support and strengthen the body. Organic Dried Ningxia Wolfberries are also a great snack.

### Directions

- Blend until thick and creamy.
- Chill in the fridge or freezer for ½ hour.
- This is wonderful on organic, einkorn pancakes or waffles with yogurt or over rice milk ice cream with sliced bananas.
- This can also be used as the filling to a precooked einkorn pie crust and then topped with yogurt and sliced bananas.
- This pudding may also be flavored with a drop of Peppermint oil, Orange oil, or a combination of both.
- This is really a delicious recipe!

## Acorn Squash Apple Crisp

*Created by Vallorie Judd*

- 1 acorn squash washed and cut in half with seeds and pulp removed
- 1 Jonagold apple or other good baking apple, peeled and cored
- ¼ cup Blue Agave or Yacon Syrup
- 1 teaspoon cinnamon
- ¼ cup Organic Dried NingXia Wolfberries

### Directions

- Take acorn squash and cut a small piece off of the bottom of it to help it sit level.
- Slice half an apple into ½ of the acorn squash; do the same for the other half.
- Mix Blue Agave or Yacon Syrup, wolfberries, and cinnamon in a bowl; and then pour half of it into each halved acorn squash.
- Divide topping and cover the top of each half of the acorn squash with the apple inside of it.
- Sprinkle extra cinnamon over the top of the oatmeal topping (see below).
- Bake for about 30 minutes or until the squash and apple are soft from baking.
- Can top with rice milk ice cream or goat yogurt.

### Topping

- ¼–½ cup butter or coconut butter (can do half and half)
- 1 cup oatmeal or ¾ cup oatmeal and ¼ cup einkorn or oat or other flour
- ½ cup Blue Agave or Yacon Syrup
- Put cinnamon oil on toothpick and stir into Blue Agave or Yacon Syrup

Seventh Edition | **Essential Oils Desk Reference** | 341

## Quinoa Oatmeal Breakfast

- 2 cups organic, old fashion rolled oatmeal
- 4 cups water
- ½ cup quinoa

### Directions

- Rinse quinoa and add to water.
- Boil for about 5 to 10 minutes.
- Add oatmeal and cook slowly for 10 minutes until thick.

### About Quinoa

Thousands of years ago, quinoa (keen-WA) was a key source of nourishment for the Incas, who grew it high in the arid Andes Mountains.

Today, it is known as a "super grain" because it's so good for you. It is rich in essential amino acids, protein, calcium, iron, potassium, and B vitamins such as riboflavin, not to mention magnesium, zinc, copper, manganese, and folate, a water-soluble B vitamin that occurs naturally in food.

The seed of a spinach-like plant, quinoa is most often creamy in color, but it also comes in pink, red, yellow, orange, or black. When cooked, it expands and releases its germ, a delicate, white fibrous ring that is pleasantly crunchy.

Look for quinoa in the health-foods or bulk-foods section of your supermarket or health food store. If the price looks a little high to you, keep in mind that quinoa triples in volume when cooked.

To make a quick, nutritious, and tasty side dish for dinner, combine ½ cup rinsed quinoa with 1 cup water in a covered saucepan and bring to a boil. Reduce to a simmer for 15 minutes, checking to be sure it does not dry out. When seeds have tripled in size and spiral-shaped white germs are prominent, toss with butter, olive or avocado oil, chopped garlic, and/or fresh herbs.

For additional recipes using essential oils and nutritious ingredients, see *The Young Living Cookbook*. The recipes were submitted by Young Living members and employees.

For more information on liver cleansing and a detailed daily protocol, consult *Re-JUVA-nate Your Health*, a book on liver cleansing by D. Gary Young, published by Life Science Publishing.

## Cooking with Essential Oils

Essential oil-enhanced cooking can be a lot of fun. A healthier lifestyle way of eating starts with your food preparation. When you have finished cooking your meats, add 2–3 drops of Anise Seed, Fennel, Basil, Rosemary, or Thyme and let the meat cool in the covered pot, so the oils can penetrate and soak into the meat.

After steaming vegetables, add 1–2 drops of Lemongrass, Melissa, Ocotea, Peppermint, Spearmint, or Lemon to enhance the enzymatic action of the food and increase the natural enzyme secretion in your GI tract (gastrointestinal tract).

When making apple pie, pumpkin pie, carrot cake, etc., add 3–4 drops of Cassia, Cinnamon, Ocotea, or other oils you desire according to taste. Essential oils kill unfriendly and unwanted microbes that can survive cooking. The essential oils also increase the ion exchange in the cells of the foods, increasing the cell surface and allowing more ATP and oxygen uptake that enhance greater enzyme function.

### ENDNOTES

1. Waitzberg DL, et al. Effect of symbiotic in constipated adult women—a randomized, double-blind, placebo-controlled study of clinical response. *Clin Nutr.* 2013 Feb;32)1):27-33.
2. Sabater-Molina M, et al. Dietary fructooligosaccharides and potential benefits on health. *J Physiol Biochem.* 2009 Sep;65(3):315-28.
3. Moroti C, et al. Effect of the consumption of a new symbiotic shake on glycemia and cholesterol levels in elderly people with type 2 diabetes mellitus. *Lipids Health Dis.* 2012 Feb 22:11:29.
4. Costa GT, et al. Fructo-oligosaccharide effects on serum cholesterol levels. An overview. *Acta Cir Bras.* 2015 May;309(5):366-70.
5. Bornet FR, Brouns F. Immune-stimulating and gut health-promoting properties of short-chain fructo-oligosaccharides. *Nutr Rev.* 2002 Oct;60(1):326-34.
6. Hsu CK, et al. Xylooligosaccarides and fructooligosaccharides affect the intestinal microbiota and precancerous colonic lesion development in rats. *J Nutr.* 2004 Jun;134(6):1523-8.
7. http://mercurypolicy.org/wp-content/uploads/2010/05/dentalmercurymidnightdealreportforweb.pdf.

# Chapter 18
## Building Blocks of Health

## Enzymes: The Key to Digestion

Enzymes are biological catalysts that speed up the chemical reactions in all living things. Without enzymes nothing would work. Our food would sit for weeks in our stomachs, and we would eventually die. Enzymes are absolutely vital to human health and are the foundation on which life is perpetuated. The purpose of enzymes is to break molecules apart or put them together, which they do very quickly and efficiently. There are specific enzymes for each chemical reaction needed to make each individual cell work properly.

Enzymes are like other proteins consisting of long chains of amino acids that are held together by peptide bonds. Amino acids are organic compounds made of carbon, hydrogen, oxygen, nitrogen, and sometimes sulfur that are bonded in various formations. There are strings of 50 or more amino acids known as proteins that are large molecules that promote growth, repair damaged tissue, strengthen the immune system, and make enzymes. Enzymes facilitate chemical reactions but are not affected by the reaction.

Many body processes that normally require high temperatures such as processing starch would have to come to the boiling point outside our stomachs. But with the catalytic enzyme action, starches are easily converted naturally to usable energy in the body.

Over 3,000 known enzymes in the body perform every type of chemical conversion imaginable. They control the body's vital metabolic processes and are present in every biological system. Enzyme conversion creates energy and builds new cells. All living cells require nutrients and enzymes to divide, grow, and perform their normal activities. Enzymes turn the food we eat into energy and facilitate the use of this energy. There are two major enzyme systems in the human body: metabolic and digestive.

**Metabolic enzymes** help run all the body systems. They speed up the chemical conversion within the cells for detoxification and the production of energy and are produced in the organs of the body such as the liver, pancreas, and gallbladder. Enzymes enable us to move, think, see, hear, and feel, which, in reality, comprise the complete control mechanism of the body. One researcher found over 98 enzymes carrying out metabolic functions in the arteries alone.

**Digestive enzymes** break down the food we eat to release the nutrients for absorption. They are perhaps the most talked-about enzymes, because food is the fuel for life. These enzymes are secreted along the digestive tract, where food is broken down and essential nutrients, vitamins, and minerals that sustain life are released to be absorbed into the blood stream and carried throughout the body.

The waste continues through the digestive tract and is discarded. However, if the waste does not move, causing constipation, then the waste begins to break down into putrefaction that the body will reabsorb as poison, creating all types of body dysfunction. Digestive enzymes include ptyalin, pepsin, trypsin, lipase, protease, and amylase. Another enzyme, cellulose, needed for the digestion of fiber, is not manufactured by the body, so it must come from the food we eat and the supplements we take.

Heat is an enemy to enzymes, and when temperatures exceed 118 degrees, the enzymes begin to break down; and at 120 degrees, the enzymes are totally destroyed, whether it is through pasteurization, sterilization, or commercial food preparation, etc., making the food difficult to digest. So naturally, that also means cooking. The body secretes its own digestive enzymes for breaking down food, but when the naturally occurring enzymes in the food have been destroyed, the body is greatly taxed in its digestive function.

Amylase, found in the saliva of adults, breaks down carbohydrates and simple sugars found in vegetables and fruits. However, it is not produced in the bodies of infants when they are born. Their digestive systems are able to produce protease, cellulase, maltase, lipase, lactase, and

Seventh Edition | **Essential Oils Desk Reference** | 343

# Enzyme Quick Reference Guide

*Please copy this page for a quick, daily reference. Keep it in the kitchen or carry it with you when traveling.*

## Open Capsules:

All capsules may be opened and enzymes sprinkled on any food or mixed in any liquid.

## Combinations:

If more than one enzyme is recommended, you may take just one or a combination and see how your body responds. Basically, any combination is acceptable.

## Key:

**Essentialzyme** (caplet)

**Essentialzymes-4** (two capsules):

**E-4 yellow capsule:** for proteins, carbohydrates, sugars, and starches

**E-4 white capsule:** for fats

## Example:

If for your evening meal you eat chicken, salad, vegetable, bread, juice, and apple pie, you will need more enzymes to digest during the night: 2 E-4 yellow, 2 Essentialzyme, 1 Allerzyme, and 6 Detoxzyme. If it seems like too many, just reduce the number. For children: 3 Mightyzyme, 1 E-4 yellow, 1 Detoxzyme

## Standard Dosages:

For each meal:
Adults: 2–4;
Children: 1–2;
Babies: ¼ to ½.

*Check with your health care professional regarding children younger than 2 years of age.*

## Choices:

The first enzyme listed is usually the first choice in combination with any others as desired.

---

**Start the Morning:** **Essentialzyme** (Adults: 2–4; Children: 1–2 or Mightyzyme 1–3; Babies: ¼ to ½)

Essentialzyme is an overall enzyme that supports the pancreas, which produces glucose the body needs throughout the day for energy.

## General Food Categories:

| | |
|---|---|
| Carbohydrates, fruits, vegetables . . . . . . . . . . . . . . . | **E-4 yellow**, Detoxzyme, Allerzyme, Mightyzyme |
| Fats . . . . . . . . . . . . . . . . . . . . . . . . . . . . . . . . . . | **E-4 white, E-4 yellow**, Essentialzyme, Mightyzyme |
| Protein of any kind . . . . . . . . . . . . . . . . . . . . . . . | **E-4 yellow**, Detoxzyme, Mightyzyme |
| Sugars, starches . . . . . . . . . . . . . . . . . . . . . . . . . | **E-4 yellow**, Allerzyme, Essentialzyme, Mightyzyme |

## Specific Foods:

| | |
|---|---|
| Eggs, meat, fish . . . . . . . . . . . . . . . . . . . . . . . . . . | **E-4 yellow**, Essentialzyme, Detoxzyme, Mightyzyme |
| Grains, oatmeal, wheat toast . . . . . . . . . . . . . . . . | **E-4 yellow**, Allerzyme, Detoxzyme, Mightyzyme |
| Meat with pasta, salad, cheese . . . . . . . . . . . . . . . | **E-4 yellow**, Essentialzyme, Allerzyme |
| Meat with salad, bread, dessert . . . . . . . . . . . . . . | **E-4 yellow**, Detoxzyme |
| Milk, yogurt, kefir . . . . . . . . . . . . . . . . . . . . . . . | **E-4 white**, Allerzyme, Mightyzyme |
| Pasta, cheese, bread . . . . . . . . . . . . . . . . . . . . . . | **Essentialzyme**, E-4 yellow, Detoxzyme |
| Rice, vegetables, fruit . . . . . . . . . . . . . . . . . . . . | **Allerzyme**, E-4 yellow, Mightyzyme |
| Salad *(no meat)*, vegetables . . . . . . . . . . . . . . . . | **E-4 yellow**, Allerzyme, Detoxzyme, Mightyzyme |
| Sweets *(ice cream, frozen Rice Dream, cookies, cake, candy bars, granola bars, apple pie)* . . . . . . . . . . | **E-4 yellow**, Allerzyme, Detoxzyme |

## Carbohydrate Categories:

| | |
|---|---|
| **Carbohydrates** *(simple: refined sugars, fruits)* . . . . . . . . | **Allerzyme**, Detoxzyme, E-4 yellow, Mightyzyme |
| **Carbohydrates** *(complex: vegetables, fruits, grains, beans, rice, bread, some milk products)* . . . . . . . | **E-4 yellow**, Allerzyme, Essentialzyme, E-4 white |

---

**Bedtime:** . . . . . . . . . . . . . . . . . . . . . . . . . . . . . . . **Detoxzyme:** 5–15 as desired; Mightyzyme: 3–4

sucrase; but they do not produce the enzyme amylase because it is at a very high level in the mother's milk and supplies the baby adequately through nursing. If the infant's body produced amylase and the baby was receiving amylase through the mother's milk, it would simply be too much and would overload the infant's system.

All animal milk contains amylase for the same purpose of nourishing their offspring. Many people choose to give their babies goat milk because it is closest to the chemical structure of human milk and is easy to digest; but, of course, the best source of amylase comes from the mother of the infant.

A vegetable source of amylase is made, but it is never as effective as true amylase. Primary sources of amylase are raw fruits and vegetables, sprouted seeds, raw nuts, whole grains, and legumes.

Children are often given a milk formula that usually comes as a powder to be mixed with water. There are many different kinds of formula powders, and perhaps some are better than others. But the formulas are all still processed and "chemicalized" with ingredients that cause various problems that parents don't link to the synthetic milk. Unfortunately, much of the public is still very uneducated in the field of health and nutrition.

Many parents, unknowingly, mix their powdered formula with chlorinated tap water—**poison!** Then they heat the bottle in the microwave—**deadly!**

Heating the bottle or food in the microwave not only kills the nutrients but also poses a hazardous danger to the child. Anything heated in a microwave oven becomes hot on the inside first and yet feels cool on the outside. So if the bottle temperature feels nice and warm, it is probably extremely hot inside. It's a horrible experience for the unsuspecting child to get lips, mouth, and throat burned from the scalding milk.

Another threat is that the bottle could become so hot that it explodes, burning the person who opens the door and touches the bottle. Microwave cooking? Don't do it! Besides, who wants to eat the plastic chemicals that have leached into the food?

How many babies on formula seem to cry a lot and keep their parents walking the floor all night? The baby can't tell you his stomach hurts and that his body does not want "that milk." How many babies have skin rashes, are not developing normally, or do not seem very happy? There can be any number of causes, but chemicals and processed foods are not healthy for anyone; and for an infant or growing baby, the negative effects can be more dramatic.

Unfortunately, too many children are not being nursed. Perhaps the mother is physically not able to nurse, she has

to get back to work, or she is just too busy. The reason does not matter; the results are the same—an amylase deficiency, which usually starts an allergic condition where the children begin to develop allergies to starches, usually proteins, and certainly sugars.

Unknowingly, parents, trying to help the child, rush to the doctor or the hospital, where more chemicals are put into this little, growing body, only to have more problems created that can become lifelong problems. If we just did things Mother Nature's way to begin with, we would not have to even be talking or writing about all this negative "stuff."

In the last couple of decades, science and technology have made it possible for us to supplement our diet with all kinds of nutritional supplements. With enzyme supplementation, children and adults alike do not have to suffer because of digestive problems and insufficient nutrient absorption.

Protease and amylase are the two most important enzymes that children need. **Ningxia wolfberries** are naturally high in protein but also contain high amounts of carbohydrates and sucrose because of the natural sugars in the different berries.

You can take a protease enzyme first because protein takes a little longer to break down than starches, carbohydrates, and even lipids.

Amylase breaks down the simple sugars that have to be in the bloodstream in order for the body to utilize protein.

By taking protease and amylase together, the body is able to digest the sugar and facilitate the assimilation of protein.

It is extremely important that children who were not nursed, or most likely drank some kind of formula, have enzyme supplementation as well. In order for children to be healthy and free of allergies, they must have amylase.

**MightyZyme**™, a chewable multienzyme for children, is easy for children to ingest. Children who were not nursed and, therefore, did not get the needed amylase should take 1-2 tablets a day until about the age of 10. At about this age, it would be good to have the child start taking the adult enzymes, which have a broader nutritional profile and are a little stronger.

Many children prefer the adult enzymes and begin taking them as early as 7 or 8 years old. However, many children have difficulty swallowing capsules, so they can be opened and emptied into yogurt, kefir, oatmeal, NingXia Red, or anything that will help them "get it down."

Below is a list of a few digestive enzymes, their actions, and the supplements in which they can be found. This will give you an idea of their critical importance in digestion, without which there will be minor and major dysfunction in the body. If any enzymes are missing or are insufficient in quantity, the body cannot perform optimally.

- **Alpha-Galactosidase** digests complex carbohydrate sugars found in vegetables, grains, nuts, seeds, and beans and prevents gas, bloating, cramping, and flatulence produced from fermented sugars (Allerzyme, Detoxzyme).

- **Amylase,** found in saliva, breaks down carbohydrates and simple sugars found in vegetables and fruits (Allerzyme, Essentialzymes-4 (yellow capsule), Detoxzyme, MightyZyme).

- **Bromelain** is the enzyme found in pineapple that promotes digestion in systems lacking sufficient digestive enzymes. It helps break down protein and the digestion of trypsin or pepsin. It can ease heartburn, nausea, and diarrhea (Allerzyme, Detoxzyme, Essentialzyme, Essentialzymes-4 (yellow capsule), MightyZyme).

- **Cellulase** is an enzyme not found in humans. It digests cellulose fiber and aids in malabsorption (Allerzyme, Detoxzyme, MightyZyme).

- **Invertase** hydrolyzes (liquefies) sucrase to glucose and fructose, promotes longer shelf life, and has broad activity range over pH 3.5 – 5.5 (Allerzyme, Detoxzyme).

- **Lactase** digests lactose, the sugar found in milk and dairy products (Allerzyme, Detoxzyme).

- **Lipase** breaks down fats in most dairy products, vegetables, nuts, oils, and meats (Allerzyme, Detoxzyme, Essentialzymes-4 (yellow and white capsules), MightyZyme).

- **Malt Diastase (Maltase)** breaks down disaccharide maltose into glucose or malt sugars (Allerzyme).

- **Pancreatin** is an enzyme composition that combines amylase, lipase, and protease to help break down starches and fats, metabolizes complex proteins, and removes dead and dying tissue (Essentialzymes-4 (white capsule), Essentialzyme).

- **Peptidase** promotes the hydrolysis of peptides into amino acids, which are the break-down product of protein absorbed in the gut (Allerzyme, Essentialzymes-4 (yellow capsule), MightyZyme).

- **Phytase** breaks down indigestible forms of phosphorus found in grains and oil seeds, releasing digestible phosphorus, calcium, and other nutrients (Detoxzyme, Essentialzymes-4 (yellow capsule), MightyZyme).

- **Protease** breaks down proteins in meats, nuts, eggs, and cheese (Allerzyme, Detoxzyme, Essentialzymes-4 (yellow capsule), MightyZyme).

- **Trypsin** is a pancreatic enzyme that hydrolyzes protein, operates at a pH of 7-12, and is used in baby food to predigest protein. It also breaks down the protein membrane surrounding cancer cells to digest and eliminate as toxic waste from the body (Essentialzyme).

**Betaine HCL (hydrochloric acid)** helps to break down fats and proteins and is found in Essentialzyme. It is important to have adequate levels of stomach acid for the absorption of protein, calcium, vitamin B12, and iron. Healthy stomach acid kills disease-causing microbes and parasites that are in the food we eat. Stomach acid decreases with age, which leaves us vulnerable to the attack of unwanted microbial invaders that bring disease and create unhealthy conditions in the body.

**Food enzymes** naturally come from the raw food we eat. However, the enzymes in a particular food are only for that specific food and have little effect on other foods. Some digestive enzymes are present in the food we eat; some are produced by the body itself.

Enzymes are very sensitive to heat, pH, and metal ions and are easily destroyed or rendered inactive. Commercially grown foods that are sprayed with chemicals are also devoid of enzymatic activity.

Enzymes are completely destroyed when cooked, boiled, heated, grilled, and baked, which means that enzymes are also destroyed in all processed food.

This means that we should avoid processed foods whenever possible, as they are devoid of the necessary enzymes for digestion and usually contain enzyme inhibitors to increase shelf life. Inhibitors block the enzymatic process, which stresses the body into an out-of-balance condition.

A lack of digestive enzymes in the food we eat forces the body to overproduce its own digestive enzymes and limits its ability to produce metabolic enzymes, which are also crucial for health and normal metabolism.

This limitation occurs because both digestive enzymes and metabolic enzymes are created from the same enzyme precursors (PST) that are produced in the liver.

The production of these precursors is limited in the human body, so when the digestive system must overproduce digestive enzymes due to an enzymeless diet, it causes a harmful underproduction of metabolic enzymes, which are involved in every process of the human body.

The immune system, circulatory system, liver, kidneys, spleen, pancreas, and even our ability to see, breathe, and think depend upon these metabolic enzymes.

When the diet is supplemented with digestive enzymes that are naturally present in whole, raw, or uncooked foods, two powerful benefits are created:

1. The body is able to extract the maximum nutritional value from the food.

2. The body can reduce its internal production of digestive enzymes, which allows for higher production of metabolic enzymes, crucial for daily metabolism, health, and detoxification.

When we put food into our mouth, amylase, in the saliva, begins to break down complex carbohydrates into simple sugars. While the food is still in our mouth, our stomach begins to produce pepsin, which, like protease, helps digest protein.

When the food enters the small intestine, the pancreas secretes pancreatic juice, which contains three enzymes that break down carbohydrates, fats, and proteins that pass into the small intestine.

The enzymes from the food mix with the nutrients and travel in the blood plasma, which is the watery liquid in which the red blood cells are suspended. This is how the body absorbs and uses the enzymes for their vast number of catalytic activities that aid the body in everything from growth to fighting infection.

**Ancient cultures** prized the natural enzymes in foods—especially meats. They probably did not know how the enzymes worked or what worked, but they knew that something happened when food was allowed to cure because it gave them more strength, endurance, and vitality.

That is why we read about the tradition of curing and why many ancient cultures "aged" or cured meats, which allowed the natural enzymes present in the flesh to predigest it, thereby easing the burden on their own digestive system and conserving their own limited pool of enzymes.

**When meat is predigested**, it places less stress on the body's own enzyme bank. Predigestion also enhances the breakdown of peptide chains and proteins into free-form amino acids, the building blocks of every major body function, from immunity to growth.

Every protein that enters the human body via digestion has to be broken down into amino acids before it can be fully utilized. Meats that are not completely digested contain large protein fragments that cannot benefit the body.

In fact, these protein fragments can cause allergic reactions if the body's antibodies mistake them for foreign microorganisms.

Even worse, these protein fragments can become trapped in the intestines, where they will ferment and promote parasite proliferation and disease.

Cathepsin, a natural enzyme present in all animal flesh, starts the aging or "curing" process to slowly digest the meat. This is not unlike the process that ripens bananas. A green banana starts out high in starch. As it ages or ripens, the natural amylase in the banana converts the starches into sugar. In effect, the amylase is digesting the banana, eventually turning it brown.

As soon as an animal is dead, cathepsin begins to predigest the meat. It begins splitting large peptide protein chains into smaller, more digestible ones. When the meat is eaten after it has been hung for two to three weeks, the digestive system now has a far easier job completing its breakdown and liberating the vital free-form amino acids, the building blocks of all bodily processes.

This explains why when an animal such as a dog or a cow is killed and left to "rot," the vultures can be seen sitting on the fence for days, just waiting until the enzymes have done their job. Then the birds have a feast and eat the dead animal to the bones.

**The history of enzymes** is rather interesting. Long before chemists determined that there was some kind of chemical reaction taking place in organic substances, common people were making soaps, fermenting wine to make vinegar, and baking breads and pastries and many other things through these enzymatic reactions. Early in the 19th century, scientists began to investigate this unusual change in substances.

The well-known French chemist Louis Pasteur (1822-1895) called these catalysts *ferments*. A few years later, the German biochemist Eduard Buchner (1860-1917) isolated these catalysts and determined that they were chemicals, which later were named enzymes.

This began the most revealing scientific journey into the world of enzymatic activity and the discovery of their purpose in all living organisms. It is fascinating to think about how this phenomenon has been observed and used from the beginning of time and was never understood or explained until modern science had the technology to give us that information.

The remarkable physical strength and endurance exhibited by the pioneers and Native Americans may have been due to their consumption of enzyme-rich raw and unprocessed foods, despite the sometimes meager rations of less than 4 ounces of food a day. We have been taught that you must eat to have strength. But there is more to it than that. You must be able to digest what you eat and assimilate the nutrients in order to sustain health and strength.

On the average, only 8 percent of the food we consume is metabolized to sustain normal bodily functions. The remainder passes through undigested. Even worse, only 1 to 2 percent of the nutrient value of the food that we consume reaches our cells.

Many people today suffer with wheat and grain allergies, perhaps caused by the fact that when the grains are cut during the harvest, they are not bundled and left standing in the fields for a few days before threshing, as was the practice many years ago.

The purpose of leaving the bundled grains standing in the field was so that the dew at night or the rain would soften the shell. Then the next day the sun would evaporate the moisture, stimulating the enzymatic process within the kernels. This began the germination to prepare the grains for digestion.

Without the germination process, the enzymes in the kernels remain inactive and, therefore, do not have the ability to digest the grain, which makes it even worse for people who have low sulfur levels and phenolic sensitivity.

Most often, the PST pathway becomes blocked and cannot digest the gluten in the grains. PST (phenol-sulfotransferase) is a Phase II enzyme that detoxifies leftover hormones and a wide variety of toxic molecules such as phenols that are produced in the body and even in the gut by bacteria, yeast, and other fungi as well as food dyes and chemicals.

A four-year study (2000-2004) conducted by the Young Life Research Clinic in Springville, Utah, found that people with gluten intolerance and even celiac disease had no allergic reaction after eating grains grown from nonhybrid seed with no chemical sprays, harvested with horses, and then left to stand in the field for 7-8 days before threshing.

Egyptian hieroglyphics depict the ancient process of grain harvesting. The grain was cut with a scythe, tied into sheaves, and left to stand in the field for several days. It was then loaded into ox carts, hauled to the threshing site, and thrown into a big stone grinder operated by an ox team. The stone rolled around on the grain, cracking the hulls. With the sifting of the wind, the chaff was blown off, and the grain was picked up by slaves and carried in baskets to the storehouse.

Stone-ground, whole wheat bread that is rich in enzymes, vitamin E, and other nutrients is, sadly, a thing of the past. Today, modern technology brings grain to us via a machine called a combine. The combine cuts the grain, almost instantly separates the kernel from the husk, and delivers the grain ready for market on the same day it was cut. It is then further processed to strip out the vitamin E and other oils. Most of it is then bleached, leaving only a tiny fraction of the grain's initial enzymes.

To maximize the enzymes in a food, the fruit of the plant needs to mature on the stalk or stem to the point of "ripening" or readiness to sprout. This is when the enzyme content of the food is the highest. Unfortunately, many fruits, vegetables, and grains are harvested when they are immature and assumed to ripen "in transit," resulting in a food that has a far lower enzyme content.

In order for grains to fully digest in the human body, they must contain a full complement of their natural enzymes. Every food has its own specific enzymes. In order for a grain to have viable enzymes, it must have time to germinate. Once it germinates, its enzymes are released from the bondage of enzyme inhibitors. This is why sprouted grains are so health-giving—the enzyme inhibitors have been deactivated and can no longer counteract the natural enzymes present in the food.

**Early signs of enzyme deficiency** can manifest with many complaints. Heartburn, gas, bloating, fatigue, headaches, stomachaches, diarrhea, constipation, chronic fatigue, yeast infections, nutritional deficiencies, pain, joint stiffness, skin eruptions, psoriasis, eczema, and colon, liver, pancreas, and intestinal problems are just a few.

Many enzymes are not only deficient but are also inactive. At the Young Life Research Clinic in Springville, Utah, D. Gary Young tested over 21 different enzyme products from 21 different manufacturers and did not find a single one that was effective in a clinical environment. The patients were closely monitored, their food intake measured, and their blood and digestive systems regularly tested and analyzed. The clinic staff found that patients were simply not obtaining value from their food because their enzymes were inactive.

## How are enzymes destroyed or rendered inactive?

1. Planting, growing, and cultivating food grown with chemical fertilizers, herbicides, and pesticides will produce a crop basically devoid of enzymes.

2. Heat begins to break down the enzymes at 118° F and are totally destroyed at 129° F.

3. Pasteurization, sterilization, microwaving, chemical processing for freezing, and any other modern processes kill the enzymes or render them inactive.

**Dr. Francis M. Pottenger, Jr.,** conducted an amazing study with over 900 cats. He fed one group of cats raw milk and meat. They lived healthy and disease free. They produced healthy litters generation after generation. He fed another group of cats pasteurized milk and cooked food. After the first generation, this group became lethargic and began to suffer from allergies, infections, and other diseases, including heart, kidney, and lung diseases. Each succeeding generation of cats that ate cooked food suffered more diseases. By the third generation, the cats were unable to reproduce.

Another study showed that after eating cooked food, the human body reacted just as if suffering from an acute illness. Within 30 minutes of eating cooked food, white blood cell counts increased dramatically, as though the body were fighting an infectious disease.

In a very interesting experiment, one group of pigs was fed enzyme-rich raw potatoes, and another group was fed enzyme-deficient cooked potatoes. The pigs eating cooked potatoes gained weight rapidly. The pigs that were eating raw potatoes did not get fat.

**Obesity** is an area of deep concern. Dr. David Galton at the Tufts University School of Medicine tested people weighing 230-240 pounds. He found that almost all of them were lacking lipase enzymes in their fatty tissues. Lipase, found abundantly in raw foods, is a fat-splitting enzyme that aids the body in digestion. Lipase activity breaks down and dissolves fat throughout the body. Without lipase, fats are kept and stored in tissues. We see this manifest around the waistline, hips, and thighs.

It is astounding to see the obesity levels of children and adults not only in America but around the world, which have reached epidemic proportions. Childhood obesity has more than tripled in the past 30 years. About 35 percent of children and teens between the ages of 2 and 19 are overweight, and almost 17 percent are obese.

According to the latest data from The State of Obesity (Robert Wood Johnson Foundation) released September 2015, 34.9 percent of adults aged 20 and over in the United States were overweight, and 2/3 of U.S. adults were overweight or obese (68.6 percent). According to the latest data from the World Health Organization, over 50 percent of both men and women in the European Region were overweight, and roughly 23 percent of women and 20 percent of men were obese.

These statistics are frightening when you look at the rapid increase in numbers. No wonder physical and mental problems as well as diseases are becoming more prominent in children and young adults. Clinics and hospitals are full of people suffering from problems due to being overweight. It is certainly possible that this overweight problem is due partly to chronic enzyme and nutrient deficiencies.

Our food is processed and devoid of nutrients and enzymes, so seeing such deterioration of our health is not surprising. Even our fresh fruits and vegetables are grown in polluted water and air and sprayed with a myriad of chemicals for pesticide and herbicide control.

There are even chemicals to induce growth and produce a perceived beautiful quality. It is hard to know the difference and impossible to see the contamination and food devoid of nutrients when we walk through a well-organized grocery store and see such beautiful produce and products on the shelves.

**We have a better chance** of buying nutritious food when we buy organic food rather than nonorganic food, but even then we don't know all the conditions under which the food is grown. The food may not be directly sprayed, but that does not change the quality of air and water. Government regulations for the organic food industry are allowing "less dangerous" chemicals to be used in organic farming, but we want to avoid all chemicals whenever possible.

Besides that, we do not know what is done to the harvest after it leaves the farm. Preserving freshness is critical to the brokers and retailers, and how long is the food kept in storage before it goes on the shelf for the buyer? These are all things to consider.

**Can we live without enzymes?** The evidence is voluminous. Our bodies would cease to function without them. It would be ideal if we could consciously eat raw, unprocessed foods rich in enzymes in order to maintain an ample reserve in the body to maintain optimal health and effectively prevent and fight disease.

Unfortunately, most of our food supply does not contain the quantity of enzymes needed for proper digestion and conversion. That is why enzymes are added to so many commercial products. When you read product labels, you will be amazed to see such phrases as "Enzyme enriched, enzymes added, enzymes for better digestion," etc. We eat too much processed and devitalized food. So what do we do? How do we solve this problem?

**Enzyme supplementation** is the modern-day solution. Science has come a long way in its ability to manufacture high quality enzymes that are absorbable and usable. Medical research shows that enzyme supplements can help fight illness, reduce or block the development of life-threatening diseases, and slow the effects of aging. There are enzymes specific to a particular need, and there are enzymes that provide overall enzymatic needs.

**The best time to ingest protein** is in the early morning or by mid-afternoon. You must have glucose in the blood to absorb protein. Because your body operates on glucose and protein primarily, it is better to put that in your body in the morning than at night when there is little or no activity. Protein at night is more difficult for the body to digest because it just sits in the stomach while the body is working to detoxify and cleanse.

**Water is the activator of your enzymes**. To activate your vegetable enzymes, you must have minerals and water. Water activates and creates enzyme saturation to the food that you have ingested. Water carries up to 18 percent oxygen, providing greater enzymatic action, so by drinking water with your meal, your food will digest better, giving you better nutrient availability, much more so than if you do not drink water with your meal.

To begin your day with breakfast, take 2 Essentialzymes-4 (yellow capsules) and 1 Essentialzyme, which help to supply both metabolic and digestive enzymes and at the same time target the carbohydrates and proteins that you've ingested for your morning meal.

**There is an old belief system** that says "Never drink with a meal." This is both correct and incorrect at the same time. All of the Young Living enzyme supplements contain raw, plant-extracted enzymes that require two things to activate them—minerals and water.

However, if you drink milk with your meal, thus saturating your food with lactose, you will need a high lactose enzyme for digestion that can create fermentation along with the other foods that you have eaten, so you will want to take 1-2 Essentialzymes-4 (white capsules). If you drink apple juice, orange juice, or other juices high in sugar with your meal, you will need a high sucrase enzyme to digest the simple carbohydrates (sugars) and proteins in the juices, so you will want to take 1-2 Essentialzymes-4 (yellow capsules).

**Essential oils** are an ingenious addition to enzyme supplementation. They support enzyme conversion with many added benefits specific to any particular oil. Many oils such as Tarragon, Ginger, Peppermint, Juniper, Rosemary, Lemongrass, Anise Seed, Fennel, and Patchouli are natural enzyme promoters in the body. They help increase the oxygen for the uptake of ATP, adenosine triphosphate, one of the most important (if not the most important) molecule that exists in the body.

ATP provides the chemical energy of fuel within the cells for all processes of human metabolism. Each enzyme supplement contains various oils for the promotion of natural enzyme activity. Enzymes and essential oils work in a synergistic way to promote a healthier digestive system.

**Enzymes** can be taken in many different quantities for many different needs. Different enzyme supplements may be combined or added for specific digestive functions. Most people are enzyme deficient, which is very detrimental to the healthy state of the body. Optimal

# Carbohydrates, Proteins, and Sugars

**This partial list** of complex and simple carbohydrates, proteins, and sugars might help you determine which supplement you want to take for different foods.

## Carbohydrates (complex)
**Essentialzyme™ and Essentialzymes-4™ (yellow capsule):**

**Vegetables:** spinach, lettuce, zucchini, asparagus, artichokes, cabbage, yams, carrots, cucumbers, potatoes, radishes, broccoli, cauliflower, onions, peas, celery, sprouts, dill pickles, eggplant

**Fruits:** grapefruit, apples, prunes, pears, plums, strawberries, oranges

**Grains:** barley, einkorn, spelt, buckwheat, whole wheat, oat bran, wild rice, brown rice, multigrain breads, lentils, granola

**Beans:** pinto, soy, garbanzo, kidney, navy

**Milk products:** skim milk, soy or almond milk, low-fat yogurt

## Carbohydrates (Simple)
**Essentialzyme™ and Essentialzymes-4™ (white capsule):**

Table sugar, corn syrup, fruit juice, cake, honey, milk, yogurt, jam, chocolate, white-flour pasta, white-flour bread, most packaged cereals

## Proteins
**Essentialzyme™ and Essentialzymes-4™ (yellow capsule):**

Meat such as beef, chicken, turkey, bison, elk, venison, fish, nuts, nut butters (almonds, peanuts, etc.)

digestion and metabolism is dependent on the presence and activation of enzymes.

It is not likely that you will do something wrong by taking too many or combining too many enzymes if you are just using common sense. The body will tell you by how you feel and by the increase in energy that you might experience.

Pay attention to an increase in clarity of thought, awareness, ability to respond faster, more energy to get things done, and not feeling tired or feeling less tired at the end of the day. These are all indicators that things are working better in the body. Minerals, vitamins, enzymes, and water must all be present and work together for a balanced process of nutrient conversion, absorption, and utilization.

**Allerzyme®** is a complex blend of enzymes used to help the body utilize nutrients, combat allergies, expel waste, and prevent gas and bloating. As children reach the age of 10, it is a good time for them to begin taking adult enzymes, which are more complete. Allerzyme (1-2 capsules daily) is a good companion for children because it specifically contains amylase and protease, along with a full complex of enzymes, such as bromelain to help prevent or alleviate symptoms of allergies, aiding in better digestive function.

**Detoxzyme®** contains amylase and bee pollen rich in amino acids, which are important for healthy body function in the promotion of enzyme development and performance. Detoxzyme is a vegetarian-based enzyme used to help digest milk products, meats, and nuts and to eliminate toxic chemicals and waste.

Detoxzyme can be taken more heavily for a detoxification program, anywhere from 4-6 capsules morning and midday and 6-10 in the evening. Your body can utilize a lot of Detoxzyme. You will know when it is enough if you start to have diarrhea.

The essential oil of Cumin has been recognized as a very powerful detoxifying agent. Combined with Anise Seed and Fennel, it creates nice stimulation of the hydrochloric acid and the pepsin that are naturally occurring in the gastrointestinal tract for more effective digestion and cleansing.

Before going to bed, take anywhere from 2 to 10 Detoxzyme, because during the night your body is going through metabolic processes of digestion and assimilation. The liver is detoxifying and "dumping" the waste into the colon to be released in the morning.

**Essentialzyme™** is a multienzyme complex originally formulated to combat degenerative disease. It digests the protein shell around cancer cells so that it can digest and remove the dead cells. It is also used to promote balanced digestion and nutrient assimilation.

It takes a combination of enzymes, minerals, proteins, lipase, and fat for building hormones. Carrot powder is very nourishing, as carrots are one of the highest enzyme foods that you can eat.

Periodically a carrot juice fast can be very beneficial for 1 to 2 days to build a ready supply of natural enzymes, giving the body an extra boost in detoxifying and cleansing. Alfalfa sprout powder contains 21 minerals, which are critical for the activation of enzymes.

Start your morning with Essentialzyme. Adults: 3-4 before eating and 3-4 after eating. More capsules can be taken if needed. Children: 1 before eating and 1 after eating or both together. It is best to drink water or herbal tea. Drinking smoothies or juices complicates and compromises the ability to digest efficiently.

**Essentialzymes-4™ (yellow capsule)** is a powerful plant enzyme complex and is very specific for the digestion of proteins in meats, eggs, cheese, and other foods high in proteins. It also assists the body in the digestion of sugars and starches found in vegetables and fruits. The essential oils of Anise Seed, Peppermint, and Rosemary are specific for stimulating the production of natural protease in the body.

When eating meals with meat such as beef, chicken, turkey, bison, etc., taking 1 Essentialzymes-4 (yellow capsule) before dinner and 1-2 Allerzyme after dinner works well in aiding digestion to prevent bloating and in helping to alleviate that heavy, lethargic feeling after eating so much.

When overcoming allergies, Essentialzymes-4 (yellow capsule) gives added benefit in breaking down carbohydrates. Take 1-2 Allerzyme for greater support in fighting allergies. If you are still eating proteins at lunchtime but adding carbohydrates like a salad combined with bread and dessert, take 1-2 Essentialzymes-4 (yellow capsules).

If you have a food allergy, a metabolic problem from gastrointestinal surgery, disease in the gastrointestinal tract, or are amylase deficient, take 1-2 Essentialzymes-4 (yellow capsules) with 3-4 Essentialzyme to meet digestive needs.

**Essentialzymes-4™ (white capsule)** contains powerful, fat-digesting enzymes for dairy products, meats, and vegetables and promotes greater nutrient absorption. It is specific for digesting the lipids or fats in foods like avocados, olives, vegetable oils, and meats. Undigested lipids can contribute to gallstones by plugging the pathway out of the gallbladder for the bile and by also causing congestion and plugging the liver, causing increased fat deposits.

This is an important supplement in fat reduction for overweight conditions. Take 1-2 capsules 2 or 3 times a day or as desired. It also contains barley grass that is a complex green that is high in minerals needed for enzyme activation.

**MightyZyme™** is formulated especially for children, providing a full spectrum of nutrients and enzymes combined with Ningxia wolfberry. Because MightyZymes are chewable and crunchy, children often think that they are a treat and are happy to eat them. They are a great snack to put in school lunches. Interestingly enough, many adults prefer MightyZyme over other supplements and eat several daily.

Although enzyme supplementation is a blessing to our modern society, not many people really know the importance of enzymes in our diet. Their function is not well understood and is often times confusing. However, more is being written about enzymes, and more people are beginning to add enzyme supplements to their diet. Many people have different ideas about how they should be used or taken, so perhaps the following suggestions will be helpful.

1. Some people open the capsules and sprinkle the enzymes onto their food, but not very hot food, to get the digestive process started.

2. Because it takes a while for a tablet or capsule to dissolve in your stomach, it is a good idea to take your enzyme tablets and capsules about 30 minutes before eating.

3. Drink plenty of water with your meal, because enzymes need water for activation.

4. Chew your food well so that the digestive enzyme cellulose can be released from the fiber; otherwise, you could experience a stomachache with gas and bloating.

5. Eat fresh fruits and vegetables to increase your enzyme intake.

6. Be careful not to eat too many foods that contain enzyme inhibitors, which neutralize some of the enzymes that your body produces. Be moderate in eating such foods as raw seeds, nuts, beans, grains, and especially peanuts and raw wheat germ. Enzyme inhibitors are found in potatoes, concentrated in the potato eyes. Lesser amounts of inhibitors are present in peas, beans, lentils, and egg whites.

7. Traditionally, seeds, nuts, beans, and grains were soaked or partially sprouted before they were eaten. These foods contain many enzyme inhibitors such as phytic acid that can tax the digestive system if eaten excessively.

   Phytic acid is important because it prevents premature germination and stores nutrients for plant growth. However, it combines with minerals such as iron, copper, calcium, magnesium, and zinc in the intestinal tract and interferes with nutrient absorption.

   Soaking these types of foods in an acid medium such as lemon juice or whey or even in water neutralizes the enzyme inhibitors and can make the vitamin and mineral content more available.

8. You can also destroy the inhibitors by cooking, but then that destroys the enzymes. The better way is by soaking, rinsing, germinating, and sprouting. This destroys the inhibitors while increasing enzyme production.

9. Another way to neutralize these inhibitors is to take extra enzymes when eating ungerminated or unsprouted seeds and nuts.

10. Fermentation also neutralizes damaging chemicals found in grains and beans. Fermentation adds many beneficial micro-organisms to foods, making them more digestible, which increases the flora in the intestinal tracts.

    A diet in unfermented whole grains can lead to mineral deficiencies and bone loss. The easiest way to cause fermentation is to put the beans, seeds, and grains in water, add whey or yogurt, and let them stand for seven or eight hours. A local health food store should carry whey or yogurt powder. Beans are even better if left in water for twelve hours.

11. Kefir is a special culture used in milk, which promotes fermentation and produces many enzymes in the process.

12. Small amounts of salt can also work as an enzyme inhibitor, so be careful. Besides the fact that salt is not the best choice to use in your diet because of the numerous health problems it can cause, it would be best to just eliminate it from your diet. Salt certainly has a place in the balance of diet, but today, white table salt is overused and becomes an enemy to the body.

**The choice is yours.** When you come to understand the critical importance of enzymes and the life-giving role they perform in our bodies, you have certainly discovered many possible explanations for health problems that you or those around you may have.

You can also see how you might prevent future health problems from arising. Knowledge gives hope, especially when products are available that can increase your potential for vibrant health and longevity.

For those who are already on a path of a healthier lifestyle, it is critical to spread this information to others who are searching for answers and to help those who do not know what questions to ask. We need to educate, strengthen, uplift people everywhere, and protect our children and the babies yet to be born.

Building Blocks of Health | Chapter 18

# Minerals: We Can't Live Without Them

**A mineral is a solid, chemical substance** that is naturally formed through geological processes. All minerals come from the ground and make their way into our bodies through the foods we eat that grow in the ground and the foods we eat that come from the animals that live off of the land. Fruits, vegetables, meats, nuts, grains, poultry, and dairy products provide a rich source of minerals that our bodies need to live and function properly in conjunction with vitamins and other nutrients such as enzymes.

The difference between vitamins and minerals is that vitamins contain carbon, classifying them as organic substances. Minerals do not contain carbon and are therefore classified as inorganic.

There are two categories of minerals: major, or large minerals, and trace minerals. The difference between them is determined by how much the body needs. The body needs a daily minimum of 100 milligrams of major minerals and less than 100 milligrams daily of trace minerals.

Minerals are a major part of every cell in all forms of life. Enzymes need minerals to build strong, healthy organisms, whether they are human, animal, or plant. All foods have minerals, but some have more than others. Plants take the minerals from the ground; we eat the plants and take the minerals from them, use the ones we need, and eliminate the ones we don't need.

We really don't give any thought to it until something starts to go wrong in our bodies. Then we start looking and asking for answers. Becoming educated about how our body works and what it needs is a key to staying healthy. But too often we wait until we have problems before we start to educate ourselves.

Unfortunately, our soil is devitalized of many nutrients and is contaminated with chemicals from the pollution in the air and water and from man-made products that are sprayed to supposedly protect our crops and help them grow. Perhaps in days gone by, we could get the minerals and vitamins we needed from rich top soil, but foods grown commercially today don't produce the quality crops that can provide the nutrients we need.

We would all do well to grow our own organic gardens, but few have the ability to do so, and often those who have the ground available are too busy. "It's just too much work." So what do we do? With a little education and awareness, we can start to improve our diet with fresh, organic fruits and vegetables and buy foods that specifically say they are grown and produced in a natural environment. This is especially true of eggs and meat products.

**Commercial food companies** have been promoting the vitamin and mineral content of their products for quite some time. We see "Fortified with vitamins and minerals" on many labels. Perhaps this list below will give you an idea of the importance of having good mineral balance in your body.

## Major Minerals

**Calcium** builds strong bones and teeth and is needed for muscle growth. It helps to normalize blood clotting and may help to prevent bone loss and osteoporosis. It is most effective in combination with vitamins A, C, D, iron, magnesium, manganese, and phosphorus. Food sources: milk products such as yogurt and cheese, whole grains, unrefined cereals, green vegetables, sardines, salmon, soybeans, and peanuts.

**Phosphorus** maintains healthy bones and teeth and is found in every cell to help make energy. Food sources: fish, poultry, beef, eggs, milk products, almonds, lentils, peanuts, pumpkin seeds, and whole wheat.

**Magnesium** helps muscles and nerves, keeps the heart rhythm smooth, and keeps bones strong. Food sources: green vegetables, legumes, nuts, seeds, whole wheat, and milk products.

**Sodium** ions regulate blood and body fluids. Sodium also maintains proper acid-base balance in the transmission of nerve impulses, smooth heart function, and good blood pressure (See Chloride). Natural food sources: barley, beets and beet greens, carrot juice, celery, kelp, some cheeses, milk from goats and cows, and buttermilk.

**Potassium** supports the muscular and nervous systems and maintains electrolyte balance between blood and body tissues (See Chloride). Food sources: prunes, prune juice, bamboo shoots, chard, sweet potato (must be cooked with whole skin), beet greens, orange juice, white beans, dates, yogurt, raisins, clams, tomato puree, blackstrap molasses, halibut, yellow tuna, Pacific rockfish, Pacific cod, winter squash, soybeans, kidney beans, lentils, plantains, apricots, prunes, and bananas.

**Sulfur** is found in all cells and especially in cartilage and keratin. It is important for healthy hair, skin, and nails and helps to maintain oxygen balance for healthy brain function. Food sources: garlic, onions, cabbage, cauliflower, asparagus, dried beans, nuts, chives, fish, and eggs.

**Chloride** is an electrolyte along with potassium and sodium that keeps the body fluids in balance. The cells need potassium on the inside and sodium on the outside.

Seventh Edition | **Essential Oils Desk Reference** | 353

Sodium and potassium have a positive electrical charge and constantly move into the cells and then out of the cells to maintain balance. Chloride has a negative charge, which balances with the sodium and potassium. This constant movement allows these minerals to carry nutrients into the cells and waste out of the cells.

Chloride helps alleviate fluid retention and keeps sodium balanced to maintain good blood pH and healthy kidney function. Chloride also helps with digestion in the production of hydrochloric acid. Food sources: seaweed, sea salt, rye, tomatoes, lettuce, celery, and olives.

## Trace Minerals

**Chromium** improves the efficiency of insulin in metabolizing carbohydrates and helps maintain normal blood pressure. Food sources: lean meats, whole grains, liver, cheese, eggs, and brewer's yeast.

**Copper** strengthens the metabolic processes in the body in combination with amino acids and vitamins. It fortifies enzymatic reactions in the utilization of iron and benefits connective tissue, hair, eyes, aging, and energy production. It supports the thyroid, smooths the heart rhythm, promotes wound healing, and prevents the buildup of cholesterol. Food sources: meat, liver, seafood, beans, whole grains, soy flour, wheat bran, almonds, avocados, barley, garlic, nuts, oats, molasses, beets, and lentils.

**Iodine** makes two thyroid hormones: triiodothyronine and thyroxine, which control and regulate basal metabolic rate, which determines how fast and efficiently the body burns calories. It is very important for proper cell metabolism. Thyroid hormones help control the mental development of children and their overall growth. Iodine is an effective antiseptic for cleaning wounds and healing the skin. Food sources: kelp (sea vegetable), vegetables grown in iodine-rich soil, yogurt, cow's milk, eggs (whole; cooked or boiled), strawberries, mozzarella cheese, and often fish and shellfish.

**Iron** is necessary for the production of hemoglobin, the primary component of red blood cells that carries oxygen to every cell of the body and removes carbon dioxide. Iron cannot work without calcium and copper to function properly and is necessary for the metabolism of B vitamins. Food sources: liver, beef, baked beans, white beans, soy beans, lima beans, black-eyed peas, fish, chicken, oatmeal, rye bread, whole wheat bread, prune juice, prunes, dried apricots, raisins, plums, spinach, peas, asparagus, Brewer's yeast, kelp, squash, molasses, wheat bran, pumpkin seeds, squash seeds, and sunflower seeds.

**Manganese**, although only needed in small amounts, is an antioxidant that fights free radicals. Manganese-activated enzymes help metabolize cholesterol, carbohydrates, and amino acids. It also helps to heal wounds and helps bones and cartilage to form properly. Manganese aids the body in the use of vitamin B1, biotin, and vitamin C. Food sources: leafy vegetables, whole grains, pecans, almonds, peanuts, brown rice, whole wheat bread, pinto beans, lima beans, navy beans, spinach, sweet potatoes, avocados, eggs, pineapple, green tea, and black tea.

**Molybdenum** is found in most plants and animal tissue. It is essential to the enzymatic action of protein synthesis and the use of iron in the body. Food sources: meats, whole grains, buckwheat, barley, wheat germ, legumes, lima beans, sunflower seeds, and dark green leafy vegetables.

**Selenium** is an important antioxidant that protects against the formation of free radical cells and works well with vitamin E. It is needed by the white blood cells to fight microorganisms and is important to the T-cells of the immune system to produce cytokines, which work as messengers between the cells. It appears that low selenium causes a risk of viral infections. It may be no coincidence that flu viruses and viruses like Bird Flu originate in a large area of China with selenium-deficient soil. Research has shown that selenium prevents and fights against cancer. Food sources: bran, broccoli, onions, tomatoes, tuna, and wheat germ.

**Zinc** is one of the most important minerals used by the body; it helps in the production of over 100 enzymes your body needs. It supports growth, builds immunity, maintains your sense of smell and taste, helps to heal wounds, and is critical for DNA syntheses. Food sources: beef, lamb, crabmeat, turkey, chicken, lobster, clams, salmon, milk, cheese, yeast, beans, whole grain cereals, brown rice, whole wheat bread, potatoes, yogurt, and pumpkin seeds.

**Minerals are extremely important,** but few people know why. The body needs iron to make hemoglobin found in red blood cells. Calcium is necessary for kidney, muscle, and nerve function. The thyroid cannot work without iodine. The thyroid controls many functions in the body, and one of them is to produce energy. How often do we hear, "If you don't have enough energy, your thyroid must be low"? Manganese, selenium, and zinc work as antioxidants and help in the healing of wounds, the growth of the skeletal system, and the protection of cell membranes. Chromium helps keep the arteries clear.

The information about minerals is voluminous, and to

Building Blocks of Health | Chapter 18

really understand their purpose and how they work takes a lot of time for study and research. But there is no doubt about their importance in maintaining a well-functioning body. Because the nutrients in so much of our food are depleted, how do our bodies get the nutrients that are needed to achieve and maintain optimal health? In the past, doctors and scientists have said that supplementation was not necessary because we could get all the nutrients we needed if we ate properly.

Today, it is a different story. Even the Food and Drug Administration (FDA) is regulating the food industry and requiring that certain vitamins and minerals be added to commercial foods. More and more, people are turning to supplementation.

**Most liquid minerals** don't taste very good. It's easy to swallow capsules or tablets, but liquid minerals are different. Some taste so awful that no one wants to consume them. However, there is one that isn't bad tasting at all—Mineral Essence. As a liquid, it is much easier and quicker for the body to assimilate and is more efficient.

**Mineral Essence**™ is an organic, liquid ionic mineral complex with more than 60 very fine ionic minerals that assimilate much easier than other mineral compounds that are taken from dirt, rocks, or other sources. Mineral Essence is uniquely formulated with essential oils to enhance its bioavailability, supplying the body with the most efficient and best-balanced mineral formula that we have found at the present time.

Minerals are essential for activating certain enzymes for digestion and metabolic function, and the minerals found in Mineral Essence are very specific for the promotion of a healthy digestive tract, reducing the risk of candida and food allergens.

Some people like to drink it in cold juice such as NingXia Red wolfberry juice or some other combination that they have discovered that helps with the taste. However, the benefits far outweigh any resistance to the taste. When one thinks of sustaining life without dysfunction or disease, Mineral Essence is certainly worth putting to the test.

## Water: The Purity of Life

Nothing is more refreshing when you are hot and thirsty than a drink of clear, cold, spring water. However, water is not only refreshing, but it is absolutely essential to life. Most of us probably don't think of water as one of the body's building blocks, but water is the second most critical substance we need for maintaining life. Without water, life ceases to exist. Water is the activator for all body functions, for growth, development, strength, and vitality. The only substance more important to the body than water is oxygen.

The human body on average is over 70 percent water. Certain vital organs and systems have an even higher concentration: the brain is over 75 percent, the blood is over 80 percent, and the liver is amazingly made up of 96 percent water. To a large degree, we are what we drink.

Water is crucial for our body's self-cleansing system. We are certainly aware of the body's normal elimination processes, but the body also eliminates waste through exhalation and perspiration, both of which require water. Our kidneys cannot cleanse efficiently if our system does not have enough water to carry the waste away.

Water ($H_2O$) plays a role in nearly every chemical reaction in the body. Aside from aiding in digestion and absorption of food, water regulates body temperature and blood circulation, carries nutrients to cells, and removes toxins and other wastes. Water also protects joints, tissues, and organs, including the spinal cord, from shock and damage.

The ideal amount of water to consume is half your body weight in ounces per day. That means if you weigh 160 pounds, you should drink 80 ounces of water or about ten, 8-ounce glasses per day. Lack of water or a state of dehydration will cause many maladies such as hypertension, asthma, allergies, migraine headaches, dizziness, and many more.

The amount of water we drink greatly affects our energy level. Over 80 percent of our population suffers from lack of energy because they don't drink enough water. Science has proven that if the average person drops as little as 5 percent in body fluids, he or she will suffer a 25 to 30 percent loss of energy. A 15 percent drop in body fluids will cause death.

The liver has to have water to metabolize fat into useable energy. Therefore, drinking pure water will help metabolize and shed stored fat, resulting in more energy and less fat.

All day long we lose water from our bodies. When we breathe, we lose moisture to the air every time we exhale— as much as two cups a day. We also lose water through evaporation from the surface of our skin, even without rigorous exercise; and, of course, we also pass water in our urine. A healthy adult can lose 8 to 10 cups of water a day. With exercise, the amount greatly increases. Many drinks

Seventh Edition | **Essential Oils Desk Reference** | 355

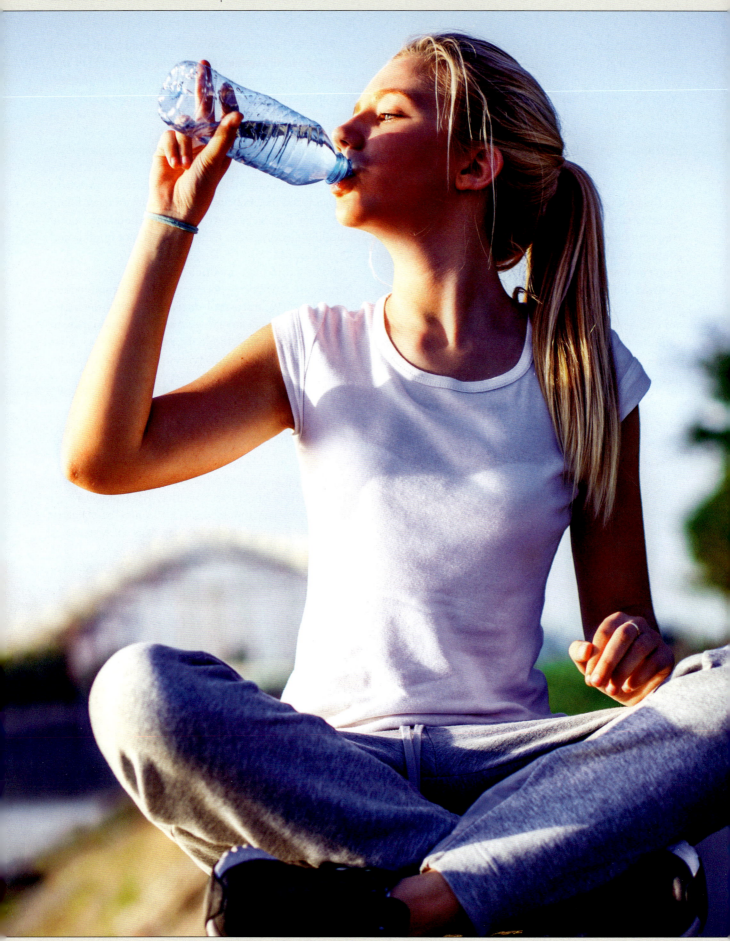

like soda, coffee, and tea contain caffeine, which has a diuretic effect, leading to increased loss of fluids through frequent urination.

The function of every cell in our body is controlled by electrical signals sent through our nervous system from the brain. Our nerves, in reality, are an elaborate system of tiny waterways. If the fluid inside our nerves thickens due to dehydration or is contaminated with synthetic chemicals or toxic heavy metals like lead, the vital signals can get distorted.

Many experts now believe that the distortion of these signals may be the root cause of many degenerative diseases and neurological illnesses, including Attention Deficit Disorder, Chronic Fatigue Syndrome, anxiety, depression, and even Alzheimer's disease.

Because water is such a major factor in brain and nervous system functions, its purity is probably the most basic component for longevity. Proper digestion and nutrient absorption depend on a healthy intake of water. We must drink plenty of pure water for our bodies to convert and assimilate the nutrients from our food and the supplements we take.

The amount of pure water we drink determines how efficiently our body is able to detoxify by excreting the body's waste. Water is the body's primary means of flushing out toxins, the key to disease prevention. Every day we are exposed to hundreds of harmful substances. Our air, food, and everything we touch contain traces of harmful chemicals. Unfortunately, we can't keep toxins from getting into our body, but we can help our body get rid of them by drinking plenty of pure water. The more pure water we drink, the more we allow our body to detoxify and purify itself.

Because water is so crucial to life, it is crucial that we drink pure water. Constantly drinking water that is contaminated will eventually lead to a miserable state of health and early death.

Finding pure drinking water is becoming a challenge. Our increasingly polluted world has made it necessary for the Environmental Protection Agency to set water standards. The EPA screens for the presence of suspended solids, oil, grease, fecal coliform bacteria, chemicals, and heavy metals. Unfortunately, 65 percent of the major source of pollution does not come from industrial sites, which can be regulated, but from storm-water runoff.

Rainfall coming in contact with pollutants from agricultural and industrial operations absorbs these chemicals and transports them into lakes and rivers. Today, about 47 percent of water pollution comes from actual industrial sites.

Excessive and uncontrolled use of chemical fertilizers and pesticides promote contaminated agricultural runoff. This not only pollutes the surface drains, but the water trickling down to lower layers of soil also causes a severe contamination of the natural aquifer.

The World Health Organization (WHO) reports that 25-30 percent of all hospital admissions are connected to water-borne bacterial and parasitic conditions, and 60 percent of infant deaths are caused by water infections.

The long-term effects on human health of pesticides and other pollutants include colon and bladder cancer, miscarriages, birth defects, deformation of bones, and sterility.

Contamination of fresh water with radionuclides, which can result from mining, testing, disposing, and manufacturing of radioactive material and transportation accidents, has led to increased incidences of cancer, developmental abnormalities, and death.

Cesspools of stagnant, dirty water, both in rural and urban areas, account for a large number of deaths caused by potentially fatal diseases like cholera, malaria, dysentery, and typhoid.

Nitrate concentration in water above 45 mg/l makes it unfit for drinking by infants. The nitrates are reduced in the body to nitrites and cause a serious blood condition called the "Blue Baby Syndrome." Higher concentrations of nitrates cause gastric cancer. Untreated and highly toxic industrial sewage is also used for irrigation near major cities, which contaminates crops and consequently affects consumers.

According to EPA reports, 40 million Americans are exposed to levels of lead in water that exceed the EPA-proposed maximum contaminant allowances. Even at low levels, lead in water causes reduced birth weight, premature births, delayed mental development, and impaired mental abilities. In 2014 between 6,000 and 12,000 children in Flint, Michigan, were exposed to high levels of lead in their drinking water.

Using information gathered from the EPA, the National Resources Defense Council (NRDC) reports that more than 45 million Americans drink tap water polluted with fecal matter, pesticides, toxic chemicals, radiation, and lead.

The tap water in some cities has parasites in it, so it is not good drinking water. Tap water contains chlorine, which kills bacteria but is very bad for you to drink. In the book *Natural Cures,* Kevin Trudeau says, "All tap water is poisonous. All tap water is loaded with chlorine and chlorine byproducts. Chlorine scars your arteries and, along with hydrogenated oil and homogenized dairy products, causes heart disease. Most tap water also has fluoride, which is one of the most poisonous and disease-causing agents [that] you can put in your body. Do not drink or use tap water except for washing your floor." Tap water is not pure drinking water.

The purpose of water is not nutrition. The purpose of water is to transport things. It brings the nutrition in and takes the waste out.

Paul Bragg, ND, PhD, says in *The Shocking Truth About Water*, "The greatest damage done by inorganic minerals—plus waxy cholesterol and salt—is to the small arteries and other blood vessels of the brain. Hardening of the arteries and calcification of the blood vessels starts on the day you start taking inorganic chemicals and minerals from tap water into our bodies."

Municipal or city water should be avoided if possible, and that includes public swimming pools as well. Most municipal waters have a high concentration of aluminum due to the use of aluminum hydroxide for water treatment. Moreover, the addition of chlorine results in the creation of cancer-causing chemicals when dissolved; organic solids are chemically altered by chlorination. While there is a trend toward replacing chlorination with peroxide treatment of water, it will be decades before peroxide is adopted as a standard.

## Chlorine

Have you noticed when you walk near an enclosed swimming pool area of a hotel that you have to hold your breath to block the horrible smell of chlorine? Chlorine is one of the most reactive and toxic elements known to man. It is very damaging to the thyroid, which is a major, regulating organ in the body. When it malfunctions, major health issues arise. When put in the public water supply as a disinfectant, chlorine creates disinfection byproducts (DBP) that can cause cancer, birth defects, and spontaneous abortions. This information makes "chlorinated sugar" (Splenda®) not quite so desirable.

Besides being used in the water supply, chlorine is also chemically bonded in the manufacture of numerous industrial chemicals. Many toxic herbicides, fungicides, and insecticides are created by attaching one or more chlorine molecules to a carbon skeleton. Once ingested or inhaled, chlorinated chemicals penetrate the fat cells and become trapped.

Some of the most common and toxic of these chemicals include a quartet of chlorinated carcinogenic chemicals known as trihalomethanes (THMs): chloroform, bromoform, bromodichloromethane, and chlorobromomethane. These trihalomethanes are created when chlorine reacts with naturally occurring organic matter in raw water.

THMs are very volatile and can mix with both air and water. From the air they can be inhaled during bathing as well as consumed with potable water. Showering, washing dishes, and flushing a toilet can also contaminate the air with trihalomethanes.

Once inhaled or ingested, THMs accumulate in the fat cells—the same way dioxins do. Once trapped inside the body, they chemically bind with and damage DNA.

A California Department of Health study surveyed 5,144 pregnant women to determine the effects of THM in the drinking water (Waller, et al., 1998). They measured levels of THM from water tests obtained from public utility records and matched these against the study group.

They found that pregnant women who consumed more than five glasses of water a day containing more than 75 ppb (parts per billion) had double the risk of spontaneous abortion. Women who drank less water or who drank water with lower levels of THM had substantially lower risk of miscarriage. Women who drank filtered water also had significantly lower risk of miscarriage.

Researchers at the University of North Carolina at Chapel Hill also examined the link between THM and miscarriages in populations living throughout central North Carolina (Savitz, et al., 1995). They found that women who suffered the highest exposure to THM in their drinking water tripled the risk of miscarriage.

Another study conducted by the U.S. Department of Health and Human Services examined the effect of THM in the water supply of 75 towns throughout the state of New Jersey (Bove, et al., 1995). When scientists compared levels of THMs to the frequency of birth defects, they found that women who consumed water exceeding 80 ppb THMs had triple the risk of giving birth to infants with neural tube defects. The authors suggested that one of the reasons for this may be due to the fact that vitamin B12 may be disrupted in the body due to chloroform, a common THM.

Another statewide study in New Jersey also linked THMs in drinking water to a doubled risk of neural tube defects (Klotz, et al., 1998).

An even larger epidemiological study by the National Institute of Public Health in Norway surveyed the effects of chlorinated water on 141,077 infants born in Norway between 1993 and 1995 (Magnus, et al., 1999). Researchers found that the higher the chlorine content of the water and the higher the organic matter in the water, the higher the risk for birth defects, including cardiac defects, respiratory tract defects, and urinary tract defects.

Murray S. Malcolm, MD, a public health physician in New Zealand, spearheaded a countrywide study that examined the role of THMs in triggering birth defects and cancer. He concluded, "A quarter of all bladder, colon, rectal cancers, and birth defects may be preventable by reducing disinfection byproducts (i.e., THMs) exposure" (Malcolm, et al., 1999; Wellington School of Medicine, New Zealand).

## A Solution

There are many ways of avoiding chlorine and the many other toxic chemicals found in water, but it isn't necessarily simple. It is most important that we avoid these chemicals in any way possible. The cost of the physical problems that contaminated water can bring can be astronomical.

Bottled water is probably one of the easiest ways to avoid contamination, but can you be certain that this water is free of chemicals and safe to drink? Regardless of cost, the bottled water you buy may simply be tap water put through a filtration process. Naturally, there are many reliable water bottling companies, but regulation in this industry is vague, and so we have to be aware all the time of the water we choose to drink.

Buying drinking water does not protect consumers from inhaling vapors. Reports from the EPA indicate that entities such as mining companies and electrical power plants release 7.8 billion pounds of toxic substances per year onto the land, into the water, and into the air, and the amount is increasing. The NRDC reports that over 940,000 Americans are sickened by contaminated tap water annually. In addition, the council reports that contaminated tap water kills 900 people each year.

Many people today are investing in a water purifier for home and business alike. There are many and varied types of purifiers. Some attach under the sink to filter the water as it comes through the tap. Other filtration systems work for the entire house and filter the water as it comes into the house from the outside. You have to weigh the cost with the perceived benefit and make the best decision you can.

Many choose to drink distilled water to be sure of getting pure water, although there has always been controversy over drinking purified versus distilled water, which almost becomes a personal preference. You can distill the water or let it stand unsealed, which allows the chlorine to evaporate over time.

Naturally, adding an essential oil will always be of great benefit to help maintain the purification of the water. Essential oils like Lemon, Clove, Orange, Cinnamon, Peppermint, etc., purify your water and taste great as well. Distilled water washes out the system. With the help of essential oils in distilled water, the body can excrete petroleum residues, metals, inorganic minerals, and other toxins.

One drop per glass is generally enough. Put the oil in a glass or container first and then fill the container with water. Since oil does not mix with water, putting the oil in first will help disperse it through the water.

Several drops of oil can be put in the end of the carbon filter of a water purification system so that when the water leaves the filter, it carries oil molecules with it as it goes into the water system of your house. This can drop nitrate levels by up to 3,000 ppm.

The inhalation of trihalomethanes in a vapor form that occurs with hot water while showering is more toxic than drinking chlorinated water. A good showerhead filter is important to be able to shower and bathe in chlorine-free water.

While carbon filters are good for removing chlorine from water, the best water distillers have preflash or preboiling chambers to flash off volatile gases such as chlorine and petroleum products. The steam should rise at least 15 inches to balance the pH and fall 15 inches to oxygenate again.

One very popular water purification system is the ion exchange used with "hard" water or water with dissolved minerals. Water is passed through a filter, exchanging charged particles (ions) in the water for charged particles in the filter. Most units use salt, with sodium and chloride ions exchanging for the contaminated ions in the water. Since the minerals are replaced with salt, at least one cold water tap needs to be left out of the system so that drinking water is not loaded with sodium.

## Types of Water Filtration Cartridges for Home Systems

Many types of filters may be purchased for home use, but only three of them are discussed below.

**A dual-gradient filter** has one layer wrapped around the other to provide finer filtration than is found in most other filters. In the second layer, the water flows through a high-powered carbon briquette filter system, not available through retail channels. The dual-gradient cartridge has three times the dirt-holding capacity of similarly sized cartridges. It removes sediment such as dirt, sand, grit, rust, etc., from the water to extend the life of the charcoal filters. In addition, the inner layers reduce the levels of fine particles.

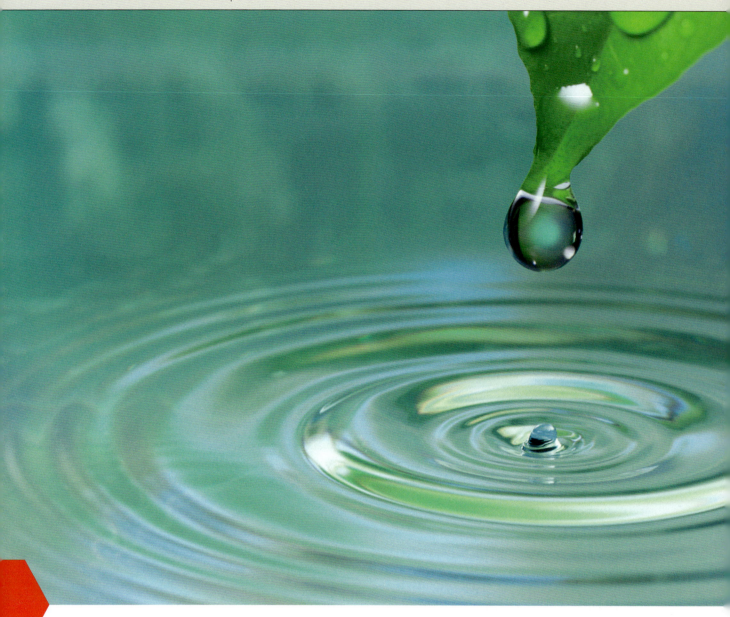

**The carbon briquette filter** system contains a superior carbon-briquette cartridge of bonded powdered charcoal. The powdered consistency of the briquette allows for increased surface contact that results in maximum absorption of chlorine. The 0.5 micron post filter greatly reduces bacteria, including giardia and cryptosporidium. This carbon filter removes trihalomethanes, which might otherwise be consumed, absorbed through the skin, or inhaled during a shower. It also reduces lead and removes pesticides, odors, and objectionable tastes.

**A UV filtration unit** is sold separately. It kills all types of viruses, bacteria, and fungi and is often combined with other types of carbon filters to add to the purification of the water and your protection.

**Water is life itself,** and pure water is critical, no matter what the cost. With anything less than pure water, the body cannot perform its metabolic functions in an efficient, healthy way. We need to study and become knowledgeable about the overwhelming damage that comes from drinking contaminated water and the undeniable benefits and health that come from drinking pure water. Think of your family, your friends, and all the children who are not aware of this crucial aspect in our lives. Make them aware so that the best choices are made to attain a vibrant life.

# Chapter 19
## Longevity and Vitality—Special Features

## Living Longer with Essential Oils

Essential oils and aromatics were some of the most highly prized natural remedies of the ancient world. References to cassia, clove, frankincense, myrrh, cinnamon, and rosemary appear in many historical manuscripts, including the Old and New Testaments, the writings of Hippocrates, Avicenna, Egyptian hieroglyphics, and other ancient writings, pictographs, and legends.

Intriguing new research offers a fascinating glimpse into the far-reaching potential of essential oils like thyme to reverse or slow the aging process by acting as powerful antioxidants that protect tissues and organs from damaging stress and deterioration.

Other essential oils such as clove and lemon have been shown to not only act as powerful antioxidants but also to protect cellular DNA from damage and to act as potent antiseptics with broad-spectrum, germ-killing properties.

Frankincense, myrrh, and balsam have been used since the beginning of mankind and even anciently were known for their spiritual and physical healing properties.

Essential oils have their own specific chemical constituents that target particular body functions for maintaining good health and emotional well-being and fighting physical and mental dysfunction as well as chronic and life-threatening diseases.

## Aging: The Power of Essential Oils

There is much controversy and many theories over the causes of aging and premature death. Some researchers believe that declining levels of hormones from the pituitary and hypothalamus are the culprits. Others point an accusing finger at the crosslinking of collagen, a key protein of the soft tissues, which constitutes a third of all protein in the body. Still others blame the buildup of lipofuscin, a brownish pigment that accumulates inside the cells, particularly nerve and heart muscle cells.[1]

However, the oxidative, stress-free theory of aging is the most persuasive and substantiated. One scientific thought is that aging is caused by cumulative, oxidative stress to the cell walls, receptors, and DNA. Rogue electrons that are generated from normal metabolic and immune functions attack proteins and disrupt DNA, eventually overloading the natural repair abilities of the body, which sometimes leads to disease and death.[2,3,4]

Many researchers have focused on damage to the DNA as the cause of aging. The DNA is a nucleic acid that contains the blueprint for genetic instructions or cellular activity used in the growth and function of all living organisms. Few scientists have understood how devastating free radical damage can be to fats—especially the unstable polyunsaturated fatty acids (PUFAs) that form the phospholipid membranes of almost every cell in the body. When these fatty membranes are attacked by free radicals, ion transport, and hormone receptors are disrupted.[5] As cell membranes become less fluid, they lose their ability to function normally. This can hasten the onset of tissue and organ damage and lead to premature death.

One of the most easy-to-understand examples of the detrimental effects of cell membrane deterioration occurs in the blood vessel walls. As the blood vessels lose their flexibility, the risk of hypertension (high blood pressure) increases, as does the incidence of arteriosclerosis.

Free radical damage seems to escalate with age because antioxidant protection declines as we grow older. Free radical scavengers such as superoxide dismutase (SOD) and glutathione peroxidase show a steady decline along with other antioxidants. This means that the older we become, the less efficient the body is in neutralizing

Seventh Edition | **Essential Oils Desk Reference** | 361

## Essential Oils vs. Fatty Oils

Fatty oils are very different from essential oils. Fatty oils, such as cottonseed, almond, olive, corn, sunflower, and canola oil, are usually pressed from a seed or fruit. They are greasy in texture and have little odor, being simple mixtures of several different fatty acids (i.e., capric, stearic, and oleic).

**CAPRIC FATTY ACID**
*(from coconut oil)*

Methyl end — Acid end

In contrast, essential oils are usually steam distilled from leaves, flowers, roots, and bark. They have strong odors and are not greasy. Because many are lighter than water, they float and tend to evaporate very easily. Essential oils are complex mosaics of hundreds of aromatic molecules (i.e., terpenes, sesquiterpenes, and phenols) that usually have a ring-like structure.

**THYMOL**
*(from thyme ess. oil)*

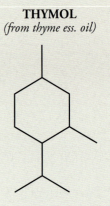

---

free radicals and combating the oxidative damage that gradually weakens and eventually destroys key organs.

Levels of polyunsaturated fats such as DHA (decosahexaenoic acid) are also crucial for healthy brain and eye function. DHA occurs in unusually high concentrations in the cerebral cortex—the most advanced part of the brain structure, where logic and reasoning take place. When DHA becomes oxidized and loses its double bonds because of free radical attacks, brain and cognitive function can deteriorate. This can lead to memory loss, dementia, and even death. By protecting fats like DHA from free radical attack, hydrolysis, or oxidation, brain health can be significantly improved.[6,7,8,9]

The root of the problem is that DHA and other long-chain PUFAs are very unstable and are vulnerable to chemical alteration and oxidation. This means that the antioxidant function of the body must work overtime to protect the PUFAs in order to sustain health. An even greater problem is that with age, the liver slows down the production of PUFAs and thus becomes less and less able to replace the dwindling supply of PUFAs needed to sustain the brain, tissues, and other organs.[10]

Therefore, the longevity of the organism is strongly linked to preserving the integrity of the polyunsaturated fats that comprise cells, nerves, and other tissues. Preventing the degradation of these fats from free radical damage can forestall the signs of accelerated aging.

### Research: Antioxidative Properties of Essential Oils

In the late 1980s, Dr. Radwan Farag of the biochemistry department of the University of Cairo was among the first to show in vitro how selected essential oils were able to significantly slow the rancidity or oxidation of fatty oils such as cottonseed oil. He dosed samples of cottonseed oil with 200 ppm of thyme oil (55.7 percent thymol and 36 percent p-cymene) and 400 ppm of clove oil (85.3 percent eugenol). After comparing the essential oil-treated samples with untreated control samples, he found that both thyme and clove oils showed significant protection against rancidity to the cottonseed oil. Thyme oil reduced rancidity by 20 percent, while clove oil reduced the rancidity by almost 30 percent.[11] A second study by Dr. Farag and his colleagues showed that essential oils such as thyme (*Thymus vulgaris*), clove (*Syzygium aromaticum*), rosemary (*Rosmarinus officinalis*), and sage (*Salvia officinalis*) arrested the oxidation of linoleic acid, a polyunsaturated omega-6 fatty acid.[12]

In addition, Dr. Farag demonstrated the safety of these essential oils in vivo. When he added thyme and clove oils to rat feed rations at up to six times the minimum

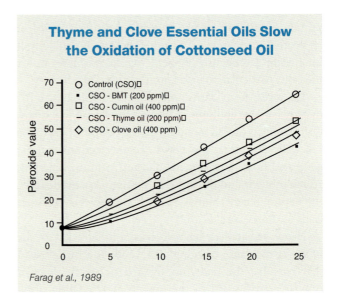

**Thyme and Clove Essential Oils Slow the Oxidation of Cottonseed Oil**

*Farag et al., 1989*

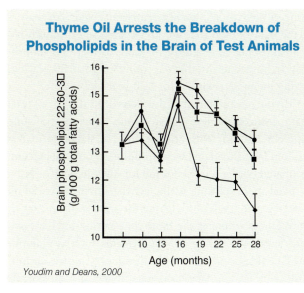
*Youdim and Deans, 2000*

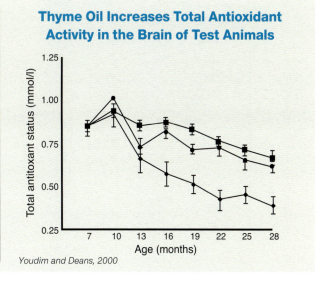
*Youdim and Deans, 2000*

concentration needed to stall fat oxidation, none of the rats studied suffered any negative side effects. Essential oil-fed rats exhibited no difference in protein, cholesterol, and liver enzyme levels (SGPT, SGOT) when compared with a control group.[13]

**Protecting Fats and Phospholipids in Animals**

Almost a decade after Farag's groundbreaking research, another series of more intensive in vivo studies was begun at the Scottish Agricultural College in the United Kingdom and the Semmelweis University of Medicine in Hungary. In these clinical trials, researchers found that daily lifelong feeding of thyme and clove oils to laboratory animals preserved key antioxidant levels in the liver, kidneys, heart, and brain. Even more importantly, essential oils arrested the oxidation and destruction of long-chain PUFAs throughout the organism.

One of the first studies to document these remarkable antioxidant effects was conducted at the Semmelweis University of Medicine in 1993. Researchers fed different groups of mice with daily doses of 0.72 mg of essential oils, including thyme (*Thymus vulgaris*), clove (*Syzygium aromaticum*), nutmeg (*Myristica fragrans*), and black pepper (*Piper nigrum*). Groups of younger mice, 6 months old, were treated for five weeks, while groups of 22-month-old mice were treated for 21 weeks. Following treatment, the livers of the animals were examined for levels of C20 and C22 polyunsaturated fatty acids, which declines substantially during the animal's lifetime.

The results were phenomenal. According to the researchers, ". . . dietary administration of the volatile oils to the aging mice had a marked effect on fatty acid distribution by virtually restoring the proportions of the polyunsaturated fatty acids within the phospholipids to the levels observed in young mice."

Another randomized, controlled animal study at Semmelweis University in 1987 showed that these same essential oils—thyme, clove, nutmeg, and pepper—restored DHA in the eyes to much younger levels. As a long-chain polyunsaturated fatty acid (PUFA) that is very fragile and easily oxidized, DHA is absolutely crucial for normal eye health. Declining levels of DHA have been directly linked to heightened risk of age-related macular degeneration, the leading cause of blindness in old age.[14,15]

In this case, dietary supplementation of just 3.9 mg per day of essential oils to laboratory animals over a 17-month period was sufficient to markedly slow DHA loss in their eyes.

## Brain Function: Essential Oils to the Rescue

The brain is another organ where DHA is essential to health. Karesh Youdim and his colleagues at the Scottish Agricultural College tested the ability of essential oils to preserve DHA levels in the brain of 100 animal subjects. Feeding them a daily dose (42.5 mg/K of body weight) of thyme oil (48 percent thymol) over the course of their lifetime (about 28 months), the researchers achieved stunning results: Thyme oil dramatically slowed age-related DHA and PUFA degeneration in the brain. In other words, the essential oil of thyme was able to partially prevent brain

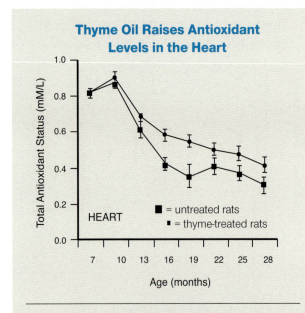

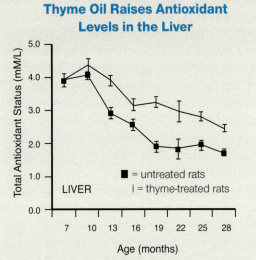

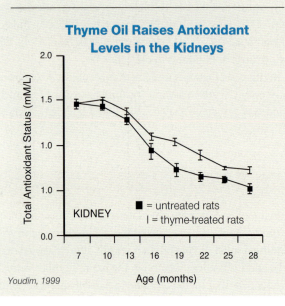

Youdim, 1999

aging through protection of essential fatty acids. An analysis of the data showed that the DHA levels in 28-month-old animals' brains were almost the same as that of 7-month-olds. In human terms, this was equivalent to an 80-year-old having the brain chemistry of a 20-year-old![16]

Thyme oil supplements also slowed the decline of total brain antioxidant levels that occurs with age. Lifelong supplementation with thyme oil in laboratory rats resulted in antioxidant levels dropping by only 29 percent, compared with a 45 percent fall for untreated animals.

Even more startling is the fact that thyme essential oil also preserved levels of PUFAs in the animals' hearts, livers, and kidneys, while at the same time raising total antioxidant levels—including key antioxidants such as glutathione peroxidase and superoxide dismutase. This was accomplished by feeding laboratory rats thyme oil supplements (42.5 mg/K of body weight) daily throughout their lives.[17]

## Clove Oil: A Powerful Antioxidant

Clove oil also has potent antioxidant-boosting properties. Animal studies conducted at LKT Laboratories in Minneapolis, Minnesota, found that five compounds within clove oil significantly increased levels of GST (glutathione S-transferase), one of the most important detoxifying enzymes in the human body that is critical for neutralizing potential cancer-causing chemicals.

Just 60 mg of each of the five compounds of b-caryophyllene, b-caryophyllene oxide (sesquiterpenoids), a-humulene and a-humulene epoxide I (terpenoids), and eugenol fed to rats over the course of six days (3 doses of 20 mg each) resulted in a doubling of GST activity in the liver and a quadrupling of GST level in the small bowel mucosa. The authors concluded that ". . . these sesquiterpenes

### How Five Constituents in Clove Oil Raise Glutathione Levels

| Compound | Liver Levels of GST | Small Bowel Levels of GST |
|---|---|---|
| Control | 0.74 | 0.25 |
| Compound 1 | 1.92 | 0.75 |
| Compound 2 | 2.13 | 1.20 |
| Compound 3 | 1.47 | 0.63 |
| Compound 4 | 1.54 | 0.81 |
| Compound 5 | 1.26 | 0.59 |

Zheng et al., 1992.

show promise as potential anti-carcinogenic agents."[18] Other research has shown that clove essential oil exhibits pronounced antitumoral and DNA-protectant effects.[19,20]

Essential oils may do more than just raise antioxidant levels and block damage to PUFAs. They may also protect cellular DNA from damage that can eventually lead to mutations and subsequent tumor growth. In a 1986 study, Yo-kota, et al., found that a diet including 5 percent eugenol, the main chemical constituent in clove oil, helped protect test animals against the mutagenic and cancer-causing effects of the chemical benzoapyrene.[21] Yokota, et al., completed five more eugenol and rat liver studies, finding in 2013 that dietary eugenol increased xenobiotic-metabolizing enzymes that are known to protect against cancer.[22]

# Fluoride: Now Classified as a Neurotoxin

**The global leader in clinical neurology, *The Lancet Neurology* journal, reported that fluoride has been added to the list of known neurotoxins such as arsenic, lead, and mercury.**

Two internationally known researchers, Philippe Grandjean, MD, PhD, Department of Environmental Health at Harvard and Philip J. Landrigan, MD, MSc, of the Department of Environmental Medicine, at the University of Southern Denmark, warned of "a pandemic of developmental neurotoxicity" in their 2014 study.[23]

Fluoride is a cumulative toxin found in drinking water and in dental products like toothpaste and mouthwash. Overuse leads to enamel-damaging fluorosis and a host of more serious health problems.

### Is Anyone Listening?

When the evidence that fluoride is more harmful than helpful is so overwhelming, we have to ask why it is still being added to the drinking water of 170 million Americans.

British newspaper *The London Observer* stated one possible answer succinctly: "If health scares about fluoride were to be recognised in the courts, the litigation, especially in the U.S., could be expected to run for decades. Consequently, scientists have been inhibited from publicising any adverse findings."[24]

Below is a prime example of how research showing fluoride dangers is first ignored, then falsely refuted, and finally, suppressed.

### Fluoride and Increased Risk of Bone Cancer for Boys

Evidence that fluoride in tap water can cause bone cancer (osteosarcoma) was first reported in 1990. Osteosarcoma is a deadly form of cancer that is usually fatal within three years. An animal study by the National Toxicology Program showed strong evidence of a link between fluoridated water and bone cancer in male rats. Several human studies followed this that also showed a link between fluoride and osteosarcoma.[25,26]

Harvard dental professor Dr. Chester Douglass stepped up with a small study (too small to be conclusive) that did not find a link between fluoridation and osteosarcoma. In 1992 Douglass submitted a proposal to the National Institutes of Health (NIH) for a more comprehensive study of this issue. He received $1.3 million for his study. During this time Douglass continually voiced concern that worry over osteosarcoma could have consequences for fluoridation health policies. No concern was expressed for cancer risks for young boys because of fluoridation.

Although Douglass' research did find a statistical link between fluoride and osteosarcoma in boys (but not in girls), he continually summarized his work as showing a *lower* risk for cancer in fluoridated areas.

One of his doctoral students, Elise Bassin, studied the relationship between fluoridation, growth spurts, and osteosarcoma. Her thesis, completed in 2001 but not published until 2006, stated: "Among males, exposure to fluoride at or above the target level was associated with an increased risk of developing osteosarcoma. The association was most apparent between ages 5-10, with a peak at six to eight years of age."[27]

WebMD wrote about Bassin's research and thought it ironic that Douglass, who led her PhD dissertation committee, warned that her results were based on a subset of exposed people. Bassin specifically looked at the subgroup of people most likely to be affected by fluoridation: children. Her analysis was limited to those who got bone cancer by the age of 20.

WebMD Health writer Daniel J. DeNoon explained why Dr. Bassin looked at this subset: "[It's] because most cases of osteosarcoma occur either during the teen years or after middle age. Fluoride collects in the bones, and it's particularly likely to accumulate in the bones during periods of rapid bone growth. So Bassin looked at fluoride exposures during childhood for 103 under-20 osteosarcoma patients and compared them with 215 matched people without bone cancer. Her study took into account how much fluoride was in the water in the communities where children actually lived and the history of municipal, well water, or bottled water use."[28]

It is of interest that if one goes by Douglass' warning to factor in all age groups (including adults), the overall risk for osteosarcoma will likely be diminished statistically. However, the fact remains that fluoride *is* a risk factor for bone cancer in young boys.

While Douglass approved Bassin's thesis and quoted from it, he did not mention that her findings were exactly opposite of his conclusion. The Fluoride Action Network [FAN] wrote that in March 2004, "In his final report to the NIH, Douglass again summarized the results of his first study as showing no significant association between fluoridation and osteosarcoma. As with his report to the NRC [National Research Council], Douglass referenced Bassin's thesis without mentioning the fact that her findings contradicted his summary."[29]

The Environmental Working Group brought an ethics charge against Douglass in 2005. After a 13-month study, The Harvard Medical School and School of Dental Medicine circled the wagons and concluded, "Douglass did not intentionally omit, misrepresent, or suppress research findings . . ."[30]

In the face of such outright erroneous reports of his findings, we have to wonder if Douglass has conflicts of interest. The FAN article on the Harvard investigation notes:

> . . . in addition to being a professor of Dentistry . . . Douglass serves as Editor of COLGATE's 'Oral Care Report.' Colgate is one of the world's largest manufacturers of fluoride toothpaste. If fluoride were found to cause osteosarcoma in children, the potential for legal litigation against Colgate would exist not only in the U.S. but also in many other countries well.
>
> Colgate, however, is not Douglass' only possible conflict of interest. Douglass, who has been a longtime proponent of fluoridation, is the Chairman of the Board of Trustees for the Delta Dental Foundation of Massachusetts, an organization that—along with its other state affiliates—actively promotes and funds water fluoridation programs in recent years."[31]

The question raised by FAN is a fair one: Is it reasonable to believe that these associations with pro-fluoride organizations make it more difficult for Douglass to report a linkage between fluoridation and childhood bone cancer? The late Dr. John Colquhoun posed the question: "How many cavities would have to be saved to justify the death of one young man from osteosarcoma?"[32]

## Fluoride Fluorosis Warning

In November 2010 the U.S. Department of Health and Human Services (HHS) released a data brief reporting that 41 percent of adolescents ages 12 to 15 had dental fluorosis from ingesting too much fluoride.[33] Fluorosis leaves white markings or spots on tooth enamel. The spots may be prominent enough to be disfiguring. The more severe forms of fluorosis actually damage tooth enamel. Besides being in drinking water, fluoride is found in dental products like toothpaste and mouth rinses, prescription fluoride supplements, and fluoride applied by dental professionals.

### Dental Fluorosis Rates in the United States
1950 through 2004

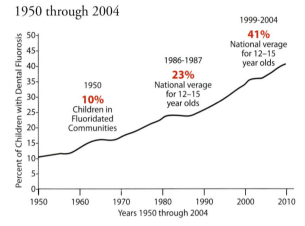

Beltran ED, et al. (2010( Prevalance and Severity of Dental Fluorosis in the United States, 199–2004. NCHS Data Brief No. 53. Figure 3.

National Research Council. (1993). Health Eddects of Ingested Fluoride. National Academy Press, Washington DC. p. 4-5.

HHS and the EPA (Environmental Protection Agency) announced on January 7, 2011, that HHS' proposed recommendation of 0.7 milligrams of fluoride per liter of water replace the current recommended range of 0.7 to 1.2 milligrams.[34]

Bill Osmunson, DDS and president of Washington Action for Safe Water, said, "Fluorosis is the first clinical sign of fluoride poisoning. Excess fluoride does not affect only teeth. It also harms bones, kidneys, thyroid, brains, and other organs. Fluoride is not a nutrient and the body has no need for any of it."[35]

## Fluoride and Endocrine Function

The U.S. National Research Council (NRC) reported that "several lines of information indicate an effect of fluoride exposure on thyroid function."[36]

How many people know that until the 1970s, European doctors prescribed fluoride to suppress thyroid function in patients with hyperthyroidism (overactive thyroid)? It was an effective medication in reducing thyroid activity at as low a dose as 2 mg a day. People with fluoridated water may be ingesting doses (up to 6.6 mg a day) that were once used by doctors to reduce thyroid activity. Could this have anything to do with an increase of hypothyroidism (underactive thyroid) in the U.S.?

The NRC concluded its review of fluoride in drinking water with this statement, ". . . evidence of several types indicates that fluoride affects normal endocrine function or response; the effects of the fluoride-induced changes vary in degree and kind in different individuals. Fluoride is therefore an endocrine disrupter in the broad sense of altering normal endocrine function or response." The report cited possible mechanisms such as inhibition of hormone secretion "by effects on things such as calcium balance and inhibition of peripheral enzymes that are necessary for activation of the normal hormone."[37]

A 2010 Chinese study on the effects of fluoride on human hypothalamus-hypophysis-testis axis hormones showed that fluoride can cause reproductive endocrine-disturbing effects, more severe in males than in females.[38]

## Fluoride and Bone Fractures

Fluoride is an equal-opportunity hydrofluoric-acid salt. It can be counted on to increase hip fractures in the elderly[39] (this study is from the *Journal of the American Medical Society*) and increased bone fractures in children with fluorosis.[40]

Remember that 41 percent of 12 to 15 year olds and 36 percent of 16 to 19 year olds have fluorosis. That means 1 out of every 3 American teenagers not only has mottled teeth but is at increased risk for bone fractures.

Dental fluorosis now affecting American youth has more dangers than a marred smile and increased risk for bone fractures. A 2011 study of fluorosis served up several vital pieces of information. First, chronic fluoride poisoning is called fluorosis. Second, researchers in Ankara, Turkey, investigated the effects of fluorosis on the cardiovascular system in children.

The conclusion is so technical that clarification from a health professional is added in brackets:

Endemic fluorosis is a risk factor for decrease in calcium and FT4 levels [FT4 is free thyroxine, the major form of thyroid hormone in the blood] increase in sodium levels and QT prolongation [prolonged QTc Syndrome is a cause of sudden death that occurs due to a cardiac arrhythmia]. These findings might be related with some cardiovascular system dysfunctions such as arrhythmias [irregular heartbeat] or syncope [temporary loss of consciousness described as fainting or passing out]. *Subjects with fluorosis should be monitored in terms of long QT and QTc intervals* [41] [Emphasis added] (Karademir S, 2011).

When an EKG is given, five peaks are tracked on a graph: P Q R S T. Electrical activity between the Q peak and the T peak is called the QT interval. A "long QT" is a genetic disorder that can lead to early death.

In a study in *Circulation*, the journal of the American Heart Association, the authors investigated 328 families with this disorder and found that by age 12 years, 50 percent of the young family members with long QT syndrome, "had experienced at least one syncopal [fainting] episode or death" (Moss AJ, 1991). Fluorosis is a risk factor for triggering either arrhythmia or sudden death in those (69 percent of whom are female) with this genetic disorder.

Recently, the EPA rejected a petition to change the source of fluoride in U.S. drinking water. William Hirzy, a chemistry researcher at American University in Washington, D.C., who worked at the EPA for 27 years, and colleagues presented research showing that fluorosilic acid is often contaminated with arsenic. Fluorosilic acid is a by-product of phosphate fertilizer manufacturing and is the fluoride form added to drinking water. Hirzy, et al., found that pharmaceutical-grade sodium fluoride contains about 100 times less arsenic than fluorosilic acid and thus carries a 100-fold lower risk of cancer. The EPA upheld Dr. Hirzy's findings on arsenic in August of 2013 but said the cost of switching to the purer form of fluoride is prohibitive.

On the website http://cof-cof.ca/hydrofluorosilicic-acid-origins/, Dr. Hirzy made this statement: "If this stuff (hydrofluorosilicic acid) gets out into the air, it's a pollutant; if it gets into the river, it's a pollutant; if it gets into the lake, it's a pollutant; but if it goes right straight into your drinking water system, it's not a pollutant. That's amazing."

Perhaps it's time to ask the FDA why Americans are forced to drink such a harmful chemical and to ask dentists why they continue to promote fluoride toothpastes.

**Essential Oils Desk Reference** | Seventh Edition

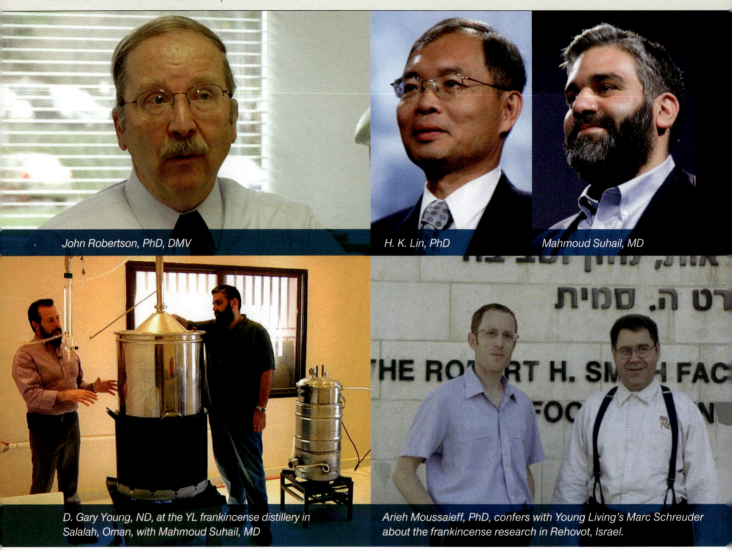

John Robertson, PhD, DMV

H. K. Lin, PhD

Mahmoud Suhail, MD

D. Gary Young, ND, at the YL frankincense distillery in Salalah, Oman, with Mahmoud Suhail, MD

Arieh Moussaieff, PhD, confers with Young Living's Marc Schreuder about the frankincense research in Rehovot, Israel.

## Frankincense: A Gift to the World

Without question, Young Living Essential Oils is the world leader in frankincense because D. Gary Young has made more than 15 trips to the Middle East to study the *Boswellia* species to find the best varieties possible to bring to market. Through his company, he has invested in trained personnel, equipment, and research to back up his own personal studies.

### Four Questions to Ask About Frankincense

Be sure to ask the following four questions before you buy frankincense essential oil:

1. Have company owners and officials actually traveled to the Middle East to meet the people and find verifiable frankincense sources?
2. Does the company own the sophisticated, technical equipment needed to test for purity? Does it employ scientists with the credentials (a PhD in chemistry) and training to use this technology correctly?
3. Does the company invest in a library of innovative, peer-reviewed research?
4. Does the company meet and work with leading botanists and cutting-edge scientists in the field of frankincense research?

Only one essential oil company can answer "yes" to every single question: Young Living Essential Oils, the World Leader in Essential Oils®.

Right now, four frankincense researchers who are conducting exciting frankincense research are H. K. Lin, PhD; Mahmoud Suhail, MD; Arieh Moussaieff, PhD; and John Robertson, PhD. The first two scientists spoke at the 2010, 2011, and 2012 Young Living conventions; and Young Living's Marc Schreuder met with the third scientist, Arieh Moussaieff.

Longevity and Vitality - Special Features | Chapter 19

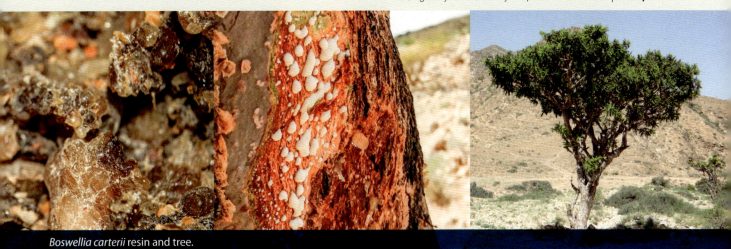

Boswellia carterii resin and tree.

John Robertson, PhD, who conducted studies on equine melanoma and will be working with researchers at Wake Forest University on human cancer studies, has been interviewed by Young Living at Virginia Tech, and has discussed collaborating with D. Gary Young.

## Cutting Edge Technology and Research

Young Living doesn't just talk about GC-MS technology; the company has purchased this expensive equipment and as of March 2016 owns 4 GC/MS, 7 GC/FID, and 1 GC/IRMS instruments. Gary Young was trained in the art of chromatography in France and at the Young Living Ecuador laboratory by the world's leading GC-MS expert, Dr. Hervé Casabianca, Director of Natural Product Research at CNRS labs in France. Young Living Global Ambassador Cole Woolley, PhD, is also a GC-MS and a Solid-Phase Microextraction (SPME) expert. This technology is extremely fast, with detection limits that can reach parts per trillion (ppt) levels for some compounds.

You will see references to frankincense studies throughout this section. Young Living has copies of all pertinent research in the field of frankincense research—not just the abstracts, but the full studies.

## Three Different Frankincense Species

One source[42] lists 42 different varieties of frankincense (*Boswellia* species). We want to share information on three of four of the most well-known species: *Boswellia carterii* from East Africa (Somalia and Yemen), *Boswellia sacra* from Oman, and *Boswellia frereana* from Somalia. The other important frankincense species is *Boswellia serrata* from India.

## *Boswellia carterii:* Frankincense

"The oleo-gum resin known as frankincense or olibanum has been obtained since ancient times from several species of Boswellia in the family Burseraceae."[43] A 2009 study discusses where the four most important frankincense species are found. "There are numerous species and varieties of frankincense trees, including *Boswellia serrata* in India, *Boswellia carterii* in East Africa [Somalia and Yemen] and China [Frankincense is believed to have been cultivated at one time in China, although the current status is unsure.], *Boswellia frereana* in Somalia, and *Boswellia sacra* in Arabia, each producing a slightly different type of resin."[44]

*Boswellia carterii* is among the most studied frankincense species. The 2009 study mentioned above with significant scientific impact is titled "Frankincense oil derived from *Boswellia carteri* induces tumor cell specific cytotoxicity." [In the scientific literature *Boswellia carterii* is also listed as *B. carteri*.] One of the study's authors, H. K. Lin, PhD, of the University of Oklahoma, has spoken at many Young Living Grand Conventions.

Dr. Lin's groundbreaking study notes: "Frankincense oil containing 1,200 mg/ml frankincense gum resin was obtained from Young Living Essential Oils (Lehi, UT)." You can confirm this by checking the second page of the study at: www.ncbi.nlm.nih.gov/pmc/articles/PMC2664784/pdf/1472-6882-9-6.pdf. Other essential oil companies falsely make this claim, but the study clearly states that the frankincense oil was obtained from Young Living.

The study states: "This is the first report demonstrating that frankincense oil can discriminate between bladder cancer cells and normal urothelial cells in a cell culture system and utilizing microarray technology to identify potential biological pathways activated by frankincense oil."[45]

Seventh Edition | Essential Oils Desk Reference | 369

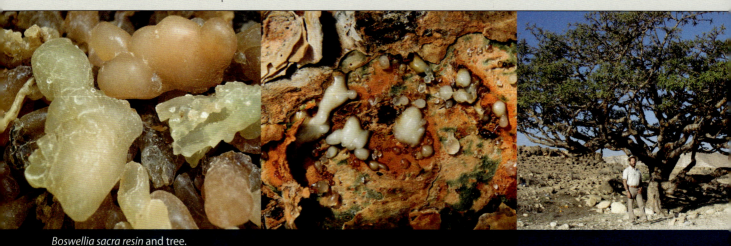

*Boswellia sacra* resin and tree.

Researchers in Tokyo, Japan, discovered that the extract of *Boswellia carterii* contains 15 triterpene acids, including 7 beta-boswellic acids, as well as the physiologically active triterpenes incensole and its acetate, and that this extract "exhibited potent cytotoxic activities against three human neuroblastoma cells."[46]

Another of the current 59 *Boswellia carteri/carterii* studies found in a search of PubMed (September 2016), the National Library of Medicine, explains how a purified mixture of boswellic acids from *B. carteri* resin exhibits not only anti-inflammatory properties but immunomodulatory activity.[47]

### *Boswellia sacra*: Sacred Frankincense

In Juliet Highet's book on frankincense, she writes: "The international aromatic trade has a grading system for frankincense depending upon size, colour, degree of transparency, and of course fragrance, but it is generally acknowledged that *the* premium resin comes from *Boswellia sacra*."[48]

Ahmed Al-Harrasi and Salim Al-Saidi are scientists at the Department of Chemistry, College of Science, Sultan Qaboos University in Oman. Gary Young has met with Dr. Al-Harrasi in Muscat, Oman; and Young Living's Seed to Seal® spokesperson and global ambassador, Cole Woolley, has also met with Dr. Harrasi multiple times in Oman, both at the university and where the frankincense trees grow in Dhofar.

Dr. Harrasi's study, "Phytochemical Analysis of the Essential Oil from Botanically Certified Oleogum Resin of *Boswellia sacra* (Omani Luban)," explains that: "*Boswellia sacra* is a tree indigenous to the Dhofar region of the Sultanate of Oman."[49]

Mahmoud Suhail, MD, Young Living's partner in the Omani frankincense venture and a noted researcher, said, "*Boswellia sacra* is the only frankincense species native to Arabia." This is documented by the Royal Botanical Gardens in England, the premier scientific botanical institution, at http://www.kew.org/ceb/sepasal/bsacra.htm (Omanis proudly consider Oman to be Arabia).

Dr. Suhail also cited a book commissioned by His Majesty Sultan Qaboos Bin Said, Sultan of Oman, *Plants of Dhofar: The Southern Region of Oman, Traditional, Economic and Medicinal Uses,* which states:

"Several species of *Boswellia* including *B. sacra*, *B. papyrifera* (from tropical NE Africa), *B. frereana* (from Somalia) and *B. serrata* (from India) produce an oleo-gum-resin which is exploited as the frankincense or olibanum of commerce—the different species each producing a distinct type and quality of the resin. Only one species, *B. sacra*, is found in Arabia."[50]

Omani frankincense, *Boswellia sacra,* is regarded the world over as the rarest, most sought-after aromatic in existence. After careful negotiations with Omani officials, Gary Young was granted permission to build a Young Living distillery in Oman. Until this partnership, no Omani frankincense had been officially exported except that purchased by Saudi royals.

*Boswellia sacra* has been the focus of research conducted by Young Living Essential Oils' scientists and their colleagues documenting that sacra and carterii are separate species,[51] a case report showing that *B. sacra* may provide a non-surgical treatment for basal cell carcinoma,[52] that *B. sacra* induces human pancreatic cancer cell death in cultures,[53] and that *B. sacra* induces cancer cell death in human breast cancer cells.[54]

Imagine the joy it brought Gary Young to be the one to reintroduce Omani frankincense to the world. Young Living is distilling *Boswellia sacra* essential oil in partnership with Mahmoud Suhail, MD, in Salalah, Oman.

### The Science Behind Spirituality

During one of his overseas trips in 2009, Young Living researcher Marc Schreuder made a vital connection with

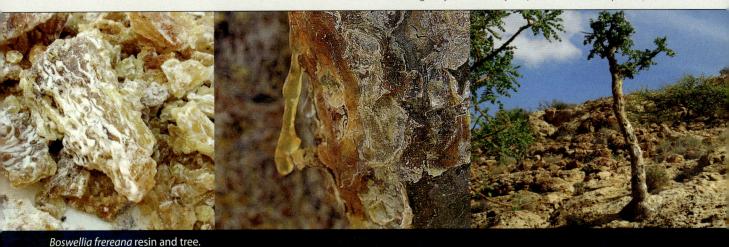

Boswellia frereana resin and tree.

an Israeli scientist named Arieh Moussaieff, who created headlines around the world when he and an international team of researchers discovered unique capabilities of a diterpene of certain *Boswellia* species.

Incensole acetate may be the reason frankincense has been part of religious and cultural ceremonies dating back to ancient times. Moussaieff's team discovered that this diterpene triggered an ion channel in the brain with heretofore unknown effects. The areas of the brain affected are known to be involved in emotions. The diterpene, incensole acetate, had anti-anxiety and antidepressant effects.

One of the media headlines was quite instructive: "Incense is psychoactive: Scientists identify the biology behind the ceremony." If you inhale frankincense with this diterpene, you will be calmed down if you are anxious, and if you are depressed, you will feel happier. What better steps to take to commune with Deity? Incensole acetate is found in *B. carterii* and *B. sacra*.

Dr. Moussaieff's studies have shown indeed that incensole acetate is responsible for the remarkable spiritual effects of frankincense.[55] But he also discovered a neuroprotective activity of incensole acetate.[56] An article about Dr. Moussaieff's work stated:

> In his doctoral work at the Hebrew University of Jerusalem, Moussaieff isolated the active compounds in the [frankincense] resin. When tested on mouse models of human head injury, he found that some of these substances provide protection for the nervous system. He later noted the resin's anti-depression and anti-anxiety properties and, investigating further, found that they act on a previously unknown pathway in the brain that regulates emotion.

Young Living's Frankincense *(Boswellia carterii)* and Sacred Frankincense *(Boswellia sacra)* contain incensole acetate.

### *Boswellia frereana:* Frereana Frankincense

*Boswellia frereana* is a rather unusual frankincense species. It is not found in Oman but grows only in Somalia, a country with a troubled history. Independent testing has questioned whether some frereana currently being sold by one essential oil company is truly a pure, quality essential oil. Gary Young traveled to Somalia in November 2013 to investigate sourcing. He made contact with harvesters who would like to sell their best frereana resins to Young Living.

While in great demand as incense, frereana does not have the same chemical configuration as other frankincense species. It does not contain boswellic acids. It does not contain incensole acetate. It does, however, contain unique constituents that have definite yet differing (from other frankincense species) anti-inflammatory activities.

Unfortunately, *Boswellia frereana* has not been the focus of many research studies. Of the five frereana studies found on PubMed, only two discuss its benefits. These two studies both show efficacy against inflammatory conditions. A 2006 study by Frank and Unger in the *Journal of Chromatography A* reported that "frankincense from *B. frereana* also potently inhibited the activity of CYP enzymes [involved in inflammation] but did not contain any of the characteristic boswellic acids."[57]

The second study was published in 2010 in the journal *Phytotherapy Research*. The researchers noted that "This is the first report detailing the anti-inflammatory efficacy of *B. frereana* in auricular cartilage."[58]

Now that Young Living has done the groundwork to obtain the best frereana Somalia has to offer, the next step will be to research this unique and distinctive frankincense species. No other essential oil company invests in scientific research like Young Living does.

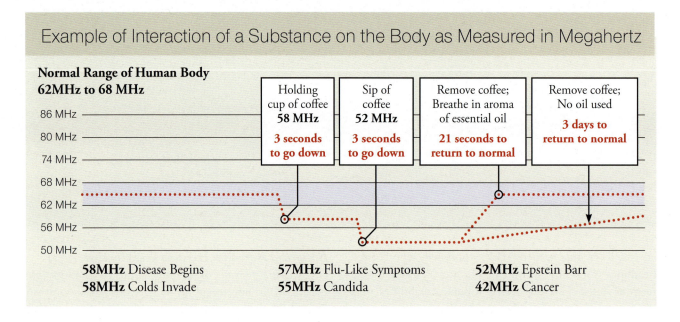

## Frequency: Our Electrical Energy

"Because science has long taught us to rely on what we can see and touch, we often don't notice that our spirit, thoughts, emotions, and body are all made of energy. Everything is vibrating. In fact, each of us has a personal vibration that communicates who we are to the world and helps shape our reality," said Penny Pierce, author of *Frequency: The Power of Personal Vibration,* 2009.

When studying the topics of vibration, frequency, and energy, it is a wise man or woman who realizes he or she does not know everything. Who is to argue with the German biophysicist Fritz-Albert Popp (author of 150 scientific studies), who proposed that all living things emit light energy, and that includes humans. Dr. Popp has written:

> We know today that man, essentially, is a being of light. And the modern science of photobiology . . . is presently proving this. In terms of healing the implications are immense. We are still on the threshold of fully understanding the complex relationship between light and life, but we can now say emphatically, that the function of our entire metabolism is dependent on light (http://www.biontologyarizona.com/dr-fritz-albert-popp/).

Certainly, more than one gifted energy worker has been able to "see" light and energy shooting up from certain essential oils like Young Living's Frankincense.

The original publication of the *Essential Oil Desk Reference* (1999) (EODR) included information on biofrequency and disease. Many people copied and disseminated the information, most often without acknowledging this as Bruce Tainio's work. Unfortunately, he did not continue with his studies, and so no further research has been conducted.

The theory of biofrequency continues to be investigated by researchers, and much of the information from the 1999 EODR deserves to be reviewed in light of recent scientific advances.

A groundbreaking study reported on research that has been "conducted with energetic measurements of essential oils using Raman spectroscopy which is based on the incidence of a monochromatic light source, which, upon reaching the oil in question undergoes scattering of light, allowing researchers to obtain information about the chemical compound indicating that *the components show energy bands* (Gnatta JR, 2016). [Emphasis added]

Science is proving long-held theories.

### Biofrequency and Disease

Frequency is defined as a measurable rate of electrical energy that is constant between any two points. When there is frequency, there is electromagnetic potential. We are being influenced by the magnetic action (or attraction) of the frequencies that surround us each day, and these frequencies influence our state of well-being. Everything has an electrical frequency measured in megahertz.

Longevity and Vitality - Special Features | **Chapter 19**

# Frequencies of Single Essential Oils and Blends

**SINGLE ESSENTIAL OILS**

| | |
|---|---|
| Angelica | 85 MHz |
| Basil | 52 MHz |
| Frankincense | 147 MHz |
| Galbanum | 56 MHz |
| German Chamomile | 105 MHz |
| Helichrysum | 181 MHz |
| Idaho Tansy | 105 MHz |
| Juniper | 98 MHz |
| Lavender | 118 MHz |
| Melissa (lemon balm) | 102 MHz |
| Myrrh | 105 MHz |
| Peppermint | 78 MHz |
| Ravintsara | 134 MHz |
| Rose | 320 MHz |
| Sandalwood | 96 MHz |

**ESSENTIAL OIL BLENDS**

| | |
|---|---|
| Abundance | 78 MHz |
| Acceptance | 102 MHz |
| Aroma Life | 84 MHz |
| Aroma Siez | 64 MHz |
| Awaken | 89 MHz |

| | |
|---|---|
| Brain Power | 78 MHz |
| Christmas Spirit | 104 MHz |
| Citrus Fresh | 90 MHz |
| Clarity | 101 MHz |
| Dragon Time | 72 MHz |
| Dream Catcher | 98 MHz |
| EndoFlex | 138 MHz |
| En-R-Gee | 106 MHz |
| Envision | 90 MHz |
| Exodus II | 180 MHz |
| Forgiveness | 192 MHz |
| Gathering | 99 MHz |
| Gentle Baby | 152 MHz |
| Grounding | 140 MHz |
| Harmony | 101 MHz |
| Hope | 98 MHz |
| Humility | 88 MHz |
| ImmuPower | 89 MHz |
| Inner Child | 98 MHz |
| Inspiration | 141 MHz |
| Into the Future | 88 MHz |
| Joy | 188 MHz |
| JuvaFlex | 82 MHz |

| | |
|---|---|
| Live With Passion | 89 MHz |
| Magnify Your Purpose | 99 MHz |
| Melrose | 48 MHz |
| Mister | 147 MHz |
| Motivation | 103 MHz |
| M-Grain | 72 MHz |
| PanAway | 112 MHz |
| Peace & Calming | 105 MHz |
| Present Time | 98 MHz |
| Purification | 46 MHz |
| Raven | 70 MHz |
| R.C. | 75 MHz |
| Release | 102 MHz |
| Relieve It | 56 MHz |
| Sacred Mountain | 176 MHz |
| SARA | 102 MHz |
| Sensation | 88 MHz |
| Surrender | 98 MHz |
| Thieves | 150 MHz |
| 3 Wise Men | 72 MHz |
| Trauma Life | 92 MHz |
| Valor | 47 MHz |
| White Angelica | 89 MHz |

Robert O. Becker, MD, documents the electrical frequency of the human body in his book *The Body Electric*.

A "frequency generator" was developed in the early 1920s by Royal Raymond Rife, MD. He found that by using certain frequencies, he could destroy a cancer cell or virus. He found that these frequencies could prevent the development of disease, and others would destroy disease.

Nikola Tesla said that if you could eliminate certain outside frequencies that interfered with our own electrical frequencies, we would have greater disease resistance.

Bjorn Nordenstrom, a radiologist from Stockholm, Sweden, wrote the book *Biologically Closed Circuits*. He discovered in the 1980s that by putting an electrode inside a tumor and running a milliamp D.C. (Direct Current) through the electrode, he could dissolve the cancer tumor and stop its growth. He found electropositive and electronegative energy fields in the human body.

Bruce Tainio of Tainio Technology in Cheney, Washington, developed new equipment to measure the biofre-quency of humans and foods. He used this biofrequency monitor to determine the relationship between frequency and disease.

Measuring in megahertz, it was found that:
- Processed/canned food had a zero MHz frequency
- Fresh foods 20–27 MHz
- Dry herbs from 15–22 MHz
- Fresh herbs from 20–27 MHz
- Essential oils started at 52 MHz and went as high as 320 MHz (which is the frequency of rose oil).

Fresh foods and herbs can be higher in frequency if grown organically and eaten freshly picked. It is believed that a healthy body typically has a frequency ranging from 62 to 78 MH, while disease may begin at 58 MHz. According to Dr. Rife's theories, every disease has a frequency, and a substance with a higher frequency will alter the disease that is at a lower frequency.

Seventh Edition | **Essential Oils Desk Reference** | 373

Clinical research shows that essential oils have the highest frequency of any natural substance known to man and can create an environment in which microbes cannot live. That would certainly indicate that the oil frequencies are several times greater than frequencies of herbs and foods.

Truly, the chemistry and frequencies of essential oils have the ability to help man maintain an optimal health frequency.

For years, research has been conducted on the use of electrical energy to reverse disease. Scientists in the field of natural healing have believed there has to be a more natural way to increase the body's electrical frequency. This led to the research and subsequent discovery of electrical frequencies in essential oils.

Patients felt better emotionally when oils were diffused in their homes. It seemed that, within seconds, these patients were calmer and less anxious with a little exposure and inhalation. Certain oils acted within 1-3 minutes; others acted within seconds. It is fascinating to think that an oil applied to the bottom of the feet can travel to the brain and take effect within 1 minute. The more results that have been seen, the more research that has been initiated.

## Unhealthy Substances Cause Frequency Changes

In one test, the frequencies of two individuals—the first a 26-year-old male and the second a 24-year-old male—were measured at 66 MHz each.

The first individual held a cup of coffee (without drinking any), and his frequency dropped to 58 MHz in 3 seconds. He put the coffee down and inhaled an aroma of essential oils. Within 21 seconds, his frequency had returned to 66 MHz.

The second individual took a sip of coffee, and his frequency dropped to 52 MHz in the same 3 seconds. However, no essential oils were used during the recovery time, and it took 3 days for his frequency to return to its normal 66 MHz.

One surprising aspect of this study measured the influence that thoughts have on the body's electrical frequency. Negative thoughts lowered the measured frequency by 12 MHz, and positive thoughts raised the measured frequency by 10 MHz. It was also found that prayer and meditation increased the measured frequency levels by 15 MHz.

## Raising Your Frequency

It has been demonstrated that we can change lower, depressed feelings and negative attitudes with the application of essential oils that carry frequencies in the higher range, resulting in a positive change of attitude and mood, thereby uplifting our spirits.

Essential oils and oil blends with higher frequency ranges work in the emotional and spiritual regions. Essential oils and blends that have a lower frequency have a more profound effect on making structural/physical changes. Oils with a frequency of 78 and below are believed to work specifically with harmonizing and balancing the physical body. Single oils may be added to a blend to increase effect.

Inhaling essential oils is particularly beneficial because the sense of smell is the only one of our senses that directly affects the amygdala, part of the limbic system of the brain, where emotions and memory are stored and released. This is why essential oils can have immediate and profound physiological and psychological effects.

This testing of the oils created a lot of interest and perhaps a better understanding of the functionality of the oils in relationship to their frequency. The frequencies should not be considered absolute, because any outside interference can minutely alter the number. However, these are as accurate as was possible at that time, and they are certainly within range and accurate to their point of usage and frequency potential.

## Frequency of the Human Body

The following frequency charts will stimulate your curiosity and intellectual mind. To some people, they will make absolute sense, and to others, no sense. We do not often hear it taught that sickness, disease, depression, negative thoughts, and emotions are of a low frequency; and it is perhaps a new thought for many people.

Few people relate to the idea that devitalized and processed food; consumer products made with chemicals; the consumption of drugs, alcohol, and tobacco; and polluted air and water envelope us in an environment of low frequencies.

It has been said that the lower the frequency, the closer we come to sickness, disease, and eventually death. The higher the frequency, the closer we come to God and a life of happiness, health, and prosperity.

Frequency is a fascinating subject, and these charts are great food for thought, whether it be in your realm of belief or mere supposition. Open your mind to greater awareness and the vast possibilities of how you might increase the frequency to which the vibration of your body and soul harmonically resonate.

Longevity and Vitality - Special Features | Chapter 19

## Normal Human Frequency

The normal body frequency ranges between 62 and 78 MHz and appears to drop somewhat during sleep, but it is still maintained within those markers.

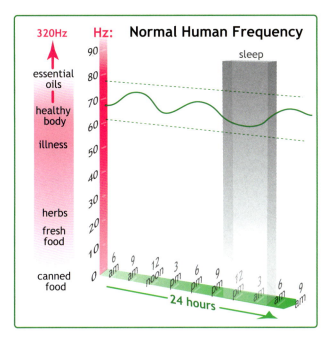

Daily activity and emotions will always cause frequency to vary. However, with proper diet, exercise, pure water, enough rest, a positive attitude, and an environment of peace and harmony, whether at work or at home, the body should be able to stay consistently within the proper and balanced range of frequency.

## Frequency Fluctuation Causes Cellular Breakdown

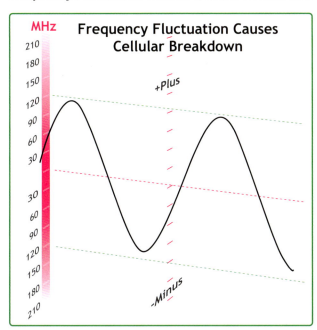

As the body picks up more negative energy particles, the frequency fluctuation begins to cause cellular breakdown. When the frequency exceeds the normal energy cycle on the negative side, a greater electrical charge is produced, causing negative attitudes, depression, and unhappy experiences. Frequencies too far off from normal will cause a cellular breakdown that leads to disease.

## Alternating Static and Incoherent Frequencies

Static and incoherent frequencies fracture the human, animal, and plant electrical fields, resulting in cellular degeneration, disease, and death.

Research was conducted with plants with classical, harmonic, beautiful music versus hard rock, noisy, nonharmonic music. With the beautiful music, the plants thrived; and with the other music, they died. It is the same with the human body.

A noisy room with a lot of talking, laughing, and loud music tends to be a very unproductive environment, creating tension and agitation. Road rage has become an evil that has developed because of a vast number of cars stuck and not moving on roadways, with thousands of car engines racing, horns blaring, and people staring at tall buildings and billboards, feeling trapped, angry, and wanting to fight—a very destructive, incoherent frequency.

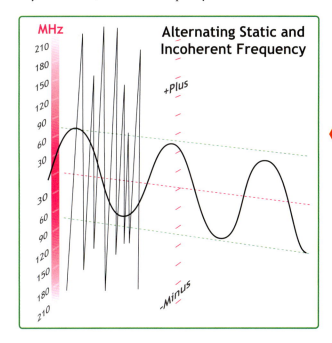

Why is it that people want to flee to the mountains, away from tall buildings, computers, cell phones, and other people? Has society become immune and so unaware that people just continue to live in oblivion, wondering why they are tired, unmotivated, and sick?

Seventh Edition | Essential Oils Desk Reference

There is so much peace and harmony in the environment of God's creations, away from man's cement and asphalt, electrical wiring, gadgets of all kinds, and millions of people scurrying thousands of different directions, all at the same time.

We live in an environment of incoherent frequency. No wonder there is so much more disease, depression, frustration, and irritation than there ever was even 50 years ago.

## Negative Magnetic Field

The shaded areas indicate the negative electromagnetic field that accumulates negatively charged magnetic particles. Daily radiation from cell phones, computers, electrical appliances and gadgets, cars, and x-ray equipment used at the dentists' and doctors' offices all contribute to this toxic build up.

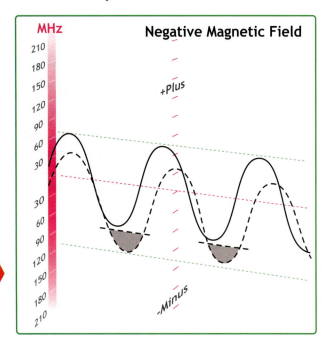

These magnetic particles travel in the airways and spread dramatically throughout the environment. Too much magnetic accumulation in the body without daily cleansing and protection results in untold cellular damage that leads to body malfunction, deterioration, disease, and death.

## Spiritual Frequencies

As spiritual frequency increases, the negative curve decreases. Man must maintain a connection with the earth in order to remain grounded and to keep the physical body on the earth plane.

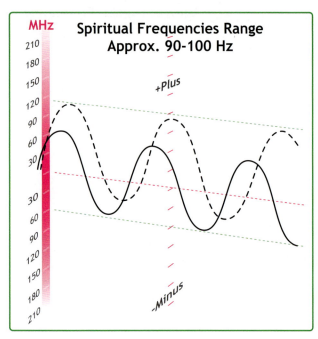

Frequency most likely elevates during times of heightened spiritual or intuitive awareness. Visions, out-of-body experiences, going beyond life for a short time (as when someone dies and then is revived a short time later) will carry higher frequencies when the spirit is in tune with spiritual dimensions. The exact copy on the minus side is the pseudo effect called spiritualism, where deception is so strong.

Longevity and Vitality - Special Features | Chapter 19

# Microbes: How Essential Oils Fight Them

Another method by which aromatics and essential oils may exert a life-lengthening effect is through their ability to inhibit the growth of bacteria, fungi, and viruses. Some bacteria, such as *Chlamydia pneumoniae,* have been implicated as one of the true causes of heart disease. Viruses, such as HIV and hepatitis, have resulted in liver failure and premature death. Fungi, like *Candida albicans,* have been implicated in cancer due to their secretion of mycotoxins.

One of the most comprehensive studies to probe the powerful antimicrobial effects of essential oils was the research directed by D. Gary Young and conducted with Sue Chao at Weber State University. Using disc diffusion assays, they tested the killing power of 67 different Young Living essential oils against a variety of yeast, molds, gram negative bacteria, and gram positive bacteria. Cinnamon, Clove, Thyme, Peppermint, Oregano, and Mountain Savory exerted the strongest antimicrobial properties.[59]

In further tests the following year, they successfully proved the ability of Thyme, Oregano, and Clove essential oils to destroy colonies of *Streptococcus pneumoniae,* the bacteria responsible for many types of throat, sinus, and lung infections.[60]

# Microwave Cooking: The Scientific Facts

Microwave ovens can be found in almost every home and restaurant because they are extremely convenient for thawing, cooking, and heating food. Yet what is the price for this convenience?

In a study conducted by Dr. Radwan Farag, dean of the Biochemistry Department at Cairo University, he discovered that just 2 seconds of microwave energy destroys all the enzymes in food, thus increasing our enzyme deficiency and altering the frequency of the food. It appears that heating food-containing proteins in the microwave for 10 minutes changes the molecular structure of the food, creating a new, harmful type of protein. Surely, the price is just too high in loss of health for this convenience.

Experiments conducted in the 1940s showed some of the dangers of microwave energy. This type of energy was actually discovered in the 1800s but was not considered for cooking until the invention of the microwave oven.

Microwaves were first used during World War II for early radar projects. It was during a radar research project in the mid-1940s that Dr. Percy Spencer of Raytheon Corporation noticed the candy bar in his pocket had melted after testing a vacuum. This piqued his curiosity, which gave him the idea to put popcorn kernels near the tube. The popcorn popped all over the office, which brought about the invention of the microwave oven, with Raytheon filing the first microwave cooking patent.

**Microwaves are a form of electromagnetic energy,** like radio waves. They are short waves of electromagnetic energy that travel at the speed of light. We have all heard about microwave towers, but what are they? Microwave towers are used to relay long-distance telephone signals, television programs, and computer information across the earth and to satellites in space. But we are most familiar with the microwave as a convenience for cooking food.

A microwave oven contains a magnetron, which is a tube in which electrons pass through a magnetic field to produce micro wave-length radiation, which interacts with the molecules in food. In the microwave oven, the wave energy changes the polarity of molecules from positive to negative millions of times every second. This friction produces extreme heat, and in the food it causes "structural isomerism," or structural damage, of the food molecules.

**This decreases the nutritional value** of food up to 60 to 90 percent. Vitamin B12, which is needed for red blood cell formation, is greatly reduced. In addition, microwave cooking kills 97 percent of the flavonoids in the food, which are some of the body's nutrient soldiers that fight disease, inflammation, and microbes. Furthermore, vitamins C and E, essential minerals, and enzymes are virtually destroyed.

This leaves the cells extremely vulnerable to viruses, fungi, and other micro-organisms. The ability of the cells to repair themselves is suppressed so that rather than producing water and carbon dioxide in the process of cell repair, hydrogen peroxide and carbon monoxide are produced. Imagine eating food filled with carbon monoxide.

A study published in the November 2003 issue of *The Journal of the Science of Food and Agriculture* found that broccoli cooked in the microwave with a little water lost

Seventh Edition | **Essential Oils Desk Reference** | 377

up to 97 percent of the beneficial antioxidant chemicals it contains. By comparison, steamed broccoli lost only 11 percent or fewer of its antioxidants.

In 1991, there was a lawsuit against a hospital in Oklahoma because a microwave was used to warm the blood for a hip-surgery patient, who died after receiving the blood transfusion. Warming blood for a transfusion is routine; unfortunately, using a microwave causes enough changes in the blood to be deadly.

The effects of microwaving breast milk have also been researched. John Kerner, MD, and Richard Quin, MD, from Stanford University, said, "Microwaving human milk, even at a low setting, can destroy some of its important disease-fighting capabilities."

Dr. Kerner subsequently wrote in the April 1992 edition of *Pediatrics* that "Microwaving itself may in fact cause some injury to the milk above and beyond the heating."

In addition, a radio announcement at the University of Minnesota said, "Microwaves are not recommended for heating a baby's bottle. Heating the bottle in a microwave can cause slight changes in the milk, and even though the bottle will feel cool on the outside, the inside could be so hot that it could burn the baby's mouth and throat. In infant formulas, there may be a loss of some vitamins. In expressed milk, some protective properties may be destroyed."

A study using ultra-high-performance liquid chromatography/tandem mass spectrometry discovered chemicals that leached from baby bottles. Low levels of BPA were found in three bottles after they had been heated in a microwave oven. A chemical, 4-n-NP, not reported to be leachable, was found in two brand name baby-feeding bottles (Wang J, 2010).

Dr. Lita Lee of Hawaii reported in the December 9, 1989, *Lancet*:

**Microwaving baby formulas** converted certain trans-amino acids into their synthetic cis-isomers. Synthetic isomers, whether cis-amino acids or trans-fatty acids, are not biologically active. Further, one of the amino acids, L-proline, was converted to its d-isomer, which is known to be neurotoxic (poisonous to the nervous system) and nephrotoxic (poisonous to the kidneys). It's bad enough that many babies are not nursed, but now they are given fake milk (baby formula) made even more toxic via microwaving.

Microwave ovens have been known to leak radiation, which can disrupt the delicate balance in cellular growth. Our bodies are regulated by electrical frequencies and electromagnetic fields. Microwave radiation can disrupt these frequencies and damage normal body functions.

Radiation suppresses the immune system, and the constant eating of microwave-cooked food causes memory loss, lowers IQ and mental capacity, and causes emotional problems, most likely due to a disruption in hormone production.

Because the body is electrochemical in nature, any force that disrupts or changes human electrochemical events will affect the physiology of the body. This is further described in Robert O. Becker's book *The Body Electric* and in Ellen Sugarman's book *Warning: The Electricity Around You May Be Hazardous to Your Health.*

Another danger to consider is the heating of the plastic in which some food is wrapped, which can increase the carcinogens in the food. Studies have shown that plastic wraps and containers do leak chemicals and toxic agents into the food they are holding. Ethylhexyl, DEHA [Bis(2-ethylhexyl) adipate)], and xenoestrogen are all substances that studies have shown migrate into your food from plastic when it is microwaved.

Dr. Edward Fujimoto, the manager of the Wellness Program at the Castle Hospital, said that we should not be heating foods that contain fat in the microwave using plastic containers. He said that the combination of fat, high heat, and plastics releases dioxins into the food and ultimately into the cells of the body. Dioxins are carcinogens and highly toxic to the cells of our bodies.

**There is a simple experiment** you can do at home to see for yourself what happens by just using water slightly heated in a microwave oven. Plant some seeds in two pots. Water one pot with water that has been microwaved for just 15 seconds. Water the other with regular tap water. Even with chlorinated tap water, the seeds will germinate and the plants will grow. The seeds that received microwaved water will not sprout. If microwaved water can stop plants from growing, imagine what microwaved food can do to your body.

**In 1980, a research project** with 20 volunteers was conducted with microwave cooking. Ten volunteers in group A and 10 in group B fasted on liquids for 10 days. Then both groups were fed the same foods for another 10 days with only one exception: The food for group A was steamed, while the food for group B was microwaved. After 10 days, stool samples were taken and analyzed. Group A stools appeared to be normally digested, while group B stools were of a plastic texture. Ultrasound scans showed adhesive food particles stuck to the stomach wall. In the stool sample, altered enzymes were found, as well as protein with altered molecular structure that could not be absorbed.

Longevity and Vitality - Special Features | **Chapter 19**

In test subjects who ate microwaved food, the following changes in blood chemistry were observed:

- Decrease in hemoglobin values
- Decrease in the ratio of HDL cholesterol (good cholesterol) and LDL (bad cholesterol)
- Decrease in lymphocytes (white blood cells, the ones that kill germs)
- Increase in luminous power by luminous bacteria exposed to blood of volunteers. In actuality, radioactive energy was passed on from the microwaved food to the blood cells of those who ate the food.

This implies that a person who eats microwaved food for an extended period could become anemic due to destruction of hemoglobin, could have an increase in heart disease because of decrease in good cholesterol and an increase in bad cholesterol, and could become subject to a number of contagious diseases due to a weakened immune system.

**In 1989, Swiss biologist** Dr. Hans Ulrich Hertel worked as a food scientist for many years with one of the major Swiss food companies that does business on a global scale. He was the first scientist to carry out a clinical study on the effects microwaved nutrients have on the blood and physiology of the human body. Because he began questioning certain processing procedures that denatured the food, he was fired from his job.

Hertel's scientific study was conducted with Dr. Bernard H. Blanc of the Swiss Federal Institute of Technology and the University Institute for Biochemistry. Eight people participated in the study for eight weeks. They lived in a controlled environment and intermittently ate raw foods, conventionally cooked foods, and microwaved foods. Blood samples were tested after each meal.

**Microwave oven manufacturers** insist that microwaved and irradiated foods do not have any significantly higher "radiolytic" compounds than do broiled, baked, or other conventionally cooked foods. **However, scientific clinical evidence shows that this is simply a lie.**

In America, neither universities nor the federal government have conducted any tests concerning the effects on our bodies from eating microwaved foods. It seems a bit strange that they are more concerned with studies on what happens if the door on a microwave oven doesn't close properly. Since people ingest this altered food, should there not be a concern for how the same damaged molecules will affect our own human biological cell structure?

**Hiding the truth** seems to be prevalent in the commercial world. At the same time Doctors Hertel and Blanc were publishing their research, an article appeared in the 19th issue of *Journal Franz Weber,* which stated:

> ...the consumption of food cooked in microwave ovens had cancerous effects on the blood. The violent deformations that can occur in the human body when exposed to microwaves are also seen in the food molecules cooked in microwaves.
>
> Studies conducted on food thawed, cooked and heated in microwaves showed that many food molecules became carcinogens. The glucoside and galactoside present in frozen foods converted into carcinogenic substances. Plant alkaloids in vegetables were converted into carcinogens. Milk and cereals heated in microwaves also had some of their amino acids converted into carcinogens.

On the cover of the magazine was a picture of the Grim Reaper holding a microwave oven in one of his hands.

**The research paper** by Doctors Hertel and Blanc followed the article, which must have created a lot of furor with the manufacturers of microwave ovens and those making money from the sale of them.

As soon as Doctors Hertel and Blanc's research was published in 1991, a powerful trade organization, the Swiss Association of Dealers for Electro-apparatuses for Households and Industry, known as FEA, struck swiftly in 1992. They forced the President of the Court of Seftigen, Canton of Bern, to issue a "gag order" against Doctors Hertel and Blanc.

In March 1993, Dr. Hertel was convicted for "interfering with commerce" and prohibited from further publishing his results. However, Dr. Hertel stood his ground and fought this decision over the years.

Eventually this decision was reversed in a judgment delivered in Strasbourg on August 25, 1998. The European Court of Human Rights held that there had been a violation of Hertel's rights in the 1993 decision.

The European Court of Human Rights also ruled that the "gag order" issued by the Swiss court in 1992 against Dr. Hertel, prohibiting him from declaring that microwave ovens are dangerous to human health, was contrary to the right of freedom of expression. In addition, Switzerland was ordered to pay Dr. Hertel compensation of 40,000 French Francs.

**After World War II**, the Russians also experimented with microwave ovens. Since 1957 their research has been carried out mainly at the Institute of Radio Technology at Klinsk, Byelorussia.

In 1976, during the Cold War, the Soviet Union banned the use of microwave ovens, based on research they had conducted revealing the damage it does to food. Although the research was never formally presented, it had become well-known throughout the international community that the Soviets understood the dangers of the microwave oven. Obviously, they knew something that the rest of the world didn't know.

According to U.S. researcher William Kopp, who gathered much of the results of Russian and German research—and was apparently prosecuted for doing so (*J. Nat. Sci*, 1998; 1:42-3)—the following effects were observed by Russian forensic teams:

1. Heating prepared meats in a microwave sufficiently for human consumption created:
   - d-Nitrosodiethanolamine (a well-known cancer-causing agent)
   - Destabilization of active protein biomolecular compounds
   - Creation of a binding effect to radioactivity in the atmosphere
   - Creation of cancer-causing agents within protein-hydrolysate compounds in milk and cereal grains

2. Microwave emissions also caused alteration in the catabolic (breakdown) behavior of glucoside- and galactoside-elements within frozen fruits when thawed in this way.

3. Microwaves altered catabolic behavior of plant-alkaloids when raw, cooked, or frozen vegetables were exposed for even very short periods.

4. Cancer-causing free radicals were formed within certain trace-mineral molecular formations in plant substances, especially in raw root vegetables.

5. Ingestion of microwaved foods caused a higher percentage of cancerous cells in blood.

6. Due to chemical alterations within food substances, malfunctions occurred in the lymphatic system, causing degeneration of the immune system's capacity to protect itself against cancerous growth.

7. The unstable catabolism of microwaved foods altered their elemental food substances, leading to disorders in the digestive system.

8. Those ingesting microwaved foods showed a statistically higher incidence of stomach and intestinal cancers, plus a general degeneration of peripheral cellular tissues with a gradual breakdown of digestive and excretory system function.

9. Microwave exposure caused significant decreases in the nutritional value of all foods studied, particularly:
   - A decrease in the bioavailability of B-complex vitamins, vitamin C, vitamin E, essential minerals, and lipotropics
   - Destruction of the nutritional value of nucleoproteins in meats
   - Lowering of the metabolic activity of alkaloids, glucosides, galactosides, and nitrilosides (all basic plant substances in fruits and vegetables)
   - Marked acceleration of structural disintegration in all foods

The Russians later lifted the ban, and currently, no countries have a ban on the use of the microwave oven.

No FDA or officially released government studies have proven current microwaving usage to be harmful, but we all know that the validity of studies can be—and are sometimes deliberately—limiting, and many of these studies are later proven to be inaccurate.

**According to OSHA**, the United States Department of Labor, Occupational Safety & Health Administration, adverse effects due to microwave radiation from cellular phones, radio transmissions, and radar traffic devices are topics of controversy and ongoing research. But what does that mean? What keeps the government from conducting studies and releasing their findings to the public? Are they protecting the public or the dollar?

**The FDA,** Food and Drug Administration, claims that radiation emissions from microwave ovens do not pose a public health risk and that radiation injury is extremely rare. The agency states that unless the microwave oven has a damaged latch, seal, or hinges, there is little concern over leaking microwave radiation. That may be true, but what does that have to do with the effects of the function of a microwave oven?

Over the past few years, manufacturers have certainly improved the technology and design of microwave ovens, but even the most advanced technology cannot change the damaging effects of radiation to our food and subsequently our bodies.

Tests by the U.S. National Institute of Environmental Health Sciences determined that inhaling the artificial butter of microwave popcorn could pose a health risk. According to the Global Health Center, microwave cooking may adversely affect the molecular makeup of certain foods.

According to the United States Department of Health and Human Services, a microwave oven can pose a serious danger to small children as young as 18 months who are able to open a microwave oven and remove scalding hot liquids. According to an article posted on the agency's website, children have been seriously burned after opening a microwave oven, which has the potential of heating liquids to a dangerously hot temperature, which can result in severe burns.

**We should all be searching** and finding out the facts for ourselves. If you type in "microwaves" on the Internet, you will find that only good, positive things come up touting the "great value" of microwaves. However, if you type in "dangers of microwaves," you will be astounded at all the research, tests, documentation, and personal stories that come up contrary to the "great value" perceived by the public.

**Dr. Sabina DeVita,** a well-known psychologist from Toronto, Canada, who for years has been studying the damaging effects of electromagnetic or radiation poisoning on the human body, says that electromagnetic pollution has become an occupational hazard of our high-tech 21st century and will probably continue to get worse as technology becomes more and more sophisticated as we move farther into the century. We are not only exposed to the radiation from the microwave oven but also to that of radios, televisions, computers, cell phones, and every electrical appliance that we conveniently use every day.

**So what is our answer?** We can avoid some of it, but not all of it, so what can we do to protect ourselves? There is one possibility that we probably have not thought of, and that is the use of essential oils, which have been used since the beginning of time for beautifying, healing, and protecting, both physically and spiritually.

Their therapeutic qualities have been lost to the synthetic world of perfumes, soaps, lotions, potions, creams, cosmetics, and, of course, the vast food industry. Only in the last decade have essential oils reemerged from their mysterious past as viable products for natural healing and wellness. Studies are being conducted in universities and research laboratories all over the world. Even allopathic medicine is starting to take notice.

Through all the scientific research, it has been discovered that essential oils are one of the highest known sources of antioxidants that can prevent free radical damage. They contain bioelectric frequencies that are several times greater than that of herbs and food, making them profoundly effective in raising the frequencies of the human body and aiding in the prevention of disease.

Dr. DeVita, in her book *Electromagnetic Pollution* (available through Life Science Publishing), states that because of the high frequency, high oxygenating molecules, fast delivery system to the cells, immune-building, antimicrobial properties, etc., essential oils become a necessary adjunct to protecting ourselves against free radical damage as well as the potential ravages of our electromagnetically polluted environment.

She strongly recommends certain essential oil blends that could be helpful in counteracting the effects of electromagnetic radiation. Many of the essential oils enhance the frequency of the energy field, thus helping to maintain a healthy electrical balance. As with all oils, one has to experiment to see which oils seem to resonate with the body.

**Certain essential oil blends** to consider are Valor, Harmony, Grounding, Brain Power, Melrose, Clarity, ImmuPower, Present Time, and many others. Single oils such as Royal Hawaiian Sandalwood, Tea Tree (Melaleuca Alternifolia), Myrtle, Palo Santo, Idaho Balsam Fir, Sacred Frankincense, and Frankincense can also help.

In June 2010 the blend The Gift, formulated with some of the oils written about in ancient scripture, including Sacred Frankincense from Oman, came on the market. This very special oil comes to us with a history from the very center of antiquity. We are learning to deeply appreciate it as we discover more and more about its powerful properties that the people of long ago already knew, and now we can add it to our arsenal of protection. Dr. Sabina's advice is well founded and would serve us in a most remarkable and gratifying way.

Many people are writing about and speaking out about the dangers of microwave usage and the dangers of radiation poisoning, but the information is still suppressed, and the general public is very unaware.

Unfortunately, convenience often takes precedence over common sense, but the price we pay for "lack of knowledge" is devastating.

Find out for yourself; the information is there for those who seek it. Inform those around you in your sphere of influence, and let us stop this deception and destruction.

# MSM—Sulfur: An Important Mineral

MSM (methylsulfonylmethane) is a natural, sulfur-bearing nutrient that occurs widely in nature (found in everything from mother's breast milk to fresh vegetables). It is an exceptional source of nutritional sulfur—a mineral that is vital to protein synthesis and sound health.

Why is sulfur so important to the body? Because sulfur is a mineral which, like vitamin C, is constantly being used up and depleted. When we fail to replenish our reserves of nutritional sulfur, we become more vulnerable to disease and degenerative conditions. Some possible signs of sulfur deficiency are:

- Poor nail and hair growth
- Eczema
- Dermatitis
- Poor muscle tone
- Acne/Pimples
- Gout
- Rheumatism
- Arthritis
- Weakening of the nervous system
- Constipation
- Impairment of mental faculties
- Lowered libido

MSM is more than just another essential nutrient. According to research compiled by Ronald Lawrence, PhD, MD, and Stanley Jacob, MD, MSM represents a safe, natural solution for chronic headaches, back pain, tendonitis, fibromyalgia, rheumatism, arthritis, athletic injuries, muscle spasms, asthma, and allergies.

In a book entitled *The Miracle of MSM,* available through Life Science Publishing, both Dr. Jacobs and Dr. Lawrence discuss how MSM has benefited hundreds of patients. A UCLA neuropsychiatrist, Dr. Lawrence is convinced that MSM will revolutionize how millions of people deal with inflammatory autoimmune diseases such as rheumatism, asthma, bursitis, and tendonitis, as well as auto-immune diseases like arthritis, lupus, scleroderma, and allergies.

Other doctors have also seen their patients dramatically improve using 2 to 4 grams of MSM daily. According to David Blyweiss, MD, of the Institute of Advanced Medicine in Lauderhill, Florida, many patients experience a 50 percent improvement in their arthritis symptoms, along with less fatigue, better sleep, and better ability to exercise.

Dr. Lawrence has also used MSM to improve the condition of patients who were virtually crippled with arthritis and back pain. One patient was able to get out of bed for the first time after just two weeks on MSM, and after two months of MSM use, he could walk to the grocery store.

Another of Dr. Lawrence's patients was a 70-year-old woman who was suffering from severe arthritis. In this case, MSM actually postponed the need for double knee replacement. In fact, after only two months on oral MSM, she was walking again with much less pain and stiffness.

Numerous other MSM users have experienced results equivalent to cortisone—but without side effects like immune suppression, fluid retention, and weakness.

According to Stanley Jacobs, MD, there may be no pharmaceutical back pain therapy better—or safer—than MSM. "MSM has an important role to play in the nonsurgical treatment of back pain," he said. "I have seen several hundred patients for back pain secondary to osteoarthritis, disc degeneration, spinal misalignments, or accidents. For such pain-related conditions, MSM is usually beneficial."

"I have been recommending MSM for more than six months," said Richard Shaefer, a chiropractor from Wheeling, Illinois. "The results have been excellent. I consistently see major reduction in pain and inflammation in arthritic joints, along with improved range of motion. I can't think of a single individual who isn't getting some kind of positive effect."

MSM may have other benefits aside from its pain and inflammation-reducing properties. Numerous patients have reported a surge in energy levels along with thicker hair, nails, and skin. Some have even reported a softening or disappearance of scar tissue.

One user reported a marked increase in stamina and energy after starting on MSM. "For a long while I have had the blahs," complained Lou Salyer of Tucson, Arizona. "I had no stamina. I had to force myself to get things done around the house. After two days on MSM, it was like a blast of energy. I am amazed at how much I get done now."

MSM may also do much more than relieve pain. "Prior to taking MSM (30 grams a day for 20 years), I would have a cold or flu two or three times a year," stated Dr. Jacobs. "Since I've been taking MSM, I've not had a single cold or the flu. I can't say that MSM prevented my cold or the flu, but it is a fascinating observation."

MSM contains an exceptionally bioavailable source of sulfur, one of the most neglected minerals needed by the human body. Carl Pfeiffer, MD, PhD, a world-renowned expert on nutritional medicine, agrees, "Sulfur is the forgotten essential element."

Found in such foods as garlic and asparagus, the sulfur within MSM is a critical part of the amino acids cysteine and methionine, which form the building blocks of the nails, hair, and skin. Sulfur is also found in therapeutic mineral baths and hot springs that have brought relief to arthritis sufferers for centuries. Sulfurzyme is a unique combination of MSM, protein-building compounds, and Ningxia wolfberry. Together, they create a new concept in balancing the immune system and supporting almost every major function of the body.

MSM is very closely related to DMSO, a powerful pain reliever that was the subject of a *60 Minutes* report in April 1980. DMSO has been approved by the FDA for interstitial cystitis, a painful urinary tract condition.

Of particular importance is MSM's ability to equalize water pressure inside the cells—a considerable benefit for those plagued with bursitis, arthritis, and tendonitis. These kinds of inflammatory outbreaks are created when the water pressure inside the cells jumps past the pressure outside the cells, creating pressure and pain. MSM acts as a sort of cellular safety valve, affecting the protein envelope of the cell so that water transfers freely in and out of the cell. The result: rapid relief and less damage to tissues. In addition, because it elasticizes the hold between the cells, MSM can restore flexibility to inflamed tissues.

When our bodies grow older and are chronically shortchanged of key minerals like sulfur and MSM, the bonds between our cells become increasingly rigid and brittle—a condition that can lead to a loss in skin flexibility and contribute to skin wrinkles. The internal manifestations of this cellular brittleness are far less visible but have a far greater negative impact on the body. MSM's ability to reintroduce flexibility into cell structures, therefore, can have widespread, restorative effects.

# Radiation: Protecting Our Environment

**Radiation** is when energy moves away from its source through space, creating two broad types.

1. **Ionizing radiation** comes from radioactive materials and machines such as an x-ray machine that carries large amounts of energy in each particle. It can hurt and damage anything that it hits and causes chemical changes in people, animals, and vegetation.

   Radiation with sufficiently high energy can ionize atoms. That most often occurs when an electron is stripped or knocked out from an electron shell, which leaves the atom with a positive charge. Because cells are made of atoms, this ionization can result in cancer. However, that probability is dependent upon the dose rate of the radiation and the sensitivity of the organism being irradiated.

2. **Nonionizing radiation** comes from other sources and causes effects known as electromagnetic radiation, commonly known as light. Nonionizing radiation does not usually cause damage, although some types can cause chemical changes or make things hotter.

We are exposed to many types of radiations, which we refer to as "natural" or normal radiation coming from televisions, microwaves, waterbeds, cell phones, and computers, in addition to our visits to the dentist, doctor, hospital, and other various types of radiation to which we are exposed in the atmosphere, particularly when flying.

Energy travels through space in many different ways. One way is in the form of shifting electrical and magnetic fields like a stream of particles of energy called photons. Another way is by traveling in the form of tiny pieces of atoms, like neutrons or protons, and is referred to as **particle radiation**.

Scientists categorize different kinds of electromagnetic radiation or light based on wavelength and frequency such as the following:

- **Radio waves** have the highest wavelength and are used to send and receive communications.
- **Micro waves** are a type of radio wave used in a microwave oven to warm up food.
- **Radar waves** detect airplanes in the sky, ships in the ocean, and changes in the weather.
- **Infrared waves** are emitted by most objects at room temperature and are not seen by the human eye. Certain types of cameras can take pictures of hot things even on the other side of a wall.
- **Visible light** is the radiation we call "light."
- **Ultraviolet light** is the invisible light that can cause sunburn and is used to kill bacteria and make invisible ink visible.
- **X-rays and Gamma rays** are extremely strong rays used in medicine to photograph the interior of the body and treat cancer. However, in too large amounts, they are very dangerous to life.

We could say that we live in a world of radiation, if we think specifically about the sun and the light that it gives to our earth. Although the energy from the sun is necessary for our health, too much can be dangerous and even deadly. The pain of a sunburn is excruciating, as those who have had this experience know. Too much of a good thing can turn into something dangerous and unwanted.

We are inundated constantly with radiation from varying levels. It has been said that those who have been exposed to high levels of radiation could have some allergic reaction in the formation of unusual rashes on the skin. We know that radiation is very damaging, because of the many scientific studies and research conducted, besides the stories told by those who have actually had this experience.

However, not only do we have this mild exposure on a daily basis, but now many governments have built nuclear plants for atomic power, national defense, communication, and research. Few of us even understand the use of atomic energy, radiation, and the technical advances that have been made in nuclear energy in the last decade. Sadly, with all this technical advancement comes the threat of even greater radiation exposure and poisoning. Unfortunately, when it comes to risks and toxic exposure levels, the government and medical community will likely downplay the threat.

The last report of the U.S. Nuclear Regulatory Commission (November 6, 2015) stated that there are 100 nuclear plants in the United States today. Wikipedia has not updated since a 2010 survey of energy accidents showing there have been at least 56 accidents at nuclear reactors in the United States (defined as incidents that either resulted in the loss of human life or more than $50,000 of property damage). Also, contaminated, radioactive water was dumped into nearby water supplies, from which many people suffered because of their exposure to an unknown invader.

One independent website listed two more recent incidents. The first, with information from a May 2013 *Scientific American* article stating that "60 of 177 underground tanks constructed to contain radioactive waste generated by the ill-fated plant were found to be leaking. Controversy surrounding the project, run by contractor Bechtel National, Inc. led to the reassignment of Chief project engineer Gary Brunson, and the filing of whistleblower complaints alleging that safety concerns were suppressed by Bechtel were filed by Nuclear and Environmental Safety Manager Donna Busche and former Deputy Chief Process Engineer Walter Tamosaitis."

This website also reported on February 14, 2014, that "a 55-gallon drum of radioactive waste burst open at the Waste Isolation Pilot Plant outside Carlsbad, New Mexico, leading to radiological contamination of 21 employees and forcing a temporary shutdown of the facility. The

## Environmental Protection Kits

The QuadShield and EndoShield kits each combine four powerful products to help people protect themselves against daily radiation bombardment of cell phones, computers, electrical appliances, and other potential dangers.

The QuadShield kit contains Longevity Softgels, the essential oil blend Melrose, and the nutritional supplements Super C (or Chewable), and Thyromin. The EndoShield kit contains Longevity Softgels and the essential oil blends Melrose, EndoFlex, and Citrus Fresh.

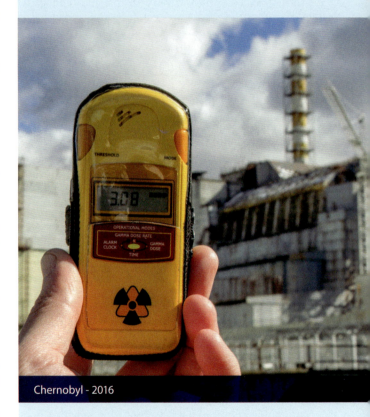
Chernobyl - 2016

The Japanese earthquake of March 11, 2011, has taught the world that nuclear power plants are vulnerable to natural disasters, as well as from years of use that have caused deterioration and weakness.

Of the 104 nuclear power plants in the United States, six are identical to the damaged Fukushima plant, 17 others are very similar, and several are close to major earthquake faults.

The "giant" that has been sleeping since the days of the Three Mile Island and Chernobyl disasters has awakened.

Longevity and Vitality - Special Features | **Chapter 19**

# Environmental Protection Kits

## QuadShield™

**Longevity Softgel**—The essential oils in Longevity Softgels increase the oxygen and ATP (adenosine triphosphate) cellular fuel for increasing cell life and immunity for stronger resistance against damage from environmental pollution.
- **Children and teens ages 10–18:** 1-2 capsules daily
- **Adults:** 2–4 capsules daily

**Melrose**—This blend is formulated with two species of Melaleuca oil: *M. alternifolia* and *M. quinquenervia*, also known as Niaouli, which were found through research by Daniel Pénoël, MD, and Pierre Franchomme, PhD, to prevent cellular damage from environmental pollution and potential daily radiation exposure.
- **Children ages 1–3:** 1 drop in yogurt or other liquid
- **Children ages 4–7:** 2 drops in yogurt or other liquid
- **Children 8 and older:** 6 drops per capsule 1–3 times daily or in yogurt or other liquid
- **Adults:** 20 drops per capsule, 1–2 capsules, 1–3 times daily or in yogurt or other liquid

**Super C (or Chewable)**—Super C provides the body with 2,166 percent of the recommended dietary intake of the powerful antioxidant vitamin C and is enhanced with minerals, bioflavonoids, and pure Orange, Lemon, and other essential oils. It is a natural antioxidant and free radical scavenger that supports the immune system and protects healthy cells from becoming damaged by the effects of environmental pollution.
- **Children ages 1–3:** 1–2 MightyVites daily
- **Children ages 4–7:** 2–3 MightyVites or Super C Chewables daily
- **Children 8 and older:** 3–4 MightyVites or Super C Chewables daily
- **Adults:** 4–6 tablets daily

**Thyromin**—Thyromin contains ingredients that give support and nutrition to both the thyroid and adrenal glands for a healthier glandular system.
- **Children:** continue to use MightyVites 2–4 daily
- **Adults:** only 1 capsule, 3 times daily

**NingXia Red**—Drink 4–6 oz. of NingXia Red for a delicious and healthy addition to your diet.

## EndoShield™

**Longevity Softgel**—The essential oils in Longevity Softgels increase the oxygen and ATP (adenosine triphosphate) cellular fuel for increasing cell life and immunity for stronger resistance against damage from environmental pollution.
- **Children and teens ages 10–18:** 1–2 capsules daily
- **Adults:** 2–4 capsules daily

**Melrose**—This blend is formulated with two species of Melaleuca oil: *M. alternifolia* and *M. quinquenervia*, also known as Niaouli, which were found through research by Daniel Pénoël, MD, and Pierre Franchomme, PhD, to prevent cellular damage from environmental pollution and potential daily radiation exposure.
- **Children ages 1–3:** 1 drop in yogurt or other liquid
- **Children ages 4–7:** 2 drops in yogurt or other liquid
- **Children 8 and older:** 6 drops per capsule 1–3 times daily or in yogurt or other liquid
- **Adults:** 20 drops per capsule, 1–2 capsules, 1–3 times daily or in yogurt or other liquid

**EndoFlex**—This blend contains oils very specific to the thyroid while at the same time addressing the entire endocrine system. Myrtle oil stimulates and promotes good thyroid health when combined with Spearmint, encouraging better circulation, stronger metabolism, and production of digestive enzymes. Geranium contains esters that protect the thyroid, which may explain why it is so heralded in French publications as a general tonic for the body. It supports the thyroid in being able to uptake iodine from food.
- **Children ages 1–3:** 1 drop in yogurt or other liquid
- **Children ages 4–7:** 2 drops in yogurt or other liquid
- **Children 8 and older:** 6 drops per capsule 2 times daily or in yogurt or other liquid
- **Adults:** 20 drops per capsule, 1–2 capsules, 1–3 times daily or in yogurt or other liquid

**Citrus Fresh**—This blend combines six citrus oils that are naturally antioxidant, antibacterial, and increase the uptake of vitamin C.
- **Children ages 1–3:** 1 drop in yogurt or other liquid
- **Children ages 4–7:** 2 drops in yogurt or other liquid
- **Children 8 and older:** 6 drops per capsule 2 times daily or in yogurt or other liquid
- **Adults:** 20 drops per capsule, 1–2 capsules, 1–3 times daily or in yogurt or other liquid

**NingXia Red**—Drink 4–6 oz. of NingXia Red for a delicious and healthy addition to your diet.

**Essential Oils Desk Reference** | Seventh Edition

cause was determined to be a switch from using clay kitty litter (a standard usage in the industry) to organic kitty litter, whose organic content interacted with the nuclear waste. More than 500 additional drums packed with the wrong type of litter were sealed in heavier containers to prevent their bursting. Numerous other safety issues were cited in the U.S. Department of Energy's official report on the accident" [http://www.lutins.org/nukes.html].

According to the United Nations and the International Atomic Energy Agency, the former Soviet Union's Chernobyl nuclear plant exploded in 1986, killing 56 and eventually leading to the deaths of more than 4,000 from radiation exposure. It is impossible to know what other deaths and illnesses were a result of this exposure, but the radiation caused the deaths of thousands of people and damage to thousands of acres of land, contaminating and destroying plants, trees, crops, and other vegetation growing on numerous farms.

We have a more recent example. "Following a major earthquake, a 15-metre tsunami disabled the power supply and cooling of three Fukushima Daiichi reactors, causing a nuclear accident on 11 March 2011. All three cores largely melted in the first three days. The accident was rated 7 on the INES scale, due to high radioactive releases over days 4 to 6, eventually a total of some 940 PBq (I-131 eq). Four reactors were written off due to damage in the accident" (World Nuclear Association) [http://www.world-nuclear.org/information-library/safety-and-security/safety-of-plants/fukushima-accident.aspx].

Regardless of the contaminated soil, water we drink, food we eat, or air we breathe, it is virtually impossible to escape the effects of the contamination if you are in its silent path. The increase of illness and disease cannot be counted, but the onset of cancer was measurable to some degree and increased dramatically in those affected areas.

Many experts and scientists talk about how air currents can carry the radioactive material from the point of origination around the world. Based on the history of the 1986 Chernobyl nuclear explosion from which thousands of people died, there is a great concern from the people of the world, especially those directly facing the air pathways carrying radioactive material.

D. Gary Young spent two years studying the effects of the Chernobyl disaster and following the path of the radiation in Canada and the United States. He saw the negative effects in his microscopy blood testing, while charting the increased rate of cancer and other related illnesses in those areas.

It is difficult to run and hide from this invisible and odorless danger that can silently fall upon us. What can we do to provide protection for ourselves, families, and loved ones in our homes, work, and outdoor environments?

**Diffusing essential oils** is a very simple and effective way to help safeguard your home. You can start with several different essential oil blends such as Purification, Melrose, and Exodus II. These are three distinct essential oil blends that are very effective in cleansing the air of impurities.

The following information gives you a guideline as to how you can begin diffusing. See additional information in this reference manual about diffusing or go to YoungLiving.com.

There are many different types of diffusers. Some diffuse just with cold air, and others diffuse oil in water that humidifies as well. Some are elaborate and some are simple.

- Diffusing is a matter of choice, and everyone is different. It is fun to try different oils and see what works best.

- Diffuse different essential oil singles or blends throughout the day.

- If you have two diffusers, in one you can diffuse a single oil such as Sacred Frankincense, and in the other, diffuse the blend of Melrose.

- Later, when you want to change oils, you can diffuse a different combination such as Palo Santo in one and Purification in the other.

- Melrose is a particularly powerful blend because it contains two Melaleuca oils that may protect cells from radiation damage, according to Dr. Daniel Pénoël, co-author of the essential oil publication *l'aromathérapie exactement*.

- You can also use other single oils such as Clove, Oregano, Peppermint, Cinnamon Bark, Frankincense, Mountain Savory, etc., and blends such as Exodus II, Raven, and Thieves.

- Another sensible precaution is to wear an inexpensive dust mask while you are outside or traveling. Use Purification, Melrose, Exodus II, or your favorite oil; dilute with water in a small spray bottle; and spray the dust mask. Some oils if used directly, undiluted, may slightly burn or sting the tender skin of the lips or nose, especially of children. Carrying a small spritzer bottle in your pocket enables you to respray the mask and the area in which you are working.

- Using an incense burner, you will further protect your environment by burning Frankincense Resin—an ancient method of purifying the air—throughout your

**386** | **Chapter 19** | Longevity and Vitality - Special Features

Longevity and Vitality - Special Features | **Chapter 19**

home and work environment. You can even burn the Frankincense Resin and diffuse the Frankincense oil at the same time or alternate different oils with the resin burning. We cannot protect our homes too much.

Internally there are also things that you can do to give added protection and strength to your body. Using a gelatin capsule, 00 size, fill the capsule with the number of oil drops recommended and the rest with V-6 or another vegetable oil and take with water one or two times daily or as you desire. Many people will completely fill the capsule with oil when they know how their body will respond.

Enzyme capsules can be emptied into juice or yogurt, especially for smaller children who have a difficult time swallowing capsules.

Below are some of the products you can choose from, and you must determine how much you can take and what is best suited for your body. You may take more or less according to your desire. Some oils and supplements you may want to take every day, and some you may want to alternate. You be the judge.

## Products

**Allerzyme:** 1-2 capsules 3 times a day to digest non-nutritious substances that cause imbalance and irritation

**ComforTone:** 2-3 capsules before breakfast and bedtime to support digestive and colon health

**Detoxzyme:** 3-5 capsules at night to work at digesting toxins while sleeping

**Digest & Cleanse:** 1 softgel capsule 1-3 times daily

**DiGize:** 1-2 capsules of oil daily to help digest and eliminate poisons

**EndoFlex:** 1-2 capsules of oil daily to support the thyroid, often compromised because of the radiation

**Essentialzyme:** 1 caplet 3 times a day to keep general digestion continually working for better nutrient absorption and usability

**Essentialzymes-4:** 2 capsules (1 dual-dose blister pack) 2 times daily with largest meals to aid in the digestion of fats, proteins, fiber, and carbohydrates

**Exodus II:** 1-2 capsules of oil daily to support the immune system

**ICP:** 1-2 teaspoons in the morning in water; a good fiber blend that binds with toxins and helps with elimination; high in rutin from buckwheat, helps to protect against radiation, and stimulates new bone marrow production

**ImmuPro:** 1 tablet before bed to support a healthy immune system

**Inner Defense:** 1 softgel daily or as needed for immune support

**JuvaPower:** 1-2 teaspoons at night to help cleanse the colon

**JuvaSpice:** Sprinkle on salads and use in cooking; has the same nutrient and protective properties as JuvaPower

**KidScents MightyVites and MightyZyme:** Formulated especially for children to provide an all-natural spectrum of critical nutrients for immunity, protection, and vitality

**LavaDerm Cooling Mist:** A spray containing lavender and spikenard essential oils that is very effective in reducing the burning and pain from the slightest to third-degree burns; spray directly on burn; if no pain, it may be rubbed on the skin with your hand. With any kind of a burn, it can be sprayed directly on the burn every 2 or 3 minutes as necessary.

**Life 9:** 1 capsule every night or as needed as a probiotic support for a healthy immune system

**Longevity Softgels:** 1-2 gel caps 2 times daily for immune and glandular support

**Melrose:** 6-20 drops per capsule or in kefir or yogurt 1-3 times a day to prevent radiation damage to normal cells; digests toxic material

**Mineral Essence:** 1 dropper-full per day; protects from mineral depletion, as minerals work as a catalyst for enzyme conversion

**MultiGreens:** 2-4 capsules daily, as green vegetables and kelp are a good source of iodine

**NingXia Red:** 4-6 oz. daily to strengthen body systems

**Sulfurzyme:** Sulfur helps with metal detoxification and free radical neutralization

**Super C or Super C Chewable:** 1-2 tablets daily to strengthen the immune system

**Thyromin:** 1 capsule 3 times a day for thyroid support, which is easily damaged by radiation; capsule may be opened and emptied into yogurt, kefir, or other drink for children who cannot swallow capsules; may have a synergistic, protective effect on your hormonal and immune systems.

Seventh Edition | **Essential Oils Desk Reference** | **387**

## General Guidelines

- **Foods to eat:** Green vegetables and fresh fruits

- **Foods to avoid:** During a particular time of disaster, **do not eat any animal flesh such as red meat, poultry, or fish** for 30 days or more to avoid any contamination there may be to this type of food

- **Water:** 3 liters of **pure water** daily, as well as fresh fruit juices

- **Superoxide dismutase (SOD)** is a very strong intracellular, antioxidant ingredient that helps free radical scavengers as they attack contaminates that try to invade the body.

- **Vitamins C and E** are very supporting to overall health and protect against whole-body radiation exposure.

- **Be sure to eat foods containing antioxidants** that offer protection and especially protect your DNA from damage. These foods should be part of your diet. Lipoic acid and the antioxidants from berries have been proven scientifically to protect your body against radiation damage.

   Recent animal research conducted by the United States Department of Agriculture showed that blueberry and strawberry extracts helped prevent brain damage from radiation exposure. The polyphenols of each different fruit protected different areas of the brain—supporting a variety of dietary berry intake.

- **NingXia Red** is perfect with its many antioxidant berries important for our protection.

- **Seaweeds, seaweed extracts, and miso soup** are good sources of iodine to help detoxify your body of radiation. Baking soda, iodine, glutathione, and clay work as natural chelators.

- **Essential oils** such as Patchouli, Hyssop, Ledum or essential oil blends such as GLF, DiGize, JuvaCleanse, Longevity, Melrose, and Thieves digest and chelate toxins naturally.

- **ICP, JuvaPower, and ComforTone** are very effective for absorbing toxins and digesting waste and help with elimination from the body. Besides that, these natural products have numerous other benefits without toxic overuse and side effects.

- **Many people ask about potassium iodide tablets or tinctures** to protect the thyroid in an emergency situation where there is a high level of radiation exposure. Potassium iodide floods the thyroid and blocks the uptake of radioactive iodine from inhalation and ingestion. Following the 1986 nuclear disaster among the residents of Belarus, the Russian Federation, and Ukraine, up to 2005 more than 6,000 cases of thyroid cancer had been reported in children and adolescents who were exposed to the radiation.

   Many pros and cons often make decisions difficult. People who have iodine sensitivity, dermatitis herpetiformis, hypocomplementemic vasculilitis, and thyroid disorders like Graves' disease should avoid potassium iodide. Therefore, it is better to research the facts in order to make the best choice about whether to take potassium iodide.

- **Sodium bicarbonate or baking soda** taken internally helps block possible damage to the kidneys from uranium exposure, as this is where it often shows up first. Sodium bicarbonate helps alkalinize the urine. It was used at Los Alamos National Laboratory in New Mexico to clean contaminated soil because it binds with uranium and separates it from the dirt. The United States Army also recommends bicarbonate to protect the kidneys from radiation damage.

- **AlkaLime** is specifically formulated with the essential oils of Lemon and Lime to help bring the body into proper pH balance. It settles an upset stomach and calms nauseated feelings that are associated with trauma, contamination, and radiation exposure.

- **Magnesium salts,** magnesium chloride in the form of magnesium bath flakes, or sea salts high in magnesium help to guard against contamination. Keep 5 to 10 pounds of magnesium salts in storage for immediate and emergency use. In 1 cup of salt, mix a few drops of **Purification, Melrose, The Gift** (which includes Sacred Frankincense), or an oil of choice, and then add to bath water. Soaking in the water for 15 to 30 minutes is enjoyable and relaxing while detoxifying contaminates from daily radiation exposure.

- **Chlorella and spirulina powders** help flush radioactive substances from the body and were used heavily by the Russians after the Chernobyl nuclear plant disaster.

- **MultiGreens** is a natural, energizing supplement that contains kelp, spirulina, amino acids, and detoxifying nutrients that synergistically work with the essential oils of Rosemary, Lemon, Lemongrass, and Melissa that cleanses, builds, and stimulates the immune system. The "specific" kelp contains natural iodine that protects the thyroid from daily radiation.

Longevity and Vitality - Special Features | **Chapter 19**

- **Cilantro** helps move heavy metals and radioactive material out of the brain cells for detoxification and elimination.

- **GLF** is a gallbladder and liver flush that aids in eliminating the negative effects of toxins in the body.

- **Radiation exposure** is a real threat to the people of the world, but the responsibility of protection lies with each individual. We are in a time when we must protect ourselves, families, friends, loved ones, and community. We need to help others learn how

to protect themselves using natural products that strengthen the immune system, cleanse the body, and protect against daily pollution, contamination, and dangerous radiation.

- **Essential oils are simple and easy to use.** The benefits are tremendous and can be life giving and long lasting. This natural God-given protection that Mother Nature affords us is ours for the taking. It is without risk or side effects and offers immense benefits that only our bodies can determine when given the opportunity.

# Secrets of Longevity: Living to 100

**The study of longevity** has been a passion of D. Gary Young for over two decades. He has traveled the world studying the cultures of different people known for their longevity. In his research he discovered that these different cultures had two unusual commonalities. The Georgian people in the Caucasus region, in Inner-Mongolia in the Ningxia Province in China, the Hunzakut people in Northern Pakistan, the people of Vilcabamba in southern Ecuador, the people of the Republic of Azerbaijan in the Talish Mountains region in Eurasia, and the Tarahumara natives of Copper Canyon in the southern state of Chihuahua, Mexico, all practiced fasting on a regular basis and lived to be over 120 years of age.

After in-depth studies of the dietary habits of these cultures, he found another common denominator: they lived a very active lifestyle and ate a mineral-rich diet, exceptionally high in antioxidant foods such as wolfberries and apricots. In particular, he found that Chinese wolfberries (*Lycium barbarum* L.) and the potassium-rich apricots of Hunzaland were two foods routinely consumed by people in these regions reaching 110 and 120 years of age.

Fasting allows the body to slow down the secretion of digestive enzymes, thereby permitting an increase in metabolic enzymes that help the body to repair and revitalize tissue that has been damaged or destroyed. Fasting, with time, enables the body to rebuild and spurs an increase in human growth hormone, which impedes premature aging.

The human body has the potential to live for 100 years and beyond. However, devitalized and enzyme-deficient foods deplete our enzyme reserves and overly stress the organs and the body's physical processes. As enzymes continue to decrease, the body's resistance to degenerative disease also decreases.

D. Gary Young, in his book *Longevity Secrets,* discusses

important, scientific, antiaging properties found in these foods, which may be due to their extremely high content of important minerals such as magnesium and potassium, as well as their rich supply of potent natural antioxidants. Research indicates that foods high in antioxidants such as wolfberries, blueberries, strawberries, raspberries, and spinach can dramatically increase glutathione levels and actually reverse the signs of aging.

A new test developed by USDA researchers at Tufts University in Boston, Massachusetts, has been able to identify the highest known antioxidant foods. Known as ORAC (oxygen radical absorbance capacity), this test is the first of its kind to measure both time and degree of free radical inhibition.

The Ningxia wolfberry was documented to have the highest ORAC score of any food tested. A special variety grown on the Yellow River in the Ningxia Province of central China, the Ningxia cultivar is very different from any other type of wolfberry. Among the 17 types of wolfberry identified, the Ningxia wolfberry has by far the highest levels of immune-stimulating polysaccharides. It also possesses over 33 times the antioxidant power of oranges and an amazing 120 times the antioxidant potential of carrots. In addition, the Chinese wolfberry is one of the most nutrient-dense foods known, rich in many vitamins and minerals, including calcium, magnesium, B vitamins, and vitamin C. A diet high in antioxidants can combat the free radical damage in the body associated with premature aging and degenerative diseases.

**A limited caloric intake** of the people living in the remote Hunza Valley in northern Pakistan contributes to their longevity. The Hunzakuts, as they call themselves, commonly live past ages 100, 110, and even 120. They also share another remarkable trait: the near absence of degenerative disease.

Seventh Edition | **Essential Oils Desk Reference** | 389

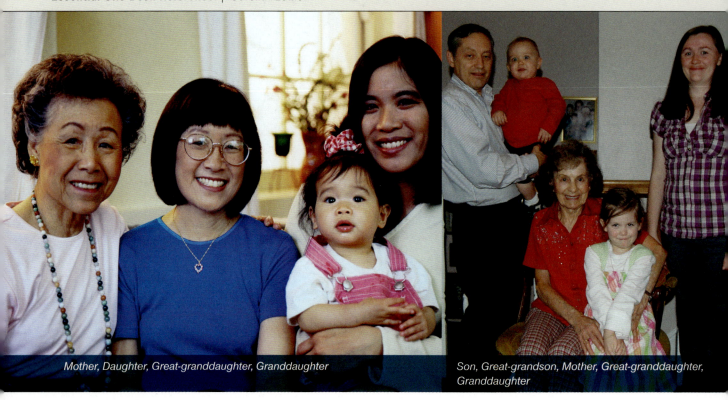

Mother, Daughter, Great-granddaughter, Granddaughter

Son, Great-grandson, Mother, Great-granddaughter, Granddaughter

The diet of the Hunza people is known to be high in potassium and low in sodium. Apricots, barley, millet, and buckwheat are the main staples of their diet along with mineral-rich water with a pH of 8.5. But there is yet another unusual factor that may protect the health of the Hunza people and increase their longevity: their limited food intake.

Because the land provides just enough food to cover their basic caloric needs, the Hunzakuts rarely indulge in overeating. In fact, prior to the construction of the Karakoram Highway, they annually endured near-fasting conditions for several weeks each spring, a time when the previous year's food supply was depleted, and the current year's harvests had not yet begun.

Restricted caloric intake such as fasting can have powerful effects on longevity because it increases blood levels of growth hormone, which is one of the most significant antiaging hormones to be identified during the last two decades. Secreted by the pituitary gland, growth hormone production steadily declines with age. By age 70, the human body produces less than one tenth of the growth hormone it did at age 20.

Clinical studies have repeatedly shown that growth hormone production is stimulated by low glucose levels. Because fasting depresses glucose levels, it leads to a surge in natural growth hormone production (Khansari, et al., 1991).

A university study showed that older adults are the fastest growing segment of the U.S. population and a greater proportion of them are obese. Seven randomized controlled studies revealed that calorie restriction combined with exercise is effective for weight loss (Locher, et al., 2016). Calorie restriction was tested among healthy non-obese adults and was found to be safe and well tolerated (Romashkan, et al., 2016).

Unfortunately, the historical cultures of "longevity and superior health and endurance" are fading away and will only be something we read about in history books. The world is more connected than ever before through the high technology of cell phones, television, media production, and satellite proliferation. The advancement of processed and prepackaged food has infiltrated every country in the world.

The use of synthetic and nature-identical chemicals in the industries of food, body care products, cosmetics, perfumes, household cleaners, drugs, and over-the-counter medicines have gradually brought a decline in health and longevity. Literally every aspect of our lives is contaminated through the food we put in our bodies, the creams and lotions we put on our bodies, the water we drink, and the air we breathe.

We are becoming a world of the sick and obese as the fast-food industry proliferates, we eat frozen dinners, and just "add water" or "pop the pizza in the oven" for a quick

Longevity and Vitality - Special Features | **Chapter 19**

meal. We open millions of cans of vegetables and fruits, eat sugar and chemically colored and preserved desserts, and gulp down snacks devoid of nutritional substance. It is sad to see that so many people are content to eat this way and then wonder why they feel awful, have no energy, and are just plain sick.

How sad to see babies and children alike grow with mental and physical deficiencies because society is not teaching anything better to parents, teachers, and those who could have an influence. For those who do see what is happening and want to help change things, the vision is immense. Correct information is the key, and we can all get involved in whatever way is possible. We need to help people become educated, so they can change their habits before they find themselves fighting an unhealthy condition and trying to save the lives of children heading down the wrong path.

It's up to us how we choose to become involved. Money talks and if you can become involved with a health-focused company or even build a business in a company that is teaching correct principles, you will have the best of both worlds. Build your business and become the master of your own time and money. You will have the products that you need and the money to educate and disseminate information. After all, word of mouth is one of the most effective ways to spread the news.

Now is the time to act, so join with thousands of others in the world whose mission is to bring health and a better way of life to those in the world they can touch.

# Sweeteners: Making the Right Choice

Many of today's health concerns are caused by so-called modern conveniences. Increased use of sugars and artificial sweeteners raises the question, "What's the difference between sugars; synthetic sweeteners; and natural, low-glycemic sweeteners?"

## Sugars

Do you remember when "treats" were for special occasions? For many families, eating sweets now begins at breakfast and continues all day long. Instead of a hearty serving of oatmeal, today's children are growing up on bowls of miniature chocolate doughnuts or sugar-coated cereals. Sweet snacks, drinks, and desserts continue until bedtime—and children aren't the only ones guzzling and gulping down sugar. How often have you seen an adult leave a convenience store toting a 64-ounce soft drink?

Nothing stresses the human body as much as refined sugar. Called a "skeletonized food" and a "castrated carbohydrate" by Edward Howell, PhD, and a "metabolic freeloader" by Ralph Golan, MD, sugar actually drains the body of vitamins, minerals, and nutrients in the process of being burned for energy. Sugar also stresses the pancreas, forcing it to pump out a surge of unneeded digestive enzymes.

Sugar also undermines and retards immune response. One study measured the effects of 100 grams of sugar (sucrose) on neutrophils, a form of white blood cell that comprises a central part of immunity. Within one hour of ingestion, neutrophil activity dropped 50 percent and remained below normal for another four hours (Castleman, 1997).

Population studies have also linked sugar consumption with diabetes and heart disease. According to researcher John Yudkin, the reason sugar elevates the risk of heart disease is due to an automatic, built-in safety switch inside the body. To protect itself from being immediately poisoned from excess sugar, the body converts it into fats, like triglycerides. So instead of killing you quickly, the body defends itself by clogging its arteries, thereby killing you on the installment plan.

## High-Fructose Corn Syrup

Ever on the lookout for a cheaper sweetener, scientists figured out how to take corn syrup, add genetically modified enzymes, and in a long chemical process, create a corn sweetener with more fructose than is found in nature (e.g., honey). The high-fructose corn syrup (HFCS) blend that is used in soft drinks, for instance, is 55 percent fructose. For low-calorie "diet" products, a blend has been concocted that has a 90-10 fructose to glucose ratio. This refined blend is intensely sweet.

Between 1970 when HFCS was introduced in the U.S. and 2000, consumer consumption jumped from less than 1 pound per person to over 60 pounds yearly. "Coincidentally," something else jumped during that time frame: obesity.

Researchers at Louisiana State University and the University of North Carolina studied food consumption patterns using USDA tables from 1967 to 2000 and found that HFCS consumption increased more than 1,000 percent between 1970 and 1990. They concluded that ". . . overconsumption of HFCS in calorically sweetened

Seventh Edition | **Essential Oils Desk Reference** | 391

beverages may play a role in the epidemic of obesity."[61]

A December 2013 animal study published in the journal *Nutrition & Diabetes,* found that HFCS induced more severe adipose inflammation and insulin resistance than an even higher-calorie-containing 'Western' high-fat diet and concluded that "HFCS has detrimental effects on metabolism, suggesting that dietary guidelines on HFCS consumption need to be revisited."[62]

There is yet more bad health news about HFCS. In October 2008, *The New York Times* reported that in a study tracking over 9,000 people, those who drank two or more sugary sodas a day (a major source of high-fructose corn syrup) were at a 40 percent higher risk for kidney damage, while the risk for women soda drinkers nearly doubled. NYT writer Tara Parker-Pope noted that a study published in the *Journal of Hepatology* ". . . suggested a link between consumption of high-fructose corn syrup in sodas and fatty liver disease."[63] Parker-Pope also wrote about a smaller study in *The Journal of Nutrition* that suggested that fructose bypasses the normal regulation of sugar and is turned to fat more quickly than other sugars.

It seems that people are beginning to awaken to the problems with this highly-processed sweetener. A 2010 NYT article reported market research showing that ". . . 58 percent of Americans say they are concerned that high-fructose corn syrup poses a health risk."[64] The Corn Refiners Association is fighting back. An advertising blitz in 2008 emphasized that ". . . HFCS is made from corn, has no artificial ingredients, and is fine in moderation." Because HFCS is in a staggering amount of food, the U.S. *Time Magazine* wryly noted, ". . . unless you're making a concerted effort to avoid it, it's pretty difficult to consume high-fructose corn syrup in moderation."[65]

### Petition for a Name Change

Because the public perceives high-fructose corn syrup (HFCS) as dangerous, a backlash has developed. Marion Nestle, a New York University professor of nutrition, said that you have to feel sorry for the corn refiners since "High-fructose corn syrup is the new trans fat."[66]

Seattle's PCC Natural Markets banned all products containing HFCS. Jason's Deli, a restaurant chain with 200 restaurants in 27 states, replaced all items that contain HFCS, except for some soft drinks. In May 2010, Hunt's ketchup returned to regular sugar because of buyer preference. Snapple, Gatorade, and Starbucks' baked goods also avoid HFCS now. Ocean Spray Cranberry Juice and Wheat Thins crackers also promote "no HFCS."

The backlash is beginning to be significant. After being scolded by a blogger, Chick-Fil-A has removed HFCS and

artificial colors from its sauces and dressings; and by the end of 2014, HFCS will be gone from sandwich buns as well.

In September of 2010, The Corn Refiners Association petitioned the FDA to start calling HFCS "corn sugar." The president of the organization believes that HFCS is confusing to consumers and thinks that the "term 'corn sugar' succinctly and accurately describes what this natural ingredient is and where it comes from—corn." HFCS is hardly "natural." We like what one health writer suggested for its new name: "enzymatically altered corn glucose."

In a win for health-conscious consumers, in March of 2012 the FDA rejected the Corn Refiners Association bid to rename HFCS as "corn sugar."

Regardless of the failed name change, sales of high fructose corn syrup are in decline. A February 2016 report by the USDA reported: "Domestic use of high-fructose corn syrup (HFCS) declined 0.8 percent in the 2014/15 fiscal year (October 1-September 30) to 7.2 million short tons, continuing a decade-long decline. Since 2004/05, domestic use has fallen by 19.1 percent, and it is down 21.8 percent since its peak in 2001/01." http://www.ers.usda.gov/data-products/chart-gallery/detail.aspx?chartId=56605.

### Synthetic Sweeteners

Health dangers are also found in the use of artificial sweeteners. Seventy-five percent of the adverse reactions reported to the U.S. Food and Drug Administration come from a single substance: the artificial sweetener aspartame. But a newer artificial sweetener, sucralose, may be challenging those numbers with a whole host of new adverse reactions.

### Sucralose (Splenda™)

Perhaps it is enough to explain that Splenda is chlorinated sugar. The structure of sugar molecules is changed by substituting three chlorine atoms for three hydroxyl groups. How healthy does that sound? However, few human studies have been published. The FDA's "Final Rule" report stated, "Sucralose was weakly mutagenic [capable of causing mutations] in a mouse lymphoma mutation assay," and other reports by the FDA were "inconclusive."

Dr. Mercola's website posted this about sucralose: "According to Consumers Research Magazine, 'Some concern was raised about sucralose being a chlorinated molecule. Some chlorinated molecules serve as the basis for pesticides such as DDT and accumulate in body fat. However, Johnson & Johnson emphasized that sucralose passes through the body unabsorbed.'" However, the

FDA's "Final Report" states that 11 percent to 27 percent of sucralose is absorbed by humans, and the rest is excreted unchanged in feces. According to the Japanese Food Sanitation Council, as much as 40 percent of ingested sucralose is absorbed.

Dr. Mercola concludes, "Considering that Splenda bears more chemical similarity to DDT than it does to sugar, are you willing to bet your health on this data? Remember that fat soluble substances, such as DDT, can remain in your fat for decades and devastate your health."[67]

The big news is that in January of 2016, a study was published in the *International Journal of Occupational and Environmental Health* showing that mice fed sucralose daily throughout their lives developed leukemia and other blood cancers. The nonprofit watchdog group Center for Science in the Public Interest had downgraded Splenda from "safe" to "caution" and now recommends that consumers *avoid* Splenda.

A 2008 animal study warns us: "[T]here are two major points to take home. First, relatively low amounts of Splenda (100mg/kg/day) may cause *weight gain*. And second, Splenda at moderate levels (300mg/kg/day and up) has adverse effects on your gut, affecting both levels of gut flora and proteins. Why does this matter? Changes in gut bacteria can lead to problems with your immune system and ability to absorb nutrients" [http://www.precisionnutrition.com/research-review-splenda-is-it-safe].

It is darkly humorous that two makers of artificial sweeteners went to court because the makers of NutraSweet believed that Splenda received an unfair advantage with its sneaky slogan "Made from sugar so it tastes like sugar." McNeil Nutritionals later changed the slogan to "Starts with sugar, tastes like sugar, but is not sugar." But the "unfair" slogan did its job. Between 2000 and 2004, the percentage of U.S. households using Splenda jumped from 3 to 20 percent. In a one-year period, Splenda sales topped $177 million compared with $62 million spent on aspartame-based Equal and $52 million on saccharin-based Sweet'N Low®.[68]

Is Sucralose natural? Far from it! Is it safe? Science now tells us, NO!

## Aspartame

Aspartame is marketed today as NutraSweet®, Equal®, and Equal® Spoonful. With so many Americans on one diet or another, the market for aspartame is simply enormous—and it matters not that aspartame users are suffering from symptoms ranging from headaches, numbness, and seizures to joint pain, chronic fatigue syndrome, multiple sclerosis, and epilepsy.

The 1996 book by Dr. Russell L. Blaylock, professor of neurosurgery at the Medical University of Mississippi, *Excitotoxins: The Taste That Kills*, explains that aspartame is a neurotransmitter, facilitating the transmission of information from one neuron to another. Aspartame allows too much calcium into brain cells, killing certain neurons, earning aspartame the name of "excitotoxin."

With aspartame now in over 9,000 products such as instant breakfasts, breath mints, cereals, frozen desserts, "lite" gelatin desserts, and even multivitamins, it is no surprise that there is a virtual epidemic of memory loss, Alzheimer's disease, and multiple sclerosis. In a move much like a telephone company selling your phone number to telephone solicitors and then charging you to block their calls, G. D. Searle (the Monsanto company that manufactures aspartame) is searching for a drug to combat memory loss caused by excitatory amino acid damage, most often caused by aspartame.

Do you fly the friendly skies? You may be interested to know that both the Air Force's magazine, *Flying Safety*, and *Navy Physiology*, the Navy's publication, detailed warnings about pilots being more susceptible to seizures after consuming aspartame. The Aspartame Consumer Safety Network notes that 600 pilots have reported acute reactions to aspartame, including grand mal seizures in the cockpit. Many other publications have warned about aspartame ingestion while flying, including a paper presented at the 57th Annual Meeting of the Aerospace Medical Association.

A final note: The Center for Science in the Public Interest (CSPI) may only currently urge "caution" for Splenda, but for saccharin, aspartame, and acesulfame potassium (Sunett and Sweet One), it says "avoid."

## Natural, Low-Glycemic Sweeteners

Natural, low-glycemic sweeteners are excellent alternatives to the sugar dilemma and include the six kinds mentioned below.

## Blue Agave Nectar

The blue agave cactus grows in Central America. It produces a sweetener that is about 68 percent fructose, 22 percent glucose, and 4 percent fructooligosaccharides. Because of its heavy fructose concentration, Blue Agave is 32 percent sweeter than table sugar but has a low glycemic index (about 34). This means that when consumed, Blue Agave has a minimal impact on blood sugar levels following consumption. It is well suited for people with candida infections.

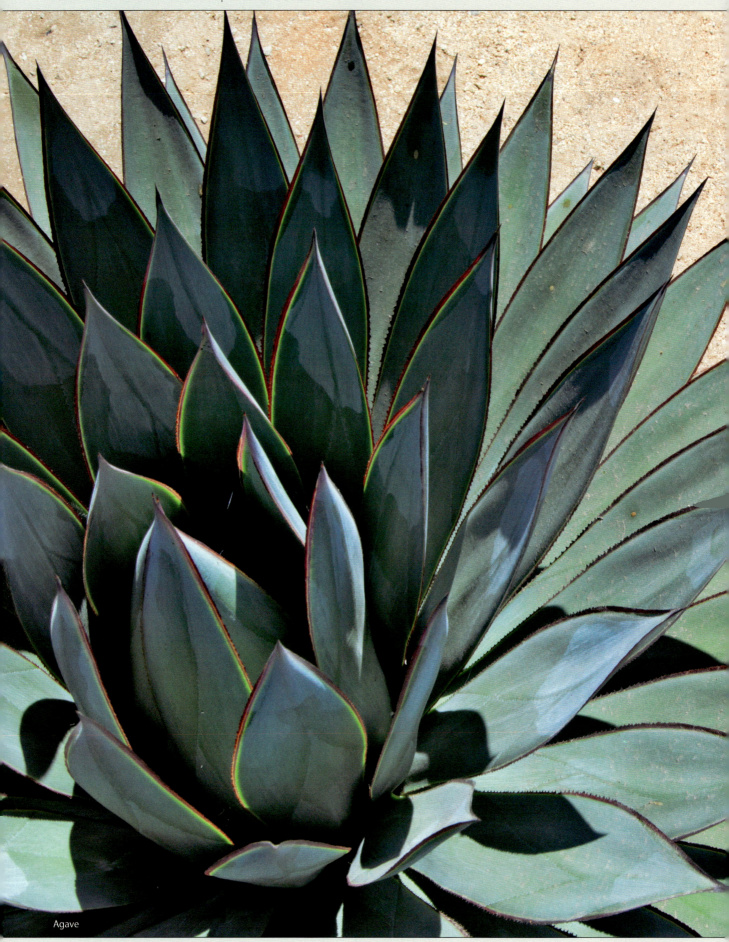
Agave

Longevity and Vitality - Special Features | **Chapter 19**

## FOS

FOS is a supernutrient documented to rebuild intestinal flora, improve mineral absorption, and more; its attributes are shown below.

- Has a minimal impact on blood sugar levels
- Has a glycemic index of 0
- Is an ideal sweetener for diabetics
- Increases populations of beneficial bifidobacteria in the colon
- Reduces populations of harmful bacteria, such as *Clostridium perfringens*
- Improves calcium and magnesium absorption
- Improves liver function

A naturally sweet, indigestible fiber derived from chicory roots, FOS (fructooligosaccharides) is one of the best-documented classes of natural nutrients for promoting the growth of *Lactobacilli* and *bifidobacteria* (beneficial bacteria), a key to sound health. FOS has also been clinically studied for its ability to increase magnesium and calcium absorption; lower blood glucose, cholesterol, and LDL levels; and inhibit production of the reductase enzymes that can contribute to cancer. Because FOS can increase magnesium absorption, it can also lead to lowered blood pressure and better cardiovascular health.

FOS is one of the most powerful prebiotics to be researched in the last decade (a "prebiotic" feeds intestinal flora; a "probiotic" adds more actual cultures to existing intestinal flora). The subject of over 400 clinical studies (as of December 26, 2013), FOS is one of the best-documented, natural nutrients for improving the healthy balance of bacteria in intestines and stimulating the growth of the beneficial *bifidobacteria*—also called "friendly flora"—that reside in the colon.

How important to good health are these so-called "friendly flora" that populate our intestines? They are our front-line defense against invading, disease-causing organisms, combating premature aging caused by the toxin-producing bacteria and fungi that reside in our intestines.

### FOS Builds Up Friendly Flora

| Subjects | Dose g/day | Duration | Fecal Bifidobacteria # bacteria (log) per gram | | Reference |
|---|---|---|---|---|---|
| 9 | 1 | 14 | 9.8 | 10.2 | Tokunaga, 92 |
| 9 | 3 | 14 | 9.9 | 10.4 | Tokunaga, 92 |
| 9 | 5 | 14 | 9.7 | 10.3 | Tokunaga, 92 |
| 20 | 12.5 | 12 | 7.9 | 9.1 | Bouhnik, 93 |
| 38 | 8 | 14 | 5.2 | 6.2 | Rochat, 94 |
| 12 | 4 | 25 | 9.5 | 9.8 | Buddington, 96 |

Start of Study    End of Study

## Seven Reasons Why Bifidobacteria Are Vital to Health

1. They produce substances that stop the growth of harmful, toxic, gram-negative and -positive bacteria in the intestines (Tejero-Sariñena S, 2013).

2. They occupy space on the intestinal wall that could be populated by pathogenic organisms. When bifidobacteria increase in numbers, they crowd out invasive, toxin-generating microorganisms.

3. They slow down the production of damaging protein-breakdown products, such as ammonia. This lowers blood ammonia levels that can be toxic to the human body (Biagi G, 2013).

4. They produce B vitamins and folic acid (D'Aimmo MR, 2013; LeBlanc JG, 2013).

5. They produce digestive enzymes, like phosphatases and lysozymes (Minagawa E, 1985).

6. They stimulate the immune system and promote immune attack against cancer cells (Vitaliti G, 2013; Chong ES, 2013; Harata G, 2010).

7. They increase the absorption of essential minerals, magnesium, and calcium. As we age, magnesium levels in the body decline, contributing to high blood pressure and diabetes.

Technically a fiber rather than a sugar, FOS is totally unlike conventional sugars because it feeds the beneficial *bifidobacteria* while selectively starving the parasitical yeast, fungi, and bacteria that contribute to disease. Most toxin-producing microorganisms in the intestines are unable to use FOS as food. Conventional sugars, like sucrose and lactose on the other hand, work in just the opposite fashion: they tend to feed harmful bacteria more readily than they feed beneficial bacteria.

### FOS Increases Mineral Absorption

Besides building up the beneficial bacteria in the body, FOS has also been shown to improve blood sugar control, liver function, and calcium and magnesium absorption.

A 2010 animal study conducted at the Shandong Centre for Tuberculosis Control in China found that a FOS diet increased magnesium and calcium absorption substantially. A study at the University of Murcia in Spain obtained similar results (Sabater-Molina M, 2009).

Magnesium is one of the most important nutrients we obtain from our diet, being involved in over 300 enzyme reactions in the body. As we age, our magnesium levels drop markedly, which creates a deficiency that increases the risk of angina, atherosclerosis, cardiac arrhythmias, depression, and diabetes (González W, 2013; Hruby A, 2013; Blaszczyk U, 2013; Serefko A, 2013). A Medical University of Ohio study suggested that correcting magnesium deficiencies may prolong life (Rowe WJ, 2012).

FOS also improves liver health. A Louvain Drug Research Institute study at Catholic University in Brussels, Belgium, reported that dietary fructooligosaccharides reduced hepatic triglyceride accumulation and thus provide an advantage in the management of liver disease (Pachikian BD, 2013).

FOS may be the ideal nutrient for diabetics. Because FOS is an indigestible sugar, it triggers no spikes in blood sugar levels the way sucrose and glucose do. About 40 to 60 percent as sweet as sugar, FOS is found in low quantities in many types of foods. However, to obtain just a quarter teaspoon of FOS from foods in your diet, you would have to consume 13 bananas, 16 tomatoes, or 16 onions. Chicory roots have one of the highest amounts of FOS of any plant, and most natural FOS supplements are commercially derived from water-extraction of the roots.

*Recommended Usage*

To obtain the best results from FOS, daily intake should range between 5 and 10 grams a day. Dosages above 15 grams may cause gas or intestinal cramping from excess bifidobacteria populations.

## Fructose

Do NOT confuse fructose with high-fructose corn syrup! Fructose is a natural sweetener that has one of the lowest glycemic indexes of any food. A glycemic index measures the impact that a food has on blood sugar levels two to three hours after ingestion. The lower the glycemic level, the lower the rise in blood sugar levels.

With a glycemic index of only 20, fructose has one of the lowest of any food and many times lower than standard breads and processed grains. Fructose has a glycemic index that is only a third that of glucose, a fourth of the glycemic index of white bread, and a fifth of the glycemic index of boiled potatoes.

## Maple Syrup – Grade B

The U.S. and Canada have slightly different grading systems for maple syrup. What is classified as Grade B maple syrup in the U.S. is the same as Grade C maple syrup in Canada. This grade is the best sweetener and the most balanced sugar. It is processed from the last tapping of the maple sap, so it is richer in invert sugars and minerals.

Grade B maple syrup is also a lower-glycemic-index food, resulting in a slow, gradual rise in blood sugar levels. The best maple syrup is currently produced in Vermont because it is strictly regulated for purity and authenticity by government law. Some unscrupulous marketers in other areas have been known to add refined sugars to colored, diluted, genuine maple syrup to produce a cheaper product. Also a number of years ago, there was a problem with some Canadian and U.S. producers inserting formaldehyde pellets in their sugar maple trees to keep tap holes open longer, increasing yields.

## Stevia

For over 1,600 years, the natives of Paraguay in South America have used this intensely sweet herb as a health agent and sweetener. Known as *Stevia rebaudiana* by botanists and yerba dulce (honey leaf) by the Guarani Indians, stevia has been incorporated into many native medicines, beverages, and foods for centuries. The Guarani used stevia separately or combined with herbs like yerba mate and lapacho.

Fifteen times sweeter than sugar, stevia was introduced to the West in 1899, when M. S. Bertoni discovered natives using it as a sweetener and medicinal herb. However, stevia was very slow to gain popularity in Europe or the United States and was only gradually adopted by several countries throughout Far East Asia.

With Japan's ban on the import of synthetic sweeteners in the 1960s, stevia began to be seriously researched by the Japanese National Institute of Health as a natural sugar substitute. After almost a decade of studies examining the safety and antidiabetic properties of the herb, Japan became a major producer, importer, and user of stevia. Japanese food companies began including stevia in hundreds of products, and eventually stevia use spread through Asia. Stevioside, the super sweet glycoside derived from stevia that is 300 times sweeter than sugar, was even used to sweeten Diet Coke sold in Japan.

Stevia has now gained widespread popularity as a low-calorie sweetener throughout the United States, South America, and Asia. Both the stevia leaf and stevioside are used in Taiwan, China, Korea, and Japan, with many of these same countries growing and harvesting large amounts of the raw herb.

In 1994, the U.S. Food and Drug Administration permitted the importation and use of stevia as a dietary supplement. But the FDA would not approve stevia for use as a food additive until the Coca-Cola Company expressed interest in approval of rebiana, its stevia-derived sweetener. In May 2008, Coca-Cola and Cargill introduced Truvia, a stevia sweetener containing erythritol and rebiana. Now stevia is considered GRAS.

Stevia, however, is more than just a noncaloric sweetener. Several modern clinical studies have documented the ability of stevia to lower and balance blood sugar levels, support the pancreas, protect the liver, and combat infectious microorganisms (Ritu, Nandini, 2016; Rizzo, et al., 2013; Chen, et al., 2006; Gamboa, Chaves, 2012; Belda-Galbis, et al., 2014).

Research has also documented stevia's powerful antioxidant and oxidative DNA damage preventive activity (Shivanna, et al., 2013; Ghanta, et al., 2007).

Regarding stevia and diabetes, one seminal study, (Oviedo, et al., 1971) showed that oral administration of a stevia leaf extract reduced blood sugar levels by over 35 percent. Another study (Suzuki, et al., 1977) documented similar results. Clearly, these and other clinical evaluations indicate that stevia holds significant promise for the treatment of diabetes.

## Yacon

Yacon is a tubular, perennial plant that looks similar to a yam or sweet potato, only with a black skin, that is indigenous of Ecuador and Peru and provides interesting nutritional products such as yacon syrup, yacon tea, and sweet candy-like snacks. These products are very popular, especially among diabetics, because the sugar they contain is not absorbed by humans.

Beyond the healthy sweetening of yacon are even more health benefits because it contains FOS. According to Wikipedia, "This form of sugar, known as FOS (fructooligosaccharide), a special kind of fructose, leaves the body undigested. The syrup is also a prebiotic, which means that it feeds the friendly bacteria in the colon that boost the immune system and help digestion.[69] (See "FOS Increases Mineral Absorption" above.)

Yacon has recently been transplanted to New Zealand and is being studied by the universities as perhaps the world's greatest-kept secret as a sweetener that has a zero glycemic index (a measure to show the impact of sugar on the pancreas), no negative effects on the body, safe for diabetics, safe for hypoglycemics, and safe for people with candida.

A Brazilian university study regarded yacon as a functional food because it "improves the growth of bifidobacteria in the colon, enhances mineral absorption and gastrointestinal metabolism and plays a role in the regulation of serum cholesterol" (Delgado GT, 2013).

Because yacon grows in the ground as a tubular in the Andes Mountains, its roots are able to take advantage of the thousands of years of volcanic ash build-up that has a tremendous high mineral content. As the yacon grows, it takes up many of these minerals and converts them into a usable form within the natural sugars. Besides its high mineral content, it is also high in amino acids and vitamin A, as in carrots, making yacon very similar in profile to the Ningxia wolfberry. Yacon has also been studied as an antidiabetic treatment and is now being studied as a preventive for digestive cancers.

**What about refined sugars and laboratory-made sweeteners?** There is so much research available about them that one cannot deny their dangers, with obesity and heart disease on the top of the list. We have to be responsible, make tough decisions, and discipline ourselves. We must not allow sugar, synthetic sweeteners, or foods made with these substances to be on our "sweet" list any more.

Unfortunately, sugar and these synthetic sweeteners are used in a great many food recipes. It is impossible to know if these ingredients have been used in the food prepared for us to eat in restaurants, at school or work, as snacks and pastries at parties, or even when invited to dinner in a friend's home. But if we avoid these dangerous and other undesirable ingredients whenever possible and read the labels before buying groceries at a store, including a health food store, the smaller amounts that we do ingest that we cannot detect and avoid will be digested and eliminated by a healthy body.

Is it easy to make any food sweet naturally? Yes. Even certain fruits make tasty, sweet food dishes. Strawberries, boysenberries, peaches, apples, and other fruits can be used as sweeteners in cooking and baking cakes, cookies, breads, and other recipes made at home. Dark colored fruits mixed with Blue Agave, Yacon Syrup, or maple syrup easily color and sweeten cream cheese for a delicious frosting.

The health food industry has used these types of foods for sweetening and coloring for years, but now other food processors and manufacturers outside the health food industry are catching on, and the public is responding positively. We do not need unhealthful sweetening substances. We are so fortunate that Mother Nature has given us so many nutritious alternatives. Let's satisfy our sweet tooth and enjoy our sweets in a naturally sweet way.

# ENDNOTES

1. Hayflick L. *How and Why We Age*. Ballantine Books, New York, 1994.
2. Harmon D. Ageing: a theory based on free radical and radiation chemistry. *J. Gerontology* 11, 1956:298-300.
3. Harmon D. Free radical theory of ageing: Effect of free radical inhibitors on the mortality rate of male LAF mice. *J. Gerontology* 23, 1968:476-482.
4. Harmon D. Free radical theory of ageing: Effect of the amount and degree of unsaturation of dietary fat on mortality rate. *J. Gerontology* 26, 1971:451-457.
5. Stubbs CD and Smith AD. The modification of mammalian membrane polyunsaturated fatty acid composition in relation to membrane fluidity and function. *Biochimica et Biophysica Acta* 779, 1984:89-137.
6. Barja de Quiroga G, et al. Antioxidant defenses and peroxidation in liver and brain of aged rats. *Biochemical Journal* 272, 1990:247-250.
7. Lamptey MS and Walker BL. A possible dietary role for linolenic acid in the development of the young rat. *Journal of Nutrition* 106, 1976:86-93.
8. Okuyama H. Minimum requirements of n-3 and n-6 essential fatty acids for the function of the central nervous system and for the prevention of chronic disease. *Proceedings of the Society for Experimental Biology and Medicine 200*, 1992:174-176.
9. Yamamoto, et al. Effects of dietary alpha-linolenate/linolenate balance of brain lipid composition and learning ability of rats. *Journal of Lipid Research* 28, 1987:144-151.
10. Bourre, et al. Function of dietary polyunsaturated fatty acids in the nervous system. *Prostaglandins, Leukotrienes, and Essential Fatty Acids* 48, 1993:5-15.
11. Farag R, et al. Antioxidant activity of some spice essential oils on linoleic acid oxidation in aqueous media. *JAOCS*, June 1989;66:792-799.
12. Farag R, et al. Inhibitory effects of individual and mixed pairs of essential oils on the oxidation and hydrolysis of cottonseed oil and butter. *FASC*, 1989;40:275-279.
13. Farag R, et al. Safety evaluation of thyme and clove essential oils as natural antioxidants. *Afr J Agr Sci*. 1991;18:169-17.
14. Rotstein, et al. Effects of aging on the composition and metabolism of docosahexaenoate-containing lipids of retina. *Lipids*, 1987 Apr;22(4):253-60.
15. Neuringer M and Connor WE. N-3 fatty acids in the brain and retina: evidence for their essentiality. *Nutrition Reviews* 44:285-294.
16. Youdim KA, et al. Effect of thyme oil and thymol dietary supplementation on the antioxidant status and fatty acid composition of the ageing rat brain. *Br J Nutr*. 2000 Jan;83(1):87-93.
17. Youdim KA and Deans SG. Dietary supplementation of thyme (Thymus vulgaris L.) essential oil during the lifetime of the rat: its effects on the antioxidant status in liver, kidney and heart tissues. *Mech Ageing Dev*. 1999 Sep 8;109(3):163-75.
18. Zheng GQ, et al. Sesquiterpenes from clove (Eugenia caryophyllata) as potential anticarcinogenic agents. *J Nat Prod*. 1992 Jul;55(7):999-1003.
19. Rompelberg, et al. Antimutagenicity of eugenol in the rodent bone marrow micronucleus test. *Mutat Res*. 1995 Feb;346(2):69-75.
20. Sukumaran, et al. Inhibition of tumour promotion in mice by eugenol. *Indian J Physiol Pharmacol*. 1994 Oct;38(4):306-8.
21. Yokota H, et al. Suppressed mutagenicity of benzo[a]pyrene by the liver S9 fraction and microsomes from eugenol-treated rats. *Mutat Res*. 1986 Dec;172(3):231-6.
22. Iwano H, Yokota H, Effect of dietary eugenol on xenobiotic metabolism and mediation of UDP-glucuronosyltransferase and cytochrome P450 1A1 expression in rat liver. *Int J Food Sci Nutr*. 2013 Oct 21.
23. Grandjean P, Landrigan PJ. *Lancet Neurol*. 2014 Mar;13(3):330-8.
24. Woofinden B. Fluoride water 'causes cancer': Boys at risk from bone tumours, shock research reveals, *The London Observer*, June 12, 2005.
25. Takahashi K, Akiniwa K, Narita K. Regression analysis of cancer incidence rates and water fluoride in the U.S.A. based in IACRI/IARC (WHO) data (1978-1992), *J Epidemiol*. 2001 Jul;11(4):170-9.
26. Cohn PD. An Epidemiological Report on Drinking Water and Fluoridation, *New Jersey Department of Health, Environmental Health Services*, Nov. 1992.
27. Bassin EB, Wypij D, Davis RB, Mittleman MA. Age-specific fluoride exposure in drinking water and osteosarcoma (United States), *Cancer Causes Control*. 2006 May;17(4):421-8.
28. DeNoon DJ. Does Fluoridation Up Bone Cancer Risk? Study Examines Boyhood Drinking of Fluoridated Water and Possible Links to Osteosarcoma, WebMD Health News, April 6, 2006, http://www.webmd.com/cancer/news/20060406/does-fluoridation-up-bone-cancer-risk.
29. Fluoride Action Network's Statement on Harvard Investigation, August 16, 2006, http://www.fluoridealert.org/harvard/.
30. http://fluoridealert.org/researchers/harvard/conflicts/.
31. http://www.slweb.org/f-bone.cancer.html
32. http://www.cdc.gov/nchs/data/databriefs/db53.htm.
33. https://yosemite.epa.gov/opa/admpress.nsf/6427a6b7538955c585257359003f0230/86964af577c37ab285257811005a8417!OpenDocument.
34. Washington Action for Safe Water, Press-Release-HHS, January 24, 2011. US government proposed regulation of fluoridation does not go far enough. http://washingtonsafewater.com/.
35. National Research Council. Fluoride in Drinking Water: A Scientific Review of EPA's Standards. *National Academies Press*, Washington, DC. 2006.
36. Ibid.

37. Hao P, et al. Effect of fluoride on human hypothalamus-hypophysis-testis axis, *Wei Sheng Yan Jiu*, 2010 Jan;39(1):53-5.
38. Danielson C, et al. Hip fractures and fluoridation in Utah's elderly population, *JAMA*, 1992 Aug 12;268(6):746-8.
39. Alarcón-Herrera MT, et al. Well Water Fluoride, Dental Fluorosis, and Bone Fractures in the Guadiana Valley of Mexico, *Fluoride* Vol. 34, No. 2, 139-149, 2001 Research Report.
40. Karademir S, et al. Effects of fluorosis on QT dispersion, heart rate variability and echocardiographic parameters in children, *Anadolu Kardiyol Derg*. 2011 Feb. 23. doi: 10.5152/akd.2011.038.
41. http://zipcodezoo.com/Key/Plantae/Boswellia_Genus.asp.
42. Hepper FN. Arabian and African Frankincense Trees, *J. of Egyptian Archaeology*, Vol. 55, Aug. 1969:66-72.
43. Frank MB, Yang Q, Lin HK, et al. Frankincense oil derived from Boswellia carteri induces tumor cell specific toxicity, *BMC Complement Altern Med.*, 2009 Mar 18;9:6.
44. Ibid.
45. Akihista T, et al. Cancer chemopreventive effects and cytotoxic activities of the triterpene acids from the resin of Boswellia carteri, *Biol Pharm Bull*. 2006 Sep;29(9):1976-9.
46. Chevrier M, et al. Boswellia carteri Extract Inhibits TH1 Cytokines and Promotes TH2 Cytokines in Vitro, *Clin Diagn Lab Immunol*. 2005 May;12(5):575-89.
47. Highet J. *Frankincense: Oman's Gift to the World*, Prestel Publishing, 2006:66.
48. Al-Harrasi A, Al-Saidi S. Phytochemical Analysis of the Essential Oil from Botanically Certified Oleogum Resin of Boswellia sacra (Omani Luban), *Molecules* 2008, 13, 2181-2189.
49. Miller AG, Morris M. *Plants of Dhofar: The Southern Region of Oman, Traditional, Economic and Medicinal Uses*, The Office of The Advisor for Conservation of The Environment, Diwan of Royal Court, Sultanate of Oman, 1988:78.
50. Woolley CL, et al. Chemical differentiation of Boswellia sacra and Boswellia carterii essential oils by gas chromatography and chiral gas chromatography-mass spectrometry. *J Chromatography A*. 2012 Oct 26;1261:158-63.
51. Fung KM, et al. Management of basal cell carcinoma of the skin using frankincense (Boswellia sacra) essential oil: a case report. *OA Altern. Med*. 2013 Jun 01;1(2):14.
52. Ni X, et al. Frankincense essential oil prepared from hydrodistillation of Boswellia sacra gum resins induces human pancreatic cancer cell death in cultures and in a xenograft murine model. *BMC Complement Altern Med*. 2012 Dec 13;12:253.
53. Suhail MM, et al. Boswellia sacra essential oil induces tumor cell-specific apoptosis and suppresses tumor aggressiveness in cultured human breast cancer cells. *BMC Complement Altern Med*. 2011 Dec 15;11:129.
54. Moussaieff A, et al. Incensole acetate, an incense component, elicits psychoactivity by activating TRPV3 channels in the brain. *FASEB J*. 2008 Aug;22(8):3024-34.
55. Moussaieff A, et al. Incensole acetate, a novel anti-inflammatory compound isolated from Boswellia carterii. *J Cereb Blood Flow Metab*. 2008 Jul;28(7):1341-52.
56. Frank A, Unger M. Analysis of frankincense from various Boswellia species with inhibitory activity on human drug metabolising cytochrome P450 enzymes using liquid chromatography mass spectrometry after automated on-line extraction. *J Chromatog A*. 2006 1112: 255-262.
57. Blain EJ, et al. Boswellia frereana (Frankincense) Suppresses Cytokine-Induced Matrix Metalloproteinase Expression and Production of Pro-Inflammatory Molecules in Articular Cartilage. *Phytother Res*. 2010 Jun;24(6):905-12.
58. Chao, et al. Screening for Inhibitory Activity of Essential Oils on Selected Bacteria, Fungi, and Viruses. *Journal of Essential Oil Research*, 1997.
59. Chao, et al. Antimicrobial Effects of Essential Oils on Streptococcus pneumoniae. *JEOR*, 2001.
60. Bray GA, Nielsen SJ, Popkim BM. Consumption of high-fructose corn syrup in beverages may play a role in the epidemic of obesity, *Am J Clin Nutr*. 2004 Apr;79(4):537-43.
61. Ma X, et al. Ghrelin receptor regulates HFCS-induced adipose inflammation and insulin resistance. *Nutr Diabetes*. 2013 Dec 23;3.
62. Parker-Pope T. Still Spooked by High-Fructose Corn Syrup, *The New York Times*, October 30, 2008.
63. Parker-Pope T. A New Name for High-Fructose Corn Syrup, *The New York Times*, September 14, 2010.
64. McLaughlin, Lisa (September 17, 2008). Is High-Fructose Corn Syrup Really Good for You? *Time Magazine*. http://www.time.com/time/health/article/0,8599, 1841910,00.html.
65. Parker-Pope T. A New Name for High-Fructose Corn Syrup, *The New York Times*, September 14, 2010.
66. Mercer D. Corn syrup producers see decline in U.S. sales, MSNbc.com, June 2, 2010, http://www.msnbc.msn.com/id/37468418/ns/business-consumer_news/print/1/displaymode/1098/.
67. http://articles.mercola.com/sites/articles/archive/2000/12/03/sucralose-dangers.aspx.
68. http://www.nbcnews.com/id/18041155/ns/business-us_business/t/splenda-court-over-claims-its-sugar/#.V63oKbBRHX4.
69. http://en.wikipedia.org/wiki/Yac%C3%B3n.

# Section 5
## Personal Usage

**PERSONAL USAGE DIRECTORY** ...........................400

**CHAPTER 20** Personal Usage ...........................405

# Personal Usage Directory

| | |
|---|---|
| Abscesses and Boils | 544 |
| Absentmindedness | 429 |
| Abuse, Mental And Physical | 415 |
| Acidosis | 415 |
| Acne | 545 |
| Addictions | 416 |
| Addison's Disease | 416 |
| Adrenal gland disorders | 416 |
| Age-Related Macular Degeneration | 472 |
| Agitation | 418 |
| AIDS | 418 |
| Alcoholism | 419 |
| Alkalosis | 419 |
| Allergic Rhinitis | 420 |
| Allergies | 419 |
| Alopecia Areata | 484 |
| ALS (Lou Gehrig's Disease) | 519 |
| Aluminum Toxicity | 487 |
| Alzheimer's | 429 |
| Analgesic | 420 |
| Anemia | 438 |
| Aneurysm | 438 |
| Angina | 438 |
| Anorexia Nervosa | 467 |
| Anthrax | 420 |
| Antibiotic Reactions | 421 |
| Antiseptics | 422 |
| Apnea | 422 |
| Appetite | 468 |
| Arteriosclerosis | 439 |
| Arthritis | 422 |
| Asthma | 501 |
| Athlete's Foot | 477 |
| Attention Deficit Disorder | 424 |
| Autism | 425 |
| Backache | 556 |
| Back Injuries and Pain | 556 |
| Bad Breath | 485 |
| Baldness | 484 |
| Bedbug Bites | 492 |
| Bedbugs | 426 |

| | |
|---|---|
| Bee Stings | 491 |
| Bell's Palsy | 516 |
| Benign Prostate Hyperplasia | 532 |
| Binge Eating Disorder | 468 |
| Bites | 492 |
| Black Widow Spider Bite | 492 |
| Bladder/Urinary Tract Infection | 426 |
| Bleeding | 439 |
| Bleeding Gums | 525 |
| Blisters | 545 |
| Bloating | 427, 463 |
| Blocked Tear Ducts | 472 |
| Blood Circulation, Poor | 439 |
| Blood Clots | 440 |
| Blood Detoxification | 440 |
| Blood Platelets (Low) | 441 |
| Blood Pressure, High | 441 |
| Boils | 546 |
| Bone Pain | 428 |
| Bone Problems | 427 |
| Bone-related Pain | 529 |
| Brain Disorders | 429 |
| Breast Cancer | 437 |
| Breastfeeding | 432 |
| Broken Bones | 427 |
| Bronchitis | 501 |
| Brown Recluse Spider Bite | 492 |
| Bruised Muscles | 512 |
| Bruising | 441 |
| Bulimia | 468 |
| Bunions | 477 |
| Burns | 546 |
| Bursitis | 433 |
| Calluses | 478 |
| Cancer | 433 |
| Candida Albicans | 479 |
| Candidiasis | 479 |
| Canker Sores | 448 |
| Cardiovascular Conditions and Problems | 438 |
| Carpal Tunnel Syndrome | 517 |
| Cartilage Injury | 454 |

**400** | **Chapter 20** | *Personal Usage Guide*

| | | | |
|---|---|---|---|
| Cataracts | 473 | Diarrhea | 460 |
| Cellulite | 448 | Digestive Problems | 459 |
| Cerebral Palsy | 449 | Diphtheria | 464 |
| Cervical Cancer | 437 | Disinfectants | 422 |
| Chapped, Cracked, or Dry Skin | 547 | Diverticulitis/Diverticulosis | 461 |
| Charley Horse | 513 | Dizziness | 465 |
| Chemical Sensitivity Reaction | 449 | Dry, Cracked Nipples | 432 |
| Chicken Pox | 450 | Dry Nose | 523 |
| Chigger and Tick Bites | 492 | Dysentery | 461 |
| Cholecystitis | 481 | Earache | 465 |
| Cholera | 450 | Ear Infection | 466 |
| Cholesterol, High | 442 | Ear problems | 465 |
| Chronic Fatigue Syndrome | 451 | Eating disorders | 467 |
| Chronic Pain | 529 | Eczema/Dermatitis | 549 |
| Clogged Pores | 547 | Edema | 469 |
| Colds | 452 | Embolism | 440 |
| Cold Sores | 451 | Endocrine System | 470 |
| Colitis | 452 | Endometriosis | 508 |
| Colon Cleanse | 450 | Environmental Protection Kits | 534 |
| Coma | 453 | Epilepsy | 470 |
| Concentration | 430 | Epstein-Barr Virus | 471 |
| Confusion | 430 | Excessive Bleeding | 508 |
| Congestive Heart Failure | 443 | Excessive Sexual Desire (Both Sexes) | 539 |
| Conjunctivitis | 473 | Eye Disorders | 471 |
| Connective Tissue Damage | 454 | Fainting | 474 |
| Constipation | 459 | Fatigue | 474 |
| Convulsions | 431 | Fever | 475 |
| Corns and Calluses | 478 | Fibrillation | 443 |
| Coughs, Congestive and Dry | 560 | Fibroids | 475 |
| Cramps | 513 | Fibromyalgia | 476 |
| Cramps, Stomach | 460 | Flatulence | 462 |
| Crohn's Disease | 456 | Food Allergies | 420 |
| Cushing's Syndrome | 417 | Food Poisoning | 476 |
| Cuts, Scrapes, and Wounds | 548 | Foot Conditions | 477 |
| Cystitis | 426 | Frigidity (Women) | 538 |
| Cysts | 457 | Fungal Infections | 478 |
| Dandruff | 484 | Fungal Skin Infections | 550 |
| Dental Visits | 526 | Gallbladder Infection | 481 |
| Depression | 457 | Gallstones | 481 |
| Diabetes | 458 | Ganglion Cysts | 457 |
| Diaper Rash | 549 | Gangrene | 482 |

Seventh Edition | **Essential Oils Desk Reference** | **401**

# Personal Usage Directory *(continued)*

| | |
|---|---|
| Gas | 462 |
| Gastritis | 482 |
| Genital Human Papillomavirus (HPV) | 540 |
| Genital Warts/Blisters | 540 |
| Giardia | 462 |
| Gingivitis and Periodontitis | 526 |
| Gonorrhea and Syphilis | 541 |
| Gout | 482 |
| Graves' Disease | 563 |
| Hair and Scalp Problems | 483 |
| Hair Loss | 484 |
| Halitosis | 485 |
| Hashimoto's Disease | 564 |
| Hay Fever | 420 |
| Headache | 485 |
| Hearing Impairment | 466 |
| Heart Attack | 443 |
| Heartburn | 463 |
| Heart Health | 444 |
| Heart Stimulant | 444 |
| Heart Vita Flex | 444 |
| Heavy Metals | 487 |
| Hematoma | 440 |
| Hemorrhagic Strokes | 446 |
| Hemorrhaging | 439 |
| Hemorrhoids | 488 |
| Hepatitis | 499 |
| Herniated Disc/Disc Deterioration | 557 |
| Herpes Simplex Type 1 | 451 |
| Herpes Simplex Type 2 | 539 |
| Herpes Zoster | 450, 541 |
| Hiccups | 488 |
| Hives | 489 |
| Hormonal Edema (Cyclic) | 509 |
| Huntington's Chorea | 520 |
| Hyperactivity | 489 |
| Hypertension | 441 |
| Hyperthyroid (Graves' Disease) | 563 |
| Hypoglycemia | 564 |
| Hypothyroid (Hashimoto's Disease) | 564 |
| Hysterectomy | 509 |

| | |
|---|---|
| Impacted Bowel | 459 |
| Impotence | 537 |
| Indigestion | 463 |
| Infected Breast | 432 |
| Infection (Bacterial and Viral) | 489 |
| Infectious Parotitis | 511 |
| Infertility (Men) | 537 |
| Infertility (Women) | 538 |
| Inflammation | 490 |
| Inflammation Due to Infection | 512 |
| Inflammation Due to Injury | 512 |
| Inflammation of Veins | 445 |
| Influenza | 490 |
| Insect Bites and Stings | 491 |
| Insect Repellent | 493 |
| Insomnia | 494 |
| Intestinal Worms | 530 |
| Irregular Periods | 509 |
| Irritable Bowel Syndrome | 463, 495 |
| Itching | 550 |
| Jaundice | 499 |
| Joint Stiffness or Pain | 495 |
| Kidney Disorders | 496 |
| Kidney Failure | 496 |
| Kidney Inflammation | 496 |
| Kidney Stones | 497 |
| Lack of Libido/Desire (Women) | 538 |
| Lack of Libido (Men) | 537 |
| Laryngitis | 561 |
| Leukemia | 437 |
| Lice | 498 |
| Ligament Sprain or Tear | 455 |
| Liver Diseases | 498 |
| Liver Spots | 501 |
| Loss of Smell | 523 |
| Lumbago (Lower Back Pain) | 557 |
| Lung Cancer | 437 |
| Lung Infections | 501 |
| Lupus | 504 |
| Lyme Disease | 505 |
| Lymphatic System | 505 |

**402** | **Chapter 20** | Personal Usage Guide

| | | | |
|---|---|---|---|
| Malaria | 506 | Oral Infection Control | 527 |
| Male Hormone Imbalance | 507 | Osteoarthritis | 422 |
| Mastitis | 432 | Osteoporosis | 428 |
| MCT (Mixed Connective Tissue) | 506 | Ovarian and Uterine Cysts | 457 |
| Measles | 507 | Pain | 528 |
| Melanoma | 437 | Pancreatitis | 529 |
| Memory | 431 | Parasites, Intestinal | 530 |
| Menopause | 510 | Parkinson's Disease | 522 |
| Menstrual and Female Hormone Conditions | 508 | Periodontitis | 526 |
| Menstrual Cramps | 510 | Phlebitis | 445 |
| Mental Fatigue | 431, 474 | Physical Fatigue | 474 |
| Migraine | 486 | Pink Eye | 473 |
| Moles | 550 | Plaque | 445 |
| Mononucleosis | 471 | Pleurisy | 502 |
| Morning Sickness | 515 | PMS | 510 |
| Mosquito Bites | 493 | Pneumonia | 502 |
| Motion Sickness | 516 | Pointer Technique | 557 |
| Mouth Ulcers | 526 | Poison Oak/Poison Ivy/Poison Sumac | 551 |
| Mucus | 511 | Polio | 531 |
| Multiple Sclerosis (MS) | 521 | Polyps, Nasal | 524 |
| Mumps | 511 | Postpartum Depression | 458 |
| Muscles | 512 | Pregnancy | 531 |
| Muscle Spasms/Weakness | 513 | Premenstrual Syndrome (PMS) | 510 |
| Muscular Dystrophy | 514 | Prostate Cancer | 437 |
| Myocardial Infarction | 443 | Prostate Problems | 532 |
| Nails, Brittle or Weak | 514 | Prostatitis | 533 |
| Narcolepsy | 515 | Psoriasis | 551 |
| Nasopharyngitis | 542 | Pyorrhea | 527 |
| Nausea | 515 | Radiation Exposure Damage | 533 |
| Neck Pain and Stiffness | 557 | Restless Legs Syndrome | 522 |
| Nephritis | 496 | Rheumatic Fever | 535 |
| Nerve Disorders | 516 | Rheumatoid Arthritis | 423 |
| Nervous System, Autonomic | 518 | Rhinitis | 543 |
| Neuralgia | 517 | Ringworm | 479 |
| Neuritis | 517 | Rocky Mountain Spotted Fever | 505 |
| Neurologic Diseases | 519 | Sagging Skin | 552 |
| Neuropathy | 518 | Scabies | 552 |
| Nose and Sinus Problems | 523 | Scalp Problems | 483 |
| Nosebleeds | 524 | Scar Tissue | 536 |
| Obesity | 525 | Schizophrenia | 523 |
| Oral Care, Teeth and Gums | 525 | Sciatica | 558 |

Seventh Edition | **Essential Oils Desk Reference** | **403**

# Personal Usage Directory *(continued)*

| | | | | |
|---|---|---|---|---|
| Scleroderma | 455 | Teeth Grinding | 528 |
| Scoliosis | 559 | Teething | 528 |
| Scorpion Sting | 493 | Tendonitis | 455 |
| Scurvy | 536 | Tension (Stress) Headache | 487 |
| Seizures | 536 | Throat Infections and Problems | 560 |
| Sexual Dysfunction | 536 | Thrombotic Strokes | 446 |
| Sexually Transmitted Diseases | 539 | Thrombus | 440 |
| Shingles | 541 | Thrush | 480 |
| Shock | 542 | Thyroid Problems | 563 |
| Sinus Congestion | 543 | Ticks | 492 |
| Sinus Headache | 486 | Tinnitus | 467 |
| Sinus Infections | 542 | Tonsillitis | 563 |
| Sinusitis / Rhinitis | 543 | Toothache and Teething Pain | 528 |
| Skin Cancer | 437 | Toxemia | 565 |
| Skin Candida | 479 | Toxic Liver | 500 |
| Skin Disorders and Problems | 544 | Trauma, Emotional | 565 |
| Skin Ulcers | 553 | Trigger Finger | 566 |
| Sleep Disorders | 554 | Tuberculosis | 503 |
| Smoking Cessation | 554 | Tumors | 437 |
| Snake Bites | 555 | Typhoid Fever | 566 |
| Snoring | 555 | Ulcerative Colitis | 453 |
| Solar Lentigines | 501 | Uterine Cancer | 437 |
| Sore Feet | 478 | Uterine Cysts | 457 |
| Sore Muscles | 513 | Vaginal Yeast Infection | 480 |
| Sore Throat | 561 | Varicose Veins | 447 |
| Spastic Colon Syndrome | 463 | Vascular Cleansing | 447 |
| Spider Veins | 447 | Viral Colitis | 453 |
| Spina Bifida | 555 | Vitiligo | 553 |
| Spine Injuries and Pain | 556 | West Nile Virus | 493 |
| Sprain | 559 | Whooping Cough | 504 |
| Stenosing Tenosynovitis | 566 | Wrinkles | 553 |
| Stings | 491 | Yeast | 478, 480, 550 |
| Stomachache | 464 | | |
| Stomach Ulcers | 464 | | |
| Strep Throat | 562 | | |
| Stress | 560 | | |
| Stretch Marks | 553 | | |
| Strokes | 446 | | |
| Sunburn | 546 | | |
| Swelling | 427 | | |
| Tachycardia | 446 | | |

**404** | **Chapter 20** | Personal Usage Guide

# Chapter 20
## Personal Usage

## Taking Charge of Your Health

Today's air, food, water, and other environmental factors are immensely deficient. They greatly affect our health and well-being and certainly need to be evaluated and changed as necessary. In addition, exercise should be a routine part of our weekly activities, although most of us simply do not make the time. To do so takes discipline and commitment but would definitely have a positive effect on our health.

Emotional and spiritual feelings and attitudes that negatively affect one's life are perhaps the most difficult to recognize. An unhealthy state of being, disease, and even death can be brought on by negative thoughts and emotions.

Many people, including social workers and health practitioners, believe that negative emotions are the precursor to both mental and physical dysfunction of the body, resulting in mental illness and disease. Surely, that is not true in all cases, but it is definitely something to consider.

We must look at all of these things in an effort to bring balance to our lives, overcome body dysfunction and disease, and find happiness and fulfillment.

### 1. What causes poor nutrition?
- Poor nutrition is caused by a poor diet, especially eating fast food. Over 40,000 chemicals are found in our food today, which includes prepared and processed foods.
- Contaminated water and water treated with chemicals like chlorine and fluoride inhibit proper thyroid function and slow down metabolism, circulation, and immune function.
- Poor digestion and assimilation caused by nutritionally deficient foods lacking in the necessary enzymes and minerals critical for digestion cause many problems, with constipation as the number one complaint.

### 2. What is environmental pollution?
- Air pollution
- Chemicals in the home and work environment
- Changes in ozone
- Electromagnetic and radiation pollution from computers, cell phones, televisions, electrical appliances, etc.

### 3. Why do we have poor physical fitness?
- No exercise
- Obesity from bad diet
- No or low self-discipline
- Premature aging
- Fragile bones and weak muscles

### 4. What causes a negative attitude?
- Depression
- Low energy
- Low self-esteem
- Few or no goals
- Little or no motivation

### 5. Why are we spiritually depressed?
- No specific belief system
- Fear
- Sense of being lost
- Poor relationship with self, spouse, children, extended family, friends, and most importantly: Our Creator, or God

We have control over many things—more than those over which we have no control. We can change our diet, change our attitude, start working out to improve our fitness, change what we can in our own personal environment, and start turning to that great universal power for understanding and direction.

We have wonderful nutritional supplements available to us, and we have God's beautiful essential oils to uplift, energize, motivate, and help propel us onto a greater path

Seventh Edition | **Essential Oils Desk Reference** | 405

of success in every walk of life. What we do and how we do it is our choice.

Essential oils are God's medicine today and for the future and can be used in many different ways. Their use and application have become vast and creative, depending on the oil.

Although their topical use is perhaps the most common, dietary use of essential oils may be one of the most effective ways of unlocking their health benefits. Many essential oils are used for food flavoring and are classified as "GRAS" by the U.S. Food and Drug Administration, meaning they are "generally regarded as safe" for human consumption. In addition, Young Living has classified many single oils and blends as Vitality supplements for dietary use.

Essential oils have been used for centuries for religious ceremonies, in cosmetics for beautification of the body, and medicinally for many maladies, endowing them with a long history of safe use.

Research indicates that certain essential oils act as potent antioxidants that can actually raise antioxidant levels in the body and prevent premature aging.

According to researcher Jean Valnet, MD, an essential oil applied directly on the skin can pass into the bloodstream and diffuse throughout the tissues in 20 minutes or less.

Inhalation can have a direct influence on both the body and mind due to its ability to stimulate the brain's limbic system, a group of subcortical structures, including the hypothalamus, the hippocampus, and the amygdala. This can produce powerful effects that can affect everything from emotional balance and energy levels to appetite control and heart and immune functions.

Some researchers believe that inhalation also enhances the body's immune system. Disease and trauma foster emotional negativity that essential oils often dissipate. Oils with immune-stimulating properties can increase the body's resistance, whether used topically or taken orally, helping to build a healthy environment that prevents the onset of disease.

# Addressing Your Overall Health

Addressing the overall health of the body is important when considering a specific solution. Although essential oils have powerful, therapeutic effects, they are not, by themselves, a total solution. They must be accompanied by a program of internal cleansing, proper diet, and supplementation. This may also include lifestyle changes such as exercise, meditation or yoga, and stress-free situations.

## Cleanse

Cleansing the colon and liver is the first and most important step to take when dealing with any disease. Many imbalances may be corrected by cleansing alone. Products that cleanse the body include the Cleansing Trio (ComforTone, Essentialzyme, and ICP), JuvaTone, JuvaCleanse, JuvaCleanse Vitality, JuvaFlex, JuvaFlex Vitality, GLF, GLF Vitality, Detoxzyme, Digest & Cleanse, DiGize, DiGize Vitality, and ParaFree (see Cleansing and Diet, Chapter 17).

**Note:** It would be difficult, if not impossible, for infants or children under age 8 to try a colon and liver cleanse. Instead, use 3 drops of DiGize in a teaspoon of V-6 Vegetable Oil Complex, rub around the navel, and place moderately warm packs on the stomach. Apply 2-3 drops of DiGize, Fennel, or Peppermint on the bottoms of the feet.

Put 1 drop of any of the same oils in a glass of water or juice for a child over the age of 4 to drink. Those same drops could also be mixed in a teaspoon of yogurt or kefir that any child can easily swallow.

## Balance and Build

After cleansing, it is easier to balance and nourish the systems of the body. This includes rebuilding and nourishing beneficial intestinal flora and re-mineralizing the blood and tissues. Products that build the body include Mineral Essence, Essentialzyme, Essentialzymes-4, Multi-Greens, Power Meal, Power Meal, Slique Shake, MegaCal, Master Formula, NingXia Red, NingXia Zyng, Life 9, Balance Complete, Pure Protein Complete, OmegaGize[3], Sulfurzyme, Super B, Super C, Super C Chewables, KidScents MightyVites, KidScents MightyZyme, etc.

## Nourish and Support

Supporting the endocrine and immune systems comprises the third phase. Products include Exodus II, Thieves, ImmuPro, Mineral Essence, Essentialzyme, Essentialzymes-4, Life 9, KidScents MightyVites, KidScents MightyZyme, Super B, Super C, Master Formula, Thyromin, EndoGize, NingXia Red, Prostrate Health, Progessence Plus, Power Meal, Slique Shake, Balance Complete, Pure Protein Complete, and others.

**Note:** For children or adults who have difficulty swallowing capsules and tablets, Essentialzymes-4, may be emptied into other food products such as yogurt, oatmeal, NingXia Red, etc., and ingested.

_Personal Usage Guide_ | **Chapter 20**

# Getting Started

## Methods of Application

Essential oils are very concentrated, natural substances—easily 100 times more concentrated than the natural herbs and plants from which they are distilled. For this reason, it is important to dilute certain essential oils before using them therapeutically.

Other essential oils are so mild that dilution is simply not necessary, even for use on infants.

The five standard methods of application are aromatic, dietary, oral, topical, and retention.

## Mixing Single Oils and Blends

The essential oil singles and blends listed for a specific condition may be used either separately or together. Combining two single oils or one single oil with a blend may often produce a synergistic, stronger effect than when using them individually.

Usually 1-3 drops of either a single oil or a blend is sufficient, mixing up to 3 or 4 oils in any given combination at a time.

## Using an Essential Oil

The essential oils recommended for specific conditions are not the only oils you can use; these oils are merely a starting point. Other oils not listed can also be just as effective. You have to use the oils to determine what works best for you.

However, the essential oils are listed in a preferred order. Start with the first single oil, blend, or supplement in the list. If results are not apparent after a little while, try another single oil, blend, supplement, or combination on the next application. Sometimes you have to keep experimenting until you find what works for you. This is because one particular oil may be more compatible with one person's body chemistry than with another person's chemistry (see further explanation at the beginning of the Usage Guide).

Essential oils can be used topically for massage, acupuncture, Raindrop Technique, and Vita Flex on the bottoms of the feet. In most cases, 3-4 drops are sufficient to produce significant effects, unless using a specific protocol.

Most single oils and blends should be diluted 50/50 when putting them on the skin. Oils that definitely should be diluted are oils such as Cistus, Clove, Cypress, Lemongrass, Mountain Savory, Oregano, Rosemary, Thyme, etc. For some people, an oil like Basil might be too "hot" if put neat on the skin; for others, Basil will not be "hot" at all. That is why it is best to always do a skin test before applying any oil. When in doubt, dilute.

When diluting the oils, use V-6 Vegetable Oil Complex for either topical or internal application, particularly if you have not used essential oils previously. Use no more than 10 to 20 drops during one topical application.

## Precautions

When using topically, first do a skin test by putting 1 drop of the desired essential oil on the inside of the upper arm. If cosmetics and personal care products made with synthetic chemicals or soaps and cleansers containing synthetic or petroleum-based chemicals have been used on the skin, then the skin may be uncomfortably sensitive.

If any redness or irritation results, the skin should be thoroughly cleansed; then the oil may be reapplied. If skin irritation persists, try using a different oil or oil blend.

You may want to consider starting an internal cleansing program for 30 days before using essential oils. Use ICP, ComforTone, JuvaPower, Essentialzyme, Essentialzymes-4, Digest & Cleanse, Detoxzyme, and other cleansing supplements.

## Internal Use

Many essential oils are taken internally as dietary supplements. Some people put 1-3 drops in water to drink, but others use cold NingXia Red or another juice of their choice.

If you prefer to swallow a capsule, you can fill a "00" capsule with oil using an eyedropper. Fill with the number of drops desired and the rest of the capsule with V-6 Vegetable Oil Complex or any other organic vegetable oil. If you are uncertain, consult with someone who is experienced in taking oils internally.

Always drink more water when using essential oils because they can accelerate the detoxification process in the body. If you are not taking in adequate fluids, the toxins could recirculate, causing nausea, headaches, etc.

---

**Consult Your Health Care Professional**

_Consult your health care professional about any serious disease or injury. Do not attempt to self-diagnose or prescribe any natural substances such as essential oils for health conditions that require professional attention._

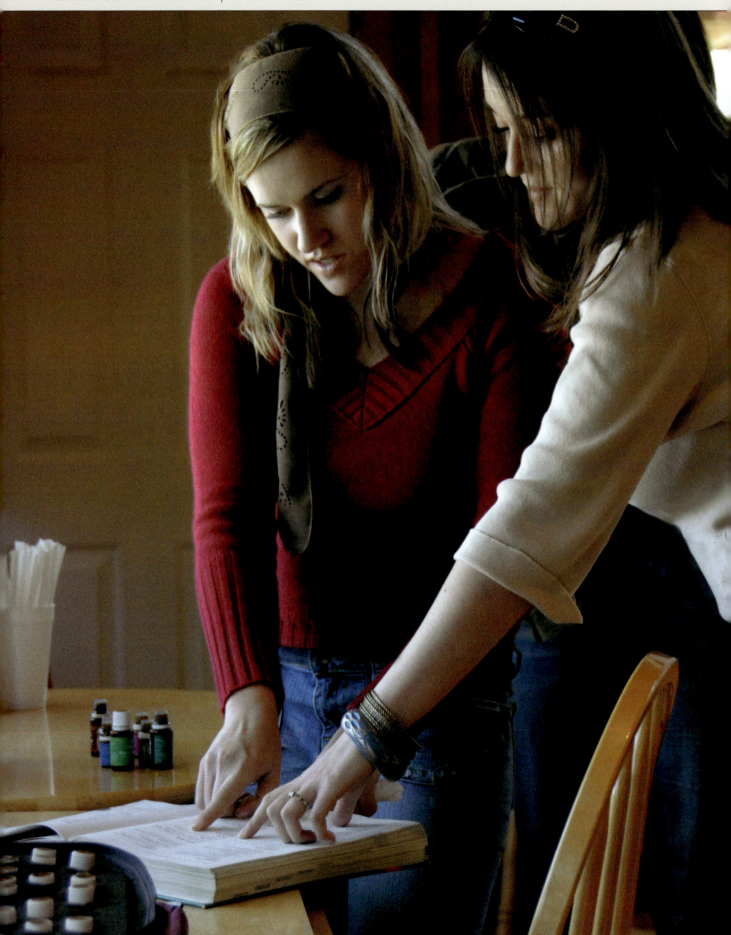

Personal Usage Guide | **Chapter 20**

# Developing Your Program

It is usually best to use one or two application methods at a time. If you were to use all 10 applications for a sore throat at once, it would take more time and probably be inconvenient, costly, and unnecessary.

First, you must decide which oils and supplements you want to use for your program. Choose up to three or four oils, be certain how many drops you are going to use, undiluted or diluted, and if diluted, what the dilution ratio is that you want to try.

**For example:** If you have sore shoulder muscles, you could decide to use the following:

**Your Oils and Creams:**
- PanAway: dilution 50/50
- Aroma Siez: dilution 50/50
- Helichrysum: neat
- V-6 Vegetable Oil Complex
- Ortho Sport Massage Oil
- Cool Azul: dilution 50/50
- Cool Azul Pain Relief Cream
- Cool Azul Sports Gel
- Deep Relief Roll-On to carry with you

**Your Supplements:**
- Mineral Essence: 2 droppers in 2 ounces of NingXia Red in water in the morning
- ICP: 2 tablespoons in water in the morning

- Essentialzyme: 2 each morning, 1 in the evening
- BLM/AgilEase: 2 capsules daily with water
- Power Meal, Slique Shake: 1 packet in water or juice 2 times daily
- Detoxzyme: 4-6 in the evening before or after dinner
- MegaCal: 1 teaspoon in water at night
- ImmuPro: 1-2 before going to bed (Do not exceed 2 daily.)

Make sure you understand the proper essential oil dilution level. Have your V-6 Vegetable Oil Complex or massage oil that you are going to use for the dilution together with all of the essential oils.

Write down your program so that it is easy to follow each day, and make sure you have enough so that you do not run out and then have to stop your program while you wait for your next order to arrive.

### Be Consistent with Your Regimen

Therapeutic-grade essential oils are powerful, natural healing substances that work extremely well with the body's own defenses to solve problems. However, they are not drugs and may not always work in seconds or even minutes. Essential oils will enhance and speed up the benefits of Dietary and Oral supplements, but it is still a "natural" process. Sometimes it can take hours or even days to see the improvement.

# Personal Usage Recommendations

In "Recommendations," products are listed in order beginning with the first, or preferred, recommendation. In other words, **the first one or two oils listed would be the first ones that you would try**. However, any single oil or blend listed would have application.

**Note:** You will see what you might think are tiresome repetitions: "Lemon, Lemon Vitality, Thieves, Thieves Vitality" under Recommendations. Young Living gives you both versions to solve a compliance issue. Aromatic and Topical use must be separate from a Dietary and Oral Supplement use as all three uses cannot be included on the same label. Thus, Vitality oils can be suggested for Dietary and Oral Supplement use and are completely FDA compliant.

Whenever you are working with natural products, you never know which product will work the best for you until you try it. Your body will tell you. Different oils work for different people. You have to experiment until you make

that determination based on your body's chemistry and need.

Supplements vary considerably in their use, so follow the instructions on the label. You may want to try the first three or four products recommended to see how your body responds. You may find that your body responds to one product over another.

In the case of enzymes, read the chapter on enzymes and minerals, the chapter on nutritionals, and consult the Enzyme Quick Reference Guide, located in both chapters.

As always, just follow the guidelines and use common sense. Trust your body, focus on your intuitive feelings and what you have learned, and you will make the right choice.

**No matter what you take, your body will benefit as long as you do not "go overboard." You are the best one to decide what is best for your body. Just start slowly and enjoy your new rejuvenation and vitality.**

Seventh Edition | **Essential Oils Desk Reference** | **409**

# Application Guidelines

## Aromatic

### Diffuse

- Diffuse your choice of oils for ½ hour every 4-6 hours or as desired.

- Undiluted oils may be diffused in a cold-air diffuser. Cold air diffusers are not designed to handle vegetable oils because they are thicker and may clog the diffuser mechanism.

- Put 8-10 drops of oil on a cotton ball or tissue and put it in an air vent in your house, vehicle, hotel room, etc.

- If diffusing while sleeping, set your timer for the desired length of time for automatic shut off.

### Direct

- Put 2-3 drops of oil in the palm of one hand, rub palms together, cup hands over your nose and mouth, and inhale throughout the day as needed.

- Applying a single drop under the nose is helpful and refreshing.

- If you touch the skin near your eyes, they may water or sting, but it will dissipate in a few minutes. Dilute with V-6 Vegetable Oil Complex or other pure vegetable oil. **Never rinse with water.** However, the essential oils will not cause any damage and will slowly stop burning.

### Steam

- Run hot, steaming water into a sink or large bowl. Water should be at least 2 inches deep to retain heat for a few minutes.

- Add 3-6 drops of oil to the hot water; then drape a towel over your head, covering the hot water so that you enclose your face over the steam.

- Inhale vapors deeply through the nose as they rise with the steam. Add more hot water to continue vaporizing, if desired. Repeat 2 to 4 times during the day.

## Dietary and Oral

- Vitality™ dietary essential oil singles and blends can be added to food for delicious, concentrated flavor or used in capsules for their supporting properties. Follow the directions on the labels.

- Generally, take 1 capsule with desired oil 2 times daily.

- Take 2-3 drops of oil in a spoonful of Blue Agave, Yacon Syrup, maple syrup, coconut oil, milk, juice, or water. Honey and yogurt are too acidic.

- Put the desired amount of oils in a small glass of rice milk, almond milk, goat milk, carrot juice, NingXia Red, or water and then drink it.

- Dilute all essential oils 20:80 before giving them to small children for oral application.

### Filling Capsules

Use a clean medicine dropper to fill the larger half of an empty "00" gelatin capsule half-way with oil. Then fill the remainder with V-6 Vegetable Oil Complex or a high quality, cold-pressed, vegetable oil; put the other half of the gel cap on; and swallow with water.

If your hand is steady, you can simply hold the bottle and let the oil drip from the bottle into the capsule.

Take the capsule(s) immediately, as it will become soft quickly, making it hard to pick up.

### Dosages

There are two sizes of capsules: (1) a "00" size capsule holds 400 mg, and (2) a "0" size capsule holds 200 mg.

The "00" size capsule is easier to use because it is bigger, there is less chance of spilling, and you can fill it with whatever amount you want.

If the "00" is not available, then use the "0" size. You just have to be more careful when filling, and you may have to swallow more capsules.

# Application Guidelines (continued)

## Topical

- You may apply single oils or blends neat on feet and spine or diluted, depending on the oil or oils being used. Follow the instructions on the label.

- Apply neat or undiluted to specific area.

- Dilute 50/50: Add 1 part essential oil to 1 part V-6 Vegetable Oil Complex.

- Dilute 20/80: Add 1 part essential oil to 4 parts V-6 Vegetable Oil Complex.

## Bath Salts

- Put 10-15 drops of essential oil into ½ cup of Epsom salts or baking soda. Add warm water, mix, and pour into warm bathwater. Soak in the tub for 20 to 30 minutes before using soap or shampoo.

- Special showerheads are available that are designed to hold salt mixtures for a revitalizing shower.

## Body Massage

- You can use any dilution of essential oils desired with V-6 Vegetable Oil Complex. It depends on the oil or oils being used. Usually, a few drops of oil are sufficient with a massage oil.

- You can also apply oils directly to the skin and then apply a massage oil such as Relaxation, Sensation, Cel-Lite Magic, Dragon Time, Ortho Ease, or Ortho Sport for a full-body massage.

- Ortho Ease and Ortho Sport massage oils have a stronger therapeutic action and help immensely with sore and aching muscles and joints.

- Oil blends such as Valor, Valor II, White Angelica, or RutaVaLa do not need to be diluted. Oil blends such as PanAway, Raven, and Relieve It are "hot" and should always be diluted.

- Read the instructions or ask for advice if you are just beginning to use the oils in massage.

## Compress

- After applying oils to the skin, soak a hand towel in warm water, wring it out, and lay it over the targeted skin area.

- Then cover the wet towel with a dry towel to hold the heat in for 10-15 minutes or until the wet towel is no longer warm.

- If the individual becomes uncomfortable or has a hot sensation, remove towel and apply V-6 Vegetable Oil Complex.

- A cool towel instead of a warm towel can be used to create a cold compress.

## Vita Flex/Auricular/Lymphatic Pump

Apply 1-3 drops neat to the Vita Flex points on the feet as directed. Children love it. See Section 4 for more information.

## Raindrop Technique

Have a Raindrop Technique 1-2 times weekly. See Section 4 for more information.

## Retention

- **Rectal:** Mix a 40/60 ratio (4 parts essential oil to 6 parts V-6 Vegetable Oil Complex), insert 1-2 tablespoons in the rectum with a bulb syringe, and retain up to 8 hours or overnight.

- **Vaginal:** Tampon: Mix a 40/60 ratio (4 parts essential oil to 6 parts V-6 Vegetable Oil Complex), put 1-2 tablespoons on a tampon, and insert into the vagina for internal infection. Put oil on a sanitary pad for external lesions. Retain up to 8 hours or overnight. Use only tampons or sanitary pads made with non-perfumed, non-scented, organic cotton.

# Quick Usage Guide

## Body Defense: Antiviral, Antibacterial, Anti-inflammatory, and Disease

**Singles:** Northern Lights Black Spruce, Carrot Seed, Carrot Seed Vitality, Cinnamon Bark, Cinnamon Bark Vitality, Frankincense, Frankincense Vitality, Idaho Balsam Fir, Idaho Blue Spruce, Cistus, Clove, Clove Vitality, Dalmatia Sage, Dorado Azul, Jade Lemon, Jade Lemon Vitality, Laurus Nobilis, Laurus Nobilis Vitality, Lemon, Lemon Vitality, Lime, Lime Vitality, Oregano, Oregano Vitality, Sage, Sage Vitality, Ocotea, Palo Santo, Spearmint, Spearmint Vitality, Tangerine, Tangerine Vitality, Thyme, Thyme Vitality, Eucalyptus Blue, Hinoki, Yuzu

**Blends:** Thieves, Thieves Vitality, Breathe Again Roll-On, SniffleEase, Melrose, Purification, R.C., Raven, Sacred Mountain, ImmuPower, The Gift

**Nutritionals:** BLM, AgilEase, ImmuPro, Inner Defense, NingXia Red, NingXia Zyng, ParaFree

**Body Care:** Thieves AromaBright Toothpaste, Thieves Dentarome Plus Toothpaste, Thieves Dentarome Ultra Toothpaste, Thieves Fresh Essence Plus Mouthwash, Thieves Spray, Thieves Cough Drops, Thieves Hard Lozenges

## Bones, Joints, and Muscles

**Singles:** Basil, Basil Vitality, Black Pepper, Black Pepper Vitality, Copaiba, Copaiba Vitality, Frankincense, Frankincense Vitality, Helichrysum, Idaho Balsam Fir, Idaho Blue Spruce, Lemongrass, Lemongrass Vitality, Marjoram, Marjoram Vitality, Roman Chamomile, Northern Lights Black Spruce, Black Spruce, Wintergreen

**Blends:** Aroma Siez, Cool Azul, Deep Relief Roll-On, M-Grain, PanAway, Relieve It

**Nutritionals:** PowerGize, BLM, AgilEase, Balance Complete, Master Formula, MegaCal, Mineral Essence, Power Meal, Slique Shake, Slique Bars, Slique CitraSlim, Sulfurzyme

**Body Care:** Cool Azul Pain Relief Cream, Cool Azul Sports Gel, Ortho Ease Massage Oil, Ortho Sport Massage Oil

## Digestive Dysfunction, Constipation, Bloating, Gas, and Cleansing

**Singles:** Carrot Seed, Carrot Seed Vitality, Coriander, Coriander Vitality, Dill, Dill Vitality, Eucalyptus Radiata, Fennel, Fennel Vitality, Sage, Sage Vitality, Ginger, Ginger Vitality, Grapefruit, Grapefruit Vitality, Ledum, Lemon, Lemon Vitality, Lime, Lime Vitality, Tea Tree, Peppermint, Peppermint Vitality, Idaho Blue Spruce, Tarragon, Tarragon Vitality, Hinoki, Basil, Basil Vitality, Dalmatia Juniper, Juniper

**Blends:** DiGize, DiGize Vitality, TummyGize, EndoFlex, EndoFlex Vitality, GLF, GLF Vitality, JuvaCleanse, JuvaCleanse Vitality, JuvaFlex, JuvaFlex Vitality, Longevity, Longevity Vitality

**Nutritionals:** AlkaLime, ComforTone, Digest & Cleanse, ICP, JuvaPower, JuvaSpice, JuvaTone, Life 9, Essentialzyme, Essentialzymes-4, Allerzyme, Detoxzyme, KidScents MightyZyme

**Body Care:** Cel-Lite Magic Massage Oil

## Emotional and Spiritual

**Singles:** Bergamot, Bergamot Vitality, Clary Sage, Frankincense, Frankincense Vitality, Lavender, Lavender Vitality, Jade Lemon, Jade Lemon Vitality, Lemon, Lemon Vitality, Orange, Orange Vitality, Sage, Sage Vitality, Patchouli, Pine, Sacred Frankincense, Tsuga, Ylang Ylang, Idaho Blue Spruce, Hinoki, Spearmint, Spearmint Vitality

**Blends:** 3 Wise Men, Amoressence, Abundance, Acceptance, Australian Blue, AromaEase, AromaSleep, Believe, Chivalry, Divine Release, Egyptian Gold, Evergreen Essence, Freedom, Forgiveness, Gathering, Gentle Baby, German Chamomile, Gratitude, Grounding, Harmony, Hope, Humility, Inner Child, Inner Harmony, Inspiration, Into the Future, InTouch, Reconnect, Joy, Lady Sclareol, Live with Passion, Live Your Passion, Light the Fire, Motivation, Peace & Calming, Peace & Calming II, Present Time, Release, RutaVaLa, SARA, SclarEssence, SclarEssence Vitality, Sensation, Surrender, The Gift, Transformation, Trauma Life, Valor, Valor II, White Angelica, White Light

Personal Usage Guide | Chapter 20

# Quick Usage Guide *(continued)*

**Nutritionals:** CortiStop, EndoGize, FemiGen, PD 80/20

**Body Care:** Dragon Time Massage Oil, Prenolone Plus Body Cream, Progessence Plus, Regenolone Moisturizing Cream

## Fortifying and Maintaining the Body—Antioxidants

**Singles:** Cinnamon Bark, Cinnamon Bark Vitality, Clove, Clove Vitality, Idaho Blue Spruce, Juniper, Jade Lemon, Jade Lemon Vitality, Lemon, Lemon Vitality, Lime, Lime Vitality, Nutmeg, Nutmeg Vitality, Orange, Orange Vitality, Oregano, Oregano Vitality, Peppermint, Peppermint Vitality, Rosemary, Rosemary Vitality, Thyme, Thyme Vitality

**Blends:** Citrus Fresh, Citrus Fresh Vitality, En-R-Gee, Longevity, Hope, ImmuPower, Joy, Motivation

**Nutritionals:** Balance Complete, EndoGize, Essentialzyme, Essentialzymes-4, Inner Defense, JuvaTone, Master Formula, MegaCal, KidScents MightyVites, KidScents MightyZyme, MindWise, Mineral Essence, MultiGreens, NingXia Red, NingXia Zyng, OmegaGize³, Power Meal, Slique Shake, Prostate Health, Pure Protein Complete, Super B, Super C, Super C Chewable, Thyromin, JuvaPower, JuvaSpice

## Memory, Confusion, Lack of Mental Clarity, Brain Fog

**Singles:** Frankincense, Frankincense Vitality, Hinoki, Lavender, Lavender Vitality, Peppermint, Peppermint Vitality, Rosemary, Rosemary Vitality, Sacred Frankincense

**Blends:** Awaken, Brain Power, GeneYus, Citrus Fresh, Citrus Fresh Vitality, Clarity, Common Sense, Dream Catcher, Envision, Gathering, Into the Future, Joy

**Nutritionals:** Essentialzyme, Essentialzymes-4, Detoxzyme, Master Formula, MegaCal, MindWise, NingXia Red, NingXia Zyng, Thyromin, Ultra Young

## Overweight, Metabolism

**Singles:** Fennel, Fennel Vitality, Grapefruit, Grapefruit Vitality, Jade Lemon, Jade Lemon Vitality, Lemon, Lemon Vitality, Nutmeg, Nutmeg Vitality, Ocotea, Patchouli, Spearmint, Spearmint Vitality

**Blends:** DiGize, DiGize Vitality, TummyGize, EndoFlex, EndoFlex Vitality, GLF, GLF Vitality, Joy, JuvaFlex, JuvaFlex Vitality, Motivation, SclarEssence, SclarEssence Vitality

**Nutritionals:** Balance Complete, Allerzyme, ComforTone, Detoxzyme, Digest & Cleanse, EndoGize, Essentialzyme, Essentialzymes-4, ICP, JuvaPower, JuvaTone, NingXia Red, NingXia Zyng, PD 80/20, Pure Protein Complete, Power Meal, Slique Shake, Slique Bars, Slique CitraSlim, Thyromin, JuvaSpice, Ultra Young

## Protection—Antioxidants

**Singles:** Cinnamon Bark, Cinnamon Bark Vitality, Clove, Clove Vitality, Copaiba, Copaiba Vitality, Dorado Azul, Eucalyptus Blue, Frankincense, Frankincense Vitality, Sacred Frankincense, Idaho Blue Spruce, Helichrysum, Tea Tree, Melissa, Mountain Savory, Mountain Savory Vitality, Ocotea, Oregano, Oregano Vitality, Palo Santo, Ravintsara, Roman Chamomile, Thyme, Thyme Vitality

**Blends**: Aroma Life, TummyGize, DiGize, DiGize Vitality, Exodus II, Melrose, PanAway, Purification, R.C., Raven, The Gift, Thieves, Thieves Vitality

**Nutritionals:** Longevity Softgels, Master Formula, Super C, Super C Chewable

**Body Care:** LavaDerm Cooling Mist, Protec

Seventh Edition | **Essential Oils Desk Reference** | 413

# Quick Usage Guide *(continued)*

## Skin Care

**Note:** After applying essential oils on the skin, use a skin cream to sooth the natural drying effect of some oils: ART (Age Refining Technology) Beauty Masque, ART Creme Masque, ART Gentle Cleanser, ART Light Moisturizer, ART Refreshing Toner, ART Renewal Serum, ART Sheerlumé Brightening Cream, Boswellia Wrinkle Cream, Genesis Hand & Body Lotion, Lavender Hand & Body Lotion, Sandalwood Moisture Cream, Sensation Hand & Body Lotion

**Singles:** Frankincense, Frankincense Vitality, Sacred Frankincense, Idaho Blue Spruce, German Chamomile, German Chamomile Vitality, Helichrysum, Jasmine, Lavender, Lavender Vitality, Myrrh, Myrtle, Roman Chamomile, Rose, Royal Hawaiian Sandalwood, Vetiver, Western Red Cedar, Ylang Ylang, Dalmatia Bay Laurel, Laurus Nobilis, Laurus Nobilis Vitality

**Blends:** 3 Wise Men, Gentle Baby, Highest Potential, Owie, Sensation, Valor, Valor II

**Nutritionals:** Sulfurzyme, Master Formula, Mineral Essence, MultiGreens

**Body Care:** ClaraDerm, Progessence Plus, Regenolone Moisturizing Cream, Prenolone Plus Body Cream, Rose Ointment, Essential Beauty Serum

## Stress

**Singles:** Dill, Dill Vitality, Lavender, Lavender Vitality, Roman Chamomile, Jade Lemon, Jade Lemon Vitality, Lemon, Lemon Vitality, Lime, Lime Vitality, Sage, Sage Vitality, Orange, Orange Vitality, Yuzu, Rosemary, Rosemary Vitality, Valerian, Vetiver, Hinoki, Dalmatia Sage, Sage, Sage Vitality

**Blends:** AromaSleep, Divine Release, Evergreen Essence, Freedom, InTouch, Reconnect, Harmony, Joy, Peace & Calming, Peace & Calming II, Release, RutaVaLa, RutaVaLa Roll-On, Sacred Mountain, Stress Away Roll-On, Tranquil Roll-On, Trauma Life, T.R. Care, Valor, Valor II, White Angelica, White Light

**Nutritionals:** ImmuPro (at bedtime), Master Formula, MegaCal, Mineral Essence, Sleep Essence, Super B, Thyromin

**Body Care:** Relaxation Massage Oil, Sensation Massage Oil

Personal Usage Guide | **Chapter 20**

# Personal Usage

## ABUSE, MENTAL AND PHYSICAL

The trauma from mental and physical abuse can result in self-defeating behavior that can undermine success later in life. Through their powerful effect on the limbic system of the brain (the center of stored memories and emotions), essential oils can help release pent-up trauma, emotions, or memories. All memories alter the RNA and DNA and create a blueprint in the DNA. This is why trauma imprinting can be passed from generation to generation. Always start with Frankincense.

### Recommendations

**Singles:** Sacred Frankincense, Frankincense, Frankincense Vitality, Idaho Balsam Fir, Royal Hawaiian Sandalwood, Melissa, Ylang Ylang, Amazonian Ylang Ylang, Dalmatia Sage, Sage Vitality

**Blends:** Divine Release, Freedom, Trauma Life, T.R. Care, SARA, Release, Acceptance, Forgiveness, Amoressence, Surrender, Humility, InTouch, Reconnect, SleepyIze, White Angelica, White Light, Inner Child, Harmony, Hope, Inner Harmony, Tranquil Roll-On, Valor, Valor II, Valor Roll-On, Peace & Calming, Peace & Calming II, The Gift, Oola Faith, Oola Family, Oola Field, Oola Finance, Oola Fitness, Oola Friends, Oola Fun, Oola Grow, Common Sense, Abundance, 3 Wise Men

**Nutritionals:** OmegaGize[3], NingXia Red, EndoGize, Mineral Essence, Master Formula, MindWise

### Application and Usage

**Aromatic:** Refer to *Application Guidelines* on page 410.

**Topical:** For guidelines on applying oils to the skin, refer to *Application Guidelines* on page 410.

### Specific Types of Abuse:

**Physical Abuse:** Apply 2-3 drops of SARA and Forgiveness over the abuse area and around the navel. Follow with 1-2 drops of Release over the Vita Flex points on the feet, especially the liver point of the right foot, under the nose, and directly over the liver. Then apply Trauma Life or T.R. Care.

**Parental, Sexual, or Ritual Abuse:** Apply 1-3 drops of SARA over the area where abuse took place; then Forgiveness, Trauma Life, T.R. Care, Release, Joy, Present Time.

**Spousal Abuse:** Apply SARA, Forgiveness, Trauma Life, T.R. Care, Release, Valor, Valor II, Joy, Amoressence, Envision, Hope.

**Feelings of Revenge:** Apply 1-2 drops of Surrender on the sternum over the heart, 2-3 drops of Present Time on the thymus, and 2-3 drops of Forgiveness over the navel.

**Suicidal:** Apply 2 drops of Hope on the rim of the ears. Melissa, Brain Power, GeneYus, Surrender, RutaVaLa, Common Sense, or Present Time may also be beneficial.

**Protection and Balance:** Apply 1-2 drops of White Angelica on each shoulder and 1-2 drops of Harmony on energy points or chakras. Finish with Valor followed by Sacred Frankincense or Frankincense to set the DNA blueprint.

## ACIDOSIS *(See also Heartburn, Fungus)*

Acidosis is a condition where the pH of the blood serum becomes excessively acidic. This condition should not be confused with an acid stomach. Acidic blood can stress the liver and eventually lead to many forms of chronic and degenerative diseases. Dietary and Oral changes will help in raising the serum pH (making it more alkaline). Cleansing is an essential Dietary and Oral step in balancing pH.

### Recommendations

**Singles:** Peppermint, Peppermint Vitality, Fennel, Fennel Vitality, Tarragon, Tarragon Vitality, Jade Lemon, Jade Lemon Vitality, Lemon, Lemon Vitality

**Blends:** DiGize, DiGize Vitality, EndoFlex, EndoFlex Vitality, TummyGize, JuvaCleanse, JuvaCleanse Vitality

**Nutritionals:** AlkaLime, Digest & Cleanse, Essentialzyme, MultiGreens, JuvaPower, MegaCal, Essentialzymes-4, Mineral Essence, Allerzyme

### Application and Usage

**Dietary and Oral:** Whether putting oils in a capsule or drinking them in a liquid, please refer to *Application Guidelines* on page 410.

- Take 1 capsule with desired oil 2 times daily.
- Take 2-3 drops of oil in a spoonful of syrup or small amount of milk, juice, or water.

Seventh Edition | **Essential Oils Desk Reference** | **415**

**Essential Oils Desk Reference** | Seventh Edition

- Take an Essentialzymes-4 yellow capsule with Peppermint Vitality until acid level is balanced; then add Essentialzyme.
- To reduce acid indigestion and prevent fermentation that can contribute to bad dreams and interrupted sleep, take 1 teaspoon of AlkaLime in water before bedtime.
- To raise pH, take 2-6 capsules of MultiGreens 3 times daily and take 1 teaspoon of AlkaLime in water 1 hour before or 2 hours after meals each day. For maintenance, take 1 teaspoon of AlkaLime once per week at bedtime.
- To stimulate enzymatic action in the digestive tract, mix together raw carrot juice, NingXia Red, alfalfa juice, and papaya juice with 1 dropper of Mineral Essence and 1 drop of DiGize Vitality.

**Topical:** For guidelines on applying oils to the skin, refer to *Application Guidelines* on page 410.

## ADDICTIONS

Many foods and plants—such as tobacco, caffeine, drugs, alcohol, breads, sugar, and other sweeteners—create chemical dependencies.

Cleansing and detoxifying the liver is a crucial first step toward breaking free of these addictions. Alkaline calcium can help bind bile acids and prevent fatty liver. A colon and tissue cleanse is also important.

A body lacking in sufficient enzymes, vitamins, minerals, and other nutrients may also play a part in some addictions. Blue Agave, Yacon Syrup, maple syrup, honey, molasses, and other natural sweeteners are good substitutes for sugar, which should be restricted in a diet.

The Thieves oil blend has been very helpful in curbing an addiction. One or two drops on the tongue are very sufficient to stop the onset of a craving.

JuvaTone, JuvaPower, and JuvaCleanse may be used long term to help detoxify the liver. They suppress the addiction and eventually change the addiction blueprint in the cells of the body.

### Recommendations

**Singles:** Orange, Orange Vitality, Ledum, Fennel, Fennel Vitality, Tarragon, Tarragon Vitality

**Blends:** GLF, GLF Vitality, GeneYus, Thieves, Thieves Vitality, Harmony, InTouch, Reconnect, SleepyIze, Peace & Calming, Peace & Calming II, JuvaCleanse, JuvaCleanse Vitality, JuvaFlex, JuvaFlex Vitality

**Nutritionals:** Detoxzyme, ComforTone, Digest & Cleanse, JuvaPower, MindWise, ICP, JuvaTone, Power Meal, Slique Shake, Slique Bars, Slique CitraSlim, MegaCal, Essentialzyme, Essentialzymes-4, Balance Complete, Blue Agave, Yacon Syrup, OmegaGize[3], Slique Tea, Slique Bars, Pure Protein Complete

### Application and Usage

**Aromatic:** Refer to *Application Guidelines* on page 410.

**Dietary and Oral:** Whether putting oils in a capsule or drinking them in a liquid, please refer to *Application Guidelines* on page 410.

- Take 1 capsule with desired oil 2 times daily.
- Take 2-3 drops of oil in a spoonful of syrup or small amount of milk, juice, or water.

**Topical:** For guidelines on applying oils to the skin, refer to *Application Guidelines* on page 410.

- Apply 1-2 drops neat (undiluted) on temples and back of neck 4 times daily or as desired.
- Place a warm compress with 1-2 drops of chosen oil over the liver.

## ADRENAL GLAND DISORDERS

The adrenal glands consist of two sections: An inner part called the medulla, which produces stress hormones, and an outer part called the cortex, which secretes critical hormones called glucocorticoids and aldosterone. Because of these hormones, the cortex has a far greater impact on overall health than the medulla.

Aldosterone and glucocorticoids are very important because they directly affect blood pressure and minerals that help regulate the conversion of carbohydrates into energy.

In cases like Addison's disease, adrenal cortex hormones fail to produce sufficient amounts or none of the critical hormones, which can lead to life-threatening fluid and mineral loss, unless these hormones are replaced.

On the other hand, Cushing's disease, or syndrome, occurs when the body has too much of the hormone cortisol or other steroid hormones.

### Addison's Disease

Addison's disease is an autoimmune disease in which the body's own immune cells begin to destroy the adrenal glands. Sulfurzyme, an important source of organic sulfur, is known to have positive effects in fighting many types of autoimmune diseases, including lupus, arthritis, and fibromyalgia.

416 | **Chapter 20** | Personal Usage Guide

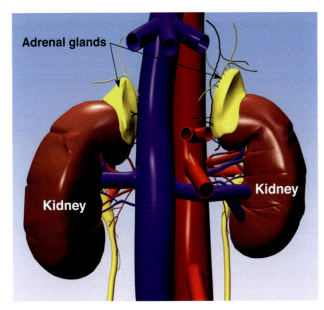

**Adrenal Glands**

**Symptoms associated with Addison's disease**

- Severe fatigue
- Lightheadedness when standing
- Nausea
- Depression/irritability
- Craving salty foods
- Loss of appetite
- Muscle spasms
- Dark, tan-colored skin

Some essential oils have chemical components or structures that have adrenal-like action, enabling them to give support to the body's own system, which may help correct those deficiencies by strengthening adrenal cortex function. The EndoFlex oil blend promotes adrenal-like activity that raises energy levels.

### Recommendations

**Singles:** Nutmeg, Nutmeg Vitality, Fennel, Fennel Vitality, German Chamomile, German Chamomile Vitality, Clove, Clove Vitality, Sacred Frankincense, Frankincense, Frankincense Vitality, Bergamot, Bergamot Vitality

**Blends:** EndoFlex, EndoFlex Vitality, En-R-Gee, GeneYus, Brain Power, Common Sense, Clarity

**Nutritionals:** Thyromin, Sulfurzyme, EndoGize, MindWise, MultiGreens, Balance Complete, MegaCal, Mineral Essence, Super B, Life 9, NingXia Red

### Application and Usage

**Aromatic:** Refer to *Application Guidelines* on page 410.

**Dietary and Oral:** Whether putting oils in a capsule or drinking them in a liquid, please refer to *Application Guidelines* on page 410.

- Take 1 capsule with desired oil 2 times daily.
- Take 2-3 drops of oil in a spoonful of syrup or small amount of milk, juice, or water.

**Topical:** For guidelines on applying oils to the skin, refer to *Application Guidelines* on page 410.

### Cushing's Syndrome (Disease)

Adrenal gland imbalance is characterized by the overproduction of adrenal cortex hormones such as cortisol. While these hormones are crucial to sound health in normal amounts, their unchecked overproduction can cause as much harm as their underproduction. This results in the following symptoms:

- Slow wound healing
- Obesity
- Low resistance
- Acne
- Infection
- Moon-shaped face
- Easily bruised skin
- Osteoporosis
- Weak or wasted muscles

Although Cushing's disease can be caused by a malfunction in the pituitary, it is usually triggered by excessive use of immune-suppressing corticosteroid medications, such as those used for asthma and arthritis. Once these are stopped, the disease often abates. The key to reducing excess cortisol is often reducing stress.

### Recommendations

**Singles:** Canadian Fleabane (Conyza), Spearmint, Spearmint Vitality, Dorado Azul, Sacred Frankincense, Frankincense, Frankincense Vitality, Idaho Balsam Fir

**Blends:** EndoFlex, EndoFlex Vitality, Exodus II, Peace & Calming, Peace & Calming II, Acceptance, Grounding, Harmony, DiGize, DiGize Vitality, TummyGize

**Nutritionals:** Ultra Young, ImmuPro, Inner Defense, PD 80/20, Mineral Essence, CortiStop, Digest & Cleanse, JuvaPower, JuvaSpice, OmegaGize[3], MindWise

**Essential Oils Desk Reference** | Seventh Edition

> ## Support the Adrenal Glands
>
> Add the following amounts of essential oils to ¼ teaspoon of massage oil and apply as a warm compress over the adrenal glands (located on top of the kidneys):
>
> - 3 drops Clove
> - 3 drops Nutmeg
> - 7 drops Rosemary

## Application and Usage

**Aromatic:** Refer to *Application Guidelines* on page 410.

**Dietary and Oral:** Whether putting oils in a capsule or drinking them in a liquid, please refer to *Application Guidelines* on page 410.

- Take 2 capsules with EndoFlex Vitality or other desired oil 2 times daily.
- Take 2-3 drops of oil in a spoonful of syrup or small amount of milk, juice, or water.

**Topical:** For guidelines on applying oils to the skin, refer to *Application Guidelines* on page 410.

- Apply warm compress over adrenal area (on back, over kidneys) with 1-2 drops of recommended oil.

## AGITATION

Agitation is caused by a weakened nervous system, lack of sleep, frustration, and is often a result of a congested liver or over stimulation of the sympathetic system.

## Recommendations

**Singles:** Lavender, Lavender Vitality, Roman Chamomile, Hinoki, Vetiver, Ocotea, Valerian, Idaho Balsam Fir, Myrrh, Sacred Frankincense, Frankincense, Frankincense Vitality, Melissa, Helichrysum, Marjoram, Marjoram Vitality, Sage, Sage Vitality

**Blends:** RutaVaLa, RutaVaLa Roll-On, Tranquil Roll-On, Stress Away Roll-On, Forgiveness, Amoressence, Peace & Calming, Peace & Calming II, AromaSleep, Surrender, Humility, InTouch, Reconnect, SleepyIze, White Angelica, White Light

**Nutritionals:** ImmuPro, Super B, JuvaTone, MegaCal, EndoGize, SleepEssence

## Application and Usage

**Aromatic:** Refer to *Application Guidelines* on page 410.

**Topical:** For guidelines on applying oils to the skin, refer to *Application Guidelines* on page 410.

- Apply 1-2 drops neat or undiluted on temples and back of neck as desired.
- You may also apply 1-2 drops on the Vita Flex brain and heart points on the bottoms of the feet.
- Applying a single drop under the nose is helpful and refreshing.
- Place a warm compress with 3-4 drops of chosen oil over the back.

## AIDS (Acquired Immune Deficiency Syndrome)

The AIDS virus attacks and infects immune cells that are essential for life. Frankincense and Myrrh have immune-building properties. Other oils like Cumin *(Cuminum cyminum)* have an inhibitory effect on viral replication.

In May 1994, Dr. Radwan Farag of Cairo University demonstrated that cumin seed oil had an 88 to 92 percent inhibition effect in vitro against HIV, the virus responsible for AIDS. Other antiviral essential oils include Oregano, Royal Hawaiian Sandalwood, Ocotea, and Tea Tree.

## Recommendations

**Singles:** Ocotea, Cumin, Cypress, Oregano, Oregano Vitality, Plectranthus Oregano, Royal Hawaiian Sandalwood, Tea Tree, Myrrh, Sacred Frankincense, Frankincense, Frankincense Vitality, Northern Lights Black Spruce, Peppermint, Peppermint Vitality, Cistus, Cumin

**Blends:** Exodus II, Thieves, Thieves Vitality, Inner Defense, InTouch, Reconnect, SleepyIze, Release, Acceptance

**Nutritionals:** NingXia Red, Power Meal, Slique Shake, ImmuPro, Longevity Softgels, Essentialzyme, Essentialzymes-4, EndoGize, Pure Protein Complete

**Body Care:** Raindrop Technique application

## Application and Usage

**Aromatic:** Refer to *Application Guidelines* on page 410.

**Dietary and Oral:** Whether putting the oils in a capsule or drinking them in a liquid, please refer to instructions at the beginning of this chapter.

- Take 2 capsules with 50:50 Cistus and Cypress 2 times daily.

**418** | **Chapter 20** | Personal Usage Guide

*Personal Usage Guide* | **Chapter 20**

- Take 2-3 drops of oil in a spoonful of syrup or small amount of milk, juice, or water.

**Topical:** For guidelines on applying oils to the skin, refer to *Application Guidelines* on page 410.

## ALCOHOLISM *(See also Addictions)*

Alcoholism, also known as alcohol dependence, includes alcohol craving and continued drinking. It includes four symptoms:

1. Craving: A strong compulsion, or need, to drink alcohol
2. Impaired control: The inability to limit drinking
3. Physical dependence: Inability to stop drinking without experiencing withdrawal symptoms such as nausea, shakiness, sweating, and anxiety
4. Tolerance: The need for increasing amounts of alcohol

### Recommendations

**Singles:** Sacred Frankincense, Frankincense, Frankincense Vitality, Lavender, Lavender Vitality, Roman Chamomile, Ledum, Helichrysum, Orange, Orange Vitality

**Blends:** JuvaCleanse, JuvaCleanse Vitality, GLF, GLF Vitality, Forgiveness, Amoressence, Release, Acceptance, Valor, Valor II, Valor Roll-On, Motivation, White Angelica, White Light, The Gift, Common Sense, InTouch, Reconnect

**Nutritionals:** JuvaTone, ICP, ComforTone, Super B, Power Meal, Slique Shake, Detoxzyme, Master Formula, Mineral Essence, Allerzyme

### Application and Usage

**Aromatic:** Refer to *Application Guidelines* on page 410.

**Dietary and Oral:** Whether putting oils in a capsule or drinking them in a liquid, please refer to *Application Guidelines* on page 410.

- Take 1 capsule with desired oil 2 times daily.
- Take 2-3 drops of oil in a spoonful of syrup or small amount of milk, juice, or water.

**Topical:** For guidelines on applying oils to the skin, refer to *Application Guidelines* on page 410.

- Apply 1-2 drops neat on temples and back of neck several times daily.
- Place a warm compress with 6-8 drops of chosen oil over the liver.

## ALKALOSIS

Alkalosis is a condition where the pH of the intestinal tract and the blood become excessively alkaline. While moderate alkalinity is essential for good health, excessive alkalinity can cause problems and result in fatigue, depression, irritability, and sickness.

The best way to lower the internal pH of the body is to eat a high protein diet (meat, eggs, dairy, seeds, nuts, legumes, etc.).

### Recommendations

**Singles:** Peppermint, Peppermint Vitality, Jade Lemon, Jade Lemon Vitality, Lemon, Lemon Vitality, Lime, Lime Vitality, Orange, Orange Vitality, Tarragon, Tarragon Vitality, Fennel, Fennel Vitality, Ginger, Ginger Vitality, Patchouli, Lemongrass, Lemongrass Vitality, Bergamot, Bergamot Vitality

**Blends:** DiGize, DiGize Vitality, GLF, GLF Vitality, EndoFlex, EndoFlex Vitality, TummyGize

**Nutritionals:** Essentialzyme, Essentialzymes-4, ICP, Allerzyme, ComforTone, Digest & Cleanse, Pure Protein Complete, Power Meal, Slique Shake, Life 9

### Application and Usage

**Aromatic:** Refer to *Application Guidelines* on page 410.

**Dietary and Oral:** Whether putting oils in a capsule or drinking them in a liquid, please refer to *Application Guidelines* on page 410.

- Take 1 capsule with desired oil 2 times daily.
- Take 2-3 drops of oil in a spoonful of syrup or small amount of milk, juice, or water.

**Topical:** For guidelines on applying oils to the skin, refer to *Application Guidelines* on page 410.

## ALLERGIES

Allergies are a result of the response to many different situations. They can be triggered by food, pollen, environmental chemicals, dander, dust, insect bites, to name just a few, and can affect the following:

- Respiration—wheezing, labored breathing
- Mouth—swelling of the lips or tongue, itching lips
- Digestive tract—diarrhea, vomiting, cramps
- Skin—rashes, dermatitis
- Nose—sneezing, congestion, bloody nose

Seventh Edition | **Essential Oils Desk Reference** | 419

**Essential Oils Desk Reference** | Seventh Edition

## Food Allergies

Food allergies are different from food intolerances. Food allergies involve an immune system reaction, whereas food intolerances involve gastrointestinal reactions and are far more common.

For example, peanuts often produce a lifelong allergy due to peanut proteins being targeted by immune system antibodies as foreign invaders. In contrast, intolerance of pasteurized cow's milk that causes cramping and diarrhea is due to the inability to digest lactose (milk sugar) because of a lack of the enzyme lactase.

Food allergies are often associated with the consumption of peanuts, shellfish, nuts, wheat, cow's milk, eggs, and soy. Infants and children are far more prone to have food allergies than adults, due to the immaturity of their immune and digestive systems.

A thorough intestinal cleansing is one of the best ways to combat most allergies. Start with ICP, ComforTone, Essentialzyme, Essentialzymes-4, JuvaTone, and Life 9.

## Hay Fever (Allergic Rhinitis)

Hay fever is an allergic reaction triggered by airborne allergens (pollen, animal hair, feathers, dust mites, etc.) that cause the release of histamines and subsequent inflammation of nasal passages and sinus-related areas. A more serious form of respiratory allergy is asthma, which manifests in the chest and lungs.

**Symptoms:** Inflammation of the nasal passages, sinuses, and eyelids that cause sneezing, runny nose, wheezing, and watery and red, itchy eyes.

## Recommendations

**Singles:** Fennel, Fennel Vitality, Eucalyptus Blue, Lavender, Lavender Vitality, Ocotea, Roman Chamomile, Peppermint, Peppermint Vitality, German Chamomile, German Chamomile Vitality, Marjoram, Marjoram Vitality, Sacred Frankincense, Frankincense, Frankincense Vitality

**Blends:** DiGize Vitality, DiGize, Harmony, JuvaCleanse, JuvaCleanse Vitality, Valor, Valor II, Valor Roll-On, R.C., Raven, TummyGize

**Nutritionals:** Allerzyme, Mineral Essence, ComforTone, Detoxzyme, Essentialzyme, ICP, JuvaPower, JuvaSpice, JuvaTone, MultiGreens, Sulfurzyme, Essentialzymes-4 yellow capsule, AlkaLime, Life 9

## Application and Usage

**Aromatic:** Refer to *Application Guidelines* on page 410.

**Dietary and Oral:** Whether putting oils in a capsule or drinking them in a liquid, please refer to *Application Guidelines* on page 410.

- Take 1 capsule with desired oil 2 times daily.
- Take 2-3 drops of oil in a spoonful of syrup or small amount of milk, juice, or water.

**Topical:** For guidelines on applying oils to the skin, refer to *Application Guidelines* on page 410.

## ANALGESIC

An analgesic is defined as a compound that binds with a number of closely related, specific receptors in the central nervous system to block the perception of pain or affect the emotional response to pain. A number of essential oils have analgesic properties.

## Recommendations

**Singles:** Clove, Helichrysum, Dorado Azul, Palo Santo, Elemi, Wintergreen, Copaiba

**Blends:** PanAway, Aroma Siez, Deep Relief Roll-On, Thieves, Inner Defense, Brain Power, Relieve It, Cool Azul

**Nutritionals:** PowerGize

**Body Care:** Cool Azul Pain Relief Cream, Cool Azul Sports Gel, Ortho Sport Massage Oil, Ortho Ease Massage Oil

## Application and Usage

**Aromatic:** Refer to *Application Guidelines* on page 410.

**Topical:** For guidelines on applying oils to the skin, refer to *Application Guidelines* on page 410.

- **Pain Relief Blend:** Mix equal parts of Wintergreen, Northern Lights Black Spruce, and Black Pepper and massage with V-6 Vegetable Oil Complex.
- You may also apply 2-3 drops on the Vita Flex liver point of the right foot.

## ANTHRAX

The anthrax bacterium *(Bacillus anthracis)* is one of the oldest and deadliest diseases known. There are three predominant types:

- External, acquired from contact with infected animal carcasses
- Internal, obtained from breathing airborne anthrax spores
- Battlefield, developed for biological warfare that is a far more lethal variety

**420** | **Chapter 20** | Personal Usage Guide

When the airborne variety of anthrax invades the lungs, it is 90 percent fatal unless antibiotics are administered at the very beginning of the infection, but anthrax often goes undiagnosed until it is too late for antibiotics.

External varieties of anthrax may be contracted by exposure to animal hides and wool. While vaccinations and antibiotics have stemmed anthrax infection in recent years, new strains have developed that are resistant to all countermeasures.

According to Jean Valnet, MD, Thyme oil may be effective for killing the anthrax bacillus.[1] Two highly antimicrobial phenols in Thyme, carvacrol and thymol, are responsible for this action.

### Recommendations

**Singles:** Ravintsara, Thyme, Thyme Vitality, Oregano, Oregano Vitality, Plectranthus Oregano, Clove, Clove Vitality, Cinnamon Bark, Cinnamon Bark Vitality, Citronella, Lemongrass, Lemongrass Vitality

**Blends:** Raven, Exodus II, Thieves, Thieves Vitality, The Gift, ImmuPower, Melrose, Longevity, Longevity Vitality

**Nutritionals:** Life 9, Inner Defense, ImmuPro, NingXia Red, Super C, Super C Chewable

**Household Care:** Thieves Household Cleaner, Thieves Waterless Hand Purifier, Thieves Foaming Hand Soap, Thieves Automatic Dishwasher Powder, Thieves Cleansing Soap, Thieves Dish Soap, Thieves Fruit & Veggie Soak (and Spray), Thieves Laundry Soap, Thieves Spray, Thieves Wipes

### Application and Usage

**Aromatic:** Refer to *Application Guidelines* on page 410.

**Dietary and Oral:** Whether putting oils in a capsule or drinking them in a liquid, please refer to *Application Guidelines* on page 410.

- Take 1 capsule 4 times daily, alternating oils.
- Take 2-3 drops of oil in a spoonful of syrup or small amount of milk, juice, or water.

**Topical:** For guidelines on applying oils to the skin, refer to *Application Guidelines* on page 410.

- Use oils neat or dilute 50:50 for hands and other exposed skin areas.

## ANTIBIOTIC REACTIONS

Synthetic antibiotic drugs indiscriminately kill both beneficial and harmful bacteria. This can result in yeast infections, including candida, diarrhea, poor nutrient assimilation, fatigue, sulfur toxicity, degenerative diseases, and many other conditions.

The average adult has 3-4 pounds of beneficial bacteria or flora constantly in the intestinal tract that support the body in healthy digestion and immune function and promote the following body functions:

- Constitutes the first line of defense against bacterial and viral infections
- Produces B vitamins
- Maintains pH balance
- Combats yeast and fungus overgrowth
- Aids in the digestive process

### Recommendations

**Singles:** Peppermint, Peppermint Vitality, Spearmint, Spearmint Vitality, Jade Lemon, Jade Lemon Vitality, Lemon, Lemon Vitality, Lime, Lime Vitality

**Blends:** JuvaCleanse, JuvaCleanse Vitality, DiGize, DiGize Vitality, Purification, Thieves, Thieves Vitality, GLF, GLF Vitality, EndoFlex, EndoFlex Vitality, TummyGize

**Nutritionals:** Life 9, Essentialzyme, Essentialzymes-4, Detoxzyme, Balance Complete, Power Meal, Slique Shake, Mineral Essence, Inner Defense, Digest & Cleanse

### Application and Usage

**Aromatic:** Refer to *Application Guidelines* on page 410.

**Dietary and Oral:** Whether putting oils in a capsule or drinking them in a liquid, please refer to *Application Guidelines* on page 410.

- Take 1 capsule with desired oil 2 times daily.
- Take 2-3 drops of oil in a spoonful of syrup or small amount of milk, juice, or water.
- Life 9: Take 2-3 capsules on an empty stomach before meals during antibiotic treatment.
- After completing antibiotic treatment, continue using Life 9 for 10-15 days.

**Topical:** For guidelines on applying oils to the skin, refer to *Application Guidelines* on page 410.

## ANTISEPTICS AND DISINFECTANTS

Antiseptics prevent the growth of pathogenic microorganisms. Many essential oils have powerful, antiseptic properties. Clove and Thyme essential oils have been documented to kill over 50 types of bacteria and 10 types of fungi.

Other potent antiseptic essential oils include Cinnamon Bark, Cassia, Tea Tree, Oregano, Plectranthus Oregano, Mountain Savory, and Dorado Azul.

### Recommendations

**Singles:** Thyme, Thyme Vitality, Thieves, Thieves Vitality, Clove, Clove Vitality, Dorado Azul, Oregano, Oregano Vitality, Plectranthus Oregano, Rosemary, Rosemary Vitality, Mountain Savory, Mountain Savory Vitality, Eucalyptus Radiata, Eucalyptus Globulus, Lavandin, Cinnamon Bark, Cassia, Ravintsara, Tea Tree, Dalmatia Sage, Sage

**Blends:** Thieves, Raven, Purification, Melrose, R.C., ImmuPower, Breathe Again Roll-On, SniffleEase

**Nutritionals:** Inner Defense, ImmuPro, Thieves Cough Drops, Thieves Hard Lozenges

**Oral Care:** Thieves AromaBright Toothpaste, Thieves Dentarome Plus Toothpaste, Thieves Dentarome Ultra Toothpaste, Thieves Fresh Essence Plus Mouthwash

**Household Care:** Thieves Foaming Hand Soap, Thieves Waterless Hand Purifier, Thieves Household Cleaner, Thieves Cleansing Soap, Thieves Automatic Dishwasher Powder, Thieves Dish Soap, Thieves Fruit & Veggie Soak (and Spray), Thieves Laundry Soap, Thieves Spray, Thieves Wipes

### Application and Usage

**Aromatic:** Refer to *Application Guidelines* on page 410.

**Topical:** For guidelines on applying oils to the skin, refer to *Application Guidelines* on page 410.

- Apply 1-2 drops diluted 50:50 and gently rub over affected areas.

## APNEA

Apnea is a temporary cessation of breathing during sleep. It can lessen the quality of sleep, resulting in chronic fatigue, lowered immune function, and lack of energy.

### Recommendations

**Singles:** Northern Lights Black Spruce, Idaho Balsam Fir, Cedarwood, Ylang Ylang, Amazonian Ylang Ylang, Lavender, Lavender Vitality, Sacred Frankincense, Frankincense, Frankincense Vitality, Royal Hawaiian Sandalwood, Dalmatia Juniper, Juniper

**Blends:** Clarity, Valor, Valor II, Valor Roll-On, Common Sense, Stress Away Roll-On, RutaVaLa, RutaVaLa Roll-On, White Angelica, White Light, Sacred Mountain, Present Time, AromaSleep, ImmuPower

**Nutritionals:** Thyromin, MultiGreens, Super B, Inner Defense, ImmuPro, Ultra Young, SleepEssence

### Application and Usage

**Aromatic:** Refer to *Application Guidelines* on page 410.

**Topical:** For guidelines on applying oils to the skin, refer to *Application Guidelines* on page 410.

- Massage 2-4 drops of oil neat on the bottoms of the feet just before bedtime.

## ARTHRITIS

More than 100 different kinds of arthritis have been identified. Two of the most common kinds are osteoarthritis and rheumatoid arthritis.

### Osteoarthritis

Osteoarthritis involves the breakdown of the cartilage that forms a cushion between two joints. As this cartilage is eaten away, the two bones of the joint start rubbing together and wearing down.

In contrast, rheumatoid arthritis is caused from a swelling and inflammation of the synovial membrane, the lining of the joint.

Natural anti-inflammatories such as German Chamomile and Wintergreen when combined with cartilage builders (boswellic acid, undenatured collagen, and hyaluronic acid) are powerful, natural cures for arthritis.

The best natural anti-inflammatories include fats rich in omega-3s and essential oils such as Nutmeg, Wintergreen, German Chamomile, and Idaho Balsam Fir.

Nutmeg, a source of myristicin, has been researched for its anti-inflammatory effects in several studies. It works by inhibiting pro-inflammatory prostaglandins when taken internally or applied topically. Clove exhibits similar action.

Chamazulene, the blue sesquiterpene in German Chamomile, also shows strong anti-inflammatory activity when used both topically and orally. Methyl salicylate is the major compound in Wintergreen, similar to the active agent in aspirin (salicylic acid). PanAway contains nature's natural analgesics from Wintergreen and Clove and is strongly anti-inflammatory. Cool Azul Pain Relief Cream and Cool Azul Sports Gel are also strongly anti-inflammatory.

Type II collagen and hyaluronic acid are the two most powerful natura l compounds for rebuilding cartilage and are the key ingredients in the supplement AgilEase.

## Recommendations

**Singles:** Wintergreen, Nutmeg, Nutmeg Vitality, Peppermint, Peppermint Vitality, Vetiver, Valerian, Palo Santo, Idaho Balsam Fir, Eucalyptus Globulus, Sacred Frankincense, Frankincense, Frankincense Vitality, Idaho Ponderosa Pine, German Chamomile, German Chamomile Vitality, Helichrysum, Dorado Azul, Northern Lights Black Spruce, Pine

**Blends:** Cool Azul, PanAway, Relieve It, Aroma Siez, Deep Relief Roll-On

**Nutritionals:** BLM, AgilEase, PowerGize, Essentialzyme, Essentialzymes-4, Sulfurzyme, ImmuPro, ICP, JuvaPower, JuvaTone, Detoxzyme, MegaCal, Longevity Softgels, Rehemogen, OmegaGize[3], Estro, EndoGize

**Body Care:** Cool Azul Pain Relief Cream, Cool Azul Sports Gel, Ortho Sport Massage Oil, Ortho Ease Massage Oil

## Application and Usage

**Aromatic:** Refer to *Application Guidelines* on page 410.

**Dietary and Oral:** Whether putting oils in a capsule or drinking them in a liquid, please refer to *Application Guidelines* on page 410.

- Detoxification of the body and strengthening the joints is important. Cleanse the colon and liver.
- Take 1 capsule with desired oil 2 times daily.
- Take 2-3 drops of oil in a spoonful of syrup or small amount of milk, juice, or water.

**Topical:** For guidelines on applying oils to the skin, refer to *Application Guidelines* on page 410.

- Dilute 5-10 drops of oil in 1 teaspoon V-6 Vegetable Oil Complex and apply on location. Essential oils can also be applied neat and then followed by application of V-6 Vegetable Oil Complex.
- Applying a single drop of oil under the nose is helpful and refreshing.
- Cool Azul Pain Relief Cream, Cool Azul Sports Gel, Ortho Sport Massage Oil, or Ortho Ease Massage Oil offer tremendous relief.

**BLM, AgilEase:** Take 2 capsules daily.

**MegaCal:** Mix 1 teaspoon in water before going to bed.

**ImmuPro:** Take 1-2 chewable tablets daily as needed, generally in the evening. Do not exceed 2 tablets per day.

**ComforTone:** Take 3 capsules 2 times daily; increase if needed.

**ICP:** Take 2 scoops in water or juice in the morning.

**JuvaPower:** Take 2 scoops in water or juice before going to bed.

**Rehemogen:** Cleans and purifies the blood, which may have toxins blocking nutrient and oxygen absorption into cells (See Circulation).

**OmegaGize[3]:** Take 1-3 capsules daily.

## Rheumatoid Arthritis

Rheumatoid arthritis is a painful, inflammatory condition of the joints marked by swelling, thickening, and inflammation of the synovial membrane lining the joint. In contrast, osteoarthritis is characterized by a breakdown of the joint cartilage, without any swelling or inflammation.

Rheumatoid arthritis is classified as an autoimmune disease because it is caused by the body's own immune system attacking the joints.

Inflammation from rheumatoid arthritis has been ameliorated by the boswellic acids found in most frankincense species.[2]

Other factors can aggravate arthritis such as:

- Deficiencies of minerals and other nutrients
- Microbes and toxins
- Lack of water intake
- Eating bread

Essential oils are effective in helping to combat pain and infection. In cases where arthritis is caused by infectious organisms, such as Lyme disease (*Borrelia burgdorferi)*, chlamydia, and salmonella, essential oils may counteract and prevent infection.

Highly antimicrobial essential oils include Mountain Savory, Mountain Savory Vitality, Rosemary, Rosemary Vitality, Tea Tree, Oregano, and Oregano Vitality. Essential oils easily pass into the bloodstream when applied topically.

MSM, the main ingredient in the supplement Sulfurzyme, has been documented to be one of the most effective, natural supplements for reducing the pain associated with rheumatism and arthritis.

MSM has been a subject of a number of clinical studies and was used extensively by Ronald Lawrence, MD, in his clinical practice to successfully treat rheumatism and arthritis.

Type II collagen and hyaluronic acid are also powerful, natural compounds for reducing inflammation, halting the progression of arthritis, and rebuilding cartilage. These are the key ingredients in the supplements BLM and AgilEase.

## Recommendations

**Singles:** Wintergreen, Peppermint, Peppermint Vitality, Sacred Frankincense, Frankincense, Frankincense Vitality, Palo Santo, Vetiver, Nutmeg, Nutmeg Vitality, Oregano, Oregano Vitality, Clove, Clove Vitality, Mountain Savory, Mountain Savory Vitality, Rosemary, Rosemary Vitality, Tea Tree, Helichrysum, Idaho Balsam Fir, Idaho Ponderosa Pine, Pine, Eucalyptus Globulus, Copaiba, Myrrh, Valerian, Dorado Azul, Northern Lights Black Spruce

**Blends:** PanAway, Relieve It, Aroma Siez, Deep Relief Roll-On

**Nutritionals:** PowerGize, BLM, AgilEase, Detoxzyme, Sulfurzyme, MegaCal, Master Formula, Mineral Essence, Essentialzyme, Essentialzymes-4, Longevity Softgels, ImmuPro, Rehemogen, EndoGize

**Body Care:** Cool Azul Pain Relief Cream, Cool Azul Sports Gel, Ortho Ease Massage Oil, Ortho Sport Massage Oil

## Application and Usage

**Aromatic:** Refer to *Application Guidelines* on page 410.

**Dietary and Oral:** Whether putting oils in a capsule or drinking them in a liquid, please refer to *Application Guidelines* on page 410.

- Take 1 capsule with desired oil 2 times daily.
- Take 2-3 drops of oil in a spoonful of syrup or small amount of milk, juice, or water.

**Topical:** For guidelines on applying oils to the skin, refer to *Application Guidelines* on page 410.

- Dilute 5-10 drops of essential oils in 1 teaspoon of V-6 Vegetable Oil Complex and apply on location. Essential oils can also be applied neat and then followed by V-6 Vegetable Oil Complex.
- Massage 2-4 drops of oil neat on the bottoms of the feet just before bedtime.
- Place a warm compress once daily with oils of your choice on the back.
- Massage with oils of your choice mixed with V-6 Vegetable Oil Complex, Relaxation Massage Oil, Sensation Massage Oil, Ortho Ease Massage Oil, or Ortho Sport Massage Oil.
- Apply Cool Azul Pain Relief Cream or Cool Azul Sports Gel.

# ATTENTION DEFICIT DISORDER (ADD AND ADHD)

Terry Friedmann, MD, in 2001 completed pioneering studies using essential oils to combat ADD and ADHD. Using twice-a-day inhalation of essential oils, including Vetiver, Cedarwood, and Lavender, Dr. Friedmann was able to achieve clinically significant results in 60 days. Researchers postulate that essential oils mitigate ADD and ADHD through their stimulation of the limbic system of the brain.

Because attention deficit disorder may be caused by mineral deficiencies in the diet, increasing nutrient intake and absorption of magnesium, potassium, and other trace minerals can also have a significant, beneficial effect in resolving ADD.

## Recommendations

**Singles:** Vetiver, Lavender, Lavender Vitality, Cedarwood, Royal Hawaiian Sandalwood, Cardamom, Cardamom Vitality, Peppermint, Peppermint Vitality, Sacred Frankincense, Frankincense, Frankincense Vitality

**Blends:** GeneYus, Brain Power, Peace & Calming, Peace & Calming II, Clarity, InTouch, Reconnect, SleepyIze

**Nutritionals:** OmegaGize[3], MindWise, Mineral Essence, NingXia Red, Power Meal, Slique Shake, Balance Complete, Essentialzyme, Essentialzymes-4, Detoxzyme, MultiGreens, Master Formula, Pure Protein Complete

## Application and Usage

**Aromatic:** Refer to *Application Guidelines* on page 410.

**Dietary and Oral:** Whether putting oils in a capsule or drinking them in a liquid, please refer to *Application Guidelines* on page 410.

- Take 1 capsule with desired oil 2 times daily.
- Take 2-3 drops of oil in a spoonful of syrup or small amount of milk, juice, or water.
- Drink 3-6 oz. of NingXia Red daily.

**Topical:** For guidelines on applying oils to the skin, refer to *Application Guidelines* on page 410.

- Apply 1-2 drops of the oil of your choice neat or diluted 4-8 times daily on the neck, brain stem, and even on the head.
- Applying a single drop under the nose is helpful and refreshing.
- Massage 2-4 drops of oil neat on the bottoms of the feet just before bedtime. Children love it.

Personal Usage Guide | **Chapter 20**

## AUTISM

Improving diet can be the key to reducing the problems associated with autism. Eliminating refined and synthetic sugars and replacing them with natural sweeteners such as Blue Agave, Yacon Syrup, natural fruit sweeteners, maple syrup, etc., has produced outstanding results in numerous cases of autism.

Autism is a neurologically based developmental disorder that is four times more common in boys than girls. It is characterized by the following:

- Social ineptness (loner)
- Nonverbal and verbal communication difficulties
- Repetitive behavior (rocking, hair twirling)
- Self-injurious behavior (head banging)
- Very limited or peculiar interests
- Reduced or abnormal responses to pain, noises, or other outside stimuli

Autism is being increasingly linked to certain vaccinations; and MMR, the one-shot combination for measles, mumps, and rubella, is most often cited by researchers. British researcher Andrew Wakefield, MD, suggests using single shots for children for measles, mumps, and rubella (instead of the combined MMR shot) until further research is done.

Dr. Wakefield's suggestions may be acceptable to people who know little about vaccinations, but the research that has been done on vaccines sends a very loud warning. Vaccinations given in combination or singularly are damaging to anyone of any age. Unfortunately, children are usually the innocent victims who suffer the most.

Until recently, children were receiving, through vaccination, large doses of thimerosal, a vaccine preservative that contains 49.6 percent mercury, which is well above the limit recommended by the EPA. Some success in reversing autism has resulted through mercury detoxification along with nutritional supplementation.

Some researchers believe that gastrointestinal disorders may be linked to the brain dysfunctions that cause autism in children (Horvath, et al., 1998). In fact, there have been several cases of successful treatment of autism using pancreatic enzymes.

Stimulation of the limbic region of the brain may also help treat autism. The aromas from essential oils have a powerful ability to stimulate this part of the brain, since the sense of smell (olfaction) is tied directly to the emotional centers. As a result, the aroma of an essential oil has the potential to exert a powerful influence on disorders such as ADD and autism.

## Recommendations

**Singles:** Vetiver, Patchouli, Lavender, Lavender Vitality, Eucalyptus Globulus, Melissa, Myrrh, Peppermint, Peppermint Vitality, Canadian Fleabane (Conyza), Cedarwood, Royal Hawaiian Sandalwood, Sacred Frankincense, Frankincense, Frankincense Vitality, Idaho Balsam Fir

**Blends:** GeneYus, Brain Power, Divine Release, Evergreen Essence, GLF, GLF Vitality, Inner Harmony, Valor, Valor II, Valor Roll-On, Clarity, Peace & Calming, Peace & Calming II, Common Sense, The Gift, InTouch, Reconnect, SleepyIze

**Nutritionals:** Essentialzyme, Essentialzymes-4, Blue Agave, MindWise, NingXia Red, ½ Super B for children, Sulfurzyme, Detoxzyme, Power Meal, Slique Shake, Balance Complete, Pure Protein Complete, AlkaLime

## Application and Usage

**Aromatic:** Refer to *Application Guidelines* on page 410.

**Dietary and Oral:** Whether putting oils in a capsule or drinking them in a liquid, please refer to *Application Guidelines* on page 410.

- Take 1 capsule with desired oil 2 times daily.
- Take 2-3 drops of oil in a spoonful of syrup or small amount of milk, juice, or water.

**Topical:** For guidelines on applying oils to the skin, refer to *Application Guidelines* on page 410.

- Apply 1-2 drops neat (undiluted) on temples and back of neck, as desired.
- Applying a single drop under the nose is helpful and refreshing.
- Massage 2-4 drops of oil neat on the bottoms of the feet just before bedtime. Children love it.

### Autism Blend

- 15 drops Sacred Frankincense, Frankincense Vitality, or Frankincense
- 12 drops Myrrh
- 10 drops Idaho Balsam Fir
- 10 drops Canadian Fleabane (Conyza)
- 4 drops Peppermint Vitality or Peppermint

Take 3 capsules daily: morning, noon, and night.

Use this blend for Raindrop Technique 2 times daily: morning and night.

Using this regimen, a 7-year-old boy with cerebral palsy and autism, after one month, was able to walk flat footed without his walker, test scores in school improved by 28 percent, and his attention span increased 30 percent, his mother reported.

Seventh Edition | **Essential Oils Desk Reference** | **425**

# BEDBUGS

Having bedbugs is a very miserable experience. Some bedbugs are so small they just look like specks of dirt that you brush off the sheets. You cannot tell they are alive unless you look at them with a microscope. They thrive in a moist, warm environment, and when you wake up in the morning, you are astounded at all the bites you have in the most unexpected places.

The itching is horrible and lasts for about one week. It is amazing that a tiny, almost microscopic bug can give such an intense bite. Essential oils are the answer to treating without dreaded chemicals. Some of the oils have a powerful ability to kill on contact. The thought of sleeping with those little, hungry critters is not a pleasant thought, and to some, it's repulsive; but knowing the bugs are dead is a positive feeling.

If you suspect bedbugs, wash all of your bedding in hot water and add 10 to 15 drops of Thieves, Palo Santo, Oregano, Plectranthus Oregano, Thyme, Citrus Fresh, Melrose, etc., and see what works best for you. After you make the bed, spray with a single oil or with one of the blends morning and night to ensure that they do not return.

If you live in a warm or hot, humid environment, then you will probably have to spray at least once every day or perhaps twice. If you see any little specks, make sure they are not biting bugs that have come to visit.

## Recommendations

These blends work for most bugs but have been tried and tested with bedbugs.

### Bedbug Killer Blend No. 1
- 20 drops Palo Santo
- 20 drops Idaho Tansy

Mix together and spray. Dilute with water as much as you think you can and still have results. You will have to experiment to determine that. Spray sheets and clothing to kill any insects that might be imbedded in the cloth or anywhere else that you might suspect their presence.

### Insect Bite Blend No. 2
- 20 drops Palo Santo
- 20 drops Idaho Tansy
- 10 drops Eucalyptus Blue
Apply on bites as needed.

### Bedbug Killer Blend No. 3
- Mix 20 drops Thieves with 2-3 cups water, shake well, and spray sheets and pillows.

# BLADDER/URINARY TRACT INFECTION (CYSTITIS)

Bladder infections and inflammation known as cystitis are caused by bacteria that travel up the urethra. This disorder is more common in women than men because of the woman's shorter urethra. If the infection travels up the ureters and reaches the kidneys, kidney infection can result.

## Symptoms of infection

- Frequent urge to urinate with only a small amount of urine passing
- Strong smelling urine
- Blood in urine
- Burning or stinging during urination
- Tenderness or chronic pain in bladder and pelvic area
- Pain intensity fluctuates as bladder fills or empties
- Symptoms worsen during menstruation

## Recommendations

**Singles:** Myrrh, Tea Tree, Juniper, Oregano, Oregano Vitality, Plectranthus Oregano, Jade Lemon, Jade Lemon Vitality, Lemon, Lemon Vitality, Lime, Lime Vitality, Melissa, Mountain Savory, Mountain Savory Vitality, Thyme, Thyme Vitality, Cistus, Rosemary, Rosemary Vitality, Clove, Clove Vitality, Palo Santo

**Blends:** Melrose, Thieves, Thieves Vitality, DiGize, DiGize Vitality, EndoFlex, EndoFlex Vitality, R.C., Purification

**Nutritionals:** K&B, ImmuPro, Inner Defense, Alka-Lime, Blue Agave

## Application and Usage

**Dietary and Oral:** Whether putting oils in a capsule or drinking them in a liquid, please refer to *Application Guidelines* on page 410.

- Take 1 capsule with desired oil 2 times daily.
- Take 2-3 drops of oil in a spoonful of syrup or small amount of milk, juice, or water.
- Use K&B tincture (2-3 droppers in distilled water) 3-6 times daily. K&B helps strengthen and tone weak bladder, kidneys, and urinary tract.
- Take ½ teaspoon of AlkaLime daily, in water only, 1 hour before or after meal.
- Drink unsweetened cranberry juice and sweeten with honey, Yacon Syrup, Blue Agave, or maple syrup.
- Drink 4 liters of purified water daily.

**Topical:** For guidelines on applying oils to the skin, refer to *Application Guidelines* on page 410.

Personal Usage Guide | Chapter 20

- Dilute 50:50 and apply a few drops on location 3-6 times daily.
- Dilute 2-4 drops of Melrose, Purification, or other oil and use in a warm compress over bladder 1-2 times daily.
- Receive a Raindrop Technique 3 times weekly.
- First Week: Use Myrrh, Thyme, Mountain Savory, Palo Santo, and Inspiration and follow with a hot compress.

## BLOATING/SWELLING
*(See also Menstrual and Female Hormone Conditions)*

Bloating is caused by many imbalances in the body. Bloating during menstrual cycle or swelling in the lower extremities is caused by pH imbalance and low estrogen. Bloating can also be caused by enzyme deficiencies, resulting in poor digestion and allergies. Swelling in the legs can be from low potassium and poor circulation, which will cause fluid retention.

It is important to determine whether it is bloating or fluid retention; there is a very significant difference.

### Recommendations

**Singles:** Juniper, Tangerine, Tangerine Vitality, Clary Sage, Sage, Sage Vitality, Cypress, Peppermint, Peppermint Vitality, Fennel, Fennel Vitality, Tarragon, Tarragon Vitality, Nutmeg, Nutmeg Vitality

**Blends:** DiGize, DiGize Vitality, GLF, GLF Vitality, Citrus Fresh, Citrus Fresh Vitality, TummyGize

**Nutritionals:** Essentialzyme, Essentialzymes-4, Mineral Essence, AlkaLime, Detoxzyme, Allerzyme, ICP, ComforTone, JuvaPower, JuvaSpice, Super B

**Body Care:** Progessence Plus

### Application and Usage

**Aromatic:** Refer to *Application Guidelines* on page 410.

**Dietary and Oral:** Whether putting oils in a capsule or drinking them in a liquid, please refer to *Application Guidelines* on page 410.

- Take 1 capsule with desired oil 2 times daily.
- Take 2-3 drops of oil in a spoonful of syrup or small amount of milk, juice, or water.
- Take 2 capsules of DiGize Vitality 3 times daily.
- Take 1 capsule of Peppermint Vitality 3 times daily.

**Topical:** For guidelines on applying oils to the skin, refer to *Application Guidelines* on page 410.

## BONE PROBLEMS

Symptoms of bone problems include pain, brittleness, and lumps. Treatment depends on the nature and cause of the problems; unexplained symptoms can be serious and should always receive medical attention.

### Broken Bones

A health professional should always be involved in the diagnosis and setting of a broken bone or a suspected broken bone.

### Recommendations

**Singles:** Thyme, Thyme Vitality, Helichrysum, Wintergreen, Peppermint, Peppermint Vitality, Northern Lights Black Spruce, Idaho Balsam Fir, Pine, Copaiba, Palo Santo, Myrrh, Lemongrass, Lemongrass Vitality, Ginger, Ginger Vitality, Vetiver

**Blends:** Cool Azul, Aroma Siez, PanAway, Relieve It, Deep Relief Roll-On

**Nutritionals:** PowerGize, BLM, AgilEase, MegaCal, PD 80/20, SuperCal, Mineral Essence, OmegaGize[3]

**Body Care:** Cool Azul Pain Relief Cream, Cool Azul Sports Gel, Ortho Ease Massage Oil, Ortho Sport Massage Oil, Regenolone, Progessence Plus

The following blends can also help relieve pain and speed the bone mending process:

### Broken Bone Blend No. 1
- 8 drops Idaho Balsam Fir
- 6 drops Helichrysum
- 1 drop Myrrh, Sacred Frankincense, or Frankincense
- 1 drop Wintergreen

### Broken Bone Blend No. 2
- 10 drops Wintergreen
- 4 drops Palo Santo
- 4 drops Vetiver
- 3 drops Pine
- 3 drops Helichrysum
- 2 drops Lemongrass

### Application and Usage

**Topical:** For guidelines on applying oils to the skin, refer to *Application Guidelines* on page 410.

- Dilute 50:50 and apply a few drops on location 3-6 times daily.

Seventh Edition | **Essential Oils Desk Reference** | 427

- Prior to casting a broken bone, mix one of the above blends and very gently apply 5-10 drops (depending on size) neat to break area. If there are any signs of skin sensitivity or irritation, apply a small amount of V-6 Vegetable Oil Complex.

**Note:** Apply extremely gently if bone break is suspected.

## Bone Pain

Bone pain can be caused from injuries, arthritis, or other more serious reasons. See your health care professional for the correct diagnosis and proper treatment.

### Recommendations

**Singles:** Wintergreen, Northern Lights Black Spruce, Copaiba, Pine, Idaho Balsam Fir, Helichrysum

**Blends:** PanAway, Cool Azul, Relieve It, Deep Relief Roll-On

**Nutritionals:** MegaCal, BLM, AgilEase, Master Formula, Essentialzyme, Essentialzymes-4

**Body Care:** Cool Azul Pain Relief Cream, Cool Azul Sports Gel, Ortho Ease Massage Oil, Ortho Sport Massage Oil, Regenolone, Progessence Plus

### Application and Usage

**Topical:** For guidelines on applying oils to the skin, refer to *Application Guidelines* on page 410.

- Dilute 50:50 and apply a few drops on location 3-6 times daily as needed.
- Poor bone and muscle development can indicate HGH, potassium, and/or mineral deficiency.

## Osteoporosis (Bone Density Loss)

Osteoporosis is primarily caused by six main factors:
- Progesterone deficiency
- Estradiol deficiency
- Testosterone deficiency
- Lack of magnesium and boron in diet
- Lack of vitamin D in diet
- Lack of Dietary and Oral calcium

Natural progesterone is the single most effective way to increase bone density in women over age 40. Clinical studies by John Lee, MD, showed dramatic increases in bone density using just 20 mg of daily, topically applied progesterone.

Calcium, magnesium, and boron are a few of the most important minerals for bone health and are usually lacking or deficient in most modern diets. Magnesium is es-

pecially important for bone strength, but most Americans consume only a fraction of the 400 mg daily value needed for bone health.

Calcium and magnesium may not be adequately metabolized when consumed because of poor intestinal flora and excess phytates in the diet (a problem with vegetarians). Phytates occur in many nuts, grains, and seeds, including rice. Enzymes like phytase are essential for increasing calcium absorption by liberating calcium from insoluble phytate complexes.

Lack of vitamin D (cholecalciferol) has become epidemic among older people and has contributed to a lack of absorption of calcium in the diet.

MegaCal, AlkaLime, and Mineral Essence are all excellent sources of calcium and magnesium, which are essential for strong bones. Mineral Essence is an excellent source of magnesium and other trace minerals.

Avoid drinking anything that is carbonated because it can leach calcium from the bones due to its phosphoric acid content.

Studies show that the majority of women who do resistance training 3-4 times a week do not develop osteoporosis.

### Recommendations

**Singles:** Wintergreen, Idaho Balsam Fir, Palo Santo, Sacred Frankincense, Frankincense, Frankincense Vitality, Thyme, Thyme Vitality, Cypress, Peppermint, Peppermint Vitality, Marjoram, Marjoram Vitality, Rosemary, Rosemary Vitality, Basil, Basil Vitality, Elemi, Northern Lights Black Spruce, Pine

**Blends:** SclarEssence, SclarEssence Vitality, PanAway, Aroma Siez, Purification, Melrose, Sacred Mountain, Relieve It

**Nutritionals:** Estro, FemiGen, EndoGize, BLM, AgilEase, MegaCal, Essentialzyme, Detoxzyme, AlkaLime, Mineral Essence, Essentialzymes-4, SuperCal, Sulfurzyme, Thyromin, PowerGize

**Body Care:** Prenolone Plus Body Cream, Progessence Plus

### Application and Usage

**Topical:** For guidelines on applying oils to the skin, refer to *Application Guidelines* on page 410.

- Massage 6-10 drops diluted 50:50 on spine (or area affected) 2-3 times daily.

Personal Usage Guide | Chapter 20

# BRAIN DISORDERS AND PROBLEMS

As the control center of the body, the brain controls speech, movement, thoughts, and memory and regulates the function of many organs. When problems occur, the results can be devastating.

## Absentmindedness

Clinical studies on Ningxia wolfberry (*Lycium barbarum*) have shown that it has an anti-senility effect.[3] Clinical studies at Tufts University and the Department of Veterans Affairs Medical Center, Denver, Colorado, and Boston, Massachusetts, found that high antioxidant foods such as spinach found in JuvaPower and blueberry found in NingXia Red dramatically improved learning and cognition.[4, 5]

### Recommendations

**Singles:** Peppermint, Peppermint Vitality, Sacred Frankincense, Frankincense, Frankincense Vitality, Rosemary, Rosemary Vitality, Cardamom, Cardamom Vitality, Canadian Fleabane (Conyza)

**Blends:** Clarity, M-Grain, Brain Power, GeneYus, Common Sense, Oola Balance, Oola Faith, Oola Family, Oola Field, Oola Finance, Oola Fitness, Oola Friends, Oola Fun, Oola Grow, InTouch, Reconnect, SleepyIze

**Nutritionals:** NingXia Red, PD 80/20, OmegaGize[3], NingXia Nitro, NingXia Zyng, Ningxia Wolfberries (Organic, Dried), Master Formula, JuvaPower, JuvaSpice, MindWise, Essentialzyme, Essentialzymes-4, Life 9

### Application and Usage

**Aromatic:** Refer to *Application Guidelines* on page 410.

**Topical:** For guidelines on applying oils to the skin, refer to *Application Guidelines* on page 410.

- Apply 1-2 drops neat (undiluted) on temples and back of neck, as desired.

## Alzheimer's

Over 4 million Americans suffer from Alzheimer's. Alzheimer's was found to nearly double in subjects with high levels of homocysteine in the Framingham Study. The Center for Disease Control and Prevention has concluded that the primary cause of Alzheimer's disease is probably not aluminum, although it could be a contributing factor in patients who were already at risk of developing the disease. In spite of this fact, people are unfortunately still being urged to get yearly flu shots, which contain aluminum as an adjuvant.

Pepper, Grapefruit, and Fennel oils have been found to stimulate brain activity.[6] Peppermint oil has been helpful in protecting against stresses and toxins in brain cells.[7]

Dr. Richard Restick, a leading neurologist in Washington, D.C., stated that maintaining normal synaptic firing would forestall many types of neurological deterioration in the body.

Essential oils high in sesquiterpenes such as Vetiver, Cedarwood, Patchouli, German Chamomile, German Chamomile Vitality, Myrrh, Melissa, and Royal Hawaiian Sandalwood are known to cross the blood-brain barrier. Frankincense and Frankincense Vitality are general cerebral stimulants.

### Recommendations

**Singles:** Melissa, Royal Hawaiian Sandalwood, Helichrysum, Ginger, Ginger Vitality, Nutmeg, Nutmeg Vitality, German Chamomile, German Chamomile Vitality, Eucalyptus Globulus, Sacred Frankincense, Frankincense, Frankincense Vitality, Patchouli, Cedarwood, Myrrh, Black Pepper, Black Pepper Vitality, Grapefruit, Grapefruit Vitality, Fennel, Fennel Vitality, Cedarwood

Helichrysum supports neurotransmitter activity and has shown the possibility of chelating aluminum. Nutmeg is a general cerebral stimulant and has adrenal cortex-like activity.

**Blends:** Brain Power, Common Sense, GeneYus, Valor, Valor II, Valor Roll-On, Clarity, Oola Balance, Oola Faith, Oola Family, Oola Field, Oola Finance, Oola Fitness, Oola Friends, Oola Fun, Oola Grow, Harmony, RutaVaLa, RutaVaLa Roll-On, InTouch, Reconnect, SleepyIze

**Nutritionals:** MindWise, MultiGreens, Power Meal, Slique Shake, Sulfurzyme, Essentialzyme, Essentialzymes-4, Mineral Essence, NingXia Red, NingXia Nitro, NingXia Zyng, Ningxia Wolfberries (Organic, Dried), Master Formula, Super C, Super C Chewable, MegaCal, OmegaGize[3]

### Application and Usage

**Aromatic:** Refer to *Application Guidelines* on page 410.

**Dietary and Oral:** Whether putting oils in a capsule or drinking them in a liquid, please refer to *Application Guidelines* on page 410.

- Take 1 capsule with desired oil 2 times daily.
- Take 2-3 drops of oil in a spoonful of syrup or small amount of milk, juice, or water.

Seventh Edition | **Essential Oils Desk Reference** | 429

**Topical:** For guidelines on applying oils to the skin, refer to *Application Guidelines* on page 410.

- Apply 1-2 drops directly onto the brain reflex centers. These points include the forehead, temples, and mastoids (the bones just behind the ears). Apply oils and mild, direct pressure to the brainstem area (center top of neck at base of skull) and work down the spine.
- Apply 1-2 drops neat to Vita Flex brain points on feet 1-2 times daily.
- Receive a Raindrop Technique once every 2 weeks.

## Concentration, Impaired

Impaired concentration is very common and may not always lead to a debilitating condition. Some common reasons why people can't concentrate are lack of sleep, lack of exercise, improper diet, and too much technology. A study in *Research in Higher Education* showed that students who texted the professor during a lecture scored 42.81 on a test following the lecture while non-texting students had a higher score of 58.67.[8]

### Recommendations

**Singles:** Peppermint, Peppermint Vitality, Basil, Basil Vitality, Jade Lemon, Jade Lemon Vitality, Lemon, Lemon Vitality, Lime, Lime Vitality, Bergamot, Bergamot Vitality, Rosemary, Rosemary Vitality, Sacred Frankincense, Frankincense, Frankincense Vitality, Dorado Azul

**Blends:** Brain Power, Clarity, GeneYus, RutaVaLa, RutaVaLa Roll-On, Harmony, Valor, Valor II, Valor Roll-On, Oola Balance, Oola Faith, Oola Family, Oola Field, Oola Finance, Oola Fitness, Oola Friends, Oola Fun, Oola Grow, Common Sense, 3 Wise Men, InTouch, Reconnect, SleepyIze

**Nutritionals:** MindWise, MegaCal, Super B, Omega-Gize[3], Digest & Cleanse, Mineral Essence, NingXia Red, NingXia Nitro, NingXia Zyng, Ningxia Wolfberries (Organic, Dried)

### Application and Usage

**Aromatic:** Refer to *Application Guidelines* on page 410.

**Dietary and Oral:** Whether putting oils in a capsule or drinking them in a liquid, please refer to *Application Guidelines* on page 410.

- Take 1 capsule with desired oil 2 times daily.
- Take 2-3 drops of oil in a spoonful of syrup or small amount of milk, juice, or water.

**Topical:** For guidelines on applying oils to the skin, refer to *Application Guidelines* on page 410.

- Apply 1-2 drops neat directly onto the brain reflex centers 2-4 times daily, as needed. These points include the forehead, temples, and mastoids (the bones just behind the ears). Apply oils and mild, direct pressure to the brainstem area (center top of neck at base of skull) and work down the spine.
- Apply 1-2 drops neat to Vita Flex brain points on feet 1-2 times daily.
- Receive a Raindrop Technique once every 2 weeks.

## Confusion

Confusion is when a person is not able to think with his or her usual level of clarity. Decision-making ability is reduced, and feeling disoriented is common. Confusion may develop gradually or arise suddenly and has multiple causes, including medical conditions, medications, injuries, environmental factors, substance abuse, stress, low hormones, and low thyroid.

### Recommendations

**Singles:** Peppermint, Peppermint Vitality, Jade Lemon, Jade Lemon Vitality, Lemon, Lemon Vitality, Rosemary, Rosemary Vitality, Basil, Basil Vitality, Sacred Frankincense, Frankincense, Frankincense Vitality, Cardamom, Cardamom Vitality

**Blends:** M-Grain, Gathering, Brain Power, Clarity, GeneYus, Oola Balance, Oola Faith, Oola Family, Oola Field, Oola Finance, Oola Fitness, Oola Friends, Oola Fun, Oola Grow, Common Sense, Harmony, InTouch, Reconnect, SleepyIze

**Nutritionals:** MindWise, MegaCal, Super B, Omega-Gize[3], Digest & Cleanse, Mineral Essence, Thyromin, NingXia Red, EndoGize

### Application and Usage

**Aromatic:** Refer to *Application Guidelines* on page 410.

**Topical:** For guidelines on applying oils to the skin, refer to *Application Guidelines* on page 410.

- Applying a single drop under the nose is helpful and refreshing.
- Dilute 50:50 and apply on location 3-6 times daily.
- Massage 2-4 drops of oil neat on the bottoms of the feet just before bedtime.

## Convulsions

Convulsions, also called seizures, are involuntary contractions of the voluntary muscles. Monitor diet and discontinue sugar, dairy products, and fried and processed foods.

### Recommendations

**Singles:** Sacred Frankincense, Frankincense, Frankincense Vitality, Palo Santo, Eucalyptus Blue, Copaiba, Copaiba Vitality, Western Red Cedar, Wintergreen

**Blends:** Brain Power, GeneYus, Valor, Valor II, Valor Roll-On, RutaVaLa, RutaVaLa Roll-On, Tranquil Roll-On, Clarity, Common Sense

**Nutritionals:** MindWise, Detoxzyme, AlkaLime, Inner Defense, Mineral Essence

### Application and Usage

**Aromatic:** Refer to *Application Guidelines* on page 410.

**Topical:** For guidelines on applying oils to the skin, refer to *Application Guidelines* on page 410.

- Apply 2-4 drops neat at base of skull, across the neck, top of spine (C1-C6 vertebrae), and bottom of feet.
- Apply 1-2 drops neat on temples and back of neck as desired.
- Place a warm compress with 1-2 drops of chosen oil on the back.

## Memory, Impaired

Many areas of the brain help create and retrieve memories. Malfunction of or damage to any of these areas can lead to memory loss.

### Recommendations

**Singles:** Rosemary, Rosemary Vitality, Peppermint, Peppermint Vitality, Cardamom, Cardamom Vitality, Basil, Basil Vitality, Vetiver, Rose, Lemon, Lemon Vitality, Lemongrass, Lemongrass Vitality, Helichrysum, Lavender, Lavender Vitality, Tangerine, Tangerine Vitality, Spearmint, Spearmint Vitality, Palo Santo

**Note:** Peppermint improves mental concentration and memory. Dr. William N. Dember conducted a study at the University of Cincinnati in 1994 showing that inhaling peppermint increased mental accuracy by 28 percent.[9]

The fragrances of diffused oils such as lemon have also been reported to increase memory retention and recall.

**Blends:** Brain Power, Clarity, M-Grain, GeneYus, En-R-Gee, Oola Balance, Oola Faith, Oola Family, Oola Field, Oola Finance, Oola Fitness, Oola Friends, Oola Fun, Oola Grow, InTouch, Reconnect, SleepyIze

**Nutritionals:** MindWise, Longevity Softgels, MultiGreens, Mineral Essence, Thyromin, NingXia Red

### Memory Blend No. 1

- 5 drops Basil or Basil Vitality
- 10 drops Rosemary or Rosemary Vitality
- 4 drops Helichrysum
- 2 drops Peppermint or Peppermint Vitality
- 2 drops Cardamom or Cardamom Vitality

### Memory Blend No. 2

- 4 drops Lavender or Lavender Vitality
- 3 drops Geranium or Geranium Vitality
- 3 drops Rosewood or Palo Santo
- 3 drops Rosemary or Rosemary Vitality
- 2 drops Tangerine or Tangerine Vitality
- 1 drop Spearmint or Spearmint Vitality

### Application and Usage

**Aromatic:** Refer to *Application Guidelines* on page 410.

**Cleansing**: Vascular cleansing may improve mental function by supporting improved blood flow, boosting distribution of oxygen and nutrients (see Vascular Cleansing).

**Dietary and Oral:** Whether putting oils in a capsule or drinking them in a liquid, please refer to *Application Guidelines* on page 410.

- Take 1 capsule with desired oil 3 times daily.
- Take 2-3 drops of oil in a spoonful of syrup or small amount of milk, juice, or water.

**Topical:** For guidelines on applying oils to the skin, refer to *Application Guidelines* on page 410.

- Applying a single drop under the nose is helpful and refreshing.
- Dilute 50:50 and apply 2-3 drops on temples, forehead, mastoids (bone behind ears), and/or brainstem (back of neck) as needed 3-6 times daily.
- Massage 2-4 drops of oil neat on the bottoms of the feet just before bedtime.

## Mental Fatigue

Some of the causes of mental fatigue are being overworked, having poor sleep patterns, lacking exercise, and having a poor diet.

## Recommendations

**Singles:** Sacred Frankincense, Frankincense, Frankincense Vitality, Rosemary, Rosemary Vitality, Vetiver, Cedarwood, Peppermint, Peppermint Vitality

**Blends:** Brain Power, Clarity, GeneYus, Valor, Valor II, Valor Roll-On, RutaVaLa, RutaVaLa Roll-On, Tranquil Roll-On, Oola Balance, Oola Faith, Oola Family, Oola Field, Oola Finance, Oola Fitness, Oola Friends, Oola Fun, Oola Grow, InTouch, Reconnect, SleepyIze

**Nutritionals:** MindWise, Thyromin, Super B, Endo-Gize, MultiGreens, NingXia Red, NingXia Zyng, NingXia Nitro, Ningxia Wolfberries (Organic, Dried), Master Formula

## Application and Usage

**Aromatic:** Refer to *Application Guidelines* on page 410.

**Cleansing**: Vascular cleansing may improve mental function by supporting improved blood flow, boosting distribution of oxygen and nutrients (see Vascular Cleansing).

**Dietary and Oral:** Whether putting oils in a capsule or drinking them in a liquid, please refer to *Application Guidelines* on page 410.

- Take 1 capsule with desired oil 3 times daily.
- Take 2-3 drops of oil in a spoonful of syrup or small amount of milk, juice, or water.

**Topical:** For guidelines on applying oils to the skin, refer to *Application Guidelines* on page 410.

- Applying a single drop under the nose is helpful and refreshing.
- Dilute 50:50 and apply 2-3 drops on temples, forehead, mastoids (bone behind ears), and/or brainstem (back of neck) as needed 3-6 times daily.
- Massage 2-4 drops of oil neat on the bottoms of the feet just before bedtime.

## BREASTFEEDING

The most common causes of sore or cracked nipples are poor breastfeeding technique, dehydration, or infection.

## Dry, Cracked Nipples

### Recommendations

**Singles:** Myrrh, Vetiver, Royal Hawaiian Sandalwood

**Blends:** Valor, Valor II, Valor Roll-on, Harmony, The Gift, Owie

**Nutritionals:** MultiGreens, Master Formula, NingXia Red

**Body Care:** Rose Ointment, KidScents Tender Tush, Essential Beauty Serum for Dry Skin

### Application and Usage

**Topical:** For guidelines on applying oils to the skin, refer to *Application Guidelines* on page 410.

- Dilute 50:50 and massage over breast and on Vita Flex points of the feet.

## Mastitis (Infected Breast)

Mastitis is an infection of the breast tissue that results in pain, swelling, redness, and warmth of the breast. It most commonly affects women who are breastfeeding.

### Recommendations

**Singles:** Myrrh, Melissa, Tea Tree, Thyme, Thyme Vitality, Patchouli, Roman Chamomile, Rosemary, Rosemary Vitality, Lavender, Lavender Vitality, Lemon, Lemon Vitality, Vetiver, Copaiba, Copaiba Vitality, Idaho Blue Spruce, Mountain Savory, Mountain Savory Vitality

**Blends:** PanAway, ImmuPower, Owie

**Nutritionals:** Longevity Softgels, ImmuPro, Inner Defense

Massage either of these blends on the breasts and under armpits 2 times daily. Wash/Cleanse breasts before breast-feeding.

**Breast Blend No. 1**
- 3 drops Thyme
- 7 drops PanAway
- 1 teaspoon V-6 Vegetable Oil Complex

**Breast Blend No. 2**
- 3 drops Lemon
- 4 drops Thyme
- 2 drops Melissa
- 1 teaspoon V-6 Vegetable Oil Complex

**Breast Blend No. 3**
- 3 drops Myrrh
- 3 drops Vetiver
- 2 drops Copaiba
- 1 drop Idaho Blue Spruce
- ½ teaspoon V-6 Vegetable Oil Complex

**Breast Blend No. 4**
- 4 drops Melissa
- 10 drops Myrrh
- 1 drop Thyme
- 1 drop Mountain Savory

### Application and Usage

**Topical:** For guidelines on applying oils to the skin, refer to *Application Guidelines* on page 410.

- Dilute 20:80 and massage over breast and on Vita Flex points of the feet.

Personal Usage Guide | Chapter 20

# BURSITIS

Bursitis is an inflammation of the bursa, which are small, fluid-filled sacs located near the joints. Bursa act as shock absorbers when muscles or tendons come into contact with bone. As the bursa become swollen, they result in pain, particularly when the affected joint is used.

Bursitis can be caused by injury, infection, or arthritis, and usually involves the joints of the knees, elbows, shoulders, and Achilles tendon. Occasionally, bursitis can occur in the base of the big toe. Bursitis may signal the beginning of arthritis.

## Recommendations

**Singles:** Wintergreen, Idaho Blue Spruce, Peppermint, Peppermint Vitality, Copaiba, Copaiba Vitality, Dorado Azul, Palo Santo, Sacred Frankincense, Frankincense, Frankincense Vitality, Idaho Balsam Fir, Basil, Basil Vitality, Lavender, Lavender Vitality, Black Pepper, Black Pepper Vitality, Elemi, Oregano, Oregano Vitality, Plectranthus Oregano, Marjoram, Marjoram Vitality

**Blends:** PanAway, Relieve It, Sacred Mountain, Deep Relief Roll-On

**Nutritionals:** Sulfurzyme, MegaCal, BLM, AgilEase

**Body Care:** Cool Azul Pain Relief Cream, Cool Azul Sports Gel, Ortho Ease Massage Oil, Ortho Sport Massage Oil

## Application and Usage

**Aromatic:** Refer to *Application Guidelines* on page 410.

**Dietary and Oral:** Whether putting oils in a capsule or drinking them in a liquid, please refer to *Application Guidelines* on page 410.

- Take 1 capsule with desired oil 2 times daily.
- Take 2-3 drops of oil in a spoonful of syrup or small amount of milk, juice, or water.

**Topical:** For guidelines on applying oils to the skin, refer to *Application Guidelines* on page 410.

- Apply 2-4 drops neat or diluted 50:50 on affected area or joint 3-5 times daily or as needed to soothe pain
- Apply a cold compress around affected joint 1-3 times daily.

# CANCER

Cancer is among the most complex and difficult of any human disease to treat. A patient diagnosed with cancer should always defer to his or her physician for primary care. Keeping this in mind, a number of individuals have achieved successful remission by following a natural protocol and some of the principles outlined in this section.

It is important to note that many natural therapies—especially those using essential oils—work best in the early stages of cancer. In fact, all clinical trials are showing that Frankincense is the number one inhibitor of many cancers. Citrus oils, high in d-limonene, including Orange, Grapefruit, and Tangerine, work better as cancer preventives than cancer treatments, although they have been tested to have powerful, anticancer properties in all stages of cancer.

A study at Charing Cross Hospital in London, England, published in 1998 achieved close to a 15 percent remission rate in patients with advanced colon and breast cancer using doses from 1 to 15 grams of d-limonene from Orange oil as their only treatment. In patients with only weeks or months to live, limonene treatment extended patients' lives by up to 18 months in some cases.[10]

## The Foundation of Natural Cancer Treatment

Natural treatment of cancer or any illness is a highly debated topic, but when you are faced with cancer, finding solutions becomes important.

## Emotions and Cancer

Cancer should always be treated first by discovering the underlying emotions that contributed to the onset of the disease. In many cases, negative emotions and trauma not only trigger the beginning of cancer but can further its metastasis. Any kind of negative emotion—anger, fear, rage, helplessness, abandonment—can cause the cancer to spread faster.

When essential oils are used as the basis of an emotional care program, they can have powerfully positive effects in improving the attitude, emotional well-being, and potential outcome of the disease. Essential oil blends such as White Angelica, White Light, Release, Grounding, Inner Child, Trauma Life, T.R. Care, Forgiveness, Joy, Common Sense, Hope, Believe, Peace & Calming, Peace & Calming II, Valor, Valor II, and SARA can form the center of any emotional care regimen (See the Chapter 16 on emotional support).

Seventh Edition | **Essential Oils Desk Reference** | 433

## Cleansing and Removing Toxins

Industrial pollutants such as benzene and lead, along with lifestyle toxins such as cigarette smoke, chemicals, heterocyclic amines from overcooked meat, and many others contribute to a vast majority of cancers. Even daily radiation from computers, cell phones, and a vast number of electrical appliances may contribute to a toxic overload within the body.

Today's fast-food industry is a major culprit in selling so much nutritionally deficient food that we eat. Processed food is fast and convenient, but is it worth the threat to our health? Cosmetics, hair sprays, dyes, soaps, paints, and household cleaners add to an endless list of pollutants in our environment and toxicity to which we are subjected.

To help lower the risk of cancer, it is important to reduce the exposure to these chemicals and change our diet and the products that we use in our environment. The chemicals should be avoided at all cost, as they can damage DNA, decrease immunity, promote oncogenes (genes that can turn normal cells into cancer cells), and accelerate cancer development.

## Cleansing and Chelation

The foundation of any cancer program should begin with a period of cleansing. Cleansing and chelation can help remove some of the toxin- and petrochemical-buildup that may have triggered the cancer initially.

Fasting can be one of the single, most powerful, anticancer tools available, particularly in the early stages. Anyone who is in advanced stages of cancer must cleanse very slowly to see how the body responds. Going without food and drinking only juices immediately could be detrimental to a sick body. Common sense needs to be used in all situations.

Essential oils that improve liver function and promote glutathione can form the center of any detoxification program. Lemon and orange oils, in studies at Johns Hopkins University, have shown to substantially increase glutathione levels in the liver and colon, which have beneficial effects in detoxification.

Chelation can be particularly important in removing carcinogenic metals from the body. Studies in Germany have shown that transition metals such as iron, mercury, lead, zinc, nickel, and cadmium can accumulate to high levels in tumors, particularly in breast cancer tissue. A series of chelations to eliminate these metals can produce tremendous benefits in the earliest stage of cancer.[11]

Rice bran is a good chelator of metals and contains anticancer phytonutrients such as gamma oryzanol and other compounds. It is also rich in immune stimulating arabinoxylans that increase cancer cell death.[12]

The Ningxia wolfberry is rich in polysaccharides that similarly amplify immunity. A number of clinical research trials have shown that wolfberry compounds can dramatically improve cancer remission, particularly when combined with immune-stimulating therapies.[13]

## Cleansing Products Suitable for Most Cancers

Many products support the body in its cleansing process. You will not be able to take all the cleansing products, so decide which ones you want to take and how much you want to take of each product. Write down your program so you can follow it consistently. Start slowly so your body can adjust and begin to cleanse.

**Cleansing:** Essentialzyme, Detoxzyme, Essentialzymes-4, JuvaPower, JuvaTone, ComforTone, TummyGize, DiGize, DiGize Vitality, GLF, GLF Vitality, Juva-Cleanse, JuvaCleanse Vitality, JuvaFlex, JuvaFlex Vitality, NingXia Red

**Emotional Support:** Divine Release, Evergreen Essence, Freedom, InTouch, Reconnect, Sacred Frankincense, Frankincense, Frankincense Vitality, Lavender, Lavender Vitality, Palo Santo, Rose, Ylang Ylang, Amazonian Ylang Ylang, Acceptance, Believe, Brain Power, Common Sense, Dream Catcher, Gathering, Envision, Forgiveness, Gratitude, Harmony, Hope, Inner Harmony, Joy, Live with Passion, Live Your Passion, Light the Fire, Motivation, Present Time, Peace & Calming, Peace & Calming II, RutaVaLa, RutaVaLa Roll-On, The Gift, Transformation, Valor, Valor II, White Angelica, White Light

## Enzymes Ramping Protocol

Essentialzyme was formulated in 1984 with this protocol for someone suffering from a degenerative disease.

**Phase 1:** Take 3 caplets 3 times daily. Increase by 1 caplet every day until you become nauseated and then discontinue Essentialzyme for 24 to 36 hours.

**Phase 2:** Take 4 caplets 3 times daily. Increase daily by 1 caplet until you become nauseated. Rest (discontinue) again for 24-36 hours.

**Phase 3:** Take 5 caplets 3 times daily. Increase daily by 1 caplet until you become nauseated. Rest for 24-36 hours.

**Phase 4:** Start again with the amount that you were taking before the nausea occurred the third time. For example: If you were taking 18 caplets, you would have been taking 6 caplets 3 times daily when you became nauseated.

Therefore, start Phase 4 again with 6 caplets 3 times daily and continue with this amount for 6 weeks.

**Phase 5:** In the 7th week, start the enzyme-ramping program all over again. This means to begin phase 1 again and increase the amount by 1 each day until nausea or vomiting starts again. Repeat and continue for 6 weeks as previously described.

If your doctor determines that you are in remission, you can maintain with 5-10 tablets daily for one year, 6 days a week.

Maintenance: Take 5-10 Essentialzyme caplets 3 times daily.

**Caution:** This is a very rigorous program, so you should consult with your doctor or health care professional before starting and have that person monitor your progress during the program.

### Why Fasting Works

New research has uncovered that insulin receptors make cancer cells different from normal cells. Cancer cells have over 10 times the number of receptors for insulin as a normal cell. Excess insulin can stimulate cancer cells disproportionately compared to well-differentiated cells. Similarly, because cancer cells are fast-growing, they require far more glucose (blood sugar) than normal cells.

The most effective way of lowering both insulin and blood glucose levels is with a fast. Bernard Jensen, ND, used a 180-day fast, made initially of only barley grass juice, to fight and eliminate metastatic prostate cancer. Even a partial fast in which refined carbohydrates are eliminated and caloric intake is reduced to 500-1,000 calories can be potentially very therapeutic.

### Determining Hormone Sensitivity

Women dealing with breast, ovarian, uterine, and cervical cancer in most cases can be estrogen receptor sensitive, yet doctors will continue to give and recommend HRT (hormone replacement therapy) made from xenoestrogens that come from petrochemicals, compounds that are known to promote and cause cancer, before determining if a patient has cancer in the early stages of development.

Premarin® is an estrogen-therapy drug created from the urine of pregnant horses. Besides animal cruelty issues, this hormone treatment is not natural to the human body and increases the risks for stroke, heart attack, and breast cancer.

We must understand the mechanism of how natural hormones are synthesized in the body. First cholesterol cascades down to pregnenolone, to progestogens, and then to androgens that divide and go to the ovaries and testes.

In the ovaries, the androgen called androstenedione, crosses the basal membrane, where it is converted to the estradiol sex hormones such as estradiol, estrone, and estriol. The ovaries produce primarily estradiol. Most free-circulating estrone stems from a conversion of estradiol in the liver, even though the ovaries produce small amounts of estrone.

The liver plays a major role as the chemistry laboratory of the body. Because the liver is the body's largest fat-storing organ, it will hold petrochemicals known as xenoestrogens that are cancer-causing agents. Xenoestrogens disrupt the conversion of estradiol and cause a division of the estrone.

This division will be either negative or positive. If estradiol converts to 16-alpha-hydroxyestrone, a cancer-causing agent, this estrone will then bind to the estrogen receptors in female and male reproductive organs. If estradiol converts to 2-hydroxyestrone, a cancer-*preventing* steroid hormone, it will bind or stick to the receptors, protecting them from the harmful estrone. This has caused a lot of controversy among the natural health and allopathic practitioners for years.

Natural hormones produced in the body are referred to as steroid hormones. Synthetic hormones are called nonsteroid hormones. Most people do not understand that plant hormones are neither steroid nor nonsteroid hormones. They are natural phytohormones that encourage the production of 2-hydroxyestrone, the cancer preventive hormone that does not bind or stick to the receptor sites contrary to the nonsteroid hormones that cause inflammation and cysts on the ovaries.

There is no evidence that phytohormones will stimulate estrogen-sensitive cancer. Phytohormones are the same as the hormone-supporting chemical compounds found in the essential oils of Fennel, Clary Sage, Melissa, Lemongrass, Sage, etc.

There is also no reason to be concerned about food unless it is a GMO food like soy. Herbs like black cohosh do not stimulate estrogen-sensitive cancer. Quite simply they are neither steroid- nor nonsteroid-stimulating hormones.

Another concern is to understand that metabolic enzymes are required to help facilitate steroid hormone conversion. When the body and liver are toxic, this becomes a serious problem, creating a metabolic enzyme deficiency. In the absence of metabolic enzymes and a toxic liver, estradiol is converted to 16-alpha-hydroxyestrone, the cancer-causing hormone.

The hormones that naturally occur in milk require metabolic hormones to ensure they are converted to 2-hydroxyestrone. When the milk goes through the pas-

**Essential Oils Desk Reference** | Seventh Edition

teurization process, it kills the enzymes necessary for the 2-hydroxyestrone conversion and converts to the cancer-causing 16-alpha-hydroxyestrone.

Essentialzyme is the metabolic enzyme, which makes it so important for daily prevention and good health.

Pasteurized milk is also a concern because milk contains steroid hormones fed to cows. When milk products are pasteurized and homogenized, whether it is milk, cheese, butter, cottage cheese, or any other product containing steroid hormones, the pasteurization destroys the natural enzymes, thus preventing the production of 2-hydroxyestrone, the cancer-preventing steroid, and instead converts it to 16-alpha-hydroxyestrone, the cancer-causing hormone.

This is where the controversy begins and the misunderstanding of estrogen-sensitive cancers becomes a problem. It is easy to see how processed and non-processed foods affect the outcome of our health.

This does not apply only to women but applies to men as well. Men have estrogen also and will respond the same way to both phytoestrogens and mycoestrogens (estrogens produced by fungi found in stored grain) that stimulate the production of 16-alpha-hydroxyestrone. If there were more focus on eating unprocessed foods; cleansing the liver of toxins, petrochemicals, and undigested pollutants; and improving and building a reserve of metabolic enzymes, there would be much less cancer.

### Cancer and Antioxidants

It is recommended to seek the advice from a health care professional before embarking on any antioxidant program. Some studies have reported that certain antioxidants can reduce the effectiveness of some types of chemotherapy such as cisplatin.

A large number of other studies have found the opposite, showing that antioxidants can improve patient remissions and prognosis. In the case of radiation treatments, a number of well-controlled studies have similarly found that antioxidants can improve patient outcomes dramatically and counter the injury and immune suppression caused by these therapies.

In fact, a 2016 human study by A. Pace and colleagues at the Regina Elena National Cancer Institute in Rome, Italy, found that vitamin E had a neuroprotective effect against the serious, adverse effects of cisplatin.[14]

Similar to DNA-protective essential oils, antioxidants produce their best results as cancer preventives and in the earliest stages of cancer. As cancer progresses, the likelihood of meaningful remissions using only antioxidants declines rapidly.

Research conducted at Brigham Young University in Provo, Utah, and the UNLV Cancer Research Institute identified some of the most inhibitory essential oils against a variety of cancer cell lines. The oils were also tested for their lack of toxicity to normal cells.

### Inflammation and Cancer

The link between cancer and inflammation has become stronger in recent years. It is well known that the salicylates in aspirin have high anti-inflammatory effects and reduce the risk of colon cancer dramatically.

The natural salicylates found in the essential oil of wintergreen are very close in structure to the acetyl salicylic acid found in aspirin. According to Erica Leibert of Harvard University, wintergreen oil is 40 percent stronger than an aspirin equivalent with very similar anti-inflammatory properties. However, it should be ingested only in very small numbers of drops.

Clove has been researched as a potential chemopreventive agent for lung cancer because of its powerful anti-inflammatory effects.[15] The biochemical alpha-humulene in the oil, also found in Idaho Balsam Fir and Copaiba, has been shown to have significant cancer prevention properties through its anti-inflammatory action.[16]

Frankincense and conifer oils like Idaho Balsam Fir containing l-limonene are coming to the forefront of attention in cancer research in various cancer-treatment study programs at Oklahoma State University, Wake Forest University, and Virginia-Maryland Regional College of Veterinary Medicine.

The l-limonene found in Frankincense, Idaho Blue Spruce, and Idaho Balsam Fir shows a remarkable ability to suppress tumor growth, particularly in melanoma. Boswellic acids found in frankincense gum resin have also been shown to have powerful, anti-inflammatory effects. Myrrh gum has been studied for its ability to combat various cancers, including breast cancer.

### Anti-inflammatory Essential Oils Suitable for Most Cancers: Frankincense, Frankincense Vitality, Clove, Clove Vitality, Idaho Balsam Fir, Palo Santo, Ledum, Myrrh, Wintergreen (topically only)

### Immunity and Cancer

Enhancing immune function is a vital component of both traditional and complementary approaches to cancer. Typically, chemotherapy and radiation can drastically break down populations of T-cells and NK (natural killer) cells that are responsible for fighting tumor growth. Certain natural compounds can restore levels of these critical immune components.

436 | **Chapter 20** | Personal Usage Guide

Personal Usage Guide | Chapter 20

**Singles:** Sacred Frankincense, Frankincense, Frankincense Vitality, Idaho Blue Spruce, Idaho Balsam Fir, Royal Hawaiian Sandalwood, Palo Santo, Hyssop, Thyme, Thyme Vitality, Clove, Clove Vitality, Tea Tree, Blue Cypress

**Blends:** Citrus Fresh, Citrus Fresh Vitality, Thieves, Thieves Vitality, Exodus II, Melrose, GLF, GLF Vitality, ImmuPower, 3 Wise Men, TummyGize, DiGize, DiGize Vitality

**Immune-Enhancing Supplements Suitable for Most Cancers:** ImmuPro, Super C, Super C Chewable, Master Formula, Essentialzyme, Detoxzyme, Essentialzymes-4, MultiGreens, NingXia Red

## Breast Cancer

### Recommendations

**Singles:** Sacred Frankincense, Frankincense, Frankincense Vitality, Royal Hawaiian Sandalwood, Myrtle, Tsuga, Sage, Sage Vitality

**Nutritionals:** NingXia Red, Super C, Essentialzyme, Essenstialzymes-4, AlkaLime

## Cervical Cancer

### Recommendations

**Singles:** Patchouli, Royal Hawaiian Sandalwood, Valerian, Sacred Frankincense, Frankincense, Frankincense Vitality, Tsuga, Hyssop, Nutmeg, Nutmeg Vitality, Tarragon, Tarragon Vitality, Sage, Sage Vitality

**Nutritionals:** NingXia Red, Super C, Essentialzyme, Essentialzymes-4, AlkaLime

## Leukemia

### Recommendations

**Singles:** Clove, Clove Vitality, Hyssop, Idaho Blue Spruce, Sacred Frankincense, Frankincense, Frankincense Vitality, Palo Santo

**Nutritionals:** NingXia Red, Super C, Essentialzyme, Essentialzymes-4, AlkaLime

## Lung Cancer

### Recommendations

**Singles:** Sacred Frankincense, Frankincense, Frankincense Vitality, Idaho Blue Spruce, Palo Santo, Royal Hawaiian Sandalwood, Clove, Clove Vitality, Thyme, Thyme Vitality, Hyssop

**Nutritionals:** NingXia Red, Super C, Essentialzyme, Essenstialzymes-4, AlkaLime

## Prostate Cancer

### Recommendations

**Singles:** Sacred Frankincense, Frankincense, Frankincense Vitality, Sage, Sage Vitality, Western Red Cedar, Thyme, Thyme Vitality, Royal Hawaiian Sandalwood, Myrtle, Dill, Dill Vitality, Idaho Blue Spruce, Sage, Sage Vitality

**Nutritionals:** Protec, NingXia Red, Super C, Essentialzyme, Essentialzymes-4, AlkaLime

## Skin Cancer (Melanoma)

### Recommendations

**Singles:** Sacred Frankincense, Frankincense, Frankincense Vitality, Thyme, Thyme Vitality, Royal Hawaiian Sandalwood, Grapefruit, Grapefruit Vitality, Hyssop, Tarragon, Tarragon Vitality

**Nutritionals:** NingXia Red, Super C, Essentialzyme, Essentialzymes-4, AlkaLime

## Tumors

### Recommendations

**Singles:** Sacred Frankincense, Frankincense, Frankincense Vitality, Western Red Cedar, Sage, Sage Vitality, Royal Hawaiian Sandalwood, Grapefruit, Grapefruit Vitality, Hyssop, Myrtle, Idaho Blue Spruce

**Nutritionals:** NingXia Red, Super C, Essentialzyme, Essentialzymes-4, AlkaLime

## Uterine Cancer

### Recommendations

**Singles:** Sacred Frankincense, Frankincense, Frankincense Vitality, Sage, Sage Vitality, Western Red Cedar, Thyme, Thyme Vitality, Royal Hawaiian Sandalwood, Myrtle, Dill, Dill Vitality, Idaho Blue Spruce

**Nutritionals:** Protec

**Essential Oils Desk Reference** | Seventh Edition

# CARDIOVASCULAR CONDITIONS AND PROBLEMS

Cardiovascular conditions are those that affect the heart and other circulatory organs.

## Anemia

Anemia is a condition caused from insufficient red blood cells. There can be many different causes of anemia, which would suggest that you should see your physician for proper diagnosis. Nutritional deficiencies of iron or vitamin B12 can contribute to this disorder as well as to improper liver function. A liver cleanse and nutritional support will certainly help in rebuilding red blood cell counts.

## Recommendations

**Singles:** German Chamomile, German Chamomile Vitality, Thyme, Thyme Vitality, Sacred Frankincense, Frankincense, Frankincense Vitality, Helichrysum, Lemon, Lemon Vitality, Lime, Lime Vitality, Mountain Savory, Mountain Savory Vitality, Rosemary, Rosemary Vitality

**Blends:** JuvaCleanse, JuvaCleanse Vitality, TummyGize, DiGize, DiGize Vitality, EndoFlex, EndoFlex Vitality, JuvaFlex, JuvaFlex Vitality

**Nutritionals:** JuvaPower, MultiGreens, Super B, Rehemogen, NingXia Red, JuvaSpice, Master Formula, Mineral Essence, MindWise (also supports cardiovascular health)

## Application and Usage

**Aromatic:** Refer to *Application Guidelines* on page 410.

**Dietary and Oral:** Whether putting oils in a capsule or drinking them in a liquid, please refer to the directions at the beginning of this chapter.

- Take 2 capsules 2 times daily filled with half Helichrysum and half Cistus.
- Take 2-3 drops of oil in a spoonful of syrup or small amount of milk, juice, or water.

**Topical:** For guidelines on applying oils to the skin, refer to *Application Guidelines* on page 410.

## Aneurysm

Aneurysms are weak spots on the blood vessel walls that balloon out and may eventually rupture. In cases of brain aneurysms, a bursting blood vessel can cause a stroke, which can result in death or paralysis. (The fatality rate is over 50 percent in the U.S.) See your physician immediately.

Some essential oils and nutritional supplements support the cardiovascular system and help with blood regulation. Cypress strengthens capillary and vascular walls. Helichrysum helps dissolve blood clots.

## Recommendations

**Singles:** Cistus, Helichrysum, Cypress, Jade Lemon, Jade Lemon Vitality, Lemon, Lemon Vitality

**Blends:** Aroma Life, JuvaCleanse, JuvaCleanse Vitality, Purification

**Nutritionals:** NingXia Red, Essentialzyme, Essentialzymes-4, Pure Protein Complete, Ningxia Wolfberries (Organic, Dried), Digest & Cleanse, Detoxzyme

**Aneurysm Blend**
- 5 drops Cistus
- 1 drop Helichrysum
- 1 drop Cypress

**Aromatic:** Refer to *Application Guidelines* on page 410.

**Dietary and Oral:** Whether putting oils in a capsule or drinking them in a liquid, please refer to *Application Guidelines* on page 410.

- Take 1 capsule with Cistus or Cypress or other desired oil 2 times daily.
- Take 2 capsules 2 times daily 50:50 with Cistus and Cypress.
- Take 2-3 drops of oil in a spoonful of syrup or small amount of milk, juice, or water.

**Topical:** For guidelines on applying oils to the skin, refer to *Application Guidelines* on page 410.

- Dilute essential oils with V-6 Vegetable Oil Complex 50:50 and massage on back of neck and head 3-5 times daily.

## Angina

Angina is a severe and crushing chest pain caused from an inadequate supply of oxygen to the heart muscle. It is a symptom of an underlying heart condition. Contact a health care professional for diagnosis.

## Recommendations

**Singles:** Clove, Clove Vitality, Marjoram, Marjoram Vitality, Helichrysum, Goldenrod, Orange, Orange Vitality, Jade Lemon, Jade Lemon Vitality, Lemon, Lemon Vitality, Lavender, Lavender Vitality, Wintergreen

**438** | **Chapter 20** | Personal Usage Guide

Personal Usage Guide | **Chapter 20**

**Blends:** Aroma Life, Peace & Calming, Peace & Calming II, Stress Away Roll-On, Valor, Valor II, Valor Roll-On, RutaVaLa, RutaVaLa Roll-On, Longevity, Longevity Vitality

**Nutritionals:** NingXia Red, Ningxia Wolfberries (Organic, Dried), OmegaGize³, MegaCal, Longevity Softgels, Essentialzyme, Essentialzymes-4, Detoxzyme, MindWise (also supports cardiovascular health)

## Application and Usage

**Aromatic:** Refer to *Application Guidelines* on page 410.

**Dietary and Oral:** Whether putting oils in a capsule or drinking them in a liquid, please refer to *Application Guidelines* on page 410.

- Take 1-2 capsules with desired oil 2 times daily.
- Take 2-3 drops of oil in a spoonful of syrup or small amount of milk, juice, or water.

**Topical:** For guidelines on applying oils to the skin, refer to *Application Guidelines* on page 410.

- Massage 1-3 drops neat over the heart area 1-3 times daily.
- Apply on left side of chest, left shoulder, and back of neck.
- Massage 1 drop each of 2 or 3 of the recommended oils on the heart Vita Flex points on foot, hand, and arm, as needed.

## Arteriosclerosis (Hardening of the Arteries)

This condition is defined as any one of a group of diseases that causes a thickening and a loss of elasticity of arterial walls. It can be caused by inflammation and is frequently an underlying cause of a heart attack or stroke.

### Recommendations

**Singles:** Clove, Clove Vitality, Helichrysum, Geranium, Lavender, Lavender Vitality, German Chamomile, German Chamomile Vitality, Dorado Azul

**Blends:** Longevity, Longevity Vitality, Aroma Life

**Nutritionals:** Longevity Softgels, OmegaGize³, MegaCal, Ningxia Wolfberries (Organic, Dried), NingXia Red, Master Formula, MindWise (also supports cardiovascular health)

## Application and Usage

**Aromatic:** Refer to *Application Guidelines* on page 410.

**Dietary and Oral:** Whether putting oils in a capsule or drinking them in a liquid, please refer to *Application Guidelines* on page 410.

- Take 1 capsule with desired oil 2 times daily.
- Take 2-3 drops of oil in a spoonful of syrup or small amount of milk, juice, or water.

**Topical:** For guidelines on applying oils to the skin, refer to *Application Guidelines* on page 410.

- Massage 1-3 drops neat over the heart area 2-3 times weekly.
- Apply on left side of chest, left shoulder, and back of neck.
- Massage 1 drop each of 2 or 3 of the recommended oils on the heart Vita Flex points on foot, hand, and arm, as needed.

## Bleeding (Hemorrhaging)

Some essential oils, when topically applied or used on pressure bandages, are excellent for slowing bleeding and initiating healing.

### Recommendations

**Singles:** Helichrysum, Geranium, Cistus, Cypress, Lavender, Myrrh

**Blends:** Purification, Trauma Life, T.R. Care, Deep Relief Roll-On

**Nutritionals:** JuvaPower, JuvaSpice, Master Formula

### Application and Usage

**Topical:** For guidelines on applying oils to the skin, refer to *Application Guidelines* on page 410.

- Apply 1-2 drops neat (undiluted) on the location of small wounds.
- You may also apply 2-3 drops on the Vita Flex points of the feet.
- Place a cold compress diluted with 1-2 drops of Helichrysum, Myrrh, etc.

## Blood Circulation, Poor

Essential oils, when used regularly, can improve circulation as much as 20 percent.

### Recommendations

**Singles:** Helichrysum, Cypress, Clove, Clove Vitality, Idaho Balsam Fir, Cistus, Idaho Blue Spruce

Seventh Edition | **Essential Oils Desk Reference** | **439**

**Blends:** Aroma Life, EndoFlex, EndoFlex Vitality, En-R-Gee, Longevity, Longevity Vitality, Valor, Valor II, Valor Roll-On

**Nutritionals:** NingXia Red, Longevity Softgels, Ningxia Wolfberries (Organic, Dried), Mineral Essence, MindWise (also supports cardiovascular health)

## Application and Usage

**Dietary and Oral:** Whether putting oils in a capsule or drinking them in a liquid, please refer to *Application Guidelines* on page 410.

- Take 1 capsule with Helichrysum, Cypress, or other desired oil 2 times daily.
- Take 2-3 drops of oil in a spoonful of syrup or small amount of milk, juice, or water.

**Topical:** For guidelines on applying oils to the skin, refer to *Application Guidelines* on page 410.

- Apply neat 2-3 drops on Vita Flex points of feet or on inside of wrists 2-3 times daily.

## Blood Clots
## (Embolism, Hematoma, Thrombus)

A blood clot, or hematoma, is a tumor-like mass of coagulated blood, caused by a break in the blood vessel or capillary wall.

Essential oils such as Helichrysum, Geranium, and Cistus are excellent for balancing blood viscosity and dissolving clots. Clove oil and citrus rind oils, such as Lemon and Grapefruit, exert a blood-thinning effect that can help speed the dissolution of the clot.

These oils are also some of the most powerful antioxidants known and can slow the formation of oxidized cholesterol in cells, which contributes to atherosclerosis. Helichrysum is effective in preventing blood clot formation and promoting the dissolution of clots.

As people age, the viscosity or thickness of the blood increases, and so does the tendency of the blood to clot excessively.

If blood clots, known as embolisms, occur in the brain, they can cause strokes; if they obstruct a coronary artery, they can cause ischemic heart attacks.

People with diabetes or high blood pressure are far more likely to die from blood clots.

Foods rich in vitamin E, vitamin A, and omega-3 fats are vital for proper blood viscosity.

## Recommendations

**Singles:** Helichrysum, Cistus, Clove, Clove Vitality, Geranium, Jade Lemon, Jade Lemon Vitality, Lemon, Lemon Vitality, Grapefruit, Grapefruit Vitality, Nutmeg, Nutmeg Vitality, Cypress, Wintergreen

**Blends:** Aroma Life, PanAway, Relieve It, Longevity, Longevity Vitality

**Nutritionals:** OmegaGize³, Super C, Super C Chewable, Mineral Essence, Longevity Softgels, Thieves, Inner Defense, NingXia Red, MindWise (also supports cardiovascular health)

**Oral Care:** Thieves toothpastes contain Clove, which has natural blood-thinning properties.

## Application and Usage

**Aromatic:** Refer to *Application Guidelines* on page 410.

**Dietary and Oral:** Whether putting the oils in a capsule or drinking them in a liquid, please refer to *Application Guidelines* on page 410.

- Take 1 capsule with desired oil 2 times daily.
- Take 2 capsules diluted 50:50 with Helichrysum and Cistus 2 times daily between meals.
- Take 2-3 drops of oil in a spoonful of syrup or small amount of milk, juice, or water.

**Topical:** For guidelines on applying oils to the skin, refer to *Application Guidelines* on page 410.

- Massage equal parts Lemon, Lavender, and Helichrysum on location with or without hot packs.
- Massage equal parts Cistus, Lavender, and Helichrysum on location.
- Place a warm compress with 1-2 drops of chosen oil on the back for 15 minutes 2 times daily.

## Blood Detoxification

When there are fewer toxins in the blood, it is easier for the blood to function properly and to continually carry the needed nutrients throughout the body and the digested waste and toxins out of the body, which is the key for staying healthy, being able to fight disease, and expelling chemicals and other pollutants.

## Recommendations

**Singles:** Helichrysum, Goldenrod, Geranium, German Chamomile, German Chamomile Vitality, Clove, Clove Vitality, Idaho Balsam Fir, Mountain Savory, Mountain Savory Vitality, Rosemary, Rosemary Vitality

**Blends:** GLF, GLF Vitality, JuvaCleanse, JuvaCleanse Vitality, DiGize, DiGize Vitality

**Nutritionals:** MultiGreens, Rehemogen, ICP, JuvaPower, JuvaSpice, Sulfurzyme, Balance Complete, Slique Tea MSM (found in Sulfurzyme) purifies the body and blood.

## Application and Usage

**Dietary and Oral:** Whether putting oils in a capsule or drinking them in a liquid, please refer to *Application Guidelines* on page 410.

- Look up the specific action of these products and decide what best targets your desired results.
- Take 1 capsule of GLF Vitality or JuvaCleanse Vitality, plus Rosemary Vitality or other desired oil 2 times daily.
- Take 2-3 drops of oil in a spoonful of syrup or small amount of milk, juice, or water.

**Topical:** For guidelines on applying oils to the skin, refer to *Application Guidelines* on page 410.

- Massage 2-3 drops neat (undiluted) on the Vita Flex points of the feet and on the inside of the wrists 2-3 times daily.

## Blood Platelets (Low)

Blood platelets (thrombocytes) are necessary for fighting infections and for blood clotting. To avoid a drastic drop in the platelet level, consume leafy vegetables, fruits like bananas and oranges, and dairy products.

## Recommendations

**Singles:** Jade Lemon, Jade Lemon Vitality, Lemon, Lemon Vitality, Thyme, Thyme Vitality, Tea Tree, Geranium, Cypress

**Blends:** Aroma Life

**Nutritionals:** JuvaTone, Rehemogen, JuvaPower, JuvaSpice

To enhance the effects of Rehemogen, use it with Juva-Tone, JuvaPower, or JuvaSpice.

## Blood Pressure, High (Hypertension)

One way to help normalize blood pressure is to cleanse the liver and colon for better circulation. Cleansing the colon will help rid the body of wastes and toxins that could be clogging the normal process of digestion. Cleansing and digestion are critical to normal body function.

## Recommendations

**Singles:** Ocotea, Helichrysum, Rosemary, Rosemary Vitality, Clove, Clove Vitality, Lavender, Lavender Vitality, Marjoram, Marjoram Vitality, Ylang Ylang,

Amazonian Ylang Ylang, Cypress, Cinnamon Bark, Cinnamon Bark Vitality

**Blends:** Aroma Life, Peace & Calming, Peace & Calming II, Citrus Fresh, Citrus Fresh Vitality, Humility, Slique Essence

**Nutritionals:** Essentialzyme, Detoxzyme, OmegaGize³, ImmuPro, Super B, Mineral Essence, Balance Complete, Essentialzymes-4, MegaCal, Ningxia Wolfberries (Organic, Dried), Slique Tea, MindWise

## Application and Usage

**Aromatic:** Refer to *Application Guidelines* on page 410.

**Dietary and Oral:** Whether putting the oils in a capsule or drinking them in a liquid, please refer to *Application Guidelines* on page 410.

- Take 1 capsule with desired oil 2 times daily.
- Take 2-3 drops of oil in a spoonful of syrup or small amount of milk, juice, or water.

**Topical:** For guidelines on applying oils to the skin, refer to *Application Guidelines* on page 410.

- Apply 1-3 drops oil diluted 20:80 for a full body massage daily.
- Rub 1-2 drops of oil on the temples and back of neck several times daily.
- Place a warm compress with 1-2 drops of chosen oil on the back.
- For 3 minutes, massage 1-2 drops each of Aroma Life and Ylang Ylang on the heart Vita Flex point and over the heart and carotid arteries along the neck.
- Notice how the blood pressure will begin to drop within 5-20 minutes. Monitor the pressure and reapply as desired.
- Increase the intake of magnesium, which acts as a smooth-muscle relaxant and as a natural calcium channel blocker for the heart, lowering blood pressure and dilating the heart blood vessels.
- Take 1 teaspoon of MegaCal before going to bed.
- Take 1-2 droppers of Mineral Essence 2 times daily.
- Take 1 Super B daily with your meal. Vitamin B3 (niacin) 20 mg daily is an excellent vasodilator found in Super B.

## Bruising *(See also Bruised Muscles)*

Some people bruise easily because the capillary walls are weak and break easily, particularly in the skin. Those who bruise easily may be deficient in vitamin C.

Seventh Edition | **Essential Oils Desk Reference** | 441

Essential oils can help speed the healing of bruises and reduce the risk of blood clot formation. Oils like Cypress help to strengthen capillary walls, while oils like Helichrysum help speed the reabsorption of the blood that has collected in the tissue.

## Recommendations

**Singles:** Helichrysum, Clove, Clove Vitality, Cistus, Geranium, Lavender, Lavender Vitality, Cypress, Roman Chamomile, Idaho Blue Spruce, Dorado Azul, Peppermint, Peppermint Vitality, Marjoram, Marjoram Vitality, Black Pepper, Black Pepper Vitality

**Blends:** Deep Relief Roll-On, PanAway, Relieve It, Cool Azul, Owie

**Nutritionals:** MultiGreens, JuvaTone, JuvaPower, JuvaSpice, Super C, Super C Chewable, NingXia Red, Slique Tea

**Body Care:** Cool Azul Pain Relief Cream, Cool Azul Sports Gel, Ortho Sport Massage Oil, Ortho Ease Massage Oil

**Bruise Blend No. 1**
- 5 drops Helichrysum
- 4 drops Lavender
- 3 drops Cypress
- 3 drops Cistus
- 3 drops Geranium

**Bruise Blend No. 2**
- 6 drops Clove
- 4 drops Black Pepper
- 3 drops Peppermint
- 2 drops Marjoram
- 2 drops Geranium
- 2 drops Cypress

## Application and Usage

**Dietary and Oral:** Whether putting oils in a capsule or drinking them in a liquid, please refer to *Application Guidelines* on page 410.

- Take 1 capsule with desired oil 2 times daily.
- Take 2-3 drops of oil in a spoonful of syrup or small amount of milk, juice, or water.
- Take 1-4 tablets of Super C Chewable daily.
- Take 2-3 capsules of MultiGreens 3 times daily.

**Topical:** For guidelines on applying oils to the skin, refer to *Application Guidelines* on page 410.

- Apply 2-3 drops neat 2-3 times daily, depending on which oil you choose. Helichrysum is especially beneficial in healing bruises when applied neat on location.

- Dilute the oil you choose 50:50 with V-6 Vegetable Oil Complex and apply 1-3 drops on bruised area 2-5 times daily.
- Apply a cold compress on location 2-4 times daily or as needed.

## Cholesterol, High

When fatty cholesterol deposits accumulate in the arteries, physical symptoms like chest pains and heart attacks may take place.

## Recommendations

**Singles:** Lemongrass, Lemongrass Vitality, Helichrysum, Rosemary, Rosemary Vitality, Clove, Clove Vitality, German Chamomile, German Chamomile Vitality, Roman Chamomile

**Blends:** Aroma Life, Longevity, Longevity Vitality, Slique Essence

**Nutritionals:** OmegaGize[3], Essentialzyme, Detoxzyme, Mineral Essence, MegaCal, JuvaPower, JuvaSpice, MultiGreens, Super C, Super C Chewable, SuperCal, Longevity Softgels, ICP, Essentialzymes-4, Balance Complete, Slique Tea, Power Meal, Slique Shake, Slique CitraSlim, Slique Bars

**Cholesterol Reducing Blend**
- 5 drops Roman Chamomile
- 5 drops Lemongrass or Lemongrass Vitality
- 4 drops Rosemary or Rosemary Vitality
- 3 drops Helichrysum

## Application and Usage

**Dietary and Oral:** Whether putting the oils in a capsule or drinking them in a liquid, please refer to *Application Guidelines* on page 410.

- Take 1 capsule with desired oil 2 times daily.
- Take 2-3 drops of oil in a spoonful of syrup or small amount of milk, juice, or water.

**Topical:** For guidelines on applying oils to the skin, refer to *Application Guidelines* on page 410.

- Apply neat or dilute 50:50, if needed, 2-4 drops at pulse points, where arteries are close to the surface (wrists, inside elbows, base of throat), 2-3 times daily.
- Also rub 6-10 drops along spine 3 times daily.
- Have a body massage 2 times weekly.

**Supplementation regimens**

1. Do a colon and liver cleanse using ICP, ComforTone, Essentialzyme, Digest & Cleanse, JuvaTone, JuvaPow-

er, JuvaFlex Vitality, or JuvaCleanse Vitality. JuvaTone is particularly useful for reducing high cholesterol.

2. Magnesium acts as a smooth muscle relaxant and supports the cardiovascular system. It acts as a natural calcium channel blocker for the heart, lowering blood pressure and dilating the heart blood vessels (Dr. T. Friedmann). Mineral Essence and MegaCal are good sources of magnesium.

## Congestive Heart Failure
*(See also Heart Attack)*

Congestive heart failure is the inability of the heart to supply enough blood to meet the demands of the body. The most common cause is coronary artery disease, a narrowing of the small blood vessels that supply oxygen and blood to the heart.

Symptoms include shortness of breath, loss of appetite, cough, fatigue, weakness, swollen abdomen, need to urinate at night, weight gain, and swollen feet and ankles.

Coenzyme Q10 (CoQ10) is one of the most effective supplements for supporting the heart muscle. MindWise nutritional supplement contains bio-identical CoQ10, as well as other valuable nutrients, and supports cardiovascular health.

### Recommendations

**Singles:** Helichrysum, Goldenrod, Clove, Clove Vitality, Marjoram, Marjoram Vitality, Cypress

**Blends:** Aroma Life, Longevity, Longevity Vitality

**Nutritionals:** MindWise, MegaCal, Mineral Essence

### Application and Usage

**Dietary and Oral:** Whether putting the oils in a capsule or drinking them in a liquid, please refer to *Application Guidelines* on page 410.

- Take 1 capsule with desired oil 2 times daily.
- Take 2-3 drops of oil in a spoonful of syrup or small amount of milk, juice, or water.

**Topical:** For guidelines on applying oils to the skin, refer to *Application Guidelines* on page 410.

- Apply 1-2 drops neat to heart Vita Flex points on foot, hand, and arm, as described under the "Heart Vita Flex" section under the topic Heart Health.
- Apply neat or dilute 50:50, if needed, 2-4 drops at pulse points, where arteries are close to the surface (wrists, inside elbows, base of throat), 2-3 times daily.
- Also rub 6-10 drops along spine 3 times daily.
- Have a body massage 2 times weekly.

## Fibrillation

This is a specific form of heart arrhythmia that occurs when the upper heart chambers contract at a rate of over 300 pulsations per minute. The lower chambers cannot keep this pace, so efficiency is reduced and not enough blood is pumped. Palpitations, a feeling that the heart is beating irregularly, more strongly, or more rapidly than normal, is the most common symptom.

### Recommendations

**Singles:** Ylang Ylang, Amazonian Ylang Ylang, Valerian, Valerian Vitality, Goldenrod, Marjoram, Marjoram Vitality, Lavender, Lavender Vitality, Rosemary, Rosemary Vitality

**Blends:** Aroma Life, Peace & Calming, Peace & Calming II

**Nutritionals:** OmegaGize[3], Mineral Essence, MegaCal, Sulfurzyme, Ningxia Wolfberries (Organic, Dried), Master Formula, MindWise (also supports cardiovascular health)

### Application and Usage

**Aromatic:** Refer to *Application Guidelines* on page 410.

**Dietary and Oral:** Whether putting the oils in a capsule or drinking them in a liquid, please refer to *Application Guidelines* on page 410.

- Take 1 capsule with desired oil 2 times daily.
- Take 2-3 drops of oil in a spoonful of syrup or small amount of milk, juice, or water.

**Topical:** For guidelines on applying oils to the skin, refer to *Application Guidelines* on page 410.

- Apply 1-3 drops neat 1-3 times daily of 2-3 of the recommended oils on the heart Vita Flex points on foot, hand, and arm as described in the "Heart Vita Flex" section under the topic Heart Health.
- Apply neat or dilute 50:50, if needed, 2-4 drops at pulse points, where arteries are close to the surface (wrists, inside elbows, base of throat), 2-3 times daily.
- Also apply to left chest, left shoulder, and back of neck.
- Also rub 6-10 drops along spine 3 times daily.
- Have a body massage 2 times weekly.

## Heart Attack (Myocardial Infarction)

A heart attack is a circulation blockage resulting in an interruption of blood supply to an area of the heart. Depending on the size of the area affected, it can be mild or severe.

**Note:** Seek medical care immediately if you suspect a heart attack.

Many people do not understand how someone who is relatively healthy, with low cholesterol levels, suffers a heart attack with no explanation. The explanation is actually inflammation, the fundamental cause of heart disease.

Inflammation of the heart is caused when blood vessels leading to the heart are clogged and damaged. This releases a protein into the bloodstream called C-reactive protein. The level of this protein indicates the degree of inflammation in the linings of the arteries. Certain essential oils have been documented to be excellent for reducing inflammation. German Chamomile contains azulene, a blue compound with highly anti-inflammatory properties. Peppermint is also highly anti-inflammatory. Other oils also have anti-inflammatory properties such as Helichrysum, Northern Lights Black Spruce, Wintergreen, and Valerian. Clove, Nutmeg, and Wintergreen are natural blood thinners and help reduce blood clotting.

Magnesium, the most important mineral for the heart, acts as a smooth muscle relaxant and supports the cardiovascular system. Magnesium will act as a natural calcium channel blocker for the heart, lowering blood pressure and dilating the heart blood vessels (according to Terry Friedmann, MD).

## Recommendations

**Singles:** Wintergreen, Peppermint, Peppermint Vitality, Lavender, Lavender Vitality, German Chamomile, German Chamomile Vitality, Helichrysum, Northern Lights Black Spruce, Valerian, Dorado Azul, Ocotea, Clove, Clove Vitality, Nutmeg, Nutmeg Vitality, Copaiba, Copaiba Vitality, Palo Santo

**Blends:** Aroma Life, PanAway, Longevity, Longevity Vitality, Peace & Calming, Peace & Calming II, Relieve It, Valor, Valor II, Valor Roll-On

**Nutritionals:** MegaCal, Longevity Softgels, Mineral Essence, OmegaGize[3], Sulfurzyme, Rehemogen, NingXia Red, MindWise (also supports cardiovascular health)

## Application and Usage

**Aromatic:** Refer to *Application Guidelines* on page 410.
**Dietary and Oral:** Whether putting the oils in a capsule or drinking them in a liquid, please refer to *Application Guidelines* on page 410.

- Take 1 capsule with desired oil 2 times daily.
- Take 2-3 drops of oil in a spoonful of syrup or small amount of milk, juice, or water.

**Topical:** For guidelines on applying oils to the skin, refer to *Application Guidelines* on page 410.

- If there is not enough time to remove shoes to get at the feet, apply the "pumping" action to left hand and arm points. Using 1-2 drops of Aroma Life on each point will increase effectiveness and may even revive an individual having a heart attack while waiting for medical attention.
- Apply 1-3 drops neat 1-3 times daily of 2-3 of the recommended oils on the heart Vita Flex points on foot, hand, and arm as described in the "Heart Vita Flex" section under the topic Heart Health.
- Apply neat or dilute 50:50, if needed, 2-4 drops at pulse points, where arteries are close to the surface (wrists, inside elbows, base of throat), 2-3 times daily.
- Also apply to left chest, left shoulder, and back of neck.
- Also rub 6-10 drops along spine 3 times daily.
- Have a body massage 2 times weekly.

## Heart Health

Heart disease is the leading cause of death in the United States. Keys to prevention include quitting smoking, controlling high blood pressure, lowering cholesterol, exercising, and maintaining a healthy weight.

## Heart Vita Flex

The foot Vita Flex point related to the heart is on the sole of the left foot, below the ring toe (fourth toe) and approximately 1 inch below the base of the toe. Massaging this point is as effective as massaging the hand and arm points together (see charts in Application).

The hand Vita Flex point related to the heart is in the palm of the left hand, 1 inch below the ring finger joint at the lifeline. A secondary heart point is on the inside of the lower end of the upper left arm, approximately 2 inches up the arm from the elbow, not on the muscle but up under the muscle. Have another person use his or her thumbs to firmly press these two points alternately for 3 minutes in a kind of pumping action. Work all three points when possible. Start with the foot first; then go to the hand and arm.

## Heart Stimulant

The effects of heart stimulants include increased heart rate and blood pressure.

## Recommendations

**Singles:** Rosemary, Rosemary Vitality, Peppermint, Peppermint Vitality, Ylang Ylang, Amazonian Ylang

444 | **Chapter 20** | Personal Usage Guide

Ylang, Goldenrod, Mandarin, Thyme, Thyme Vitality, Marjoram, Marjoram Vitality

**Blends:** Aroma Life, Peace & Calming, Peace & Calming II, Release, Joy, Sacred Mountain, RutaVaLa, RutaVaLa Roll-On, Valor, Valor II, Valor Roll-On, Stress Away Roll-On

**Nutritionals:** Master Formula

## Application and Usage

**Aromatic:** Refer to *Application Guidelines* on page 410.

**Dietary and Oral:** Whether putting the oils in a capsule or drinking them in a liquid, please refer to *Application Guidelines* on page 410.

- Take 1 capsule with desired oil 2 times daily.
- Take 2-3 drops of oil in a spoonful of syrup or small amount of milk, juice, or water.

**Topical:** For guidelines on applying oils to the skin, refer to *Application Guidelines* on page 410.

- Apply 1-3 drops neat over the heart area 1-3 times daily.
- Massage the Vita Flex points with one drop each of the 2-3 recommended oils on the heart Vita Flex points along the foot, hand, and arm as needed.

## Phlebitis (Inflammation of Veins)
*(See also Edema)*

Phlebitis refers to inflammation of a blood vein, usually due to a thrombus or blood clot. Symptoms include pain and tenderness along the course of the vein, discoloration of the skin, inflammatory swelling, joint pain, and acute edema below the inflamed site. Natural progesterone is an effective anti-inflammatory.

## Recommendations

**Singles:** Juniper, Helichrysum, Cistus, Cypress, Wintergreen, Tangerine, Tangerine Vitality, Copaiba, Copaiba Vitality, German Chamomile, German Chamomile Vitality, Geranium, Lavender, Lavender Vitality, Clove, Clove Vitality, Nutmeg, Nutmeg Vitality, Jade Lemon, Jade Lemon Vitality, Lemon, Lemon Vitality

**Blends:** Aroma Life, Longevity, Longevity Vitality

**Nutritionals:** Longevity Softgels

**Body Care:** Progessence Plus, Prenolone Plus Body Cream

### Phlebitis Blend
- 10 drops Tangerine
- 7 drops Lemon

- 5 drops Cypress
- 4 drops Juniper

## Application and Usage

**Topical:** For guidelines on applying oils to the skin, refer to *Application Guidelines* on page 410.

- The essential oil of Cypress may help strengthen vascular walls.
- You may apply single oils or blends neat or diluted, depending on the oils that are used.
- Massage 2-4 drops of oil neat on the bottoms of the feet just before bedtime.
- Apply 2-4 drops neat on location 2-4 times daily.
- Apply a cold compress on location 2-4 times daily.

## Plaque

Plaque is a cholesterol build up along the walls of the arteries, which causes the arteries to narrow. This is often when the physical symptoms of high cholesterol are noticed.

**Singles:** Rosemary, Helichrysum, Dorado Azul

**Blends:** Aroma Life, TummyGize, DiGize, DiGize Vitality

**Nutritionals:** Detoxzyme, Digest & Cleanse, JuvaPower, Life 9

## Application and Usage

**Aromatic:** Refer to *Application Guidelines* on page 410.

**Dietary and Oral:** Whether putting the oils in a capsule or drinking them in a liquid, please refer to *Application Guidelines* on page 410.

- Take 1 capsule with Helichrysum or other desired oil 2 times daily.
- Take 1-2 capsules 50:50 with Helichrysum and Cistus 2 times daily.
- Take 2-3 drops of oil in a spoonful of syrup or small amount of milk, juice, or water.

**Topical:** For guidelines on applying oils to the skin, refer to *Application Guidelines* on page 410.

- Apply 1-3 drops, diluted 50:50, on temples, forehead, mastoids, back of neck, and at base of throat just above clavicle notch.
- Applying a single drop under the nose is helpful and refreshing.
- Massage 2-4 drops of oil neat on Vita Flex brain points on the bottoms of the feet just before bedtime.

**Essential Oils Desk Reference** | Seventh Edition

# Strokes

Two principal kinds of strokes can damage the brain: hemorrhagic strokes and thrombotic strokes.

Some essential oils can be used topically to help strengthen the integrity of capillary walls. In particular, the essential oils of Helichrysum, Cistus, and Nutmeg are known to have anticlotting properties and can be used as a preventive measure to reduce the risk of thrombotic stroke.

## Hemorrhagic Strokes

A hemorrhagic stroke is caused by an aneurysm or a weakness in the blood vessel wall that balloons out and ruptures, spilling blood into the surrounding brain tissue. Strokes are very serious events, and if you suspect that you may be susceptible, immediately see a physician.

### Recommendations

**Singles:** Cypress, Cistus, Helichrysum, Nutmeg, Nutmeg Vitality, Royal Hawaiian Sandalwood

**Blends:** Brain Power, Common Sense, Clarity, GeneYus, Longevity, Longevity Vitality, Stress Away Roll-On, Peace & Calming, Peace & Calming II

**Nutritionals:** Sulfurzyme, MindWise, MegaCal, Mineral Essence, Essentialzyme, Rehemogen, Master Formula, NingXia Red

### Application and Usage

**Aromatic:** Refer to *Application Guidelines* on page 410.

**Dietary and Oral:** Whether putting the oils in a capsule or drinking them in a liquid, please refer to *Application Guidelines* on page 410.

- Take 1 capsule with Helichrysum or other desired oil 2 times daily.
- Take 1-2 capsules 50:50 with Helichrysum and Cistus 2 times daily.
- Take 2-3 drops of oil in a spoonful of syrup or small amount of milk, juice, or water.

**Topical:** For guidelines on applying oils to the skin, refer to *Application Guidelines* on page 410.

- Apply 1-3 drops, diluted 50:50, on temples, forehead, mastoids, back of neck, and at base of throat just above clavicle notch.
- Applying a single drop under the nose is helpful and refreshing.
- Massage 2-4 drops of oil neat on Vita Flex brain points on the bottoms of the feet just before bedtime.

# Thrombotic Strokes

Thrombotic strokes are caused by a blood clot lodging in a cerebral blood vessel and cutting blood supply to a part of the brain.

## Recommendations

**Singles:** Helichrysum, Cistus, Nutmeg, Nutmeg Vitality, Cypress, Royal Hawaiian Sandalwood, Juniper, Grapefruit, Grapefruit Vitality, Orange, Orange Vitality, Clove, Clove Vitality

**Blends:** Longevity, Longevity Vitality, Aroma Life, JuvaCleanse, JuvaCleanse Vitality

**Nutritionals:** Sulfurzyme, MegaCal, OmegaGize$^3$, MindWise, Essentialzyme, Pure Protein Complete, Master Formula, Mineral Essence, Essentialzymes-4, Power Meal, Slique Shake, Slique Bars, Slique CitraSlim, NingXia Red

These supplements are rich in essential minerals, fatty acids, and nutrients necessary for regenerating and rebuilding damaged nerve tissues.

## Application and Usage

**Aromatic:** Refer to *Application Guidelines* on page 410.

**Topical:** For guidelines on applying oils to the skin, refer to *Application Guidelines* on page 410.

- Applying the essential oil of Cypress may help strengthen vascular walls.
- You may apply single oils or blends neat or diluted, depending on the oils that are used.
- Apply 1-2 drops neat on temples and back of neck as desired.
- Applying a single drop under the nose is helpful and refreshing.
- Massage 2-4 drops of oil neat on the bottoms of the feet just before bedtime.

# Tachycardia

Tachycardia is another form of heart arrhythmia in which the heart rate suddenly increases to 160 beats per minute or faster. See your physician if you experience this condition. If fainting, difficulty breathing, or chest pain also occur, seek emergency care.

## Recommendations

**Singles:** Ylang Ylang, Amazonian Ylang Ylang, Rosemary, Rosemary Vitality, Royal Hawaiian Sandalwood, Wintergreen, Marjoram, Marjoram Vitality, German Chamomile, German Chamomile Vitality, Lavender, Lavender Vitality, Goldenrod

**446** | **Chapter 20** | Personal Usage Guide

**Blends:** Aroma Life, Peace & Calming, Peace & Calming II, Acceptance

**Nutritionals:** Sulfurzyme, NingXia Red, MindWise (also supports cardiovascular health)

## Application and Usage

**Aromatic:** Refer to *Application Guidelines* on page 410.

**Dietary and Oral:** Whether putting the oils in a capsule or drinking them in a liquid, please refer to *Application Guidelines* on page 410.

- Take 1 capsule with desired oil 3 times daily.
- Take 2-3 drops of oil in a spoonful of syrup or small amount of milk, juice, or water.

**Topical:** For guidelines on applying oils to the skin, refer to *Application Guidelines* on page 410.

- Massage 1-3 drops over heart area 1-3 times daily. Also apply to left chest, left shoulder, and back of neck.
- Massage 1 drop each of 2 or 3 of the recommended oils on heart Vita Flex points on foot, hand, and arm as needed.

## Varicose Veins (Spider Veins)

The blue color of varicose veins is coagulated blood in the surrounding tissue from hemorrhaging of capillaries around the veins. This blood has to be dissolved and re-absorbed.

### Recommendations

**Singles:** Helichrysum, Cypress, Cistus, Elemi, Geranium, Clove, Clove Vitality, Peppermint, Peppermint Vitality, Jade Lemon, Jade Lemon Vitality, Lemon, Lemon Vitality, Lavender, Lavender Vitality, Tangerine

    Helichrysum helps dissolve the coagulated blood in the surrounding tissue.

**Blends:** Aroma Life, Citrus Fresh, Aroma Siez

**Nutritionals:** MultiGreens, Super B, Longevity Softgels, PowerGize, Essentialzyme, Essentialzymes-4, Life 9

**Body Care:** Cool Azul Pain Relief Cream, Ortho Ease Massage Oil

## Application and Usage

**Topical:** For guidelines on applying oils to the skin, refer to *Application Guidelines* on page 410.

### Varicose Vein Blend
- 3-4 drops Geranium
- 1 drop Cistus
- 1 drop Cypress
- 1 drop Helichrysum

Apply 2-4 drops on location, massaging toward the heart, 3-6 times daily.

### Nightly Varicose Vein Regimen (Legs)

1. Apply 1-3 drops varicose vein blend, neat, on location. Rub very gently toward heart with smooth strokes along the vein, then up and over the vein until the oil is absorbed.
2. Apply 6 drops Tangerine and 6 drops Cypress to the area. Gently massage until absorbed.
3. Do the lymphatic pump procedure as described in Chapter 15.
4. Follow with a soft massage of the whole leg using 10-15 drops of Aroma Life diluted 50:50.
5. Wrap and elevate the leg. It is best to do this at night before retiring and to gradually elevate the foot off the bed, an inch more each night, until it is 4 inches higher than the head.
6. Wear support hose during the daytime. It may take up to a year to achieve desired results.

## Vascular Cleansing

Keeping your blood clean will help you stay healthy.

1. Drink plenty of water.
2. Cleanse the blood by taking blood-cleansing herbs and essential oils.
3. Cleanse the kidneys.
4. Consider fasting for one to three days.
5. Take enzymes.

**Singles:** Helichrysum, Clove, Clove Vitality, Idaho Blue Spruce, Sacred Frankincense, Frankincense, Frankincense Vitality, Dorado Azul

**Blends:** GLF, GLF Vitality, DiGize, DiGize Vitality, JuvaCleanse, JuvaCleanse Vitality, TummyGize

**Nutritionals:** Essentialzyme, Essentialzymes-4, Life 9, JuvaPower, JuvaSpice, NingXia Red

## Application and Usage

**Aromatic:** Refer to *Application Guidelines* on page 410.

**Dietary and Oral:** Whether putting the oils in a capsule or drinking them in a liquid, please refer to *Application Guidelines* on page 410.

- Take 1 capsule with Helichrysum or other desired oil 2 times daily.
- Take 1-2 capsules 2 times daily 50:50 with Helichrysum and Cistus.

- Take 2-3 drops of oil in a spoonful of syrup or small amount of milk, juice, or water.

**Topical:** For guidelines on applying oils to the skin, refer to *Application Guidelines* on page 410.

- Apply 1-3 drops, diluted 50:50, on temples, forehead, mastoids, back of neck, and at base of throat just above the clavicle notch.
- Applying a single drop under the nose is helpful and refreshing.
- Massage 2-4 drops of oil neat on Vita Flex brain points on the bottoms of the feet just before bedtime.

## CANKER SORES *(See also Mouth Ulcers)*

These are technically known as aphthous ulcers, are not regarded as an infectious disease, and are not caused by the herpes virus.

Canker sores tend to occur because of stress, illness, weakened immune system, and injury caused by such things as hot food, rough brushing of teeth, or dentures. They appear under the tongue more commonly than cold sores.

## Recommendations

**Singles:** Melissa, Clove, Clove Vitality, Lavender, Lavender Vitality, Royal Hawaiian Sandalwood, Cypress, Thyme, Thyme Vitality

**Blends:** Thieves, Thieves Vitality, Melrose

**Nutritionals:** Inner Defense, ImmuPro, AlkaLime

**Oral Care:** Thieves Spray, Thieves Fresh Essence Mouthwash

## Application and Usage

### Dietary and Oral

- Gargle with Thieves mouthwash 2-4 times daily.
- Take maple syrup 2-4 times daily.

**Topical:** For guidelines on applying oils to the skin, refer to *Application Guidelines* on page 410.

- Gently apply 1 drop of oil neat with fingertip to canker sore 4-8 times daily.

## CELLULITE

Cellulite is one of the harder types of fats to dissolve in the body. It's an accumulation of old fat cell clusters that solidifies and hardens as the surrounding tissue loses its elasticity.

Excess fat is undesirable for two reasons:
1. The extra weight puts an extra load on all body systems, particularly the heart and cardiovascular system, as well as the joints (knees, hips, spine, etc.).
2. Toxins and petrochemicals (pesticides, herbicides, and metals) tend to accumulate in fatty tissue. This can contribute to hormone imbalance, neurological problems, and a higher risk of cancer.

Essential oils such as Ledum, Tangerine, and Grapefruit may help reduce fat cells. Cypress enhances circulation to support the elimination of fatty deposits. The essential oils of Lemongrass and Spearmint also may help fat metabolism. Cel-Lite Magic Massage Oil contains many of these oils and may help reduce cellulite deposits.

Cellulite is slow to dissolve, so target areas should be worked for a month or more in conjunction with weight training, a weight-loss program, and drinking purified water—one-and-a-half times the body weight in ounces each day. Be patient. You should begin to see results in 4-6 weeks when using the oils in combination with a muscle-building and weight-loss regimen.

## Recommendations

**Singles:** Grapefruit, Grapefruit Vitality, Spearmint, Spearmint Vitality, Ledum, Lavender, Lavender Vitality, Rosemary, Rosemary Vitality, Helichrysum, Jade Lemon, Jade Lemon Vitality, Patchouli, Lemon, Lemon Vitality, Tangerine, Tangerine Vitality, Cypress, Fennel, Fennel Vitality, Juniper, Orange, Orange Vitality, Lemongrass, Lemongrass Vitality

**Blends:** EndoFlex, EndoFlex Vitality, Digest & Cleanse

**Nutritionals:** Thyromin, Power Meal, Slique Shake, Slique Bars, Slique CitraSlim, OmegaGize[3], Essentialzyme, Essentialzymes-4, Life 9, Balance Complete

Thyromin balances and boosts metabolism.

**Body Care:** Cel-Lite Magic Massage Oil

## Application and Usage

**Topical:** For guidelines on applying oils to the skin, refer to *Application Guidelines* on page 410.

- Dilute 50:50 and massage 3-6 drops vigorously on cellulite locations at least 3 times daily, especially before exercising.

### Cellulite Blend No. 1
- 10 drops Grapefruit
- 5 drops Lavender
- 3 drops Helichrysum
- 3 drops Patchouli
- 4 drops Cypress

Use as bath salt 2-4 times weekly.

**Cellulite Blend No. 2 (Bath)**
- 5 drops Juniper
- 3 drops Cypress
- 3 drops Orange
- 3 drops Rosemary

Mix the above blend together with 2 tablespoons Epsom salts or Bath Gel Base and dissolve in warm bath water. Massage with Cel-Lite Magic after bath.
- Apply 3-5 drops of Grapefruit neat 1-2 times daily to increase fat-reducing action in areas of fat rolls, puckers, and dimples.

# CEREBRAL PALSY

The effects of cerebral palsy vary greatly, causing impaired movement associated with exaggerated reflexes or rigidity of the limbs and trunk, abnormal posture, involuntary movements, unsteadiness of walking, or a combination of these.

It is caused most often by abnormal development in the brain before birth or injury during delivery. Individuals stricken with cerebral palsy often have other conditions related to developmental brain abnormalities such as intellectual disabilities, vision and hearing problems, or seizures.

**Signs and symptoms**
- Stiff muscles and exaggerated reflexes (spasticity)
- Stiff muscles with normal reflexes (rigidity)
- Lack of muscle coordination, tremors, or involuntary movements
- Slow development of motor skills such as pushing with arms, sitting up, or crawling
- Reaching with only one hand or dragging a leg while crawling
- Difficulty eating and swallowing, excessive drooling
- Slow speech development or difficulty speaking
- Difficulty in picking up toys, spoons, etc.

Medical researchers have not found an answer but offer different therapies and medication in an effort to help. Natural medicine offers help with the same desire of seeing improvement. Because essential oils cross the blood brain barrier, they can stimulate brain activity in a nontoxic way, and one can hope and wait to see what possible benefits will appear.

Different people have tried different things that have resulted in the information below. By investigating further with supplements and natural remedies, many new things will be discovered. The risk is minimal and the gain could be slight to immense.

## Recommendations

**Singles:** Sacred Frankincense, Frankincense, Frankincense Vitality, Myrrh, Idaho Balsam Fir, Peppermint, Peppermint Vitality, Canadian Fleabane (Conyza)

**Blends:** PanAway, Aroma Siez, Relieve It, Deep Relief Roll-On

**Nutritionals:** BLM, AgilEase, Sulfurzyme, Essentialzymes-4, Power Meal, Slique Shake, Pure Protein Complete, MultiGreens, Mineral Essence, Essentialzyme, Super B, NingXia Red, PowerGize

**Body Care:** Cool Azul Pain Relief Cream, Cool Azul Sports Gel, Ortho Ease Massage Oil, Ortho Sport Massage Oil

## Application and Usage

**Aromatic:** Refer to *Application Guidelines* on page 410.
**Dietary and Oral:** Whether putting oils in a capsule or drinking them in a liquid, please refer to *Application Guidelines* on page 410.

- Take 1 capsule with desired oil 2 times daily.
- Take 2-3 drops of oil in a spoonful of syrup or small amount of milk, juice, or water.

**Topical:** For guidelines on applying oils to the skin, refer to *Application Guidelines* on page 410.

- Use blend for Raindrop Technique 2 times daily: morning and night.

### Cerebral Palsy Blend
Take 3 capsules daily: morning, noon, and night:
- 15 drops Frankincense Vitality
- 12 drops Myrrh
- 10 drops Idaho Balsam Fir
- 10 drops Canadian Fleabane (Conyza)
- 4 drops Peppermint Vitality

Using this regimen, a 7-year-old boy with cerebral palsy and autism, after one month, was able to walk flat footed without his walker, test scores in school improved by 28 percent, and his attention span increased 30 percent, his mother reported.

# CHEMICAL SENSITIVITY REACTION

Environmental poisoning and chemical sensitivity are becoming a major cause of discomfort and disease. Strong chemical compounds, such as insecticides, herbicides, and formaldehyde found in paints, glues, cosmetics, and finger nail polish, enter the body easily. Symptoms include indigestion, upper and lower gas, poor assimilation, poor

**Essential Oils Desk Reference** | Seventh Edition

electrolyte balance, rashes, hypoglycemia, and allergic reaction to foods and other substances, along with emotional mood swings, fatigue, irritability, lack of motivation, and lack of discipline and creativity.

## Recommendations

**Singles:** Wintergreen, Sacred Frankincense, Frankincense, Frankincense Vitality, Jade Lemon, Jade Lemon Vitality, Lemon, Lemon Vitality, Lime, Lime Vitality, Royal Hawaiian Sandalwood, Copaiba, Copaiba Vitality, Eucalyptus Globulus

**Blends:** PanAway, Citrus Fresh, Citrus Fresh Vitality, Inner Child, Christmas Spirit

**Resins:** Frankincense Gum Resin

**Nutritionals:** Detoxzyme, JuvaPower, JuvaSpice, JuvaTone, Balance Complete, ICP, ComforTone, Essentialzyme, Essentialzymes-4, Life 9, Allerzyme

## Application and Usage

**Aromatic:** Refer to *Application Guidelines* on page 410.

**Dietary and Oral:** Whether putting oils in a capsule or drinking them in a liquid, please refer to *Application Guidelines* on page 410.

- Take 1 capsule with desired oil 2 times daily.
- Take 2-3 drops of oil in a spoonful of syrup or small amount of milk, juice, or water.

**Topical:** For guidelines on applying oils to the skin, refer to *Application Guidelines* on page 410.

- Dilute oil 50:50 and apply on affected areas 2-4 times daily.

**For headache relief, take the following:**

- 4 Essentialzyme
- 1/8 teaspoon M-Grain diluted 50:50 in vegetable oil

Drink 2-3 large glasses of water immediately after taking these products.

## CHICKEN POX (HERPES ZOSTER)
*(See also Cold Sores, Blisters)*

Chicken pox (also known as shingles, *Varicella zoster*, or *Herpes zoster*) is caused by a virus that is closely related to the herpes simplex virus. This virus is prone to hiding along nerves under the skin and may cause recurring infection through life.

When *Herpes zoster* infection occurs in children, it is known as chicken pox; when infection occurs or recurs in adults, it is known as shingles.

A childhood bout with chicken pox may leave the virus dormant in sensory (skin) nerves. If the immune system is taxed by severe emotional stress, illness, or long-term use of cortico-steroids, the dormant viruses may become active and start to infect the pathway of the skin nerves.

## Recommendations

**Singles:** Lemongrass, Lemongrass Vitality, Lavender, Lavender Vitality, Tea Tree, Royal Hawaiian Sandalwood, Melissa, Clove, Clove Vitality, Cypress, Blue Cypress, Geranium, Wintergreen

**Blends:** Thieves, Thieves Vitality, Australian Blue, Melrose

**Nutritionals:** Inner Defense, ImmuPro, Balance Complete, Power Meal, Slique Shake, SuperCal, PD 80/20

**Body Care:** Thieves Spray, Ortho Ease Massage Oil, LavaDerm Cooling Mist

## Application and Usage

**Aromatic:** Refer to *Application Guidelines* on page 410.

**Dietary and Oral:** Whether putting oils in a capsule or drinking them in a liquid, please refer to *Application Guidelines* on page 410.

- Take 1 capsule with desired oil 2 times daily.
- Take 2-3 drops of oil in a spoonful of syrup or small amount of milk, juice, or water.

**Topical:** For guidelines on applying oils to the skin, refer to *Application Guidelines* on page 410.

- Add 20 drops of essential oils (using any of the above oils) to 1 tablespoon of calamine lotion or V-6 Vegetable Oil Complex and lightly dab on spots (lesions).

## CHOLERA

Cholera is an acute diarrheal disease caused by an enterotoxin produced by a gram negative bacterium called *Vibrio cholerae*. Severe cases are marked by vomiting, muscle cramps, and constant watery diarrhea, which can result in serious fluid loss, saline depletion, acidosis, and shock. The disease is typically found in India and Southeast Asia and is spread by feces-contaminated water and food. If you suspect cholera, you should immediately seek professional medical advice.

A study done in 2000 shows that lemon—freshly squeezed juice, peel, and essential oil—act as a biocide against *Vibrio cholerae* with no harmful side effects.[17]

## Recommendations

**Singles:** Jade Lemon, Jade Lemon Vitality, Lemon, Lemon Vitality, Lime, Lime Vitality, Clove, Clove Vitality, Thyme, Thyme Vitality, Rosemary, Rosemary Vitality, Oregano, Oregano Vitality

**Blends:** DiGize, DiGize Vitality, Citrus Fresh, Citrus Fresh Vitality, ImmuPower, TummyGize

**Nutritionals:** Digest & Cleanse, Inner Defense, Immu-Pro

## Application and Usage

**Aromatic:** Refer to *Application Guidelines* on page 410.

**Dietary and Oral**: Whether putting oils in a capsule or drinking them in a liquid, please refer to *Application Guidelines* on page 410.

- Take 1 capsule with desired oil 2 times daily.
- Take 2-3 drops of oil in a spoonful of syrup or small amount of milk, juice, or water.

**Topical:** For guidelines on applying oils to the skin, refer to *Application Guidelines* on page 410.

## CHRONIC FATIGUE SYNDROME

The cause of chronic fatigue syndrome is somewhat of a mystery, but scientists believe it may be caused by a combination of factors, including immune system problems, hormone imbalances, genetic factors, psychiatric or emotional conditions, brain abnormalities, and viruses, including Epstein-Barr virus, human herpes virus 6, and mouse leukemia viruses. However, no primary cause has been found.

### Recommendations

**Singles:** Peppermint, Peppermint Vitality, Jade Lemon, Jade Lemon Vitality, Lemon, Lemon Vitality, Lime, Lime Vitality, Orange, Orange Vitality

**Blends:** Awaken, DiGize, DiGize Vitality, Evergreen Essence, Joy, InTouch, Reconnect, SleepyIze, Citrus Fresh, Citrus Fresh Vitality, TummyGize

**Nutritionals:** Detoxzyme, EndoGize, ImmuPro, Inner Defense, PD80/20, Super B, Thyromin, Ultra Young, NingXia Red, NingXia Nitro, NingXia Zyng

**Body Care:** Progessence Plus

### Application and Usage

**Aromatic:** Refer to *Application Guidelines* on page 410.

**Dietary and Oral:** Whether putting oils in a capsule or drinking them in a liquid, please refer to *Application Guidelines* on page 410.

- Take 1 capsule with desired oil 2 times daily.
- Take 2-3 drops of oil in a spoonful of syrup or small amount of milk, juice, or water.

**Topical:** For guidelines on applying oils to the skin, refer to *Application Guidelines* on page 410.

## COLD SORES
## (Herpes Simplex Type 1)

Cold sores are also known as *Herpes labialis*. Diets high in the amino acid lysine can reduce the incidence of herpes. Conversely, the amino acid arginine can worsen herpes outbreaks.

Studies have shown neat applications of Melissa to be effective against herpes simplex type I and type II. The healing period was shortened, the spread of infection was prevented, and symptoms such as itching, tingling, and burning were lessened.

The University of Maryland Medical Center reported that a large study involving three German hospitals and one dermatology clinic showed that when lemon balm (*Melissa officinalis*) was used to treat the *primary* infection of HSV I, which produces most cold sores, not a single recurrence was noted.

Peppermint and Tea Tree oils have also been studied for positive effects on the pain of herpes.

## Recommendations

**Singles:** Peppermint, Peppermint Vitality, Ravintsara, Melissa, Tea Tree, Lavender, Lavender Vitality, Royal Hawaiian Sandalwood, Mountain Savory, Mountain Savory Vitality, Oregano, Oregano Vitality, Plectranthus Oregano, Thyme, Thyme Vitality, Clove, Clove Vitality

**Blends:** Thieves, Thieves Vitality, Melrose, Purification

**Nutritionals:** Inner Defense, ImmuPro, Super C, Super C Chewable, MultiGreens, ICP, ComforTone, Essentialzyme, JuvaTone, Essentialzymes-4, JuvaPower, JuvaSpice

**Body Care:** Thieves Spray, Rose Ointment

## Application and Usage

**Topical:** For guidelines on applying oils to the skin, refer to *Application Guidelines* on page 410.

- Apply single oils or blends neat or diluted, depending on the oils being used.
- Apply 1 drop neat as soon as the cold sore appears. Repeat 5-10 times daily.

**Essential Oils Desk Reference** | Seventh Edition

- If needed, dilute 50:50 with V-6 Vegetable Oil Complex or Rose Ointment to reduce discomfort of drying skin after applying essential oils to an open sore.

## COLDS (See also Lung Infections, Sinus Infections, Throat Infections)

The best treatment for a cold or flu is prevention. Because many essential oils have strong antimicrobial properties, they can be diffused to prevent the spread of airborne bacteria and viruses. Antiviral essential oils, blends, and supplements are very effective as preventive aids in avoiding colds as well as in helping the body's defenses fight colds once an infection has started. ImmuPro is a powerful immune stimulant that can also increase infection resistance and is best when taken in the evening at bedtime.

### Recommendations

**Singles:** Ravintsara, Cypress, Blue Cypress, Wintergreen, Dalmatia Bay Laurel, Peppermint, Peppermint Vitality, Thyme, Thyme Vitality, Laurus Nobilis, Laurus Nobilis Vitality, Hyssop, Oregano, Oregano Vitality, Plectranthus Oregano, Eucalyptus Blue, Northern Lights Black Spruce, Eucalyptus Radiata, Tea Tree, Frankincense, Frankincense Vitality, Rosemary, Rosemary Vitality, Clove, Clove Vitality, Lemon, Lemon Vitality, Mountain Savory, Mountain Savory Vitality

**Blends:** Raven, Thieves, Thieves Vitality, Melrose, Australian Blue, Purification, ImmuPower, Sacred Mountain, R.C., Exodus II, Breathe Again Roll-On, SniffleEase

**Nutritionals:** Inner Defense, ImmuPro, Thieves Lozenges, Super C, Super C Chewable, Longevity Softgels, Master Formula, Detoxzyme, AlkaLime

**Oral Care:** Thieves Spray, Thieves Cough Drops, Thieves Hard Lozenges, Thieves Mouth Wash

### Cold Blend No. 1
- 5 drops Rosemary or Rosemary Vitality
- 4 drops Eucalyptus Radiata
- 4 drops Peppermint or Peppermint Vitality
- 3 drops Cypress
- 2 drops Lemon or Lemon Vitality

### Cold Blend No. 2
- 5 drops Rosemary or Rosemary Vitality
- 4 drops R.C.
- 4 drops Sacred Frankincense, Frankincense, or Frankincense Vitality
- 2 drops Peppermint or Peppermint Vitality
- 1 drop Oregano or Oregano Vitality

## Application and Usage

**Aromatic:** Refer to *Application Guidelines* on page 410.

**Dietary and Oral:** Whether putting oils in a capsule or drinking them in a liquid, please refer to *Application Guidelines* on page 410.

- Take 1 capsule with desired oil 2 times daily.
- Take 2-3 drops of oil in a spoonful of syrup or small amount of milk, juice, or water.
- Take Cold Blend 3-6 times daily.
- Gargle 3-6 times daily.

**Topical:** For guidelines on applying oils to the skin, refer to *Application Guidelines* on page 410.

- Dilute 50:50 and massage 1-3 drops on each of the following areas: forehead, nose, cheeks, lower throat, chest, and upper back 1-3 times daily.
- Massage 1-3 drops on Vita Flex points on the feet 1-2 times daily.
- Receive a Raindrop Technique 1-2 times weekly.
- Bath salts (see below)

### Bath Blend for Relief of Cold Symptoms
- 15 drops Ravintsara
- 8 drops Wintergreen
- 6 drops Northern Lights Black Spruce
- 6 drops Sacred Frankincense or Frankincense
- 3 drops Laurus Nobilis
- 2 drops Eucalyptus Radiata

Stir essential oils into ½ cup Epsom salt or baking soda and then add the mixture to hot bath water while tub is filling. Soak in hot bath until water cools.

## COLITIS
### (See also Crohn's, Diverticulosis/Diverticulitis)

Also known as ileitis or proctitis, ulcerative colitis is marked by the inflammation of the top layers of the lining of the colon, the large intestine. It is different from both irritable bowel syndrome, which has no inflammation, and Crohn's disease, which usually occurs deeper in the colon wall.

The inflammation and ulcerous sores that are characteristic of ulcerative colitis occur most frequently in the lower colon and rectum and occasionally throughout the entire colon.

Symptoms include fatigue, nausea, weight loss, loss of appetite, bloody diarrhea, loss of body fluids and nutrients, frequent fevers, abdominal cramps, arthritis, liver disease, and skin rash.

Take Essentialzymes-4 along with ComforTone and wait about 2 weeks or more before adding JuvaPower.

Personal Usage Guide | **Chapter 20**

Start with a small amount and increase slowly. If any discomfort is experienced, reduce the amount taken.

## Ulcerative Colitis

### Recommendations

**Singles:** Carrot Seed, Carrot Seed Vitality, Spearmint, Spearmint Vitality, Wintergreen, Peppermint, Peppermint Vitality, Tarragon, Tarragon Vitality, Fennel, Fennel Vitality

**Blends:** DiGize, DiGize Vitality, GLF, GLF Vitality, JuvaCleanse, JuvaCleanse Vitality, TummyGize

**Nutritionals:** Digest & Cleanse, ComforTone, Alka-Lime, Life 9, JuvaPower, JuvaSpice, Detoxzyme, ICP, Essentialzyme, Essentialzymes-4, Life 9, MegaCal

### Application and Usage

**Aromatic:** Refer to *Application Guidelines* on page 410.
**Dietary and Oral:** Whether putting oils in a capsule or drinking them in a liquid, please refer to *Application Guidelines* on page 410.

- Take 2 capsules with any 2 of the oils above 2-3 times daily.
- Take 2-3 drops of oil in a spoonful of syrup or small amount of milk, juice, or water.

**Topical:** For guidelines on applying oils to the skin, refer to *Application Guidelines* on page 410.

- Apply 4-6 drops of your choice of oil, diluted 50:50, on lower abdomen 3-6 times daily.
- Massage 2-4 drops of oil neat on the bottoms of the feet just before bedtime.

## Viral Colitis

Use the remedies below for colitis that may be caused by virus rather than bacteria.

### Recommendations

**Singles:** Melissa, Lemongrass, Lemongrass Vitality, Clove, Clove Vitality, Melaleuca Quinquenervia (Niaouli), Blue Cypress, Oregano, Oregano Vitality, Plectranthus Oregano, Helichrysum, Cumin, Tea Tree, Tarragon, Tarragon Vitality, Thyme, Thyme Vitality, Roman Chamomile, German Chamomile, German Chamomile Vitality, Rosemary, Rosemary Vitality, Peppermint, Peppermint Vitality, Cinnamon Bark, Cinnamon Bark Vitality

**Blends:** Melrose, Thieves, Thieves Vitality, Purification, DiGize, DiGize Vitality, TummyGize

**Nutritionals:** Digest & Cleanse, Inner Defense, Longevity Softgels, Essentialzymes-4, Essentialzyme, Life 9

### Application and Usage

**Dietary and Oral:** Whether putting oils in a capsule or drinking them in a liquid, please refer to *Application Guidelines* on page 410.

- Take 1 capsule with desired oil 2 times daily.
- Take 2-3 drops of oil in a spoonful of syrup or small amount of milk, juice, or water.

**Topical:** For guidelines on applying oils to the skin, refer to *Application Guidelines* on page 410.

- Apply several drops diluted 50:50 over colon area 4-6 times daily.
- You may also apply 2-3 drops on the Vita Flex colon points.
- Have Raindrop Technique 1-2 times weekly.
- Place a warm compress diluted 20:80 using equal parts Helichrysum and DiGize over the colon area.
- Use the blend below in a rectal implant 3 times weekly.

**Colitis-Colon Blend**
- 3 drops Melaleuca Quinquenervia (Niaouli)
- 2 drops Oregano Vitality
- 2 drops Thyme Vitality
- 2 drops German Chamomile Vitality
- 2 drops Melissa
- 2 drops Peppermint Vitality

Mix above oils with 1 tablespoon V-6 Vegetable Oil Complex.

## COMA

Patients in a coma will likely be in a hospital or care center. Discuss with the patient's physician about rubbing essential oils on the bottoms of the patient's feet and diffusing the oils. After the patient returns home, the oils listed below could be helpful.

### Recommendations

**Singles:** Valerian, Vetiver, Royal Hawaiian Sandalwood, Blue Cypress, Black Pepper, Black Pepper Vitality, Peppermint, Peppermint Vitality, Idaho Balsam Fir, Copaiba, Copaiba Vitality, Sacred Frankincense, Frankincense, Frankincense Vitality

**Blends:** Hope, Valor, Valor II, Valor Roll-On, Surrender, The Gift, Inspiration, Brain Power, GeneYus, Trauma Life, T.R. Care, R.C.

Seventh Edition | **Essential Oils Desk Reference** | 453

**Body Care:** Progessence Plus, Regenolone Moisturizing Cream, Sensation Massage Oil

## Application and Usage

**Aromatic:** Refer to *Application Guidelines* on page 410.
- Diffuse your choice of oils for 15 minutes 4-7 times daily.

**Topical:** For guidelines on applying oils to the skin, refer to *Application Guidelines* on page 410.
- Apply 3-5 drops diluted 50:50 on temples, neck, and shoulders.
- Receive a Raindrop Technique with the above mentioned oils.

## CONNECTIVE TISSUE DAMAGE (Cartilage, Ligaments, Tendons)

Tendonitis, often called tennis elbow and golfer's elbow, is a torn or inflamed tendon. Repetitive use or infection may be the cause.

MegaCal, BLM, and AgilEase provide critical nutrients for connective tissue repair. Sulfurzyme, an outstanding source of organic sulfur, equalizes water pressure inside the cells and reduces pain.

PanAway reduces pain and Lemongrass promotes the repair of connective tissue. Lavender with Lemongrass and Marjoram with Lemongrass work well together for inflamed tendons. Deep Relief Roll-On is a convenient way to apply a blend of oils that is both pain relieving and anti-inflammatory.

When selecting oils for injuries, think through the cause and type of injury and select appropriate oils. For instance, tendonitis could encompass muscle damage, nerve damage, ligament strain/tear, inflammation, infection, and possibly an emotion. Therefore, select an oil or oils for each potential cause and apply in rotation or prepare a blend to address multiple causes. The oils in Ortho Sport and Ortho Ease massage oils reduce pain and promote healing. Cool Azul products are also great pain relievers.

## Recommendations

**Singles:** Sacred Frankincense, Frankincense, Frankincense Vitality, Lemongrass, Lemongrass Vitality, Lavender, Lavender Vitality, Marjoram, Marjoram Vitality, Eucalyptus Blue, Dorado Azul

**Blends:** PanAway, Deep Relief Roll-On, Aroma Siez, Melrose, Cool Azul

**Nutritionals:** MegaCal, BLM, AgilEase, Super B, Super C, Super C Chewable, MultiGreens, Mineral Essence, Sulfurzyme, PD 80/20, PowerGize

**Body Care:** Cool Azul Pain Relief Cream, Cool Azul Sports Gel, Ortho Ease Massage Oil, Ortho Sport Massage Oil, Regenolone Moisturizing Cream

## Application and Usage

**Topical:** For guidelines on applying oils to the skin, refer to *Application Guidelines* on page 410.

- Apply oils neat or diluted 50:50 on location 3-6 times daily.
- Massage 4-6 drops of oil on affected area. For swelling, elevate and apply ice packs.
- Place a cold compress with 1-2 drops of chosen oil on area 2-4 times daily.

## Cartilage Injury on Knee, Elbow, Etc.

People with cartilage damage often experience decreased range of motion, stiffness, joint pain, and/or swelling in the affected area.

## Recommendations

**Singles:** Wintergreen, Copaiba, Copaiba Vitality, Lemongrass, Lemongrass Vitality, Palo Santo, Peppermint, Peppermint Vitality, Idaho Balsam Fir, Marjoram, Marjoram Vitality, Eucalyptus Blue, Dorado Azul, Idaho Blue Spruce

**Blends:** PanAway, Relieve It, Aroma Siez, Deep Relief Roll-On, Cool Azul

**Nutritionals:** MegaCal, Super B, Super C, Super C Chewable, MultiGreens, Mineral Essence, BLM, AgilEase, Master Formula, Sulfurzyme, PowerGize

**Body Care:** Cool Azul Pain Relief Cream, Cool Azul Sports Gel, Ortho Ease Massage Oil, Ortho Sport Massage Oil, Regenolone Moisturizing Cream

### Cartilage Blend
- 12 drops Wintergreen
- 10 drops Marjoram
- 9 drops Lemongrass

## Application and Usage

**Topical:** For guidelines on applying oils to the skin, refer to *Application Guidelines* on page 410.

- Apply neat or diluted 50:50 on location 3-6 times daily.
- Massage 4-6 drops of oil on affected area. For swelling, elevate and apply ice packs.
- Place a cold compress with 1-2 drops of chosen oil in Ortho Ease or Ortho Sport Massage Oil on area 2-4 times daily.

Personal Usage Guide | **Chapter 20**

## Ligament Sprain or Tear

**Note:** For sprains, use cold packs. For any serious sprain or constant skeletal pain, always consult a health care professional. Anytime there is tissue damage, there is always inflammation. Reduce this first.

### Recommendations

**Singles:** Lemongrass, Lemongrass Vitality, Helichrysum, Lavender, Lavender Vitality, Elemi, Basil, Basil Vitality, Marjoram, Marjoram Vitality, Peppermint, Peppermint Vitality, Palo Santo

**Blends:** PanAway, Relieve It, Aroma Siez, Deep Relief Roll-On, Cool Azul

**Nutritionals:** BLM, AgilEase, MegaCal, Super B, Super C, MultiGreens, Essentialzyme, Essentialzymes-4, Life 9, Mineral Essence, Sulfurzyme, PowerGize

**Body Care:** Cool Azul Pain Relief Cream, Cool Azul Sports Gel, Ortho Ease Massage Oil, Ortho Sport Massage Oil, Regenolone Moisturizing Cream

### Sprain Blend
- 15 drops Aroma Siez
- 5 drops Lemongrass

### Application and Usage

**Topical:** For guidelines on applying oils to the skin, refer to *Application Guidelines* on page 410.

- Apply oils neat or diluted 50:50 on location 3-6 times daily.
- Massage 4-6 drops of oil on affected area. For swelling, elevate and apply ice packs.
- Place a cold compress with 1-2 drops of chosen oil on area 2-4 times daily.

## Tendonitis

Tendons are cords of tough, fibrous connective tissue that attach muscles to bones and are found throughout the entire human body. Tendonitis is the irritation and inflammation of those tendons.

### Recommendations

**Singles:** Lemongrass, Lemongrass Vitality, Marjoram, Marjoram Vitality, Copaiba, Copaiba Vitality, Rosemary, Rosemary Vitality, Eucalyptus Radiata, Peppermint, Peppermint Vitality, Palo Santo, Basil, Basil Vitality, Wintergreen, Vetiver, Valerian, Elemi

**Blends:** Deep Relief Roll-On, Aroma Siez, PanAway, Relieve It

**Nutritionals:** BLM, AgilEase, MegaCal, Super B, Super C, Super C Chewable, MultiGreens, Mineral Essence, Sulfurzyme, PowerGize

**Body Care:** Cool Azul Pain Relief Cream, Cool Azul Sports Gel, Regenolone Moisturizing Cream, Ortho Sport Massage Oil, Ortho Ease Massage Oil

### Tendonitis Blend No. 1
- 8 drops Wintergreen
- 4 drops Vetiver
- 4 drops Valerian

### Tendonitis Relief Blend No. 2 (for Pain Relief)
- 10 drops Rosemary
- 10 drops Eucalyptus Radiata
- 10 drops Peppermint
- 5 drops Palo Santo

### Application and Usage

**Topical:** For guidelines on applying oils to the skin, refer to *Application Guidelines* on page 410.

- Apply oils neat or diluted 50:50 on location 3-6 times daily.
- Massage 4-6 drops of oil on affected area. For swelling, elevate and apply ice packs.
- Place a cold compress with 1-2 drops of chosen oil on area 2-4 times daily.

## Scleroderma

Also known as systemic sclerosis, scleroderma is a non-infectious, chronic, autoimmune disease of the connective tissue. Caused by an overproduction of collagen, the disease can involve either the skin or internal organs and can be life threatening.

Scleroderma is far more common among women than men.

### Recommendations

**Singles:** Myrrh, Wintergreen, German Chamomile, Sacred Frankincense, Frankincense, Copaiba, Lavender, Patchouli, Royal Hawaiian Sandalwood

**Blends:** Melrose, Aroma Siez, Thieves, Purification, SclarEssence,

**Nutritionals:** PD 80/20, ICP, ComforTone, Essentialzyme, JuvaTone, JuvaPower, JuvaSpice, Thyromin, Mineral Essence, Power Meal, Slique Shake, Sulfurzyme, Detoxzyme, Longevity Softgels, PowerGize

**Body Care:** Prenolone Plus Body Cream, LavaDerm Cooling Mist

Seventh Edition | **Essential Oils Desk Reference** | 455

**Essential Oils Desk Reference** | Seventh Edition

## Application and Usage

**Topical:** For guidelines on applying oils to the skin, refer to *Application Guidelines* on page 410.

- Apply 4-6 drops diluted 50:50 on location 3 times daily. Alternate between using Blend No. 1 and Bend No. 2 each day.

**Scleroderma Blend No. 1**
- 2 drops German Chamomile
- 2 drops Myrrh
- 1 drop Lavender
- 1 drop Patchouli

**Scleroderma Blend No. 2**
- 3 drops Myrrh
- 2 drops Royal Hawaiian Sandalwood

## CROHN'S DISEASE
*(See also Colitis, Diverticulosis/Diverticulitis)*

Crohn's disease creates inflammation, sores, and ulcers on the intestinal wall. These sores occur deeper than ulcerative colitis. Unlike other forms of colitis, Crohn's disease can affect the entire digestive tract from the mouth all the way to the rectum.

### Symptoms

- Abdominal cramping
- Lower-right abdominal pain
- Diarrhea
- A general sense of feeling ill

Attacks may occur once or twice a day for life. If the disease continues for years, it can cause deterioration of bowel function, leaky gut syndrome, poor absorption of nutrients, loss of appetite and weight, intestinal obstruction, severe bleeding, and increased susceptibility to intestinal cancer.

Most researchers believe that Crohn's disease is caused by an overreacting immune system and is actually an autoimmune disease where the immune system mistakenly attacks the body's own tissues. MSM has been extensively researched for its ability to treat many autoimmune diseases and is the subject of research by University of Oregon researcher Stanley Jacobs. MSM is a key ingredient in Sulfurzyme.

### Recommendations

**Singles:** Ginger, Ginger Vitality, Nutmeg, Nutmeg Vitality, Wintergreen, German Chamomile, German Chamomile Vitality, Peppermint, Peppermint Vitality, Copaiba, Copaiba Vitality, Fennel, Fennel Vitality, Patchouli

**Blends:** ImmuPower, DiGize, DiGize Vitality, PanAway, TummyGize

**Nutritionals:** Sulfurzyme, OmegaGize$^3$, Life 9, Detoxzyme, Essentialzyme, Essentialzymes-4, AlkaLime, ICP, ComforTone, MultiGreens, Digest & Cleanse, NingXia Red, Balance Complete

## Application and Usage

**Aromatic:** Refer to *Application Guidelines* on page 410.

**Dietary and Oral:** Whether putting oils in a capsule or drinking them in a liquid, please refer to *Application Guidelines* on page 410.

- Take 1 capsule with desired oil 2 times daily.
- Take 2-3 drops of oil in a spoonful of syrup or small amount of milk, juice, or water.

**Topical:** For guidelines on applying oils to the skin, refer to *Application Guidelines* on page 410.

- Receive a Raindrop Technique 1-2 times weekly incorporating ImmuPower.
- Place a warm compress with 1-2 drops of chosen oil on the back.

### Regimen for Crohn's disease

Each phase lasts 3 days and should be added to the previous phases.

- **Phase I:** Essentialzymes-4: Take 1-2 capsules, both white and yellow, 3 times daily.
- **Phase II:** Take the Essentialzymes-4 in yogurt or liquid acidophilus and charcoal tablets. Do not use ICP, ComforTone, or Essentialzyme yet.
- **Phase III:** Drink 6 oz. raw juice (cherry, prune, celery, carrot, or NingXia Red) 2 times daily.
- **Phase IV:** Take 2 scoops Balance Complete in water or juice 2 times daily.
- **Phase V:** (Start only if there is no sign of bleeding.)
- **ComforTone:** Take 1 capsule morning and night until stools loosen.
- **ICP:** Start with 1 level teaspoon 2 times daily and gradually increase.
- **Essentialzyme:** Start with 1 caplet 3 times daily. If irritation occurs, discontinue for a few days and start again.

456 | **Chapter 20** | Personal Usage Guide

Personal Usage Guide | **Chapter 20**

# CYSTS

Cysts are closed, sac-like structures that contain fluid, gas, or semisolid material that is not a normal part of the tissue where it is located. There are hundreds of types, are common, vary in size, and can occur anywhere in the body in people of all ages. Two of the most common types of cysts are ganglion and ovarian.

## Ganglion Cysts

Ganglion cysts develop in the tissues near joints and tendons, often in the ankles, in the wrists, and behind the knees. They cause painful swelling and are often filled with a thick fluid.

### Recommendations

**Singles:** Oregano, Oregano Vitality, Plectranthus Oregano, Thyme, Thyme Vitality, Myrrh, Mountain Savory, Mountain Savory Vitality

**Blends:** Purification, Thieves

**Nutritionals:** Super C, Mineral Essence, Detoxzyme

**Body Care:** LavaDerm Cooling Mist, Thieves Spray, Cool Azul Pain Relief Cream, Cool Azul Sports Gel

### Application and Usage

**Topical:** For guidelines on applying oils to the skin, refer to *Application Guidelines* on page 410.

- Apply 2 drops of chosen oil neat the first day.
- Apply 2 drops of Thyme the second day.
- Apply on location as often as needed.

## Ovarian and Uterine Cysts *(See also Menstrual and Female Hormone Conditions)*

Ovarian cysts can be painless or painful if they grow large and affect the ovary. They may be caused by an egg sac that doesn't properly break open or dissolve as part of the menstrual cycle.

### Recommendations

**Singles:** Myrrh, Geranium, Sacred Frankincense, Frankincense, Frankincense Vitality, Sage, Sage Vitality, Tea Tree, Clary Sage, Thyme, Thyme Vitality, Rosemary, Rosemary Vitality, Oregano, Oregano Vitality

**Blends:** Dragon Time, SclarEssence, SclarEssence Vitality

**Nutritionals:** PD 80/20, EndoGize, Estro, FemiGen, Mineral Essence, Essentialzyme, Essenstialzymes-4

**Body Care:** Protec, Prenolone Plus Body Cream, Progessence Plus, Estro, FemiGen

**Female Cyst Blend No. 1**
- 9 drops Sacred Frankincense, Frankincense, or Frankincense Vitality
- 5 drops Clary Sage
- 5 drops Myrrh
- 2 drops Thyme or Thyme Vitality
- 2 drops Rosemary or Rosemary Vitality

**Female Cyst Blend No. 2**
- 4 drops Sacred Frankincense, Frankincense, or Frankincense Vitality
- 4 drops Geranium
- 2 drops Oregano or Oregano Vitality

### Application and Usage

**Topical:** For guidelines on applying oils to the skin, refer to *Application Guidelines* on page 410.

- Apply 1-3 drops on the reproductive Vita Flex points, located around the anklebone on either side of the foot. Work from the ankle bone down to the arch of the foot.
- Place a warm compress with 1-2 oils of your choice on location as needed.
- Retention: Apply 1-2 drops diluted 50:50 on a tampon and insert nightly for 4 nights. **Note:** If irritation occurs, discontinue use for 3 days before resuming.

# DEPRESSION *(See also Insomnia)*

Diffusing or directly inhaling essential oils can have an immediate, positive impact on mood. Olfaction (smell) is the only sense that can have direct effects on the limbic region of the brain. Studies at the University of Vienna have shown that some essential oils and their primary constituents (cineole) can stimulate blood flow and activity in the emotional regions of the brain.[18]

Clinical studies at the Department of Psychiatry at the Mie University of Medicine showed that lemon not only reduced depression, but it also reduced stress when inhaled.[19]

### Recommendations

**Singles:** Lavender, Lavender Vitality, Roman Chamomile, Melissa, Jasmine, Sacred Frankincense, Frankincense, Frankincense Vitality, Peppermint, Peppermint Vitality, Ylang Ylang, Amazonian Ylang Ylang, Rosemary, Rosemary Vitality, Jade Lemon, Jade Lemon Vitality, Lemon, Lemon Vitality, Lime, Lime Vitality, Cedarwood, Bergamot, Bergamot Vitality

Seventh Edition | **Essential Oils Desk Reference** | 457

**Blends:** Build Your Dream, Divine Release, Evergreen Essence, Freedom, Inner Harmony, InTouch, Reconnect, SleepyIze, Valor, Valor II, Valor Roll-On, Live with Passion, Live Your Passion, Light the Fire, Hope, Joy, Common Sense, The Gift, Oola Balance, Oola Faith, Oola Family, Oola Field, Oola Finance, Oola Fitness, Oola Friends, Oola Fun, Oola Grow, RutaVaLa, RutaVaLa Roll-On, AromaSleep, SclarEssence, SclarEssence Vitality

**Nutritionals:** MultiGreens, Life 9, Super B, Mineral Essence, Balance Complete, Thyromin, EndoGize, Ecuadorian Dark Chocolessence, Slique Bars–Chocolate-Coated, Chocolate-Coated Wolfberry Crisp Bars, NingXia Red, NingXia Zyng, NingXia Nitro

## Application and Usage

**Aromatic:** Refer to *Application Guidelines* on page 410.
**Topical:** For guidelines on applying oils to the skin, refer to *Application Guidelines* on page 410.

- Apply 1-2 drops of recommended oil neat on temples and back of neck as desired.

### Postpartum Depression

"Baby blues" are normal for a few days after childbirth. Postpartum depression can follow and feel like more of the same or feel worse than before. It can also happen months after childbirth or pregnancy loss.

### Recommendations

**Singles:** Jade Lemon, Jade Lemon Vitality, Lemon, Lemon Vitality, Lime, Lime Vitality, Sage, Sage Vitality, Melissa, Clary Sage, Cedarwood, Royal Hawaiian Sandalwood, Sacred Frankincense, Frankincense, Frankincense Vitality, Ocotea, Bergamot, Bergamot Vitality

**Blends:** Joy, Trauma Life, T.R. Care, Peace & Calming, Peace & Calming II, Hope, RutaVaLa, RutaVaLa Roll-On, Transformation, Dragon Time, Oola Balance, Oola Faith, Oola Family, Oola Field, Oola Finance, Oola Fitness, Oola Friends, Oola Fun, Oola Grow,

**Nutritionals:** Super B, EndoGize, Estro, FemiGen, Ecuadorian Dark Chocolessence, Slique Bars–Chocolate-Coated, Chocolate-Coated Wolfberry Crisp Bars, NingXia Red, NingXia Zyng, NingXia Nitro

**Body Care:** Progessence Plus, Prenolone Plus Body Cream

## Application and Usage

**Aromatic:** Refer to *Application Guidelines* on page 410.
**Dietary and Oral:** Whether putting oils in a capsule or drinking them in a liquid, please refer to *Application Guidelines* on page 410.

- Take 1 capsule with desired oil 2 times daily.
- Take 2-3 drops of oil in a spoonful of syrup or small amount of milk, juice, or water.

**Topical:** For guidelines on applying oils to the skin, refer to *Application Guidelines* on page 410.

- Apply 2-4 drops neat on temples and back of neck 2-4 times daily or as needed.
- Applying a single drop under the nose is helpful and refreshing.
- Place a warm compress with 1-2 drops of chosen oil on the back.

## DIABETES

Diabetes is the leading cause of cardiovascular disease and premature death in Westernized countries today. Diabetes causes low energy and persistently high blood glucose.

Type I diabetes usually manifests by age 30 and is often considered to be genetic. Type II diabetes generally manifests later in life and may have a nutritional origin.

Chromium has been shown to help the body metabolize sugars properly.

Wolfberry balances the pancreas and is a detoxifier and cleanser. Diabetes is not common in certain regions of China where wolfberry is consumed regularly.

Stevia leaf extract is one of the most health-restoring plants known. It is a natural sweetener, has no calories, and does not have the harmful side effects of processed sugar or sugar substitutes. Substituting stevia for sugar helps rebuild glucose tolerance and normalize blood sugar fluctuations.

Yacon Syrup contains inulin, the complex sugar that slowly breaks down into FOS (fructooligosaccharide). Inulin is not digestible so it passes through the body, with the result that it is half the calories of other sugars. FOS is well-known for its prebiotic effects and also supports microflora in the large intestine, while it promotes the absorption of calcium.

### Recommendations

**Singles:** Ocotea, Clove, Clove Vitality, Coriander, Coriander Vitality, Fennel, Fennel Vitality, Dill, Dill Vitality, Cinnamon Bark, Cinnamon Bark Vitality, Lemongrass, Lemongrass Vitality

**Blends:** EndoFlex, EndoFlex Vitality, DiGize, DiGize Vitality, Thieves, Thieves Vitality, Slique Essence, TummyGize

**Nutritionals:** MultiGreens, Yacon Syrup, MegaCal, Balance Complete, Essentialzyme, Essentialzymes-4, Master Formula, Ningxia Wolfberries (Organic, Dried), Pure Protein Complete, Slique Tea

## Application and Usage

**Aromatic:** Refer to *Application Guidelines* on page 410.

**Dietary and Oral:** Whether putting oils in a capsule or drinking them in a liquid, please refer to *Application Guidelines* on page 410.

- Take 2 capsules 50:50 Ocotea and Coriander Vitality 2 times daily.
- Take 2-3 drops of oil in a spoonful of syrup or small amount of milk, juice, or water.

**Topical:** For guidelines on applying oils to the skin, refer to *Application Guidelines* on page 410.

## DIGESTIVE PROBLEMS

Digestive problems often result in symptoms such as stomach pain, constipation, gas, cramps, bloating, and diarrhea.

### Constipation (Impacted Bowel)

The principle causes of constipation are inadequate fluid intake and low fiber consumption. Constipation can eventually lead to diverticulosis and diverticulitis, conditions common among older people.

Certain essential oils have demonstrated their ability to improve colon health through supporting intestinal flora, stimulating intestinal motility and peristalsis, fighting infections, and eliminating parasites.

### Recommendations

**Singles:** Ginger, Ginger Vitality, Fennel, Fennel Vitality, Tarragon, Tarragon Vitality, Peppermint, Peppermint Vitality

**Blends:** DiGize, DiGize Vitality, JuvaCleanse, Juva-Cleanse Vitality, TummyGize

**Nutritionals:** Digest & Cleanse, ICP, ComforTone, Detoxzyme, Life 9, MegaCal, Mineral Essence, Balance Complete, Essentialzyme, Essentialzymes-4, Omega-Gize[3], JuvaPower, JuvaSpice

## Constipation Causes Body Dysfunction

The reason constipation creates diverticulosis is because the muscles of the colon must strain to move an overly hard stool, which puts excess pressure on the colon. Eventually, weak spots in the colon walls form, creating abnormal pockets called diverticula.

These pockets can also be created by parasites that burrow and embed in the lining of the colon wall, lay eggs there, and leave waste matter that hardens on the colon walls, kinking and twisting the colon unnaturally. It is always wise to consider the possibility of parasites and their treatment when diverticula are present.

Enzymes such as Detoxzyme, Essentialzyme, Essentialzymes-4, Allerzyme, and Mightyzyme (for children) are critical to help in the digestion and softening of waste material. ICP and JuvaPower add fiber that help scrub the colon wall, absorb toxins, and help with the elimination process. ParaFree is always a good cleanse at least once a year and certainly when parasites are suspected.

## Application and Usage

**Aromatic:** Refer to *Application Guidelines* on page 410.

**Dietary and Oral:** Whether putting oils in a capsule or drinking them in a liquid, please refer to *Application Guidelines* on page 410.

- Take 1 capsule with desired oil 2 times daily.
- Take 2-3 drops of oil in a spoonful of syrup or small amount of milk, juice, or water.

**Topical:** For guidelines on applying oils to the skin, refer to *Application Guidelines* on page 410.

- Apply 6-10 drops neat or diluted 50:50 on stomach area as desired.
- Place a warm compress with 1-3 drops of recommended oil over the stomach area and Vita Flex points of the feet.

### Regimen

- **Essentialzyme:** Take 3-6 tablets 3 times daily.
- **ComforTone:** Start with 1 capsule and increase the next day to 2 capsules. Continue to increase 1 capsule each day until bowels start moving.

- **ICP:** 1 week after ComforTone, start with 1 tablespoon ICP 2 times daily and then increase to 3 times daily up to 2 tablespoons 3 times daily.
- **Balance Complete:** 3 scoops daily or as needed.
- **Drink** at least ½ cup unsweetened cherry juice, prune juice, pineapple juice, or other raw fruit or vegetable juice each morning.
- **Drink** 8 glasses of pure water daily.

## Cramps, Stomach

Stomach cramps may be caused by constipation, diarrhea, anxiety, gas, bloating, and PMS. Although stomach cramps are fairly common, paying attention to them is important.

### Recommendations

**Singles:** Ginger, Ginger Vitality, Peppermint, Peppermint Vitality, Rosemary, Rosemary Vitality, Lavender, Lavender Vitality, Bergamot, Bergamot Vitality

**Blends:** DiGize, DiGize Vitality, TummyGize

**Nutritionals:** AlkaLime, Digest & Cleanse, Life 9, Essentialzymes-4, Essentialzyme, Life 9

### Application and Usage

**Dietary and Oral:** Whether putting the oils in a capsule or drinking them in a liquid, please refer to *Application Guidelines* on page 410.

- Take 1 capsule with desired oil 2 times daily.
- Take 2-3 drops of oil in a spoonful of syrup or small amount of milk, juice, or water.

**Topical:** For guidelines on applying oils to the skin, refer to *Application Guidelines* on page 410.

- Dilute 50:50 and apply 6-10 drops over stomach area 2 times daily.
- Apply a warm compress 1-2 times daily.
- Apply 1-3 drops on stomach Vita Flex points of feet.

## Diarrhea

Diarrhea is the second most commonly reported illness in the U.S. and happens to nearly everyone. It may be caused by bacteria, viruses, food, medication, stress, or chronic medical conditions.

### Recommendations

**Singles:** Ginger, Ginger Vitality, Oregano, Oregano Vitality, Plectranthus Oregano, Mountain Savory, Mountain Savory Vitality, Clove, Clove Vitality, Jade

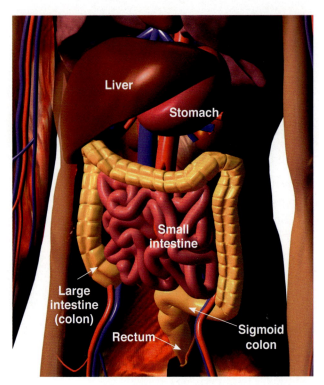

**Gastrointestinal System**

Lemon, Jade Lemon Vitality, Lemon, Lemon Vitality, Lime, Lime Vitality, Peppermint, Peppermint Vitality, Nutmeg, Nutmeg Vitality, Wintergreen

**Blends:** DiGize, DiGize Vitality, JuvaFlex, JuvaFlex Vitality, TummyGize, Thieves, Thieves Vitality

**Nutritionals:** Life 9, ComforTone, Essentialzyme, Detoxzyme, Essentialzymes-4, MegaCal, SuperCal, Inner Defense, ICP, ImmuPro

### Diarrhea Blend

- 4 drops Lemon or Lemon Vitality
- 3 drops Mountain Savory or Mountain Savory Vitality
- 2 drops Wintergreen

### Application and Usage

**Dietary and Oral:** Whether putting oils in a capsule or drinking them in a liquid, please refer to *Application Guidelines* on page 410.

- Take 1 capsule with desired oil 2 times daily.
- Take 2-3 drops of oil in a spoonful of syrup or small amount of milk, juice, or water.
- A maintenance dosage of ComforTone has helped to protect travelers going to other countries from diarrhea and other digestive discomforts.

- Nutmeg has been shown to have powerful action against diarrhea in a number of medical studies. [20,21]

**Topical:** For guidelines on applying oils to the skin, refer to *Application Guidelines* on page 410.

- Apply 6-10 drops neat on stomach area as desired.
- Dilute 50:50 and apply on location 3-6 times daily.
- Place a warm compress with 1-2 drops of chosen oil on the back.

## Diverticulosis/Diverticulitis
(See also Colitis, Crohn's Disease)

Diverticulosis is one of the most common conditions in the U.S. and is caused by a lack of fiber in the diet. Diverticulosis is characterized by small, abnormal pockets (diverticula) that bulge out through weak spots in the wall of the intestine. It is estimated that half of all Americans from age 60 to 80 have diverticulosis.

### Symptoms
- Cramping
- Bloating
- Constipation
- Fever and chills
- Cramping tenderness on lower left side of abdomen

One of the easiest ways to resolve this condition is by increasing fiber intake to 20-30 grams daily. Peppermint oil can also stimulate contractions in the colon.

While diverticulosis involves the condition of merely having colon abnormalities, diverticulitis occurs when these abnormalities or diverticula become infected or inflamed. Diverticulitis is present in 10-25 percent of people with diverticulosis.

Many of these symptoms are similar to those of irritable bowel syndrome.

### Recommendations

**Singles:** Oregano, Oregano Vitality, Plectranthus Oregano, Patchouli, Tarragon, Tarragon Vitality, Rosemary, Rosemary Vitality, Fennel, Fennel Vitality, Peppermint, Peppermint Vitality, Thyme, Thyme Vitality, Nutmeg, Nutmeg Vitality, Clove, Clove Vitality, Ocotea, Ocotea Vitality, Tangerine, Tangerine Vitality, Sacred Frankincense, Frankincense, Frankincense Vitality, Cedarwood

**Blends:** DiGize, DiGize Vitality, Melrose, Thieves, Thieves Vitality, Exodus II, ImmuPower, TummyGize

**Nutritionals:** AlkaLime, Detoxzyme, Inner Defense, Digest & Cleanse, ICP, ComforTone, Essentialzyme, Essentialzymes-4, Balance Complete, JuvaPower

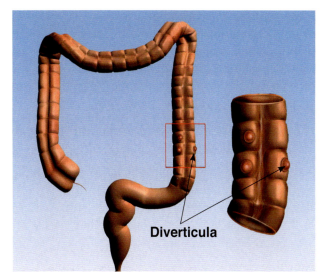

**Large Intestine**

**Diverticulitis Blend**
- 15 drops DiGize Vitality
- 5 drops Melrose

### Application and Usage

**Aromatic:** Refer to *Application Guidelines* on page 410.

**Dietary and Oral:** Whether putting oils in a capsule or drinking them in a liquid, please refer to *Application Guidelines* on page 410.

- Take 1 capsule with desired oil 2 times daily.
- Take 2-3 drops of oil in a spoonful of syrup or small amount of milk, juice, or water.

**Topical:** For guidelines on applying oils to the skin, refer to *Application Guidelines* on page 410.

- Dilute 50:50 and apply on lower abdomen 2 times daily.
- Massage 2-4 drops on the intestinal Vita Flex points on the feet 2-3 times daily.
- Retention: Rectal, nightly before retiring, retain overnight.

## Dysentery

Dysentery is a serious disorder of the digestive tract that commonly occurs throughout the world. It can be caused by viruses, bacteria, protozoa, parasitic worms, or chemical irritation of the intestines.

It is one of the oldest known gastrointestinal disorders, often called the "bloody flux," that frequently occurred in army camps, walled cities, aboard sailing vessels, and where large groups of people lived together with poor sanitation.

In the modern world, dysentery is most likely to affect people who live in less developed countries and travelers

**Essential Oils Desk Reference** | Seventh Edition

who visit those countries. It also affects immigrants from developing countries, people who live in housing with poor sanitation, military personnel serving in developing countries, people in nursing homes, and children in day care centers.

## Recommendations

**Singles:** Peppermint, Peppermint Vitality, Jade Lemon, Jade Lemon Vitality, Lemon, Lemon Vitality, Lime, Lime Vitality, Myrrh, Mountain Savory, Mountain Savory Vitality, Oregano, Oregano Vitality

**Blends:** Thieves, Thieves Vitality, DiGize, DiGize Vitality, JuvaCleanse, JuvaCleanse Vitality, JuvaFlex, JuvaFlex Vitality, TummyGize

**Nutritionals:** Inner Defense, Detoxzyme, Essentialzymes-4, ImmuPro, ICP, ComforTone, Essentialzyme, Mineral Essence, Life 9, ParaFree

**Dysentery Blend**
- 5 drops Thieves or Thieves Vitality
- 5 drops Peppermint or Peppermint Vitality

## Application and Usage

**Aromatic:** Refer to *Application Guidelines* on page 410.

**Dietary and Oral:** Whether putting oils in a capsule or drinking them in a liquid, please refer to *Application Guidelines* on page 410.

- Take 1 capsule with desired oil 3 times daily.
- Take 2-3 drops of oil in a spoonful of syrup or small amount of milk, juice, or water.

**Topical:** For guidelines on applying oils to the skin, refer to *Application Guidelines* on page 410.

## Gas (Flatulence)

Gas (flatulence) can be caused by a lack of digestive enzymes and the consumption of indigestible starches that promote bifid bacteria production in the colon.

Although increasing bifid bacteria production can lead to gas, it is highly beneficial to long-term health, as the increase of beneficial flora crowds out disease-causing microorganisms such as *Clostridium perfringens.*

Consumption of FOS (fructooligosaccharides), an indigestible sugar, can create short-term flatulence, even as it drastically improves bifidobacteria production in the small and large intestines and increases mineral absorption.

## Recommendations

**Singles:** Carrot Seed, Carrot Seed Vitality, Peppermint, Peppermint Vitality, Nutmeg, Nutmeg Vitality, Oregano, Oregano Vitality, Plectranthus Oregano,

Thyme, Thyme Vitality, Clove, Clove Vitality, Ginger, Ginger Vitality, Cumin, Fennel, Fennel Vitality

**Blends:** TummyGize, DiGize, DiGize Vitality, Thieves, Thieves Vitality, Longevity, Longevity Vitality

**Nutritionals:** AlkaLime, Detoxzyme, Life 9, Digest & Cleanse, ICP, ComforTone, Essentialzyme, Essentialzymes-4, Inner Defense, JuvaPower, ImmuPro, Longevity Softgels

## Application and Usage

**Aromatic:** Refer to *Application Guidelines* on page 410.

**Dietary and Oral:** Whether putting oils in a capsule or drinking them in a liquid, please refer to *Application Guidelines* on page 410.

- Take 1 capsule with desired oil 2 times daily.
- Take 2-3 drops of oil in a spoonful of syrup or small amount of milk, juice, or water.

**Topical:** For guidelines on applying oils to the skin, refer to *Application Guidelines* on page 410.

## Giardia

Giardia is a microscopic parasite found on surfaces or in soil, water, or food that has been contaminated with feces from infected animals or humans. It is most commonly transmitted in water.

## Recommendations

**Singles:** Basil, Basil Vitality, Patchouli, Peppermint, Peppermint Vitality, Spearmint, Spearmint Vitality

**Blends:** DiGize, DiGize Vitality, JuvaCleanse, JuvaCleanse Vitality, Melrose, Purification, TummyGize

**Nutritionals:** Detoxzyme, ParaFree, Essentialzyme, Digest & Cleanse, Mineral Essence, Essentialzymes-4

## Application and Usage

**Dietary and Oral:** Whether putting oils in a capsule or drinking them in a liquid, please refer to *Application Guidelines* on page 410.

- Take 1 capsule with desired oil 2 times daily.
- Take 10 drops of Basil Vitality, Peppermint Vitality, DiGize Vitality, or other oils desired diluted 50:50 in a capsule every 2 hours.
- Take 2-3 drops of oil in a spoonful of syrup or small amount of milk, juice, or water.

462 | **Chapter 20** | Personal Usage Guide

Personal Usage Guide | **Chapter 20**

# Heartburn

Heartburn is a burning feeling or pain in the center of the chest that may extend into your back or neck during or after eating.

Lemon juice is one of the best remedies for heartburn. Mix the juice of ½ of a squeezed lemon in 8 oz. of water and sip slowly upon awakening each morning.

Lemon juice helps the stomach stop making digestive acids, therefore alleviating heartburn or other stomach ailments.

## Recommendations

**Singles:** Basil, Basil Vitality, Fennel, Fennel Vitality, Spearmint, Spearmint Vitality, Ginger, Ginger Vitality, Jade Lemon, Jade Lemon Vitality, Lemon, Lemon Vitality, Lime, Lime Vitality, Idaho Tansy, Palo Santo, Cypress, Tarragon, Tarragon Vitality, Sage, Sage Vitality, Royal Hawaiian Sandalwood

**Blends:** DiGize, DiGize Vitality, JuvaCleanse, Juva-Cleanse Vitality, Citrus Fresh, Citrus Fresh Vitality, TummyGize

**Nutritionals:** AlkaLime, ICP, ComforTone, Essential-zymes-4, Detoxzyme, Allerzyme

## Heartburn Blend
- 8 drops Sage or Sage Vitality
- 3 drops Royal Hawaiian Sandalwood
- 2 drops Basil or Basil Vitality
- 1 drop Idaho Tansy or Palo Santo

## Application and Usage

**Aromatic:** Refer to *Application Guidelines* on page 410.
**Dietary and Oral:** Whether putting oils in a capsule or drinking them in a liquid, please refer to *Application Guidelines* on page 410.

- Take 1 capsule with desired oil 2 times daily.
- Take 2-3 drops of oil in a spoonful of syrup or small amount of milk, juice, or water.

**Topical:** For guidelines on applying oils to the skin, refer to *Application Guidelines* on page 410.

- Dilute 50:50 and apply on location 3-6 times daily.
- Place a warm compress with 1-3 drops of recommended oils over stomach.
- Apply recommended oils to the Vita Flex points of the feet.

# Indigestion (Bloating)

Indigestion causes discomfort in the upper abdomen, resulting in bloating, belching, and nausea. It often occurs during or right after eating and is medically known as dyspepsia.

## Recommendations

**Singles:** Peppermint, Peppermint Vitality, Nutmeg, Nutmeg Vitality, Fennel, Fennel Vitality, Ginger, Ginger Vitality, Cumin, Spearmint, Spearmint Vitality, Grapefruit, Grapefruit Vitality, Copaiba, Copaiba Vitality, Wintergreen

**Blends:** TummyGize, DiGize, DiGize Vitality, Juva-Cleanse, JuvaCleanse Vitality

**Nutritionals:** AlkaLime, Detoxzyme, ICP, ComforTone, JuvaPower, Essentialzyme, Essentialzymes-4, Mineral Essence, Allerzyme

## Application and Usage

**Dietary and Oral:** Whether putting the oils in a capsule or drinking them in a liquid, please refer to *Application Guidelines* on page 410.

- Take 1 capsule with desired oil 2 times daily.
- Take 2-3 drops of oil in a spoonful of syrup or small amount of milk, juice, or water.
- Take 2-4 capsules of Essentialzymes-4, Essentialzyme, or Detoxzyme before eating to help with digestion and upset stomach.
- When the stomach feels "heavy" from eating meat, Essentialzymes-4 is a beneficial companion to DiGize Vitality (See "Enzymes" in Special Issues).

**Topical:** For guidelines on applying oils to the skin, refer to *Application Guidelines* on page 410.

- Dilute 50:50 and apply on location 3-6 times daily.
- Place a warm compress with 1-3 drops of recommended oil over the stomach.

# Spastic Colon Syndrome/Irritable Bowel Syndrome

Spastic colon syndrome, often called irritable bowel syndrome, is a functional disorder where the bowel does not work as it should. It is characterized by constipation, diarrhea, gas, bloating, lower abdominal pain or discomfort, and nausea.

**Singles:** Fennel, Fennel Vitality

**Blends:** DiGize, DiGize Vitality, TummyGize

**Nutritionals:** AlkaLime, Essentialzymes-4, Life 9, Mineral Essence, NingXia Red, Slique Tea

Seventh Edition | **Essential Oils Desk Reference** | 463

## Application and Usage

**Aromatic:** Refer to *Application Guidelines* on page 410.

**Dietary and Oral:** Whether putting oils in a capsule or drinking them in a liquid, please refer to *Application Guidelines* on page 410.

- Take 1 capsule with desired oil 2 times daily.
- Take 2-3 drops of oil in a spoonful of syrup or small amount of milk, juice, or water.

**Topical:** For guidelines on applying oils to the skin, refer to *Application Guidelines* on page 410.

- Dilute 50:50 and apply on location 3-6 times daily.
- Place a warm compress with 1-3 drops of recommended oils over stomach.
- Apply recommended oils to the Vita Flex points of the feet.

## Stomachache

The term "stomachache" is used for many types of stomach or other abdominal discomfort. Some of the following symptoms may occur: pain before or after eating, bloating, heartburn, flatulence, feeling full, vomiting, loss of appetite, etc.

## Recommendations

**Singles:** Peppermint, Peppermint Vitality, Roman Chamomile, Lavender, Lavender Vitality, Blue Tansy, Cedarwood, Marjoram, Marjoram Vitality, Rose, Royal Hawaiian Sandalwood, Sacred Frankincense, Frankincense, Frankincense Vitality, Valerian

**Blends:** DiGize, DiGize Vitality, TummyGize, Trauma Life, T.R. Care, Humility, Harmony, RutaVaLa, RutaVaLa Roll-On, Valor, Valor II, Valor Roll-On, Peace & Calming, Peace & Calming II, Tranquil Roll-On

**Nutritionals:** Super B, Super C, MultiGreens, MegaCal, Mineral Essence, OmegaGize$^3$, AlkaLime, Life 9

## Application and Usage

**Aromatic:** Refer to *Application Guidelines* on page 410.

**Dietary and Oral:** Whether putting oils in a capsule or drinking them in a liquid, please refer to *Application Guidelines* on page 410.

- Take 1 capsule with desired oil 2 times daily.
- Take 2-3 drops of oil in a spoonful of syrup or small amount of milk, juice, or water.

**Topical:** For guidelines on applying oils to the skin, refer to *Application Guidelines* on page 410.

- Apply any of the desired oils diluted 50:50 on temples, neck, and shoulders 2 times daily or as needed.
- Add desired oil to bath salts and incorporate into daily bathing.

## Stomach Ulcers

Ulcers may be caused by several gastroduodenal diseases such as gastritis or gastric or peptic ulcers caused by the *Helicobacter pylori* bacteria.

## Recommendations

**Singles:** Lemongrass, Lemongrass Vitality, Copaiba, Copaiba Vitality, Jade Lemon, Jade Lemon Vitality, Lemon, Lemon Vitality, Lime, Lime Vitality, Myrtle, German Chamomile, German Chamomile Vitality, Myrrh, Patchouli, Peppermint, Peppermint Vitality

**Blends:** Thieves, Thieves Vitality, DiGize, DiGize Vitality, Melrose

**Nutritionals:** Digest & Cleanse, Inner Defense, ICP, JuvaPower, AlkaLime, Essentialzymes-4, Essentialzyme

## Application and Usage

**Aromatic:** Refer to *Application Guidelines* on page 410.

**Dietary and Oral:** Whether putting oils in a capsule or drinking them in a liquid, please refer to *Application Guidelines* on page 410.

- Take 1 capsule with desired oil 3 times daily for 20 days.
- Take 2-3 drops of oil in a spoonful of syrup or small amount of milk, juice, or water.

**Topical:** For guidelines on applying oils to the skin, refer to *Application Guidelines* on page 410.

Any calming oil applied through massage may help to decrease stress and bring a relaxing atmosphere: Dream Catcher, Gathering, Egyptian Gold, The Gift, Harmony, Inner Child, White Angelica, White Light, etc.

## DIPHTHERIA

Diphtheria is an acute infectious disease caused by toxigenic strains of *Corynebacterium diphtheriae*, acquired by contact with an infected person or carrier. It is usually confined to the upper respiratory tract and characterized by the formation of a tough, false membrane attached firmly to the underlying tissue that will bleed if forcibly removed.

In the most serious infections, the membrane begins in the tonsil area and may spread to the uvula, soft palate, and pharyngeal wall, followed by the larynx, trachea, and bronchial tree, where it may cause life-threatening bronchial obstructions. See your physician.

Personal Usage Guide | Chapter 20

## Recommendations

**Singles:** Oregano, Oregano Vitality, Plectranthus Oregano, Thyme, Thyme Vitality, Clove, Clove Vitality, Mountain Savory, Mountain Savory Vitality, Eucalyptus Radiata, Palo Santo, Northern Lights Black Spruce, Sacred Frankincense, Frankincense, Frankincense Vitality, Eucalyptus Blue, Spearmint, Spearmint Vitality, Ravintsara, Peppermint, Peppermint Vitality, Dorado Azul

**Blends:** Thieves, Thieves Vitality, Melrose, Exodus II, Raven, R.C., DiGize, DiGize Vitality

**Nutritionals:** Inner Defense, Essentialzyme, Essentialzymes-4, ICP, JuvaPower, JuvaSpice

**Oral Care:** Thieves Fresh Essence Plus Mouthwash, Thieves Cough Drops, Thieves Spray, Thieves Hard Lozenges

## Application and Usage

**Aromatic:** Refer to *Application Guidelines* on page 410.

**Dietary and Oral:** Whether putting the oils in a capsule or drinking them in a liquid, please refer to *Application Guidelines* on page 410.

- Take 1 capsule with desired oil 2 times daily.
- Take 2-3 drops of oil in a spoonful of syrup or small amount of milk, juice, or water.
- Gargle with Thieves Fresh Essence Plus Mouthwash several times daily.
- Spray throat as desired with Thieves Spray.
- Use Thieves Cough Drops and/or Thieves Hard Lozenges as desired.

**Topical:** For guidelines on applying oils to the skin, refer to *Application Guidelines* on page 410.

- Applying a single drop under the nose is helpful and refreshing.
- Apply 2-3 drops over neck and lung areas several times daily.

## DIZZINESS

Feeling dizzy is not an illness but a symptom of something else. Lightheadedness is often caused by a decrease in blood supply to the brain, while vertigo may be caused by an imbalance in the inner ear or brain. Dizziness may also be caused by dehydration or heat stroke.

## Recommendations

**Singles:** Peppermint, Peppermint Vitality, Ocotea, Ocotea Vitality, Eucalyptus Blue, Dorado Azul, Tangerine, Tangerine Vitality, Basil, Basil Vitality, Cardamom, Cardamom Vitality, Melaleuca Quinquenervia (Niaouli), Royal Hawaiian Sandalwood, Sacred Frankincense, Frankincense, Frankincense Vitality, Idaho Blue Spruce

**Blends:** Clarity, R.C., Brain Power, Common Sense, GeneYus, M-Grain, Grounding, Citrus Fresh, Citrus Fresh Vitality, Harmony

**Nutritionals:** MindWise, NingXia Red, MultiGreens, Master Formula, MegaCal, Mineral Essence

## Application and Usage

**Aromatic:** Refer to *Application Guidelines* on page 410.

**Dietary and Oral:** Whether putting the oils in a capsule or drinking them in a liquid, please refer to *Application Guidelines* on page 410.

- Take 1 capsule with desired oil 2 times daily.
- Take 2-3 drops of oil in a spoonful of syrup or small amount of milk, juice, or water.

**Topical:** For guidelines on applying oils to the skin, refer to *Application Guidelines* on page 410.

- Apply 1-2 drops neat (undiluted) on temples and back of neck, as desired.
- Applying a single drop under the nose is helpful.
- Massage 2-4 drops of oil neat on the bottoms of the feet.

## EAR PROBLEMS

Although ear problems are often caused by infections, other conditions may also cause ear pain or discomfort.

### Earache

Earaches result from inflammation and swelling of the structures that make up the ear and have a multitude of causes and a variety of symptoms.

## Recommendations

**Singles:** Helichrysum, Lavender, Lavender Vitality, Tea Tree, Roman Chamomile, Ravintsara, Peppermint, Peppermint Vitality, Eucalyptus Radiata, Basil, Basil Vitality

**Blends:** Purification, PanAway, ImmuPower, Melrose

**Nutritionals:** ImmuPro, Super C, Super C Chewable, Inner Defense

**Spray:** Thieves Spray

Seventh Edition | Essential Oils Desk Reference | 465

**Essential Oils Desk Reference** | Seventh Edition

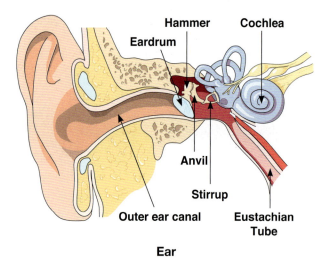

Ear

## Application and Usage

**Aromatic:** Refer to *Application Guidelines* on page 410.

**Dietary and Oral:** Whether putting the oils in a capsule or drinking them in a liquid, please refer to *Application Guidelines* on page 410.

- Take 1 capsule with desired oil 2 times daily.
- Take 2-3 drops of oil in a spoonful of syrup or small amount of milk, juice, or water.
- Gargle up to 8 times daily with Thieves Fresh Essence Plus Mouthwash.
- Spray Thieves Spray into the throat up to 5 times daily.

**Topical:** For guidelines on applying oils to the skin, refer to *Application Guidelines* on page 410.

- Apply 2 drops of oil diluted 50:50 in warm olive or fractionated coconut oil to a cotton swab. Using the swab, apply traces to the skin around the opening of the ear, but not in it. Put 2-3 drops of the diluted essential oil on a piece of cotton and place it carefully over the ear opening. Leave in overnight.
- Additional relief may be obtained by placing a warm compress over the ear.
- Massage 1-2 drops on ears and ear lobes using the Vita Flex Technique and on the Vita Flex points for the ear on the feet.

**CAUTION:** Never put essential oils directly into the ear canal. Ear pain can be very serious. Always seek medical attention if pain persists.

## Ear Infection

An ear infection often occurs in conjunction with other symptoms, which may vary in character and intensity in different individuals.

### Recommendations

**Singles:** Basil, Myrrh, Thyme, Wintergreen, Helichrysum, Mountain Savory

**Blends:** ImmuPower, Melrose, Thieves, Purification, Exodus II

**Nutritionals:** ImmuPro, Inner Defense

### Application and Usage

**Aromatic:** Refer to *Application Guidelines* on page 410.

**Topical:** For guidelines on applying oils to the skin, refer to *Application Guidelines* on page 410.

- Put Basil on the outer ear when you feel an ear infection coming on. Just the aromatic fumes will kill an ear infection (otitis media).
- Apply 2 drops of oil diluted 50:50 in warm olive oil to a cotton swab. Using the swab, apply traces to the skin around the opening of the ear, but not in it.
- Put 2-3 drops of the diluted essential oil on a piece of cotton and place it carefully over the ear opening. Leave in overnight.

**CAUTION:** Never put essential oils directly into the ear. Ear pain can be very serious. Always seek medical attention if pain persists.

## Hearing Impairment

Hearing impairment refers to people with either partial or full hearing loss.

### Recommendations

**Singles:** Helichrysum, Juniper, Geranium, Peppermint, Lavender, Basil

**Blends:** Purification, Surrender, Awaken, Magnify Your Purpose

### Application and Usage

**Aromatic:** Refer to *Application Guidelines* on page 410.

**Topical:** For guidelines on applying oils to the skin, refer to *Application Guidelines* on page 410.

- Apply single oils or blends neat or diluted, depending on the oils that are used.
- Apply 1 drop neat on a cotton ball and place it

carefully in the opening of the ear canal. Retain overnight. **DO NOT place oils directly in the ear canal.**

- Massage 1-2 drops of oil neat on each ear lobe, behind the ears, and down the jaw line along the Eustachian tube.

**Hearing Vita Flex Regimen**

- Apply 1-2 drops neat of Helichrysum on the area **outside** the opening to the ear canal with fingertip or cotton swab. **DO NOT** put oil inside the ear canal.
- After applying the Helichrysum, hold ear lobes firmly and pull in a circular motion 10 times to help stimulate absorption and circulation in the ear canal.

## Tinnitus (Ringing in the Ears)

Tinnitus is a sound in one or both ears like buzzing, whistling, or ringing and occurs without an external stimulus.

### Recommendations

**Singles:** Helichrysum, Juniper, Geranium, Rose, Peppermint, Lavender, Basil

**Blends:** Purification

**Nutritionals:** NingXia Red, Detoxzyme, Sulfurzyme

### Application and Usage

**Aromatic:** Refer to *Application Guidelines* on page 410.
**Topical:** For guidelines on applying oils to the skin, refer to *Application Guidelines* on page 410.

- Massage 1-2 drops neat on temples, forehead, and back of neck.
- Apply one drop each on tips of the toes and fingers so that the oils get into the Vita Flex pathways.

**Hearing Vita Flex Regimen:**

- Apply 1-2 drops neat of Helichrysum to the area **outside** the opening to the ear canal with fingertip or cotton swab. **DO NOT** put oil inside the ear canal.
- After applying the Helichrysum, hold ear lobes firmly and pull in a circular motion 10 times to help stimulate absorption and circulation in the ear canal.

## EATING DISORDERS *(See also Addictions)*

Eating disorders are serious psychological conditions that generally involve negative, self-critical feelings and thoughts about body weight, size, and shape. They involve eating habits that disrupt daily activities and normal body functions.

### Anorexia Nervosa

Anorexia nervosa is an eating disorder characterized by total avoidance of food and virtual self-starvation. It may or may not be accompanied by bulimia (binge-purge behavior).

While psychotherapy remains indispensable, the aroma of essential oils may alter emotions enough to effect a change in the underlying psychology or disturbed-thinking patterns that support this self-destructive behavior. This is accomplished by the ability of aroma to directly stimulate the amygdala gland, which is part of the emotional center of the brain known as the limbic system.

Many essential oils such as Lemon and Ginger when inhaled regularly can combat the emotional addiction that leads anorexics to premature death.

Many people with anorexia believe they do not deserve to be healthy or loved unless they are "slender."

Many people who are anorexic suffer life-threatening nutrient and mineral deficiencies. The lack of magnesium and potassium can actually trigger heart rhythm abnormalities and cardiac arrest. It is absolutely essential that calcium, magnesium, potassium, and other mineral deficiencies are replenished.

### Recommendations

**Singles:** Jade Lemon, Jade Lemon Vitality, Lemon, Lemon Vitality, Lime, Lime Vitality, Tangerine, Tangerine Vitality, Ginger, Ginger Vitality, Mandarin

**Blends:** Divine Release, Evergreen Essence, Freedom, Inner Harmony, InTouch, Reconnect, Valor, Valor II, Valor Roll-On, Motivation, Brain Power, Stress Away Roll-On

**Nutritionals:** Mineral Essence, Balance Complete, MegaCal, MindWise, Power Meal, Slique Shake, Slique Bars, Essentialzyme, Essentialzymes-4, OmegaGize[3], Slique Bars–Chocolate-Coated, Chocolate-Coated Wolfberry Crisp Bars

### Application and Usage

**Aromatic:** Refer to *Application Guidelines* on page 410.

**Essential Oils Desk Reference** | Seventh Edition

**Dietary and Oral**

- Whether putting the oils in a capsule or drinking them in a liquid, please refer to *Application Guidelines* on page 410.
- Take 1 capsule with desired oil 2 times daily.
- Take 2-3 drops of oil in a spoonful of syrup or small amount of milk, juice, or water.

**Topical:** For guidelines on applying oils to the skin, refer to *Application Guidelines* on page 410.

## Appetite, Loss of

Ginger has been shown to stimulate digestion and improve appetite.

## Recommendations

**Singles:** Ginger, Ginger Vitality, Spearmint, Spearmint Vitality, Orange, Orange Vitality, Nutmeg, Nutmeg Vitality, Peppermint, Peppermint Vitality

**Blends:** Citrus Fresh, Citrus Fresh Vitality, Christmas Spirit, RutaVaLa, RutaVaLa Roll-On, TummyGize, DiGize, DiGize Vitality

**Nutritionals:** Essentialzyme, Essentialzymes-4, ComforTone, MegaCal, Mineral Essence, NingXia Red, Slique Bars, Wolfberry Crisp Bars

## Application and Usage

**Aromatic:** Refer to *Application Guidelines* on page 410.

**Dietary and Oral:** Whether putting the oils in a capsule or drinking them in a liquid, please refer to *Application Guidelines* on page 410.

- Take 1 capsule with DiGize Vitality or other desired oil 2 times daily.
- Take 2-3 drops of oil in a spoonful of syrup or small amount of milk, juice, or water.

**Topical:** For guidelines on applying oils to the skin, refer to *Application Guidelines* on page 410.

- Apply 5-6 drops with massage oil 3-5 times daily or as needed.
- You may also apply 2-3 drops on the Vita Flex points on the feet.
- Applying a single drop under the nose is helpful and refreshing.

## Binge Eating Disorder

Binge eating disorder is characterized by the binge eater consuming unnaturally large amounts of food in a short period of time, which acts as a psychological release for excessive emotional stress. However, unlike a bulimic, the binge eater does not usually engage in excessive exercise, vomiting, or taking laxatives to reduce weight.

**Singles:** Sacred Frankincense, Frankincense, Frankincense Vitality, Peppermint, Peppermint Vitality

**Blends:** Divine Release, Evergreen Essence, Freedom, Inner Harmony, InTouch, Reconnect, Slique Essence, 3 Wise Men

**Nutritionals:** Slique Tea, Slique Bars–Chocolate-Coated, Chocolate-Coated Wolfberry Crisp Bars, Slique Gum, NingXia Red

**Aromatic:** Refer to *Application Guidelines* on page 410.

**Dietary and Oral:** Whether putting the oils in a capsule or drinking them in a liquid, please refer to *Application Guidelines* on page 410.

- Take 1 capsule with desired oil 2 times daily.
- Take 2-3 drops of oil in a spoonful of syrup or small amount of milk, juice, or water.

**Topical:** For guidelines on applying oils to the skin, refer to *Application Guidelines* on page 410.

## Bulimia

Bulimia is characterized by habitual binge eating and then purging.

**Singles:** Idaho Balsam Fir, Fennel, Fennel Vitality, Nutmeg, Nutmeg Vitality

**Blends:** Slique Essence, Common Sense, DiGize, DiGize Vitality, Forgiveness

**Nutritionals:** Slique Tea, Slique CitraSlim Caps, Slique Bars, Slique Bars–Chocolate-Coated, Chocolate-Coated Wolfberry Crisp Bars, Slique Gum, NingXia Red

**Aromatic:** Refer to *Application Guidelines* on page 410.

**Dietary and Oral:** Whether putting the oils in a capsule or drinking them in a liquid, please refer to *Application Guidelines* on page 410.

- Take 1 capsule with desired oil 2 times daily.
- Take 2-3 drops of oil in a spoonful of syrup or small amount of milk, juice, or water.

**Topical:** For guidelines on applying oils to the skin, refer to *Application Guidelines* on page 410.

Personal Usage Guide | Chapter 20

## EDEMA (Swelling) *(See also Phlebitis)*

Swelling, particularly around the ankles, is noticeable when fluids accumulate in the tissue. This puffiness under the skin and around the ankles is more apparent at the end of the day when fluids settle to the lowest part of the body. A potassium deficiency can make swelling worse, so the first recourse is to increase potassium intake.

### Recommendations

**Singles:** Fennel, Fennel Vitality, Juniper, German Chamomile, German Chamomile Vitality, Peppermint, Peppermint Vitality, Lavender, Lavender Vitality, Grapefruit, Grapefruit Vitality, Helichrysum, Tangerine, Tangerine Vitality, Patchouli, Geranium, Cypress, Wintergreen

**Blends:** Aroma Life, EndoFlex, EndoFlex Vitality, Di-Gize, DiGize Vitality

**Nutritionals:** Digest & Cleanse, Super C, Super C Chewable, ICP, JuvaPower, Essentialzyme, Essentialzymes-4, Detoxzyme, Life 9, MegaCal, Balance Complete

### Edema Blend (General)
- 10 drops Wintergreen
- 8 drops Tangerine or Tangerine Vitality
- 6 drops Fennel or Fennel Vitality
- 4 drops Juniper
- 3 drops Patchouli

### Edema Blend (Morning)
- 10 drops Tangerine or Tangerine Vitality
- 10 drops Cypress

### Edema Blend (Evening)
- 8 drops Geranium
- 5 drops Cypress
- 5 drops Helichrysum, Grapefruit, or Grapefruit Vitality

### Application and Usage

**Dietary and Oral:** Whether putting the oils in a capsule or drinking them in a liquid, please refer to *Application Guidelines* on page 410.

- Take 1 capsule with desired oil 2 times daily.
- Take 2-3 drops of oil in a spoonful of syrup or small amount of milk, juice, or water.

**Topical:** For guidelines on applying oils to the skin, refer to *Application Guidelines* on page 410.

- Apply 1-3 drops diluted 50:50 on affected area 2-3 times daily.

- Place a cold compress with 1-2 drops of chosen oil 1-2 times daily on the area.
- Massage 1-3 drops on bladder Vita Flex point on foot.
- Massage 15-20 drops of the General Edema Blend diluted 60:40 in V-6 Vegetable Oil Complex or other massage oil on legs, working from the feet up to the thighs. Do this for 1 week.
- Massage 15-20 drops of Morning Edema Blend diluted 60:40 in V-6 Vegetable Oil Complex or other massage oil on legs, working from the feet up to the thighs. Do this in the morning for 1 week. Repeat the same process in the evening with the Evening Edema Blend.

## EMOTIONAL TRAUMA

The effect of heavy emotional trauma can disrupt the stomach and digestive system.

### Recommendations

**Singles:** Sacred Frankincense, Frankincense, Frankincense Vitality, Idaho Blue Spruce, Idaho Balsam Fir, Jade Lemon, Jade Lemon Vitality, Lemon, Lemon Vitality, Lime, Lime Vitality, German Chamomile, German Chamomile Vitality, Rose, Lavender, Lavender Vitality, Marjoram, Marjoram Vitality, Spearmint, Spearmint Vitality, Peppermint, Peppermint Vitality, Valerian, Vetiver

**Blends:** Divine Release, Evergreen Essence, Freedom, Inner Harmony, InTouch, Reconnect, SleepyIze, Trauma Life, T.R. Care, Hope, Build Your Dream, Inner Child, Present Time, Valor, Valor II, Valor Roll-On, Release, Sacred Mountain, Christmas Spirit, 3 Wise Men, Tranquil Roll-On, Stress Away Roll-On, Harmony, Forgiveness, Amoressence, Peace & Calming, Peace & Calming II, White Angelica, White Light, The Gift, Oola Balance, Oola Faith, Oola Family, Oola Field, Oola Finance, Oola Fitness, Oola Friends, Oola Fun, Oola Grow, Grounding

**Nutritionals:** Thyromin, Ultra Young, Master Formula, EndoGize, PD 80/20

### Emotional Pain Relief Blend No. 1
- 10 drops Idaho Blue Spruce
- 5 drops Idaho Balsam Fir
- 5 drops Sacred Frankincense

### Emotional Pain Relief Blend No. 2
- 8 drops Lavender or Lavender Vitality
- 6 drops Marjoram or Marjoram Vitality
- 3 drops Spearmint or Spearmint Vitality
- 2 drops Peppermint or Peppermint Vitality

Seventh Edition | **Essential Oils Desk Reference** | 469

## Application and Usage

**Aromatic:** Refer to *Application Guidelines* on page 410.

**Dietary and Oral:** Whether putting the oils in a capsule or drinking them in a liquid, please refer to *Application Guidelines* on page 410.

- Take 1 capsule with desired oil 2 times daily.
- Take 2-3 drops of oil in a spoonful of syrup or small amount of milk, juice, or water.

**Topical:** For guidelines on applying oils to the skin, refer to *Application Guidelines* on page 410.

- Place 1-3 drops of Release over the thymus and rub in gently. Apply up to 3 times daily as needed.
- Blend equal parts Frankincense and Valor and apply 1-2 drops neat on temples, forehead, crown, and back of neck before retiring. Use for 3 nights.
- Apply 1-2 drops neat to the crown of head and forehead as needed. It is best if it is applied in a quiet, darkened room.
- Massage 1-3 drops on heart Vita Flex points 2-3 times daily.
- Rub 1-2 drops of oil on the temples and back of neck several times daily.

## ENDOCRINE SYSTEM *(See also Thyroid Problems, Cushing's Syndrome (Disease), Male Hormone Imbalance, Menstrual and Female Hormone Conditions)*

The endocrine system encompasses the hormone-producing glands of the body. These glands cluster around blood vessels and release their hormones directly into the bloodstream. The pituitary gland exerts a wide range of control over the hormonal (endocrine) system and is often called the master gland. Other glands include the pancreas, adrenals, thyroid and parathyroid, ovaries, and testes.

The limbic system lies along the margin of the cerebral cortex (brain) and is the hormone-producing system of the brain. It includes the amygdala, hippocampus, pineal, pituitary, thalamus, and hypothalamus.

Essential oils increase circulation to the brain and enable the pituitary and other glands to better secrete neural transmitters and hormones that support the endocrine and immune systems.

The thyroid is one of the most important glands for regulating the body systems. The hypothalamus plays an even more important role, since it regulates not only the thyroid but also the adrenals and the pituitary gland.

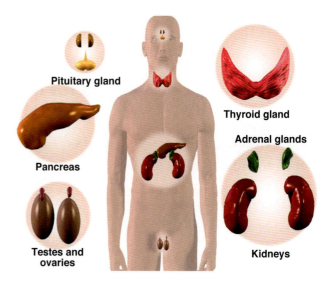

**Endocrine System**

**Singles:** Canadian Fleabane (Conyza), Myrtle, Sacred Frankincense, Frankincense, Frankincense Vitality, Fennel, Fennel Vitality, Idaho Blue Spruce, Sage, Sage Vitality

**Blends:** EndoFlex, EndoFlex Vitality, Harmony, The Gift, Shutran

**Nutritionals:** Ultra Young, Thyromin, CortiStop, Super B, NingXia Red, Master Formula

## EPILEPSY

**Note:** Epileptics should consult their health care professional before using essential oils. Use extreme caution with high ketone oils such as Basil, Rosemary, Sage, and Idaho Tansy.

### Recommendations

**Singles:** Clary Sage, Royal Hawaiian Sandalwood, Cedarwood, Sacred Frankincense, Frankincense, Frankincense Vitality, Lavender, Lavender Vitality

**Blends:** Valor, Valor II, Valor Roll-On, Brain Power, GeneYus, RutaVaLa, RutaVaLa Roll-On, Common Sense, Peace & Calming, Peace & Calming II,

**Nutritionals:** MindWise, ICP, ComforTone, Essentialzyme, Essentialzymes-4, Life 9, NingXia Red, JuvaPower, JuvaSpice, Master Formula, Super B

### Application and Usage

**Aromatic:** Refer to *Application Guidelines* on page 410.
**Topical:** For guidelines on applying oils to the skin, refer to *Application Guidelines* on page 410.

- Massage 2-4 drops on brain Vita Flex points on feet 2-3 times daily.

Personal Usage Guide | Chapter 20

# EPSTEIN-BARR VIRUS

Epstein-Barr virus is a type of herpes virus that also causes mononucleosis.

Symptoms include indigestion, upper and lower gas, poor assimilation, poor electrolyte balance, allergic reaction to foods and other substances, emotional mood swings, fatigue, irritability, and a lack of motivation, discipline, and creativity.

Hypoglycemia is a precursor and can render the body susceptible to the Epstein-Barr virus. Treat the hypoglycemia, and the symptoms of the Epstein-Barr virus may begin to disappear.

## Recommendations

**Singles:** Palo Santo, Mountain Savory, Mountain Savory Vitality, Oregano, Oregano Vitality, Plectranthus Oregano, Rosemary, Rosemary Vitality, Thyme, Thyme Vitality, Clove, Clove Vitality, Royal Hawaiian Sandalwood, Northern Lights Black Spruce, Grapefruit, Grapefruit Vitality, Nutmeg, Nutmeg Vitality, Tea Tree, Sage, Sage Vitality

**Blends:** Thieves, Thieves Vitality, ImmuPower, EndoFlex, EndoFlex Vitality, Longevity, Longevity Vitality, TummyGize, DiGize, DiGize Vitality, Exodus II

**Nutritionals:** Inner Defense, Super C, Super C Chewable, ImmuPro, Thyromin, Detoxzyme, Digest & Cleanse, ICP, JuvaPower, ComforTone, Essentialzyme, Allerzyme, Life 9, Essentialzymes-4, Master Formula

## Application and Usage

**Aromatic:** Refer to *Application Guidelines* on page 410.

**Dietary and Oral:** Whether putting the oils in a capsule or drinking them in a liquid, please refer to *Application Guidelines* on page 410.

- Take 1 capsule with desired oil 3 times daily.
- Take 2-3 drops of oil in a spoonful of syrup or small amount of milk, juice, or water.

**Topical:** For guidelines on applying oils to the skin, refer to *Application Guidelines* on page 410.

- Receive a Raindrop Technique weekly with ImmuPower, Thieves, Exodus II, and the oils of Raindrop Technique.
- Massage 2-4 drops of oil neat on the bottoms of the feet just before bedtime.

## Mononucleosis

Infectious mononucleosis is a disease caused by the Epstein-Barr virus (EBV), which is a type of herpes virus. The symptoms usually last for four weeks or more. The spleen enlarges and may even rupture in severe cases.

### Recommendations

**Singles:** Ravintsara, Hyssop, Clove, Clove Vitality, Thyme, Thyme Vitality, Sacred Frankincense, Northern Lights Black Spruce, Frankincense, Frankincense Vitality, Palo Santo, Mountain Savory, Mountain Savory Vitality, Ocotea

**Blends:** Thieves, Thieves Vitality, Inner Defense, R.C., Breathe Again Roll-On, Raven, Exodus II, ImmuPower

**Nutritionals:** ImmuPro, Super C, Super C Chewable, Longevity Softgels, ICP, ComforTone, Essentialzyme, Essentialzymes-4, Detoxzyme, Life 9

### Mononucleosis Blend

- 3 drops Thieves or Thieves Vitality
- 3 drops Thyme or Thyme Vitality
- 3 drops Mountain Savory or Mountain Savory Vitality
- 2 drops Ravintsara

### Application and Usage

**Aromatic:** Refer to *Application Guidelines* on page 410.

**Dietary and Oral:** Whether putting the oils in a capsule or drinking them in a liquid, please refer to *Application Guidelines* on page 410.

- Take 1 capsule with desired oil 3 times daily.
- Take 2-3 drops of oil in a spoonful of syrup or small amount of milk, juice, or water.

**Topical:** For guidelines on applying oils to the skin, refer to *Application Guidelines* on page 410.

- Receive a Raindrop Technique 2 times weekly.
- Massage 3-6 drops using the Vita Flex technique on the bottoms of feet 2 times daily.

# EYE DISORDERS

In 1997 Dr. Terry Friedmann, MD, eliminated his need for glasses after applying Sandalwood and Juniper on the areas around his eyes, above the eyebrows, and on the cheeks, being careful never to get oil into his eyes. He also used the supplements of MultiGreens, ICP, ComforTone, Essentialzyme, JuvaTone, and JuvaPower for a complete colon and liver cleanse.

**Caution:** Never put any essential oils in the eyes or on the eyelids.

Seventh Edition | Essential Oils Desk Reference | 471

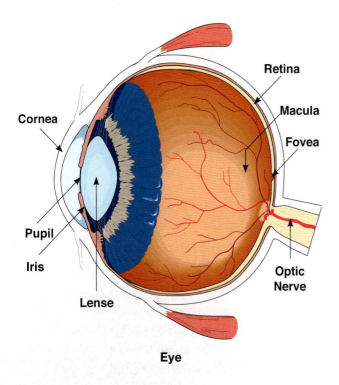

Eye

## Age-Related Macular Degeneration (AMD)

AMD is one of the most common causes of blindness among people over 60 years of age. In fact, 30 percent of all people over 70 years of age suffer to some degree from this disease. The most common form of the disease is called "dry" when macular cells degenerate irreversibly.

The "wet" form of the disease is when there is abnormal blood vessel growth that results in macula-damaging blood leaks. The disease results in a steady loss of central vision until eyesight is totally impaired.

For dry AMD, the best prevention will be foods rich in antioxidants and carotenoids. The Ningxia wolfberry, the highest known antioxidant food, is also extremely high in lutein and zeaxanthin, which are vital for preserving eye health. Other foods rich in carotenoids that are also powerful antioxidants include blueberries and spinach.

For dry AMD, Lemon Vitality may be helpful as a Dietary and Oral supplement.

Clove Vitality, one of the highest known antioxidant nutrients, may be a good nutritional defense for wet AMD only.

### Recommendations

**Singles:** Sacred Frankincense, Lemon Vitality (dry AMD only) as a Dietary and Oral supplement, Clove Vitality (wet AMD only) as a Dietary and Oral supplement

**Blends:** Longevity, Longevity Vitality

**Nutritionals:** NingXia Red, OmegaGize[3], Longevity Softgels, Power Meal, Slique Shake, Slique Bars, Slique CitraSlim, MultiGreens, Essentialzyme, Essentialzymes-4, Super C, Super C Chewable, Ningxia Wolfberries (Organic, Dried), Master Formula, MindWise

### Application and Usage

**Aromatic:** Refer to *Application Guidelines* on page 410.

**Dietary and Oral:** Whether putting the oils in a capsule or drinking them in a liquid, please refer to *Application Guidelines* on page 410.

- Take 1 capsule with desired oil 2 times daily.
- Take 2-3 drops of oil in a spoonful of syrup or small amount of milk, juice, or water.

**Topical:** For guidelines on applying oils to the skin, refer to *Application Guidelines* on page 410.

- Receive a Raindrop Technique 2 times weekly.
- Massage 3-6 drops using the Vita Flex technique on the bottoms of feet 2 times daily.

## Blocked Tear Ducts

A blocked tear duct is a partial or complete blockage in the system that carries tears away from the eye into the nose.

### Recommendations

**Singles:** Lavender, Lavender Vitality, Sacred Frankincense, Frankincense, Frankincense Vitality, Cypress, Idaho Blue Spruce

**Blends:** Inner Child, Sacred Mountain

**Nutritionals:** NingXia Red, OmegaGize[3], Longevity Softgels, Essentialzyme, Essentialzymes-4, Master Formula

### Application and Usage

**Aromatic:** Refer to *Application Guidelines* on page 410.

**Dietary and Oral:** Whether putting the oils in a capsule or drinking them in a liquid, please refer to *Application Guidelines* on page 410.

- Take 1 capsule with desired oil 3 times daily.
- Take 2-3 drops of oil in a spoonful of syrup or small amount of milk, juice, or water.

**Topical:** For guidelines on applying oils to the skin, refer to *Application Guidelines* on page 410.

- Rubbing 1 drop of Lavender oil over the bridge of the nose 2 times daily has been reported to help in some cases.

- Receive a Raindrop Technique 2 times weekly.
- Massage 3-6 drops using the Vita Flex technique on the bottoms of feet 2 times daily.

## Cataracts

Cataracts are a clouding of the eye lens that often comes with aging.

### Recommendations

**Singles:** Lavender, Lavender Vitality, Lemongrass, Lemongrass Vitality, Cypress, Sacred Frankincense, Frankincense, Frankincense Vitality, Eucalyptus Radiata, Jade Lemon, Jade Lemon Vitality, Lemon, Lemon Vitality, Clove, Clove Vitality

**Blends:** Longevity, Longevity Vitality, Melrose, En-R-Gee, Purification

**Nutritionals:** JuvaPower, OmegaGize[3], Mineral Essence, Essentialzyme, Essentialzymes-4, ImmuPro, NingXia Red, Ningxia Wolfberries (Organic, Dried)

### Eye Blend
- 10 drops Lemongrass
- 5 drops Cypress
- 3 drops Eucalyptus Radiata
- 2 drops Sacred Frankincense or Frankincense

Mix this blend with a little V-6 Vegetable Oil Complex and apply around the eyes, being careful not to touch the eyes. It is best at night because the eyes could water, just like when you cut onions.

**Note:** If essential oils should ever accidentally get into the eyes, dilute with V-6 Vegetable Oil Complex or other pure vegetable oil. **Never rinse with water.** However, the essential oils will not cause any damage and will slowly stop burning.

### Application and Usage

**Aromatic:** Refer to *Application Guidelines* on page 410.

**Dietary and Oral:** Whether putting the oils in a capsule or drinking them in a liquid, please refer to *Application Guidelines* on page 410.

- Take 1 capsule with desired oil 2 times daily.
- Take 2-3 drops of oil in a spoonful of syrup or small amount of milk, juice, or water.
- Clove Vitality is a powerful antioxidant, and when taken internally, it can slow or prevent both cataracts and AMD.
- Drink 2-6 ounces of NingXia Red daily or more if desired.

**Topical:** For guidelines on applying oils to the skin, refer to *Application Guidelines* on page 410.

- Apply 2-4 drops diluted 20:80 in a wide circle around the eye 1-3 times daily, being careful not to get any oil in the eyes or on the eyelids. This may also help with puffiness.
- Apply on temples and eye Vita Flex points on the feet and hands (the undersides of your two largest toes and your index and middle fingers).

**Note:** If essential oils should ever accidentally get into the eyes, dilute with V-6 Vegetable Oil Complex or other pure vegetable oil. **Never rinse with water.** However, the essential oils will not cause any damage and will slowly stop burning.

## Conjunctivitis / Pink Eye

Conjunctivitis (also called pink eye) is inflammation of the outermost layer of the eye and the inner surface of the eyelids. It has many causes, which may be infectious or noninfectious.

### Recommendations

**Singles:** Myrrh, Lavender, Lavender Vitality, Vetiver

**Nutritionals:** NingXia Red, Ningxia Wolfberries (Organic, Dried), OmegaGize[3], ImmuPro, Exodus II

### Application and Usage

**Aromatic:** Refer to *Application Guidelines* on page 410.

**Dietary and Oral:** Whether putting the oils in a capsule or drinking them in a liquid, please refer to *Application Guidelines* on page 410.

- Take 1 capsule with desired oil 3 times daily.
- Take 2-3 drops of oil in a spoonful of syrup or small amount of milk, juice, or water.

**Topical:** For guidelines on applying oils to the skin, refer to *Application Guidelines* on page 410.

- Apply 2-4 drops diluted 20:80 in a wide circle around the eye 1-3 times daily, being careful not to get any oil in the eyes or on the eyelids. This may also help with puffiness.
- Apply on temples and eye Vita Flex points on the feet and hands (the undersides of your two largest toes and your index and middle fingers).

**Note:** If essential oils should ever accidentally get into the eyes, dilute with V-6 Vegetable Oil Complex or other pure vegetable oil. **Never rinse with water.** However, the essential oils will not cause any damage and will slowly stop burning.

**Essential Oils Desk Reference** | Seventh Edition

## FAINTING (See also Shock)

Fainting happens when your brain does not get enough oxygen and you lose consciousness for a brief time. It can be caused by many different things. See your health care professional.

### Recommendations

**Singles:** Idaho Blue Spruce, Melissa, Peppermint, Royal Hawaiian Sandalwood, Cardamom, Spearmint, Sacred Frankincense, Frankincense

**Blends:** Clarity, Trauma Life, T.R. Care, Brain Power, GeneYus, R.C., Awaken

### Application and Usage

**Aromatic:**
- Open an oil bottle and wave it under the nose of the person who fainted.
- If you are feeling faint, open the oil bottle and inhale or put 2-3 drops of your chosen oil in your hands, rub them together, cup your hands over your nose, and inhale.

**Topical:** For guidelines on applying oils to the skin, refer to *Application Guidelines* on page 410.

## FATIGUE

Hormone imbalances may play a large role in fatigue as well as in latent viral infections (herpes virus and/or Epstein-Barr virus). Also, mineral deficiencies (especially magnesium) can play a large part in low energy.

Natural progesterone for women and DHEA for men can be instrumental in helping combat the fatigue that comes with age and declining hormone levels. Because pregnenolone is a precursor for all male and female hormones, both men and women can benefit from its supplementation.

### Mental Fatigue

Mental fatigue is excessive mental tiredness and may manifest itself in difficulty concentrating and solving problems, irritability, loss of passion for work, anxiety, sleeplessness, confusion, or frustration.

### Recommendations

**Singles:** Idaho Blue Spruce, Peppermint, Peppermint Vitality, Spearmint, Spearmint Vitality, Idaho Balsam Fir, Sacred Frankincense, Frankincense, Frankincense Vitality, Black Pepper, Black Pepper Vitality, Sage, Sage Vitality, Nutmeg, Nutmeg Vitality, Pine

**Blends:** Envision, Valor, Valor II, Oola Balance, Oola Faith, Oola Family, Oola Field, Oola Finance, Oola Fitness, Oola Friends, Oola Fun, Oola Grow, Motivation, En-R-Gee, Clarity, Common Sense, Shutran

**Nutritionals:** Power Meal, Slique Shake, Slique Bars, Slique Bars–Chocolate-Coated, Chocolate-Coated Wolfberry Crisp Bars, Slique CitraSlim, Balance Complete, MultiGreens, Mineral Essence, Longevity Softgels, NingXia Red, NingXia Nitro, NingXia Zyng, Pure Protein Complete, Essentialzyme, Essentialzymes-4, Ultra Young, Super B, EndoGize, Sleep Essence

### Application and Usage

**Aromatic:** Refer to *Application Guidelines* on page 410.

**Dietary and Oral:** Whether putting the oils in a capsule or drinking them in a liquid, please refer to *Application Guidelines* on page 410.
- Take 1 capsule with desired oil 2 times daily.
- Take 2-3 drops of oil in a spoonful of syrup or small amount of milk, juice, or water.

**Topical:** For guidelines on applying oils to the skin, refer to *Application Guidelines* on page 410.
- Apply 2-4 drops diluted 50:50 at base of throat, temples, and back of neck as needed.
- Massage 1-3 drops on corresponding Vita Flex points on feet 1-3 times daily.

### Physical Fatigue

Physical fatigue is a lack of energy that can be caused by a host of factors, including poor thyroid function, adrenal imbalance, diabetes, cancer, and other conditions.

MultiGreens is a plant-derived, high-protein energy formula that athletes use to boost endurance. Longevity Softgels increase energy and endurance. Digestion and colon problems may cause fatigue. A colon and liver cleanse unburdens the digestive system and increases energy.

### Recommendations

**Singles:** Peppermint, Peppermint Vitality, Nutmeg, Nutmeg Vitality, Lemongrass, Lemongrass Vitality, Eucalyptus Blue, Dorado Azul, Juniper, Basil, Basil Vitality, Jade Lemon, Jade Lemon Vitality, Lemon, Lemon Vitality, Lime, Lime Vitality, Rosemary, Rosemary Vitality, Thyme, Thyme Vitality, Cypress

**Blends:** Awaken, Motivation, Valor, Valor II, Valor Roll-On, En-R-Gee, Oola Balance, Oola Faith, Oola Family, Oola Field, Oola Finance, Oola Fitness, Oola Friends, Oola Fun, Oola Grow, Hope, EndoFlex, EndoFlex Vitality

**474** | **Chapter 20** | Personal Usage Guide

Personal Usage Guide | **Chapter 20**

**Nutritionals:** Thyromin, MultiGreens, Power Meal, Slique Shake, Slique Bars, Slique CitraSlim, EndoGize, Longevity Softgels, Super B, NingXia Red, Ningxia Wolfberries (Organic, Dried), Digest & Cleanse, Life 9, NingXia Nitro, NingXia Zyng, ImmuPro

## Application and Usage

**Aromatic:** Refer to *Application Guidelines* on page 410.

**Dietary and Oral:** Whether putting the oils in a capsule or drinking them in a liquid, please refer to *Application Guidelines* on page 410.

- Take 1 capsule with desired oil 3 times daily.
- Take 2-3 drops of oil in a spoonful of syrup or small amount of milk, juice, or water.

**Topical:** For guidelines on applying oils to the skin, refer to *Application Guidelines* on page 410.

- Apply 2-4 drops diluted 50:50 on temples, in clavicle notch (over thyroid), and behind ears 2-4 times daily as needed.
- Place a warm compress with 1-2 drops of chosen oil on the back.

## FEVER

Fevers are one of the most powerful healing responses of the human body and are an indication that the body is fighting an infectious disease. However, if the fever raises body temperature excessively (over 104ºF), then neurological damage can occur.

Reducing the fever is best accomplished by using anti-inflammatory essential oils internally and topically.

### Recommendations

**Singles:** Peppermint, Peppermint Vitality, Eucalyptus Blue, Nutmeg, Nutmeg Vitality, German Chamomile, German Chamomile Vitality, Idaho Balsam Fir, Copaiba, Copaiba Vitality, Myrrh, Dorado Azul

**Blends:** ImmuPower, Melrose, Raven, Clarity, M-Grain, RutaVaLa, RutaVaLa Roll-On

**Nutritionals:** Super C, Super C Chewable, ImmuPro, Longevity Softgels, Thieves Spray

**Body Care:** Cinnamint Lip Balm, Lavender Lip Balm, Grapefruit Lip Balm

### Application and Usage

**Aromatic:** Refer to *Application Guidelines* on page 410.

**Dietary and Oral:** Whether putting the oils in a capsule or drinking them in a liquid, please refer to *Application Guidelines* on page 410.

- Take 1 capsule with desired oil 2 times daily.
- Take 2-3 drops of oil in a spoonful of syrup or small amount of milk, juice, or water.

**Topical:** For guidelines on applying oils to the skin, refer to *Application Guidelines* on page 410.

- Apply 2-3 drops diluted 50:50 to forehead, temples, and back of neck.
- You may also apply 2-3 drops on the Vita Flex liver point of the right foot.

## FIBROIDS

*(See also Menstrual and Female Hormone Conditions)*

Fibroids are fairly common benign tumors of the female pelvis that are composed of smooth muscle cells and fibrous connective tissue. Fibroids are not cancerous and neither develop into cancer nor increase a woman's cancer risk in the uterus.

Fibroids can have a diameter as small as 1 mm or as large as 8 inches. They can develop in clusters or alone as a single knot or nodule.

Fibroids frequently occur in premenopausal women and are seldom seen in young women who have not begun menstruation. Fibroids usually stabilize or even regress in women who have been through menopause.

### Recommendations

**Singles:** Sacred Frankincense, Frankincense, Frankincense Vitality, Oregano, Oregano Vitality, Plectranthus Oregano, Pine, Cistus, Helichrysum, Lavender, Lavender Vitality, Geranium

**Blends:** Valor, Valor II, Valor Roll-On, EndoFlex, EndoFlex Vitality

**Nutritionals:** MultiGreens, Power Meal, Slique Shake, Balance Complete, PD 80/20, Essentialzyme, Essentialzymes-4, Life 9

**Body Care:** Cel-Lite Magic Massage Oil

### Application and Usage

**Aromatic:** Refer to *Application Guidelines* on page 410.

**Dietary and Oral:** Whether putting the oils in a capsule or drinking them in a liquid, please refer to *Application Guidelines* on page 410.

- Take 1 capsule with desired oil 2 times daily.
- Take 2-3 drops of oil in a spoonful of syrup or small amount of milk, juice, or water.

**Topical:** For guidelines on applying oils to the skin, refer to *Application Guidelines* on page 410.

Seventh Edition | **Essential Oils Desk Reference** | 475

**Essential Oils Desk Reference** | Seventh Edition

- Place a warm compress with 1-2 drops of chosen oil on the back.
- Applying a single drop under the nose is helpful and refreshing.
- Dilute 50:50 and apply on location 3-6 times daily.
- Massage 2-4 drops of oil neat on the bottoms of the feet just before bedtime.

## FIBROMYALGIA

Fibromyalgia is an autoimmune disorder of the soft tissues and appears to include problems within the pain-signaling pathways of the brain and the spinal cord. By contrast, arthritis occurs in the joints.

The symptoms of fibromyalgia include general body pain, in some places worse than others, and are usually brought on by short periods of exercise or low levels of stimulation. Diagnosis includes tenderness or pain in at least 11 of 18 specific points in muscles, tendons, and bones.

The pain is generally continuous and interrupts sleep patterns so that the fourth stage of sleep is never attained, and the body cannot rejuvenate and heal. Fibromyalgia is an acid condition in which the liver is toxic (See Liver Disorders).

The best natural remedy for fibromyalgia is to consume supplements such as flax seed and omegas, proteolytic enzymes such as bromelain and pancreatin, and MSM.

According to UCLA researcher Ronald Lawrence, MD, PhD, supplementation with MSM often offers a breakthrough in the treatment of fibromyalgia.

### Recommendations

**Singles:** Sacred Frankincense, Frankincense, Frankincense Vitality, Wintergreen, Idaho Blue Spruce, Copaiba, Copaiba Vitality, German Chamomile, German Chamomile Vitality, Nutmeg, Nutmeg Vitality, Idaho Balsam Fir

**Blends:** PanAway, Relieve It, Cool Azul, ImmuPower, Ortho Ease, Deep Relief Roll-On, Stress Away Roll-On, EndoFlex, EndoFlex Vitality

**Nutritionals:** AlkaLime, BLM, AgilEase, Sulfurzyme, Life 9, Essentialzyme, Super C, Super C Chewable, MultiGreens, ICP, ComforTone, SuperCal, Thyromin, SleepEssence, Essentialzymes-4, OmegaGize[3], EndoGize

**Body Care:** Cool Azul Pain Relief Cream, Cool Azul Sports Gel, Frankincense Gum Resin

## Application and Usage

**Aromatic:** Refer to *Application Guidelines* on page 410.

**Dietary and Oral:** Whether putting the oils in a capsule or drinking them in a liquid, please refer to *Application Guidelines* on page 410.

- Take 1-2 capsules with desired oil 2 times daily.
- Take 2-3 drops of oil in a spoonful of syrup or small amount of milk, juice, or water.

**Topical:** For guidelines on applying oils to the skin, refer to *Application Guidelines* on page 410.

- Apply a warm compress on location 3 times weekly.
- Massage into muscle tissue in a full-body massage weekly.
- Receive a Raindrop Technique and add an immune blend weekly.

## FOOD POISONING
*(See also Giardia under Digestive Problems)*

Food poisoning symptoms vary with the source and type of contamination and may include nausea, diarrhea, vomiting, congestion, coughing, abdominal pain, cramps, sore throat, and fever.

### Recommendations

**Singles:** Oregano, Oregano Vitality, Plectranthus Oregano, Thyme, Thyme Vitality, Clove, Clove Vitality, Ginger, Ginger Vitality

**Blends:** Thieves, Thieves Vitality, TummyGize, DiGize, DiGize Vitality

**Nutritionals:** Essentialzymes-4, Inner Defense, ComforTone, Digest & Cleanse, Detoxzyme, Essentialzyme, AlkaLime

**Oral Care:** Thieves Cough Drops, Thieves Hard Lozenges, Thieves Mints

### Application and Usage

**Dietary and Oral:** Whether putting the oils in a capsule or drinking them in a liquid, please refer to *Application Guidelines* on page 410.

- Take 2 capsules with desired oil 2-3 times daily.
- Take 2-3 drops of oil in a spoonful of syrup or small amount of milk, juice, or water.

Personal Usage Guide | **Chapter 20**

# FOOT CONDITIONS AND PROBLEMS

Foot problems can occur due to a variety of reasons such as injuries, medical conditions such as fungal and bacterial conditions or spurs, poorly fit shoes, or age.

## Recommendations

**Singles:** Peppermint, Lavender, Patchouli, Myrrh, Sacred Frankincense, Frankincense, Royal Hawaiian Sandalwood, Vetiver

**Blends:** Melrose, PanAway, Relieve It, Thieves, Cool Azul

**Body Care:** Cool Azul Pain Relief Cream, Cool Azul Sports Gel

## Application and Usage

**Aromatic:** Refer to *Application Guidelines* on page 410.

**Topical**: For guidelines on applying oils to the skin, refer to *Application Guidelines* on page 410.

- Dilute any of the recommended oils 50:50 and massage 6-9 drops onto each foot at night.
- Create a warm, oil-infused compress for added effect and penetration.
- Add any of the recommended oils to bath salts, mix 10 drops of essential oils per 1 tablespoon of Epsom salts, and add to hot water.

## Athlete's Foot

Athlete's foot *(Tinea pedis)* is a fungal infection of the feet. It is identical to ringworm that infects the skin elsewhere on the body (See Ringworm). This fungus thrives in a warm, moist environment.

The best remedy is to keep feet cool and dry and avoid wearing tight-fitting shoes or heavy, natural-fiber socks such as cotton. It is helpful to wear sandals, shoes, and socks woven from a light, breathable fabric.

Essential oils with antifungal properties such as Tea Tree, Melaleuca Ericifolia, and Melaleuca Quinquenervia or Melrose (a blend of Tea Tree, Melaleuca Quinquenervia, Clove, and Rosemary) can be added to bath water or Epsom salts and used in specially designed showerheads to help add antifungal protection to the water.

## Recommendations

**Singles:** Patchouli, Tea Tree, Melaleuca Ericifolia, Blue Cypress, Lemongrass (usually diluted), Lavender, Ocotea, Peppermint, Thyme, Mountain Savory, Melissa, Myrrh, Hinoki, Rosemary, Dalmatia Bay Laurel, Laurus Nobilis

**Blends:** Melrose, Thieves, Purification

**Nutritionals:** Detoxzyme, Digest & Cleanse

**Body Care:** ClaraDerm, Thieves Spray, Ortho Ease Massage Oil, Thieves Fresh Essence Plus Mouthwash on the feet

### Athlete's Foot Blend

- 8 drops Tea Tree
- 4 drops Peppermint
- 2 drops Mountain Savory
- 1 drop Myrrh

## Application and Usage

**Topical:** For guidelines on applying oils to the skin, refer to *Application Guidelines* on page 410.

- Pour ½ cup of Thieves Fresh Essence Plus Mouthwash into a pan of water for soaking the feet. It works amazingly well.

## Blisters *(See Blisters under Skin Disorders)*

## Bunions *(See also Bursitis)*

Bunions are caused from bursitis at the base of a toe and develop when the joints in the big toe no longer fit together as they should and become tender and swollen.

## Recommendations

**Singles:** Eucalyptus Radiata, Raven, Lemon, Wintergreen, Vetiver, Idaho Blue Spruce, Hinoki

**Blends:** PanAway, Cool Azul, Deep Relief Roll-On, Relieve It

**Body Care:** Cool Azul Pain Relief Cream, Cool Azul Sports Gel, Ortho Sport Massage Oil, Ortho Ease Massage Oil

### Bunion Blend

- 6 drops Eucalyptus Radiata
- 4 drops Raven
- 3 drops Lemon
- 1 drop Wintergreen
- 1 drop Vetiver

## Application and Usage

**Topical:** For guidelines on applying oils to the skin, refer to *Application Guidelines* on page 410.

- Apply 2-4 drops neat or diluted 50:50 over bunion area 2-3 times daily.

Seventh Edition | **Essential Oils Desk Reference** | 477

## Corns and Calluses

Corns and calluses are caused by friction and pressure when the bony parts of the feet rub against the shoes.

### Recommendations

**Singles:** Lavender, Helichrysum, Basil, Idaho Blue Spruce, Myrrh, Cypress, Oregano, Plectranthus Oregano, Hinoki

**Blends:** PanAway, Deep Relief Roll-On, Cool Azul, Relieve It

**Body Care:** Cool Azul Pain Relief Cream, Cool Azul Sports Gel, Ortho Sport Massage Oil, Ortho Ease Massage Oil

### Corns Blend

- 4 drops Basil
- 2 drops Myrrh
- 2 drops Cypress
- 1 drop Oregano
- 1 drop Hinoki

### Application and Usage

**Topical:** For guidelines on applying oils to the skin, refer to *Application Guidelines* on page 410.

- Apply 1 drop neat directly on the corn 2-3 times daily.

## Sore Feet

Having sore feet is very common and is usually a symptom of an underlying problem or condition. Some causes are simple and require simple fixes, while others are more complicated and require more complex treatment.

### Recommendations

**Single Oils:** Peppermint, Lavender, Patchouli, Myrrh, Sacred Frankincense, Frankincense, Royal Hawaiian Sandalwood, Vetiver, Wintergreen, German Chamomile, Idaho Blue Spruce, Copaiba, Orange

**Blends:** Melrose, PanAway, Deep Relief Roll-On, Cool Azul, Relieve It

**Personal Care:** Cool Azul Pain Relief Cream, Cool Azul Sports Gel, Ortho Sport Massage Oil, Ortho Ease Massage Oil

### Sore Feet Blend

- 5 drops Wintergreen
- 3 drops Peppermint
- 2 drops German Chamomile
- 2 drops Idaho Blue Spruce
- 1 drop Copaiba
- 1 drop Royal Hawaiian Sandalwood

### Application and Usage

**Topical:** For guidelines on applying oils to the skin, refer to *Application Guidelines* on page 410.

- Dilute 50:50 and massage 6-9 drops onto each foot at night.
- Apply a warm compress for added effect and penetration.
- Mix 10 drops essential oils in 1 tablespoon Epsom salts and add to hot water in a basin large enough for a footbath.

## FUNGAL INFECTIONS

Fungi and yeast feed on decomposing or dead tissues and exist inside our stomachs, on our skin, out on the lawn, and just about everywhere. When kept under control, the yeast and fungi populating our bodies are harmless and digest what our bodies cannot or do not use.

When we feed the naturally occurring fungi in our bodies too many simple sugars, the fungal populations can grow out of control. This condition is known as systemic candidiasis and is marked by fungi invading the blood, gastrointestinal tract, and tissues.

Reducing or eliminating simple sugars from the diet is essential to combating all fungal infections. Antibiotics should also be avoided, and alcohol is deadly.

Fungal cultures such as candida excrete large amounts of poisons called mycotoxins as part of their life cycles. These poisons in the blood flow through the liver and hopefully are digested and eliminated from the body. If there is too much poison creating a toxic overload, the body eventually weakens. These toxins can wreak enormous damage on the tissues and organs and can be an aggravating factor in many degenerative diseases such as cancer, arteriosclerosis, and diabetes.

Insufficient intake of minerals and trace minerals like magnesium, potassium, and zinc may also stimulate candida and fungal overgrowth in the body.

### Symptoms of Systemic Fungal Infection

- Fatigue/low energy
- Overweight
- Low resistance to illness
- Allergies
- Unbalanced blood sugar
- Headaches
- Irritability
- Mood swings
- Indigestion
- Colitis and ulcers
- Diarrhea/constipation
- Urinary tract infections
- Rectal or vaginal itch

---

478 | Chapter 20 | Personal Usage Guide

Personal Usage Guide | **Chapter 20**

## Recommendations

**Singles:** Melaleuca Ericifolia, Blue Cypress, Lemongrass (always dilute), Lavender, Lavender Vitality, Mastrante, Thyme, Thyme Vitality, Mountain Savory, Mountain Savory Vitality, Melissa, Myrrh, Hinoki

**Blends:** Melrose, Thieves, Thieves Vitality, Purification, DiGize, DiGize Vitality, Exodus II, Evergreen Essence

**Nutritionals:** Mineral Essence, Essentialzyme, Essentialzymes-4, Life 9, Detoxzyme, AlkaLime

**Body Care:** ClaraDerm, Thieves Spray on the skin, Thieves Fresh Essence Plus Mouthwash on the feet, Ortho Ease Massage Oil, or V-6 Vegetable Oil Complex mixed with your choice of singles or blends

## Application and Usage

**Topical:** For guidelines on applying oils to the skin, refer to *Application Guidelines* on page 410.

- Apply any of the recommended oils neat or diluted 50:50. Always dilute Lemongrass.
- Apply 5-7 drops to affected areas between toes and around toenails.
- Add any of the recommended oils to bath salts and soak affected area daily.

### Athlete's Foot *(See Athlete's Foot under Foot Conditions and Problems; see also Ringworm in this section).*

### Candida Albicans (Candidiasis)

Two of the most powerful weapons for fighting intestinal fungal infections such as candida are FOS (fructooligosaccharides) and *L. acidophilus* cultures.

FOS has been clinically documented in dozens of peer-reviewed studies for its ability to build up the healthy intestinal flora in the colon and combat the overgrowth of negative bacteria and fungi.

Acidophilus cultures have also been shown to combat fungus overgrowth in the gastrointestinal tract.

## Recommendations

**Singles:** Lemongrass, Lemongrass Vitality, Geranium, Tea Tree, Mastrante, Melaleuca Quinquenervia, Ravintsara, Thyme, Thyme Vitality, Peppermint, Peppermint Vitality, Lavender, Lavender Vitality, Rosemary, Rosemary Vitality, Palmarosa

**Blends:** Melrose, Raven, R.C., ImmuPower, Thieves, Thieves Vitality

**Nutritionals:** Detoxzyme, Life 9, Essentialzyme, Essentialzymes-4, ImmuPro, MultiGreens, Digest & Cleanse, Super C, Super C Chewable, AlkaLime

### Candida Blend

- 5 drops Lemongrass or Lemongrass Vitality
- 4 drops Thyme or Thyme Vitality
- 4 drops Tea Tree
- 2 drops Geranium

(**Note:** This blend is not recommended for those with estrogen-sensitive cancers.)

## Application and Usage

**Aromatic:** Refer to *Application Guidelines* on page 410.

**Dietary and Oral:** Whether putting the oils in a capsule or drinking them in a liquid, please refer to *Application Guidelines* on page 410.

- Take 1 capsule with desired oil 2 times daily.
- Take 2-3 drops of oil in a spoonful of syrup or small amount of milk, juice, or water.

**Topical:** For guidelines on applying oils to the skin, refer to *Application Guidelines* on page 410.

- Dilute 50:50 or 20:80, as needed, and massage 3-4 drops on thymus (at clavicle notch, center of collarbone at base of throat) to stimulate the immune system. Also apply 3-6 drops on bottoms of the feet and on the chest. Also apply 5-10 drops on stomach. Do these applications 2 times daily.
- Massage 2-4 drops on relevant Vita Flex points on feet 2-4 times daily.
- Use bath salts daily.

### Ringworm and Skin Candida

The ringworm fungus infects the skin, causing scaly, round, itchy patches. It is infectious and can be spread from an animal or human host alike.

Skin candida is a fungal infection that can erupt almost anywhere on the skin. It shows up in various places such as behind the knees, inside the elbows, behind the ears, on temple area, and between the breasts.

## Recommendations

**Singles:** Geranium, Tea Tree, Melaleuca Quinquenervia, Cypress, Lavender, Rosemary, Mastrante, Lemongrass, Lemon Myrtle, Oregano, Plectranthus Oregano, Spearmint, Peppermint, Dalmatia Bay Laurel, Laurus Nobilis

**Blends:** Melrose, Raven, R.C., Thieves, Purification

Seventh Edition | **Essential Oils Desk Reference** | 479

**Essential Oils Desk Reference** | Seventh Edition

**Body Care:** Thieves Spray, Ortho Sport Massage Oil, Ortho Ease Massage Oil

**Ringworm Blend**
- 3 drops Tea Tree
- 3 drops Spearmint
- 1 drop Peppermint
- 1 drop Rosemary

**Skin Candida Blend**
- 10 drops Tea Tree
- 4 drops Lavender
- 2 drops Geranium
- 1 drop Oregano or Plectranthus Oregano

## Application and Usage

**Topical:** For guidelines on applying oils to the skin, refer to *Application Guidelines* on page 410.

- Dilute 50:50 and massage 2-4 drops over affected area 2-4 times daily. In severe cases, use 35 percent food-grade hydrogen peroxide to clean infected areas before applying essential oils. Saturate a gauze pad with essential oils, apply to affected area, and wrap to hold in place.

## Thrush

Thrush is a fungal infection of the mouth and throat marked by creamy, curd-like patches in the oral cavity. Even though it appears in the mouth, thrush is usually a sign of systemic fungal overgrowth throughout the body. Thrush can usually be treated locally through the use of antifungal essential oils such as Clove Vitality, Cinnamon Bark Vitality, Rosemary Vitality, or Peppermint Vitality.

## Recommendations

**Singles:** Clove, Clove Vitality, Cinnamon Bark, Cinnamon Bark Vitality, Peppermint, Peppermint Vitality, Rosemary, Rosemary Vitality, Mastrante, Geranium, Orange, Orange Vitality, Lavender, Lavender Vitality

**Blends:** Melrose, Thieves, Thieves Vitality, Inner Defense, Purification

**Oral Care:** Thieves Hard Lozenges, Thieves Fresh Essence Plus Mouthwash, Thieves Spray

## Application and Usage

**Aromatic:** Refer to *Application Guidelines* on page 410.

**Dietary and Oral:** Whether putting the oils in a capsule or drinking them in a liquid, please refer to *Application Guidelines* on page 410.

- Take 1 capsule with desired oil 2-3 times daily between meals.

- Take 2-3 drops of oil in a spoonful of syrup or small amount of milk, juice, or water.
- Gargle 3-5 times daily with Thieves Fresh Essence Plus Mouthwash.

**Note:** These applications are for adults, not infants. In cases of infants with thrush, consult a medical professional first.

**Topical:** For guidelines on applying oils to the skin, refer to *Application Guidelines* on page 410.

- Dilute 50:50 or 20:80 as needed and massage 3-4 drops on the thymus (at clavicle notch, center of collarbone at base of throat) to stimulate the immune system. Also apply 3-6 drops on the bottoms of the feet and on the chest. Also apply 5-10 drops on the stomach. Do these applications 2 times daily.
- Massage 2-4 drops on relevant Vita Flex points on the bottoms of the feet 2-4 times daily.

## Vaginal Yeast Infection

Vaginal yeast infections are usually caused from overgrowth of fungi like *Candida albicans*. These naturally occurring intestinal yeast and fungi are normally kept under control by the immune system, but when excess sucrose is consumed or antibiotics are used, these organisms convert from relatively harmless yeast into an invasive, harmful fungus that secretes toxins as part of its life cycle.

Vaginal yeast infections are just one symptom of systemic fungal infestation. While the yeast infection can be treated locally, the underlying problem of systemic candidiasis may still remain, unless specific Dietary and Oral and health practices are used.

Diet and cleansing are two major factors in overcoming this problem. Sugar, milk products, breads, and medications such as antibiotics all contribute to the growth of candida. A cleansing program should be considered with various supplements and essential oils (See chapter on Cleansing).

## Recommendations

**Singles:** Tea Tree, Myrrh, Melissa, Oregano, Oregano Vitality, Plectranthus Oregano, Thyme, Thyme Vitality, Mastrante, Rosemary, Rosemary Vitality, Palo Santo, Mountain Savory, Mountain Savory Vitality, Idaho Blue Spruce, Hinoki

**Blends:** Melrose, Thieves, Exodus II, Purification, 3 Wise Men, Inspiration

**Nutritionals:** ICP (a.m.), JuvaPower (p.m.), Comfor-Tone, Detoxzyme, Essentialzyme, Essentialzymes-4, Life 9 (for 60 days)

480 | **Chapter 20** | Personal Usage Guide

**Body Care:** ClaraDerm

**Vaginal Yeast Infection Blend**
- 7 drops Tea Tree
- 5 drops Mountain Savory
- 2 drops Myrrh

## Application and Usage

**Dietary and Oral:** Whether putting the oils in a capsule or drinking them in a liquid, please refer to *Application Guidelines* on page 410.

- Take 1 capsule with desired oil 2-3 times daily between meals.
- Take 2-3 drops of oil in a spoonful of syrup or small amount of milk, juice, or water.
- Stop eating sugar.

**Retention**
- Mix an 80:20 ratio (8 parts chosen essential oil to 2 parts V-6 Vegetable Oil Complex), put 1-2 tablespoons on a tampon, and insert into the vagina daily for internal infection.
- Alternate approach: Douche with 1 tablespoon Thieves Fresh Essence Plus Mouthwash overnight 3 times a week. If it stings a little, dilute with a little V-6 Vegetable Oil Complex.

## GALLBLADDER INFECTION (Cholecystitis)

The gallbladder stores the bile created by the liver and releases it through the biliary ducts into the duodenum to promote digestion. Bile is extremely important for fat digestion and the absorption of vitamins A, D, and E.

When the bile flow is obstructed due to gallstones or inflamed due to infection, serious consequences can ensue, including poor digestion, jaundice, and severe abdominal pain.

### Recommendations

**Singles:** Carrot Seed, Carrot Seed Vitality, Jade Lemon, Jade Lemon Vitality, Lemon, Lemon Vitality, Lime, Lime Vitality, Cistus, Myrrh, Ledum, Hyssop, Juniper, German Chamomile, Oregano, Oregano Vitality, Plectranthus Oregano, Cumin

**Blends:** GLF, GLF Vitality, Thieves, Thieves Vitality, Citrus Fresh, JuvaFlex, JuvaFlex Vitality, JuvaCleanse, JuvaCleanse Vitality, PanAway, DiGize, DiGize Vitality

**Nutritionals:** Inner Defense, Sulfurzyme, JuvaTone, Essentialzyme, Essentialzymes-4, Longevity Softgels, Life 9

## Application and Usage

**Topical:** For guidelines on applying oils to the skin, refer to *Application Guidelines* on page 410.

- Apply 6-10 drops of any of the recommended oils or oil blends over gallbladder area 2-3 times daily.
- Apply a warm, oil-infused compress over gallbladder area 2-3 times daily.
- Apply 1-3 drops of suggested oils over liver and use Vita Flex massage.
- Use Vita Flex massage on the feet 2-3 times daily.

## GALLSTONES

When bile contains excessive cholesterol, bilirubin, or bile salts, gallstones can form. Stones made from hardened cholesterol account for the vast majority of gallstones, while stones made from bilirubin, the brownish pigment in bile, constitute only about 20 percent of gallstones.

Gallstones can block both bile flow and the passage of pancreatic enzymes. This can result in inflammation in the gallbladder (cholecystitis), pancreas (pancreatitis), and jaundice. In some cases, gallstones can be life threatening, depending on where they are lodged.

Several Japanese studies show that limonene, a key constituent in orange, lemon, and tangerine oils, can effectively dissolve gallstones with no negative side effects.[22, 23]

### Recommendations

**Singles:** Carrot Seed, Carrot Seed Vitality, Jade Lemon, Jade Lemon Vitality, Lemon, Lemon Vitality, Lime, Lime Vitality, Helichrysum, Sacred Frankincense, Frankincense, Frankincense Vitality, Orange, Orange Vitality, Grapefruit, Grapefruit Vitality, Mandarin, Tangerine, Tangerine Vitality, Juniper, Rosemary, Rosemary Vitality, Idaho Balsam Fir

**Blends:** GLF, GLF Vitality, Citrus Fresh, Citrus Fresh Vitality, JuvaCleanse, JuvaCleanse Vitality

**Nutritionals:** Essentialzyme, Essentialzymes-4, Life 9, JuvaPower, JuvaSpice, ComforTone, ICP, JuvaTone

## Application and Usage

**Dietary and Oral:** Whether putting the oils in a capsule or drinking them in a liquid, please refer to *Application Guidelines* on page 410.

- Take 1 capsule with desired oil 2 times daily for 2 weeks.
- Take 2-3 drops of oil in a spoonful of syrup or small amount of milk, juice, or water.

**Topical:** For guidelines on applying oils to the skin, refer to *Application Guidelines* on page 410.

- Dilute 50:50 and massage 6-10 drops over gallbladder 2 times daily.
- Apply a compress 2-3 times daily.
- You may also apply 1-3 drops on the Vita Flex liver and digestive points of the right foot 2-3 times daily.

## GANGRENE

**Note:** As with all serious medical conditions, consult your health care professional immediately if you suspect gangrene.

Gangrene is the death or decay of living tissue caused by a lack of blood supply. A shortage of blood can result from a blood clot, arteriosclerosis, frostbite, diabetes, infection, or some other obstruction in the arterial blood supply. Gas gangrene, also known as acute or moist gangrene, occurs when tissues are infected with clostridium bacteria. Unless the body is given antibiotics to treat the disease or the limb is amputated, gangrene can be fatal.

The part of the body affected by gangrene displays the following symptoms:

- Coldness
- Dark in color or even black
- Looks rotten or decomposed
- Putrid smell
- Fever
- Anemia

Dr. René Gattefossé suffered gas gangrene as a result of burns from a chemical explosion at the turn of the century. He successfully engineered his own recovery solely with the use of pure lavender oil.

### Recommendations

**Singles:** Myrrh, Lavender, Thyme, Peppermint, Oregano, Plectranthus Oregano, Rosemary, Sacred Frankincense, Frankincense, Mountain Savory, Cistus, Cypress, Vetiver, Copaiba

**Blends:** Exodus II, Thieves, ImmuPower, Melrose

**Nutritionals:** Super C, Super C Chewable, Inner Defense, ImmuPro, Mineral Essence, Essentialzyme, Essentialzymes-4, MultiGreens, Detoxzyme

### Application and Usage

**Topical:** For guidelines on applying oils to the skin, refer to *Application Guidelines* on page 410.

- Apply 2-4 drops diluted 20:80 on the affected area 3-5 times daily.
- Apply a warm compress 3 times daily every other day.

## GASTRITIS

Gastritis occurs when the stomach's mucosal lining becomes inflamed and the cells become eroded. This can lead to bleeding ulcers and severe digestive disturbances. Gastritis is caused by excess acid production in the stomach, alcohol consumption, stress, and fungal or bacterial infections.

Symptoms of gastritis are weight loss, abdominal pain, and cramping.

### Recommendations

**Singles:** Peppermint, Peppermint Vitality, Jade Lemon, Jade Lemon Vitality, Lemon, Lemon Vitality, Lime, Lime Vitality, Fennel, Fennel Vitality, Patchouli, Tarragon, Tarragon Vitality, Spearmint, Spearmint Vitality

**Blends:** DiGize, DiGize Vitality, Purification, JuvaCleanse, JuvaCleanse Vitality, TummyGize, Slique Essence

**Nutritionals:** AlkaLime, Essentialzymes-4, Essentialzyme, Detoxzyme, Life 9, Digest & Cleanse, Balance Complete

### Application and Usage

**Dietary and Oral:** Whether putting the oils in a capsule or drinking them in a liquid, please refer to *Application Guidelines* on page 410.

- Take 1 capsule with desired oil 2 times daily.
- Take 2-3 drops of oil in a spoonful of syrup or small amount of milk, juice, or water.

**Supplementation regimen for gastritis:**

- **AlkaLime:** Take ½ teaspoon each morning.
- **Essentialzymes-4:** Take 3-4 yellow capsules 3 times daily.
- **ComforTone and ICP:** Begin after 2 weeks of using the products listed above.
- **MegaCal:** Take 1 tablespoon each morning in 8 oz. warm water.

## GOUT *(See also Joint Stiffness/Pain)*

Gout is a disease marked by abrupt, temporary bouts of joint pain and swelling that are most evident in the joint of the big toe. It can also affect the wrist, elbow, knee, ankle, hand, and foot. As the disease progresses, pain and swelling in the joints become more frequent and chronic, with deposits called tophi appearing over many joints, including on the elbows and strangely on the ears.

Personal Usage Guide | **Chapter 20**

Ears are a body extremity, colder, with slower blood circulation. All are factors to attract gout attacks. If you have ear tophi, you almost certainly have chronic gout.

Gout is characterized by accumulation of uric acid crystals in the joints caused by excess uric acid in the blood. Uric acid is a byproduct of the breakdown of protein that is normally excreted by the kidneys into the urine. To reduce uric acid concentrations, it is necessary to support the kidneys, adrenals, and immune functions. It is also necessary to detoxify by cleansing and drinking plenty of fluids.

Excess alcohol, allergy-producing foods, or strict diets can cause outbreaks of gout. Foods rich in purines such as wine, anchovies, and animal liver can also cause gout.

## Recommendations

**Singles:** Juniper, Helichrysum, Dalmatia Juniper, Jade Lemon, Jade Lemon Vitality, Lemon, Lemon Vitality, Lime, Lime Vitality, Idaho Blue Spruce, Roman Chamomile, Tea Tree, Sacred Frankincense, Frankincense, Frankincense Vitality

**Blend:** GLF, GLF Vitality, JuvaCleanse, JuvaCleanse Vitality, Cool Azul

**Nutritionals:** AlkaLime, BLM, AgilEase, MultiGreens, ICP (a.m.), ComforTone, Essentialzyme, JuvaPower (p.m.), JuvaTone

**Body Care:** Cool Azul Pain Relief Cream, Cool Azul Sports Gel, Ortho Ease Massage Oil, Ortho Sport Massage Oil

### Gout Blend
- 10 drops Lemon
- 5 drops Idaho Blue Spruce
- 4 drops Juniper
- 3 drops Tea Tree
- 2 drops Roman Chamomile

## Application and Usage

**Dietary and Oral:** Whether putting the oils in a capsule or drinking them in a liquid, please refer to *Application Guidelines* on page 410.

- Take 1 capsule with desired oil 1 time daily for 10 days, rest 4 days, repeat as needed.
- Take 2-3 drops of oil in a spoonful of syrup or small amount of milk, juice, or water.

**Topical:** For guidelines on applying oils to the skin, refer to *Application Guidelines* on page 410.

- Gently massage 1-3 drops neat on affected joints 2-3 times daily.

# HAIR AND SCALP PROBLEMS

Sulfur is the single most important mineral for maintaining the strength and integrity of the hair and hair follicle.

## Recommendations

**Singles:** Lavender, Lavender Vitality, Cedarwood (dry scalp), Peppermint (oily scalp), Peppermint Vitality, Rosemary, Rosemary Vitality, Clary Sage, Sage, Sage Vitality, Basil, Basil Vitality, Juniper, Dalmatia Juniper, Ylang Ylang, Royal Hawaiian Sandalwood, Geranium, Lemon, Lemon Vitality, Cypress, Patchouli

**Blends:** Melrose, Thieves, Thieves Vitality, Citrus Fresh, Citrus Fresh Vitality, Purification, Inspiration, The Gift

**Nutritionals:** Sulfurzyme, AlkaLime, Super B, Pure Protein Complete, Essentialzymes-4, Essentialzyme, Balance Complete

**Hair Care:** Lavender Mint Daily Shampoo, Lavender Mint Daily Conditioner, Copaiba Vanilla Moisturizing Shampoo, Copaiba Vanilla Moisturizing Conditioner, Lavender Shampoo, Lavender Conditioner

### Dry Scalp Blend
- 6 drops Cedarwood
- 4 drops Lavender
- 2 drops Royal Hawaiian Sandalwood or Geranium
- 2 drops Patchouli

### Oily Scalp Blend
- 6 drops Peppermint
- 4 drops Lemon
- 2 drops Lavender

### Scalp Rinse Blend to Restore Acid Mantle
- 1 drop Rosemary
- 1 teaspoon pure apple cider vinegar
- 8 oz. water

Rub 1-2 drops of oil on hair to prevent static electricity.

## Application and Usage

**Dietary and Oral:** Whether putting the oils in a capsule or drinking them in a liquid, please refer to *Application Guidelines* on page 410.

- Take 1 capsule with desired oil 2 times daily.
- Take 2-3 drops of oil in a spoonful of syrup or small amount of milk, juice, or water.

**Topical:** For guidelines on applying oils to the skin, refer to *Application Guidelines* on page 410.

- Apply 1 teaspoon diluted 20:80 onto the scalp and rub vigorously for 2-3 minutes. Leave on scalp for 60-90 minutes.

Seventh Edition | **Essential Oils Desk Reference** | 483

**Essential Oils Desk Reference** | Seventh Edition

- Mix 2-4 drops of essential oils with 1-2 teaspoons of shampoo to wash hair after exercising.

## Baldness/Hair Loss (Alopecia Areata)

Male pattern baldness is often a result of hormonal imbalances such as excess conversion of testosterone to dihydrotestosterone through the enzyme 5-alpha reductase. It can also be caused by an inflammatory condition called alopecia areata.

Alopecia is an inflammatory hair loss disease that is the second-leading cause of baldness in the U.S. A double-blind study conducted at the Aberdeen Royal Infirmary in Scotland found that certain essential oils were extremely effective in combating this disease.[24]

Essential oils are excellent for cleansing, nourishing, and strengthening the hair follicle and shaft. Rosemary (cineole chemotype) encourages hair growth. The Arabian people for centuries have used frankincense resin water to rinse their hair and massage their scalp to maintain a healthy head of hair and stimulate regrowth.

Thyroid balance also prevents hair loss.

### Recommendations

**Singles:** Lavender, Lavender Vitality, Cypress, Sacred Frankincense, Frankincense, Frankincense Vitality, Peppermint, Peppermint Vitality, Canadian Fleabane (Conyza), Royal Hawaiian Sandalwood, Black Pepper, Black Pepper Vitality, Rosemary, Rosemary Vitality, Thyme, Thyme Vitality, Cedarwood, Juniper, Dalmatia Juniper, Eucalyptus Blue, Palo Santo, Clary Sage

**Blends:** Melrose, Longevity, Longevity Vitality, Mister, M-Grain, Transformation, JuvaCleanse, JuvaCleanse Vitality

**Nutritionals:** Prostate Health, PD 80/20, EndoGize, Master Formula, Sulfurzyme, Balance Complete, Mineral Essence, Essentialzyme, Essentialzymes-4, Allerzyme, Thyromin

### Hair Loss Prevention Blend No. 1
- 10 drops Cedarwood
- 10 drops Royal Hawaiian Sandalwood
- 10 drops Lavender or Lavender Vitality
- 8 drops Rosemary or Rosemary Vitality
- 1 drop Juniper or Juniper Vitality

### Hair Loss Prevention Blend No. 2
- 5 drops Lavender or Lavender Vitality
- 4 drops Cypress
- 3 drops Rosemary or Rosemary Vitality
- 2 drops Clary Sage
- 2 drops Palo Santo

### Hair Loss Prevention Blend No. 3
- 5 drops Lavender or Lavender Vitality
- 5 drops Sacred Frankincense, Frankincense, or Frankincense Vitality
- 2 drops Clary Sage
- 3 drops Eucalyptus Blue
- 1 drop Peppermint or Peppermint Vitality

### Hair Loss Prevention Blend No. 4
- 4 drops Rosemary or Rosemary Vitality
- 4 drops Thyme or Thyme Vitality
- 4 drops Lavender or Lavender Vitality
- 4 drops Cedarwood
- 2 drops Sacred Frankincense, Frankincense, or Frankincense Vitality

## Application and Usage

**Dietary and Oral:** Whether putting the oils in a capsule or drinking them in a liquid, please refer to *Application Guidelines* on page 410.

- Take 1 capsule with desired oil 2 times daily.
- Take 2-3 drops of oil in a spoonful of syrup or small amount of milk, juice, or water.

**Topical:** For guidelines on applying oils to the skin, refer to *Application Guidelines* on page 410.

- Dilute 50:50 oil of choice and V-6 Vegetable Oil Complex and massage 1 teaspoon into scalp vigorously and thoroughly for 2-3 minutes before retiring.
- Dilute 5 drops of your essential oil in 20 drops of V-6 Vegetable Oil Complex, grape seed oil, or coconut oil and massage into scalp before going to bed.
- Add 10 drops of any of the above blends to 1 teaspoon of coconut oil and massage into the scalp where it is balding; then rub gently into the remainder of the scalp. This works best when done at night. It may also help to alternate blends.
- Mix 2-4 drops of essential oils with 1-2 teaspoons of shampoo. Massage into the scalp vigorously and thoroughly for 2-3 minutes and then leave the shampoo on the scalp for 15 minutes. This is an excellent time to do an exercise routine. Rinse hair afterward.

## Dandruff

Dandruff may be caused by allergies, parasites (fungal), and/or chemicals. The mineral selenium has been shown to help prevent dandruff.

Tea Tree has been shown to be effective in treating dandruff and other fungal infections.[25]

Personal Usage Guide | Chapter 20

## Recommendations

**Singles:** Tea Tree, Lemon, Cedarwood, Lavender, Rosemary, Peppermint, Copaiba, Eucalyptus Blue, Sacred Frankincense, Frankincense, Vetiver, Dorado Azul

**Blends:** Citrus Fresh, Melrose, Thieves, The Gift

**Nutritionals:** Mineral Essence, NingXia Red

**Hair Care:** Lavender Mint Daily Shampoo, Lavender Mint Daily Conditioner, Copaiba Vanilla Moisturizing Shampoo, Copaiba Vanilla Moisturizing Conditioner, Lavender Shampoo, Lavender Conditioner

### Dandruff Blend
- 5 drops Lemon
- 2 drops Lavender
- 2 drops Peppermint
- 1 drop Rosemary

## Application and Usage

**Topical:** For guidelines on applying oils to the skin, refer to *Application Guidelines* on page 410.

- Add a few drops of a single oil or blend to your shampoo and massage it into your scalp or add a few drops of the oils of your choice to the Bath & Shower Gel Base for your own custom shampoo.
- Apply 1 teaspoon of the shampoo mixture to the scalp and rub vigorously for 2-3 minutes and then leave shampoo on scalp for 15 minutes. Mix 2-4 drops of the essential oils with 1 teaspoon shampoo to wash hair afterward.

**Dietary and Oral:** Whether putting the oils in a capsule or drinking them in a liquid, please refer to *Application Guidelines* on page 410.

- Take 1 dropper of Mineral Essence and 2 ounces of NingXia Red in water in the morning.

## HALITOSIS (BAD BREATH) *(See also Oral Care, Teeth and Gums; Candida; Fungal Infections)*

Persistent bad breath or gum disease may be a sign of poor digestion, candida, yeast infestation, or other health problems.

## Recommendations

**Singles:** Clove, Clove Vitality, Peppermint, Peppermint Vitality, Jade Lemon, Jade Lemon Vitality, Lemon, Lemon Vitality, Lime, Lime Vitality, Tea Tree, Spearmint, Spearmint Vitality, Mandarin, Cinnamon Bark, Cinnamon Bark Vitality, Rosemary, Rosemary Vitality, Wintergreen, Ocotea

**Blends:** Thieves, Thieves Vitality, Melrose, Purification, TummyGize, DiGize, DiGize Vitality, Slique Essence

**Nutritionals:** Detoxzyme, Allerzyme, Digest & Cleanse, Mineral Essence, Life 9, ICP, ComforTone, Slique Gum

**Oral Care:** Thieves AromaBright Toothpaste, Thieves Dentarome Plus Toothpaste, Thieves Dentarome Ultra Toothpaste, Thieves Spray, Thieves Hard Lozenges, Thieves Mints, KidScents Slique Toothpaste, Thieves Dental Floss, Thieves Mints, Thieves Cough Drops

### Bad Breath Blend No. 1
- 3 drops Peppermint Vitality
- 2 drops Lemon Vitality
- 2 drops Clove Vitality
- 1 drop Tea Tree

### Bad Breath Blend No. 2
- 4 drops Spearmint Vitality
- 2 drops Mandarin
- 2 drops Cinnamon Bark Vitality

## Application and Usage

**Dietary and Oral:** Whether putting the oils in a capsule or drinking them in a liquid, please refer to *Application Guidelines* on page 410.

- Take 1 capsule with desired oil 2 times daily.
- Take 2-3 drops of oil in a spoonful of syrup or small amount of milk, juice, or water.
- Dilute essential oils and blends in 2 teaspoons of Blue Agave nectar and 4 oz. of hot water. Gargle as needed (2-4 times daily).

**Topical:** For guidelines on applying oils to the skin, refer to *Application Guidelines* on page 410.

- Swab 4-8 drops of the singles or blends above diluted 50:50 inside cheeks and on tongue, gums, and teeth 2-4 times daily as needed.

## HEADACHE *(See Stress, Hypoglycemia, Liver Disorders, Menstrual and Female Hormone Conditions)*

Headaches are usually caused by hormone imbalances, circulatory problems, stress, sugar imbalance (hypoglycemia), structural (spinal) misalignments, and blood pressure concerns.

Placebo-controlled, double-blind, crossover studies at the Christian-Albrecht University in Kiel, Germany, found that essential oils (particularly peppermint alone and in combination with eucalyptus) were just as effective in blocking pain from tension-type headaches as acetaminophen (i.e., Tylenol®).[26, 27]

Seventh Edition | **Essential Oils Desk Reference** | 485

Essential oils also promote circulation, reduce muscle spasms, and decrease inflammatory response.

## Recommendations

**Singles:** Peppermint, Peppermint Vitality, Clove, Clove Vitality, Copaiba, Copaiba Vitality, Eucalyptus Globulus, Eucalyptus Blue, Dorado Azul, Mastrante, German Chamomile, German Chamomile Vitality, Lavender, Lavender Vitality, Myrrh, Roman Chamomile, Rosemary, Rosemary Vitality, Spearmint, Spearmint Vitality, Valerian, Wintergreen

**Blends:** Brain Power, Clarity, GeneYus, Deep Relief Roll-On, M-Grain, PanAway, Stress Away Roll-On, Relieve It, R.C., Raven, Tranquil Roll-On

**Body Care:** Prenolone Plus Body Cream, Progessence Plus

### General Headache Blend No. 1
- 4 drops Wintergreen
- 3 drops German Chamomile or German Chamomile Vitality
- 2 drops Lavender or Lavender Vitality
- 2 drops Copaiba or Copaiba Vitality
- 1 drop Clove or Clove Vitality

### General Headache Blend No. 2
- 6 drops Peppermint or Peppermint Vitality
- 4 drops Eucalyptus Globulus
- 2 drops Myrrh

## Application and Usage

**Aromatic:** Refer to *Application Guidelines* on page 410.

**Dietary and Oral:** Whether putting the oils in a capsule or drinking them in a liquid, please refer to *Application Guidelines* on page 410.

- Take 1 capsule with desired oil 2 times daily.
- Place 1 drop on the tongue and then push it against the roof of the mouth.
- Take 2-3 drops of oil in a spoonful of syrup or small amount of milk, juice, or water.

**Topical:** For guidelines on applying oils to the skin, refer to *Application Guidelines* on page 410.

- Dilute 50:50 and apply 1-3 drops on the back of the neck, behind the ears, on the temples, on the forehead, and under the nose. Be careful to keep away from eyes and eyelids.
- Massage 2-4 drops of oil neat on the bottoms of the feet just before bedtime.
- Place a warm compress with 1-2 drops of chosen oil on the back.

## Migraine (Vascular-type Headache)

The vast majority of migraine headaches may be due to colon congestion or poor digestion. The combination of ICP, ComforTone, and Essentialzyme is most important for cleansing the colon. Eyestrain and decreased vision can accompany migraine headaches. Dried wolfberries contain large amounts of lutein and zeaxanthin, which are vital for healthy vision.

## Recommendations

**Singles:** Basil, Copaiba, Eucalyptus Globulus, Mastrante, German Chamomile, Helichrysum, Lavender, Marjoram, Peppermint, Rosemary, Wintergreen

**Blends:** M-Grain, Thieves, Clarity, PanAway, The Gift, R.C., Raven, Stress Away Roll-On, Tranquil Roll-On

**Nutritionals:** Essentialzyme, Essentialzymes-4, NingXia Red, Balance Complete, ComforTone, Ningxia Wolfberries (Organic, Dried), ICP, MegaCal

## Application and Usage

**Aromatic:** Refer to *Application Guidelines* on page 410.

**Topical:** For guidelines on applying oils to the skin, refer to *Application Guidelines* on page 410.

- Apply 1-2 drops neat to temples, at the base of the neck, in the center of the forehead, and at the nostril openings. Also massage on thumbs and big toes.
- Place a warm compress with 1-2 drops of chosen oil on the back of the neck or on the back.

## Sinus Headache (See also Sinus Infections)

Signs and symptoms of migraines and sinus headaches can be confused. With both kinds, the pain often gets worse when you bend forward and can be accompanied by various nasal signs and symptoms. However, sinus headaches are usually not associated with nausea or vomiting or aggravated by bright light or noise, which are common features of migraines.

## Recommendations

**Singles:** Dorado Azul, Peppermint, Eucalyptus Blue, Eucalyptus Radiata, Tea Tree, Mastrante, Geranium, Lavender, Rosemary

**Blends:** R.C., Breathe Again Roll-On, SniffleEase, Melrose, Purification, Raven, RutaVaLa, RutaVaLa Roll-On, Stress Away Roll-On

**Nutritionals:** Super C, Super C Chewable, ImmuPro, Mineral Essence, Detoxzyme

486 | Chapter 20 | Personal Usage Guide

**Sinus Headache Blend**
- 9 drops Rosemary
- 5 drops Tea Tree
- 4 drops Geranium
- 3 drops Peppermint
- 2 drops Eucalyptus Blue
- 2 drops Lavender

## Application and Usage

**Aromatic:** Refer to *Application Guidelines* on page 410.

**Topical:** For guidelines on applying oils to the skin, refer to *Application Guidelines* on page 410.

- Apply 1-2 drops neat or diluted 2-5 times daily or as needed.
- Massage 2-4 drops neat on the bottoms of the feet just before bedtime.

### Tension (Stress) Headache *(See also Stress)*

Tension headaches are the most common type of headaches among adults and are commonly referred to as stress headaches. They are usually triggered by some type of internal or environmental stress. In some people tension headaches are caused by tightened muscles in the scalp and in the back of the neck and may be caused by anxiety, fatigue, overexertion, hunger, inadequate rest, poor posture, mental or emotional stress, or depression.

## Recommendations

**Singles:** Valerian, Cardamom, Cardamom Vitality, Tangerine, Tangerine Vitality, Jasmine, Palmarosa, Mastrante, Geranium, Sacred Frankincense, Frankincense, Frankincense Vitality, Peppermint, Peppermint Vitality, Lavender, Lavender Vitality, Roman Chamomile, Bergamot, Bergamot Vitality

**Blends:** Divine Release, Evergreen Essence, Freedom, Valor, Valor II, Aroma Siez, M-Grain, Peace & Calming, Peace & Calming II, Hope, Sacred Mountain, Trauma Life, T.R. Care, Inner Harmony, InTouch, Reconnect, SleepyIze, PanAway, Stress Away Roll-On, RutaVaLa, RutaVaLa Roll-On, Tranquil Roll-On, Valor, Valor II, Valor Roll-On

**Nutritionals:** MegaCal, Essentialzymes-4, Balance Complete, NingXia Red, Mineral Essence, ICP, ComforTone, SleepEssence, Essentialzyme, PowerGize

## Application and Usage

**Aromatic:** Refer to *Application Guidelines* on page 410.

**Topical:** For guidelines on applying oils to the skin, refer to *Application Guidelines* on page 410.

- Apply 1-2 drops diluted 50:50 around the hairline, on the back of the neck, and across the forehead. Be careful not to use too much, as it will burn if any oil drips near the eyes. If this should occur, dilute with a pure vegetable oil—never with water.

# HEAVY METALS

We absorb heavy metals from air, water, food, skin care products, mercury fillings in teeth, etc. These chemicals lodge in the fatty tissues of the body, which, in turn, give off toxic gases that may cause allergic symptoms. Cleansing the body of these heavy metals is extremely important to have a healthy immune function, especially if one has amalgam fillings. Drink at least 64 ounces of distilled water daily to flush toxins and chemicals out of the body (see Circulation).

## Recommendations

**Singles:** Helichrysum, Jade Lemon, Jade Lemon Vitality, Lemon, Lemon Vitality, Lime, Lime Vitality, Orange, Orange Vitality, Tangerine, Tangerine Vitality, Clove, Clove Vitality, Patchouli

**Blends:** GLF, GLF Vitality, Thieves, Thieves Vitality, JuvaCleanse, JuvaCleanse Vitality, DiGize, DiGize Vitality

**Nutritionals:** MultiGreens, Detoxzyme, Essentialzyme, ComforTone, MegaCal, JuvaPower, Super C, Super C Chewable, Mineral Essence, Life 9, ICP

## Aluminum Toxicity

Aluminum is a very toxic metal that can cause serious neurological damage in the human body—even in minute amounts. Aluminum has been implicated as a possible cause of many maladies in the body, especially Alzheimer's disease.

People unwittingly ingest aluminum from their cookware, beverage cans, antacids, and even deodorants and other cosmetic compounds. The first step toward reducing aluminum toxicity in the body is to avoid these types of aluminum-based products. Read the labels and see for yourself.

## Recommendations

**Singles:** Helichrysum, Jade Lemon, Jade Lemon Vitality, Lemon, Lemon Vitality, Lime, Lime Vitality, Orange, Orange Vitality, Tangerine, Tangerine Vitality, Clove, Clove Vitality, Patchouli

**Blends:** GLF, GLF Vitality, Thieves, Thieves Vitality, JuvaCleanse, JuvaCleanse Vitality, DiGize, DiGize Vitality

**Nutritionals:** JuvaTone, ICP (a.m.), Detoxzyme, Essentialzyme, MegaCal, ComforTone, JuvaPower (p.m.)

## Application and Usage

**Aromatic:** Refer to *Application Guidelines* on page 410.

**Dietary and Oral:** Whether putting the oils in a capsule or drinking them in a liquid, please refer to *Application Guidelines* on page 410.

- Begin by cleansing the liver, blood, and colon to rid the body of toxins and waste.
- Take 1 capsule with desired oil 2 times daily.
- Take 2-3 drops of oil in a spoonful of syrup or small amount of milk, juice, or water.

**Topical:** For guidelines on applying oils to the skin, refer to *Application Guidelines* on page 410.

## HEMORRHOIDS

Symptoms of hemorrhoids are bleeding during bowel movements, rectal pain, and itching.

### Recommendations

**Singles:** Myrrh, Helichrysum, Cypress, Cistus, Basil, Basil Vitality, Jade Lemon, Jade Lemon Vitality, Lemon, Lemon Vitality, Lime, Lime Vitality, Peppermint, Peppermint Vitality

**Blends:** Melrose, Purification, Aroma Siez, Aroma Life, PanAway

**Nutritionals:** Essentialzymes-4, MultiGreens, Longevity Softgels, MegaCal, Digest & Cleanse, ICP, ComforTone, Essentialzyme, JuvaPower

**Body Care:** Rose Ointment, KidScents Tender Tush

### Hemorrhoid Blend No. 1
- 4 drops Basil
- 1 drop Cistus
- 1 drop Cypress
- 1 drop Helichrysum

Mix with Rose Ointment for dilution and easier application.

### Hemorrhoid Blend No. 2
- 4 drops Myrrh
- 3 drops Cypress
- 2 drops Helichrysum

Mix with Rose Ointment for dilution and easier application.

## Application and Usage

**Dietary and Oral:** Whether putting the oils in a capsule or drinking them in a liquid, please refer to *Application Guidelines* on page 410.

- Take 1 capsule with desired oil 2 times daily.
- Take 2-3 drops of oil in a spoonful of syrup or small amount of milk, juice, or water.

**Topical:m** For guidelines on applying oils to the skin, refer to *Application Guidelines* on page 410.

- Apply single oils or blends neat or diluted, depending on the oils that are used.
- Use a rectal implant of your choice of the above formulas; place in rectum with a small syringe 1 time every other day for 6 days. It is best done at night to be able to retain as long as possible.
- Apply 3-5 drops diluted 50:50 on location. This may sting but usually brings relief with 1 or 2 applications.

## HICCUPS

People have been curious about the cause of hiccups for years. There are many ideas, but scientifically, everyone is still waiting for an explanation. Some say hiccups are caused by irritated nerves of the diaphragm, possibly from eating too much or from indigestion.

One technique that often works for stopping hiccups is to put 1 drop of Cypress and 1 drop of Tarragon on the end of the index finger and then place that finger on the neck against the esophagus in the clavicle notch in the center, curl inward and down like you are curling down inside the throat, and release.

Tarragon or Cypress applied topically or taken as a Dietary and Oral supplement may relax intestinal spasms, nervous digestion, and hiccups. It's worth a try.

### Recommendations

**Singles:** Carrot Seed, Carrot Seed Vitality, Tarragon, Tarragon Vitality, Cypress, Spearmint, Peppermint, Peppermint Vitality

**Blends:** DiGize, DiGize Vitality, JuvaFlex, JuvaFlex Vitality, TummyGize

**Nutritionals:** AlkaLime, Digest & Cleanse, MegaCal

### Application and Usage

**Dietary and Oral:** Whether putting the oils in a capsule or drinking them in a liquid, please refer to *Application Guidelines* on page 410.

- Take 1 capsule with desired oil 2 times daily.
- Take 2-3 drops of oil in a spoonful of syrup or small amount of milk, juice, or water.

**Topical:** For guidelines on applying oils to the skin, refer to *Application Guidelines* on page 410.

- Apply 3-5 drops diluted 50:50 to chest and stomach areas.

## HIVES

Hives are a generalized itching or dermatitis that can be due to allergies, damaged liver, chemicals, or other factors.

### Recommendations

**Singles:** Myrrh, German Chamomile, Roman Chamomile, Ravintsara, Lavender, Eucalyptus Radiata, Tea Tree, Peppermint, Myrrh

**Blends:** RutaVaLa, RutaVaLa Roll-On, Stress Away Roll-On, Tranquil Roll-On, Peace & Calming, Peace & Calming II

**Nutritionals:** SuperCal, MegaCal, Mineral Essence, Sulfurzyme, Master Formula, MultiGreens, Super B

**Body Care:** KidScents Tender Tush, Rose Ointment

### Application and Usage

**Topical:** For guidelines on applying oils to the skin, refer to *Application Guidelines* on page 410.

- Apply 2-4 drops diluted 50:50 on location as needed.
- Place a cold compress on location as needed.

## HYPERACTIVITY
*(See also Attention Deficit Disorder)*

Hyperactivity behavior usually refers to a group of characteristics, including inability to concentrate, being easily distracted, being impulsive, being aggressive, fidgeting, constant moving, too much talking, and difficulty participating in quiet activities.

### Recommendations

**Singles:** Lavender, Vetiver, Hinoki, Idaho Blue Spruce, Roman Chamomile, Peppermint, Ocotea, Valerian, Cedarwood

**Blends:** RutaVaLa, RutaVaLa Roll-On, Peace & Calming, Peace & Calming II, Stress Away Roll-On, Tranquil Roll-On, Sacred Mountain, Grounding, Gathering

**Nutritionals:** Super B, Master Formula, MegaCal, Ultra Young

## Application and Usage

**Aromatic:** Refer to *Application Guidelines* on page 410.

- Diffuse 5 times daily for up to 30 days, stop for 5 days, and then repeat, if necessary.

**Topical:** For guidelines on applying oils to the skin, refer to *Application Guidelines* on page 410.

- Apply 2-4 drops neat on toes and balls of feet as needed.

## INFECTION (Bacterial and Viral)

Diffusing essential oils is one of the best ways to prevent the spread of airborne bacteria and viruses. Many essential oils, such as Oregano, Plectranthus Oregano, Mountain Savory, and Rosemary, exert highly antimicrobial effects and can effectively eliminate many kinds of pathogens.

Viruses and bacteria have a tendency to hibernate along the spine. The body may hold a virus in a suspended state for a long period of time. When the immune system is compromised, these viruses may be released and then manifest as illness.

Raindrop Technique along the spine using Oregano and Thyme helps reduce inflammation and kill the microorganisms. However, other oils may also be used, which also have strong antiviral and antibacterial properties. ImmuPower, R.C., and Purification all work well in the Raindrop Technique application method.

Mountain Savory, Ravintsara, Eucalyptus Blue, Palo Santo, Sacred Frankincense or Frankincense, and Thyme, etc., applied along the spine through the Raindrop Technique application, may be beneficial for many infections, particularly chest-related (See Colds, Lung, Sinus, and Throat Infection).

### Recommendations

**Singles:** Palo Santo, Ocotea, Sacred Frankincense, Frankincense, Frankincense Vitality, Mountain Savory, Mountain Savory Vitality, Ravintsara, Eucalyptus Blue, Rosemary, Rosemary Vitality, Lemongrass, Lemongrass Vitality, Clove, Clove Vitality, Melissa, Tea Tree, Oregano, Oregano Vitality, Plectranthus Oregano, Thyme, Thyme Vitality, Geranium, Dorado Azul, Northern Lights Black Spruce

**Blends:** Thieves, Thieves Vitality, Purification, Melrose, R.C., ImmuPower, Exodus II, Raven, The Gift, Breathe Again Roll-On, SniffleEase

**Nutritionals:** Inner Defense, Super C, Super C Chewable, NingXia Red, Longevity Softgels, MultiGreens, ImmuPro, OmegaGize[3], Life 9, Ningxia Wolfberries (Organic, Dried)

## Application and Usage

**Aromatic:** Refer to *Application Guidelines* on page 410.

**Dietary and Oral:** Whether putting the oils in a capsule or drinking them in a liquid, please refer to *Application Guidelines* on page 410.

- Take 1 capsule with desired oil 2 times daily.
- Take 2-3 drops of oil in a spoonful of syrup or small amount of milk, juice, or water.

**Topical:** For guidelines on applying oils to the skin, refer to *Application Guidelines* on page 410.

- Apply 4-6 drops on location diluted 20:80 2-3 times daily.
- Receive a Raindrop Technique treatment 1-2 times weekly.

## INFLAMMATION *(See also Muscles)*

Inflammation can be caused by a variety of conditions, including bacterial infection, poor diet, chemicals, hormonal imbalance, and physical injury.

Certain essential oils have been documented to be excellent for reducing inflammation such as German Chamomile, which contains azulene, a blue compound with highly anti-inflammatory properties. Other oils with anti-inflammatory properties include Peppermint, Tea Tree, Clove, Mountain Savory, Palo Santo, Dorado Azul, and Wintergreen.

Some oils are better suited for certain types of inflammation, for example:

- Myrrh, Vetiver, Cistus, and Helichrysum work well for inflammation due to tissue and capillary damage and bruising.
- German Chamomile and Tea Tree are helpful with inflammation due to bacterial infection.
- Ravintsara, Hyssop, Myrrh, Thyme are appropriate for inflammation caused by viral infection.

## Recommendations

**Singles:** Wintergreen, Vetiver, German Chamomile, German Chamomile Vitality, Idaho Blue Spruce, Myrrh, Ravintsara, Hinoki, Copaiba, Copaiba Vitality, Palo Santo, Helichrysum, Cistus, Clove, Clove Vitality, Nutmeg, Nutmeg Vitality, Lavender, Lavender Vitality, Thyme, Thyme Vitality, Frankincense, Frankincense Vitality, Roman Chamomile, Sacred Frankincense, Hyssop, Peppermint, Peppermint Vitality, Tea Tree, Eucalyptus Blue, Eucalyptus Globulus, Mountain Savory, Mountain Savory Vitality, Dorado Azul

**Blends:** Purification, PanAway, Cool Azul, Aroma Siez, Melrose, Relieve It, Deep Relief Roll-On

**Nutritionals:** PowerGize, ImmuPro, Super C, Super C Chewable, Power Meal, Slique Shake, Slique CitraSlim

**Body Care:** Cool Azul Pain Relief Cream, Cool Azul Sports Gel, Ortho Ease Massage Oil, Ortho Sport Massage Oil

### Anti-inflammation Blend No. 1

- 6 drops Eucalyptus Blue
- 6 drops Tea Tree
- 4 drops German Chamomile or German Chamomile Vitality
- 2 drops Peppermint or Peppermint Vitality
- 2 drops Idaho Blue Spruce

### Anti-inflammation Blend No. 2

- 6 drops Myrrh
- 6 drops Eucalyptus Globulus
- 4 drops Clove or Clove Vitality
- 3 drops Palo Santo
- 1 drop Vetiver

## Application and Usage

**Dietary and Oral:** Whether putting the oils in a capsule or drinking them in a liquid, please refer to *Application Guidelines* on page 410.

- Take 1 capsule with desired oil 2 times daily.
- Take 2-3 drops of oil in a spoonful of syrup or small amount of milk, juice, or water.

**Topical:** For guidelines on applying oils to the skin, refer to *Application Guidelines* on page 410.

- Apply 2-4 drops diluted 50:50 2 times daily.
- Place a cold compress 1-3 times daily as needed.

## INFLUENZA

Having the flu may seem like just having a cold with a sore throat, runny nose, and sneezing. However, colds usually develop slowly, whereas the flu generally comes on suddenly. Although a cold can be a nuisance, you usually feel much worse with the flu.

Common symptoms of the flu include nasal congestion, headache, dry cough, fatigue and weakness, aching muscles, chills and sweats, and high fever.

## Recommendations

**Singles:** Mountain Savory, Mountain Savory Vitality, Oregano, Oregano Vitality, Plectranthus Oregano, Eucalyptus Radiata, Peppermint, Peppermint Vitality, Clove, Clove Vitality, Tea Tree, Eucalyptus Blue, Dorado Azul, Frankincense, Frankincense Vitality, Idaho Blue Spruce, Ravintsara, Wintergreen

**Blends:** ImmuPower, TummyGize, DiGize, DiGize Vitality, Exodus II, Thieves, Thieves Vitality, Raven, R.C., Breathe Again Roll-On, SniffleEase

**Nutritionals:** Digest & Cleanse, Inner Defense, Alka-Lime, Life 9, Essentialzyme, Essentialzymes-4, Detoxzyme, ICP, JuvaPower

**Oral Care:** Thieves Cough Drops, Thieves Hard Lozenges, Thieves Mints

## Application and Usage

**Aromatic:** Refer to *Application Guidelines* on page 410.

**Dietary and Oral:** Whether putting the oils in a capsule or drinking them in a liquid, please refer to *Application Guidelines* on page 410.

- Take 1 capsule with desired oil 3 times daily.
- Take 2-3 drops of oil in a spoonful of syrup or small amount of milk, juice, or water.

**Topical:** For guidelines on applying oils to the skin, refer to *Application Guidelines* on page 410.

- Apply 2-4 drops diluted 50:50 on chest, stomach, or lower back 2 times daily or as needed.
- Receive Raindrop Technique 1-2 times weekly.
- Place a warm compress on lower abdomen 1-2 times daily.
- Take a warm bath with custom bath salts, using the following influenza blend:

**Blend for Influenza or Colds**
- 15 drops Ravintsara
- 6 drops Sacred Frankincense or Frankincense
- 6 drops Idaho Blue Spruce
- 3 drops Dorado Azul
- 2 drops Eucalyptus Radiata
- 1 drop Wintergreen

Stir above essential oils thoroughly into ¼ cup Epsom salt or baking soda and then add salt and oil mixture to hot bath water while tub is filling. Soak in hot bath for 20 to 30 minutes or until water cools.

## INSECT BITES AND STINGS

Essential oils are ideal for treating most kinds of insect bites because of their outstanding antiseptic and oil-soluble properties. Essential oils such as Lavender and Peppermint reduce insect bite-induced itching and infection.

## Recommendations

**Singles:** Lavender, Citronella, Eucalyptus Globulus, Eucalyptus Radiata, Eucalyptus Blue, Tea Tree, Pepper-

mint, Rosemary, Copaiba, Dorado Azul, Palo Santo, Idaho Tansy, German Chamomile, Thyme

**Blends:** Bite Buster, PanAway, Purification, Melrose, Thieves

**Stings and Bites Blend No. 1**
- 10 drops Lavender
- 4 drops Eucalyptus Radiata
- 3 drops German Chamomile
- 2 drops Thyme

Spray sheets and clothing to kill any insects that might be imbedded in the cloth.

**Insect Bite Blend No. 2**
- 20 drops Palo Santo
- 20 drops Idaho Tansy
- 10 drops Eucalyptus Blue

Rub a small amount on skin or use in spray bottle.

## Application and Usage

**Topical:** For guidelines on applying oils to the skin, refer to *Application Guidelines* on page 410.

- Apply 1-2 drops of the sting and bite blends neat or diluted 50:50 on location 2-4 times daily.

## Bee Stings

Bee stings can be painful and annoying, but they rarely cause problems, unless you are allergic to the venom—then they can be fatal.

## Recommendations

**Singles:** Lavender, Peppermint, Palo Santo, German Chamomile, Idaho Balsam Fir, Vetiver

**Blends:** Bite Buster, Purification, PanAway, Melrose, Deep Relief Roll-On

**Bee Sting Blend**
- 2 drops Lavender
- 1 drop Peppermint
- 1 drop German Chamomile
- 1 drop Vetiver

**Bee Sting Regimen**
- Flick or scrape stinger out with a knife or hard plastic like a credit card, taking care not to squeeze the venom sac.
- Apply 1-2 drops of the Bee Sting Blend on location. Repeat every 15 minutes for 1 hour.
- Apply any of the recommended blends 2-3 times daily until redness abates.

**Essential Oils Desk Reference** | Seventh Edition

## Bites

Essential oils are ideal for treating most kinds of insect bites because of their outstanding antiseptic and oil-soluble properties. Essential oils such as Lavender and Peppermint reduce insect bite-induced itching and infection.

### Recommendations

**Singles:** Lavender, Eucalyptus Radiata, German Chamomile, Citronella, Thyme, Eucalyptus Globulus, Tea Tree, Peppermint, Rosemary, Idaho Tansy, Palo Santo, Copaiba, Dorado Azul

**Blends:** Bite Buster, PanAway, Purification, Melrose

### Stings and Bites Blend No. 1

- 10 drops Lavender
- 4 drops Eucalyptus Radiata
- 3 drops German Chamomile
- 2 drops Thyme

### Application and Usage

**Topical:** For guidelines on applying oils to the skin, refer to *Application Guidelines* on page 410.

- Apply 1-2 drops of the Stings and Bites Blend neat or diluted 50:50 on location 2-4 times daily.

## Bedbug Bites

Bedbug bites can be difficult to distinguish from other insect bites. However, bedbug bites are usually:
- Found on the face, neck, arms, and hands
- Arranged in a rough line or in a cluster
- Itchy
- Red, often with a darker red spot in the middle

**Singles:** Palo Santo, Eucalyptus Blue, Idaho Tansy

**Blends:** Bite Buster, Purification, Thieves

### Insect Bite Blend No. 2

- 20 drops Palo Santo
- 20 drops Idaho Tansy
- 10 drops Eucalyptus Blue

## Black Widow Spider Bite

A bite from a female black widow spider can cause pain and affect the victim's nervous system, but it is rarely fatal. If you know you have been bitten by a black widow spider, seek emergency medical treatment immediately.

**Singles:** Myrrh, Lemon

**Blends:** Purification, Thieves, Melrose, PanAway, The Gift

**Nutritionals:** Inner Defense

**Topical:** For guidelines on applying oils to the skin, refer to *Application Guidelines* on page 410.

- Put on 1 drop of any oil you have such as Purification, Melrose, The Gift, Lemon, etc.

## Brown Recluse Spider Bite

The bite of this spider causes a painful redness and blistering, which progresses to a gangrenous slough of the affected area. Seek immediate medical attention.

**Singles:** Myrrh, Sacred Frankincense, Frankincense, Rosemary, Ocotea

**Blends:** Purification, Thieves, PanAway

**Nutritionals:** Inner Defense

### Spider Bite Blend

- 1 drop Sacred Frankincense or Frankincense
- 1 drop Myrrh
- 1 drop Melrose

**Topical:** For guidelines on applying oils to the skin, refer to *Application Guidelines* on page 410.

- Apply 1 drop of any of the above blends every 10 minutes until you reach professional medical treatment.
- Put on 1 drop of any oil you have such as Purification, Melrose, The Gift, Lemon, etc.

## Chigger and Tick Bites

It is important that ticks and chiggers be removed before treating the bite. People have tried many different ways of getting rid of these invaders. Sometimes chiggers can be removed or killed by covering the bite with clear fingernail polish.

A common method for removing ticks is to touch them gently with a recently blown-out match head. The heat often causes ticks to let go so that they can just be brushed off.

Essential oils work quickly to remove ticks and chiggers. Mix Thyme or Oregano in a 50:50 dilution and apply 1-2 drops on the bite area. The phenols in these oils will usually cause them to let go and squirm to get away from the oil. When they do, they can be brushed off and killed.

Applying a single drop of Peppermint, Abundance, Exodus II, or any other oil or blend that is considered to be "hot" will cause the tick or chigger to come out of the skin. A "hot" oil is one that is high in phenols that can burn the skin when applied neat. In this case, the objective is to "get the critter out."

For most people, a little stinging does not matter. After

492 | **Chapter 20** | Personal Usage Guide

Personal Usage Guide | **Chapter 20**

the tick or chigger is removed, apply 1-2 drops of any of the oils listed below on the bite location.

## Recommendations

**Singles:** Peppermint, Oregano, Plectranthus Oregano, Clove, Tea Tree, Lavender, Rosemary, Myrrh, Sacred Frankincense, Frankincense, Idaho Balsam Fir

**Blends:** Purification, Exodus II, Abundance, Melrose, Thieves, R.C., The Gift

## Application and Usage

**Topical:** For guidelines on applying oils to the skin, refer to *Application Guidelines* on page 410.

- Apply 1-6 drops neat or diluted, depending on size of affected area, 3-5 times daily.

## Mosquito Bites

For most people, a mosquito bite causes minor irritation. For those who are allergic to bites, their skin breaks out in hives, the chest and throat feel tight, they develop a dry cough, their eyes itch, and they often have nausea, vomiting, abdominal pain, and dizziness.

If you suspect you have a mosquito bite allergy, let your health care professional see your red, swollen bite.

## Recommendations

**Singles:** Peppermint, Tea Tree, Lavender, Rosemary, Myrrh, Sacred Frankincense, Frankincense, Idaho Balsam Fir, Dalmatia Bay Laurel, Laurus Nobilis

**Blends:** Purification, Melrose, Thieves, R.C., The Gift, Bite Buster, Owie

## Application and Usage

**Topical:** For guidelines on applying oils to the skin, refer to *Application Guidelines* on page 410.

- Apply 1-6 drops neat or diluted, depending on size of affected area, 3-5 times daily.

## West Nile Virus

Most people infected with West Nile virus have no signs or symptoms, and mild symptoms usually go away in a few days. However, if you experience symptoms or signs of a serious infection like a high fever, severe headache, stiff neck, or an altered mental state, see your health care professional immediately. A serious West Nile virus infection generally requires hospitalization.

## Recommendations

**Singles:** Peppermint, Tea Tree, Lavender, Rosemary, Myrrh, Sacred Frankincense, Frankincense, Idaho Balsam Fir, Oregano, Plectranthus Oregano, Thyme, Northern Lights Black Spruce, Dalmatia Bay Laurel, Laurus Nobilis

**Blends:** Purification, Melrose, Thieves, R.C., The Gift

## Application and Usage

**Topical:** For guidelines on applying oils to the skin, refer to *Application Guidelines* on page 410.

- Apply 1-6 drops neat or diluted, depending on size of affected area, 3-5 times daily.

## Scorpion Sting

Several species of scorpions are found in the United States and Canada, but most do not produce a significant toxicity by stinging and are not as toxic as those found in South America and other parts of the world. A sting may cause swelling and a lot of discomfort but is rarely fatal. However, a person who has been stung by a scorpion should see a doctor as soon as possible. Follow these first-aid measures:

- If breathing and heartbeat stop, start CPR immediately.
- Apply an ice pack or cold water to the bite area to help slow the spread of the venom.
- Seek medical care.

## Recommendations

**Singles:** Lemongrass, Sacred Frankincense, Frankincense

**Blends:** Purification

## Application and Usage

**Topical:** For guidelines on applying oils to the skin, refer to *Application Guidelines* on page 410.

- Apply 1-6 drops neat or diluted 50:50, depending on size of affected area, 3-5 times daily.

## INSECT REPELLENT

An insect repellent is a substance applied to skin, clothing, or other surfaces that discourages insects from landing on those surfaces. Repellents help prevent the outbreak of insect-borne diseases such as West Nile fever, Lyme disease, dengue fever, bubonic plague, and malaria.

Seventh Edition | **Essential Oils Desk Reference** | 493

## Insect Repellents

- **Mosquito-repellent:** Palo Santo, Lemon, Idaho Tansy, Citronella

- **Moth repellent:** Patchouli, Palo Santo

- **Horse-fly repellent:** Idaho Tansy, Citronella

- **Aphids repellent:** Mix 10 drops Spearmint and 15 drops Orange essential oils in 2 quarts salt water, shake well, and spray on plants.

- **Cockroach repellent:** Mix 10 drops Peppermint and 5 drops Cypress in ½ cup salt water. Shake well and spray where roaches live.

- **Silverfish repellent:** Eucalyptus Radiata, Thieves

- To repel insects, essential oils can be diffused or put on cotton balls or cedar chips (for use in closets or drawers).

- Experiment with your own combination of oils and make new discoveries.

## Recommendations

**Singles:** Palo Santo, Idaho Tansy, Peppermint, Tea Tree, Geranium, Lemon, Rosemary, Lemongrass, Thyme, Spearmint, Citronella, Oregano, Basil

**Blends:** Purification, Melrose, Thieves, Bite Buster, DiGize

### Insect Repellent Blend No. 1
- 9 drops Idaho Tansy or Palo Santo
- 6 drops Peppermint
- 6 drops Citronella

### Insect Repellent Blend No. 2
- 6 drops Idaho Tansy
- 6 drops Palo Santo

Mix together and use undiluted or diluted with a little water.

### Ed & Steven Geiger's Bug Spray
- 1 gallon distilled water
- 1 ounce organic catnip made into a tea, strained, and cooled
- 1 teaspoon Bath Gel Base
- 40 drops Purification
- 40 drops Idaho Tansy or Palo Santo
- 40 drops DiGize
- 20 drops Rosemary
- 8 drops Peppermint
Optional: Add Lemongrass and/or Oregano

### Chérie Ross's Formula for Flea, Tick, and Insect Repellent

- 1 gallon distilled or pure water
- 4 heaping tablespoons organic dried catnip
- 2½ tablespoons organic Neem oil
- 2 teaspoons Thieves Household Cleaner or Bath Gel Base
- 80 drops Purification
- 80 drops Lemongrass
- 40 drops Idaho Tansy
- 40 drops Palo Santo
- 40 drops Ocotea or Basil
- 20 drops Peppermint (optional for high temperatures)

Steep the catnip in the gallon of water for 20-30 minutes. Cool to room temperature. Strain if needed. Add all remaining ingredients into Thieves Household Cleaner or Bath Gel Base. Then mix together and put into spray bottle. Use as needed.

## Application and Usage

**Topical:** For guidelines on applying oils to the skin, refer to *Application Guidelines* on page 410.

- Apply 1-6 drops neat or diluted, depending on size of affected area, 3-5 times daily.

## INSOMNIA
*(See also Depression, Thyroid Problems)*

After age 40, sleep quality and quantity deteriorate noticeably as melatonin production in the brain declines. Supplemental melatonin has been researched to dramatically improve sleep/wake cycles and combat age-related insomnia.

Insomnia may also be caused by bowel or liver toxicity, poor heart function, negative memories and trauma, depression, mineral deficiencies, hormone imbalance, or underactive thyroid.

The fragrance of many essential oils can exert a powerful, calming effect on the mind through their influence on the limbic region of the brain. Historically, lavender sachets or pillows were used for babies, children, and adults alike.

## Recommendations

**Singles:** Lavender, Lavender Vitality, Valerian, Cedarwood, Orange, Orange Vitality, Roman Chamomile, Dorado Azul

**Blends:** AromaSleep, RutaVaLa, RutaVaLa Roll-On, Peace & Calming, Peace & Calming II, Harmony, Dream Catcher, Valor, Valor II, Valor Roll-On, Gentle Baby, Tranquil Roll-On, Trauma Life, T.R. Care, Stress Away Roll-On

**Nutritionals:** ImmuPro, MegaCal, PD 80/20, Life 9, OmegaGize³, SleepEssence, Stress Away, MindWise

**Body Care:** Progessence Plus, Prenolone Plus Body Cream

### Insomnia Blend
- 12 drops Orange or Orange Vitality
- 8 drops Lavender or Lavender Vitality
- 4 drops Dorado Azul
- 3 drops Valerian
- 2 drops Roman Chamomile

## Application and Usage

**Aromatic:** Refer to *Application Guidelines* on page 410.

**Dietary and Oral:** Whether putting the oils in a capsule or drinking them in a liquid, please refer to *Application Guidelines* on page 410.

- Take 1 capsule with desired oil 2 times daily.
- Take 1 capsule of Lavender Vitality oil or any desired oil undiluted or diluted 50:50 1 hour before bedtime.
- Take 2-3 drops of oil in a spoonful of syrup or small amount of milk, juice, or water.

**Topical:** For guidelines on applying oils to the skin, refer to *Application Guidelines* on page 410.

- Apply 1-3 drops neat to shoulders, stomach, and on bottoms of feet.
- Mix 6-8 drops of oils with ¼ cup Epsom salt or baking soda in hot water and add to hot bath water while tub is filling. Soak in bathtub for 20 to 30 minutes or until water cools.
- Rub 1-2 drops of oil on the temples and back of neck several times daily.
- Place a warm compress with 1-2 drops of chosen oil on the back.

## IRRITABLE BOWEL SYNDROME

Irritable bowel syndrome (IBS) is a common disorder of the intestines marked by the following symptoms:
- Cramps
- Gas and bloating
- Constipation
- Diarrhea and loose stools

It may be caused by a combination of stress and a high-fat diet. Fatty foods increase the intensity of the contractions in the colon, thereby increasing symptoms.

Chocolate and milk products, in particular, seem to have the most negative effects on those suffering.

Irritable bowel syndrome is not the same as colitis, mucous colitis, spastic colon, and spastic bowel. Unlike colitis, it does not involve any inflammation and is actually called "functional disorder" because it presents no obvious, outward signs of disease.

A number of medical studies have documented that peppermint oil, in capsules, is beneficial in treating irritable bowel syndrome and decreasing pain.[28, 29, 30]

## Recommendations

**Singles:** Tarragon, Tarragon Vitality, Peppermint, Peppermint Vitality, Fennel, Fennel Vitality, Nutmeg, Nutmeg Vitality, Juniper, Ocotea

**Blends:** DiGize, DiGize Vitality, JuvaFlex, JuvaFlex Vitality, TummyGize

**Nutritionals:** Detoxzyme, OmegaGize³, Digest & Cleanse, Life 9, AlkaLime, JuvaPower. After symptoms stop, then start Essentialzymes-4, Essentialzyme, and ICP.

## Application and Usage

**Aromatic:** Refer to *Application Guidelines* on page 410.

**Dietary and Oral:** Whether putting the oils in a capsule or drinking them in a liquid, please refer to *Application Guidelines* on page 410.

- Take 1 capsule with desired oil 3 times daily.
- Take 2-3 drops of oil in a spoonful of syrup or small amount of milk, juice, or water.

**Topical:** For guidelines on applying oils to the skin, refer to *Application Guidelines* on page 410.

## JOINT STIFFNESS OR PAIN

Joint stiffness is caused by inflammation in the lining of the joint. Specific causes may be rheumatoid arthritis, osteoarthritis, bone diseases, cancer, joint trauma, or overuse of the joint. However, no matter what causes it, joint pain and stiffness can be very bothersome.

## Recommendations

**Singles:** Wintergreen, Lemongrass, Palo Santo, Idaho Blue Spruce, Elemi, Idaho Balsam Fir, German Chamomile, Peppermint, Pine

**Blends:** PanAway, Aroma Siez, Cool Azul, Relieve It, Deep Relief Roll-On

**Nutritionals:** BLM, AgilEase, PowerGize, MegaCal, Sulfurzyme, OmegaGize³, MultiGreens

**Resins:** Myrrh or Frankincense Gum Resin (ingest 2 crystals 2 times daily)

**Body Care:** Cool Azul Pain Relief Cream, Cool Azul Sports Gel, Regenolone Moisturizing Cream, Ortho Ease Massage Oil, Ortho Sport Massage Oil

**Joint Pain Blend No. 1**
- 10 drops Black Pepper
- 5 drops Marjoram
- 5 drops Idaho Blue Spruce
- 2 drops Rosemary

**Joint Pain Blend No. 2**
- 7 drops Idaho Balsam Fir
- 4 drops Wintergreen
- 3 drops Vetiver
- 2 drops German Chamomile

## Application and Usage

**Topical:** For guidelines on applying oils to the skin, refer to *Application Guidelines* on page 410.

- Massage 3-6 drops diluted 50:50 on location. Repeat as needed to control pain.
- Apply to appropriate Vita Flex points on the feet. Repeat as needed.

# KIDNEY DISORDERS

The kidneys remove waste products from the blood and help control blood pressure. They filter over 200 quarts of blood each day and remove over 2 quarts of waste products and water that flow into the bladder as urine through tubes called ureters.

Strong kidneys are essential for good health. Inefficient or damaged kidneys can result in waste accumulating in the blood and causing serious damage.

High blood pressure can be a cause and a result of chronic kidney failure, since kidneys are central to blood regulation (See Blood Pressure, High).

Symptoms of poor kidney function:
- Infrequent or inefficient urinations
- Swelling, especially around the ankles
- Labored breathing due to fluid accumulation in the chest

## Recommendations

**Singles:** Grapefruit, Grapefruit Vitality, Jade Lemon, Jade Lemon Vitality, Lemon, Lemon Vitality, Geranium, Juniper

**Blends:** DiGize, DiGize Vitality, GLF, GLF Vitality, JuvaFlex, JuvaFlex Vitality, Citrus Fresh, Citrus Fresh Vitality, TummyGize

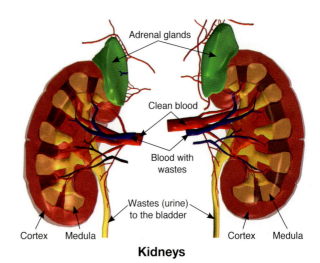

**Kidneys**

**Nutritionals:** K&B, Digest & Cleanse

## Application and Usage

**Aromatic:** Refer to *Application Guidelines* on page 410.

**Dietary and Oral:** Whether putting the oils in a capsule or drinking them in a liquid, please refer to *Application Guidelines* on page 410.

- Take 1 capsule with desired oil 2 times daily.
- Take 2-3 drops of oil in a spoonful of syrup or small amount of milk, juice, or water.

**Topical:** For guidelines on applying oils to the skin, refer to *Application Guidelines* on page 410.

- Apply 6-8 drops diluted 50:50 on the back over the kidney area as needed.
- Applying a single drop under the nose is helpful and refreshing.
- Massage 2-4 drops of oil neat on the bottoms of the feet just before bedtime. Children with kidney disorders may especially benefit from this application.
- Place a warm compress with 1-2 drops of chosen oil on the back 1-2 times daily.

## Kidney Inflammation/Infection (Nephritis)

Kidney inflammation can be caused by structural defects, poor diet, or bacterial infection from *Escherichia coli, Staphylococcus aureus,* Enterobacter, and Klebsiella bacteria. Abnormal proteins trapped in the glomeruli (tiny filtering units in the kidneys), called glomerulonephritis, can also cause inflammation and damage to these tiny filtering units.

This disease can be acute (flaring up in a few days) or chronic (taking months or years to develop). The mildest forms may not show any symptoms except through a

Personal Usage Guide | Chapter 20

urine test. At more advanced stages, urine appears smoky as small amounts of blood are passed and eventually turn red as more blood is excreted—the signs of impending kidney failure.

As with all serious conditions, you should immediately consult a health care professional if you suspect a kidney infection of any kind.

Symptoms may include the following:
- Feeling of discomfort in lower back
- Drowsiness
- Nausea
- Smokey or red-colored urine

Damage to the glomeruli caused by bacterial infections is called pyelonephritis. To reduce infection, drink a gallon of water mixed with 8 oz. of unsweetened cranberry juice daily and use the products listed below.

## Recommendations

**Singles:** Cumin, Cistus, Sacred Frankincense, Frankincense, Frankincense Vitality, Juniper, Myrrh, Helichrysum, Lemongrass, Lemongrass Vitality, Rosemary, Rosemary Vitality, Geranium, Thyme, Thyme Vitality

**Blends:** Melrose, Purification, Longevity, Longevity Vitality, Thieves, Thieves Vitality, 3 Wise Men

**Nutritionals:** K&B, Mineral Essence, ICP, JuvaPower, Inner Defense, Super C, Super C Chewable, Life 9, Digest & Cleanse

## Application and Usage

**Aromatic:** Refer to *Application Guidelines* on page 410.

**Dietary and Oral:** Whether putting the oils in a capsule or drinking them in a liquid, please refer to *Application Guidelines* on page 410.

---

## A Simple Way to Strengthen the Kidneys

- Take 3 droppers of K&B in 4 oz. distilled water 3 times daily.
- Drink 8 oz. water with about 10 percent unsweetened cranberry juice and the fresh juice of ½ lemon.
- Drink plenty of other liquids, preferably distilled water.

---

## Detoxifying the Kidneys

The Chinese wolfberry has been used in China for centuries as a kidney tonic and detoxifier. Essential oils can also assist in the detoxification due to various chemical constituents and unique, lipid-soluble properties.

**Kidney Detoxifying Recipe:**
- 6 drops German Chamomile
- 6 drops Juniper
- 2 drops Fennel

Put 5 drops of the recipe in a gel capsule and then fill the capsule with V-6 Vegetable Oil Complex; take 2 times daily. You may also apply the recipe neat in a compress over the kidneys.

**Supplements:** K&B, MultiGreens, Sulfurzyme, Detoxzyme, Essentialzyme, ICP, JuvaPower

---

- Take 2 capsules with desired oil 2 times daily for 10 days.
- Take 2-3 drops of oil in a spoonful of syrup or small amount of milk, juice, or water.

**Topical:** For guidelines on applying oils to the skin, refer to *Application Guidelines* on page 410.

- Massage 2-4 drops of oil neat on the bottoms of the feet Vita Flex points just before bedtime.
- Place a cold compress with 1-2 drops of chosen oil over the kidney area 1-2 times daily.

## Kidney Stones
*(See also Bladder / Urinary Tract Infection)*

Kidney stones can create intense pain and dangerous infection. You should always consult a qualified health care professional before beginning any treatment for kidney stones.

A kidney stone is a solid piece of material that forms in the kidney from mineral or protein-breakdown products in the urine. Occasionally, larger stones can become trapped in a ureter, bladder, or urethra, which can block urine flow, causing intense pain.

There are four types of kidney stones:
- Stones made from calcium (the most common type)
- Stones made from magnesium and ammonia (a struvite stone)
- Stones made from uric acid
- Stones made from cystine (the rarest)

Seventh Edition | **Essential Oils Desk Reference** | 497

**Essential Oils Desk Reference** | Seventh Edition

Symptoms may include the following:
- Persistent, penetrating pain in side or lower back
- Blood in the urine
- Fainting

It is important to drink plenty of water (at least six 8 oz. glasses daily) to help pass a kidney stone.

## Recommendations

**Singles:** Carrot Seed, Carrot Seed Vitality, Helichrysum, Jade Lemon, Jade Lemon Vitality, Lemon, Lemon Vitality, Sacred Frankincense, Frankincense, Frankincense Vitality, Geranium, Juniper, Orange, Orange Vitality, Jade Lemon, Jade Lemon Vitality, Lemon, Lemon Vitality

**Blends:** Citrus Fresh, Citrus Fresh Vitality, Purification

**Nutritionals:** K&B, Essentialzymes-4, Essentialzyme, Detoxzyme

**Liquids:** Apple Cider Vinegar

## Application and Usage

**Aromatic:** Refer to *Application Guidelines* on page 410.

**Dietary and Oral:** Whether putting the oils in a capsule or drinking them in a liquid, please refer to *Application Guidelines* on page 410.

- Take 2 capsules with desired oil 2 times daily.
- Take 2-3 drops of oil in a spoonful of syrup or small amount of milk, juice, or water.

**Topical:** For guidelines on applying oils to the skin, refer to *Application Guidelines* on page 410.

- Massage 2-4 drops neat to the kidney Vita Flex points of the feet just before bedtime.
- Apply 6-10 drops of recommended oils neat over kidney area 1-2 times daily.
- Place a warm compress with 1-2 drops of chosen oil over the back.

## LICE

The most commonly recommended remedy for lice (pediculosis) and their eggs (nits) is lindane (gamma benzene hexachloride), a highly toxic polychlorinated chemical that is structurally very similar to hazardous banned pesticides such as DDT and chlordane. It is so dangerous that Dr. Guy Sansfacon, head of the Quebec Poison Control Centre in Canada, has requested that lindane be banned.

Essential oils offer a safe, effective alternative. A 1996 study by researchers in Iceland showed the effectiveness against head lice of the essential oils of anise seed, cinnamon leaf, thyme, tea tree, peppermint, and nutmeg in shampoo and rinse solutions.[31]

## Recommendations

**Singles:** Tea Tree, Palo Santo, Lavender, Peppermint, Thyme, Geranium, Nutmeg, Rosemary, Cinnamon Bark

**Blends:** Purification, Thieves

**Head Lice Blend**
- 4 drops Thyme
- 2 drops Lavender
- 2 drops Geranium

## Application and Usage

**Topical:** For guidelines on applying oils to the skin, refer to *Application Guidelines* on page 410.

- You may apply single oils or blends neat or diluted, depending on the oils that are used. Add 1 teaspoon of oil diluted 50:50 to shampoo and massage onto entire scalp.
- Cover with a disposable shower cap and leave on for at least ½ hour.
- Rinse well using 1 cup of Thieves Fresh Essence Plus Mouthwash massaged into hair and scalp. Leave on for 10 minutes before rinsing out.

## LIVER DISEASES AND DISORDERS

The liver is one of the most important organs, playing a major role in detoxifying the body. When the liver is damaged, frequently due to excess alcohol consumption, viral hepatitis, or poor diet, an excess of toxins can build up in the blood and tissues that can result in degenerative disease and death.

Jaundice (abnormal yellow color of the skin), may be the only visible sign of liver disease.

Symptoms of a stressed or diseased liver:
- Nausea
- Loss of appetite
- Dark-colored urine
- Yellowish or gray-colored bowel movements
- Abdominal pain or ascites, an unusual swelling of the abdomen caused by an accumulation of fluid, itching, dermatitis, or hives
- Disturbed sleep caused by the buildup of unfiltered toxins in the blood
- General fatigue and loss of energy
- Lack of sex drive

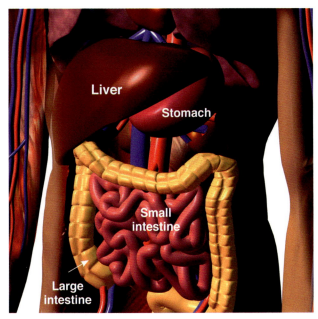

liver

## Hepatitis

Viral hepatitis is a serious, life-threatening disease of the liver that can result in scarring (cirrhosis) and eventual organ destruction and death. A qualified health professional should be seen immediately if you suspect hepatitis.

There are several different kinds of hepatitis: Hepatitis A (spread by contaminated food, water, or feces) and Hepatitis B and C (spread by contaminated blood or semen).

An unpublished 2003 study conducted by Roger Lewis, MD, at the Young Life Research Clinic in Springville, Utah, evaluated the efficacy of Helichrysum, Ledum, and Celery Seed in treating cases of advanced Hepatitis C. In one case a 20-year-old male diagnosed with Hepatitis C had a viral count of 13,200. After taking 2 capsules (approximately 750 milligrams each) of GLF, a blend of Helichrysum, Ledum, Celery Seed, and JuvaCleanse daily for one month with no other intervention, the patient's viral count dropped more than 80 percent to 2,580.

Hepatitis symptoms include jaundice, weakness, loss of appetite, nausea, brownish or tea colored urine, abdominal discomfort, fever, and whitish bowel movements.

### Recommendations

**Singles:** Carrot Seed, Carrot Seed Vitality, German Chamomile, German Chamomile Vitality, Helichrysum, Ledum, Celery Seed, Celery Seed Vitality, Ravintsara, Peppermint, Peppermint Vitality, Myrrh

**Blends:** GLF, GLF Vitality, JuvaCleanse, JuvaCleanse Vitality, JuvaFlex, JuvaFlex Vitality

**Nutritionals:** ImmuPro, MultiGreens, JuvaPower, JuvaSpice, JuvaTone, Essentialzymes-4, Detoxzyme, Life 9, ICP, ComforTone, Essentialzyme, Master Formula

**Note:** Avoid grapefruit juice and any medications that stress the liver.

### Application and Usage

**Aromatic:** Refer to *Application Guidelines* on page 410.

**Dietary and Oral:** Whether putting the oils in a capsule or drinking them in a liquid, please refer to *Application Guidelines* on page 410.

- Take 2 capsules with desired oil 3 times daily.
- Take 2-3 drops of oil in a spoonful of syrup or small amount of milk, juice, or water.

**Topical:** For guidelines on applying oils to the skin, refer to *Application Guidelines* on page 410.

- Apply 1-3 drops diluted 50:50 on carotid arteries on the right and left side of the throat just under the jaw bone on either side 2-5 times daily. Carotid arteries are an excellent place to apply oils for fast absorption.
- Apply 1-3 drops on the Vita Flex liver point of the right foot 1-3 times daily.
- Receive a Raindrop Technique 2-3 times weekly.
- Place a warm compress with 1-2 drops of chosen oil over the liver 1-2 times daily.

### Daily hepatitis regimen

- Begin with a colon cleanse using ICP, ComforTone, and Essentialzyme.
- After 3 days, add 1-2 tablets of JuvaTone 3 times daily.
- ImmuPro: Take 1-2 tablets before going to bed. Do not exceed 2 daily.
- MultiGreens: Take 1-3 capsules 3 times daily.

## Jaundice

Jaundice is the yellowish staining of the skin and the whites of the eyes that is caused by too much bilirubin being produced for the liver to remove it from the blood.

### Recommendations

**Singles:** Carrot Seed, Carrot Seed Vitality, German Chamomile, German Chamomile Vitality, Ledum, Celery Seed, Celery Seed Vitality, Ravintsara, Peppermint, Peppermint Vitality, Myrrh

**Blends:** JuvaCleanse, JuvaCleanse Vitality, JuvaFlex, JuvaFlex Vitality, GLF, GLF Vitality

## Protecting Your Liver

- Avoid alcoholic beverages.
- Avoid unnecessary use of prescription drugs. Even over-the-counter pain relievers can have toxic effects on the liver in moderately high doses.
- Consume a diet high in selenium found in plant food, Brazil nuts, tuna, meat, eggs, etc. Selenium helps proteins make important antioxidant enzymes that prevent cellular damage from free radicals.
- Avoid mixing pharmaceutical drugs, especially with alcohol.
- Avoid exposure to industrial chemicals whenever possible.
- Eat a healthy diet of vegetables and fruits; fruits are naturally cleansing.
- Nutritionals: Detoxzyme, Essentialzyme, and Ningxia wolfberry, which is widely used in China as a liver tonic and detoxifier.

**Nutritionals:** JuvaPower, JuvaSpice, MultiGreens, JuvaTone, ImmuPro, Essentialzymes-4, Detoxzyme, Life 9, ICP, ComforTone, Essentialzyme, Master Formula

**Note:** Avoid grapefruit juice and any medications that stress the liver.

### Application and Usage

**Aromatic:** Refer to *Application Guidelines* on page 410.

**Dietary and Oral:** Whether putting the oils in a capsule or drinking them in a liquid, please refer to *Application Guidelines* on page 410.

- Take 2 capsules with desired oil 3 times daily.
- Take 2-3 drops of oil in a spoonful of syrup or small amount of milk, juice, or water.

**Topical:** For guidelines on applying oils to the skin, refer to *Application Guidelines* on page 410.

- Apply 1-3 drops diluted 50:50 on carotid arteries on the right and left side of the throat just under the jaw bone on either side 2-5 times daily. Carotid arteries are an excellent place to apply oils for fast absorption.
- Apply 1-3 drops on the Vita Flex liver point of the right foot 1-3 times daily.

- Receive a Raindrop Technique 2-3 times weekly.
- Place a warm compress with 1-2 drops of chosen oil over the liver 1-2 times daily.

## Toxic Liver

The liver is important in transforming and eliminating chemicals and is susceptible to becoming toxic from these substances.

### Recommendations

**Singles:** Carrot Seed, Carrot Seed Vitality, Orange, Orange Vitality, Ledum, Celery Seed, Celery Seed Vitality, Jade Lemon, Jade Lemon Vitality, Lemon, Lemon Vitality, Lime, Lime Vitality, Cardamom, Cardamom Vitality, Geranium, German Chamomile, German Chamomile Vitality, Rosemary, Rosemary Vitality

**Blends:** GLF, GLF Vitality, JuvaFlex, JuvaFlex Vitality, Release, JuvaCleanse, JuvaCleanse Vitality, Citrus Fresh, Citrus Fresh Vitality

**Nutritionals:** JuvaTone, JuvaPower, JuvaSpice, Longevity Softgels, Sulfurzyme, Digest & Cleanse, ICP, ComforTone, Essentialzyme, Life 9, K&B

### Liver Support Blend
- 10 drops Orange or Orange Vitality
- 5 drops Rosemary or Rosemary Vitality
- 3 drops Celery Seed or Celery Seed Vitality
- 2 drops German Chamomile or German Chamomile Vitality

### Application and Usage

**Aromatic:** Refer to *Application Guidelines* on page 410.

**Dietary and Oral:** Whether putting the oils in a capsule or drinking them in a liquid, please refer to *Application Guidelines* on page 410.

- Take 1 capsule with desired oil 2 times daily.
- Take 2-3 drops of oil in a spoonful of syrup or small amount of milk, juice, or water.

**Topical:** For guidelines on applying oils to the skin, refer to *Application Guidelines* on page 410.

- Apply 1-3 drops on the liver Vita Flex point of the right foot.
- Massage 2-4 drops of oil neat on the bottoms of the feet just before bedtime.
- Place a warm compress with 1-2 drops of chosen oil over the liver 1-2 times daily.
- Have Raindrop Technique 1-2 times weekly.

## LIVER SPOTS (Solar Lentigines)

Liver spots (also called age spots and solar lentigines) are flat brown, gray, or black spots and vary in size. They usually are found on the face, arms, shoulders, and hands—the areas that receive the greatest exposure to the sun.

### Recommendations

**Singles:** Royal Hawaiian Sandalwood, Blue Cypress, Lavender, Nutmeg

**Blends:** DiGize, GLF

**Liver Spot Blend**
- 20 drops Avocado Oil
- 6 drops Royal Hawaiian Sandalwood
- 4 drops Blue Cypress
- 4 drops Lavender
- 4 drops Nutmeg

### Application and Usage

**Topical:** For guidelines on applying oils to the skin, refer to *Application Guidelines* on page 410.

- Apply 2-4 drops neat of the liver spot blend over affected area 3 times daily for 2 weeks.

## LUNG INFECTIONS AND PROBLEMS

The lungs provide us with oxygen and remove carbon dioxide through respiration. Breathing brings irritants and contaminants into the lungs, making them susceptible to damage and infection.

### Asthma *(See also Allergies)*

During an asthma attack, the bronchial air tubes in the lungs become swollen and clogged with thick, sticky mucus. The muscles of the air tubes will also begin to constrict or tighten.

This results in very difficult or labored breathing. If an attack is severe, it can actually be life-threatening.

Many asthma attacks are triggered by an allergic reaction to pollen, skin particles, dandruff, cat and dog dander, dust mites, as well as from foods such as eggs, milk, flavorings, dyes, preservatives, and other chemicals. Asthma can also be triggered by respiratory infection, exercise, stress, and psychological factors.

### Recommendations

**Singles:** Dorado Azul, Eucalyptus Radiata, Sacred Frankincense, Frankincense, Frankincense Vitality, Eucalyptus Blue, Ravintsara, Palo Santo

**Blends:** R.C., Breathe Again Roll-On, SniffleEase, Valor, Valor II, Raven, Inspiration, Sacred Mountain

**Nutritionals:** Detoxzyme, ICP, JuvaPower, MultiGreens, ImmuPro, Essentialzyme, Essentialzymes-4, Kid-Scents MightyZyme

**Body Care:** Ortho Ease Massage Oil, Relaxation Massage Oil, Sensation Massage Oil

### Application and Usage

**Aromatic:** Refer to *Application Guidelines* on page 410.

**Dietary and Oral:** Whether putting the oils in a capsule or drinking them in a liquid, please refer to *Application Guidelines* on page 410.

- Take 1-2 capsules of Dorado Azul, Eucalyptus Blue, or other desired oil 2 times daily.
- Take 2-3 drops of oil in a spoonful of syrup or small amount of milk, juice, or water.

**Topical:** For guidelines on applying oils to the skin, refer to *Application Guidelines* on page 410.

- Apply 1-2 drops mixed with Ortho Ease, Relaxation, or Sensation massage oils on temples and back of neck as desired.
- You may also apply 2-3 drops on the Vita Flex points on the feet.

### Bronchitis *(See also Asthma)*

Bronchitis is characterized by inflammation of the bronchial tube lining accompanied by a heavy mucus discharge. Bronchitis can be caused by an infection or exposure to dust, chemicals, air pollution, or cigarette smoke.

When bronchitis occurs regularly over long periods (i.e., 3 months out of the year for several years), it is known as chronic bronchitis. It can eventually lead to emphysema.

Symptoms may include the following:
- Persistent, hacking cough
- Mucus discharge from the lungs
- Difficulty breathing

Avoiding air pollution is an easy way to reduce bronchitis symptoms. In cases where bronchitis is caused by a bacteria or virus, the aroma of high antimicrobial essential oils may help combat the infection. Heavy mucus may increase after eating foods containing processed sugar or flour or high levels of fat.

### Recommendations

**Singles:** Northern Lights Black Spruce, Dorado Azul, Myrtle, Ravintsara, Eucalyptus Blue, Palo Santo, Rosemary, Rosemary Vitality, Eucalyptus Radiata, Eucalyptus Globulus, Lavender, Lavender Vitality,

Myrrh, Thyme, Thyme Vitality, Wintergreen, Pine, Oregano, Oregano Vitality, Plectranthus Oregano, Tea Tree, Idaho Balsam Fir, Copaiba, Copaiba Vitality, Clove, Clove Vitality, Peppermint, Peppermint Vitality, Dalmatia Bay Laurel, Laurus Nobilis, Laurus Nobilis Vitality

**Blends:** Raven, R.C., Melrose, Purification, PanAway, Thieves, Thieves Vitality, Breathe Again Roll-On, SniffleEase, Exodus II

**Nutritionals:** Super C, Super C Chewable, Life 9, Longevity Softgels, Digest & Cleanse, Inner Defense

**Oral Care:** Thieves Cough Drops, Thieves Hard Lozenges, Thieves Fresh Essence Plus Mouthwash, Thieves Spray

### Bronchitis Blend No. 1
- 6 drops Ravintsara
- 5 drops Clove or Clove Vitality
- 4 drops Myrrh
- 2 drops Palo Santo

### Bronchitis Blend No. 2
- 10 drops Dorado Azul
- 6 drops Eucalyptus Blue
- 5 drops Lavender or Lavender Vitality
- 3 drops Eucalyptus Globulus

**Note:** Essential oil blends work especially well in respiratory applications.

## Application and Usage

**Aromatic:** Refer to *Application Guidelines* on page 410.

**Dietary and Oral:** Whether putting the oils in a capsule or drinking them in a liquid, please refer to *Application Guidelines* on page 410.

- Take 1 capsule with desired oil 2 times daily.
- Take 2-3 drops of oil in a spoonful of syrup or small amount of milk, juice, or water.

**Topical:** For guidelines on applying oils to the skin, refer to *Application Guidelines* on page 410.

- Apply 2-6 drops neat or diluted 50:50 to the neck and chest as needed.
- Massage 2-3 drops on the lung Vita Flex points of the feet 2-4 times daily.
- Place a warm compress with 1-2 drops of chosen oil on the neck, chest, and upper back areas 1-3 times daily.
- Rectal: Using any of the recommended blends, combine 20 drops with 1 tablespoon olive oil. Insert into rectum with bulb syringe and retain

throughout the night. Repeat nightly for 2-3 days.
- Gargle a mixture of essential oils and water 4-8 times daily.

## Pleurisy

This is an inflammation of the pleura, the outer membranes covering the lungs and the thoracic cavity.

### Recommendations

**Singles:** Ravintsara, Eucalyptus Blue, Dorado Azul, Eucalyptus Radiata, Wintergreen, Myrrh, German Chamomile, German Chamomile Vitality

**Blends:** PanAway, Raven, Exodus II, Thieves, Thieves Vitality

**Nutritionals:** Sulfurzyme, Super C, Super C Chewable, OmegaGize[3], Mineral Essence, Essentialzyme, Essentialzymes-4, Digest & Cleanse, ICP, JuvaPower, JuvaSpice

**Oral Care:** Thieves Cough Drops, Thieves Hard Lozenges, Thieves Fresh Essence Plus Mouthwash, Thieves Spray

### Application and Usage

**Aromatic:** Refer to *Application Guidelines* on page 410.

**Topical:** For guidelines on applying oils to the skin, refer to *Application Guidelines* on page 410.

- Massage 5-7 drops of oil diluted 20:80 on neck and chest 2-3 times daily.
- Place a warm compress with 1-2 drops of oil on the neck, chest, and upper back areas daily.
- Apply 1-3 drops on the lung Vita Flex points on the feet daily.
- Receive a Raindrop Technique 1-2 times weekly.

## Pneumonia

Pneumonia is a lung infection caused by bacteria or viruses. It starts when you breathe germs into your lungs and is likely to occur after having a cold or the flu.

### Recommendations

**Singles:** Thyme, Thyme Vitality, Ravintsara, Eucalyptus Radiata, Eucalyptus Globulus, Mountain Savory, Mountain Savory Vitality, Clove, Clove Vitality, Oregano, Oregano Vitality, Plectranthus Oregano, Tea Tree, Eucalyptus Blue, Dorado Azul, Peppermint, Peppermint Vitality, Northern Lights Black Spruce

**Blends:** Raven, Melrose, R.C., Thieves, Thieves Vitality, Breathe Again Roll-On, SniffleEase

**Nutritionals:** Inner Defense, Super C, Super C Chewable, Longevity Softgels, MultiGreens, ImmuPro, Digest & Cleanse, Life 9

**Oral Care:** Thieves Spray, Thieves Cough Drops, Thieves Hard Lozenges, Thieves Fresh Essence Plus Mouthwash

**Pneumonia Blend**
- 10 drops Eucalyptus Globulus
- 8 drops Ravintsara
- 2 drops Oregano or Oregano Vitality
- 2 drops Dorado Azul

## Application and Usage

**Aromatic:** Refer to *Application Guidelines* on page 410.

**Dietary and Oral:** Whether putting the oils in a capsule or drinking them in a liquid, please refer to *Application Guidelines* on page 410.

- Take 1 capsule with desired oil 2 times daily.
- Take 2-3 drops of oil in a spoonful of syrup or small amount of milk, juice, or water.
- Gargle a mixture of essential oils and water 4-8 times daily.

**Topical:** For guidelines on applying oils to the skin, refer to *Application Guidelines* on page 410.

- Apply 2-6 drops neat or diluted 50:50 to the neck and chest as needed.
- Massage 2-3 drops on the lung Vita Flex points of the feet 2-4 times daily.
- Place a warm compress with 1-2 drops of chosen oil on the neck, chest, and upper back areas 1-3 times daily.
- Rectal: Using any of the recommended blends, combine 20 drops with 1 tablespoon olive oil. Insert into rectum with bulb syringe and retain throughout the night. Repeat nightly for 5-6 days.

## Tuberculosis

Tuberculosis (TB) is a highly contagious lung disease caused by *Mycobacterium tuberculosis*. The germs are spread via coughs, sneezes, and physical contact.

The most worrisome aspect of this disease is its latency. Those infected may harbor the germ for years, yet display no outward or visible signs of infection. However, when the immune system becomes challenged or weakened due to stress, candida, diabetes, corticosteroid use, or other factors, the bacteria can become activated and develop into full-blown TB.

Because many essential oils have broad-spectrum, antimicrobial properties, they can be diffused to prevent the spread of airborne bacteria like *Mycobacterium tuberculosis*. Essential oils and blends like Thieves, Purification, Raven, R.C., and Sacred Mountain are extremely effective for killing this type of germ.

Many essential oils have also been shown to stimulate the immune system. Lemon oil has been shown to increase lymphocyte production—a pivotal part of the immune system.

## Recommendations

**Singles:** Melissa, Lemon, Lemon Vitality, Oregano, Oregano Vitality, Plectranthus Oregano, Thyme, Thyme Vitality, Eucalyptus Blue, Dorado Azul, Sacred Frankincense, Frankincense, Frankincense Vitality, Palo Santo, Ravintsara, Rosemary, Rosemary Vitality, Cinnamon Bark, Cinnamon Bark Vitality, Eucalyptus Radiata, Eucalyptus Globulus, Clove, Clove Vitality, Mountain Savory, Mountain Savory Vitality, Peppermint, Peppermint Vitality, Spearmint, Spearmint Vitality, Myrtle, Idaho Balsam Fir, Myrrh

**Blends:** Exodus II, Thieves, Thieves Vitality, Raven, Melrose, R.C., ImmuPower, Purification, Sacred Mountain, Breathe Again Roll-On, SniffleEase

**Nutritionals:** Inner Defense, ImmuPro, Super C, Super C Chewable, Longevity Softgels, MultiGreens, ICP, ComforTone, Essentialzyme, Essentialzymes-4, NingXia Red

**Oral Care:** Thieves Cough Drops, Thieves Hard Lozenges, Thieves Fresh Essence Plus Mouthwash, Thieves Spray

## Application and Usage

**Aromatic:** Refer to *Application Guidelines* on page 410.

**Dietary and Oral:** Whether putting the oils in a capsule or drinking them in a liquid, please refer to *Application Guidelines* on page 410.

- Take 1 capsule with desired oil 2 times daily.
- Take 2-3 drops of oil in a spoonful of syrup or small amount of milk, juice, or water.

**Topical:** For guidelines on applying oils to the skin, refer to *Application Guidelines* on page 410.

- Apply 6-10 drops of oil, diluted 50:50, on chest and upper back 1-3 times daily.
- Apply a warm compress with chosen oils on chest and upper back 2 times daily.

## Tuberculosis-Specific Regimen
- Alternate diffusing Raven and R.C. combined with Eucalyptus Globulus as often as possible during the day.

### Retention Blend No. 1
- 15 drops Frankincense or Sacred Frankincense
- 5 drops Clove
- 4 drops Myrrh
- 2 drops Oregano

### Retention Blend No. 2
- 10 drops Dorado Azul
- 5 drops Eucalyptus Blue
- 5 drops Myrrh
- 2 drops Oregano

Mix blend with 2 tablespoons of V-6 Vegetable Oil Complex. Using a bulb syringe, insert into rectum and retain overnight. Do this nightly for 7 nights, rest for 4 nights, and then repeat.
- Take 2 Inner Defense 3 times daily for 10 days.
- Rub 4-6 drops Thieves on the bottoms of the feet nightly.
- Massage Melrose (15 drops) up the spine daily. Apply compress on back and chest 2 times daily.
- Receive a Raindrop Technique weekly.
- **For cough:** Mix 10 drops Myrrh and 1 drop Peppermint Vitality in water and gargle; dissolve Thieves Cough Drops in mouth as needed.

## Whooping Cough

Whooping cough is a contagious disease affecting the respiratory system, particularly in children. The lungs become infected as the air passages become clogged with thick mucus. Over the course of several days, the condition worsens, resulting in long coughing bouts (up to 1 minute). The continual coughing makes breathing difficult and labored. Watch carefully and seek medical attention if needed.

Whooping cough usually affects children, so always dilute the essential oils in V-6 Vegetable Oil Complex or other cold-pressed vegetable oil before topically applying. Start with low concentrations until response is observed. Diffuse intermittently and observe reaction.

### Recommendations

**Singles:** Rosemary, Rosemary Vitality, Lavender, Lavender Vitality, Basil, Basil Vitality, Wintergreen, Thyme, Thyme Vitality, Oregano, Oregano Vitality, Mastrante, Plectranthus Oregano, Tea Tree, Northern Lights Black Spruce, Nutmeg, Nutmeg Vitality, Peppermint, Peppermint Vitality, Eucalyptus Blue, Dorado Azul

**Blends:** Thieves, Thieves Vitality, Melrose, Raven, R.C., Breathe Again Roll-On, SniffleEase

**Nutritionals:** Super C, Super C Chewable, Longevity Softgels, Essentialzyme, Essentialzymes-4, Detoxzyme, MultiGreens, ImmuPro, Sulfurzyme, Digest & Cleanse, Inner Defense, Master Formula

**Oral Care:** Thieves Cough Drops, Thieves Spray, Thieves Fresh Essence Plus Mouthwash, Thieves Hard Lozenges, Thieves Mints

### Application and Usage

**Aromatic:** Refer to *Application Guidelines* on page 410.

**Topical:** For guidelines on applying oils to the skin, refer to *Application Guidelines* on page 410.

- Apply 2-4 drops diluted 50:50 on neck and chest as needed.
- Massage 2-4 drops of oil neat on the bottoms of the feet and on Vita Flex points just before bedtime. Children may especially benefit from this application.
- Place a warm compress with 1-2 drops of chosen oil on the neck, chest, and upper back area 1-3 times daily.

## LUPUS
*(See also Mixed Connective Tissue Disease)*

Lupus is an autoimmune disease that has several different varieties:

*Lupus vulgaris* is characterized by brownish lesions that may form on skin and/or face and become ulcerous and form scars.

Discoid *Lupus erythematosus* is characterized by scaly, red patches on the skin or butterfly-shaped lesions on the face. It is milder than the systemic type.

Systemic *Lupus erythematosus* is more serious—and more common—than discoid lupus. It inflames the connective tissue in any part of the body, including the joints, muscles, skin, blood vessels, membranes surrounding the lungs and heart, and occasionally the kidneys and brain.

Because lupus is an autoimmune disease, it has been successfully treated using MSM, a form of organic sulfur, which can be found in Sulfurzyme.

### Recommendations

**Singles:** Myrrh, Wintergreen, Lavender, Lavender Vitality, Basil, Basil Vitality, Eucalyptus Globulus, Thyme, Thyme Vitality, Nutmeg, Nutmeg Vitality

**Blends:** Valor, Valor II, Valor Roll-On, PanAway, R.C., Breathe Again Roll-On, EndoFlex, EndoFlex Vitality

**Nutritionals:** Thyromin, Sulfurzyme, Essentialzyme, Essentialzymes-4, MultiGreens, Master Formula

### Lupus Blend
- 10 drops Lavender or Lavender Vitality
- 4 drops Eucalyptus Globulus
- 3 drops Myrrh
- 3 drops Nutmeg or Nutmeg Vitality

## Application and Usage

**Aromatic:** Refer to *Application Guidelines* on page 410.

**Dietary and Oral:** Whether putting the oils in a capsule or drinking them in a liquid, please refer to *Application Guidelines* on page 410.

- Take 1 capsule with 5 drops of desired oil 2 times daily.
- Take 2-3 drops of oil in a spoonful of syrup or small amount of milk, juice, or water.

**Topical:** For guidelines on applying oils to the skin, refer to *Application Guidelines* on page 410.

- Apply 1-2 drops neat on temples and back of neck as desired.
- Have Raindrop Technique 1-2 times weekly.
- Have body massage using desired essential oils once every other day.

### Lupus Daily Regimen
1. Bath Salts: Using lupus blend above, add 30 drops to ½ cup Epsom salt or baking soda and add to hot bath. Soak for 20-30 minutes or until water cools.
2. Vita Flex: Massage PanAway on bottoms of the feet and follow 2 hours later with a foot massage using Thieves.
3. Topical: Massage 10-15 drops Basil over liver and on feet 2-3 times daily.
4. Sulfurzyme: Take 1-2 tablespoons of powder or 5 capsules 1-2 times daily.
5. Essentialzyme: Take 2-6 caplets 2 times daily.
6. MultiGreens: Take 2-4 capsules 2 times daily.

# LYME DISEASE / ROCKY MOUNTAIN SPOTTED FEVER

Lyme disease is a bacterial infection caused by the bite of an infected tick. It is caused by the microorganism *Borrelia burgdorferi*. Some researchers believe that "stealth viruses" may also be involved in Lyme disease. While the suggested oils of Eucalyptus Blue and Dorado Azul are antibacterial, all other oils listed are both antibacterial and antiviral, which will fight either type of infection.

Rocky Mountain Spotted Fever is caused by the bacterium *Rickettsia rickettsii* and is also transmitted to humans by the bite of an infected tick.

Typical symptoms are headache, fever, muscle pain, abdominal pain, and vomiting. A rash may develop after a few days. Both illnesses can be severe or even fatal if not treated in the first few days of symptoms. Seek medical attention as soon as possible after being bitten by a tick.

## Recommendations

**Singles:** Melissa, Oregano, Oregano Vitality, Plectranthus Oregano, Myrrh, Eucalyptus Blue, Dorado Azul, Thyme, Thyme Vitality, Clove, Clove Vitality, Northern Lights Black Spruce

**Blends:** PanAway, Melrose, Thieves, Thieves Vitality, Exodus II

**Nutritionals:** Inner Defense, Power Meal, Slique Shake, Essentialzyme, Essentialzymes-4, Life 9, Detoxzyme

## Application and Usage

**Aromatic:** Refer to *Application Guidelines* on page 410.

**Dietary and Oral:** Whether putting the oils in a capsule or drinking them in a liquid, please refer to *Application Guidelines* on page 410.

- Take 1 capsule with desired oil 3 times daily.
- Take 2-3 drops of oil in a spoonful of syrup or small amount of milk, juice, or water.

**Topical:** For guidelines on applying oils to the skin, refer to *Application Guidelines* on page 410.

- Apply 1-2 drops of oil neat on temples and back of neck, as desired.
- Massage 2-4 drops of oil neat on bottoms of the feet just before bedtime.

# LYMPHATIC SYSTEM

Essential oils have long been known to aid in stimulating and detoxifying the lymphatic system, which filters lymph, fights infection, recycles plasma proteins, and drains fluid back into the circulatory system from the tissues in order to prevent dehydration. It plays a crucial role in maintaining good health.

## Recommendations

**Singles:** Myrtle, Grapefruit, Grapefruit Vitality, Lemongrass, Lemongrass Vitality, Tangerine, Tangerine Vitality, Orange, Orange Vitality, Rosemary, Rosemary Vitality, Cypress, Hyssop, Myrrh

**Blends:** DiGize, DiGize Vitality, Aroma Life, En-R-Gee, Citrus Fresh, Citrus Fresh Vitality

**Nutritionals:** ImmuPro, Super C, Super C Chewable, Longevity Softgels, MultiGreens, Digest & Cleanse, Life 9

**Body Care:** Cel-Lite Magic Massage Oil, Regenolone Moisturizing Cream

### Lymphatic System Blend
- 3 drops Cypress
- 2 drops Grapefruit
- 1 drop Orange

## Application and Usage

**Aromatic:** Refer to *Application Guidelines* on page 410.

**Dietary and Oral:** Whether putting the oils in a capsule or drinking them in a liquid, please refer to *Application Guidelines* on page 410.

- Take 1 capsule with 5 drops of Lymphatic System Blend 2 times daily.
- Take 2-3 drops of oil in a spoonful of syrup or small amount of milk, juice, or water.

**Topical:** For guidelines on applying oils to the skin, refer to *Application Guidelines* on page 410.

- Apply 2-4 drops of lymphatic system blend above or other recommended oils diluted 50:50 on sore lymph glands and under arms 2-3 times daily.
- Have Raindrop Technique weekly or as needed.
- Place a warm compress with 1-2 drops of chosen oil over affected areas 1-2 times daily.
- Massage lymphatic system blend above over lymph gland areas and then apply Cel-Lite Magic Massage Oil and Grapefruit or Cypress oil that help detoxify chemicals stored in body fat.

## MCT (Mixed Connective Tissue Disease)
*(See also Lupus)*

MCT is an autoimmune disease similar to lupus in which the connective tissue in the body becomes inflamed and painful. This condition is usually due to poor assimilation of protein and mineral deficiencies.

### Recommendations

**Singles:** Rosemary, Nutmeg, Clove, Basil, Marjoram, Peppermint, Wintergreen

**Blends:** Relieve It, Valor, Valor II, Valor Roll-On, ImmuPower, PanAway, Cool Azul

**Nutritionals:** Sulfurzyme, Essentialzyme, Detoxzyme, Pure Protein Complete, Mineral Essence, JuvaPower, JuvaSpice, ICP, MultiGreens, MegaCal, OmegaGize[3]

**Body Care:** Cool Azul Pain Relief Cream, Cool Azul Sports Gel, Ortho Ease Massage Oil

### MCT Blend for Aches and Discomfort
- 10 drops Basil
- 8 drops Wintergreen
- 6 drops Cypress
- 3 drops Peppermint

## Application and Usage

**Aromatic:** Refer to *Application Guidelines* on page 410.

**Topical:** For guidelines on applying oils to the skin, refer to *Application Guidelines* on page 410.

- Massage 4-8 drops diluted 50:50 on affected locations 2-3 times daily.
- Apply 1-3 drops on the Vita Flex points of the feet.
- Have Raindrop Technique weekly or as needed.

### MCT/Lupus Regimen
- Rub 2-4 drops of ImmuPower over the liver and on the liver Vita Flex Points on the bottom of the right foot 2-3 times daily. This has been reported to help fight lupus, which is similar to MCT.

## MALARIA

Malaria is a serious disease contracted from several species of Anopheles mosquitoes. While malaria is largely confined to the continents of Asia and Africa, an increasing number of cases have arisen in North and South America. If not treated, malaria can be fatal. If malaria is suspected, seek medical attention. Symptoms are fever, chills, and anemia.

The best defense against malaria is to use insect repellents effective against Anopheles mosquitoes. Once a person has contracted the disease, one of the few natural aids to healing it is natural quinine. Essential oils such as Melaleuca Quinquenervia (Niaouli) can help amplify immune response.

### Recommendations

**Singles:** Ocotea, Melaleuca Quinquenervia (Niaouli), Jade Lemon, Jade Lemon Vitality, Lemon, Lemon Vitality, Lime, Lime Vitality, Thyme, Thyme Vitality, Sacred Frankincense, Frankincense, Frankincense Vitality, Rosemary, Rosemary Vitality, Sage, Sage Vitality, Fennel, Fennel Vitality, Geranium, Yarrow

**Blends:** Thieves, Thieves Vitality, Melrose, ImmuPower

**Nutritionals:** Inner Defense, Digest & Cleanse, Multi-Greens, JuvaPower

**Body Care:** Prenolone Plus Body Cream, Thieves Spray (for protection from nerve damage)

## Application and Usage

**Aromatic:** Refer to *Application Guidelines* on page 410.

**Dietary and Oral:** Whether putting the oils in a capsule or drinking them in a liquid, please refer to *Application Guidelines* on page 410.

- Take 1 capsule with desired oil 2 times daily.
- Take 2-3 drops of oil in a spoonful of syrup or small amount of milk, juice, or water.
- Mix 3-6 drops Lemon Vitality in 1 teaspoon Blue Agave or Yacon Syrup and 8 oz. of water, shake, and sip regularly to build the immune system.

**Topical:** For guidelines on applying oils to the skin, refer to *Application Guidelines* on page 410.

- Apply 1-2 drops neat or diluted 50:50 on temples and back of neck, as desired.
- Applying a single drop under the nose is helpful and refreshing.
- Massage 2-4 drops of oil neat on the bottoms of the feet just before bedtime.

## MALE HORMONE IMBALANCE

As men age, their DHEA and testosterone levels decline. Conversely, levels of dihydrotestosterone (DHT) increase, contributing to prostate enlargement and hair loss.

Because pregnenolone is the master hormone from which all hormones are created. Men can directly benefit from transdermal pregnenolone creams as a way of jump-starting sagging DHEA levels.

Herbs such as saw palmetto and *Pygeum africanum* can prevent the conversion of testosterone into DHT, thereby reducing prostate enlargement and slowing hair loss.

### Recommendations

**Singles:** Idaho Blue Spruce, Rosemary, Rosemary Vitality, Sage, Sage Vitality, Fennel, Fennel Vitality, Geranium, Clary Sage, Yarrow, Sacred Frankincense, Frankincense, Frankincense Vitality

**Blends:** Shutran, Mister, SclarEssence, SclarEssence Vitality

**Nutritionals:** EndoGize, Prostate Health, Protec

**Body Care:** Prenolone Plus Body Cream

## Application and Usage

**Aromatic:** Refer to *Application Guidelines* on page 410.

**Dietary and Oral:** Whether putting the oils in a capsule or drinking them in a liquid, please refer to *Application Guidelines* on page 410.

- Take 1 capsule with desired oil 1 time daily only.
- Take 2-3 drops of oil in a spoonful of syrup or small amount of milk, juice, or water.

**Topical:** For guidelines on applying oils to the skin, refer to *Application Guidelines* on page 410.

- Applying a single drop under the nose is helpful and refreshing.
- Dilute 50:50 and apply on location 3-6 times daily.
- Massage 2-4 drops of oil neat on the bottoms of the feet just before bedtime.

## MEASLES

Measles, also called rubella, is a highly contagious—but rare—respiratory infection caused by a virus. It causes a total-body skin rash and flu-like symptoms, including a fever, cough, and runny nose.

Since measles is caused by a virus, symptoms typically go away on their own without medical treatment once the virus has run its course. A person with measles should get plenty of fluids and rest and avoid spreading the infection to others.

The first symptoms of the infection are sometimes a hacking cough, runny nose, high fever, and watery, red eyes. Another indicator is Koplik's spots, small red spots with blue-white centers inside the mouth.

The measles rash typically has a red or reddish brown, blotchy appearance and first usually shows up on the forehead, then spreads downward over the face, neck, and body and then down to the feet.

### Recommendations

**Singles:** Lavender, Lavender Vitality, Roman Chamomile, Tea Tree, Clove, Clove Vitality, Northern Lights Black Spruce, Thyme, Thyme Vitality, German Chamomile, German Chamomile Vitality, Ravintsara, Dalmatia Bay Laurel, Laurus Nobilis, Laurus Nobilis Vitality

**Blends:** Thieves, Thieves Vitality, Melrose

**Nutritionals:** ImmuPro, Super C, Super C Chewable, Longevity Softgels, Life 9, Digest & Cleanse, Inner Defense

**Measles Blend**
- 10 drops Lavender or Lavender Vitality
- 10 drops German Chamomile or German Chamomile Vitality
- 5 drops Ravintsara
- 5 drops Tea Tree

## Application and Usage

**Aromatic:** Refer to *Application Guidelines* on page 410.

**Dietary and Oral:** Whether putting the oils in a capsule or drinking them in a liquid, please refer to *Application Guidelines* on page 410.

- Take 1 capsule with 5 drops of desired oil 2-3 times daily.
- Take 2-3 drops of oil in a spoonful of syrup or small amount of milk, juice, or water.

**Topical:** For guidelines on applying oils to the skin, refer to *Application Guidelines* on page 410.

- Apply 2-3 drops diluted 50:50 on location 3-5 times daily or as needed.
- Mix 6-9 drops of any of the recommended oils in bath salts and soak at least 30 minutes daily.
- Mix 6-9 drops of any of the recommended oils in 8 oz. water, shake well, and use to sponge down the patient 1-2 times daily.

# MENSTRUAL AND FEMALE HORMONE CONDITIONS
*(See also Ovarian and Uterine Cysts)*

Natural hormones such as natural progesterone and pregnenolone are the most effective treatment for menstrual difficulties and irregularities. The most effective method of administration is transdermal delivery in a cream. Just 20 mg applied to the skin twice daily is equivalent to 1,000 mg taken internally.

As women reach menopause, progesterone production declines, and a state of estrogen dominance often arises. The most commonly prescribed drugs are conjugated estrogens (from horse urine) or synthetic medroxyprogesterone. The molecules in these animal and synthetic hormones are foreign to the human body and can dramatically increase the risk for ovarian and breast cancer with time.

## Endometriosis

This occurs when the uterine lining develops on the outer wall of the uterus, ovaries, fallopian tubes, vagina, intestines, or on the abdominal wall. These fragments cannot escape like the normal uterine lining that is shed during menstruation.

Because of this, fibrous cysts often form around the misplaced uterine tissue. Symptoms can include abdominal or back pain during menstruation or pain that often increases after the period is over. Other symptoms may include heavy periods and pain during intercourse.

## Recommendations

**Singles:** Fennel, Fennel Vitality, Clary Sage, Sage, Sage Vitality, Helichrysum

**Blends:** Thieves, Thieves Vitality, Melrose, SclarEssence, SclarEssence Vitality, Lady Sclareol

**Nutritionals:** ImmuPro, EndoGize, FemiGen, Super C, Super C Chewable, PD 80/20, ICP, Estro, ComforTone, Essentialzyme, Essentialzymes-4

**Body Care:** Prenolone Plus Body Cream, Progessence Plus

## Application and Usage

**Aromatic:** Refer to *Application Guidelines* on page 410.

**Dietary and Oral:** Whether putting the oils in a capsule or drinking them in a liquid, please refer to *Application Guidelines* on page 410.

- Take 1 capsule with desired oil 2 times daily.
- Take 2-3 drops of oil in a spoonful of syrup or small amount of milk, juice, or water.
- Colon and liver cleanse: ICP, ComforTone, Detoxzyme, Essentialzyme, JuvaPower

**Topical:** For guidelines on applying oils to the skin, refer to *Application Guidelines* on page 410.

- Apply a hot compress containing Melrose on the stomach.
- Massage 2-4 drops of Thieves blend neat on the bottoms of the feet.

## Excessive Bleeding

The most common causes of heavy menstrual bleeding are hormonal imbalances, uterine fibroids or polyps, lack of ovulation, use of an intrauterine device, miscarriage, use of anticoagulants, or endometriosis.

## Recommendations

**Singles:** Helichrysum, Cypress, Cistus

**Blends:** PanAway, Deep Relief Roll-On, Relieve It, Cool Azul

**Nutritionals:** OmegaGize[3], JuvaTone, Rehemogen

**Body Care:** Progessence Plus, Prenolone Plus Body Cream, Cool Azul Pain Relief Cream

**Excessive Bleeding Blend**
- 10 drops Cypress
- 5 drops Helichrysum
- 5 drops Cistus

## Application and Usage

**Aromatic:** Refer to *Application Guidelines* on page 410.

**Dietary and Oral:** Whether putting the oils in a capsule or drinking them in a liquid, please refer to *Application Guidelines* on page 410.

- Take 1 capsule with desired oil 2 times daily.
- Take 2-3 drops of oil in a spoonful of syrup or small amount of milk, juice, or water.
- Drink 1/10 teaspoon cayenne in 8 oz. warm water to help regulate bleeding during periods.

**Topical:** For guidelines on applying oils to the skin, refer to *Application Guidelines* on page 410.

- Apply 4-6 drops diluted 50:50 to the forehead, crown of the head, bottoms of the feet, lower abdomen, and lower back 1-3 times daily.
- Place a warm compress with 1-2 drops of chosen oil on lower back and abdomen.

## Hormonal Edema (Cyclic)

This type of edema usually fluctuates with the female menstrual cycle. A good progesterone hormone cream might be the way to begin; however, before starting any hormone therapy, you should see your doctor or health care professional and ask for a hormone blood panel to evaluate your needs.

## Recommendations

**Singles:** Clary Sage, Sage, Sage Vitality, Geranium, Tangerine, Tangerine Vitality

**Blends:** SclarEssence, SclarEssence Vitality, Lady Sclareol, Dragon Time, EndoFlex, EndoFlex Vitality

**Nutritionals:** Thyromin, PD 80/20, Ultra Young, FemiGen, EndoGize

**Body Care:** Progessence Plus, Prenolone Plus Body Cream

## Hysterectomy

A hysterectomy is a surgical removal of all or part of a woman's uterus.

## Recommendations

**Singles:** Sage, Sage Vitality, Clary Sage

**Blends:** Dragon Time, Lady Sclareol, SclarEssence, SclarEssence Vitality

**Nutritionals:** PD 80/20, EndoGize, FemiGen

**Body Care:** Progessence Plus, Prenolone Plus Body Cream

## Application and Usage

**Aromatic:** Refer to *Application Guidelines* on page 410.

**Topical:** For guidelines on applying oils to the skin, refer to *Application Guidelines* on page 410.

- Massage 2-4 drops of oil neat on the bottoms of the feet just before bedtime.
- Place a warm compress with 1-2 drops of chosen oil over the lower back and abdomen.

## Irregular Periods

Menstrual cycles that vary more than a few days in length from month to month are considered to be irregular. All women have variations occasionally, but true irregularity persists over several months.

## Recommendations

**Singles:** Peppermint, Peppermint Vitality, Clary Sage, Sage, Sage Vitality, Roman Chamomile, Fennel, Fennel Vitality, Jasmine, Canadian Fleabane (Conyza)

**Blends:** EndoFlex, EndoFlex Vitality, SclarEssence, SclarEssence Vitality, Inner Child, Peace & Calming, Peace & Calming II

**Body Care:** Progessence Plus, Prenolone Plus Body Cream

**Period Regulator Blend No. 1**
- 16 drops Clary Sage
- 11 drops Sage
- 9 drops Canadian Fleabane (Conyza)
- 5 drops Peppermint
- 5 drops Jasmine

**Period Regulator Blend No. 2**
- 10 drops Roman Chamomile
- 10 drops Fennel Vitality

## Application and Usage

**Aromatic:** Refer to *Application Guidelines* on page 410.

**Topical:** For guidelines on applying oils to the skin, refer to *Application Guidelines* on page 410.

- Apply 4-6 drops diluted 50:50 to forehead, crown of the head, bottoms of the feet, lower abdomen, and lower back 1-3 times daily.

- Massage 3-6 drops on the reproductive Vita Flex points of the feet 2-3 times daily.
- Place a warm compress on the lower back and lower abdomen daily.

## Menopause

As women age, their levels of progesterone decline and contribute to osteoporosis, increased risk of breast and uterine cancers, mood swings, depression, and many other conditions. Estrogen levels can also decline and increase women's risk of heart disease.

Between the ages of 45 and 55, these hormones decline to a point where menstruation ceases. Replacing these declining levels using topically applied progesterone or pregnenolone creams may be the most effective way to replace and boost declining hormone levels.

Pregnenolone may be especially effective as it is the precursor hormone from which the body creates both progesterone and estrogens.

## Recommendations

**Singles:** Geranium, Clary Sage, Sage, Sage Vitality, Bergamot, Bergamot Vitality

**Blends:** Dragon Time, Lady Sclareol, Transformation, SclarEssence, SclarEssence Vitality

**Nutritionals:** PD 80/20, EndoGize

**Body Care:** Progessence Plus, Prenolone Plus Body Cream

## Application and Usage

**Aromatic:** Refer to *Application Guidelines* on page 410.

**Topical:** For guidelines on applying oils to the skin, refer to *Application Guidelines* on page 410.

- Apply 4-6 drops diluted 50:50 to forehead, crown of the head, bottoms of the feet, lower abdomen, and lower back 1-3 times daily.
- Massage 3-6 drops on the reproductive Vita Flex points of the feet.
- Place a warm compress on the lower back and lower abdomen daily.

## Menstrual Cramps

Menstrual cramps (dysmenorrhea) are throbbing, dull, or cramping pains in the lower abdomen that many women experience just before and during their menstrual periods. The pain may be just annoying, or it may be severe enough to interfere with daily activities. Treating the underlying cause is important to reducing pain.

## Recommendations

**Singles:** Valerian, Lavender, Lavender Vitality, Clary Sage, Basil, Basil Vitality, Rosemary, Rosemary Vitality, Sage, Sage Vitality, Roman Chamomile, Cypress, Tarragon, Tarragon Vitality, Vetiver, Idaho Blue Spruce

**Blends:** Dragon Time, EndoFlex, EndoFlex Vitality

**Nutritionals:** PD 80/20, EndoGize, Deep Relief Roll-On, Relieve It, PanAway, NingXia Red

**Body Care:** Prenolone Plus Body Cream, Regenolone Moisturizing Cream

**Menstrual Cramp Relief Blend**
- 10 drops Dragon Time
- 5 drops Hops (*Humulus lupulus*)

## Application and Usage

**Aromatic:** Refer to *Application Guidelines* on page 410.

**Dietary and Oral:** Whether putting the oils in a capsule or drinking them in a liquid, please refer to *Application Guidelines* on page 410.

- Take 1 capsule with desired oil 2 times daily for 2 weeks prior to menses.
- Take 2-3 drops of oil in a spoonful of syrup or small amount of milk, juice, or water.
- If migraine headaches accompany periods, a colon and liver cleanse may reduce symptoms.

**Topical:** For guidelines on applying oils to the skin, refer to *Application Guidelines* on page 410.

- Place a warm compress over the uterus area 2-3 times weekly.
- Massage 2-4 drops on the reproductive Vita Flex points of the feet.
- Apply 2-3 drops of the recommended oils above to the lower back and stomach area several times daily as needed.

## Premenstrual Syndrome (PMS)

PMS is one of the most common hormone-related conditions in otherwise healthy women.

Women can experience a wide range of symptoms for 10 to 14 days before menstruation and even 2 to 3 days into menstruation. These symptoms include mood swings, fatigue, headaches, breast tenderness, abdominal bloating, anxiety, depression, confusion, memory loss, sugar cravings, cramps, low back pain, irritability, weight gain, acne, and oily skin and hair.

Causes are hormonal, nutritional, and psychological. The stress of the Western culture can also be a cause.

510 | **Chapter 20** | Personal Usage Guide

Personal Usage Guide | Chapter 20

## Recommendations

**Singles:** Rose, Clary Sage, Idaho Blue Spruce, Sage, Sage Vitality, Fennel, Fennel Vitality, Ylang Ylang, Amazonian Ylang Ylang, Neroli, Bergamot, Bergamot Vitality

**Blends:** SclarEssence, SclarEssence Vitality, Dragon Time, Mister, EndoFlex, EndoFlex Vitality, Acceptance, Aroma Siez, Lady Sclareol, Transformation

**Nutritionals:** PowerGize, MultiGreens, Super B, Sulfurzyme, Mineral Essence, ImmuPro, PD 80/20, Thyromin, EndoGize

**Body Care:** Prenolone Plus Body Cream, Progessence Plus

## Application and Usage

**Aromatic:** Refer to *Application Guidelines* on page 410.

**Dietary and Oral:** Whether putting the oils in a capsule or drinking them in a liquid, please refer to *Application Guidelines* on page 410.

- Take 1 capsule with desired oil 2 times daily.
- Take 2-3 drops of oil in a spoonful of syrup or small amount of milk, juice, or water.
- Place 1 drop of EndoFlex Vitality on the tongue and then hold the tongue on the roof of the mouth 2-4 times daily.

**Topical:** For guidelines on applying oils to the skin, refer to *Application Guidelines* on page 410.

- Apply 4-6 drops diluted 50:50 to forehead, crown of the head, bottoms of the feet, lower abdomen, and lower back 1-3 times daily.
- Massage 2-4 drops on reproductive Vita Flex points of the feet.
- Place a warm compress on the lower back and lower abdomen daily.

# MUCUS (EXCESS)

Many oils are natural expectorants, helping tissues discharge mucus, soft and hard plaque, and toxins.

## Recommendations

**Singles:** Lavender, Lavender Vitality, Jade Lemon, Jade Lemon Vitality, Lemon, Lemon Vitality, Lime, Lime Vitality, Cypress, Peppermint, Peppermint Vitality, Tea Tree, Pine, Thyme, Thyme Vitality, Eucalyptus Globulus, Rosemary, Rosemary Vitality

**Blends:** TummyGize, DiGize, DiGize Vitality, Raven, 3 Wise Men, Purification, R.C., Breathe Again Roll-On, SniffleEase

**Nutritionals:** Allerzyme, Detoxzyme, Essentialzyme, Essentialzymes-4, ImmuPro, Inner Defense, Life 9

### Expectorant Blend

- 3 drops Lemon
- 3 drops Eucalyptus Globulus
- 2 drops Pine

## Application and Usage

**Aromatic:** Refer to *Application Guidelines* on page 410.

**Note:** Some studies conclude that the expectorant effect of essential oils is obtained faster and stronger through aroma than through ingestion

**Topical:** For guidelines on applying oils to the skin, refer to *Application Guidelines* on page 410.

- Apply 2-4 drops, diluted 50:50, on the T4 and T5 thoracic vertebrae at the neck to the shoulder intersection 3-5 times daily.
- Massage recommended oils on Vita Flex points of the feet 2-4 times daily.

**Dietary and Oral:** Whether putting the oils in a capsule or drinking them in a liquid, please refer to *Application Guidelines* on page 410.

- Take 1 capsule with desired oil 2 times daily.
- Take 2-3 drops of oil in a spoonful of syrup or small amount of milk, juice, or water.

# MUMPS (INFECTIOUS PAROTITIS)

Mumps is an acute, contagious, viral disease marked by painful swelling and inflammation of the salivary glands. The causative agent is a paramyxovirus that is spread by direct contact, airborne droplets, and urine.

## Recommendations

**Singles:** Dorado Azul, Thyme, Thyme Vitality, Tea Tree, Ravintsara, Melissa, Myrrh, Blue Cypress, Northern Lights Black Spruce, Wintergreen

**Blends:** R.C., Raven, Breathe Again Roll-On, SniffleEase, Thieves, Thieves Vitality, Deep Relief Roll-On, PanAway, Relieve It, Cool Azul, JuvaCleanse, JuvaCleanse Vitality

**Nutritionals:** ImmuPro, Super C, Super C Chewable, Exodus II, Inner Defense, Essentialzyme, Detoxzyme, JuvaPower, JuvaSpice, Sulfurzyme, Power Meal, Slique Shake, Balance Complete, Pure Protein Complete

**Body Care:** Cool Azul Pain Relief Cream

Seventh Edition | **Essential Oils Desk Reference** | 511

**Essential Oils Desk Reference** | Seventh Edition

## Application and Usage

**Aromatic:** Refer to *Application Guidelines* on page 410.

**Dietary and Oral:** Whether putting the oils in a capsule or drinking them in a liquid, please refer to *Application Guidelines* on page 410.

- Take 1 capsule with desired oil 2 times daily.
- Take 2-3 drops of oil in a spoonful of syrup or small amount of milk, juice, or water.

**Topical:** For guidelines on applying oils to the skin, refer to *Application Guidelines* on page 410.

- Apply 2-4 drops diluted 50:50 behind the ears 4 times daily.
- Receive a Raindrop Technique 1-2 times weekly.
- Place a warm compress 1-3 times daily around the throat and jaw.

## MUSCLES

The body has more than 600 muscles that are grouped into three categories—smooth, cardiac, and skeletal—and are all made of a type of elastic tissue.

### Bruised Muscles *(See also BRUISING)*

A bruise is a skin discoloration and occurs when small blood vessels break and leak their contents into the tissue beneath the skin. The main symptoms of a bruise are pain, skin discoloration, and swelling.

### Recommendations

**Singles:** Helichrysum, Copaiba, Geranium, German Chamomile, Wintergreen, Cypress, Basil, Peppermint, Lavender

**Blends:** Cool Azul, Aroma Siez, PanAway, Peace & Calming, Peace & Calming II, Deep Relief Roll-On, Relieve It

**Nutritionals:** PowerGize, MegaCal, Mineral Essence, NingXia Red, Sulfurzyme, BLM, AgilEase, Super B

**Body Care:** Cool Azul Pain Relief Cream, Cool Azul Sports Gel, Ortho Ease Massage Oil, Ortho Sport Massage Oil, Relaxation Massage Oil

### Application and Usage

**Topical:** For guidelines on applying oils to the skin, refer to *Application Guidelines* on page 410.

- Apply 2-4 drops diluted 50:50 to bruised area 3 times daily.
- Sequence of application for bruising:

- When a bruise displays black and blue discoloration and pain, start with Helichrysum, Geranium, or Wintergreen.
- When the pain and inflammation decrease, use Cypress, then Basil, and then Aroma Siez to help the muscle relax.
- Follow with Peppermint to stimulate nerve response and reduce inflammation.
- Finish with cold packs.

## Inflammation Due to Infection

Inflammation is the first response of the immune system to irritation or infection and is characterized by swelling, heat, redness, pain, and dysfunction of the organs involved. Treatment depends on the type of infection.

### Recommendations

**Singles:** Ravintsara, Thyme, Myrrh, Hyssop, Blue Cypress

**Nutritionals:** BLM, AgilEase, Longevity Softgels, ImmuPro, Detoxzyme, Essentialzyme, Essentialzymes-4, Digest & Cleanse

**Body Care:** Cool Azul Pain Relief Cream, Cool Azul Sports Gel

### Application and Usage

**Topical:** For guidelines on applying oils to the skin, refer to *Application Guidelines* on page 410.

- Massage 2-4 drops diluted 50:50 on inflamed muscle 3 times daily.
- Place a cold compress on location up to 1-3 times daily.

## Inflammation Due to Injury

Tissue damage is usually accompanied by inflammation. Reduce inflammation by massaging with anti-inflammatory oils to minimize further tissue damage and speed healing.

### Recommendations

**Singles:** Wintergreen, German Chamomile, Nutmeg, Palo Santo, Peppermint, Lavender, Myrrh, Marjoram, Clove, Thyme, Copaiba, Lemongrass, Vetiver, Yarrow

**Blends:** PanAway, Aroma Siez, Deep Relief Roll-On, Relieve It, Cool Azul

**Nutritionals:** BLM, AgilEase, PowerGize, Mineral Essence, MegaCal, Sulfurzyme, Detoxzyme, Allerzyme, MultiGreens, Life 9

512 | Chapter 20 | Personal Usage Guide

**Muscle Injury Blend**
- 10 drops German Chamomile
- 8 drops Lavender
- 6 drops Marjoram
- 3 drops Yarrow
- 2 drops Peppermint

## Application and Usage

**Topical:** For guidelines on applying oils to the skin, refer to *Application Guidelines* on page 410.

- Massage 2-4 drops diluted 50:50 on inflamed muscle 3 times daily.

## Muscle Spasms, Cramps, and Charley Horses

Magnesium and calcium deficiency may contribute to muscle cramps.

## Recommendations

**Singles:** Idaho Blue Spruce, Idaho Balsam Fir, Dorado Azul, Wintergreen, Ravintsara, Basil, Rosemary, Fennel, Marjoram, Elemi, Nutmeg, Copaiba, Black Pepper, Palo Santo

**Blends:** PanAway, Cool Azul, Relieve It, Aroma Siez, Deep Relief Roll-On

**Nutritionals:** PowerGize, MegaCal, Mineral Essence, BLM, AgilEase, Sulfurzyme, Life 9

**Body Care:** Cool Azul Pain Relief Cream, Ortho Sport Massage Oil, Ortho Ease Massage Oil, Cool Azul Sports Gel, Relaxation Massage Oil, Regenolone Moisturizing Cream

## Application and Usage

**Aromatic:** Refer to *Application Guidelines* on page 410.

**Topical:** For guidelines on applying oils to the skin, refer to *Application Guidelines* on page 410.

**Blend for Muscle Spasms**
- 2 drops Ravintsara
- 5 drops Aroma Siez
- 2 drops Black Pepper

Apply 2-4 drops diluted 50:50 on cramped muscle 3 times daily. Alternate with cold and hot packs when applying the blend for muscle spasms.

## Muscle Weakness

To overcome temporary muscle weakness, eat a balanced diet, replace lost fluids, engage in only light activities, and slowly start exercising again. However, muscles

## Tired and Fatigued Muscles

Tired muscles may be lacking in minerals such as calcium and magnesium. Mega Cal and Mineral Essence are excellent sources of both trace and macro minerals and are good for all muscle conditions. Enzymes including Essentialzyme, Essentialzymes-4, and Allerzyme all help with the needed enzymatic conversion of minerals for absorption.

that slowly become weaker for no apparent reason could indicate a disease or condition in the body. Check with your health care professional.

## Recommendations

**Singles:** Idaho Balsam Fir, Ravintsara, Dorado Azul, Palo Santo, Northern Lights Black Spruce, Juniper, Nutmeg, Lemongrass

**Blends:** En-R-Gee, The Gift, Sacred Mountain

**Nutritionals:** BLM, AgilEase, Power Meal, Slique Shake, MultiGreens, Balance Complete, Pure Protein Complete, MegaCal, JuvaPower, JuvaSpice, PowerGize

## Application and Usage

**Topical:** For guidelines on applying oils to the skin, refer to *Application Guidelines* on page 410.

- Massage 4-6 drops diluted 50:50 into weak muscles 3 times daily.

## Sore Muscles

Whenever you engage in a more strenuous activity than you normally do, you may create microscopic tears (microtrauma) in your muscle tissue. The more tears you create, the more soreness you feel later on as the muscles are being repaired. The soreness is a result of both the damage to the muscles and the chemical waste products produced by the muscles when they are being used.

## Recommendations

**Singles:** Rosemary, Wintergreen, Black Pepper, Eucalyptus Blue, Ginger, Northern Lights Black Spruce, Pine, Marjoram, Peppermint, Lemongrass, Helichrysum, Idaho Balsam Fir, Basil, Vetiver, Elemi, Cypress, Dorado Azul.

**Blends:** PanAway, Deep Relief Roll-On, Cool Azul, Peace & Calming, Peace & Calming II, M-Grain, Aroma Siez

**Essential Oils Desk Reference** | Seventh Edition

## Make Your Own High-powered Massage Oil

Add either of these recipes to 4 oz. of V-6 Vegetable Oil Complex to create a custom, muscle-toning formula.

**Massage Oil Recipe No. 1:**
- 10 drops Eucalyptus Blue
- 10 drops Idaho Balsam Fir
- 10 drops Marjoram
- 8 drops Elemi
- 8 drops Vetiver
- 5 drops Helichrysum
- 5 drops Cypress
- 5 drops Peppermint

**Massage Oil Recipe No. 2:**
- 20 drops Eucalyptus Blue
- 15 drops Marjoram
- 10 drops Juniper
- 10 drops Cypress
- 6 drops Dorado Azul

**Nutritionals:** PowerGize, MegaCal, Mineral Essence, Power Meal, Slique Shake, Sulfurzyme

**Body Care:** Cool Azul Pain Relief Cream, Cool Azul Sports Gel, Ortho Sport Massage Oil, Ortho Ease Massage Oil

**Sore Muscle Blend No. 1**
- 5 drops Idaho Balsam Fir
- 4 drops Marjoram
- 4 drops Basil
- 2 drops Rosemary

**Sore Muscle Blend No. 2**
- 5 drops Pine
- 4 drops Rosemary
- 4 drops Ginger
- 1 drop Vetiver

### Application and Usage

**Topical:** For guidelines on applying oils to the skin, refer to *Application Guidelines* on page 410.

- Massage 4-6 drops diluted 50:50 into sore muscles up to 3 times daily.
- Place a warm compress on location up to 1-3 times daily.

## MUSCULAR DYSTROPHY

Muscular dystrophy is a group of disorders that involve loss of muscle tissue and muscle weakness that get progressively worse. All or only specific groups of muscles may be affected.

### Recommendations

**Singles:** Palo Santo, Pine, Lavender, Marjoram, Lemongrass, Vetiver, Idaho Balsam Fir

**Blends:** PanAway, Aroma Siez, Relieve It, Deep Relief Roll-On, Cool Azul

**Nutritionals:** BLM, AgilEase, PowerGize, Sulfurzyme, Essentialzymes-4, Power Meal, Slique Shake, Pure Protein Complete, MultiGreens, Mineral Essence, Essentialzyme, Super B

**Body Care:** Cool Azul Pain Relief Cream, Cool Azul Sports Gel, Ortho Ease Massage Oil, Ortho Sport Massage Oil

### Application and Usage

**Topical:** For guidelines on applying oils to the skin, refer to *Application Guidelines* on page 410.

- Massage 4-6 drops diluted 50:50 along spine 3 times daily.

## NAILS, BRITTLE OR WEAK

Poor or weak nails, often containing ridges, indicate a sulfur, calcium, and/or vitamin A deficiency; disease; infection; trauma; unhealthy diet; use of nail polish and remover; use of detergents; or excessive exposure to water.

### Recommendations

**Singles:** Myrrh, Lemon, Lemon Vitality, Sacred Frankincense, Frankincense, Frankincense Vitality, Wintergreen, Idaho Balsam Fir

**Blends:** Citrus Fresh, Citrus Fresh Vitality, DiGize, DiGize Vitality, GLF, GLF Vitality

**Nutritionals:** Sulfurzyme, MegaCal, Mineral Essence, Master Formula, Essentialzyme, Essentialzymes-4, NingXia Red, Ningxia Wolfberries (Organic, Dried)

### Nail Strengthening Blend
- 4 drops Wheat Germ Oil
- 2 drops Sacred Frankincense or Frankincense
- 2 drops Myrrh
- 2 drops Lemon
- 1 drop Wintergreen

514 | Chapter 20 | Personal Usage Guide

Personal Usage Guide | Chapter 20

## Application and Usage

**Dietary and Oral:** Whether putting the oils in a capsule or drinking them in a liquid, please refer to *Application Guidelines* on page 410.

- Take 1 capsule with desired oil 2 times daily.
- Place a few drops of oil on the tongue 1-4 times as needed.
- Take 2-3 drops of oil in a spoonful of syrup or small amount of milk, juice, or water.

**Topical:** For guidelines on applying oils to the skin, refer to *Application Guidelines* on page 410.

- Apply 1-3 drops of oil neat on nails and at base of nails daily for 30 days.
- Apply 1 drop of the blend on each nail 2-3 times daily for 30 days.

## NARCOLEPSY *(See also Thyroid Problems)*

Narcolepsy is a chronic ailment consisting of uncontrollable, recurrent attacks of drowsiness and sleep during the daytime. Narcolepsy may be aggravated by hypothalamus dysregulation or thyroid hormone deficiency.

### Recommendations

**Singles:** Peppermint, Lemon, Canadian Fleabane (Conyza), Rosemary, Black Pepper

**Blends:** Clarity, Brain Power, Awaken, Common Sense, GeneYus, Motivation, M-Grain

**Nutritionals:** Thyromin, MultiGreens, Mineral Essence, MindWise, Essentialzyme, Essentialzymes-4, Life 9, Sulfurzyme, JuvaPower, Power Meal, Slique Shake

### Application and Usage

**Aromatic:** Refer to *Application Guidelines* on page 410.

**Topical:** For guidelines on applying oils to the skin, refer to *Application Guidelines* on page 410.

- Apply 1-2 drops diluted 50:50 on temples, behind ears, back of neck, on forehead, and under nostrils as needed.

## NAUSEA

Patchouli oil contains compounds that are extremely effective in preventing vomiting due to their ability to reduce the gastrointestinal muscle contractions associated with vomiting.[32] Peppermint has also been found to be effective in many kinds of stomach upset, including nausea.

### Recommendations

**Singles:** Patchouli, Peppermint, Peppermint Vitality, Ginger, Ginger Vitality, Nutmeg, Nutmeg Vitality, Ocotea

**Blends:** TummyGize, DiGize, DiGize Vitality, JuvaCleanse, JuvaCleanse Vitality, GLF, GLF Vitality

**Nutritionals:** AlkaLime, Detoxzyme, Essentialzymes-4, Essentialzyme, Digest & Cleanse, MegaCal, Life 9

### Application and Usage

**Aromatic:** Refer to *Application Guidelines* on page 410.

**Dietary and Oral:** Whether putting the oils in a capsule or drinking them in a liquid, please refer to *Application Guidelines* on page 410.

- Take 1 capsule with desired oil 2 times daily.
- Place a few drops of oil on the tongue 1-4 times as needed.
- Take 2-3 drops of oil in a spoonful of syrup or small amount of milk, juice, or water.

**Topical:** For guidelines on applying oils to the skin, refer to *Application Guidelines* on page 410.

- Massage 1-3 drops diluted 50:50 behind each ear (mastoids) and over navel 2-3 times hourly.
- Place a warm compress with 1-2 drops of chosen oil over the back or the stomach as needed.
- Rub 1-2 drops of oil on the temples and back of neck several times daily.

## Morning Sickness

The medical definition for "morning sickness" is "nausea and vomiting of pregnancy." Sometimes the symptoms are worse in the morning, but they can strike at any time; and for many women, they last all day long. The intensity varies from woman to woman.

### Recommendations

**Singles:** Peppermint, Peppermint Vitality, Ginger, Ginger Vitality, Spearmint, Spearmint Vitality, Lavender, Lavender Vitality, Jade Lemon, Jade Lemon Vitality, Lemon, Lemon Vitality, Lime, Lime Vitality, Patchouli

**Blends:** DiGize, DiGize Vitality, Gentle Baby

**Nutritionals:** Essentialzymes-4, Essentialzyme, Life 9, Detoxzyme, AlkaLime, Power Meal, Slique Shake, MegaCal

Seventh Edition | **Essential Oils Desk Reference** | 515

## Application and Usage

**Aromatic:** Refer to *Application Guidelines* on page 410.

**Dietary and Oral:** Whether putting the oils in a capsule or drinking them in a liquid, please refer to *Application Guidelines* on page 410.

- Take 1 capsule with desired oil 2 times daily.
- Place a few drops of oil on the tongue 1-4 times as needed.
- Take 2-3 drops of oil in a spoonful of syrup or small amount of milk, juice, or water.

**Topical:** For guidelines on applying oils to the skin, refer to *Application Guidelines* on page 410.

- Massage 1-3 drops diluted 50:50 behind each ear (mastoids) and over navel 2-3 times hourly.
- Place a warm compress on stomach as needed.

### Motion Sickness

Motion sickness is a bodily response to real or perceived movement. The inner ear senses movement, while your eyes tell you that you are standing still. This confuses the brain and causes dopamine levels to increase, which causes motion sickness. Common symptoms are nausea, vomiting, dizziness, and fatigue.

## Recommendations

**Singles:** Peppermint, Peppermint Vitality, Ginger, Ginger Vitality, Patchouli, Spearmint, Spearmint Vitality, Lavender, Lavender Vitality, Rose, Sacred Frankincense, Frankincense, Frankincense Vitality, Palo Santo

**Blends:** Valor, Valor II, Valor Roll-On, Harmony, TummyGize, DiGize, DiGize Vitality, Tranquil Roll-On, Peace & Calming, Peace & Calming II

**Nutritionals:** Essentialzymes-4, Essentialzyme, Detoxzyme, MegaCal, Mineral Essence, EndoGize

### Motion Sickness Preventive Blend
- 2 drops Peppermint Vitality
- 2 drops Ginger Vitality
- 2 drops Patchouli
- 5 drops V-6 Vegetable Oil Complex

## Application and Usage

**Aromatic:** Refer to *Application Guidelines* on page 410.

**Dietary and Oral:** Whether putting the oils in a capsule or drinking them in a liquid, please refer to *Application Guidelines* on page 410.

- Take 1 capsule with desired oil 2 times daily.

- Place a few drops of oil on the tongue 1-4 times as needed.
- Take 2-3 drops of oil in a spoonful of syrup or small amount of milk, juice, or water.

**Topical:** For guidelines on applying oils to the skin, refer to *Application Guidelines* on page 410.

- Massage 1-3 drops diluted 50:50 behind each ear (mastoids) and over navel 2-3 times hourly.
- Place a warm compress on stomach as needed.
- Rub 6-10 drops of the blend on chest and stomach 1 hour before traveling.

## NERVE DISORDERS
*(See also Neurological Diseases)*

Nerve disorders usually involve peripheral or surface nerves and include Bell's palsy, carpal tunnel syndrome, neuralgia, neuritis, and neuropathy. In contrast, neurological diseases are usually associated with deep neurological disturbances in the brain. These conditions include ALS (Lou Gehrig's disease), MS, and Parkinson's disease.

MegaCal and Mineral Essence used with OmegaGize3 and MindWise help provide calcium, magnesium, and natural lipids, including healthy omega-3 fatty acids, necessary to maintain nerve signal transmissions along neurological pathways.

Sulfur deficiency is often present in nerve problems. Sulfur requires calcium and vitamins B and C for the body to metabolize. Super B, Super C, and Sulfurzyme work well together to help repair nerve damage and the myelin sheath.

**CAUTION:** Never use hot packs for neurological problems. Always use cold packs to reduce pain and inflammation.

### Bell's Palsy

This is a type of neuritis, marked by paralysis on one side of the face and inability to open or close the eyelid.

## Recommendations

**Singles:** Peppermint, Rosemary, Vetiver, Cypress, Royal Hawaiian Sandalwood, Helichrysum, Pine

**Blends:** Aroma Siez, RutaVaLa, RutaVaLa Roll-On, Deep Relief Roll-On, PanAway, Relieve It, PowerGize

**Nutritionals:** MultiGreens, Sulfurzyme, Super B, Super C, Super C Chewables, MegaCal, Mineral Essence, MindWise, Ultra Young, OmegaGize[3]

**Body Care:** Cool Azul Pain Relief Cream, Cool Azul Sports Gel, Ortho Ease Massage Oil

Personal Usage Guide | Chapter 20

## Application and Usage

**Aromatic:** Refer to *Application Guidelines* on page 410.

**Topical:** For guidelines on applying oils to the skin, refer to *Application Guidelines* on page 410.

- Use 1-2 drops neat to massage on the facial nerve in front and behind the ears and on any areas of pain 3-5 times daily until symptoms end.

## Carpal Tunnel Syndrome

Nerves pass through a tunnel formed by wrist bones (known as carpals) and a tough membrane on the underside of the wrist that binds the bones together. The tunnel is rigid, so if the tissues within it swell, they press and pinch the nerves and create a painful condition known as carpal tunnel syndrome, which is often the result of a combination of factors that increase pressure on the median nerve and tendons in the carpal tunnel, rather than a problem with the nerve itself.

Often the problem is due to a genetic factor in which the carpal tunnel is smaller in some people than in others. Other possible factors are trauma or injury to the wrist that causes swelling, such as a fracture or sprain; overactivity of the pituitary gland; work stress; hypothyroidism; rheumatoid arthritis; repeated use of vibrating hand tools; fluid retention during pregnancy or menopause; mechanical problems in the wrist joint; or the development of a cyst or tumor in the canal. Sometimes other causes or no causes can be identified.

Repeated motions can result in repetitive motion disorders such as tendonitis or bursitis, but there is little clinical data to prove that such repetitive or forceful movements of the hand and wrist during leisure activities or work can cause carpal tunnel syndrome.

A similar, but less common condition can occur in the ankle (tarsal tunnel syndrome) or elbow.

## Recommendations

**Singles:** Wintergreen, Helichrysum, Marjoram, Peppermint, Vetiver, Basil, Cypress, Lemongrass, Myrrh

**Blends:** PanAway, Cool Azul, Relieve It, Aroma Siez, Deep Relief Roll-On

**Nutritionals:** Sulfurzyme, MegaCal, Mineral Essence, Ultra Young, PD 80/20, BLM, AgilEase, PowerGize

**Body Care:** Cool Azul Pain Relief Cream, Cool Azul Sports Gel, Regenolone Moisturizing Cream, Ortho Ease Massage Oil, Ortho Sport Massage Oil

## Carpal Tunnel Blend

- 5 drops Wintergreen
- 2 drops Marjoram
- 3 drops Cypress
- 1 drop Peppermint
- 3 drops Myrrh

## Application and Usage

**Topical:** For guidelines on applying oils to the skin, refer to *Application Guidelines* on page 410.

- Apply 2-4 drops neat or diluted 50:50 to affected area 3-5 times daily, as needed.
- Place a cold compress on location 2-3 times daily.

## Neuralgia

Neuralgia is pain from a damaged nerve. It can occur in the face, spine, or elsewhere. This recurring pain can be traced along a nerve pathway. Carpal tunnel syndrome is a specific type of neuralgia. The primary symptom is temporary sharp pain in the peripheral nerve(s).

## Recommendations

**Singles:** Wintergreen, Helichrysum, Peppermint, Marjoram, Nutmeg, Tea Tree, Roman Chamomile, Rosemary

**Blends:** Cool Azul, RutaVaLa, RutaVaLa Roll-On, Relieve It, Peace & Calming, Peace & Calming II, Deep Relief Roll-On, PanAway

**Nutritionals:** PD 80/20, BLM, AgilEase, Sulfurzyme, Super B, Super C, Super C Chewable, MindWise, OmegaGize[3]

**Body Care:** Cool Azul Pain Relief Cream, Cool Azul Sports Gel, Regenolone Moisturizing Cream, Prenolone Plus Body Cream, Ortho Ease Massage Oil, Ortho Sport Massage Oil

## Application and Usage

**Topical:** For guidelines on applying oils to the skin, refer to *Application Guidelines* on page 410.

- Apply 2-4 oil drops neat or diluted 50:50 to affected area 3-5 times daily, as needed.
- Place a cold compress on location 2-3 times daily.

## Neuritis

Neuritis is a painful inflammation of the peripheral nerves. It is usually caused by prolonged exposure to cold temperature, heavy-metal poisoning, diabetes, vitamin deficiencies (beriberi and pellagra), and infectious diseases such as typhoid fever and malaria.

Symptoms may include pain, burning, numbness, tingling, muscle weakness, or paralysis.

Seventh Edition | **Essential Oils Desk Reference** | 517

## Recommendations

**Singles:** Lavender, Nutmeg, Copaiba, Helichrysum, Canadian Fleabane (Conyza), Juniper, Vetiver, Valerian, Thyme, Yarrow, Clove

**Blends:** Cool Azul, PanAway, Relieve It, Valor, Valor II, Valor Roll-On, Aroma Siez, Deep Relief Roll-On, RutaVaLa, RutaVaLa Roll-On

**Nutritionals:** PowerGize, Sulfurzyme, Super B, Super C, Super C Chewable, PD 80/20, OmegaGize[3], Ultra Young, MindWise

**Body Care:** Cool Azul Pain Relief Cream, Cool Azul Sports Gel, Regenolone Moisturizing Cream, Prenolone Plus Body Cream

## Application and Usage

**Aromatic:** Refer to *Application Guidelines* on page 410.

**Topical:** For guidelines on applying oils to the skin, refer to *Application Guidelines* on page 410.

- Apply 2-4 drops neat or diluted 50:50 to affected area 3-5 times daily as required.
- Place a cold compress on location 2-3 times daily.

## Neuropathy

Neuropathy refers to actual damage to the peripheral nerves, usually from an autoimmune condition.

Damage to these peripheral nerves (other than spinal or those in the brain) generally starts as tingling in hands and feet and slowly spreads along limbs to the trunk.

Numbness, sensitive skin, neuralgic pain, and weakening of muscle power can all develop in varying degrees. Most common causes include complications from diabetes (diabetic neuropathy), alcoholism, vitamin B12 deficiency, tumors, too many painkillers, exposure to and absorption of chemicals, metals, pesticides, etc.

B vitamins and minerals such as magnesium, calcium, potassium, and organic sulfur are important in repairing nerve damage and quenching pain from inflamed nerves.

Canadian Fleabane *(Conyza)* may boost production of pregnenolone and human growth hormone. Pregnenolone aids in repairing damage to the myelin sheath.[33] Juniper also may help in supporting nerve repair.

If paralysis is a problem, a regeneration of up to 60 percent may be possible. If, however, the nerve damage is too severe, treatment may not help. If the damage starts to reverse, there will be pain. Apply a few drops of PanAway neat on location.

Symptoms include tingling or numbness, gangrene.

## Recommendations

**Singles:** Sacred Frankincense, Frankincense, Lavender, Cedarwood, Idaho Blue Spruce, Peppermint, Roman Chamomile, Vetiver, Valerian, Geranium, Yarrow, Goldenrod, Helichrysum, Canadian Fleabane (Conyza), Nutmeg

**Blends:** Cool Azul, Aroma Siez, Peace & Calming, Peace & Calming II, PanAway, RutaVaLa, RutaVaLa Roll-On, Deep Relief Roll-On

**Nutritionals:** PowerGize, Ultra Young, Super B, OmegaGize[3], Sulfurzyme, Longevity Softgels, Mineral Essence, MegaCal, Super B, Super C, Super C Chewable, MultiGreens, PD 80/20, MindWise

**Body Care:** Prenolone Plus Body Cream, Cool Azul Pain Relief Cream, Cool Azul Sports Gel, Ortho Ease Massage Oil, Ortho Sport Massage Oil

### Neuropathy Blend No. 1
- 3 drops Sacred Frankincense or Frankincense
- 3 drops Geranium
- 3 drops Lavender

### Neuropathy Blend No. 2
- 3 drops Geranium
- 3 drops Canadian Fleabane (Conyza)
- 3 drops Cedarwood
- 2 drops Peppermint

## Application and Usage

**Aromatic:** Refer to *Application Guidelines* on page 410.

**Topical:** For guidelines on applying oils to the skin, refer to *Application Guidelines* on page 410.

- Apply 2-4 drops neat or diluted 50:50 to affected area 3-5 times daily, as required.
- Place a cold compress on location 2-3 times daily.

# NERVOUS SYSTEM, AUTONOMIC

The autonomic nervous system controls involuntary activities such as heartbeat, breathing, digestion, glandular activity, and contraction and dilation of blood vessels.

The autonomic nervous system is composed of two parts that balance and complement each other: the parasympathetic and sympathetic nervous systems.

## To Stimulate Parasympathetic Nervous System

The parasympathetic nervous system has relaxing effects and is responsible for secreting acetylcholine, which slows the heart and speeds digestion.

Personal Usage Guide | **Chapter 20**

## Recommendations

**Singles:** Lavender, Lavender Vitality, Valerian, Patchouli, Marjoram, Marjoram Vitality, Ylang Ylang, Amazonian Ylang Ylang, Rose, Vetiver, Idaho Blue Spruce, Dalmatia Sage, Sage, Sage Vitality

**Blends:** Peace & Calming, Peace & Calming II, Harmony, Valor, Valor II, Valor Roll-On, RutaVaLa, RutaVaLa Roll-On

**Nutritionals:** NingXia Red, MegaCal, MindWise, Sulfurzyme, Mineral Essence, Super B, Super C, Super C Chewable

## Application and Usage

**Aromatic:** Refer to *Application Guidelines* on page 410.

**Dietary and Oral:** Whether putting the oils in a capsule or drinking them in a liquid, please refer to *Application Guidelines* on page 410.

- Take 1 capsule with desired oil 2 times daily.
- Take 2-3 drops of oil in a spoonful of syrup or small amount of milk, juice, or water.

**Topical:** For guidelines on applying oils to the skin, refer to *Application Guidelines* on page 410.

- Have Raindrop Technique 2 times a week.

## To Stimulate Sympathetic Nervous System

The sympathetic nervous system has stimulatory effects and is responsible for secreting stress hormones like adrenaline and noradrenaline.

## Recommendations

**Singles:** Fennel, Fennel Vitality, Ginger, Ginger Vitality, Eucalyptus Radiata, Peppermint, Peppermint Vitality, Rosemary, Rosemary Vitality, Black Pepper, Black Pepper Vitality

**Blends:** Clarity, Brain Power, GeneYus

**Nutritionals:** Super B, Super C, Super C Chewable, Sulfurzyme, Mineral Essence, MindWise, Essentialzymes-4, Essentialzyme, MegaCal

## Application and Usage

**Aromatic:** Refer to *Application Guidelines* on page 410.

**Dietary and Oral:** Whether putting the oils in a capsule or drinking them in a liquid, please refer to *Application Guidelines* on page 410.

- Take 1 capsule with desired oil 2 times daily.

- Take 2-3 drops of oil in a spoonful of syrup or small amount of milk, juice, or water.

**Topical:** For guidelines on applying oils to the skin, refer to *Application Guidelines* on page 410.

- Have Raindrop Technique 2 times a week.

## NEUROLOGIC DISEASES
*(See also Nerve Disorders)*

Neurologic diseases are disorders of the spinal cord, brain, and nerves throughout your body. Together they control all of the functions of the body. There are more than 600 neurologic diseases.

**CAUTION:** Never use hot packs for neurological problems. Always use cold packs to reduce pain and inflammation. In other words, reduce the temperature of the damaged site.

### ALS (Lou Gehrig's Disease)

Lou Gehrig's disease is another name for Amyotrophic Lateral Sclerosis (ALS), a degenerative nerve disorder. ALS affects the nerve fibers in the spinal cord that control voluntary movement.

Muscles require continuous stimulation by their associated nerves to maintain their tone. Removal or deadening of these nerves results in muscular atrophy. The lack of control forces the muscles to spasm, resulting in twitching and cramps. The sensory pathways are unaffected, so feeling is never lost in the afflicted muscles.

Juniper may support nerve function. Frankincense may help clear the emotions of fear and anger, which is common with people who have these neurologic diseases. When these diseases are contracted, people often become suicidal.

Hope, Joy, Gathering, and Forgiveness will help individuals work through the psychological and emotional aspects of the disease.

Sulfur deficiency is often prevalent in neurological diseases. Sulfur requires calcium and vitamin C for the body to metabolize. Super B and Sulfurzyme work well together to help repair nerve damage and the myelin sheath.

### Recommendations

**Singles:** Rosemary, Rosemary Vitality, Royal Hawaiian Sandalwood, Sacred Frankincense, Frankincense, Frankincense Vitality, Helichrysum, Cypress, Sage, Sage Vitality, Juniper, Clove, Clove Vitality, Cardamom, Cardamom Vitality, Eucalyptus Blue, Ylang Ylang, Amazonian Ylang Ylang

Seventh Edition | **Essential Oils Desk Reference** | 519

**Blends:** Hope, Joy, Gathering, Brain Power, Clarity, GeneYus, Forgiveness, Common Sense

**Nutritionals:** PD 80/20, BLM, AgilEase, Sulfurzyme, MindWise, MultiGreens, MegaCal, Super C, Super C Chewable, Super B, Longevity Softgels, OmegaGize[3]

**Body Care:** Prenolone Plus Body Cream, Cool Azul Pain Relief Cream

## ALS Blend

- 3 drops Rosemary or Rosemary Vitality
- 2 drops Clove or Clove Vitality
- 1 drop Eucalyptus Blue
- 1 drop Ylang Ylang (or Amazonian Ylang Ylang)
- 1 drop Sacred Frankincense, Frankincense, or Frankincense Vitality

## Application and Usage

**Aromatic:** Refer to *Application Guidelines* on page 410..

**Dietary and Oral:** Whether putting the oils in a capsule or drinking them in a liquid, please refer to *Application Guidelines* on page 410.

- Take 1 capsule with desired oil 2 times daily.
- Take 2-3 drops of oil in a spoonful of syrup or small amount of milk, juice, or water.

**Topical:** For guidelines on applying oils to the skin, refer to *Application Guidelines* on page 410.

- Apply 1-3 drops diluted 50:50 on the brain reflex points on the forehead, temples, and mastoids (just behind ears).
- Use a direct pressure application and massage 6-10 drops diluted 50:50 from the base of the skull, down the neck, and down the spine.
- Place a few drops of oil on a loofah brush and rub along the spine vigorously. (Always use a natural bristle brush, since the oils may dissolve plastic bristles.)
- Receive a Raindrop Technique 3 times monthly.

## Huntington's Chorea

Huntington's chorea is a degenerative nerve disease that generally becomes manifest in middle age. It is marked by uncontrollable body movements, which are followed—and occasionally preceded—by mental deterioration.

**Note:** Huntington's chorea should not be confused with Sydenham's chorea, often called St. Vitus Dance, chorea minor, or juvenile chorea that affects children, especially females, usually appearing between the ages of 7 and 14. The jerking symptoms eventually disappear.

## Recommendations

**Singles:** Peppermint, Peppermint Vitality, Ocotea, Juniper, Basil, Basil Vitality, Royal Hawaiian Sandalwood, Sacred Frankincense, Frankincense, Frankincense Vitality, Geranium, Palo Santo, Eucalyptus Blue

**Blends:** Aroma Siez, RutaVaLa, RutaVaLa Roll-On, EndoFlex, EndoFlex Vitality, Awaken, Christmas Spirit, Citrus Fresh, Citrus Fresh Vitality, Tranquil Roll-On

**Nutritionals:** PowerGize, Sulfurzyme, BLM, AgilEase, MultiGreens, NingXia Red, Ningxia Wolfberries (Organic, Dried), Power Meal, Slique Shake, Super C, Super C Chewable, Super B, MegaCal, MindWise, OmegaGize[3], Master Formula, Balance Complete, Mineral Essence, Essentialzyme, Allerzyme

## Application and Usage

**Aromatic:** Refer to *Application Guidelines* on page 410.

**Dietary and Oral:** Whether putting the oils in a capsule or drinking them in a liquid, please refer to *Application Guidelines* on page 410.

- Take 1 capsule with desired oil 2 times daily.
- Take 2-3 drops of oil in a spoonful of syrup or small amount of milk, juice, or water.

**Topical:** For guidelines on applying oils to the skin, refer to *Application Guidelines* on page 410.

- Apply 1-3 drops diluted 50:50 on the brain reflex points on the forehead, temples, and mastoids just behind ears.
- Use a direct pressure application and massage 6-10 drops diluted 50:50 from the base of the skull, down the neck, and down the spine.
- Place a few drops of oil on a loofah brush and rub along the spine vigorously. Always use a natural bristle brush, since the oils may dissolve plastic bristles.
- Receive a Raindrop Technique 3 times monthly.

**Nerve Blend**
- 5 drops Juniper
- 3 drops Aroma Siez
- 2 drops Peppermint or Peppermint Vitality
- 1 drop Basil or Basil Vitality

Personal Usage Guide | **Chapter 20**

## Multiple Sclerosis (MS)

Multiple sclerosis is a progressive, disabling autoimmune disease of the nervous system, brain, and spinal cord in which inflammation occurs in the central nervous system. Eventually, the myelin sheaths protecting the nerves are destroyed, resulting in a slowing or blocking of nerve transmission.

MS is an autoimmune disease in which the body's own immune system attacks the nerves. Some researchers believe that MS is triggered by a virus, while others make a case that it has a strong genetic or environmental component.

### Symptoms

- Muscle weakness in extremities
- Deteriorating coordination and balance
- Numbness or prickling sensations
- Poor attention or memory
- Speech impediments
- Incontinence
- Tremors
- Dizziness
- Hearing loss

### Recommendations

**Singles:** Juniper, Geranium, Sacred Frankincense, Frankincense, Frankincense Vitality, Rosemary, Rosemary Vitality, Basil, Basil Vitality, Helichrysum, Royal Hawaiian Sandalwood, Peppermint, Peppermint Vitality, Thyme, Thyme Vitality, Marjoram, Marjoram Vitality, Cypress

**Blends:** PanAway, Cool Azul, Valor, Valor II, Valor Roll-On, Aroma Siez, RutaVaLa, RutaVaLa Roll-On, Acceptance, Awaken

**Nutritionals:** BLM, AgilEase, PowerGize, OmegaGize[3], Sulfurzyme, MultiGreens, Power Meal, Slique Shake, Essentialzyme, Essentialzymes-4, Mineral Essence, MegaCal, Super C, Super C Chewable, Super B, NingXia Red, MindWise

**Body Care:** Cool Azul Pain Relief Cream, Cool Azul Sports Gel, Progessence Plus, Regenolone Moisturizing Cream, Ortho Sport Massage Oil, Ortho Ease Massage Oil

### MS Blend

- 4 drops Geranium
- 4 drops Rosemary or Rosemary Vitality
- 2 drops Helichrysum
- 2 drops Juniper

## Maintaining Multiple Sclerosis (MS) Status Quo

One of the simplest ways to keep MS symptoms from becoming more severe is to keep the body cool and avoid any locations or physical activities that heat the body (including hot showers or exercise). Cold baths and relaxed swimming are two of the best activities for relieving symptoms.

Applying heat is the worst thing to do for MS. If an MS patient is experiencing increasingly severe symptoms, lower the patient's body temperature (by up to 3 degrees F) by having the patient lie on a table, covering the patient with a sheet, ice, shower curtain, and blankets (in that order) for 10 to 15 minutes or longer if possible. The individual can tell you how he or she feels. Work the feet with oils and watch for benefits.

### Application and Usage

**Aromatic:** Refer to *Application Guidelines* on page 410.

**Dietary and Oral:** Whether putting the oils in a capsule or drinking them in a liquid, please refer to *Application Guidelines* on page 410.

- Take 1 capsule with desired oil 2 times daily.
- Take 2-3 drops of oil in a spoonful of syrup or small amount of milk, juice, or water.

**Topical:** For guidelines on applying oils to the skin, refer to *Application Guidelines* on page 410.

- Apply 1-3 drops diluted 50:50 on the brain reflex points on the forehead, temples, and mastoids just behind the ears.
- Apply direct pressure and massage 6-10 drops diluted 50:50 from the base of the skull, down the neck, and down the spine.
- Place a few drops of oil on a loofah brush and rub along the spine vigorously. Always use a natural bristle brush, since the oils may dissolve plastic bristles.
- Receive a Raindrop Technique 3-4 times monthly.

### MS Daily Regimen

1. Apply neat 4-6 drops of Helichrysum, Geranium, Juniper, Royal Hawaiian Sandalwood, Rosemary, and Peppermint Raindrop-style along the spine. Lightly massage oils in the direction of the MS paralysis. For example, if it is in the lower part of

Seventh Edition | **Essential Oils Desk Reference** | **521**

the spine, massage down; if it is in the upper part of the spine, massage up. Follow the application with 30 minutes of cold packs (change cold packs as needed).

2. Apply 4-6 drops of Valor on the spine. If the MS affects the legs, rub down the spine; if it affects the neck, rub up the spine.

3. Apply 2-3 drops each of Cypress, Royal Hawaiian Sandalwood, and Marjoram to the back of the neck and then cover with 2-3 drops of Aroma Siez.

To give additional emotional support to the person with MS symptoms, use Acceptance and Awaken. Be patient. Overcoming MS is a long-term endeavor.

## Parkinson's Disease

Parkinson's disease is a deterioration of specific nerve centers in the brain that affects more men than women by a ratio of 3:2.

### Symptoms
- Tremors, an involuntary shaking of hands, head, or both
- Rigidity, slowed movement, and loss of balance
- Stooped posture
- Continuous rubbing together of thumb and forefinger
- Mask-like face
- Trouble swallowing
- Depression
- Difficulty performing simple tasks

These symptoms may all be seen at different stages of the disease. The tremors are most severe when the affected part of the body is not in use. There is no pain or other sensation, other than a decreased ability to move. Symptoms appear slowly in no particular order and may end before they interfere with normal activities.

Restoring dopamine levels in the brain can reduce symptoms of Parkinson's. Sulfurzyme provides a source of organic sulfur, a vital nutrient for nerve and myelin sheath formation.

### Recommendations

**Singles:** Helichrysum, Lavender, Lavender Vitality, Peppermint, Peppermint Vitality, Cedarwood, Myrrh, Basil, Basil Vitality, Royal Hawaiian Sandalwood

**Blends:** GLF, GLF Vitality, Peace & Calming, Peace & Calming II, Valor, Valor II, Valor Roll-On, Brain Power, Shutran

**Nutritionals:** PowerGize, Sulfurzyme, Super B, PD 80/20, BLM, AgilEase, MindWise, Mineral Essence, Power Meal, Slique Shake, JuvaPower, JuvaSpice, Super C, Super C Chewable, Life 9, OmegaGize[3], Essentialzyme, Essentialzymes-4

## Application and Usage

**Aromatic:** Refer to *Application Guidelines* on page 410.

**Dietary and Oral:** Whether putting the oils in a capsule or drinking them in a liquid, please refer to *Application Guidelines* on page 410.

- Take 1 capsule with desired oil 2 times daily.
- Take 2-3 drops of oil in a spoonful of syrup or small amount of milk, juice, or water.

**Topical:** For guidelines on applying oils to the skin, refer to *Application Guidelines* on page 410.

- Apply 1-3 drops diluted 50:50 on the brain reflex points on the forehead, temples, and mastoids just behind the ears.
- Use a direct pressure application and massage 6-10 drops diluted 50:50 from the base of the skull, down the neck, and down the spine.
- Place a few drops of oil on a loofah brush and rub along the spine vigorously. Always use a natural bristle brush, since the oils may dissolve plastic bristles.
- Receive a Raindrop Technique 3 times monthly.

**CAUTION:** Never use hot packs for neurological problems. Always use cold packs to reduce pain and inflammation. In other words, reduce the temperature of the affected area.

## Restless Legs Syndrome
*(See also Attention Deficit Disorder)*

Restless legs syndrome (Willis-Ekbom disease) is a neurologic disorder characterized by an irresistible urge to move the body to stop odd or uncomfortable sensations. It commonly affects the legs but can also affect the torso, arms, and even phantom limbs.

### Recommendations

**Singles:** Valerian, Lavender, Lavender Vitality, Basil, Basil Vitality, Marjoram, Marjoram Vitality, Cypress, Roman Chamomile

**Blends:** RutaVaLa, RutaVaLa Roll-On, Aroma Siez, Peace & Calming, Peace & Calming II, Tranquil Roll-On, Stress Away Roll-On, Valor, Valor II, Valor Roll-On

**Nutritionals:** ImmuPro, Mineral Essence, MultiGreens, MegaCal, OmegaGize[3], SleepEssence, Thyromin, MindWise, PowerGize, BLM, AgilEase

## Application and Usage

**Aromatic:** Refer to *Application Guidelines* on page 410.

**Dietary and Oral:** Whether putting the oils in a capsule or drinking them in a liquid, please refer to *Application Guidelines* on page 410.

- Take 1 capsule with desired oil 2 times daily.
- Take 2-3 drops of oil in a spoonful of syrup or small amount of milk, juice, or water.

**Topical:** For guidelines on applying oils to the skin, refer to *Application Guidelines* on page 410.

- Apply 2-4 drops neat as desired.
- Massage 2-4 drops of oil on the Vita Flex points of the feet before retiring.
- Receive a Raindrop Technique 1 time a week.

### Schizophrenia

This is a neurologic disease that involves identity confusion. Onset is typically between the late teens and early 30's. Abnormal neurological findings may show a broad range of dysfunction, including slow reaction time, poor coordination, abnormalities in eye tracking, and impaired sensory gating.

Typically, schizophrenia involves dysfunction in one or more areas such as interpersonal relations, work, education, or self-care. Some cases are believed to be caused by viral infection.

## Recommendations

**Singles:** Cardamom, Cardamom Vitality, Cedarwood, Vetiver, Melissa, Rosemary, Rosemary Vitality, Valerian, Peppermint, Peppermint Vitality, Sacred Frankincense, Frankincense, Frankincense Vitality

**Blends:** Brain Power, GeneYus, Valor, Valor II, Valor Roll-On, M-Grain, Clarity, Common Sense

**Nutritionals:** Mineral Essence, MegaCal, MindWise, NingXia Red, Super B, Power Meal, Slique Shake, JuvaPower, JuvaSpice, Master Formula, Ningxia Wolfberries (Organic, Dried)

## Application and Usage

**Aromatic:** Refer to *Application Guidelines* on page 410.

- Diffuse your choice of oils for ½ hour every 4-6 hours or as desired.

**Dietary and Oral:** Whether putting the oils in a capsule or drinking them in a liquid, please refer to *Application Guidelines* on page 410.

- Take 1 capsule with desired oil 2 times daily.
- Take 2-3 drops of oil in a spoonful of syrup or small amount of milk, juice, or water.

**Topical:** For guidelines on applying oils to the skin, refer to *Application Guidelines* on page 410.

- Receive a Raindrop Technique treatment 1 time a week.

# NOSE AND SINUS PROBLEMS

Millions of people have chronic sinus troubles, and millions more suffer from rhinitis, a term for stuffy nose. One of the most effective treatments for nasal and sinus problems is a saltwater nose rinse.

## Dry Nose

Dry nose refers to a lack of moisture in the nasal passage, which can occasionally cause the skin inside the nose to itch, crack, and bleed.

### Recommendations

**Singles:** Myrrh, Lavender, Lemon, Peppermint

**Blends:** R.C., Raven, Breathe Again Roll-On, SniffleEase

**Ointments:** Boswellia Wrinkle Cream, Rose Ointment

**Dry Nose Blend**
- 2 drops Lavender
- 1 drop Myrrh

### Application and Usage

**Aromatic:** Refer to *Application Guidelines* on page 410.

**Topical:** For guidelines on applying oils to the skin, refer to *Application Guidelines* on page 410.

- Apply 1-2 drops diluted 50:50 to the nostril walls with a cotton swab 2 times daily.
- Massage 2-4 drops of oil neat on the bottoms on the Vita Flex points of the feet just before bedtime.

## Loss of Smell

The senses of smell and taste are strongly connected. Some of the common causes of loss of smell and taste are cigarette smoke, medications like antibiotics and blood pressure medicines, the common cold, pollutants, allergies, blocked nasal passages, tooth and gum diseases, chemotherapy, Alzheimer's disease, surgery, tumors, Parkinson's disease, polyps, or even a head injury.

## Nasal Irrigation Regimen

Rosemary and Tea Tree oils can be used in a saline solution for very effective nasal irrigation that clears and decongests sinuses. As recommended by Daniel Pénoël, MD, the saline solution is prepared as follows:

- 10 drops Rosemary
- 6 drops Thyme
- 2 drops Cypress
- 8 tablespoons ultra-fine salt

The essential oils are mixed thoroughly in the fine salt and stored in a sealed container. For each nasal irrigation session, 1 teaspoon of this salt mixture is dissolved into 1½ cups distilled water.

This solution is then placed in the tank of an oral irrigator or neti pot to irrigate the nasal cavities, which is done while bending over a sink. This application has brought surprisingly positive results in treating latent sinusitis and other nasal congestion problems.

## Recommendations

**Singles**: Peppermint, Thyme, Myrtle, Eucalyptus Globulus

**Blends:** R.C., Raven, Exodus II, Joy, Highest Potential, The Gift, Sensation

**Nutritionals:** NingXia Red

## Application and Usage

**Aromatic:** Refer to *Application Guidelines* on page 410.

**Topical:** For guidelines on applying oils to the skin, refer to *Application Guidelines* on page 410.

## Nosebleeds

Nosebleeds usually are not serious. However, if bleeding does not stop in a short time or is excessive or frequent, consult your health care professional.

## Recommendations

**Singles:** Helichrysum, Cistus, Cypress, Dorado Azul, Geranium

**Blends:** GLF, JuvaCleanse

**Nutritionals:** Mineral Essence, Sulfurzyme, Master Formula

### Nosebleed Blend
- 3 drops Helichrysum or Geranium
- 2 drops Cistus
- 2 drops Cypress

## Application and Usage

**Topical:** For guidelines on applying oils to the skin, refer to *Application Guidelines* on page 410.

- Apply 2-4 drops neat to the bridge and sides of the nose and back of the neck. Repeat as needed.
- Applying a single drop under the nose is helpful and refreshing.
- Dilute 50:50 and apply on location 3-6 times daily.
- Massage 2-4 drops of oil neat on the bottoms on the Vita Flex points of the feet just before bedtime. Children love it.

### Nosebleed Regimen
- Put 1 drop of Geranium on a tissue paper and wrap the paper around a chip of ice about the size of a thumb nail, push it up under the top lip in the center to the base of the nose. Hold from the outside with lip pressure. This usually will stop bleeding in a very short time.

## Polyps, Nasal

Nasal polyps are soft, painless, noncancerous growths on the lining of the nasal passages or sinuses. They hang down like grapes or teardrops and result from chronic inflammation due to allergies, asthma, recurring infection, drug sensitivity, or certain immune disorders.

Small polyps may not cause problems, but larger growths or groups of polyps can block the nasal passages, lead to breathing problems, cause frequent infections, or cause a lost sense of smell.

## Recommendations

**Singles:** Citronella, Helichrysum, Sacred Frankincense, Frankincense

**Blend:** Purification, Citrus Fresh, Melrose

## Application and Usage

**Topical:** For guidelines on applying oils to the skin, refer to *Application Guidelines* on page 410.

- Apply 1-2 drops diluted 50:50 on a cotton swab and carefully apply on the inside nostrils 1-3 times daily.

Personal Usage Guide | **Chapter 20**

## OBESITY *(See also Depression)*

Hormone treatments using natural progesterone (for women) and testosterone (for men) may be one of the most powerful treatments for obesity. In women, progesterone levels drop dramatically after menopause, and this can result in substantial weight gain, particularly around the hips and thighs. Using transdermal creams or serums to replace declining progesterone can result in a substantial decline in body fat.

Diffusing or directly inhaling essential oils can have an immediate positive impact on moods and appetites. Olfaction is the only sense that can have a direct effect on the limbic region of the brain. Studies at the University of Vienna have shown that some essential oils and their primary constituents can stimulate blood flow and activity in the emotional centers of the brain.[18]

Fragrance influences can penetrate the amygdala in the center of the brain in such a manner that frequent smelling of pleasing aromas can significantly reduce appetite. Dr. Alan Hirsch, in his landmark studies, showed dramatic weight loss in research subjects using aromas from peppermint oil and vanilla absolute to curb food cravings.[34]

### Recommendations

**Singles:** Peppermint, Peppermint Vitality, Roman Chamomile, Nutmeg, Nutmeg Vitality, Clove, Clove Vitality, Grapefruit, Grapefruit Vitality, Fennel, Fennel Vitality, Cinnamon Bark, Cinnamon Bark Vitality, Lavender, Lavender Vitality, Sacred Frankincense, Frankincense, Frankincense Vitality, Vanilla, Bergamot, Bergamot Vitality

**Blends:** Build Your Dream, Valor, Valor II, Valor Roll-On, JuvaCleanse, JuvaCleanse Vitality, Slique Essence, Oola Balance, Joy, The Gift, 3 Wise Men, Sacred Mountain, White Angelica, White Light, Gathering

**Nutritionals:** JuvaPower, Thyromin, Detoxzyme, OmegaGize[3], Power Meal, Slique Shake, Slique CitraSlim, Slique Bars, Slique Bars (Chocolate-Coated), Slique Gum, Balance Complete, Digest & Cleanse, Pure Protein Complete, Chocolate-Coated Wolfberry Crisp Bars

**Body Care:** Progessence Plus, Prenolone Plus Body Cream, Cel-Lite Magic Massage Oil

### Application and Usage

**Aromatic:** Refer to *Application Guidelines* on page 410.

**Dietary and Oral:** Whether putting the oils in a capsule or drinking them in a liquid, please refer to *Application Guidelines* on page 410.

- Take 1 capsule with desired oil 2 times daily.
- Take 2-3 drops of oil in a spoonful of syrup or small amount of milk, juice, or water.

**Topical:** For guidelines on applying oils to the skin, refer to *Application Guidelines* on page 410.

- Applying a single drop under the nose is helpful and refreshing.
- Massage 2-4 drops of oil neat on the bottoms of the feet just before bedtime.

## ORAL CARE, TEETH AND GUMS

Poor oral hygiene has not only been linked to bad breath (halitosis) but also to cardiovascular disease. Some of the same bacteria that populate the mouth have now been implicated in arteriosclerosis.

Essential oils make excellent oral antiseptics, analgesics, and anti-inflammatories. Clove essential oil has been used in mainstream dentistry for decades to numb the gums and help prevent infections. Similarly, menthol (found in Peppermint essential oil), methyl salicylate (found in Wintergreen essential oil), thymol (found in Thyme essential oil), and eucalyptol (found in Eucalyptus and Rosemary essential oils) are approved OTC drug products for combating gingivitis and periodontal disease.

### Bleeding Gums

Bleeding gums can be a sign that you have, or are at risk for, gum disease. However, persistent gum bleeding may be caused by serious medical conditions such as leukemia or bleeding and platelet disorders. Bleeding gums are mainly due to inadequate plaque removal from the teeth at the gum line, which will lead to gingivitis, or inflamed gums.

### Recommendations

**Singles:** Clove, Clove Vitality, Eucalyptus Globulus, Sacred Frankincense, Frankincense, Frankincense Vitality, Rosemary, Rosemary Vitality, Helichrysum, Wintergreen, Cinnamon Bark, Cinnamon Bark Vitality, Mountain Savory, Mountain Savory Vitality, Myrrh, Peppermint, Peppermint Vitality, Thyme, Thyme Vitality

**Blends:** Thieves, Thieves Vitality, Melrose, PanAway, Relieve It, Slique Essence

**Nutritionals:** Slique Gum, KidScents Slique Toothpaste, Super C

**Oral Care:** Thieves AromaBright Toothpaste, Thieves Dentarome Plus Toothpaste, Thieves Dentarome

Seventh Edition | **Essential Oils Desk Reference** | 525

Ultra Toothpaste, Thieves Fresh Essence Plus Mouthwash, Thieves Dental Floss, Thieves Hard Lozenges, Thieves Mints

### Blend for Combating Gum Bleeding

- 2 drops Myrrh
- 2 drops Helichrysum
- 1 drop Thieves Vitality or Thieves
- 1 drop Frankincense Vitality, Frankincense, or Sacred Frankincense

### Application and Usage

**Dietary and Oral:** Whether putting the oils in a capsule or drinking them in a liquid, please refer to *Application Guidelines* on page 410.

- Take 1 capsule with desired oil 2 times daily.
- Take 2-3 drops of oil in a spoonful of syrup or small amount of milk, juice, or water.
- Gargle 3-10 times daily with Thieves Fresh Essence Plus Mouthwash or as needed.
- Brush teeth and gums after every meal with a Thieves Toothpaste.

**Topical:** For guidelines on applying oils to the skin, refer to *Application Guidelines* on page 410.

- Apply 1-2 drops diluted 50:50 on gums 2-3 times daily.

## Dental Visits

Prior to visiting the dentist, rub 1 drop each of Helichrysum, Clove, and PanAway on gums and jaw. Clove may interfere with bonding of crowns, so keep it off the teeth if this procedure is planned.

**General Oral Infection:** For general oral infection of any kind, roll a piece of gauze tightly into a string about ¼ inch thick. Put drops of Thieves blend on it; if it feels too "hot," add V-6. Put the string between the teeth and the lip and leave it all night, allowing it to "wick up," or absorb, the infection. Change as often as needed.

## Gingivitis and Periodontitis

Periodontal diseases are infections of the gum and bone that hold the teeth in place. Gingivitis affects the upper areas of the gum where it bonds to the visible enamel, while periodontitis is a more internal infection affecting the gum at the root level of the tooth. In advanced stages, these diseases can lead to painful chewing problems and even tooth loss.

Oils such as Peppermint, Wintergreen, Clove, Thyme, and Eucalyptus can kill bacteria and effectively combat a variety of gum infections.

### Recommendations

**Singles:** Clove, Clove Vitality, Tea Tree, Thyme, Thyme Vitality, Mountain Savory, Mountain Savory Vitality, Wintergreen, Peppermint, Peppermint Vitality, Oregano, Oregano Vitality, Plectranthus Oregano, Helichrysum, Eucalyptus Globulus, Eucalyptus Radiata

**Blends:** Thieves, Thieves Vitality, Exodus II, PanAway, Slique Essence, ImmuPower, Cool Azul

**Nutritionals:** Super C, Super C Chewable, Longevity Softgels, OmegaGize³, Inner Defense, ImmuPro

**Oral Care:** Thieves AromaBright Toothpaste, KidScents Slique Toothpaste, Thieves Dentarome Plus Toothpaste, Thieves Dentarome Ultra Toothpaste, Thieves Fresh Essence Plus Mouthwash, Thieves Hard Lozenges, Thieves Mints, Thieves Spray, Thieves Dental Floss, Slique Gum

### Application and Usage

**Dietary and Oral:** Whether putting the oils in a capsule or drinking them in a liquid, please refer to *Application Guidelines* on page 410.

- Take 1 capsule with desired oil 2 times daily.
- Take 2-3 drops of oil in a spoonful of syrup or small amount of milk, juice, or water.
- Gargle 3-10 times daily with Thieves Fresh Essence Plus Mouthwash or as needed.
- Brush teeth and gums after every meal with a Thieves Toothpaste.

**Topical:** For guidelines on applying oils to the skin, refer to *Application Guidelines* on page 410.

## Mouth Ulcers (See Canker Sores)

Mouth ulcers are sores or open lesions in the mouth and are caused by many disorders such as canker sores, oral cancer, thrush, fever blisters, or gingivostomatitis.

### Recommendations

**Singles:** Carrot Seed, Carrot Seed Vitality, Tea Tree, Thyme, Thyme Vitality, Myrrh, Lavender, Lavender Vitality, Peppermint, Peppermint Vitality, Ocotea, Oregano, Oregano Vitality

**Blends:** Thieves, Thieves Vitality, Exodus II, ImmuPower

**Nutritionals:** AlkaLime, ImmuPro, Inner Defense

**Oral Care:** Thieves AromaBright Toothpaste, KidScents Slique Toothpaste, Thieves Dentarome Plus Toothpaste, Thieves Dentarome Ultra Toothpaste, Thieves Fresh Essence Plus Mouthwash, Thieves Hard Lozenges, Thieves Mints, Thieves Spray, Slique Gum

## Application and Usage

**Dietary and Oral:** Whether putting the oils in a capsule or drinking them in a liquid, please refer to *Application Guidelines* on page 410.

- Take 1 capsule with desired oil 2 times daily.
- Take 2-3 drops of oil in a spoonful of syrup or small amount of milk, juice, or water.
- Gargle 3-10 times daily with Thieves Fresh Essence Plus Mouthwash or as needed.
- Brush teeth and gums after every meal with a Thieves Toothpaste.
- Gargle with Thieves Fresh Essence Plus Mouthwash or Thieves Spray and add 1-2 drops of Thieves Vitality, Clove Vitality, and Exodus II to strengthen the therapeutic action.

**Topical:** For guidelines on applying oils to the skin, refer to *Application Guidelines* on page 410.

- Apply 1-2 drops diluted 50:50 on gums 2 times daily.

## Oral Infection Control

Oral infection control procedures are precautions taken in dental offices and other health care settings to prevent the spread of disease.

## Recommendations

**Singles:** Clove, Clove Vitality, Myrrh, Oregano, Oregano Vitality, Plectranthus Oregano, Thyme, Thyme Vitality, Helichrysum, Eucalyptus Radiata

**Blends:** PanAway, Thieves, Thieves Vitality, R.C., Slique Essence, ImmuPower

**Nutritionals:** Inner Defense, ImmuPro, Mineral Essence, Essentialzyme, Essentialzymes-4, Life 9, Detoxzyme, MegaCal, Power Meal, Slique Shake

**Oral Care:** Fresh Essence Plus Mouthwash, Thieves Spray, Thieves AromaBright Toothpaste, KidScents Slique Toothpaste, Thieves Dentarome Plus Toothpaste, Thieves Dentarome Ultra Toothpaste, Thieves Hard Lozenges, Thieves Mints, Slique Gum

## Application and Usage

**Topical:** For guidelines on applying oils to the skin, refer to *Application Guidelines* on page 410.

- Apply 1-2 drops diluted 50:50 on gums and around teeth. Repeat as needed.
- Just before a tooth extraction, rub 1-2 drops of Helichrysum, Thieves Vitality, and R.C. around the gum area.
- Rubbing R.C. on gums may also help to bring back feeling after numbness from anesthesia.

## Pyorrhea

Essential oils are some of the best treatments against gum diseases such as gingivitis and pyorrhea. For example: The active constituent in clove oil is eugenol, which is used as a dental disinfectant and is one of the best-studied germ killers available.

## Recommendation

**Singles:** Clove, Clove Vitality, Thyme, Thyme Vitality, Oregano, Oregano Vitality, Wintergreen; (dilute all 50:50)

**Blends:** Thieves, Exodus II, ImmuPower; (dilute all if desired)

**Nutritionals:** Mineral Essence, Essentialzyme, Essentialzymes-4, Detoxzyme, MegaCal, Power Meal, Slique Shake, Inner Defense, ImmuPro

**Oral Care:** Thieves Fresh Essence Plus Mouthwash, Thieves Spray, Thieves AromaBright Toothpaste, KidScents Slique Toothpaste, Thieves Dentarome Ultra Toothpaste, Thieves Dentarome Plus Toothpaste, Thieves Hard Lozenges, Thieves Mints, Thieves Dental Floss

## Application and Usage

**Dietary and Oral:** Use any of the recommended single oils or blends with toothpaste on toothbrush or alone. Generally, 1-2 drops are very sufficient. For some people, the recommended oils will seem very "hot." Even one drop mixed with toothpaste may seem very strong, but within a minute the "hot" feeling is gone, and the mouth feels very clean and refreshed. Many people like using one drop of Slique Essence or Thieves directly on the toothbrush without using any toothpaste.

- Gargle 4-6 times daily with Thieves Fresh Essence Plus Mouthwash or as needed.
- Mix 1-2 drops of Clove Vitality or any other recommended oil of choice in a glass of water and gargle.
- Spray mouth several times daily with Thieves Spray.

**Topical:** For guidelines on applying oils to the skin, refer to *Application Guidelines* on page 410.

- Put 1-2 drops of Thieves on your toothbrush directly or put 1-2 drops of Thieves on your Dentarome toothpaste.
- Put 1 drop of Thieves directly on affected tooth and gum area, as needed.

## Teeth Grinding

Teeth grinding (bruxism) is a condition in which you grind, clench, or gnash your teeth, consciously or unconsciously. If it is frequent and severe enough, it can lead to jaw disorders, headaches, damaged teeth, and other problems.

### Recommendations

**Singles:** Valerian, Lavender, Lavender Vitality, Roman Chamomile

**Blends:** Peace & Calming, Peace & Calming II, RutaVaLa, RutaVaLa Roll-On, Stress Away Roll-On, Tranquil Roll-On, ImmuPower

**Nutritionals:** Mineral Essence, MegaCal, ImmuPro, SleepEssence, Inner Defense

**Oral Care:** Thieves Spray, Thieves AromaBright Toothpaste, KidScents Slique Toothpaste, Thieves Dentarome Plus Toothpaste, Thieves Dentarome Ultra Toothpaste, Thieves Fresh Essence Plus Mouthwash, Slique Gum

### Application and Usage

**Aromatic:** Refer to *Application Guidelines* on page 410.

**Topical:** For guidelines on applying oils to the skin, refer to *Application Guidelines* on page 410.

- Massage 1-3 drops neat of Lavender, RutaVaLa, and Valerian on bottoms of feet each night before retiring.

## Toothache and Teething Pain

A toothache is a pain in or around a tooth, and treatment for a toothache depends on the cause.

### Recommendations

**Singles:** Clove, Clove Vitality, Sacred Frankincense, Frankincense, Frankincense Vitality, German Chamomile, German Chamomile Vitality, Tea Tree

**Blends:** Thieves, Thieves Vitality, PanAway, Cool Azul, Slique Essence

**Oral Care:** Thieves Spray, Thieves AromaBright Toothpaste, KidScents Slique Toothpaste, Thieves Dentarome Plus Toothpaste, Thieves Dentarome Ultra Toothpaste, Thieves Fresh Essence Plus Mouthwash, Slique Gum

### Application and Usage

**Dietary and Oral:** Whether putting the oils in a capsule or drinking them in a liquid, please refer to *Application Guidelines* on page 410.

- Take 1 capsule with desired oil 2 times daily.
- Take 2-3 drops of oil in a spoonful of syrup or small amount of milk, juice, or water.
- Gargle 4-6 times daily or as needed with Thieves Fresh Essence Plus Mouthwash.

**Note:** All essential oils should be diluted 20:80 before being used orally on small children.

**Topical**: For guidelines on applying oils to the skin, refer to *Application Guidelines* on page 410.

- Apply oil neat or diluted 50:50 on affected tooth and gum area as needed.

## PAIN

One of the most effective essential oils for blocking pain is Helichrysum. A study in 1994 showed that Peppermint is extremely effective in blocking calcium channels and substance P, important factors in the transmission of pain signals.[35] Other essential oils also have unique pain-relieving properties, including Helichrysum, Sacred Frankincense, Frankincense, Eucalyptus Blue, Vetiver, Dorado Azul, Palo Santo, Valerian, and Idaho Balsam Fir.

MSM, a source of organic sulfur, has also been proven to be extremely effective for alleviating pain, especially tissue and joint pain. The subject of a best-selling book by Dr. Ronald Lawrence and Dr. Stanley Jacobs, MSM is redefining the treatment of pain, especially associated with arthritis and fibromyalgia. Sulfurzyme is an excellent source of MSM.

Natural pregnenolone can also blunt pain.

### How MSM Works to Control Pain

When fluid pressure inside cells is higher than outside, pain is experienced. MSM, found in Sulfurzyme, equalizes fluid pressure inside cells and helps balance the protein envelope of the cell so that water transfers freely in and out.

Personal Usage Guide | **Chapter 20**

## Bone-related Pain

Bone pain emanates from the bone tissue and occurs as a result of disease and/or physical conditions. Each type of bone pain has many potential sources or causes.

### Recommendations

**Singles:** Helichrysum, Wintergreen, Idaho Balsam Fir, Copaiba, Peppermint, Vetiver, Dorado Azul, Palo Santo, Idaho Blue Spruce, Pine, Cypress

**Blends:** PanAway, Relieve It, Deep Relief Roll-On, Cool Azul

**Nutritionals:** Sulfurzyme, MegaCal, BLM, AgilEase, Mineral Essence, Master Formula, MultiGreens, Super B, Super C, Super C Chewable

**Body Care:** Cool Azul Pain Relief, Cool Azul Sports Gel, Ortho Ease Massage Oil, Ortho Sport Massage Oil, Regenolone Moisturizing Cream

### Application and Usage

**Dietary and Oral:** Whether putting the oils in a capsule or drinking them in a liquid, please refer to *Application Guidelines* on page 410.

- Take 1 capsule with desired oil 2 times daily.
- Take 2-3 drops of oil in a spoonful of syrup or small amount of milk, juice, or water.
- Gargle 4-6 times daily or as needed with Thieves Fresh Essence Plus Mouthwash.

**Topical:** For guidelines on applying oils to the skin, refer to *Application Guidelines* on page 410.

- Apply 2-4 drops diluted 50:50 on location, as needed.
- Massage several drops onto the Vita Flex points of the feet and repeat as needed.

## Chronic Pain

To pinpoint the most effective essential oil single, blend, or product for quenching pain, it may be necessary to try each of the products in these categories to find those that are most effective for your particular pain situation.

### Recommendations

**Singles:** Helichrysum, Wintergreen, Clove, Clove Vitality, Peppermint, Peppermint Vitality, Dorado Azul, Palo Santo, Idaho Blue Spruce, Elemi, Oregano, Oregano Vitality, Plectranthus Oregano, Idaho Balsam Fir, Copaiba, Copaiba Vitality, Sacred Frankincense, Frankincense, Frankincense Vitality, Northern Lights Black Spruce

### Essential Oils for Pain Control

PanAway is powerful for pain reduction. When applied on location or to the Vita Flex points on the feet, it can act within seconds. Alternate with Relieve It. These two blends are a powerful combination for deep-tissue pain as well as bone-related pain. Deep Relief Roll-On is extremely helpful at home, at work, or when traveling.

**Blends:** PanAway, Deep Relief Roll-On, Cool Azul, Relieve It, Aroma Siez, Release, Sacred Mountain

**Nutritionals:** PowerGize, Sulfurzyme, SuperCal, MegaCal, BLM, AgilEase

**Body Care:** Cool Azul Pain Relief Cream, Cool Azul Sports Gel, Ortho Sport Massage Oil, Ortho Ease Massage Oil, Regenolone Moisturizing Cream

### Application and Usage

**Dietary and Oral:** Whether putting the oils in a capsule or drinking them in a liquid, please refer to *Application Guidelines* on page 410.

- Take 1 capsule with desired oil 2 times daily.
- Take 2-3 drops of oil in a spoonful of syrup or small amount of milk, juice, or water.
- Gargle 4-6 times daily or as needed with Thieves Fresh Essence Plus Mouthwash.

**Note:** All essential oils should be diluted 20:80 before being used orally on small children.

**Topical:** For guidelines on applying oils to the skin, refer to *Application Guidelines* on page 410.

- Apply 2-4 drops diluted 50:50 on location, as needed.
- Place 1-2 drops oil with a warm compress on location, as needed.

## PANCREATITIS

Pancreatitis is an inflammation of the pancreas that can be either acute or chronic.

Acute pancreatitis can be brought on by a sudden blockage in the main pancreatic duct caused by enzymes unable to function properly with pancreas function and literally begin digesting the pancreas unless remedied. If there is not good flow of the enzymatic process whereby nutrients are able to be absorbed and waste eliminated, the enzymes begin to fight against that blockage.

Seventh Edition | **Essential Oils Desk Reference** | 529

**Essential Oils Desk Reference** | Seventh Edition

Chronic pancreatitis occurs more gradually, with attacks recurring over weeks or months.

**Symptoms**

- Abdominal pain
- Muscle aches
- Vomiting
- Jaundice
- Abdominal swelling
- Sudden hypertension
- Rapid weight loss
- Fever

In the case of acute pancreatitis, a total fast for at least 4-5 days is one of the safest and most effective methods of alleviating the problem. In the case of infection, fasting should be combined with immune stimulation by using Exodus II combined with vitamin C and Super B vitamin complex.

## Recommendations

**Singles:** Geranium, Peppermint, Peppermint Vitality, Oregano, Oregano Vitality, Plectranthus Oregano, Vetiver, Mountain Savory, Mountain Savory Vitality, Orange, Orange Vitality

**Blends:** DiGize, DiGize Vitality, Exodus II, Thieves, Thieves Vitality, ImmuPower

**Nutritionals:** MultiGreens, Super B, Digest & Cleanse, OmegaGize[3], Super C, Super C Chewable, Essentialzyme, Essentialzymes-4, Detoxzyme, ImmuPro, Inner Defense

## Application and Usage

**Dietary and Oral:** Whether putting the oils in a capsule or drinking them in a liquid, please refer to *Application Guidelines* on page 410.
- Take 1 capsule with desired oil 3 times weekly.
- Take 2-3 drops of oil in a spoonful of syrup or small amount of milk, juice, or water.

**Topical:** For guidelines on applying oils to the skin, refer to *Application Guidelines* on page 410.

- Receive a Raindrop Technique 2 times a week.
- Retention: Use an enema with the recommended oils 3 times per week.

## PARASITES, INTESTINAL (WORMS)

Many types of parasites use up nutrients while giving off toxins; this can leave the body depleted, nutritionally deficient, and susceptible to infectious disease.

Occasionally, parasites can lie dormant in the body and then become active due to ingestion of a particular food or drink. This can result in the appearance and disappearance of symptoms, even though parasites are always present.

---

### DiGize and ParaFree for Parasite Control

The essential oil blend DiGize and ParaFree softgel capsules are excellent for parasite removal.

**DiGize:** Add 6 drops to 1 tsp. V-6 Vegetable Oil Complex or to 4 oz. rice, almond, or goat milk and take as a dietary supplement 2 times a day, or take 15 drops in a capsule 3 times a day for 7 days. DiGize can also be diluted in massage oil and applied on abdomen.

**ParaFree:** Take 5 softgels, 2-3 times daily for 21 days; then rest for 7 days. Repeat up to 3 times to achieve desired results.

---

The parasite *Cryptosporidium parvum* may be present in many municipal or tap waters. To remove this parasite, the water must be distilled or filtered using a 0.3 micron filter.

**Symptoms**

- Fatigue
- Weakness
- Diarrhea
- Blood in stools
- Chronic pain
- Weight loss
- Gas and bloating
- Cramping
- Nausea
- Irregular bowel movements

The first step to controlling parasites is beginning a fasting and cleansing program. A colon cleanse is particularly important.

## Recommendations

**Singles:** Tarragon, Tarragon Vitality, Fennel, Fennel Vitality, Basil, Basil Vitality, Peppermint, Peppermint Vitality, Ginger, Ginger Vitality, Nutmeg, Nutmeg Vitality, Tea Tree, Rosemary, Rosemary Vitality, Cumin

**Blends:** Thieves, Thieves Vitality, DiGize, DiGize Vitality, JuvaFlex, JuvaFlex Vitality, JuvaCleanse, JuvaCleanse Vitality

**Nutritionals:** ParaFree, Digest & Cleanse, Inner Defense, Life 9, ICP, ComforTone, Detoxzyme, JuvaPower, Essentialzyme, Essentialzymes-4

### Retention Blend for Parasite Killing
- 4 drops Ginger
- 4 drops DiGize
- 16 drops V-6 Vegetable Oil Complex

530 | Chapter 20 | Personal Usage Guide

Personal Usage Guide | **Chapter 20**

## Application and Usage

**Dietary and Oral:** Whether putting the oils in a capsule or drinking them in a liquid, please refer to *Application Guidelines* on page 410.

- Take 1 capsule with desired oil 2 times daily.
- Take 2-3 drops of oil in a spoonful of syrup or small amount of milk, juice, or water.

**Topical**: For guidelines on applying oils to the skin, refer to *Application Guidelines* on page 410.

- Place a warm compress with recommended oils over intestinal area 2 times weekly.
- Massage up to 6 drops on the small intestine and colon Vita Flex points of the feet daily (instep area on both feet).

**Retention:** Add the blend for parasite killing to an enema and insert nightly for 7 nights; then rest for 7 nights. Repeat this cycle 3 times to eliminate all stages of parasite development.

## POLIO

Polio (poliomyelitis) is an acute, infectious disease, usually manifested in epidemics and caused by a virus. It creates an inflammation of the gray matter of the spinal cord and is characterized by fever, sore throat, headache, vomiting, and sometimes stiffness of the neck and back. If it develops into the major illness, it can involve paralysis and atrophy of groups of muscles, ending in contraction and permanent deformity.

If polio is suspected, seek medical attention.

### Recommendations

**Singles:** Sacred Frankincense, Frankincense, Frankincense Vitality, Ravintsara, Blue Cypress, Wintergreen, Tea Tree, Melissa, Northern Lights Black Spruce, Peppermint, Peppermint Vitality, Royal Hawaiian Sandalwood, Palo Santo, Oregano, Oregano Vitality, Plectranthus Oregano, Thyme, Thyme Vitality, Myrrh, Lemon, Lemon Vitality, Mountain Savory, Mountain Savory Vitality

**Blends:** The Gift, Aroma Siez, ImmuPower, Valor, Valor II, Valor Roll-On

**Nutritionals:** ImmuPro, Life 9, PowerGize, Inner Defense

**Oral Care:** Thieves Cough Drops, Thieves Hard Lozenges, Thieves Mints

### Polio Blend

- 15 drops Myrrh
- 10 drops Ravintsara
- 10 drops Wintergreen
- 7 drops Sacred Frankincense, Frankincense Vitality or Frankincense
- 8 drops Blue Cypress
- 6 drops Lemon

## Application and Usage

**Aromatic:** Refer to *Application Guidelines* on page 410.

**Dietary and Oral:** Whether putting the oils in a capsule or drinking them in a liquid, please refer to *Application Guidelines* on page 410.

- Take 1 capsule with desired oil 2 times daily.
- Take 2-3 drops of oil in a spoonful of syrup or small amount of milk, juice, or water.

**Topical:** For guidelines on applying oils to the skin, refer to *Application Guidelines* on page 410.

- Apply 1-2 drops neat or undiluted as desired.
- Applying a single drop under the nose is helpful and refreshing.
- Receive a Raindrop Technique 3 times weekly.

## PREGNANCY

Essential oils can be invaluable companions during pregnancy. Oils like Lavender and Myrrh may help reduce stretch marks and improve the elasticity of the skin. Geranium and Gentle Baby have similar effects and can be massaged on the perineum (tissue between vagina and rectum) to lower the risk of tearing or the need for an episiotomy (an incision in the perineum) during birth.

### Recommendations

**Singles:** Lavender, Myrrh, Rose, Geranium, Helichrysum, German Chamomile, Neroli, Royal Hawaiian Sandalwood, Frankincense, Sacred Frankincense

**Blends:** Gentle Baby, Amoressence, Forgiveness, Valor, Valor II, Valor Roll-On, Grounding, Peace & Calming, Peace & Calming II, Highest Potential, Joy, Sacred Mountain, White Angelica, White Light

**Body Care:** ClaraDerm, Tender Tush

**Labor Blend** (Use only after labor has started.)

- 5 drops Ylang Ylang (or Amazonian Ylang Ylang)
- 4 drops Helichrysum
- 2 drops Fennel Vitality
- 2 drops Peppermint
- 2 drops Clary Sage

Seventh Edition | **Essential Oils Desk Reference** | 531

## Essential Oils and Pregnancy

As always, when using essential oils, common sense is most important when deciding how to use them.

During pregnancy most oils are safe and bring peace and contentment. When rubbing them over the stomach, many women have said that they have felt a positive response from the unborn infant. Energy sensitivity is very high during this time and is something to be aware of and enjoyed. Gentle Baby, Valor, White Angelica, RutaVaLa, Magnify Your Purpose, Joy, Harmony, Highest Potential, Gathering, DiGize, and Dream Catcher are just a few that are enjoyable for both mother and baby throughout the pregnancy.

Oils such as Basil, Clary Sage, Fennel, Hyssop, Nutmeg, Rosemary, Sage, Tansy, and Tarragon should be used carefully with a good understanding as to their benefits and how to use them.

Some essential oils such as Fennel and Clary Sage may help to accelerate labor once it has begun. Take 1-2 capsules 2 times daily when labor is imminent. Always consult a health professional before using essential oils during pregnancy, other than the ones recommended in this book.

A few drops of Vetiver and Valerian mixed together with 1 tablespoon of V-6 Vegetable Oil Complex may help reduce the pain of contractions when applied on the lower back.

### Application and Usage

**Aromatic:** Refer to *Application Guidelines* on page 410.
- Diffuse Gentle Baby, Joy, or Valor to reduce stress before and after the birth. Expectant fathers will also find this helps to reduce anxiety during delivery.

**Topical:** For guidelines on applying oils to the skin, refer to *Application Guidelines* on page 410.
- Massage 2-4 drops Labor Blend from above diluted 50:50 on reproductive Vita Flex points on the sides of the ankles. Apply **ONLY** after labor has started.
- Massage 2-4 drops Labor Blend from above on lower stomach and lower back.

## PROSTATE PROBLEMS

Natural progesterone is one of the best natural remedies for prostate inflammation (BPH) that can obstruct urinary flow and lead to impotence. Transdermal creams are the most effective means of hormone delivery.

Scientists are tracing the higher incidence of hormone-dependent cancers, including cancer of the breast, prostate, and testes, to exposure to endocrine disrupters in the environment. Contamination from 39 petrochemicals like DDT, PCB, pesticides, the phthalate DBP, recombinant bovine growth hormone (rBGH) in milk, and synthetic steroids in meat are all implicated in interfering with hormone receptors, rendering them unable to function properly, eventually leading to cancer.

For prostate problems, Peppermint acts as an anti-inflammatory to the prostate. Saw palmetto, *Pygeum africanum*, and pumpkin seed oil also help reduce prostate swelling.

### Recommendations

**Singles:** Myrrh, Idaho Balsam Fir, Oregano, Oregano Vitality, Plectranthus Oregano, Sage, Sage Vitality, Yarrow, Thyme, Thyme Vitality, Wintergreen

**Blends:** Mister, EndoFlex, EndoFlex Vitality, Australian Blue

**Nutritionals:** Prostate Health, Master Formula, Longevity Softgels, PD 80/20

**Retention:** Protec

**Body Care:** Prenolone Plus Body Cream

### Application and Usage

**Aromatic:** Refer to *Application Guidelines* on page 410.

**Topical:** For guidelines on applying oils to the skin, refer to *Application Guidelines* on page 410.

- Apply 2-4 drops diluted 20:80 between the rectum and scrotum 2 times daily. Mister works especially well applied there.
- Massage 4-6 drops on the Vita Flex reproductive points on the feet 2 times daily.
- Retention: Rectal, nightly for 7 days, rest 7 days, then repeat.

### Benign Prostate Hyperplasia (BPH)

Almost all males over age 50 have some degree of prostate hyperplasia, a condition that worsens with age. BPH can severely restrict urine flow and result in frequent, small urinations.

532 | Chapter 20 | Personal Usage Guide

Two herbs that are extremely effective for treating this condition are saw palmetto and pumpkin seed oil. The hormone-like activity of some essential oils can support a nutritional regimen to reduce BPH swelling.

## Recommendations

**Singles:** Sacred Frankincense, Frankincense, Frankincense Vitality, Myrrh, Idaho Balsam Fir, Sage, Sage Vitality, Blue Cypress

**Blends:** Mister, EndoFlex, EndoFlex Vitality, Australian Blue, Chivalry

**Nutritionals:** Prostate Health, Master Formula, Longevity Softgels, Mineral Essence

**Retention:** Protec

**Body Care:** Prenolone Plus Body Cream

### BPH Blend
- 10 drops Frankincense or Sacred Frankincense
- 5 drops Myrrh
- 3 drops Sage

## Application and Usage

**Aromatic:** Refer to *Application Guidelines* on page 410.

**Dietary and Oral:** Whether putting the oils in a capsule or drinking them in a liquid, please refer to *Application Guidelines* on page 410.

- Take 1 capsule with desired oil 3 times daily.
- Take 2-3 drops of oil in a spoonful of syrup or small amount of milk, juice, or water.

**Topical:** For guidelines on applying oils to the skin, refer to *Application Guidelines* on page 410.

- PSA counts typically rise when BPH occurs. The following regimen reduced PSA (prostate specific antigen) counts 70 percent in 2 months. Use the following applications simultaneously:
- Mix the BPH Blend found above with 1 tablespoon olive oil and use 3 times weekly as an overnight rectal retention enema.
- Apply 2-4 drops of the BPH Blend diluted 50:50 between the rectum and scrotum 1-3 times daily.
- Massage 1-3 drops of the BPH Blend on the reproductive Vita Flex points on the feet 2 times daily.

## Prostatitis

Prostatitis is an inflammation of the prostate that can present symptoms similar to benign prostate hyperplasia: frequent urinations, restricted flow, etc.

## Recommendations

**Singles:** Peppermint, Peppermint Vitality, Clary Sage, Palo Santo, Yarrow, German Chamomile, German Chamomile Vitality, Wintergreen, Rosemary, Rosemary Vitality, Myrtle, Thyme, Thyme Vitality, Tsuga, Blue Cypress

**Blends:** Australian Blue, Mister, Aroma Siez, DiGize, DiGize Vitality

**Nutritionals:** Prostate Health, PowerGize, Longevity Softgels, ImmuPro, Mineral Essence, JuvaPower, JuvaSpice, ICP

**Retention:** Protec

**Body Care:** Prenolone Plus Body Cream

## Application and Usage

**Dietary and Oral:** Whether putting the oils in a capsule or drinking them in a liquid, please refer to *Application Guidelines* on page 410.

- Take 1 capsule with desired oil 2 times daily.
- Take 2-3 drops of oil in a spoonful of syrup or small amount of milk, juice, or water.

**Topical:** For guidelines on applying oils to the skin, refer to *Application Guidelines* on page 410.

- Apply 1-3 drops diluted 20:80 to the area between the rectum and the scrotum daily.
- Massage 4-6 drops on the reproductive Vita Flex points on the feet daily.
- Retention: Rectal 3 times per week at night.

# RADIATION EXPOSURE DAMAGE

Many cancer treatments use radiation therapy that can severely damage both the skin and vital organs. Using gentle, antioxidant essential oils topically, as well as proper nutrients internally, is helpful in minimizing radiation damage.

Daily radiation from cell phones, computers, air travel, televisions, all types of electronic equipment, and kitchen appliances bombards us constantly. The more we can do to protect ourselves as well as cleanse on a regular basis, the better health we can maintain.

## Environmental Protection Kits

The QuadShield and EndoShield kits each combine four powerful products to help people protect themselves against daily radiation bombardment of cell phones, computers, electrical appliances, and other potential dangers.

The QuadShield kit contains Longevity Softgels, the essential oil blend Melrose, and the nutritional supplements Super C (or Chewable), and Thyromin. The EndoShield kit contains Longevity Softgels and the essential oil blends Melrose, EndoFlex, and Citrus Fresh.

## QuadShield™

**Longevity Softgel** —The essential oils in Longevity Softgels increase the oxygen and ATP (adenosine triphosphate) cellular fuel for increasing cell life and immunity for stronger resistance against damage from environmental pollution.

- **Children and teens ages 10–18:** 1-2 capsules daily
- **Adults:** 2–4 capsules daily

**Melrose**—This blend is formulated with two species of Melaleuca oil: *M. alternifolia* and *M. quinquenervia*, also known as Niaouli, which were found through research by Daniel Pénoël, MD, and Pierre Franchomme, PhD, to prevent cellular damage from environmental pollution and potential daily radiation exposure.

- **Children ages 1–3:** 1 drop in yogurt or other liquid
- **Children ages 4–7:** 2 drops in yogurt or other liquid
- **Children 8 and older:** 6 drops per capsule 1–3 times daily or in yogurt or other liquid
- **Adults:** 20 drops per capsule, 1–2 capsules, 1–3 times daily or in yogurt or other liquid

**Super C (or Chewable)** —Super C provides the body with 2,166 percent of the recommended dietary intake of the powerful antioxidant vitamin C and is enhanced with minerals, bioflavonoids, and pure Orange, Lemon, and other essential oils. It is a natural antioxidant and free radical scavenger that supports the immune system and protects healthy cells from becoming damaged by the effects of environmental pollution.

- **Children ages 1–3:** 1–2 MightyVites daily
- **Children ages 4–7:** 2–3 MightyVites or Super C Chewables daily
- **Children 8 and older:** 3–4 MightyVites or Super C Chewables daily
- **Adults:** 4–6 tablets daily

**Thyromin**—Thyromin contains ingredients that give support and nutrition to both the thyroid and adrenal glands for a healthier glandular system.

- **Children:** continue to use MightyVites 2–4 daily
- **Adults:** only 1 capsule, 3 times daily

**NingXia Red**—Drink 4–6 oz. of NingXia Red for a delicious and healthy addition to your diet.

## EndoShield™

**Longevity Softgel**—The essential oils in Longevity Softgels increase the oxygen and ATP (adenosine triphosphate) cellular fuel for increasing cell life and immunity for stronger resistance against damage from environmental pollution.

- **Children and teens ages 10–18:** 1–2 capsules daily
- **Adults:** 2–4 capsules daily

**Melrose**—This blend is formulated with two species of Melaleuca oil: *M. alternifolia* and *M. quinquenervia*, also known as Niaouli, which were found through research by Daniel Pénoël, MD, and Pierre Franchomme, PhD, to prevent cellular damage from environmental pollution and potential daily radiation exposure.

- **Children ages 1–3:** 1 drop in yogurt or other liquid
- **Children ages 4–7:** 2 drops in yogurt or other liquid
- **Children 8 and older:** 6 drops per capsule 1–3 times daily or in yogurt or other liquid
- **Adults:** 20 drops per capsule, 1–2 capsules, 1–3 times daily or in yogurt or other liquid

**EndoFlex** —This blend contains oils very specific to the thyroid while at the same time addressing the entire endocrine system. Myrtle oil stimulates and promotes good thyroid health when combined with Spearmint, encouraging better circulation, stronger metabolism, and production of digestive enzymes. Geranium contains esters that protect the thyroid, which may explain why it is so heralded in French publications as a general tonic for the body. It supports the thyroid in being able to uptake iodine from food.

- **Children ages 1–3:** 1 drop in yogurt or other liquid
- **Children ages 4–7:** 2 drops in yogurt or other liquid
- **Children 8 and older:** 6 drops per capsule 2 times daily or in yogurt or other liquid
- **Adults:** 20 drops per capsule, 1–2 capsules, 1–3 times daily or in yogurt or other liquid

**Citrus Fresh**—This blend combines six citrus oils that are naturally antioxidant, antibacterial, and increase the uptake of vitamin C.

- **Children ages 1–3:** 1 drop in yogurt or other liquid
- **Children ages 4–7:** 2 drops in yogurt or other liquid
- **Children 8 and older:** 6 drops per capsule 2 times daily or in yogurt or other liquid
- **Adults:** 20 drops per capsule, 1–2 capsules, 1–3 times daily or in yogurt or other liquid

**NingXia Red**—Drink 4–6 oz. of NingXia Red for a delicious and healthy addition to your diet.

## Recommendations

**Singles:** Sacred Frankincense, Frankincense, Frankincense Vitality, Idaho Balsam Fir, Blue Cypress, Royal Hawaiian Sandalwood, Hyssop, Oregano, Oregano Vitality, Plectranthus Oregano, Tea Tree, Melaleuca Quinquenervia

**Blends:** Melrose, Longevity, Longevity Vitality, Valor, Valor II, Stress Away Roll-On

**Nutritionals:** QuadShield or EndoShield products, Super C, Super C Chewable, Power Meal, Slique Shake, Slique Bars, Slique CitraSlim, ImmuPro, NingXia Red, Mineral Essence, Essentialzyme, Longevity Softgels, OmegaGize³, Ultra Young, Ningxia Wolfberries (Organic, Dried)

## Application and Usage

**Aromatic:** Refer to *Application Guidelines* on page 410.

**Dietary and Oral:** Whether putting the oils in a capsule or drinking them in a liquid, please refer to *Application Guidelines* on page 410.

- Take 1 capsule with desired oil 2 times daily.
- Take 2-3 drops of oil in a spoonful of syrup or small amount of milk, juice, or water.

**Topical:** For guidelines on applying oils to the skin, refer to *Application Guidelines* on page 410.

- Apply 1-2 drops diluted 50:50 on affected area 1-2 times daily.
- Massage 2-4 drops of oil neat on the bottoms of the feet just before bedtime.

# RHEUMATIC FEVER

Rheumatic fever results from a streptococcus infection that primarily strikes children (usually before age 14). It can lead to inflammation that damages the heart muscle and valve.

Rheumatic fever is caused by the same genus of bacteria that causes strep throat and scarlet fever. Diffusing essential oils can help reduce the likelihood of contracting the disease. Essential oils such as Mountain Savory, Rosemary, Tea Tree, Thyme, Palo Santo, Sacred Frankincense, Frankincense, Eucalyptus Blue, and Oregano have powerful antimicrobial effects.

In cases where a person is already infected, the use of essential oils in the Raindrop Technique may be appropriate.

## Recommendations

**Singles:** Oregano, Oregano Vitality, Plectranthus Oregano, Clove, Clove Vitality, Tea Tree, Mountain Savory, Mountain Savory Vitality, Peppermint, Peppermint Vitality, Thyme, Thyme Vitality, Rosemary, Rosemary Vitality, Black Pepper, Black Pepper Vitality, Eucalyptus Blue, Sacred Frankincense, Frankincense, Frankincense Vitality, Palo Santo, Cistus

**Blends:** Thieves, Thieves Vitality, Melrose, Exodus II, ImmuPower

**Nutritionals:** Inner Defense, ImmuPro, Super C, Super C Chewable, Sulfurzyme, Longevity Softgels, Master Formula, NingXia Red, Essentialzyme, Essentialzymes-4, Life 9, Mineral Essence

## Application and Usage

**Aromatic:** Refer to *Application Guidelines* on page 410.

**Topical:** For guidelines on applying oils to the skin, refer to *Application Guidelines* on page 410.

- Apply 3-5 drops diluted 50:50 on the bottoms of the feet and on carotid artery spots under the earlobes.
- Receive a Raindrop Technique 1 time weekly.

# ROCKY MOUNTAIN SPOTTED FEVER
*(See Lyme Disease / Rocky Mountain Spotted Fever)*

## SCAR TISSUE

Scar tissue is the fibrous connective tissue that forms a scar and can be found on any tissue on the body where an injury, surgery, cut, or disease has taken place and then healed. It is thicker, paler, and denser than the surrounding tissue because it has a limited blood supply.

### Recommendations

**Singles:** Sacred Frankincense, Frankincense, Royal Hawaiian Sandalwood, Cypress, Elemi, Yarrow, Rose, Cistus, Myrrh, Helichrysum, Lavender

**Blends:** Gentle Baby, Australian Blue, 3 Wise Men

**Nutritionals:** Super C, Super C Chewable, Sulfurzyme, Power Meal, Slique Shake, MegaCal, Mineral Essence, Essentialzyme, Essentialzymes-4, Life 9

**Body Care:** KidScents Tender Tush, Regenolone Body Cream, Rose Ointment, Boswellia Wrinkle Cream

### Scar Prevention Blend
- 4 drops Myrrh
- 3 drops Lavender
- 2 drops Helichrysum
- 1 drop Royal Hawaiian Sandalwood

### Application and Usage

**Topical:** For guidelines on applying oils to the skin, refer to *Application Guidelines* on page 410.

- Apply 2-6 drops neat of the scar prevention blend around and over the wound daily until healed.

## SCURVY

This condition is due to a deficiency of vitamin C in the diet and marked by weakness, anemia, spongy gums, bleeding of the gums and nose, and a hardening of the muscles of the calves and legs.

### Recommendations

**Singles:** Orange, Orange Vitality, Jade Lemon, Jade Lemon Vitality, Lemon, Lemon Vitality, Lime, Lime Vitality, Spearmint, Spearmint Vitality, Lavender, Lavender Vitality, Tangerine, Tangerine Vitality

**Blends:** Citrus Fresh, Citrus Fresh Vitality, Thieves, Thieves Vitality, GLF, GLF Vitality, Deep Relief Roll-On

**Nutritionals:** Super C Chewable, Super C, Power Meal, Slique Shake, Balance Complete, Pure Protein Complete, NingXia Red, Mineral Essence, Essentialzyme, Essentialzymes-4, Detoxzyme, Super B, Master Formula

## SEIZURES

Many seizures can be reduced or alleviated by removing all forms of sugar, artificial colors and flavors, and processed food from the diet and chemicals of all types. Avoid using personal care products with ammonia-based compounds such as quaterniums and polyquaterniums.

### Recommendations

**Singles:** Peppermint, Sacred Frankincense, Frankincense, Royal Hawaiian Sandalwood, Melissa, Jasmine, Basil

**Blends:** RutaVaLa, RutaVaLa Roll-On, R.C., Valor, Valor II, Valor Roll-On, Breathe Again Roll-On, Aroma Siez, Exodus II, Peace & Calming, Peace & Calming II, Trauma Life, T.R. Care, Stress Away Roll-On

**Nutritionals:** Mineral Essence, MultiGreens, Essentialzyme, Essentialzymes-4, Life 9, BLM, AgilEase, PowerGize, Super B, Longevity Softgels, Power Meal, Slique Shake, Sulfurzyme, OmegaGize[3], Balance Complete, MindWise, Master Formula, Yacon Syrup in place of sugars

### Application and Usage

**Aromatic:** Refer to *Application Guidelines* on page 410.

**Topical:** For guidelines on applying oils to the skin, refer to *Application Guidelines* on page 410.

- Massage 10 drops into scalp diluted 50:50 up to 3 times daily to help reduce risk of seizure.
- Supplement with Seizure Regimen below:

### Seizure Regimen (do all of the following)
- Diffuse Peace & Calming or Peace & Calming II for 30 minutes 3-4 times daily.
- Massage 4-6 drops Valor or Valor II on bottoms of feet daily.
- Massage 4-6 drops Joy over heart daily.
- Receive a Raindrop Technique 2 times monthly.

## SEXUAL DYSFUNCTION

There is an extensive, historical basis that fragrance may amplify desire and create a mood that can overcome frigidity or impotence. In fact, aromas such as rose and jasmine have been used since antiquity to attract the opposite sex and create a romantic atmosphere.

Modern research has shown that the aroma of some essential oils can stimulate the emotional center of the brain. This may explain why essential oils have the potential to help people overcome impotence or frigidity based on emotional factors or inhibitions.

## Dysfunction (Men)
*(See also Prostate Problems, Trauma)*

Causes of male sexual dysfunction are divided into two types: physical or psychological problems.

## Impotence (Men)

Impotence, the inability to perform sexually, may be caused by physical limitations due to an accident or injury or by psychological factors such as inhibitions, trauma, stress, etc.

Male impotence is often linked to problems with the prostate or prostate surgery.

If impotence is related to psychological trauma or unresolved emotional issues, it may be necessary to deal with these issues before any meaningful progress can be made.

### Recommendations

**Singles:** Idaho Blue Spruce, Goldenrod, Sacred Frankincense, Frankincense, Myrrh, Ginger, Nutmeg, Jasmine, Ylang Ylang

**Blends:** Shutran, Build Your Dream, Freedom, InTouch, Reconnect, Valor, Valor II, Valor Roll-On, Mister, SclarEssence, Inner Harmony

**Nutritionals:** EndoGize, Prostate Health, Ultra Young, Protec, PowerGize

### Application and Usage

**Aromatic:** Refer to *Application Guidelines* on page 410.

**Topical:** For guidelines on applying oils to the skin, refer to *Application Guidelines* on page 410.

- Apply 2-3 drops neat to Vita Flex points on feet or lower abdomen. Do not apply on sensitive skin in crotch area.

## Infertility (Men)

Male infertility is the inability of a male to achieve pregnancy in a fertile female. It is commonly due to deficiencies in the semen.

### Recommendations

**Singles:** Idaho Blue Spruce, Sage, Sage Vitality, Sacred Frankincense, Frankincense, Frankincense Vitality, Clary Sage, Goldenrod

**Blends:** Mister, SclarEssence, SclarEssence Vitality, Shutran

**Nutritionals:** EndoGize, MultiGreens, Prostate Health, Sulfurzyme, Essentialzyme, Essentialzymes-4, Life 9, Super B, Mineral Essence, Thyromin, Ultra Young

**Retention:** Protec

### Application and Usage

**Topical:** For guidelines on applying oils to the skin, refer to *Application Guidelines* on page 410.

- Apply 2-4 drops neat or diluted on the reproductive Vita Flex points of hands and feet inside of wrists, around the front of the ankles in line with the anklebone, on the lower sides of the anklebone, and along the Achilles tendon 1-3 times daily.
- Rub 4-6 drops of Protec on the lower abdomen near the pubic bone and in the area between the scrotum and the rectum.
- Alternatively, use 1 tablespoon of Protec in overnight rectal retention.

## Lack of Libido (Men)

Lack of libido in men is a much more common complaint than our culture would seem to indicate. The leading reasons men don't want to have sex are medications, usually antidepressants and antihypertensive drugs, drug or alcohol abuse, or low testosterone.

### Recommendations

**Singles:** Idaho Blue Spruce, Pine, Ocotea, Myrrh, Black Pepper, Ylang Ylang, Ginger, Nutmeg

**Blends:** Light the Fire, SclarEssence, Valor, Valor II, Valor Roll-On, Mister, Light the Fire, Live with Passion, Live Your Passion, Transformation, The Gift, En-R-Gee, Shutran

**Nutritionals:** EndoGize, MultiGreens, Prostate Health, Sulfurzyme, Essentialzyme, Essentialzymes-4, Life 9, Super B, Mineral Essence, Thyromin, Ultra Young

**Body Care:** Prenolone Plus Body Cream

### Application and Usage

**Aromatic:** Refer to *Application Guidelines* on page 410.

**Topical:** For guidelines on applying oils to the skin, refer to *Application Guidelines* on page 410.

- Massage 4-6 drops diluted 50:50 on neck, shoulders, and lower abdomen 1-3 times daily.

## Dysfunction (Women)

Sexual dysfunction can be a result of a physical or psychological problem.

## Frigidity (Women)

Frigidity is a condition in which women have a lack of libido and tend to become unresponsive to sexual intercourse or are unable to achieve an orgasm. It may leave a woman unhappy, unsatisfied, and depressed.

### Recommendations

**Singles:** Jasmine, Rose, Ylang Ylang, Clary Sage, Nutmeg

**Blends:** En-R-Gee, The Gift, Joy, Valor, Valor II, Valor Roll-On

**Nutritionals:** EndoGize, Thyromin, Mineral Essence, Super B, PD 80/20, MegaCal, ImmuPro

**Body Care:** Progessence Plus, Prenolone Plus Body Cream

- Ylang Ylang helps balance sexual emotion and sex drive problems. Its aromatic influence elevates sexual energy and enhances relationships.
- Clary Sage can help with lack of sexual desire, particularly in women, by regulating and balancing hormones.
- Nutmeg supports the nervous system to help overcome frigidity.

### Application and Usage

**Aromatic:** Refer to *Application Guidelines* on page 410.

**Topical:** For guidelines on applying oils to the skin, refer to *Application Guidelines* on page 410.

- Massage 4-6 drops diluted 50:50 on neck, shoulders, and lower abdomen up to 1-3 times daily.

## Infertility (Women)

Natural progesterone creams when used from the middle to the end of the cycle starting on the day after ovulation, usually day 15 or later, may improve fertility. Some essential oils have hormone-like qualities that can support or improve fertility processes.

### Recommendations

**Singles:** Clary Sage, Ylang Ylang, Sage, Sage Vitality, Fennel, Fennel Vitality, Yarrow, Geranium

**Blends:** Dragon Time, Acceptance, Mister, SclarEssence, SclarEssence Vitality, Lady Sclareol, EndoFlex, EndoFlex Vitality

**Nutritionals:** PD 80/20, MultiGreens, Mineral Essence, SuperCal, Thyromin, EndoGize, FemiGen, Estro, MultiGreens: Take 3-8 capsules 2-3 times daily.

**Body Care:** Progessence Plus, Prenolone Plus Body Cream

### Application and Usage

**Dietary and Oral:** Whether putting the oils in a capsule or drinking them in a liquid, please refer to *Application Guidelines* on page 410.

- Take 1 capsule with desired oil 2 times daily.
- Take 2-3 drops of oil in a spoonful of syrup or small amount of milk, juice, or water.

**Topical:** For guidelines on applying oils to the skin, refer to *Application Guidelines* on page 410.

- Apply 2-4 drops neat or diluted 50:50 on the lower back and lower abdomen areas 2-3 times daily.
- Apply 2-4 drops on the reproductive Vita Flex points of hands and feet inside of wrists, around the front of the ankles in line with the anklebone, on the lower sides of the anklebone, and along the Achilles tendon 1-3 times daily.
- Rub daily 10 drops Progessence Plus or ½ teaspoon Prenolone Plus Body Cream on lower back area and the lower bowel area near the pubic bone.

## Lack of Libido/Desire (Women)

A woman's sexual desires naturally fluctuate over the years and are affected by a range of physical and emotional factors. Most physical causes of low libido are a result of hormonal imbalance.

### Recommendations

**Singles:** Clary Sage, Nutmeg, Nutmeg Vitality, Geranium, Ylang Ylang, Rose, Idaho Balsam Fir, Lemongrass, Lemongrass Vitality, Jasmine, Sacred Frankincense, Frankincense, Frankincense Vitality, Sage, Sage Vitality

**Blends:** Light the Fire, SclarEssence, SclarEssence Vitality, Sensation, Lady Sclareol, Joy, Build Your Dream, Valor, Valor II, Valor Roll-On, Live with Passion, Live Your Passion

**Nutritionals:** EndoGize, MultiGreens, Estro, Sulfurzyme, PD 80/20, Thyromin, FemiGen

**Body Care:** Progessence Plus, Prenolone Plus Body Cream

- Ylang Ylang helps balance sexual emotion and sex drive problems. Its aromatic influence elevates sexual energy and enhances relationships.
- Clary Sage can help with lack of sexual desire, particularly with women, by regulating and balancing hormones.
- Nutmeg supports the nervous system to help overcome frigidity.

Personal Usage Guide | Chapter 20

## Application and Usage

**Aromatic:** Refer to *Application Guidelines* on page 410.

**Dietary and Oral:** Whether putting the oils in a capsule or drinking them in a liquid, please refer to *Application Guidelines* on page 410.

- Take 1 capsule with desired oil diluted 50:50 2 times daily.
- Take 2-3 drops of oil in a spoonful of syrup or small amount of milk, juice, or water.

**Topical:** For guidelines on applying oils to the skin, refer to *Application Guidelines* on page 410.

- Massage 4-6 drops diluted 50:50 on neck, shoulders, and lower abdomen up to 1-3 times daily or apply 2-3 drops neat to Vita Flex points.

## Excessive Sexual Desire (Both Sexes)

Excessive sexual desire is a psychological disorder in which the person is unable to manage his or her sex life and may feel compelled to continually seek sexual activity. Some professionals speculate that it is a form of obsessive-compulsive disorder or a manifestation of the manic phase of bipolar disorder. Excessive sexual desire is best diagnosed and treated by a health care professional.

### Recommendations

**Singles:** Rose, Myrrh, Marjoram, Marjoram Vitality, Valerian, Lavender, Lavender Vitality

**Blends:** Peace & Calming, Peace & Calming II, Acceptance, Surrender, Joy, Harmony, Gathering

### Application and Usage

**Aromatic:** Refer to *Application Guidelines* on page 410.

**Dietary and Oral:** Whether putting the oils in a capsule or drinking them in a liquid, please refer to *Application Guidelines* on page 410.

- Take 1 capsule with desired oil diluted 50:50 2 times daily.
- Take 2-3 drops of oil in a spoonful of syrup or small amount of milk, juice, or water.

**Topical:** For guidelines on applying oils to the skin, refer to *Application Guidelines* on page 410.

- Massage 4-6 drops diluted 50:50 on neck, shoulders, and lower abdomen up to 1-3 times daily.

## SEXUALLY TRANSMITTED DISEASES
*(See also Infections)*

Sexually transmitted diseases are infections that you can get from having sex with someone who has the infection and are caused by bacteria, parasites, and viruses.

### Herpes Simplex Type 2

*Herpes genitalis* is transmitted by sexual contact and results in sores or lesions. Four to seven days after contact with an infected partner, tingling, burning, or persistent itching usually heralds an outbreak. One or two days later, small pimple-like bumps appear over reddened skin. The itching and tingling continue, and the pimples turn into painful blisters, which burst, bleeding with yellowish pus. Five to seven days after the first tingling, scabs form, and healing begins.

Antiviral essential oils have generally been very effective in treating herpes lesions and reducing their onset. Oils such as Tea Tree, Melissa, and Rosemary have been successfully used for this purpose by Daniel Pénoël, MD, in his clinical practice. A study at the University of Buenos Aires found that sandalwood essential oil inhibited the replication of herpes simplex viruses 1 and 2.41.[36]

Those with herpes should avoid diets high in the amino acid l-arginine, substituting instead l-lysine. Lysine retards the growth of the virus. Foods such as amaranth and plain yogurt are good sources of lysine.

### Recommendations

**Singles:** Royal Hawaiian Sandalwood, Melissa, Ravintsara, Dorado Azul, Tea Tree, Blue Cypress, Rosemary, Rosemary Vitality, Northern Lights Black Spruce, Sage

**Blends:** Melrose, Thieves, Thieves Vitality, Exodus II, Purification

**Nutritionals:** ImmuPro, Sulfurzyme, Super C, Super C Chewable, ICP, Essentialzyme, Essentsialzymes-4, Life 9, Mineral Essence, ComforTone

**Body Care:** Thieves Spray, Rose Ointment

**Herpes Blend No. 1 (Topical)**
- 4 drops Dorado Azul
- 2 drops Tea Tree
- 1 drop Ravintsara

**Herpes Blend No. 2 (Vaginal)**
- 4 drops Dorado Azul
- 3 drops Ravintsara
- 2 drops Sage
- 1 drop Lavender

Seventh Edition | **Essential Oils Desk Reference** | 539

## Application and Usage

**Aromatic:** Refer to *Application Guidelines* on page 410.

**Dietary and Oral:** Whether putting the oils in a capsule or drinking them in a liquid, please refer to *Application Guidelines* on page 410.

- Take 1 capsule with desired oil diluted 50:50 2 times daily.
- Take 2-3 drops of oil in a spoonful of syrup or small amount of milk, juice, or water.

**Topical:** For guidelines on applying oils to the skin, refer to *Application Guidelines* on page 410.

- Apply single oils or blends neat or diluted, depending on the oils that are used.
- Use Herpes Blend No. 2 diluted 20:80 and put a few drops on a tampon or sanitary pad for nightly applications. If it continues to sting after 5 minutes, remove and change the dilution to 10:90.
- Apply Herpes Blend No.1 on lesions as soon as they appear. Apply 1-2 drops neat 2-3 times daily, alternating between Herpes Blend No. 1 and Melrose each day.
- Receive a Raindrop Technique 1-2 times monthly, as needed.

## Genital Human Papillomavirus (HPV)

Infection by genital HPV is very common. At least half of the people who are sexually active will contract the virus, yet many will not know it because they will not have any symptoms. There are more than 100 types of HPV, and some types are associated with genital warts, although the warts are not always visible. The longer the virus is in the body, the higher the risk of developing health problems such as cervical cancer or anal cancer.

## Recommendations

**Singles:** Melissa, Dorado Azul, Ravintsara, Palo Santo, Tea Tree, Lavender, Lavender Vitality, Royal Hawaiian Sandalwood

**Blends:** Melrose, Thieves, Thieves Vitality, ImmuPower, Hope

**Nutritionals:** ImmuPro, Inner Defense, Life 9

**Body Care:** Thieves Spray

## Application and Usage

**Aromatic:** Refer to *Application Guidelines* on page 410.

**Dietary and Oral:** Whether putting the oils in a capsule or drinking them in a liquid, please refer to *Application Guidelines* on page 410.

- Take 1 capsule with desired oil diluted 50:50 2 times daily.
- Take 2-3 drops of oil in a spoonful of syrup or small amount of milk, juice, or water.

**Topical:** For guidelines on applying oils to the skin, refer to *Application Guidelines* on page 410.

- Apply 1-3 drops neat or dilute 50:50 and apply on location 3-6 times daily.
- Massage 2-4 drops of oil neat on the bottoms of the feet or on the Vita Flex points of the feet just before bedtime.
- Use Thieves Spray on location.

**Retention:** Put 2-3 drops of oil of your choice on a tampon and insert nightly.

## Genital Warts/Blisters (Herpes Simplex Type 2)

Genital warts are a form of viral infection caused by the human papillomavirus (HPV), of which there are more than 100 different types.

One type of HPV virus is among the most common sexually transmitted diseases. Up to 24 million Americans may currently be infected with HPV, which is usually spread through sexual contact. HPV lives only in genital tissue and can later lead to cervical cancer in women.

## Recommendations

**Singles:** Melissa, Dorado Azul, Ravintsara, Palo Santo, Tea Tree, Lavender, Lavender Vitality, Royal Hawaiian Sandalwood

**Blends:** Melrose, Thieves, Thieves Vitality, ImmuPower, Hope

**Nutritionals:** ImmuPro, Inner Defense, Life 9

**Body Care:** Thieves Spray

## Application and Usage

**Aromatic:** Refer to *Application Guidelines* on page 410.

**Dietary and Oral:** Whether putting the oils in a capsule or drinking them in a liquid, please refer to *Application Guidelines* on page 410.

- Take 1 capsule with desired oil diluted 50:50 2 times daily.
- Put 2-3 drops of oil in a spoonful of Blue Agave, Yacon Syrup, maple syrup, coconut oil, milk, etc.

- Put the desired amount of oils in a glass of rice milk, almond milk, goat milk, carrot juice, NingXia Red, or even water and then drink it.

**Topical:** For guidelines on applying oils to the skin, refer to *Application Guidelines* on page 410.

- Apply 1-3 drops neat or dilute 50:50 and apply on location 3-6 times daily.
- Massage 2-4 drops of oil neat on the bottoms of the feet or on the Vita Flex points of the feet just before bedtime.
- Use Thieves Spray on location.

**Retention:** Put 2-3 drops of the oil of your choice on a tampon and insert nightly.

## Gonorrhea and Syphilis

Gonorrhea is a very common sexually transmitted disease caused by a bacterium (*Neisseria gonorrhoeae*) that can grow and multiply easily in the warm, moist areas of the reproductive tract. It can also grow in the eyes, mouth, throat, and anus.

Syphilis, also a common sexually transmitted disease, is caused by a bacterium (*Treponema pallidum*) and has often been called "the great imitator" because so many of the signs and symptoms are the same as those of other diseases. Sores occur mainly on the external genitals, vagina, anus, or in the rectum. Sores can also occur on the lips and in the mouth.

**Note:** Seek immediate professional medical attention if you suspect you may have either of these diseases.

### Recommendations

**Singles:** Melissa, Thyme, Thyme Vitality, Mountain Savory, Mountain Savory Vitality, Cinnamon Bark, Cinnamon Bark Vitality, Oregano, Oregano Vitality

**Blends:** Melrose, Exodus II, Thieves, Thieves Vitality, ImmuPower

**Nutritionals:** Inner Defense, ImmuPro, Life 9

**Sprays:** Thieves Spray

### Application and Usage

**Dietary and Oral:** Whether putting the oils in a capsule or drinking them in a liquid, please refer to *Application Guidelines* on page 410.

- Take 1 capsule with desired oil 2 times daily for 15 days.
- Take 2-3 drops of oil in a spoonful of syrup or small amount of milk, juice, or water.

**Topical:** For guidelines on applying oils to the skin, refer to *Application Guidelines* on page 410.

## SHINGLES (Herpes Zoster)

Shingles is a short-lived viral infection of the nervous system that starts with fatigue, fever, chills, and intestinal upset. The affected skin areas become sensitive and prone to blistering. One attack usually provides immunity for life. However, for many people, particularly the elderly, pain can persist for months, even years.

**Note:** Occurrences of shingles around the eyes or on the forehead can cause blindness. Consult an ophthalmologist (eye doctor) immediately if such outbreaks occur.

### Recommendations

**Singles:** Melissa, Blue Cypress, Elemi, Tea Tree, Oregano, Plectranthus Oregano, Geranium, German Chamomile, Mountain Savory, Royal Hawaiian Sandalwood, Thyme, Peppermint, Ravintsara, Northern Lights Black Spruce, Dalmatia Bay Laurel, Laurus Nobilis, Dalmatia Sage, Sage

**Blends:** Thieves, Australian Blue, Exodus II

**Nutritionals:** SuperCal, Sulfurzyme, PD 80/20, MegaCal, Mineral Essence, Essentialzyme

### Shingles Blend No. 1
- 10 drops German Chamomile
- 5 drops Lavender
- 4 drops Royal Hawaiian Sandalwood
- 2 drops Geranium

### Shingles Blend No. 2
- 10 drops Royal Hawaiian Sandalwood
- 5 drops Blue Cypress
- 4 drops Peppermint
- 2 drops Ravintsara

### Application and Usage

**Aromatic:** Refer to *Application Guidelines* on page 410.

**Topical:** For guidelines on applying oils to the skin, refer to *Application Guidelines* on page 410.

- Apply 6-10 drops neat or diluted 50:50 on affected area, back of the neck, and down the spine 1-3 times daily.
- Apply a compress alternating warm and cold on the spine 1-3 times daily.
- Layering in Raindrop Technique style, apply 3-4 drops each of Oregano (or Plectranthus Oregano), Mountain Savory, and Thyme along the spine.
- Apply 15-20 drops V-6 Vegetable Oil Complex to the spine, massage briefly over the other oils, cover the skin with a dry towel, and apply a warm pack for 15-20 minutes.

- **Note:** Be cautious about warming. If the back becomes too hot, remove the warm pack immediately and add V-6 Vegetable Oil Complex to cool.
- Remove the warm pack and towel, and then layer 4-8 drops each of Tea Tree, Elemi, and Peppermint along the spine.
- Put the dry towel back over the skin and apply an ice pack for 30 minutes.

## SHOCK (See also Fainting, Burns)

Shock can be described as a state of profound depression of the vital processes associated with reduced blood volume and pressure. The blood rushes to the vital organs after trauma.

It may be caused by the sudden stimulation of the nerves and convulsive contraction of the muscles caused by the discharge of electricity. Other causes include sudden trauma, terror, surprise, horror, or disgust.

**Symptoms or signs**
- Irregular breathing
- Low blood pressure
- Dilated pupils
- Cold and sweaty skin
- Weak and rapid pulse
- Dry mouth
- Muscle weakness
- Dizziness or fainting

Any injury that results in the sudden loss of substantial amounts of fluids can trigger shock.

Shock can also be caused by allergic reactions (anaphylactic shock), infections in the blood (septic shock), or emotional trauma (neurogenic shock).

To help someone in shock while waiting for first responders, first cover the victim with a blanket and elevate the feet, unless there is a head or upper torso injury. Inhaling any one of many different essential oils can also help—especially in cases of emotional shock.

## Recommendations

**Singles:** Peppermint, Idaho Balsam Fir, Basil, Sacred Frankincense, Frankincense, Eucalyptus Blue, Dorado Azul, Cardamom, Rosemary, Melissa, Ocotea

**Blends:** Trauma Life, T.R. Care, Evergreen Essence, Freedom, Clarity, 3 Wise Men, Build Your Dream, Valor, Valor II, Valor Roll-On, R.C., Harmony, InTouch, Reconnect, Present Time, Inner Harmony

## Application and Usage

**Aromatic:** Refer to *Application Guidelines* on page 410.

**Topical:** For guidelines on applying oils to the skin, refer to *Application Guidelines* on page 410.

- When applying essential oil to the temples, be careful to not get the oil too close to the eyes.
- Apply 1-2 drops diluted 50:50 on temples, back of the neck, and under the nose neat as desired.
- You may also apply 2-3 drops on the Vita Flex points of the feet.
- Applying a single drop under the nose is helpful and refreshing.

# SINUS INFECTIONS

A sinus infection is an inflammation of the sinuses and nasal passages. Sinus problems are among the most common chronic ailments.

## Nasopharyngitis

Nasopharyngitis is an inflammatory condition of the mucous membranes of the back of the nasal cavity where it connects to the throat and the Eustachian tubes.

### Recommendations

**Singles:** Peppermint, Ravintsara, Eucalyptus Blue, Thyme, Rosemary, Blue Cypress, Dorado Azul, Eucalyptus Radiata, Tea Tree

**Blends:** Raven, R.C., Exodus II, Thieves, Breathe Again Roll-On

**Nutritionals:** Super C, Super C Chewable, ImmuPro, Digest & Cleanse, Inner Defense

**Oral Care:** Thieves Fresh Essence Plus Mouthwash, Thieves Spray

### Application and Usage

**Aromatic:** Refer to *Application Guidelines* on page 410.

**Dietary and Oral:** Whether putting the oils in a capsule or drinking them in a liquid, please refer to *Application Guidelines* on page 410.

- Take 1 capsule with desired oil 2 times daily.
- Take 2-3 drops of oil in a spoonful of syrup or small amount of milk, juice, or water.
- Gargle 2-5 times daily with Thieves Fresh Essence Plus Mouthwash or with water that contains 1-2 drops of another oil.
- Put 1 drop of Thieves or Tea Tree at the very back of the tongue and hold it in the mouth, mixing it

with saliva for several minutes, and then swallow. This can be very effective if started at the very first indication of infection and repeated 3-4 times for the first hour, then once an hour until symptoms subside.

- Spray inside mouth with Thieves Spray as often as desired.
- Put 1 drop of Exodus II on tongue and swish it around in your mouth before swallowing.

**Special Note:** In most sinus infections, including naso-pharyngitis, rhinitis, sinus congestion, and sinusitis, the nasal irrigation regimen can be extremely effective.

**Topical:** For guidelines on applying oils to the skin, refer to *Application Guidelines* on page 410.

- Apply 1-2 drops diluted 50:50 just under jawbone on right and left sides 4-8 times daily.
- You may also apply 2-3 drops on the Vita Flex points of the feet

## Sinus Congestion

Sinus congestion is extremely annoying, and symptoms can last for several days. The most common symptom is difficulty breathing because of blocked nasal passages due to excessive mucus. As a result, the sinuses become inflamed and produce other symptoms such as headaches, fatigue, coughing, sinus pressure or pain, and loss of smell.

## Nasal Irrigation Regimen:

Rosemary and Tea Tree oils can be used in a saline solution for very effective nasal irrigation that clears and decongests sinuses. As recommended by Daniel Pénoël, MD, the saline solution is prepared as follows:

- 10 drops Rosemary
- 6 drops Tea Tree
- 8 tablespoons ultra-fine salt

The essential oils are mixed thoroughly in the fine salt and stored in a sealed container. For each nasal irrigation session, 1 teaspoon of this salt mixture is dissolved into 1½ cups distilled water.

This solution is then placed in the tank of an oral irrigator or neti pot to irrigate the nasal cavities, which is done while bending over a sink. This application has brought surprisingly positive results in treating latent sinusitis and other nasal congestion problems.

## Recommendations

**Singles:** Eucalyptus Blue, Peppermint, Dorado Azul, Eucalyptus Globulus, Palo Santo, Eucalyptus Radiata, Ravintsara, Myrrh, Idaho Balsam Fir, Thyme, Fennel, Fennel Vitality, Rosemary, Rosemary Vitality

**Blends:** Raven, DiGize, DiGize Vitality, Thieves, Thieves Vitality, Exodus II, Breathe Again Roll-On, SniffleEase, Melrose, R.C., Christmas Spirit

**Nutritionals:** Super C, Super C Chewable, ImmuPro, Inner Defense

**Oral Care:** Thieves AromaBright Toothpaste, Thieves Dentarome Plus Toothpaste, Thieves Dentarome Ultra Toothpaste, KidScents Slique Toothpaste, Thieves Hard Lozenges, Thieves Mints, Thieves Fresh Essence Plus Mouthwash, Thieves Spray

## Application and Usage

**Aromatic:** Refer to *Application Guidelines* on page 410.

**Dietary and Oral:** Whether putting the oils in a capsule or drinking them in a liquid, please refer to *Application Guidelines* on page 410.

- Take 1 capsule with desired oil 2 times daily.
- Take 2-3 drops of oil in a spoonful of syrup or small amount of milk, juice, or water.
- Gargle with Thieves Fresh Essence Plus Mouthwash 4-6 times daily, as desired.

**Topical:** For guidelines on applying oils to the skin, refer to *Application Guidelines* on page 410.

- Apply 1-2 drops neat on the temples and back of the neck, as desired.
- Applying a single drop of chosen oil or a swipe of Breathe Again Roll-On under the nose is helpful and refreshing.
- Dilute 50:50 and apply on location 3-6 times daily.
- Massage 2-4 drops of oil neat on the bottoms of the feet just before bedtime. Children love it.

**Nasal Irrigation Regimen** *(see box on left)*
- Place a warm compress with 1-2 drops of chosen oil on the back.

## Sinusitis / Rhinitis

Sinusitis is an inflammation of the sinuses and nasal passages. It can cause pressure in the eyes, cheek area, nose, or on one side of the head. A person with a sinus infection may also have a headache, cough, fever, bad breath, and nasal congestion.

Seventh Edition | **Essential Oils Desk Reference** | 543

Essential oils such as Eucalyptus Radiata and Ravintsara strengthen the respiratory system, open the pulmonary tract, and fight respiratory infection.

## Recommendations

**Singles:** Eucalyptus Blue, Peppermint, Peppermint Vitality, Eucalyptus Radiata, Ravintsara, Tea Tree, Idaho Balsam Fir, Thyme, Thyme Vitality, Northern Lights Black Spruce, Fennel, Fennel Vitality, Rosemary, Rosemary Vitality

**Blends:** R.C., Melrose, Raven, Thieves, Thieves Vitality, Exodus II, Breathe Again Roll-On, SniffleEase

**Nutritionals:** Super C, Super C Chewable, ImmuPro, Inner Defense

**Oral Care:** Thieves AromaBright Toothpaste, Thieves Dentarome Plus Toothpaste, Thieves Dentarome Ultra Toothpaste, Thieves Fresh Essence Mouthwash, Thieves Hard Lozenges, Thieves Mints, Thieves Spray

## Application and Usage

**Aromatic:** Refer to *Application Guidelines* on page 410.

**Dietary and Oral:** Whether putting the oils in a capsule or drinking them in a liquid, please refer to *Application Guidelines* on page 410.

- Take 1 capsule with desired oil 2 times daily.
- Take 2-3 drops of oil in a spoonful of syrup or small amount of milk, juice, or water.
- Gargle 2-6 times daily with Thieves Fresh Essence Plus Mouthwash.

**Topical:** For guidelines on applying oils to the skin, refer to *Application Guidelines* on page 410.

- Massage 1-3 drops neat on forehead, nose, cheeks, lower throat, chest, and upper back 3-5 times daily. Be careful not to get oils in or near eyes or eyelids.
- Apply 1-2 drops neat on temples and back of neck as desired.
- Apply 1-3 drops on the Vita Flex points of feet 2-4 times daily.
- Use the Raindrop Technique 1-2 times weekly.
- Bath salts: Mix 4-5 drops of oil with 1 cup of salt in hot water to dissolve salts. Pour into bathtub and then soak for 15-20 minutes or until water cools.
- Place a warm compress with 1-2 drops of chosen oil on the back.

**Nasal Irrigation Regimen** *(see box on previous page)*

# SKIN DISORDERS AND PROBLEMS

Essential oils can have powerful antioxidant and antibacterial benefits for the skin. Essential oils used on the skin are often combined with a vegetable carrier oil to:

- Slow evaporation, allowing more time for the oils to penetrate the skin.
- Maintain the lipid barrier of the skin because most essential oils will tend to dry the skin.
- Enhance the effect of the essential oils because many oils work well synergistically in a vegetable oil. Many skin conditions are related to dysfunctions of the liver. It may be necessary to cleanse, stimulate, and condition the liver and colon for 30-90 days before the skin begins to improve.

## Abscesses and Boils

Skin abscesses are small pockets of pus that collect under the skin, usually caused by a bacterial or fungal infection.

Any number of essential oils may help reduce inflammation and combat infection, helping to bring an abscess or boil to a head so that the pus will come out and the healing can begin.

## Recommendations

**Singles:** Oregano, Plectranthus Oregano, Clove, Myrrh, Tea Tree, Sacred Frankincense, Frankincense, Lavender, Rosemary, Thyme, Patchouli, Dalmatia Bay Laurel, Laurus Nobilis (Bay Laurel)

**Blends:** Melrose, Purification, Thieves

**Nutritionals:** JuvaTone, ComforTone, Essentialzyme, Essentialzymes-4, Life 9, Digest & Cleanse, Inner Defense

## Application and Usage

**Topical:** For guidelines on applying oils to the skin, refer to *Application Guidelines* on page 410.

- Apply 2-3 drops neat (undiluted), depending on which oil you choose.
- Dilute the oil you choose 50:50 with V-6 Vegetable Oil Complex and apply on location 3-6 times daily or as needed.

544 | Chapter 20 | Personal Usage Guide

Personal Usage Guide | Chapter 20

## Acne

Acne results from an excess accumulation of dirt and sebum (oil) produced in the follicles and pores of the skin. As the pores and hair follicles become congested, bacteria begin to feed on the sebum. This leads to inflammation, infection, and the formation of a pimple or a blackhead around the hair follicle.

One of the most common forms of acne, *Acne vulgaris,* occurs primarily in adolescents due to hormone imbalances that stimulate the production of sebum.

Acne may be caused by a hormone imbalance, poor diet, and the use of chemicals found in cleaning products, soaps, cosmetics, lotions, and creams.

Stress may also play a role. According to research conducted by Dr. Toyoda in Japan, acne and other skin problems are a direct result of physical and emotional stress.[37] Essential oils are outstanding for treating acne because of their ability to dissolve sebum, kill bacteria, and preserve the acid mantle of the skin. Natural hormone creams such as Prenolone Plus Body Cream or the gentle Progessence Plus may help with hormone imbalance problems directly affecting the skin.

### Recommendations

**Singles:** Tea Tree, Geranium, Vetiver, Royal Hawaiian Sandalwood, Patchouli, Lavender, German Chamomile, Roman Chamomile, Cedarwood, Eucalyptus Radiata, Melaleuca Quinquenervia (Niaouli)

**Blends:** Melrose, Purification, Harmony, Shutran

**Nutritionals:** Mineral Essence, Detoxzyme, Multi-Greens, ICP, ComforTone, Essentialzyme, Essentialzymes-4, Life 9, Ningxia Wolfberries (Organic, Dried), OmegaGize³, Digest & Cleanse, Balance Complete

**Body Care:** Boswellia Wrinkle Cream, ART Gentle Cleanser, ART Refreshing Toner, Satin Facial Scrub (Mint), Progessence Plus, Prenolone Plus Body Cream, Royal Hawaiian Sandalwood Soaps, Shutran Bar Soap, Melaleuca-Geranium Moisturizing Soap

### Application and Usage

**Dietary and Oral:** Whether putting the oils in a capsule or drinking them in a liquid, please refer to *Application Guidelines* on page 410.

- Take 1 capsule with desired oil 2 times daily.
- Take 2-3 drops of oil in a spoonful of syrup or small amount of milk, juice, or water.
- Remove sugar and dairy from your diet

## Tips for Clearing Acne

- Eliminate dairy products, fried foods, chemical additives, and sugar from diet.
- Avoid using makeup or chlorinated water.
- Avoid using plastics that may exude estrogenic chemicals.
- Topically apply essential oils such as Tea Tree to problem areas. It was shown to be equal to benzoyl peroxide in the treatment of acne, according to research published in the *Medical Journal of Australia*.
- Begin a cleansing program with the Cleansing Trio, Sulfurzyme, Detoxzyme, Essentialzyme, ICP, and JuvaPower.

**Topical:** For guidelines on applying oils to the skin, refer to *Application Guidelines* on page 410.

- Gently massage 3-5 drops neat or diluted with V-6 Vegetable Oil Complex into the oily areas 1-3 times daily. Alternate the oils daily for maximum effect.

## Blisters

Blisters are caused when fluid is trapped under the skin caused by physical injury, chemical burns, sunburns, allergies, and microbial infestation caused by fungal and viral diseases such as herpes simplex, athletes foot, etc.

### Recommendations

**Singles:** Tea Tree, Myrrh, Lavender, Roman or German Chamomile, Helichrysum, Dalmatia Bay Laurel, Laurus Nobilis (Bay Laurel)

**Blends:** Melrose, Purification, Valor, Valor II, Owie

**Body Care:** LavaDerm Cooling Mist, Rose Ointment, Genesis Hand & Body Lotion

### Application and Usage

**Topical:** For guidelines on applying oils to the skin, refer to *Application Guidelines* on page 410.

- Dilute 50:50 and apply to blistered area 3-6 times daily.
- Spray LavaDerm as often as every 30 minutes as desired.
- Gently apply a little Rose Ointment or lotion to keep skin soft and moist.

Seventh Edition | Essential Oils Desk Reference | 545

## Boils

Boils and carbuncles (a group of boils) are caused by bacterial infection that creates a pus-filled hair follicle. They can be easily treated with antiseptic essential oils, including Tea Tree and Clove.

### Recommendations

**Singles:** Tea Tree, Myrrh, Clove, Thyme, Oregano

**Blends:** Melrose, Purification, Thieves

### Application and Usage

**Topical:** For guidelines on applying oils to the skin, refer to *Application Guidelines* on page 410.

- Dilute 2-3 drops of any oil above 50:50 and apply on location 3-6 times daily.

## Burns *(See also Shock)*

There are three types of burns:

**First-degree burns** only damage the outer layer of the skin. Sunburn is typically a first-degree burn.

**Second-degree burns** damage both the outer layer and the underlying layer known as the dermis, manifested by blisters.

**Third-degree burns** not only destroy or damage skin but can even damage underlying tissues.

Burns can be caused by sunlight, chemicals, electricity, radiation, and heat. Thermal burns are the most common type.

Aloe vera gel (contained in LavaDerm) is used extensively in the treatment of burns and has been studied for its anti-inflammatory and tissue-regenerating properties.

Helichrysum, Lavender, Idaho Balsam Fir, and Frankincense oils support tissue regeneration and reduce scarring and skin discoloration.

Severe burns can result in dehydration and mineral loss. Inflammation often accompanies burns, so Dietary and Oral protocols should be used to lessen inflammation.

If the burn is large or severe, the individual may go into shock. Inhaling oils may help reduce the shock.

After a burn has started to heal and is drying and cracking, use Rose Ointment or a body lotion with a few drops of Lavender oil to keep skin soft and to promote faster healing.

**Seek medical attention for serious burns as necessary.**

## FIRST-DEGREE BURNS (Sunburn)

The best prevention for sunburn is to avoid prolonged exposure to the sun. When you do go outdoors, always wear sun block or lotion with a SPF greater than 15—especially during the summer and when you expect to be outdoors for a prolonged period of time.

Certain natural vegetable oils and essential oils have been found to provide some protection against the sun. Sesame oil can block or reduce about 30 percent of the burning rays, coconut and olive oils can reduce about 20 percent, and aloe vera inhibits about 20 percent. Helichrysum essential oil has been researched for its ability to effectively screen out some of the sun's rays.

### Chérie Ross's Sunscreen Blend No. 1
- 10 drops Helichrysum
- 5 drops Lavender
- 3 drops Roman Chamomile
- 1 oz. Sesame Oil
- ½ oz. Coconut Oil
- ½ oz. Olive Oil

Mix and apply before going out in the sun.

### Chérie Ross's Sunscreen Blend No. 2
- 30 drops Lavender
- 4 oz. Avocado Oil

Mix and apply before going out in the sun.

In the event of a sunburn, LavaDerm Cooling Mist, and Lavender and Idaho Balsam Fir essential oils can offer excellent pain-relieving and healing benefits.

## Recommendations

**Singles:** Lavender, Idaho Balsam Fir, Helichrysum, Rose, Melaleuca Quinquenervia (Niaouli), German Chamomile, Vetiver

**Blends:** Gentle Baby, Australian Blue, Melrose, Valor, Valor II, Valor Roll-On

**Nutritionals:** Longevity Softgels, Sulfurzyme, MegaCal, OmegaGize[3], Rose Ointment

**Body Care:** LavaDerm Cooling Mist

## Application and Usage

**Topical:** For guidelines on applying oils to the skin, refer to *Application Guidelines* on page 410.

- For fast relief of first-degree burns, spray burn immediately with LavaDerm Cooling Mist and continue misting as necessary to cool the area. Spray as often as needed for the first several hours and follow with 2-3 drops of Lavender or Idaho Balsam Fir.

Personal Usage Guide | **Chapter 20**

## The Deadly Dehydration of Burns

Burns tend to swell and blister because of fluid loss from the damaged blood vessels. This is why it is important to keep the burn well hydrated and to drink plenty of water.

In cases of serious burns, fluid loss can become so severe that it sends the victim into shock and requires intravenous transfusions of saline solution to bring up blood pressure.

- Apply 1-3 drops neat or diluted 50:50 on burn location to cool tissue and reduce inflammation.
- Apply 3-6 times daily or as needed.

### SECOND-DEGREE BURNS (Blisters)

- Spray burn immediately with LavaDerm Cooling Mist and continue misting when necessary to cool the area. Spray as often as needed for the first several hours and follow with 2-3 drops of Lavender or Idaho Balsam Fir.
- Thereafter, apply LavaDerm every 15-30 minutes during the first day. Apply 2-4 drops of Lavender or Melaleuca Quinquenervia as needed immediately after each LavaDerm misting.
- On days 2 through 5, mist every hour and follow with 2-4 drops Lavender or Melaleuca Quinquenervia.
- Continue using LavaDerm 3 to 6 times daily until healed. Apply Rose Ointment to keep tissue soft.
- Mineral Essence: Put 2 droppers full in 3 liters of water and drink throughout the day.

### THIRD-DEGREE BURNS

- Spray LavaDerm Cooling Mist immediately to hydrate the skin.
- **Seek medical attention immediately.**

## Chapped, Cracked, or Dry Skin

Dry skin results from loss of the protective lipid layer on the skin surface. It results from exposure to low humidity environments and is often more prevalent during the winter. Dry skin may also crack, creating an opportunity for infection.

### Recommendations

**Singles:** Neroli, Rose, Cedarwood, Roman Chamomile, Palmarosa, Geranium, Lavender, Myrrh, Royal Hawaiian Sandalwood

**Blends:** Gentle Baby, Owie

**Body Care:** LavaDerm Cooling Mist, Essential Beauty Serum for Dry Skin, Tender Tush, Boswellia Wrinkle Cream, Sandalwood Moisture Cream, Rose Ointment, KidScents Lotion, Royal Hawaiian Sandalwood Soaps, Shutran Bar Soap, Melaleuca-Geranium Moisturizing Soap, Dragon Time Bath and Shower Gel, Evening Peace Bath and Shower Gel, Morning Start Bath and Shower Gel, Sensation Bath and Shower Gel

**Lip Care:** Lavender Lip Balm, Cinnamint Lip Balm, Grapefruit Lip Balm, Vanillamint Lip Balm

### Application and Usage

**Topical**: For guidelines on applying oils to the skin, refer to *Application Guidelines* on page 410.

- Apply 2-3 drops of oil diluted 20:80 in a natural, unperfumed lotion base (V-6 Vegetable Oil Complex or avocado oil) or other high-grade, emollient oil; apply on location as often as needed.
- Combine 3-5 drops of essential oils with 1 teaspoon of Sensation, KidScents Lotion, or Genesis Hand & Body Lotion to create a very effective lotion for rehydrating the skin of chapped hands and maintaining the natural pH balance of the skin.
- Bath and shower gels, such as Dragon Time, Evening Peace, Morning Start, and Sensation are formulated to help balance the acid mantle of the skin. The bar soaps are rich in moisturizers.

## Clogged Pores

Most skin blemishes begin as clogged pores. To have clean pores, you should maintain a regular skin care routine. If you keep your pores unclogged and clean, you will have fewer breakouts and more beautiful skin.

### Recommendations

**Singles:** Lemon, Orange, Geranium, Cypress, Lavender

**Blends:** Melrose, Purification, Inner Child

**Skin Care:** ART Gentle Cleanser, Satin Facial Scrub (Mint), Orange Blossom Facial Wash

### Application and Usage

**Topical**: For guidelines on applying oils to the skin, refer to *Application Guidelines* on page 410.

- Apply 2-4 drops neat to affected area and gently remove with cotton ball.
- Use ART Refreshing Toner and moisturizing bar soaps.

Seventh Edition | **Essential Oils Desk Reference** | **547**

- Satin Facial Scrub, Mint is a gentle exfoliator designed to clarify skin and reduce acne. If its texture is too abrasive for your skin, mix it with Orange Blossom Facial Wash. This is excellent for those with severe or mild acne.
- Spread scrub over face and let dry for perhaps five minutes to draw out impurities, purifying and toning the skin at the same time. Put a hot towel over face for greater penetration.
- Wash off with warm water by gently patting skin with warm face cloth. If you do not have time to let the mask dry, gently massage in a circular motion for 30 seconds, then rinse.
- Afterward, apply Sandalwood Moisture Cream or Boswellia Wrinkle Cream. This also works well underneath foundation makeup.

## Cuts, Scrapes, and Wounds

When selecting essential oils for surface injuries, determine the needs of the entire body, not just of the cut. Think through the cause and type of injury and select oils for each aspect of the trauma. For instance, a wound could encompass muscle damage, nerve damage, ligament damage, inflammation, infection, bone injury, fever, and possibly an emotion. Therefore, select an oil or blend that is specific to each need.

## Recommendations

**Single Oils:** Lavender, Tea Tree, Helichrysum, Rosemary, Eucalyptus Globulus, Dorado Azul, Cypress, Wintergreen, Thyme, Oregano, Plectranthus Oregano, German Chamomile, Mountain Savory, Sacred Frankincense, Frankincense, Myrrh, Eucalyptus Blue, Eucalyptus Radiata, Cistus

**Blends:** Melrose, Thieves, The Gift, 3 Wise Men, Aroma Siez, Aroma Life, Purification, Trauma Life, T.R. Care, Peace & Calming, Peace & Calming II, R.C., RutaVaLa, RutaVaLa Roll-On, Stress Away Roll-On, Tranquil Roll-On, Owie

**Body Care:** Thieves Spray, LavaDerm Cooling Mist

**Bruise and Scrape Blend**
(May be used on infants and children)
- 4 drops Lavender
- 1 drop Cistus
- 1 drop Myrrh

**Infected Cut Blend**
- 7 drops Geranium
- 5 drops Myrrh
- 3 drops Tea Tree

# First Aid Spray

**First Aid Recipe:**
- 5 drops Lavender
- 3 drops Tea Tree
- 2 drops Dorado Azul

Mix the recipe above thoroughly in ½ teaspoon of salt. Add this to 8 oz. of distilled water, shake vigorously, and pour into a spray bottle. Spray minor cuts and wounds before applying bandage. Repeat 2-3 times daily for 3 days. Continue the healing process by applying 1-2 drops of Tea Tree oil to the wound daily for the next few days. Apply Rose Ointment or Tender Tush to keep the scab soft and to help prevent scarring.

Animal Scents works extremely well for any animal, and it is also very effective for any person who wishes to cover a large area such as the bottoms of the feet. When working in rough conditions such as the cold outdoors, construction and building, or anything that is abrasive to the hands, add a few drops of the recipe to a tablespoon of Animal Scents or Rose Ointment and use it throughout the day to relieve the pain and ache of small cuts and scrapes on the skin.

## Application and Usage

**Topical:** For guidelines on applying oils to the skin, refer to *Application Guidelines* on page 410.

- Dilute recommended oils 50:50 and apply 2-6 drops on location 1-4 times daily.
- Apply LavaDerm Cooling Mist to the affected area.

**Note:** Peppermint can be helpful in treating wounds but may sting when applied to an open wound. To reduce discomfort, dilute with Lavender or mix in a sealing ointment before applying. When applied to a wound or cut that has a scab, a diluted Peppermint blend will soothe, cool, and reduce inflammation in damaged tissue.

## TO DISINFECT
## Recommendations

**Singles:** Tea Tree, Oregano, Plectranthus Oregano, Lemongrass, Melissa, Thyme, Mountain Savory, Lemon, Rosemary, Eucalyptus Radiata, Cinnamon Bark, Clove

**Blends:** Thieves, Melrose, Purification, Citrus Fresh

Personal Usage Guide | **Chapter 20**

## Application and Usage

**Topical:** For guidelines on applying oils to the skin, refer to *Application Guidelines* on page 410.

- Apply Thieves Spray.
- Dilute recommended oils 50:50 and apply 2-4 drops on the wound 2-5 times daily.

## TO PROMOTE HEALING

### Recommendations

**Singles:** Sacred Frankincense, Frankincense, Royal Hawaiian Sandalwood, Melissa, Lavender, Idaho Balsam Fir, Palo Santo, Patchouli, Melaleuca Quinquenervia, Myrrh, Helichrysum

**Blends:** Melrose, Purification, Gentle Baby, Valor, Owie

## Application and Usage

**Topical:** For guidelines on applying oils to the skin, refer to *Application Guidelines* on page 410.

- Dilute recommended oils 50:50 and apply 2-4 drops on the wound 2-5 times daily.

## TO REDUCE BLEEDING

### Recommendations

**Singles:** Helichrysum, Cistus, Cypress, Lemon, Geranium, Vetiver, Valerian, Sacred Frankincense, Frankincense, Myrrh, German Chamomile

**Blends:** PanAway, Relieve It, Aroma Siez

## Application and Usage

**Topical:** For guidelines on applying oils to the skin, refer to *Application Guidelines* on page 410.

- Apply a cold compress to the affected area 1-2 times until bleeding stops.

**Wound Compress Blend**
- 5 drops Geranium
- 5 drops Lemon
- 5 drops German Chamomile
- 2 drops Helichrysum

## TO REDUCE SCARRING

### Recommendations

**Singles:** Sacred Frankincense, Frankincense, Lavender, Royal Hawaiian Sandalwood, Cistus, Geranium, Helichrysum, Myrrh, Vetiver, Patchouli

**Blends:** Gentle Baby, Valor, Valor II, Melrose, Owie

**Scar Prevention Blend No. 1**
- 3 drops Royal Hawaiian Sandalwood
- 3 drops Sacred Frankincense or Frankincense
- 1 drop Vetiver

**Scar Prevention Blend No. 2**
- 10 drops Geranium
- 8 drops Helichrysum
- 6 drops Lavender
- 4 drops Patchouli

## Application and Usage

**Topical:** For guidelines on applying oils to the skin, refer to *Application Guidelines* on page 410.

- Dilute recommended oils 50:50 and apply 2-4 drops on the wound 2-5 times daily.

## Diaper Rash

Dilute all oils when being used for babies. Just 1-2 drops mixed in Tender Tush or Rose Ointment are sufficient for using on diaper rash.

### Recommendations

**Singles:** Lavender, Helichrysum, German Chamomile, Cypress

**Blends:** Gentle Baby, Purification, Valor, Owie

**Body Care:** Tender Tush, Rose Ointment, ClaraDerm, LavaDerm Cooling Mist

## Application and Usage

**Topical:** For guidelines on applying oils to the skin, refer to *Application Guidelines* on page 410.

- Apply 1-2 drops diluted 50:50 and/or ointments on location 2-4 times daily during diaper changes.

## Eczema/Dermatitis

Eczema and dermatitis are both inflammations of the skin and are most often due to allergies, including from gluten (wheat) and dairy, but they also can be a sign of liver disease.

Dermatitis usually results from external factors such as sunburn or contact with poison ivy, metals from wristwatch, earrings, jewelry, etc.; internal factors such as irritant chemicals, soaps, and shampoos; or from gluten and lactose allergies or intolerance.

In both dermatitis and eczema, the skin can become red, flaky, and itchy. Small blisters may form, and if they are broken by scratching, they can become infected.

### Recommendations

**Singles:** Lavender, German Chamomile, Myrrh, Blue

Seventh Edition | **Essential Oils Desk Reference** | 549

Cypress, Roman Chamomile, Geranium, Dalmatia Bay Laurel, Laurus Nobilis (Bay Laurel)

**Blends:** JuvaCleanse, Purification, Melrose, Australian Blue

**Nutritionals:** Detoxzyme, ICP, ComforTone, Essentialzyme, JuvaTone, JuvaPower, JuvaSpice, Essentialzymes-4, KidScents MightyZyme, Life 9

**Body Care:** Rose Ointment, KidScents Tender Tush, Regenolone Moisturizing Cream

## Application and Usage

**Topical:** For guidelines on applying oils to the skin, refer to *Application Guidelines* on page 410.

- Apply 1-2 drops diluted 50:50 on location as needed.

## Fungal Skin Infections

Fungi and yeast feed on decomposing or dead tissues that exist everywhere such as in our stomachs, on our skin, on food, outside in the lawn, in the garden, on pets, etc. When kept under control, the yeast and fungi populating our bodies are harmless and digest what our bodies cannot or do not use.

When we feed the naturally occurring fungi in our bodies with simple sugars, the fungi are more likely to grow out of control. This condition is known as systemic candidiasis, which invades the blood, gastrointestinal tract, and tissues.

## Recommendations

**Singles:** Tea Tree, Lemongrass, Oregano, Plectranthus Oregano, Lavender, Northern Lights Black Spruce, Patchouli, Melaleuca Quinquenervia

**Blends:** Melrose, Purification

**Nutritionals:** Life 9, Digest & Cleanse, ICP, ComforTone, Essentialzyme, Mineral Essence

**Skin Care:** ClaraDerm

**Antifungal Skin Blend**
- 10 drops Patchouli
- 5 drops Lemongrass
- 4 drops Melaleuca Quinquenervia
- 2 drops Tea Tree

## Application and Usage

**Topical:** For guidelines on applying oils to the skin, refer to *Application Guidelines* on page 410.

- Apply 2-4 drops of oil diluted 50:50 on location 3-5 times daily.

---

### Tea Tree *(Melaleuca alternifolia)*

During World War II, tea tree oil (*Melaleuca alternifolia*) was found to have very strong antibacterial properties and worked well in preventing infection in open wounds.

Melrose is a blend containing two types of Melaleuca oil: Tea Tree (*M. alternifolia*) and Niaouli (*M. quinquenervia),* plus Rosemary and Clove, making it an exceptional antiseptic and tissue regenerator.

---

## Itching

Itching can be due to dry skin, impaired liver function, insects, allergies, or overexposure to chemicals or sunlight.

## Recommendations

**Singles:** Peppermint, Patchouli, Lavender, Oregano, Plectranthus Oregano, Vetiver, Nutmeg, German Chamomile

**Blends:** Aroma Siez, Purification, Melrose, Thieves, DiGize, Owie, JuvaFlex, JuvaCleanse

**Nutritionals:** Digest & Cleanse, Life 9, JuvaTone, ComforTone, Essentialzyme, Essentialzymes-4, Detoxzyme, ICP, JuvaPower, JuvaSpice, PowerGize

**Body Care:** KidScents Tender Tush, Rose Ointment, Regenolone Moisturizing Cream, LavaDerm Cooling Mist, ClaraDerm

## Application and Usage

**Topical:** For guidelines on applying oils to the skin, refer to *Application Guidelines* on page 410.

- Apply 1-2 drops neat on location several times daily as needed.
- Dilute 50/50 and apply on location 3-6 times daily.
- Spray LavaDerm Cooling Mist or ClaraDerm if condition is evident on the skin.

## Moles

Moles appear as small, dark brown spots; come in many colors; and can develop virtually anywhere on your body. Most moles are harmless, but monitoring them is important in detecting skin cancer.

## Recommendations

**Singles:** Oregano, Plectranthus Oregano, Thyme, Tea Tree, Frankincense, Sacred Frankincense

**Blends:** Melrose, Purification

Personal Usage Guide | **Chapter 20**

## Application and Usage

**Topical:** For guidelines on applying oils to the skin, refer to *Application Guidelines* on page 410.

- To dry up moles, apply 1-2 drops of Oregano neat (undiluted) on the mole 2-3 times daily.
- Other oils may be used that may also show benefit.

## Poison Oak/Poison Ivy/Poison Sumac

Poison ivy, poison oak, and poison sumac are plants that contain an irritating, oily sap called urushiol, which triggers an allergic reaction when it comes into contact with skin. An itchy rash can appear within hours of exposure or several days later and usually develops into oozing blisters.

## Recommendations

**Singles:** Peppermint, Myrrh, Patchouli, Vetiver, Eucalyptus Blue, German Chamomile, Roman Chamomile, Rose, Lemon, Idaho Tansy, Palo Santo, Tea Tree, Rosemary, Basil

**Blends:** Melrose, Purification, R.C., JuvaCleanse, Owie

**Nutritionals:** Detoxzyme, ComforTone, Mineral Essence, Digest & Cleanse, ICP, JuvaPower, JuvaSpice, OmegaGize[3]

**Body Care:** Rose Ointment, KidScents Tender Tush, Sandalwood Moisture Cream, Boswellia Wrinkle Cream, ART Light Moisturizer, Thieves Spray, Lava-Derm Cooling Mist, ClaraDerm

## Application and Usage

**Topical:** For guidelines on applying oils to the skin, refer to *Application Guidelines* on page 410.

- Apply 4-6 drops of oil diluted 50:50 to affected areas 2 times daily.
- Apply a cold compress on affected area 2 times daily.

## Psoriasis

Psoriasis is a noninfectious skin disorder that is marked by skin patches or flaking skin that can occur in limited areas such as the scalp or that can cover up to 80-90 percent of the body.

The overly rapid growth of skin cells is the primary cause of psoriasis. In some cases, skin cells grow four times faster than normal, resulting in the formation of silvery layers that flake off.

## The pH Balance Makes a Difference

Psoriasis, eczema, dermatitis, dry skin, allergies, and similar problems indicate an excessive acidic pH in the body. The more acid that is in the blood and skin, the less therapeutic effect the oils will have.

People who have a negative reaction to essential oils are usually highly acidic. An alkaline balance must be maintained in the blood and skin for the oils to work the best. AlkaLime and MultiGreens are both helpful for this balancing (See Fungus).

### Symptoms

- It occurs on elbows, chest, knees, and scalp.
- Slightly elevated reddish lesions are covered with silver-white scales.
- The disease can be limited to one small patch or can cover the entire body.
- Rashes subside after exposure to sunlight.
- Rashes recur over a period of years.

**Stop eating sugar!**

## Recommendations

**Singles:** Roman Chamomile, Tea Tree, Patchouli, Helichrysum, Rose, Melissa, German Chamomile, German Chamomile Vitality, Lavender, Lavender Vitality, Vetiver, Royal Hawaiian Sandalwood

**Blends:** Melrose, Gentle Baby, JuvaCleanse, JuvaCleanse Vitality, JuvaFlex, JuvaFlex Vitality

**Nutritionals:** ICP, ComforTone, Essentialzyme, Essentialzymes-4, Life 9, Balance Complete, AlkaLime, JuvaTone, JuvaPower, Sulfurzyme

**Body Care:** KidScents Tender Tush, Rose Ointment

**Psoriasis Blend**
- 4 drops Rosewood or Palo Santo
- 2 drops Patchouli
- 2 drops Roman Chamomile
- 2 drops Vetiver
- 2 drops Royal Hawaiian Sandalwood

## Application and Usage

**Aromatic:** Refer to *Application Guidelines* on page 410.

**Dietary and Oral:** Whether putting the oils in a capsule or drinking them in a liquid, please refer to *Application Guidelines* on page 410.

Seventh Edition | **Essential Oils Desk Reference** | 551

**Essential Oils Desk Reference** | Seventh Edition

## Essential Oils Skin Rejuvenation

**Rejuvenate and heal**
- Rose, Sandalwood, Myrrh, Frankincense, Vetiver

**Prevent and retard wrinkles**
- Lavender, Myrrh, Frankincense, Sandalwood

**Regenerate**
- Geranium, Helichrysum, Melrose Sandalwood

**Restore skin elasticity**
- Sandalwood with Lavender
- Ylang Ylang with Lavender
- Patchouli with Ylang Ylang

**Combat premature aging of the skin**

Mix the following recipe into 1 tablespoon V-6 Vegetable Oil Complex, any high-grade vegetable oil, or unscented skin lotion and apply on location 2 times daily.

**Skin Rejuvenating Recipe**
- 6 drops Sandalwood
- 4 drops Geranium
- 3 drops Lavender
- 2 drops Sacred Frankincense

---

- Take 1 capsule with desired oil 1 time daily.
- Take 2-3 drops of oil in a spoonful of syrup or small amount of milk, juice, or water.

**Topical:** For guidelines on applying oils to the skin, refer to *Application Guidelines* on page 410.

- Apply 2-4 drops neat to affected area 2 times daily.
- Add 6-10 drops to 1 teaspoon of regular skin lotion and apply daily or as needed.
- Place a warm compress with 1-2 drops of chosen oil on the back 3 times weekly.

## Sagging Skin

Sagging skin is a common problem for many people, especially as they get older. It occurs as the skin loses its elasticity over time.

### Recommendations

**Singles:** Lavender, Helichrysum, Patchouli, Cypress, Tangerine, Royal Hawaiian Sandalwood, Geranium

**Blends:** Humility, Inspiration, Joy

**Nutritionals:** Super C, Super C Chewable, ICP, ComforTone, Essentialzyme, Essentialzymes-4, Life 9, Mineral Essence, JuvaPower, JuvaSpice

**Body Care:** ART Refreshing Toner, Boswellia Wrinkle Cream, Cel-Lite Magic Massage Oil

**Skin Firming Blend (Morning)**
- 3 drops Tangerine
- 3 drops Cypress

**Skin Firming Blend (Evening)**
- 8 drops Patchouli
- 5 drops Cypress
- 5 drops Geranium
- 1 drop Royal Hawaiian Sandalwood

### Application and Usage

**Topical:** For guidelines on applying oils to the skin, refer to *Application Guidelines* on page 410.

- Apply 4-6 drops neat or diluted 50:50 on affected area 2 times daily. Use the morning blend before dressing in the morning and the evening blend before bed at night.
- Strength training with weights can also help tighten sagging skin.

## Scabies

Scabies are caused by eight-legged insects known as itch mites—tiny parasites that burrow into the skin, usually in the fingers and genital areas. The most common variety, *Sarcoptes scabiei,* can quickly infest other people. Although it lives for only one to two months, the female continually lays eggs once it digs into the skin.

The most common remedy for scabies and lice is lindane (gamma benzene hexachloride), a highly toxic polychlorinated chemical that is structurally very similar to hazardous banned pesticides such as DDT and chlordane. It is so dangerous that Dr. Guy Sansfacon, head of the Quebec Poison Control Centre in Canada, has requested that lindane be banned.

Natural, plant-derived essential oils have the same activity as commercial pesticides but are far safer. Essential oils have been studied for their ability to not only repel insects but also to kill them and their eggs as well. Because most oils are nontoxic to humans, they make excellent treatments to combat scabies infestations.

### Recommendations

**Singles:** Palo Santo, Peppermint, Citronella, Rosemary, Palmarosa, Lavandin, Eucalyptus Globulus, Black Pepper, Ginger, Oregano, Plectranthus Oregano, Thyme, Mountain Savory

**Blends:** Purification, Melrose, Thieves, Exodus II, ImmuPower

---

**552** | **Chapter 20** | Personal Usage Guide

## Application and Usage

**Topical:** For guidelines on applying oils to the skin, refer to *Application Guidelines* on page 410.

- Apply 2-4 drops of recommended oils neat or diluted 50:50 if needed on location 3 times daily.
- To treat hair or scalp, add 3-5 drops of essential oil to 1 teaspoon of shampoo and massage into wet hair. Leave for 5 minutes, then rinse.

## Skin Ulcers

Skin ulcers are open sores that are often accompanied by the sloughing-off of inflamed tissue. They can be caused by problems with blood circulation, irritation from exposure to corrosive material, exposure to heat, cold, or trauma.

### Recommendations

**Singles:** Helichrysum, Roman Chamomile, Patchouli, Lavender, Clove, Myrrh

**Blends:** Thieves, Purification, Relieve It, Melrose

**Nutritionals:** Super C, ICP, ComforTone, Essentialzyme, Essentialzymes-4, Life 9, NingXia Red, Inner Defense, Digest & Cleanse, Power Meal, Slique Shake, ImmuPro

**Body Care:** KidScents Tender Tush, Rose Ointment

### Application and Usage

**Topical:** For guidelines on applying oils to the skin, refer to *Application Guidelines* on page 410.

- Apply 4-6 drops neat or diluted 50:50 on affected area 2 times daily.

## Stretch Marks

Stretch marks are most commonly associated with pregnancy but can also occur during growth spurts and periods of weight gain.

### Recommendations

**Singles:** Sacred Frankincense, Frankincense, Elemi, Geranium, Lavender, Myrrh

**Blends:** Gentle Baby, Sensation, Valor, Valor II, White Angelica, White Light

**Nutritionals:** Sulfurzyme, MegaCal, Super B, Super C, Super C Chewable, Essentialzyme, Essentialzymes-4, Life 9, Ultra Young, Master Formula

**Body Care:** KidScents Tender Tush, Rose Ointment

## Application and Usage

**Topical:** For guidelines on applying oils to the skin, refer to *Application Guidelines* on page 410.

- Apply 3-6 drops of oil neat or diluted 50:50 2 times daily.

## Vitiligo

Vitiligo is a condition in which your skin loses melanin, the pigment that determines the color of your skin, hair, and eyes and occurs when the cells that produce melanin die or no longer form melanin, causing slowly enlarging white patches of irregular shapes to appear on your skin.

The cause has not yet been determined, but there are theories that it may be due to an immune system disorder, heredity possibilities, nutritional deficiencies, overuse of chemicals, and perhaps environmental pollution that affects the proper function of the body that produces melanin.

Some people have reported a single event such as sunburn or emotional distress that triggered the condition. However, none of these theories has been proved to be a definite cause of vitiligo.

### Recommendations

**Singles:** Royal Hawaiian Sandalwood, Myrrh, Vetiver, Patchouli

**Blends:** Brain Power, Dream Catcher, Humility, Deep Relief Roll-On

**Nutritionals:** Essentialzyme, Essentialzymes-4, Life 9, Detoxzyme, ICP, JuvaPower, Mineral Essence, MindWise, Digest & Cleanse, Inner Defense, ImmuPro, SleepEssence

### Application and Usage

**Topical:** For guidelines on applying oils to the skin, refer to *Application Guidelines* on page 410.

- Apply 2-4 drops of desired oil neat 2 times daily.
- A cleansing diet might be helpful. Cleansing the liver and digestive system facilitates greater nutritional absorption and waste elimination for proper body function and vibrant health.

## Wrinkles

Although wrinkles are a natural part of aging, sun exposure is the major cause. Exposure to heat, wind, and dust, as well as smoking, may also contribute to wrinkling.

### Recommendations

**Singles:** Sacred Frankincense, Frankincense, Myrrh, Vetiver, Helichrysum, Cypress, Rose, Lavender, Patchouli,

**Essential Oils Desk Reference** | Seventh Edition

## Essential Oils and Skin Vitality

Tea Tree, Dorado Azul, and Lemongrass can help clear acne and balance oily skin conditions. Lemongrass is the predominant ingredient in Morning Start Bath and Shower Gel, which can be used to balance the pH of the skin, decongest the lymphatics, and stimulate circulation.

Geranium, Royal Hawaiian Sandalwood, Neroli, Palmarosa

**Blends:** Gentle Baby, Sensation, 3 Wise Men, White Angelica, Highest Potential

**Nutritionals:** MegaCal, Longevity Softgels, NingXia Red, OmegaGize[3], Master Formula, Sulfurzyme, Super B, Ningxia Wolfberries (Organic, Dried), MindWise

**Body Care:** Boswellia Wrinkle Cream, Wolfberry Eye Cream, ART Gentle Cleanser, ART Refreshing Toner, Rose Ointment, Sandalwood Moisture Cream, ART Light Moisturizer, ART Sheerlumé Brightening Cream

**Wrinkle-Reducing Blend**

- 6 drops Sacred Frankincense or Frankincense
- 5 drops Royal Hawaiian Sandalwood
- 4 drops Geranium
- 3 drops Lavender

### Application and Usage

**Topical:** For guidelines on applying oils to the skin, refer to *Application Guidelines* on page 410.

- Mix 3-4 drops of oil 50:50 in V-6 Vegetable Oil Complex or add to the ART skin care lotions or moisturizing creams and apply as needed.
- Rose Ointment was developed to keep the skin soft and moist and to supply healing nutrients. It is a natural emollient and contains no chemicals or synthetic ingredients that can cause skin irritation.

**Note:** Be careful not to get lotion or oils near the eyes.

## SLEEP DISORDERS

Melatonin is the most powerful natural remedy for restoring both quality and quantity of sleep. It improves the length of the time the body sustains deep, stage 4 sleep, the time when the immune system and growth hormone production reaches its maximum.

ImmuPro not only contains melatonin, but it also contains mineral and polysaccharide complexes to restore natural sleep rhythm and eliminate insomnia.

Valerian has been shown to be effective in calming the mind, enabling one to fall asleep easier.

### Recommendations

**Singles:** Lavender, Goldenrod, Valerian, Roman Chamomile, Orange, Mandarin

**Blends:** AromaSleep, RutaVaLa, RutaVaLa Roll-On, Tranquil Roll-On, Peace & Calming, Peace & Calming II, Surrender, Trauma Life, T.R. Care, Hope, Humility, Stress Away Roll-On

**Nutritionals:** SleepEssence, ImmuPro, Essentialzyme, MegaCal, Mineral Essence, OmegaGize[3], Life 9, Thyromin (take just before getting into bed), MindWise

### Application and Usage

**Aromatic:** Refer to *Application Guidelines* on page 410.

**Topical:** For guidelines on applying oils to the skin, refer to *Application Guidelines* on page 410.

- Apply 1-2 drops neat on temples and back of neck, as desired.
- Applying a single drop under the nose is helpful.
- Dilute 50:50 and apply on location 3-6 times daily.
- Massage 2-4 drops of oil neat on the bottoms of the feet just before bedtime. Children love it.

## SMOKING CESSATION *(See also Addictions)*

Smoking is a difficult habit to break because it involves many aspects of a person's emotions and social life as well as a physical addiction to nicotine. Smoking cessation (quitting smoking) is a vital part of cancer prevention.

### Recommendations

**Singles:** Cinnamon Bark, Cinnamon Bark Vitality, Clove, Clove Vitality, Nutmeg, Nutmeg Vitality, Peppermint, Peppermint Vitality, Roman Chamomile, Clary Sage, Sage, Sage Vitality

**Blends:** Thieves, Thieves Vitality, Harmony, JuvaCleanse, JuvaCleanse Vitality, Peace & Calming, Peace & Calming II, GLF, GLF Vitality

**Nutritionals:** ICP, ComforTone, Essentialzyme, Essentialzymes-4, Life 9, JuvaTone, JuvaPower, JuvaSpice

### Application and Usage

**Aromatic:** Refer to *Application Guidelines* on page 410.
- Inhale the oils that work best for you whenever the urge for a cigarette arises.

**554** | **Chapter 20** | Personal Usage Guide

**Dietary and Oral:** Whether putting the oils in a capsule or drinking them in a liquid, please refer to *Application Guidelines* on page 410.

- Take 1 capsule with desired oil 2 times daily.
- Take 2-3 drops of oil in a spoonful of syrup or small amount of milk, juice, or water.
- Cleanse colon and liver with ICP, ComforTone, Essentialzyme, and JuvaTone.
- Put 1 drop of Thieves on the tongue every time you have the urge to smoke.
- JuvaTone, JuvaPower, and JuvaSpice detoxify the liver, which in turn help to reduce cravings for nicotine and caffeine. Take 3 tablets of JuvaTone 3 times daily and 2 tablespoons of JuvaPower or JuvaSpice daily.

**Topical:** For guidelines on applying oils to the skin, refer to *Application Guidelines* on page 410.

## SNAKE BITES

**CAUTION:** Seek medical attention immediately if you are bitten by a poisonous snake.

### Recommendations

**Singles:** Clove, Eucalyptus Blue, Idaho Balsam Fir, Copaiba, Lemon, Patchouli, Sacred Frankincense, Frankincense, Thyme, Tea Tree

**Blends:** Purification, Melrose, Thieves

**Sprays:** Thieves Spray

### Application and Usage

**Topical:** For guidelines on applying oils to the skin, refer to *Application Guidelines* on page 410.

- Apply 2-3 drops diluted 50:50 on location every 15 minutes until professional medical help is available.

## SNORING *(See also Apnea)*

Just about everyone snores occasionally, but it can affect the quantity and quality of your sleep, which can lead to fatigue, irritability, and increased health problems, in addition to relationship problems with your partner.

### Recommendations

**Singles:** Idaho Balsam Fir, Royal Hawaiian Sandalwood, Rose, Lavender, Lavender Vitality, Valerian, Western Red Cedar, Ylang Ylang

**Blends:** RutaVaLa, RutaVaLa Roll-On, Stress Away Roll-On, The Gift, Harmony, Sacred Mountain, Valor, Valor II, Transformation

**Nutritionals:** SleepEssence, MegaCal, Mineral Essence, Detoxzyme, Essentialzyme, Essentialzymes-4, Life 9, ImmuPro

### Application and Usage

**Dietary and Oral:** Whether putting the oils in a capsule or drinking them in a liquid, please refer to *Application Guidelines* on page 410.

- Take 1 capsule with desired oil 2 times daily.
- Take 2-3 drops of oil in a spoonful of syrup or small amount of milk, juice, or water.

**Topical:** For guidelines on applying oils to the skin, refer to *Application Guidelines* on page 410.

- Rub 4-6 drops diluted 50:50 on the bottoms of both feet at bedtime.

## SPINA BIFIDA

Spina bifida (SB) is a defect in which the spinal cord of the fetus fails to close during the first month of pregnancy. This results in varying degrees of permanent nerve damage, paralysis in lower limbs, and incomplete brain development. The exact cause is unknown, but scientists suspect that nutritional, genetic, and environmental factors such as exposure to harmful substances may play a role in its cause. Having enough folate during the mother's pregnancy greatly reduces the risk of spina bifida and other neural tube disorders.[38]

Spina bifida has three different variations:

The most severe form is myelomeningocele, when the spinal cord and its protective sheath (known as the meninges) protrude from an opening in the spine.

Meningocele is when only the meninges protrude from the opening in the spine. The mildest form is occulta, characterized by malformed vertebrae.

Symptoms of this disease range from bowel and bladder dysfunctions to excess build up in the brain of cerebrospinal fluid.

The easiest way to possibly prevent spina bifida is with folic acid supplementation (at least 400 mcg daily, found in Super B) by all women of child-bearing ages.

### Recommendations

**Singles:** Mountain Savory, Mountain Savory Vitality, Helichrysum, Thyme, Thyme Vitality, Tea Tree, Idaho Balsam Fir, Sacred Frankincense, Frankincense, Frankincense Vitality

**Blends:** Melrose, Exodus II, The Gift, Peace & Calming, Peace & Calming II, Deep Relief Roll-On, Tranquil Roll-On, Aroma Siez

**Nutritionals:** Super B, Balance Complete, Sulfurzyme, PowerGize, MegaCal, JuvaPower, JuvaSpice, Master Formula, OmegaGize[3], Essentialzyme, Essential-zymes-4, Life 9, MindWise, Power Meal, Slique Shake

## Application and Usage

**Dietary and Oral:** Whether putting the oils in a capsule or drinking them in a liquid, please refer to *Application Guidelines* on page 410.

- Take 1 capsule with desired oil 2 times daily.
- Take 2-3 drops of oil in a spoonful of syrup or small amount of milk, juice, or water.

**Topical:** For guidelines on applying oils to the skin, refer to *Application Guidelines* on page 410.

- Receive a Raindrop Technique weekly.
- Place a warm compress with 1-2 drops of chosen oil over the affected area.

## SPINE INJURIES AND PAIN

According to numerous chiropractors, the Raindrop Technique using therapeutic-grade essential oils is revolutionizing the treatment of many types of back pain, spine inflammation, and vertebral misalignments.

The following essential oils, blends, and supplements are for supporting the structural integrity of the spine and reducing discomfort:

## Recommendations

**Singles:** Idaho Blue Spruce, Dorado Azul, Wintergreen, Marjoram, Marjoram Vitality, Idaho Balsam Fir, Helichrysum, Palo Santo, Peppermint, Peppermint Vitality, Basil, Basil Vitality, Copaiba, Copaiba Vitality

**Blends:** PanAway, Cool Azul, Aroma Siez, Relieve It, Valor, Valor II, Valor Roll-On, Deep Relief Roll-On

**Nutritionals:** PowerGize, MegaCal, SuperCal, Longevity Softgels, BLM, AgilEase, Essentialzyme, Mineral Essence, Power Meal, Slique Shake, Sulfurzyme

**Body Care:** Cool Azul Pain Relief Cream, Cool Azul Sports Gel, Ortho Sport Massage Oil, Ortho Ease Massage Oil

## Application and Usage

**Dietary and Oral:** Whether putting the oils in a capsule or drinking them in a liquid, please refer to *Application Guidelines* on page 410.

- Take 1 capsule with desired oil 2 times daily.
- Take 2-3 drops of oil in a spoonful of syrup or small amount of milk, juice, or water.

> Chiropractors have found that by applying Valor on the bottoms of the feet, spinal manipulations are easier to do and last 75 percent longer.

**Topical:** For guidelines on applying oils to the skin, refer to *Application Guidelines* on page 410.

- Apply 6-10 drops diluted 50:50 on location 2 times daily or as needed.
- Place a warm compress with 1-2 drops of desired oil daily (if area is not inflamed).
- Receive a Raindrop Technique 3 times a month.

## Back Injuries and Pain (Backache)
*(See also Muscles)*

According to numerous chiropractors, the Raindrop Technique using therapeutic-grade essential oils has added tremendous benefit to the treatment of many types of back pain, inflammation, and vertebral misalignments.

## Recommendations

**Singles:** Lavender, Idaho Balsam Fir, Helichrysum, Wintergreen, German Chamomile, Basil, Copaiba, Marjoram, Peppermint

**Blends:** Cool Azul, Aroma Siez, PanAway, Relieve It, Deep Relief Roll-On

**Nutritionals:** BLM, AgilEase, PowerGize, MegaCal, Master Formula, Power Meal, Slique Shake, MultiGreens, NingXia Red

**Body Care:** Cool Azul Pain Relief Cream, Cool Azul Sports Gel, Regenolone Moisturizing Cream, Ortho Sport Massage Oil, Ortho Ease Massage Oil

### Backache Blend
- 5 drops Wintergreen
- 3 drops Lavender
- 3 drops Idaho Balsam Fir
- 2 drops Marjoram

## Application and Usage

**Topical:** For guidelines on applying oils to the skin, refer to *Application Guidelines* on page 410.

- Apply 2-4 drops neat on specific area 1-3 times daily or as needed.
- Apply 2-4 drops on Vita Flex area of foot.
- Use warm compress with 1-2 drops of chosen oil on the back daily.
- Apply Raindrop Technique 2 times weekly for 3 weeks.
- Massage with Ortho Ease or Ortho Sport Massage Oil.

Personal Usage Guide | Chapter 20

## Herniated Disc/Disc Deterioration

A herniated disc is an abnormal rupture of the central portion of a disc of the spine. For this situation, it is best to consult a specialist.

However, many essential oils can give temporary pain relief.

### Recommendations

**Singles:** Basil, Tarragon, Idaho Blue Spruce, Sacred Frankincense, Frankincense, Idaho Balsam Fir, Helichrysum, Wintergreen, Vetiver, Valerian

**Blends:** PanAway, Cool Azul, Relieve It, Aroma Siez, Deep Relief Roll-On

**Nutritionals:** Sulfurzyme, BLM, AgilEase, PowerGize, MegaCal, Power Meal, Slique Shake, Master Formula, Essentialzyme, Mineral Essence, OmegaGize[3]

**Body Care:** Cool Azul Pain Relief Cream, Cool Azul Sports Gel, Regenolone Moisturizing Cream, Ortho Sport Massage Oil, Ortho Ease Massage Oil

### Application and Usage

**Topical:** For guidelines on applying oils to the skin, refer to *Application Guidelines* on page 410.

- Dilute 50:50 and apply on location for pain relief.
- Place a cold compress on location as needed.
- Receive a Raindrop Technique 2 times weekly.
- Stimulate vertebrae with "pointer technique" *(see box at right with explanation).*

## Lumbago (Lower back pain)

Chronic lower back pain can have many causes, including a damaged or pinched nerve (neuralgia) or a congested colon.

### Recommendations

**Singles:** Basil, Basil Vitality, Helichrysum, German Chamomile, German Chamomile Vitality, Elemi, Peppermint, Peppermint Vitality, Copaiba, Copaiba Vitality, Marjoram, Marjoram Vitality, Wintergreen

**Blends:** Relieve It, Cool Azul, PanAway, Deep Relief Roll-On, Stress Away Roll-On

**Nutritionals:** MegaCal, BLM, AgilEase, ICP, ComforTone, Essentialzyme, Essentialzymes-4, Life 9, OmegaGize[3], PowerGize

**Body Care:** Cool Azul Pain Relief Cream, Cool Azul Sports Gel, Regenolone Moisturizing Cream, Ortho Sport Massage Oil, Ortho Ease Massage Oil

## Pointer Technique for Nerve Damage

The "pointer technique" uses a pointer with a rounded tip like a pen to stimulate specific locations on the skin after the essential oils have been applied to the area. It works very well on the Vita Flex points of the foot but may be quite ticklish. The pointer stimulation promotes greater blood flow to a particular area, increasing the nutrient supply and healing properties.

If there is nerve damage, apply 4-6 drops of Peppermint, or other desired oil, along the spine. Use a gentle, rocking motion on the tissue between each vertebra, between each rib on the vertebra knuckles starting at the base of the spine all the way up on each side of the spine to the neck. Use medium pressure with the rocking motion for 1-10 seconds at each location. Then follow the same procedure once more along the spine next to each vertebra.

### Application and Usage

**Topical:** For guidelines on applying oils to the skin, refer to *Application Guidelines* on page 410.

- Apply 6-10 drops of oil diluted 50:50 on location 2 times daily. Also apply around navel.
- Apply 2-3 drops of desired oil on stomach and intestine and on Vita Flex points of the feet.
- Place a warm compress on lower back 1-2 times daily. If inflamed, use a cool compress.
- Receive a complete Raindrop Technique 3 times each month.

## Neck Pain and Stiffness

Neck pain and stiffness can be caused by a variety of factors, including stress, injury, tension, everyday activities, or other health problems, some of which may have serious consequences.

### Recommendations

**Singles:** Basil, Marjoram, Idaho Blue Spruce, Helichrysum, Idaho Balsam Fir, Peppermint, Wintergreen, Cypress, Nutmeg, Copaiba, Elemi, Dorado Azul

**Blends:** Cool Azul, Relieve It, PanAway, Deep Relief Roll-On

Seventh Edition | **Essential Oils Desk Reference** | 557

**Nutritionals:** Mineral Essence, MegaCal, Master Formula, Balance Complete, BLM, AgilEase, OmegaGize[3]

**Body Care:** Cool Azul Pain Relief Cream, Cool Azul Sports Gel, Regenolone Moisturizing Cream, Ortho Sport Massage Oil, Ortho Ease Massage Oil

**Neck Stiffness Blend**
- 5 drops PanAway
- 5 drops Marjoram
- 3 drops Peppermint

**Neck Pain Blend**
- 7 drops Basil
- 5 drops Wintergreen
- 4 drops Cypress
- 2 drops Peppermint

## Application and Usage

**Topical:** For guidelines on applying oils to the skin, refer to *Application Guidelines* on page 410.

- Apply 4-6 drops diluted 50:50 to neck area and massage 1-3 times daily as needed.
- Place a warm compress on neck area daily or as needed. With inflammation, use a cool compress.

## Sciatica

Sciatica is characterized by pain in the buttocks and down the back of the thigh. The pain worsens during coughing, sneezing, or with flexing and stretching the back. The pain is caused by pressure on the sciatic nerve as it leaves the spine in the lower pelvic region due to spinal misalignment and/or nerve inflammation.

The sciatic nerve is the largest in the body, with branches throughout the legs and feet; sciatica pain can be intense and immobilizing. Acute sciatica has a sudden onset and is usually triggered by a misaligned vertebra pressing against the sciatic nerve due to accident, injury, pregnancy, or inflammation.

### Symptoms
- Lower back pain
- Swelling or stiffness in a leg
- Loss of sensation in a leg
- Muscle wasting in a leg

Sulfurzyme, Super B, and OmegaGize[3] work well together to help rebuild nerve damage and the myelin sheath.

### Recommendations

**Singles:** Helichrysum, Tarragon, Vetiver, Peppermint, Nutmeg, Thyme, Idaho Blue Spruce, Basil, Rosemary, Copaiba, Copaiba Vitality

# See the Whole Picture to Produce the Best Results

When selecting oils, particularly for injuries, think through the cause and type of injury and then select oils for each segment.

For instance, a broken bone could encompass muscle damage, nerve damage, ligament strain or tear, inflammation, infection, and bone injury. The emotion of shock, anger, guilt, or suffering from long-time pain is another dimension of the injury that needs to be dealt with through understanding and help on an emotional level. All factors of the injury need to be considered in order to choose the oils that would offer the most benefits.

Select the single oils for each perceived problem, or select a blend that may address all of the needs, and then apply gently in a rotating motion. It would be best to apply the oils first to the feet using the Vita Flex Technique, if that is possible.

**Blends:** Cool Azul, Aroma Siez, Relieve It, PanAway, Deep Relief Roll-On

**Nutritionals:** Sulfurzyme, PowerGize, Super B, Essentialzyme, Master Formula, OmegaGize[3], MegaCal, Mineral Essence

**Body Care:** Cool Azul Pain Relief Cream, Cool Azul Sports Gel, Regenolone Moisturizing Cream, Ortho Sport Massage Oil, Ortho Ease Massage Oil

## Application and Usage

**Dietary and Oral:** Whether putting the oils in a capsule or drinking them in a liquid, please refer to *Application Guidelines* on page 410.

- Take 1 capsule with desired oil 2 times daily.
- Take 2-3 drops of oil in a spoonful of syrup or small amount of milk, juice, or water.

**Topical:** For guidelines on applying oils to the skin, refer to *Application Guidelines* on page 410.

- Apply 6-10 drops diluted 50:50 on location 2 times daily or as needed.
- Place a warm compress on affected area 1-2 times daily; cold compress if inflamed.
- Massage 2-3 drops into Vita Flex points of the feet 2-4 times daily.

- Receive a complete Raindrop Technique 3 times monthly.
- Walk backwards for 20 minutes daily with no shoes.

## Scoliosis

Scoliosis is an abnormal lateral or side-to-side curvature or twist in the spine. It is different from hyperkyphosis (hunchback) or hyperlordosis (swayback), which involve excessive front-to-back accentuation of existing spine curvatures.

While some cases of scoliosis can be attributed to congenital deformities such as MS, cerebral palsy, Down syndrome, or Marfan syndrome, the vast majority of scoliosis types are of unknown origin.

Some medical professionals believe that scoliosis may be caused by persistent muscle spasms that pull the vertebrae of the spine out of alignment. Others feel—and there is a growing body of research documenting this hypothesis—that it begins with hard-to-detect inflammation along the spine caused by latent viruses.

### Symptoms
- When bending forward, the left side of the back is higher or lower than the right side (the patient must be viewed from the rear).
- One hip may appear to be higher or more prominent than the other.
- Uneven shoulders or scapulas (shoulder blades).
- When the arms are hanging loosely, the distance between the left arm and left side is different than the distance between the right arm and right side.

The Raindrop Technique is proving to be an effective therapy for helping scoliosis, easing pain, and reducing misalignment.

### Recommendations

**Singles:** Oregano, Oregano Vitality, Plectranthus Oregano, Thyme, Thyme Vitality, Basil, Basil Vitality, Wintergreen, Cypress, Marjoram, Marjoram Vitality, Peppermint, Peppermint Vitality

**Blends:** Valor, Valor II, Valor Roll-On, Aroma Siez, PanAway, Cool Azul

**Nutritionals:** PowerGize, Mineral Essence, MegaCal, Power Meal, Slique Shake, Sulfurzyme, BLM, AgilEase, Master Formula, NingXia Red

**Body Care:** Cool Azul Pain Relief Cream, Cool Azul Sports Gel, Ortho Ease Massage Oil, Ortho Sport Massage Oil

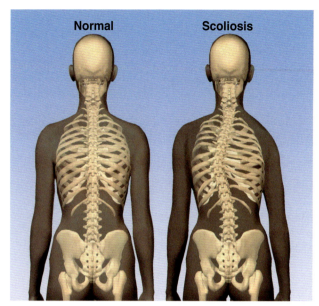

Scoliosis

### Application and Usage

**Dietary and Oral:** Whether putting the oils in a capsule or drinking them in a liquid, please refer to *Application Guidelines* on page 410.

- Take 1 capsule with desired oil 2 times daily.
- Take 2-3 drops of oil in a spoonful of syrup or small amount of milk, juice, or water.

**Topical:** For guidelines on applying oils to the skin, refer to *Application Guidelines* on page 410.

- Apply 3-6 drops diluted 50:50 along the spine daily or as needed.
- Receive a Raindrop Technique 2-3 times a week.

## SPRAIN

A sprain is an injury to a ligament caused by excessive stretching. The ligament can have a partial tear or be completely torn apart. Sprained ligaments swell rapidly and are painful. Usually, the greater the pain, the more severe the injury is.

### Recommendations

**Singles:** Basil, Dorado Azul, Idaho Blue Spruce, Peppermint, Copaiba, Idaho Balsam Fir, Helichrysum, Wintergreen

**Blends:** PanAway, Cool Azul, Relieve It, Aroma Siez, Deep Relief Roll-On

**Nutritionals:** PowerGize, BLM, AgilEase, Sulfurzyme, Mineral Essence, MegaCal, Essentialzyme, Super C, Power Meal, Slique Shake, Super B

**Body Care:** Cool Azul Pain Relief Cream, Cool Azul Sports Gel, Prenolone Plus Body Cream, Ortho Sport Massage Oil, Ortho Ease Massage Oil

## Application and Usage

**Dietary and Oral:** Whether putting the oils in a capsule or drinking them in a liquid, please refer to *Application Guidelines* on page 410.

- Take 1 capsule with desired oil 2 times daily.
- Take 2-3 drops of oil in a spoonful of syrup or small amount of milk, juice, or water.

**Topical:** For guidelines on applying oils to the skin, refer to *Application Guidelines* on page 410.

- Apply 4-6 drops diluted 50:50 on location 3-5 times daily.
- Place a cold compress on location 2 times daily.

## STRESS

Stress can be either good or bad. However, long-term stressful situations can produce a lasting, low-level stress that's hard on people. The nervous system pumps out extra stress hormones over an extended period, which can wear out the body's reserves and the adrenals, leaving a person feeling depleted or overwhelmed, weakening the body's immune system, and causing other problems.

## Recommendations

**Singles:** Lavender, Lavender Vitality, Roman Chamomile, Blue Tansy, Cedarwood, Marjoram, Marjoram Vitality, Rose, Royal Hawaiian Sandalwood, Sacred Frankincense, Frankincense, Frankincense Vitality, Valerian, Sage, Sage Vitality

**Blends:** Valor, Valor II, Valor Roll-On, Peace & Calming, Peace & Calming II, Tranquil Roll-On Trauma Life, T.R. Care, Humility, Harmony, RutaVaLa, RutaVaLa Roll-On, The Gift, Common Sense

**Nutritionals:** Super B, Super C, MultiGreens, Master Formula, MegaCal, OmegaGize3, MindWise, Corti-Stop Women's

## Application and Usage

**Aromatic:** Refer to *Application Guidelines* on page 410.

**Dietary and Oral:** Whether putting the oils in a capsule or drinking them in a liquid, please refer to *Application Guidelines* on page 410.

- Take 1 capsule with desired oil 2 times daily.
- Take 2-3 drops of oil in a spoonful of syrup or small amount of milk, juice, or water.

**Topical:** For guidelines on applying oils to the skin, refer to *Application Guidelines* on page 410.

- Dilute 50:50 and apply on temples, neck, and shoulders 2 times daily or as needed.
- Use bath salts daily.

## THROAT INFECTIONS AND PROBLEMS
*(See also Colds, Coughs, Infections, Lung Infections)*

Throat infection is one of the most common conditions in the world. It is broadly divided into two types, viral and bacterial throat infections.

### Coughs, Congestive and Dry

Coughs are classified into two categories, acute and chronic. An acute cough is one that has been present for less than three weeks and is divided into infectious and noninfectious causes.

Chronic coughs are those that have been present for more than three weeks and are categorized as conditions within the lungs, conditions within the chest cavity but outside of the lungs, conditions along the passages that transmit air from the lungs to the environment, and digestive causes.

## Recommendations

**Singles:** Eucalyptus Blue, Eucalyptus Globulus, Peppermint, Peppermint Vitality, Tea Tree, Eucalyptus Radiata, Myrrh, Goldenrod, Ledum, Lemon, Lemon Vitality, Mastrante, Northern Lights Black Spruce, Ravintsara, Cedarwood, Marjoram, Marjoram Vitality, Hyssop, Copaiba, Copaiba Vitality, Idaho Balsam Fir, Cypress, Melissa, Wintergreen

**Blends:** Raven, R.C., Breathe Again Roll-On, SniffleEase, Thieves, Thieves Vitality, Melrose, Peace & Calming, Peace & Calming II, Exodus II

**Nutritionals:** Inner Defense, Life 9, ImmuPro, Super C, Super C Chewable,

**Oral Care:** Thieves Cough Drops, Thieves Fresh Essence Mouthwash, Thieves Hard Lozenges, Thieves Mints, Thieves Spray

**Cough Blend**
- 10 drops Eucalyptus Globulus
- 1 drop Wintergreen
- 1 drop Peppermint Vitality

The Cough Blend may be ingested, applied topically, and/or diffused as you wish.

Personal Usage Guide | **Chapter 20**

### Dry Cough Tea Blend
- 3 drops Eucalyptus Radiata
- 2 drops Lemon Vitality
- teaspoon Blue Agave or maple syrup
- 4 oz. heated distilled or purified water

Sip slowly. Repeat as often as needed for relief.

### Application and Usage

**Aromatic:** Refer to *Application Guidelines* on page 410.

**Dietary and Oral:** Whether putting the oils in a capsule or drinking them in a liquid, please refer to *Application Guidelines* on page 410.

- Take 1 capsule with desired oil 2 times daily.
- Take 2-3 drops of oil in a spoonful of syrup or small amount of milk, juice, or water.
- Gargle with Thieves Fresh Essence Plus Mouthwash throughout the day as desired.
- Use Thieves Spray as desired.
- Dissolve Thieves Cough Drops in your mouth as desired.

**Topical:** For guidelines on applying oils to the skin, refer to *Application Guidelines* on page 410.

- Place a warm compress with 1-2 drops of chosen oil on the chest, throat, and upper back 2 times daily.
- Apply 1-3 drops to lung Vita Flex points 1-3 times daily.
- Receive a Raindrop Technique 1-2 times weekly.

## Laryngitis

Laryngitis is inflammation and swelling of the larynx, also known as the voice box. Laryngitis is usually caused by a virus, sometimes caused by a bacterial infection, or occurs in people who overuse their voice.

**Singles:** Eucalyptus Radiata, Jade Lemon, Jade Lemon Vitality, Lemon, Lemon Vitality, Lime, Lime Vitality, Eucalyptus Blue, Palo Santo, Oregano, Oregano Vitality, Plectranthus Oregano, Sacred Frankincense, Frankincense, Frankincense Vitality, Ravintsara, Thyme, Thyme Vitality, Myrrh, Cedarwood, Eucalyptus Globulus, Northern Lights Black Spruce, Peppermint, Peppermint Vitality

**Blends:** R.C., Thieves, Thieves Vitality, Melrose, Raven, Purification, Exodus II, Breathe Again Roll-On

**Nutritionals:** Super C, Super C Chewable, Longevity Softgels, MultiGreens, ImmuPro, OmegaGize[3]

**Oral Care:** Thieves Cough Drops, Thieves Spray, Thieves Fresh Essence Plus Mouthwash, Thieves Hard Lozenges, Thieves Mints

### Application and Usage

**Aromatic:** Refer to *Application Guidelines* on page 410.
- Receive a Raindrop Technique 2-3 times weekly.

**Dietary and Oral:** Whether putting the oils in a capsule or drinking them in a liquid, please refer to *Application Guidelines* on page 410.

- Take 1 capsule with desired oil 2 times daily.
- Take 2-3 drops of oil in a spoonful of syrup or small amount of milk, juice, or water.
- Put 2 drops of Melrose and 1 drop of Lemon Vitality in ½ teaspoon of Blue Agave, Yacon Syrup, or maple syrup, etc., hold in the back of the mouth for 1-2 minutes, and then swallow. Repeat as needed.
- Place a few drops on or under your tongue 2-6 times daily or as often as needed.
- Gargle with a mixture of essential oils and water 4-8 times daily.
- Spray throat with Thieves Spray as often as desired.
- Gargle with Thieves Fresh Essence Plus Mouthwash as needed.
- Dissolve Thieves Cough Drops or Thieves Hard Lozenges in your mouth as desired.

**Topical:** For guidelines on applying oils to the skin, refer to *Application Guidelines* on page 410.

- Apply 1-3 drops diluted 50:50 to throat, chest, and back of neck 2-4 times daily.
- Apply 1-3 drops of selected oil to lung Vita Flex points of the feet 1-3 times daily.

## Sore Throat

Sore throats are caused by many things such as viruses, bacteria, smoking, breathing polluted air, and allergies to pet dander, pollens, and molds.

### Recommendations

**Singles:** Tea Tree, Ravintsara, Cypress, Eucalyptus Radiata, Eucalyptus Globulus, Jade Lemon, Jade Lemon Vitality, Lemon, Lemon Vitality, Lime, Lime Vitality, Sacred Frankincense, Frankincense, Frankincense Vitality, Thyme, Thyme Vitality, Oregano, Oregano Vitality, Plectranthus Oregano, Northern Lights Black Spruce, Peppermint, Peppermint Vitality, Myrrh, Wintergreen, Cypress

**Blends:** Thieves, Thieves Vitality, Melrose, Raven, ImmuPower, R.C.

**Nutritionals:** Inner Defense, Super C, Super C Chewable, ImmuPro, Longevity Softgels, OmegaGize[3]

Seventh Edition | **Essential Oils Desk Reference** | 561

**Oral Care:** Thieves Cough Drops, Thieves Hard Lozenges, Thieves Fresh Essence Mouthwash, Thieves Spray, Thieves Mints

**Sore Throat Blend No. 1**
- 2 drops Thyme Vitality
- 2 drops Cypress
- 1 drop Eucalyptus Radiata
- 1 drop Peppermint Vitality
- 1 drop Myrrh
- 1 teaspoon honey

**Sore Throat Blend No. 2**
- 5 drops Lemon Vitality
- 2 drops Eucalyptus Globulus
- 2 drops Wintergreen
- 1 drop Peppermint Vitality

## Application and Usage

**Aromatic:** Refer to *Application Guidelines* on page 410.

**Dietary and Oral:** Whether putting the oils in a capsule or drinking them in a liquid, please refer to *Application Guidelines* on page 410.

- Take 1 capsule with desired oil 2 times daily.
- Take 2-3 drops of oil in a spoonful of syrup or small amount of milk, juice, or water.
- Place a drop on or under the tongue 2-6 times daily or as often as needed.
- Gargle 4-8 times daily with a mixture of essential oils and water.
- Dissolve Thieves Cough Drops or Thieves Hard Lozenges in your mouth as desired.

**Topical:** For guidelines on applying oils to the skin, refer to *Application Guidelines* on page 410.

- Apply 1-3 drops diluted 50:50 to the throat, chest, and back of the neck 2-4 times daily.
- Apply 1-3 drops on the lung Vita Flex points of the foot 1-3 times daily.
- Receive a Raindrop Technique weekly.
- Place a warm compress with 1-2 drops of chosen oil on the throat and chest area 2-3 times daily.

## Strep Throat

Strep throat is a bacterial throat infection caused by Group A streptococcus and is generally more severe than a viral throat infection. If left untreated, strep throat can lead to kidney inflammation and rheumatic fever.

### Recommendations

**Singles:** Oregano, Oregano Vitality, Plectranthus Oregano, Thyme, Thyme Vitality, Eucalyptus Globulus,

Sacred Frankincense, Frankincense, Frankincense Vitality, Lavender, Lavender Vitality, Myrrh, Dorado Azul, Eucalyptus Blue, Mountain Savory, Mountain Savory Vitality, Ocotea, Clove, Clove Vitality, Cinnamon Bark, Cinnamon Bark Vitality

**Blends:** Thieves, Thieves Vitality, Exodus II, Melrose, Raven, R.C., ImmuPower

**Nutritionals:** Inner Defense, ImmuPro, Super C, Longevity Softgels, Super C Chewable, MultiGreens, ICP, ComforTone, Essentialzyme, Life 9, OmegaGize[3]

**Oral:** Thieves Spray, Thieves Cough Drops, Thieves Hard Lozenges, Thieves Fresh Essence Mouthwash, Thieves Mints

**Strep Throat Blend**
- 6 drops Lavender Vitality
- 2 drops Oregano Vitality
- 1 drop Cinnamon Bark Vitality
- 1 drop Thyme Vitality

## Application and Usage

**Aromatic:** Refer to *Application Guidelines* on page 410.

**Dietary and Oral:** Whether putting the oils in a capsule or drinking them in a liquid, please refer to *Application Guidelines* on page 410.

- Take 1 capsule with desired oil 2 times daily.
- Take 2-3 drops of oil in a spoonful of syrup or small amount of milk, juice, or water.
- Place a drop of oil on or under the tongue 2-6 times daily or as often as needed.
- Gargle with a mixture of essential oils and water 4-8 times daily.
- Spray throat with Thieves Spray as often as desired.
- Dissolve Thieves Cough Drops or Thieves Hard Lozenges in your mouth as desired.

**Topical:** For guidelines on applying oils to the skin, refer to *Application Guidelines* on page 410.

- Apply 1-3 drops diluted 50:50 to the throat, chest, and back of the neck 2-4 times daily.
- You may also apply 1-3 drops on the lung Vita Flex points of the foot 1-3 times daily.
- Place a warm compress with 1-2 drops of chosen oil on the throat and chest area 2-3 times daily.
- Receive a Raindrop Technique weekly.

### Regimen for Strep Throat
- ImmuPro: Take 1-2 before going to bed. Do not exceed 2 daily.
- Longevity Softgels: Take 2-4 softgels daily.

Personal Usage Guide | Chapter 20

- Super C: Take 2-3 tablets 2 times daily or chew Super C Chewable as desired.
- Receive a Raindrop Technique with ImmuPower and/or Exodus II along sides of spine weekly.
- Spray throat with Thieves Spray every 2 hours.

## Tonsillitis

The tonsils are infection-fighting lymphatic tissues at the back of the throat. When they become infected with streptococcal bacteria, they become inflamed, causing a condition known as tonsillitis.

It became popular in the 1960's and 1970's to have the tonsils removed when they became infected. However, tonsillectomies have become much less frequent, as researchers have discovered the important role tonsils play in protecting and fighting infectious diseases and optimizing immune response.

The pharyngeal tonsils located at the back of the throat (known as the adenoids) can also become infected—a condition known as adenoiditis.

### Recommendations

**Singles:** Clove, Clove Vitality, Tea Tree, Myrrh, Dorado Azul, Cassia, Ocotea, Goldenrod, Oregano, Oregano Vitality, Plectranthus Oregano, Mountain Savory, Mountain Savory Vitality, Ravintsara, Thyme, Thyme Vitality

**Blends:** Thieves, Thieves Vitality, Melrose, Exodus II, ImmuPower

**Nutritionals:** Inner Defense, ImmuPro, Super C Chewable, Super C, Detoxzyme, Mineral Essence

**Oral Care:** Thieves Spray, Thieves Cough Drops, Thieves Fresh Essence Mouthwash, Thieves Hard Lozenges, Thieves Mints

### Application and Usage

**Aromatic:** Refer to *Application Guidelines* on page 410.

**Dietary and Oral:** Whether putting the oils in a capsule or drinking them in a liquid, please refer to *Application Guidelines* on page 410.

- Take 1 capsule with desired oil 2 times daily.
- Take 2-3 drops of oil in a spoonful of syrup or small amount of milk, juice, or water.
- Place a drop on or under the tongue 2-6 times daily or as often as needed.
- Gargle a mixture of essential oils and water 4-8 times daily.
- Dissolve Thieves Cough Drops or Thieves Hard Lozenges in your mouth as desired.

**Topical:** For guidelines on applying oils to the skin, refer to *Application Guidelines* on page 410.

- Apply 1-3 drops diluted 50:50 to the throat, chest, and back of the neck 2-4 times daily.
- You may also apply 1-3 drops on the lung Vita Flex points of the feet 1-3 times daily.
- Place a warm compress with 1-2 drops of chosen oil on the throat and chest area 2-3 times daily.
- Use the Raindrop Technique weekly.

## THYROID PROBLEMS

*(See also Depression, Narcolepsy, Male Hormone Imbalance, Menstrual and Female Hormone Conditions)*

The thyroid is the energy gland of the human body and produces T3 and T4 thyroid hormones that control the body's metabolism. The thyroid also controls other vital functions such as digestion, circulation, immune function, hormone balance, and emotions.

The thyroid gland is controlled by the pituitary gland, which signals the thyroid when to produce the thyroid hormone.

The hypothalamus gland sends chemical signals to the pituitary gland to monitor hormone levels in the blood stream.

A lack of the thyroid hormone does not necessarily mean that the thyroid is not functioning properly. In some instances, the pituitary gland may be malfunctioning because of its failure to release sufficient TSH (thyroid stimulating hormone) to stimulate the thyroid to make thyroid hormones.

Other cases of thyroid hormone deficiency may be due to the hypothalamus failing to release sufficient TRH (thyrotropin-releasing hormone).

In cases where thyroid hormone deficiency is caused by a malfunctioning pituitary or hypothalamus, supplements or essential oils such as Cedarwood may help stimulate the pituitary or hypothalamus.

People with type-A blood have more of a tendency to have weak thyroid function.

### Hyperthyroid (Graves' Disease)

When the thyroid becomes overactive and produces excess thyroid hormone, the following symptoms may occur:

- Anxiety
- Restlessness
- Insomnia
- Premature gray hair
- Diabetes mellitus
- Arthritis
- Vitiligo (loss of skin pigment)

Seventh Edition | **Essential Oils Desk Reference** | 563

Graves' disease, unlike Hashimoto's disease, is an autoimmune disease that results in an excess of thyroid hormone production. MSM has been studied for its ability to reverse many kinds of autoimmune diseases. MSM is a key component of Sulfurzyme.

## Recommendations

**Singles:** Myrrh, Idaho Blue Spruce, Lemongrass, Lemongrass Vitality, Wintergreen, German Chamomile, German Chamomile Vitality, Bergamot, Bergamot Vitality, Cedarwood

**Blends:** EndoFlex, EndoFlex Vitality, Brain Power, Clarity, Common Sense

**Nutritionals:** Sulfurzyme, MultiGreens, Mineral Essence, MegaCal, MindWise, Essentialzyme, Detoxzyme, Essentialzymes-4, Life 9, OmegaGize[3], Thyromin (only in the morning), Ultra Young

## Application and Usage

**Aromatic:** Refer to *Application Guidelines* on page 410.

**Dietary and Oral:** Whether putting the oils in a capsule or drinking them in a liquid, please refer to *Application Guidelines* on page 410.

- Take 1 capsule with desired oil 2 times daily.
- Take 2-3 drops of oil in a spoonful of syrup or small amount of milk, juice, or water.

**Topical:** For guidelines on applying oils to the skin, refer to *Application Guidelines* on page 410.

## Hypoglycemia

Hypoglycemia may be caused by low thyroid function. Excessive consumption of sugar or honey will also cause reactive hypoglycemia, in which a rapid rise in blood sugar is followed by a steep drop to abnormally low levels.

In some cases, hypoglycemia may be a precursor to candida, allergies, chronic fatigue syndrome, depression, and chemical sensitivities.

Signs of hypoglycemia (low blood sugar) include:

- Fatigue, drowsiness, and sleepiness after meals
- Headache or dizziness if times between meals are too long
- Craving for sweets
- Allergic reaction to foods
- Palpitations, tremors, sweats, rapid heartbeat
- Inattentiveness, mood swings, irritability, anxiety, nervousness, inability to cope with stress, and feelings of emotional depression

- Lack of motivation, discipline, and creativity
- Hunger that cannot be satisfied

Often people with some of these symptoms are misdiagnosed as suffering either chronic fatigue or neurosis. Instead, they may be hypoglycemic.

To treat chronic hypoglycemia, it is important to treat the underlying cause such as candida or yeast overgrowth (See Fungal Infections).

Essential oils may reduce hypoglycemic symptoms by helping to normalize sugar cravings, supporting and stabilizing sugar metabolism in the body.

## Recommendations

**Singles:** Lavender, Lavender Vitality, Coriander, Coriander Vitality, Dill, Dill Vitality, Fennel, Fennel Vitality, Cinnamon Bark, Cinnamon Bark Vitality

**Nutritionals:** MultiGreens, NingXia Red, Life 9, Digest & Cleanse, Essentialzyme, Essentialzymes-4, ICP, JuvaPower, JuvaSpice, Ningxia Wolfberries (Organic, Dried)

## Application and Usage

**Aromatic:** Refer to *Application Guidelines* on page 410.

**Dietary and Oral:** Whether putting the oils in a capsule or drinking them in a liquid, please refer to *Application Guidelines* on page 410.

- Take 1 capsule with desired oil 1 time daily (Coriander Vitality, Dill Vitality, and Fennel Vitality work best through ingestion).
- Take 2-3 drops of oil in a spoonful of syrup or small amount of milk, juice, or water.

**Topical:** For guidelines on applying oils to the skin, refer to *Application Guidelines* on page 410.

- Rub 1-2 drops of oil on the temples and back of neck several times daily.
- Place a warm compress with 1-2 drops of chosen oil on the back.

## Hypothyroid (Hashimoto's Disease)

This condition occurs when the thyroid is underactive and produces insufficient thyroid hormone. Approximately 40 percent of the U.S. population suffers from milder forms of this disorder to some degree, and these people tend to suffer from hypoglycemia (low blood sugar). In its severe form, it is referred to as Hashimoto's disease.

Hashimoto's disease, like Graves' disease, is an autoimmune condition that affects the thyroid differently, however, by limiting its ability to produce thyroid hormone.

Personal Usage Guide | Chapter 20

**The following symptoms may occur:**

- Fatigue
- Yeast infections (candida)
- Lack of energy
- Reduced immune function
- Poor resistance to disease
- Recurring infections
- Low sex hormones

## Recommendations

**Singles:** Lemongrass, Lemongrass Vitality, Spearmint, Spearmint Vitality, Ledum, Myrtle, Peppermint, Peppermint Vitality, Myrrh, Clove, Clove Vitality

**Blends:** EndoFlex, EndoFlex Vitality, Brain Power, Clarity

**Nutritionals:** Thyromin, MultiGreens, Sulfurzyme, Ultra Young, Essentialzyme, Essentialzymes-4, Life 9, Detoxzyme, MegaCal, MindWise

## Application and Usage

**Aromatic:** Refer to *Application Guidelines* on page 410.

**Dietary and Oral:** Whether putting the oils in a capsule or drinking them in a liquid, please refer to *Application Guidelines* on page 410.

- Take 1 capsule with desired oil 2 times daily.
- Take 2-3 drops of oil in a spoonful of syrup or small amount of milk, juice, or water.

**Topical:** For guidelines on applying oils to the skin, refer to *Application Guidelines* on page 410.

- Apply 3-5 drops neat or diluted 50:50 over the thyroid, the front of the neck, and on both sides of the trachea 1-3 times daily.
- Apply 1-3 drops on the thyroid Vita Flex points of the feet located on the inside edge of the ball of the foot just below the base of the big toe.

## TOXEMIA

Toxins or bacteria that accumulate in the bloodstream create a condition called toxemia.

## Recommendations

**Singles:** Clove, Clove Vitality, Tangerine, Tangerine Vitality, Jade Lemon, Jade Lemon Vitality, Lemon, Lemon Vitality, Lime, Lime Vitality, Cypress, Orange, Orange Vitality, Patchouli

**Blends:** Purification, Thieves, Thieves Vitality, Melrose, Citrus Fresh, Citrus Fresh Vitality

**Nutritionals:** Rehemogen, ICP, ComforTone, Essentialzyme, Essentialzymes-4, Life 9, Super C, JuvaTone, JuvaPower, JuvaSpice, Detoxzyme, Super C Chewable

## Application and Usage

**Aromatic:** Refer to *Application Guidelines* on page 410.

**Dietary and Oral:** Whether putting the oils in a capsule or drinking them in a liquid, please refer to *Application Guidelines* on page 410.

- Take 1 capsule with desired oil 3 times daily.
- Take 2-3 drops of oil in a spoonful of syrup or small amount of milk, juice, or water.
- Best results may be achieved by eliminating certain foods such as all sugar, white flour, breads, pasta, fried foods, and chlorinated water.

**Topical:** For guidelines on applying oils to the skin, refer to *Application Guidelines* on page 410.

- Dilute 50:50 and apply on location 2-3 times daily or as needed.
- Massage 2-4 drops of oil neat on the bottoms of the feet just before bedtime.

## TRAUMA, EMOTIONAL

Emotional trauma can be generated from events that involve loss, abuse, bereavement, accidents, or misfortunes. The scents of essential oils have the ability to cross the blood brain barrier, simulating the amygdala that controls the emotional and memory center of the brain. Certain essential oils help facilitate the processing and release of emotional trauma in a simple way that minimizes psychological turmoil.

## Recommendations

**Singles:** Sacred Frankincense, Frankincense, Idaho Blue Spruce, Idaho Balsam Fir, Western Red Cedar, Northern Lights Black Spruce, Royal Hawaiian Sandalwood, Rose, Palo Santo, Ocotea, Cedarwood

**Blends:** Evergreen Essence, Freedom, The Gift, Trauma Life, T.R. Care, Peace & Calming, Peace & Calming II, Hope, RutaVaLa, RutaVaLa Roll-On, Harmony, InTouch, Reconnect, Inner Harmony, Gathering, Amoressence, Forgiveness, Release, Envision, Build Your Dream, Valor, Valor II, Valor Roll-On, Joy, Oola Balance, Oola Faith, Oola Family, Oola Field, Oola Finance, Oola Fitness, Oola Friends, Oola Fun, Oola Grow, Highest Potential, 3 Wise Men, Sacred Mountain

Seventh Edition | **Essential Oils Desk Reference** | 565

**Nutritionals:** Super C, Super C Chewable, Mineral Essence, MegaCal, Essentialzyme, Essentialzymes-4, Life 9, OmegaGize³, Balance Complete, NingXia Red

## Application and Usage

**Aromatic:** Refer to *Application Guidelines* on page 410.
**Topical:** For guidelines on applying oils to the skin, refer to *Application Guidelines* on page 410.

- Apply 2-4 drops of oil diluted 50:50 or neat to the temples, forehead, crown, and shoulders 1-3 times daily.

## TRIGGER FINGER (Stenosing Tenosynovitis)

Tendonitis, often called "tennis elbow" and "golfer's elbow," is a torn or inflamed tendon. Tenosynovitis, sometimes called "trigger finger," is an inflamed tendon being restricted by its sheath (particularly in thumbs and fingers). Repetitive use or infection may be the cause.

When selecting oils for injuries, think through the cause and type of injury and select appropriate oils. For instance, tendonitis could encompass muscle damage, nerve damage, ligament strain/tear, inflammation, infection, and possibly an emotion. The emotional distress may be anger or guilt.

Therefore, select a single oil or blend for each potential cause or to address multiple causes.

**Singles:** Lemongrass (promotes the repair of connective tissue), Royal Hawaiian Sandalwood, Helichrysum, Frankincense, Lavender, Marjoram

**Blends:** Cool Azul, PanAway, Relieve It, Deep Relief Roll-On

**Nutritionals:** MegaCal, BLM, AgilEase, Sulfurzyme
- MegaCal builds and strengthens bones. Mix 1 teaspoon in water and drink. Taken at night, MegaCal promotes peaceful sleep.
- BLM and AgilEase provide critical nutrients for connective tissue and muscle repair and strengthens the bones. Take 1 capsule 1-3 times daily.
- Sulfurzyme equalizes water pressure inside the cells and reduces pain. Mix 1-2 teaspoons in water and drink 2 times daily.

**Body Care:** Cool Azul Pain Relief Cream, Cool Azul Sports Gel, Ortho Sport Massage Oil, Ortho Ease Massage Oil

The oils in the body care products reduce pain and promote healing.

## Application and Usage

**Aromatic:** Refer to *Application Guidelines* on page 410.

**Topical:** For guidelines on applying oils to the skin, refer to *Application Guidelines* on page 410.

- Massage finger with Lavender and Lemongrass.
- Massage Marjoram with Lemongrass for inflamed tendons.
- Single oils or blends may be used singularly or together.

## TYPHOID FEVER

Typhoid fever is an infectious disease caused by a bacterium known as *Salmonella typhi*. Usually contracted through infected food or water, typhoid is common in lesser-developed countries.

Some people infected with typhoid fever display no visible symptoms of disease, while others become seriously ill. Both people who recover from typhoid fever and those who remain symptomless are carriers for the disease and can infect others through the bacteria they shed in their feces.

To avoid contracting typhoid fever—especially when traveling overseas—it is essential to drink purified or distilled water and to thoroughly cook foods. Fresh vegetables can be carriers of the bacteria, especially if they have been irrigated with water that has come into contact with human waste.

### Symptoms
- Sustained, high fever (101° to 104° F)
- Stomach pains
- Headache
- Rash of reddish spots
- Impaired appetite
- Weakness

### Recommendations

**Singles:** Clove, Clove Vitality, Thyme, Thyme Vitality, Ravintsara, Cinnamon Bark, Cinnamon Bark Vitality, Cassia, Peppermint, Peppermint Vitality, Black Pepper, Black Pepper Vitality, Mountain Savory, Mountain Savory Vitality, Oregano, Oregano Vitality, Plectranthus Oregano, Tea Tree

**Blends:** Thieves, Thieves Vitality, Melrose, Exodus II

**Nutritionals:** Inner Defense, ImmuPro, Super C, Super C Chewable, NingXia Red

Personal Usage Guide | Chapter 20

## Application and Usage

**Aromatic:** Refer to *Application Guidelines* on page 410.

**Dietary and Oral:** Whether putting the oils in a capsule or drinking them in a liquid, please refer to *Application Guidelines* on page 410.

- Take 1 capsule with desired oil 2 times daily for 10 days.
- Take 2-3 drops of oil in a spoonful of syrup or small amount of milk, juice, or water.

**Topical:** For guidelines on applying oils to the skin, refer to *Application Guidelines* on page 410.

- Apply 4-6 drops of oil diluted 50:50 on lower abdomen 2-4 times daily.

## ENDNOTES

1. Valnet J, MD. "The Practice of Aromatherapy: A Classic Compendium of Plant Medicines & Their Healing Properties," *Healing Arts Press*. 1990:197.

2. Ammon HP. "Boswellic acids in chronic inflammatory diseases," *Planta Med.* 2006 Oct;72(12):1100-16.

3. Yu MS, et al. "Neuroprotective effects of anti-aging oriental medicine *Lycium barbarum* against beta-amyloid peptide neurotoxicity," *Exp Gerontol.* 2005 Aug-Sep;40(8-9):716-27.

4. Galli RL, et al. "Fruit polyphenolics and brain aging: nutritional interventions targeting age-related neuronal and behavioral deficits," *Ann N Y Acad Sci.* 2002 Apr; 959:128-32.

5. Bickford PC, et al. "Antioxidant-rich diets improve cerebellar physiology and motor learning in aged rats," *Brain Res.* 2000 Jun 2; 866(1-2):211-7.

6. Haze S, Sakai K, Gozu Y. "Effects of fragrance on sympathetic activity in normal adults," *Jpn J Pharmacol.* 2002 Nov;903):247-53.

7. Koo HN, et al. "Inhibition of heat shock-induced apoptosis by peppermint oil in astrocytes," *J Mol Neurosci.* 2001 Dec;17(3):391-6.

8. Ellis Y, et al. "The effect of multi-tasking on the grade performance of business students," *Research in Higher Education.* June 2010. Vol. 8:1-10.

9. Dember WN, et al. "Olfactory Stimulation and Sustained Attention," *Compendium of Olfactory Research,* Ed. Avery N. Gilbert, Kendall Hunt Publishing, 1995:39-46.

10. Vigushin DM, et al. "Phase I and pharmacokinetic study of D-limonene in patients with advanced cancer," Cancer Research Campaign Phase I/II Clinical Trials Committee. *Cancer Chemother Pharmacol.* 1998;42(2):111-7.

11. Ionescu JG, et al. "Increased levels of transition metals in breast cancer tissue," *Neuro Endocrinol Lett.* 2006 Dec;27 Suppl 1:36-9.

12. Ghoneum M, Gollapudi S. "Modified arabinoxylan rice bran (MGN-3/Biobran) enhances yeast-induced apoptosis in human breast cancer cells in vitro," *Anticancer Res.* 2005 Mar-Apr;25 (2A):859-70.

13. Cao GW, Yang WG, Du P. "Observation of the effects of LAK/IL-2 therapy combining with *Lycium barbarum* polysaccharides in the treatment of 75 cancer patients," *Zhonghua Zhong Liu Za Zhi.* 1994 *Psychosomatics.* 2002 Nov-Dec;43(6):508-9.

14. Pace A, et al. "Vitamin E neuroprotection for cisplatin neuropathy: a randomized, placebo-controlled trial," *Neurology.* 2010 Mar 2;74(9):762-6.

15. Banerjee S., Panda CKL, Das S. "Clove (*Syzygium aromaticum* L.), a potential chemopreventive agent for lung cancer," *Carcinogenisis.* 2006 Aug;27(8):1645-54. Epub 2006 Feb 25.

16. Legault J, et al. "Antitumor activity of balsam fir oil: production of reactive oxygen species induced by alpha-humulene as possible mechanism of action," *Planta Med.* 2003 May;69(5):402-7.

17. de Castillo MC, et al. "Bactericidal activity of lemon juice and lemon derivatives against *Vibrio cholerae," Biol Pharm Bull.* 2000 Oct;23(10):1235-8.

18. Nasel C, et al. "Functional imaging of effects of fragrances on the human brain after prolonged Aromatic," *Chem Senses.* 1994 Aug;19(4):359-64.

19. Komori T, et al. "Effects of citrus fragrance on immune function and depressive states," *Neuroimmunomodulation.* 1995 May-Jun;2(3):174-80.

20. Barrowman JA, et al. "Diarrhoea in thyroid medullary carcinoma: role of prostaglandins and therapeutic effect of nutmeg," *Br Med J.* 1975 Jul 5;3(5974):11-12.

21. Fawell WN, Thompson G. "Nutmeg for diarrhea of medeatinullary carcinoma of thyroid," *N Eng J Med.* 1973 Jul 12;289(2):108-9.

22. Igimi H, et al. "Medical dissolution of gallstones. Clinical experience of d-limonene as a simple, safe, and effective solvent," *Dig Dis Sci.* 1991 Feb;36(2):200-8.

23. Igimi H, et al. "A useful cholesterol solvent for medical dissolution of gallstones," *Gastroenterol Jpn.* 1992 Aug;27(4):536-45.

24. Hay IC, Jamieson M, Ormerod AD. "Randomized trial of aromatherapy. Successful treatment for alopecia areata," *Arch Dermatol.* 1998 Nov;134(11):1349-52.

25. Nenoff P, Haustein UF, Brandt W. "Antifungal activity of the essential oil of *Tea Tree* (tea tree oil) against pathogenic fungi in vitro," *Skin Pharmacol.* 1996;9(6):388-94.

26. Göbel H, et al. "*Effectiveness of Oleum menthae piperitae and paracetamol in therapy of headache of the tension type,*" *Nervenarzt.* 1996 Aug; 67(8):672-81.

27. Göbel H, Schmidt G, Soyka D. "*Effect of peppermint and eucalyptus oil preparations on neurophysiological and experimental algesimetric headache parameters,*" *Cephalalgia.* 1994 Jun; 14(3):228-34; discussion 182.

28. Weydert JA, et al. "Systematic review of treatments for recurrent abdominal pain," *Pediatrics.* 2003 Jan;111(1):e1-11.

29. Logan AC, Beaulne TM. "The treatment of small intestinal bacterial overgrowth with enteric-coated peppermint oil: a case report," *Altern Med Rev.* 2002 Oct;7(5):410-7.

30. Sagduyu K. "Peppermint oil for irritable bowel syndrome," *Psychosomatics.* 2002 Nov-Dec;43(6):508-9.

31. Veal L. "The potential effectiveness of essential oils as a treatment for headlice, *Pediculus humanus capitis," Complement Ther Nurs Midwifery.* 1996 Aug;2(4):97-101.

32. Yang Y. "Anti-emetic principles of *Pogostemon cablin* (Blanco) Benth." *Phytomedicine.* 1999 May;6(2):89-93.

33. Zhu TS, Glaser M. "Regulatory role of cytochrome P40scc and pregnenolone in myelination by rat Schwann cells." *Mol Cell Biochem.* 2006 June;313(1-20:79-89.

34. Hirsch AR, Gomez R. "Aromatic of odorants for weight reduction," *Int. J. Obes.* Vol. 18, Supplement 2, August 1994:79.

35. Göbel H, Schmidt G, Soyka D. "Effect of peppermint and eucalyptus oil preparations on neurophysiological and experimental algesimetric headache parameters," *Cephalalgia.* 1994 Jun;14(3):228-34; discussion 182.

36. Benencia F, Courrèges MC. "Antiviral activity of sandalwood against herpes simplex viruses-1 and -2." *Phytomedicine.* 1999 May;6(2):119-23.

37. Toyoda M, Morohashi M. "Pathenogenesis of acne," *Med Electron Microsc.* 2001 Mar;34(1):29-40.

38. http://www.mayoclinic.org/diseases-conditions/spina-bifida/basics/prevention/con-20035356.

Seventh Edition | **Essential Oils Desk Reference** | 567

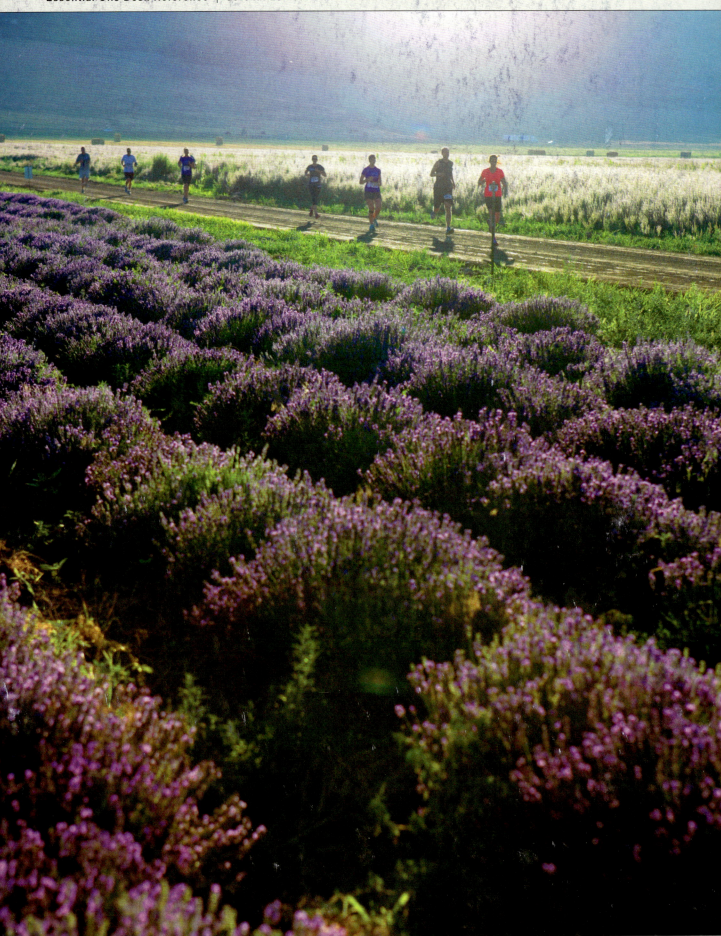

# Section 6
## Appendix & Index

| | | |
|---|---|---|
| **APPENDIX A** | Common and Botanical Plant Names | 571 |
| **APPENDIX B** | Single Oil Data | 575 |
| **APPENDIX C** | Essential Oil Blends Data | 591 |
| **APPENDIX D** | Flash Points for Essential Oils | 597 |
| **APPENDIX E** | Product Usage for Body Systems | 601 |
| **INDEX** | | 613 |

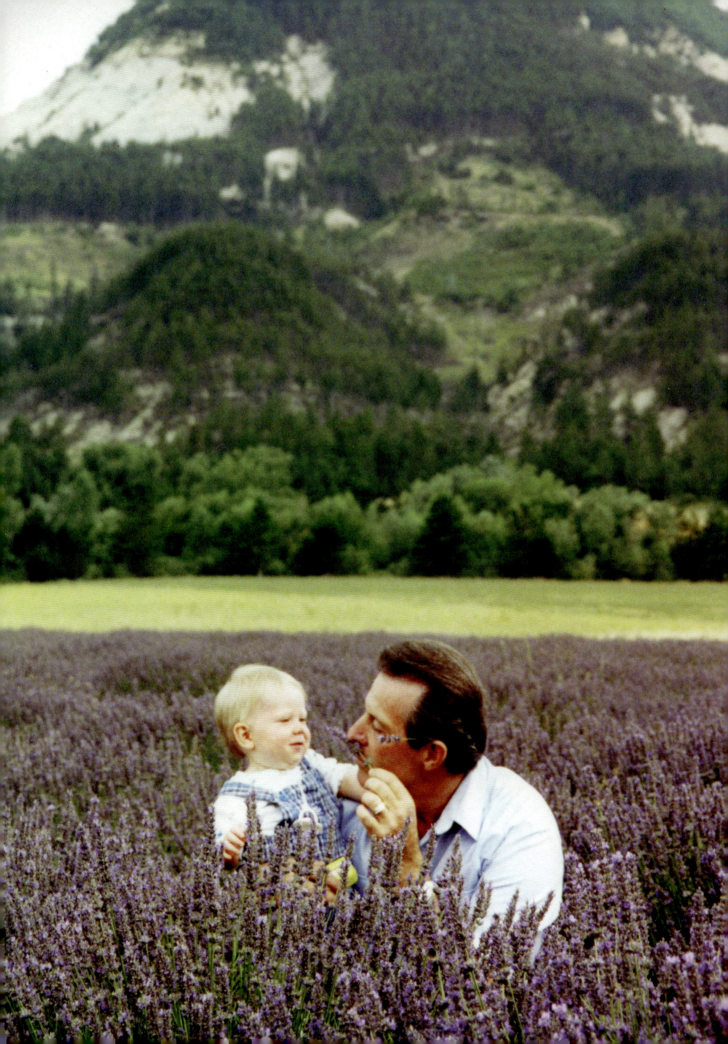

# Appendix A
## Common and Botanical Plant Names

### Botanical Name First

*Abies balsamea* ......... Idaho Balsam Fir (Balsam Canada)
*Abies concolor* ...................................... White Fir
*Achillea millefolium* ................................. Yarrow
*Acorus calamus* .................................... Calamus
*Anethum graveolens* ................................... Dill
*Anethum graveolens* ........................... Dill Vitality
*Angelica archangelica* ............................. Angelica
*Aniba rosaeodora* ................................ Rosewood
*Anthemis nobilis* ...................... Roman Chamomile
*Apium graveolens* ............................... Celery Seed
*Apium graveolens* ....................... Celery Seed Vitality
*Artemisia dracunculus* ........................... Tarragon
*Artemisia dracunculus* ................... Tarragon Vitality
*Artemisia pallens* ................................. Davana
*Backhousia citriodora* ....................... Lemon Myrtle
*Boswellia carterii* ........................... Frankincense
*Boswellia carterii* ................... Frankincense Vitality
*Boswellia frereana* ............... Frereana Frankincense
*Boswellia sacra* ................... Sacred Frankincense
*Bursera graveolens* ........................... Palo Santo
*Callitris intratropica* ....................... Blue Cypress
*Cananga odorata* ............................ Ylang Ylang
*Cananga odorata Equitoriana* ...... Amazonian Ylang Ylang
*Canarium luzonicum* ............................. Elemi
*Cedrus atlantica* .............................. Cedarwood
*Chamaecyparis formosensis* ................... Hong Kuai
*Chamaecyparis obtusa* ........................... Hinoki
*Chamaemelum nobile* ............... Roman Chamomile
*Chamomilla recutita* ..... German Chamomile (Matricaria)
*Cinnamomum aromaticum* ..................... Cassia
*Cinnamomum camphora* ..................... Ravintsara
*Cinnamomum verum* ........... Cinnamon Bark Vitality
*Cinnamomum zeylanicum* (Syn. *C. verum*).... Cinnamon Bark
*Cistus ladanifer* (Syn. *C. ladaniferus*).............. Cistus
*Cistus ladaniferus* .............. Rose of Sharon (Cistus)
*Citrus aurantifolia*................................. Lime
*Citrus aurantifolia*.......................... Lime Vitality
*Citrus aurantium amara* ..... Neroli (Bitter Orange)
*Citrus aurantium amara* ..................... Petitgrain
*Citrus aurantium bergamia* .................. Bergamot

*Citrus aurantium bergamia* ............. Bergamot Vitality
*Citrus hystrix*.......................... Citrus Hystrix
*Citrus junos*............................... Yuzu
*Citrus limon* ................................ Lemon
*Citrus limon* ............................. Lemon Vitality
*Citrus limon eureka* var. *formosensis* ........... Jade Lemon
*Citrus limon eureka* var. *formosensis* .... Jade Lemon Vitality
*Citrus paradisi*............................. Grapefruit
*Citrus paradisi*..................... Grapefruit Vitality
*Citrus reticulata* ..............................Mandarin
*Citrus reticulata* ..............................Tangerine
*Citrus reticulata* ................... Tangerine Vitality
*Citrus sinensis* ............................... Orange
*Commiphora erythraea*............. Biblical Sweet Myrrh
*Commiphora gileadensis*.................. Balm of Gilead
*Commiphora myrrha* ........................... Myrrh
*Conyza canadensis*................... Canadian Fleabane
*Copaifera officinalis*........... Copaiba (Balsam Copaiba)
*Copaifera officinalis*.................. Copaiba Vitality
*Coriandrum sativum* ..................... Coriander
*Coriandrum sativum* ............... Coriander Vitality
*Cuminum cyminum* ...........................Cumin
*Cupressus sempervirens*..................... Cypress
*Cymbopogon citratus* ........................Xiang Mao
*Cymbopogon flexuosus* ...................... Lemongrass
*Cymbopogon flexuosus* ............... Lemongrass Vitality
*Cymbopogon martini*.................. Palmarosa
*Cymbopogon nardus*........................ Citronella
*Cymbopogon winterianus,* Java Type ........... Citronella
*Daucus carota* ......................... Carrot Seed
*Daucus carota* ..................... Carrot Seed Vitality
*Dorado Azul Guayfolius officinalis*..... Dorado Azul (Ecuador)
*Elettaria cardamomum* ................... Cardamom
*Elettaria cardamomum* ........... Cardamom Vitality
*Eucalyptus bicostata*.................. Eucalyptus Blue
*Eucalyptus citriodora* ............ Eucalyptus Citriodora
*Eucalyptus globulus* ............ Eucalyptus Globulus
*Eucalyptus radiata*................. Eucalyptus Radiata
*Eucalyptus staigeriana*... ......... Eucalyptus Staigeriana
*Eugenia caryophyllus* ...........................Clove

| | |
|---|---|
| *Ferula galbaniflua* | Galbanum |
| *Foeniculum vulgare* | Fennel |
| *Foeniculum vulgare* | Fennel Vitality |
| *Gaultheria procumbens* | Wintergreen |
| *Helichrysum italicum* | Helichrysum |
| *Hyptis suaveolens* | Dorado Azul |
| *Hyssopus officinalis* | Hyssop |
| *Jasminum officinale* | Jasmine |
| *Juniperus osteosperma* | Juniper |
| *Juniperus oxycedrus* | Dalmatia Juniper |
| *Laurus nobilis* | Dalmatia Bay Laurel |
| *Laurus nobilis* | Laurus Nobilis (Bay Laurel) |
| *Laurus nobilis* | Laurus Nobilis Vitality |
| *Lavandula angustifolia* | Lavender |
| *Lavandula angustifolia* | Lavender Vitality |
| *Lavandula intermedia* | Lavandin |
| *Leptospermum scoparium* | Manuka |
| *Lippia alba* | Mastrante |
| *Matricaria recutita* | German Chamomile (Matricaria) |
| *Matricaria recutita* | German Chamomile Vitality |
| *Melaleuca alternifolia* | Tea Tree |
| *Melaleuca ericifolia* | Melaleuca Ericifolia |
| *Melaleuca viridiflora* | Melaleuca Quinquenervia (Niaouli) |
| *Melissa officinalis* | Melissa |
| *Mentha piperita* | Peppermint |
| *Mentha piperita* | Peppermint Vitality |
| *Mentha spicata* | Spearmint |
| *Mentha spicata* | Spearmint Vitality |
| *Micromeria fruticosa* | Micromeria |
| *Myristica fragrans* | Nutmeg |
| *Myristica fragrans* | Nutmeg Vitality |
| *Myrtus communis* | Myrtle |
| *Nardostachys jatamansi* | Spikenard |
| *Nymphaea lotus* | White Lotus |
| *Ocimum basilicum* | Basil |
| *Ocimum basilicum* | Basil Vitality |
| *Ocotea quixos* | Ocotea |
| *Ocotea quixos* | Ishpingo |
| *Origanum majorana* | Marjoram |
| *Origanum majorana* | Marjoram Vitality |
| *Origanum majorana* (Syn. *O. vulgare*) | Oregano |
| *Origanum vulgare* | Oregano Vitality |
| *Pelargonium graveolens* | Geranium |
| *Picea mariana* | Black Spruce |
| *Picea mariana* | Northern Lights Black Spruce |
| *Picea pungens* | Idaho Blue Spruce |
| *Pimpinella anisum* | Anise |
| *Pinus ponderosa* | Idaho Ponderosa Pine |
| *Pinus sylvestris* | Pine |
| *Piper nigrum* | Black Pepper |
| *Piper nigrum* | Black Pepper Vitality |
| *Plectranthus amboinicus* | Plectranthus Oregano |
| *Pogostemon cablin* | Patchouli |
| *Prunus amygdalus dulcis* | Sweet Almond Oil |
| *Pseudotsuga menziesii* | Douglas Fir |
| *Rhododendrum groenlandicum* | Ledum |
| *Rosa damascena* | Rose |
| *Rosmarinus officinalis* | Rosemary |
| *Rosmarinus officinalis* | Rosemary Vitality |
| *Ruta graveolens* | Ruta |
| *Salvia lavandulaefolia* | Spanish Sage |
| *Salvia officinalis* | Dalmatia Sage |
| *Salvia officinalis* | Sage |
| *Salvia sclarea* | Clary Sage |
| *Santalum album* | Sandalwood |
| *Santalum paniculatum* | Royal Hawaiian Sandalwood™* |
| *Satureja montana* | Mountain Savory |
| *Satureja montana* | Mountain Savory Vitality |
| *Solidago canadensis* | Goldenrod |
| *Styrax benzoin* | Onycha |
| *Syzygium aromaticum* | Clove |
| *Syzygium aromaticum* | Clove Vitality |
| *Tanacetum annuum* | Blue Tansy |
| *Tanacetum vulgare* | Idaho Tansy |
| *Thuja plicata* | Western Red Cedar |
| *Thymus vulgaris* | Thyme |
| *Thymus vulgaris* | Thyme Vitality |
| *Tsuga canadensis* | Tsuga |
| *Valeriana officinalis* | Valerian |
| *Vanilla planifolia* | Vanilla |
| *Vetiveria zizanoides* (Syn. *Vetiveria zizanioides*) | Vetiver |
| *Zingiber officinale* | Ginger |
| *Zingiber officinale* | Ginger Vitality |

*Registered trademark of Jawmin, LLC

# Common Name First

Amazonian Ylang Ylang . . . . . . . *Cananga odorata Equitoriana*
Angelica . . . . . . . . . . . . . . . . . . . . *Angelica archangelica*
Anise . . . . . . . . . . . . . . . . . . . . *Pimpinella anisum*
Balsam Canada (Idaho Balsam Fir). . . . . . . . . *Abies balsamea*
Balsam Copaiba(Copaiba) . . . . . . . . . . . .*Copaifera officinalis*
Balm of Gilead . . . . . . . . . . . . . . . *Commiphora gileadensis*
Basil . . . . . . . . . . . . . . . . . . . . *Ocimum basilicum*
Basil Vitality. . . . . . . . . . . . . . . . . . *Ocimum basilicum*
Bay Laurel (Laurus Nobilis) . . . . . . . . . . . *Laurus nobilis*
Bergamot . . . . . . . . . . . . . . . . . .*Citrus aurantium bergamia*
Bergamot Vitality. . . . . . . . . . . . . .*Citrus aurantium bergamia*
Biblical Sweet Myrrh . . . . . . . . . . . . *Commiphora erythraea*
Black Pepper. . . . . . . . . . . . . . . . . . . . . *Piper nigrum*
Black Pepper Vitality . . . . . . . . . . . . . . . . *Piper nigrum*
Black Spruce. . . . . . . . . . . . . . . . . . . . *Picea mariana*
Blue Cypress. . . . . . . . . . . . . . . . . *Callitris intratropica*
Blue Tansy . . . . . . . . . . . . . . . . . . *Tanacetum annuum*
Calamus . . . . . . . . . . . . . . . . . . . *Acorus calamus*
Canadian Fleabane. . . . . . . . . . . . . . *Conyza canadensis*
Cardamom. . . . . . . . . . . . . . . . . . *Elettaria cardamomum*
Cardamom Vitality. . . . . . . . . . . . . . *Elettaria cardamomum*
Carrot Seed . . . . . . . . . . . . . . . . . . . . .*Daucus carota*
Carrot Seed Vitality . . . . . . . . . . . . . . . . .*Daucus carota*
Cassia. . . . . . . . . . . . . . . . . . *Cinnamomum aromaticum*
Cedarwood . . . . . . . . . . . . . . . . . . . *Cedrus atlantica*
Celery Seed . . . . . . . . . . . . . . . . . . *Apium graveolens*
Celery Seed Vitality . . . . . . . . . . . . . . *Apium graveolens*
Cinnamon Bark . . . *Cinnamomum zeylanicum* (Syn. *C. verum*)
Cinnamon Bark Vitality. . . . . . . . . . . . *Cinnamomum verum*
Cistus . . . . . . . . . . . . . *Cistus ladanifer* (Syn. *C. ladaniferus*)
Citronella. . . . . . . . . . . . . . . . . . *Cymbopogon nardus*
Citronella . . . . . . . . . . . *Cymbopogon winterianus*, Java Type
Citrus Hystrix . . . . . . . . . . . . . . . . . . . *Citrus hystrix*
Clary Sage . . . . . . . . . . . . . . . . . . . . *Salvia sclarea*
Clove . . . . . . *Syzygium aromaticum* (Syn. *Eugenia caryophyllus*)
Clove Vitality . . *Syzygium aromaticum* (Syn. *Eugenia caryophyllus*)
Copaiba (Balsam Copaiba). . . . . . . . . . .*Copaifera officinalis*
Copaiba Vitality. . . . . . . . . . . . . . . .*Copaifera officinalis*
Coriander. . . . . . . . . . . . . . . . . . .*Coriandrum sativum*
Coriander Vitality . . . . . . . . . . . . . .*Coriandrum sativum*
Cumin . . . . . . . . . . . . . . . . . . . *Cuminum cyminum*
Cypress . . . . . . . . . . . . . . . . . *Cupressus sempervirens*
Dalmatia Bay Laurel . . . . . . . . . . . . . .*Laurus nobilis*
Dalmatia Juniper . . . . . . . . . . . . . . .*Juniperus oxycedrus*
Dalmatia Sage . . . . . . . . . . . . . . . . *Salvia officinalis*
Davana. . . . . . . . . . . . . . . . . . . . *Artemesia pallens*
Dill . . . . . . . . . . . . . . . . . . . . .*Anethum graveolens*
Dill Vitality . . . . . . . . . . . . . . . . .*Anethum graveolens*
Dorado Azul . . . . . . . . . . . . . . . . .*Hyptis suaveolens*
Dorado Azul (Ecuador) . . . .*Dorado Azul Guayfolius officinalis*
Douglas Fir . . . . . . . . . . . . . . . . . *Pseudotsuga menziesii*

Elemi . . . . . . . . . . . . . . . . . . . . . *Canarium luzonicum*
Eucalyptus Blue . . . . . . . . . . . . . . . *Eucalyptus bicostata*
Eucalyptus Citriodora . . . . . . . . . . . . .*Eucalyptus citriodora*
Eucalyptus Globulus . . . . . . . . . . . . . *Eucalyptus globulus*
Eucalyptus Radiata. . . . . . . . . . . . . . .*Eucalyptus radiata*
Eucalyptus Staigeriana . . . . . . . . . . . .*Eucalyptus staigeriana*
Fennel . . . . . . . . . . . . . . . . . . . .*Foeniculum vulgare*
Fennel Vitality . . . . . . . . . . . . . . . .*Foeniculum vulgare*
Frankincense . . . . . . . . . . . . . . . . . *Boswellia carterii*
Frankincense Vitality . . . . . . . . . . . . . *Boswellia carterii*
Frereana Frankincense . . . . . . . . . . . . . *Boswellia frereana*
Galbanum . . . . . . . . . . . . . . . . . .*Ferula galbaniflua*
Geranium . . . . . . . . . . . . . . . *Pelargonium graveolens*
German Chamomile (Matricaria) . . . . . .*Chamomilla recutita*
(Syn. *Matricaria recutita*)
German Chamomile Vitality . . . . . . . . . . *Matricaria recutita*
Ginger . . . . . . . . . . . . . . . . . . . . .*Zingiber officinale*
Ginger Vitality . . . . . . . . . . . . . . . . .*Zingiber officinale*
Goldenrod . . . . . . . . . . . . . . . . . .*Solidago canadensis*
Grapefruit . . . . . . . . . . . . . . . . . . . *Citrus paradisi*
Grapefruit Vitality . . . . . . . . . . . . . . . *Citrus paradisi*
Helichrysum . . . . . . . . . . . . . . . . . *Helichrysum italicum*
Hinoki . . . . . . . . . . . . . . . . . . .*Chamaecyparis obtusa*
Hong Kuai. . . . . . . . . . . . . . *Chamaecyparis formosensis*
Hyssop. . . . . . . . . . . . . . . . . . . . *Hyssopus officinalis*
Idaho Balsam Fir (Balsam Canada). . . . . . . . . *Abies balsamea*
Idaho Blue Spruce . . . . . . . . . . . . . . . . *Picea pungens*
Idaho Ponderosa Pine. . . . . . . . . . . . . . . *Pinus ponderosa*
Idaho Tansy . . . . . . . . . . . . . . . . . . *Tanacetum vulgare*
Ishpingo. . . . . . . . . . . . . . . . . . . . . *Ocotea quixos*
Jade Lemon . . . . . . . . . . .*Citrus limon eureka* var. *formosensis*
Jade Lemon Vitality . . . . . .*Citrus limon eureka* var. *formosensis*
Jasmine. . . . . . . . . . . . . . . . . . . .*Jasminum officinale*
Juniper . . . . . . . . . . . . . . . . . *Juniperus osteosperma*
Laurus Nobilis (Bay Laurel) . . . . . . . . . . . . .*Laurus nobilis*
Laurus Nobilis Vitality . . . . . . . . . . . . . . .*Laurus nobilis*
Lavandin . . . . . . . . . . . . . . . . . .*Lavandula intermedia*
Lavender . . . . . . . . . . . . . . . . . *Lavandula angustifolia*
Lavender Vitality . . . . . . . . . . . . . *Lavandula angustifolia*
Ledum . . . . . . . . . . . . . *Rhododendrum groenlandicum*
Lemon . . . . . . . . . . . . . . . . . . . . . .*Citrus limon*
Lemon Vitality. . . . . . . . . . . . . . . . . . .*Citrus limon*
Lemon Myrtle . . . . . . . . . . . . . . . . *Backhousia citriodora*
Lemongrass . . . . . . . . . . . . . . . . .*Cymbopogon flexuosus*
Lemongrass Vitality . . . . . . . . . . . . .*Cymbopogon flexuosus*
Lime . . . . . . . . . . . .*Citrus latifolia* (Syn. *C. aurantifolia*)
Lime Vitality . . . . . . . . . . . . . . . . . *Citrus aurantifolia*
Mandarin. . . . . . . . . . . . . . . . . . . *Citrus reticulata*
Manuka . . . . . . . . . . . . . . *Leptospermum scoparium*
Marjoram . . . . . . . . . . . . . . . . . . *Origanum majorana*
Marjoram Vitality . . . . . . . . . . . . . . .*Origanum majorana*

Mastrante . . . . . . . . . . . . . . . . . . . . . . . . . . . . . . . *Lippia alba*
Matricaria (German Chamomile) . . . . . . . *Chamomilla recutita*
                                        (Syn. *Matricaria recutita)*
Melaleuca Alternifolia (Tea Tree) . . . . . . *Melaleuca alternifolia*
Melaleuca Ericifolia . . . . . . . . . . . . . . . . . *Melaleuca ericifolia*
Melaleuca Quinquenervia (Niaouli) . . . . . *Melaleuca viridiflora*
Melissa . . . . . . . . . . . . . . . . . . . . . . . . . . . *Melissa officinalis*
Micromeria . . . . . . . . . . . . . . . . . . . . . . *Micromeria fruticosa*
Mountain Savory . . . . . . . . . . . . . . . . . . . *Satureja montana*
Mountain Savory Vitality . . . . . . . . . . . . . *Satureja montana*
Myrrh . . . . . . . . . . . . . . . . . . . . . . . . . . *Commiphora myrrha*
Myrtle . . . . . . . . . . . . . . . . . . . . . . . . . . . *Myrtus communis*
Neroli (Bitter Orange) . . . . . . . . . . . *Citrus aurantium amara*
Niaouli (Melaleuca Quinquenervia) . . . . *Melaleuca viridiflora*
Northern Lights Black Spruce . . . . . . . . . . . . *Picea mariana*
Nutmeg . . . . . . . . . . . . . . . . . . . . . . . . . *Myristica fragrans*
Nutmeg Vitality . . . . . . . . . . . . . . . . . . . . *Myristica fragrans*
Ocotea . . . . . . . . . . . . . . . . . . . . . . . . . . . . . *Ocotea quixos*
Onycha . . . . . . . . . . . . . . . . . . . . . . . . . . . *Styrax benzoin*
Orange . . . . . . . . . . . . . . . . . . . . . . . . . . . . *Citrus sinensis*
Orange Vitality . . . . . . . . . . . . . . . . . . . . . . *Citrus sinensis*
Oregano . . . . . . . . . . . *Origanum vulgare* (Syn. *O. majorana)*
Oregano Vitality . . . . . . . . . . . . . . . . . . . . *Origanum vulgare*
Palmarosa . . . . . . . . . . . . . . . . . . . . . . . *Cymbopogon martini*
Palo Santo . . . . . . . . . . . . . . . . . . . . . . . *Bursera graveolens*
Patchouli . . . . . . . . . . . . . . . . . . . . . . . . *Pogostemon cablin*
Peppermint . . . . . . . . . . . . . . . . . . . . . . . *Mentha piperita*
Peppermint Vitality . . . . . . . . . . . . . . . . . . *Mentha piperita*
Petitgrain . . . . . . *Citrus aurantium amara* (Syn. *Citrus sinensis)*
Pine . . . . . . . . . . . . . . . . . . . . . . . . . . . . . *Pinus sylvestris*
Plectranthus Oregano . . . . . . . . . . . . *Plectranthus amboinicus*
Ravintsara . . . . . . . . . . . . . . . . . . . . *Cinnamomum camphora*
Roman Chamomile . . . . . . . . . . . . . . . . . *Anthemis nobilis*
                                 (Syn. *Chamaemelum nobile)*
Rose . . . . . . . . . . . . . . . . . . . . . . . . . . . . . *Rosa damascena*

Rose of Sharon (Cistus) . . . . . . . . . . . . . . *Cistus ladaniferus*
Rosemary . . . . . . . . . . . . . . . . . . . . . . *Rosmarinus officinalis*
Rosemary Vitality . . . . . . . . . . . . . . . . . *Rosmarinus officinalis*
Rosewood . . . . . . . . . . . . . . . . . . . . . . . . *Aniba rosaeodora*
Royal Hawaiian Sandalwood™* . . . . . . *Santalum paniculatum*
Ruta . . . . . . . . . . . . . . . . . . . . . . . . . . . . *Ruta graveolens*
Sacred Frankincense . . . . . . . . . . . . . . . . . *Boswellia sacra*
Sage . . . . . . . . . . . . . . . . . . . . . . . . . . . *Salvia officinalis*
Sandalwood . . . . . . . . . . . . . . . . . . . . . . . *Santalum album*
Spanish Sage (Sage Lavender) . . . . . . . . . *Salvia lavandulifolia*
Spearmint . . . . . . . . . . . . . . . . . . . . . . . . . *Mentha spicata*
Spearmint Vitality . . . . . . . . . . . . . . . . . . . *Mentha spicata*
Spikenard . . . . . . . . . . . . . . . . . . . *Nardostachys jatamansi*
Tangerine . . . . . . . . . . . . . . . . . . . . . . . . *Citrus reticulata*
Tangerine Vitality . . . . . . . . . . . . . . . . . . . *Citrus reticulata*
Tarragon . . . . . . . . . . . . . . . . . . . . . . . *Artemisia dracunculus*
Tarragon Vitality . . . . . . . . . . . . . . . . . *Artemisia dracunculus*
Tea Tree . . . . . . . . . . . . . . . . . . . . . . *Melaleuca alternifolia*
Thyme . . . . . . . . . . . . . . . . . . . . . . . . . . . *Thymus vulgaris*
Thyme Vitality . . . . . . . . . . . . . . . . . . . . . *Thymus vulgaris*
Tsuga . . . . . . . . . . . . . . . . . . . . . . . . . . *Tsuga canadensis*
Valerian . . . . . . . . . . . . . . . . . . . . . . . *Valeriana officinalis*
Vanilla . . . . . . . . . . . . . . . . . . . . . . . . . *Vanilla planifolia*
Vetiver . . . . . . . . . . . *Vetiveria zizanoides* (Syn. *V. zizanioides)*
Western Red Cedar . . . . . . . . . . . . . . . . . . . *Thuja plicata*
White Fir . . . . . . . . . . . . . . . . . . . . . . . . . . *Abies concolor*
White Lotus . . . . . . . . . . . . . . . . . . . . . . *Nymphaea lotus*
Wintergreen . . . . . . . . . . . . . . . . . *Gaultheria procumbens*
Xiang Mao . . . . . . . . . . . . . . . . . . *Cymbopogon citratus*
Yarrow . . . . . . . . . . . . . . . . . . . . . . . *Achillea millefolium*
Ylang Ylang . . . . . . . . . . . . . . . . . . . . . . *Cananga odorata*
Yuzu . . . . . . . . . . . . . . . . . . . . . . . . . . . . . . *Citrus junos*

*Registered trademark of Jawmin, LLC

# Appendix B
## Single Oil Data

| Single Oil Name | Botanical Name | Products Containing Single Oil |
|---|---|---|
| Angelica | *Angelica archangelica* | Angelica, Awaken, Divine Release, Forgiveness, Grounding, Harmony, Inner Harmony, Live with Passion, Oola Balance, Oola Friends, Surrender, T-Away, T.R. Care |
| Anise | *Pimpinella anisum* | Allerzyme, Awaken, Build Your Dream, ComforTone, Detoxzyme, Digest & Cleanse, DiGize, DiGize Vitality, Dream Catcher, Essentialzyme, Essentialzymes-4, ICP, JuvaPower, JuvaSpice, MindWise, ParaFree, ParaGize, Thieves Fruit & Veggie Soak, TummyGize |
| Basil | *Ocimum basilicum* | Aroma Siez, Basil, Basil Vitality, Clarity, M-Grain, Oola Finance, Oola Fitness, Taste of Italy |
| Basil Vitality | | |
| Bergamot | *Citrus aurantium bergamia* | Acceptance, Animal Scents Ointment, AromaGuard Meadow Mist Deodorant, AromaSleep, ART Renewal Serum, Awaken, Believe, Bergamot, Bergamot Vitality, Build Your Dream, Clarity, Divine Release, Dragon Time Bath & Shower Gel, Dream Catcher, Evening Peace Bath & Shower Gel, Forgiveness, Genesis Hand & Body Lotion, GeneYus, Gentle Baby, Gratitude, Harmony, Humility, Inspiration, Joy, KidScents Lotion, KidScents Tender Tush, Lady Sclareol, Lavender-Oatmeal Bar Soap, Magnify Your Purpose, Oola Balance, Oola Faith, Oola Family, Oola Field, Oola Finance, Oola Grow, Peace & Calming II, Prenolone Plus Body Cream, Progessence Plus, Reconnect, Relaxation Massage Oil, Rose Ointment, Sandalwood Moisture Cream, Sensation, Sensation Bath & Shower Gel, Sensation Hand & Body Lotion, Sensation Massage Oil, SleepyIze, Thieves Dish Soap, Thieves Laundry Soap, T.R. Care, Valor II, White Angelica, Wolfberry Eye Cream |
| Bergamot Vitality | | |
| Biblical Sweet Myrrh | *Commiphora erythraea* | |
| Bitter Orange (See *Neroli*) | *Citrus aurantium amara* | |
| Black Pepper | *Piper nigrum* | Awaken, Black Pepper, Black Pepper Vitality, Cel-Lite Magic Massage Oil, Dream Catcher, En-R-Gee, NingXia Nitro, Relieve It |
| Black Pepper Vitality | | |

| Single Oil Name | Botanical Name | Products Containing Single Oil |
|---|---|---|
| Black Spruce | *Picea mariana* | Abundance, Awaken, Christmas Spirit, Envision, GeneYus, Grounding, Harmony, Hope, Inner Child, Inspiration, Motivation, Oola Family, Oola Field, Oola Friends, Present Time, R.C., Relieve It, Sacred Mountain, Sacred Mountain Moisturizing Soap, SniffleEase, Surrender, 3 Wise Men, T-Away, Trauma Life, Valor, Valor Moisturizing Soap, Valor Roll-On, White Angelica |
| Blue Cypress | *Callitris intratropica* | Acceptance, Australian Blue, Awaken, Blue Cypress, Brain Power, Breathe Again Roll-On, Build Your Dream, Cool Azul, Cool Azul Pain Relief Cream, Cool Azul Sports Gel, Divine Release, Dream Catcher, Essential Beauty Serum (Dry Skin), Gary's Equine Essentials Massage Oil, GeneYus, Highest Potential, Oola Friends, Oola Grow, Reconnect, Release, SARA, Sheerlumé Brightening Cream, T.R. Care |
| Blue Tansy | *Tanacetum annuum* | Acceptance, Australian Blue, Awaken, Build Your Dream, Dragon Time Bath & Shower Gel, Dream Catcher, Evening Peace Bath & Shower Gel, Highest Potential, JuvaFlex, JuvaTone, Peace & Calming, Release, SARA, T-Away, T.R. Care, Valor, Valor Moisturizing Soap, Valor Roll-On |
| Calamus | *Acorus calamus* | Exodus II |
| Canadian Fleabane | *Conyza canadensis* | Cortistop, EndoGize, Light the Fire, Ultra Young |
| Caraway | *Carum carvi* | Cool Azul, Cool Azul Pain Relief Cream, Cool Azul Sports Gel, Gary's Equine Essentials Massage Oil |
| Cardamom<br>Cardamom Vitality | *Elettaria cardamomum* | Aroma Ease, Cardamom, Cardamom Vitality, Clarity, Master Formula, Oola Family, Oola Field, Oola Finance, Transformation, TummyGize |
| Carrot Seed<br>Carrot Seed Vitality | *Daucus carota* | Animal Scents Ointment, ART Sheerlumé Brightening Cream, Carrot Seed, Carrot Seed Vitality, Rose Ointment |
| Cassia | *Cinnamomum aromaticum* | EndoGize, Exodus II, Light the Fire, Peace & Calming II, Red Shot, Slique CitraSlim, Valor II |
| Cedarwood | *Cedrus atlantica* | ART Beauty Masque, ART Intensive Moisturizer, Australian Blue, Brain Power, Cedarwood, Cel-Lite Magic Massage Oil, Egyptian Gold, Essential Beauty Serum (Dry Skin), GeneYus, Grounding, Highest Potential, Inspiration, Into the Future, InTouch, KidScents Bath Gel, KidScents Lotion, Live with Passion, Mirah Shave Oil, Oola Faith, Oola Family, Oola Fun, Oola Grow, Peppermint-Cedarwood Moisturizing Soap, Progessence Plus, Sacred Mountain, Sacred Mountain Moisturizing Soap, SARA, Shutran, Shutran Aftershave Lotion, Shutran Bar Soap, Shutran Shave Cream, Stress Away Roll-On, T.R. Care, Tranquil Roll-On |
| Celery Seed<br>Celery Seed Vitality | *Apium graveolens* | Celery Seed, Celery Seed Vitality, GLF, JuvaCleanse |

Single Oil Data | **Appendix B**

| Single Oil Name | Botanical Name | Products Containing Single Oil |
|---|---|---|
| **Cinnamon Bark**<br><br><br><br><br>**Cinnamon Bark Vitality** | *Cinnamomum zeylanicum (Syn. C. verum)* | Abundance, Christmas Spirit, Cinnamint Lip Balm, Cinnamon Bark, Cinnamon Bark Vitality, Ecuadorian Dark Chocolessence (Cinnamon Bark, Nutmeg, and Clove), Egyptian Gold, Gary's Equine Essentials Shampoo, Exodus II, Gathering, Highest Potential, Inner Defense, KidScents Slique Toothpaste, Magnify Your Purpose, Mineral Essence, Oola Finance, Oola Grow, Slique Bars, Slique Bars–Chocolate-Coated, Thieves, Thieves AromaBright Toothpaste, Thieves Automatic Dishwashing Powder, Thieves Cleansing Soap, Thieves Cough Drops, Thieves Dental Floss, Thieves Dentarome Plus Toothpaste, Thieves Dentarome Ultra Toothpaste, Thieves Dish Soap, Thieves Foaming Hand Soap, Thieves Fresh Essence Plus Mouthwash, Thieves Fruit & Veggie Soak, Thieves Fruit & Veggie Spray, Thieves Hard Lozenges, Thieves Household Cleaner, Thieves Laundry Soap, Thieves Mints, Thieves Spray, Thieves Vitality, Thieves Waterless Hand Purifier, Thieves Wipes, T.R. Care |
| **Cistus** | *Cistus ladanifer (Syn. C. ladaniferus)* | Cistus, ImmuPower, KidScents Tender Tush, Oola Balance, Oola Fitness, Owie, Peace & Calming II, PuriClean, The Gift, Valor II |
| **Citronella** | *Cymbopogon nardus* | Animal Scents Shampoo, Bite Buster, Citronella, Gary's Equine Essentials Shampoo, Oola Finance, PuriClean, Purification, RepelAroma, Thieves Fruit & Veggie Soak |
| **Citronella** | *Cymbopogon winterianus* | Animal Scents Shampoo, Gary's Equine Essentials Shampoo, Oola Finance |
| **Citrus Hystrix** | *Citrus hystrix* | Acceptance, Australian Blue, Awaken, Build Your Dream, Dream Catcher, Highest Potential, Oola Grow, Release, SARA, T-Away, T.R. Care, Trauma Life |
| **Clary Sage** | *Salvia sclarea* | Cel-Lite Magic Massage Oil, Clary Sage, Cortistop, Dragon Time, Dragon Time Bath & Shower Gel, Dragon Time Massage Oil, EndoGize, Estro, Evening Peace Bath & Shower Gel, FemiGen, Into the Future, Lady Sclareol, Lavender Conditioner, Lavender Shampoo, Live with Passion, Oola Fitness, Oola Grow, Prenolone Plus Body Cream, SclarEssence, Sensation Massage Oil, Transformation |
| **Clove**<br><br><br><br><br><br><br>**Clove Vitality** | *Syzygium aromaticum (Syn. Eugenia caryophyllus)* | Abundance, AromaGuard Meadow Mist Deodorant, AromaGuard Mountain Mint Deodorant, ART Sheerlumé Brightening Cream, Clove, Clove Vitality, Deep Relief Roll-On, Ecuadorian Dark Chocolessence (Cinnamon Bark, Nutmeg, and Clove), En-R-Gee, Essential Beauty Serum (Dry Skin), Essentialzyme, Gary's Equine Essentials Shampoo, ImmuPower, Inner Defense, K&B, KidScents Slique Toothpaste, Longevity, Longevity Softgels, Master Formula, Melrose, OmegaGize[3], Owie, PanAway, ParaFree, Progessence Plus, Thieves, Thieves AromaBright Toothpaste, Thieves Automatic Dishwashing Powder, Thieves Cleansing Soap, Thieves Cough Drops, Thieves Dental Floss, Thieves Dentarome Plus Toothpaste, Thieves Dentarome Ultra Toothpaste, Thieves Dish Soap, Thieves Foaming Hand Soap, Thieves Fresh Essence Plus Mouthwash, Thieves Fruit & Veggie Soak, Thieves Fruit & Veggie Spray, Thieves Hard Lozenges, Thieves Household Cleaner, Thieves Laundry Soap, Thieves Mints, Thieves Spray, Thieves Vitality, Thieves Waterless Hand Purifier, Thieves Wipes |

Seventh Edition | **Essential Oils Desk Reference** | 577

**Essential Oils Desk Reference** | Seventh Edition

| Single Oil Name | Botanical Name | Products Containing Single Oil |
|---|---|---|
| **Copaiba (Balsam Copaiba)**<br><br>**Copaiba Vitality** | *Copaifera officinalis* | ART Beauty Masque, Breathe Again Roll-On, Cool Azul, Cool Azul Pain Relief Cream, Cool Azul Sports Gel, Copaiba, Copaiba Vitality, Copaiba Vanilla Moisturizing Conditioner, Copaiba Vanilla Moisturizing Shampoo, Deep Relief, Deep Relief Roll-On, Gary's Equine Essentials Massage Oil, Freedom, Oola Fitness, Progessence Plus, Stress Away, Stress Away Roll-On |
| **Coriander**<br><br><br>**Coriander Vitality** | *Coriandrum sativum* | Acceptance, Animal Scents Ointment, AromaGuard Meadow Mist Deodorant, ART Renewal Serum, Awaken, Believe, Build Your Dream, Clarity, Coriander, Coriander Vitality, Dragon Time Bath & Shower Gel, Evening Peace Bath & Shower Gel, Forgiveness, Genesis Hand & Body Lotion, GeneYus, Gentle Baby, Gratitude, Harmony, Humility, Inspiration, Joy, KidScents Lotion, KidScents Tender Tush, Lady Sclareol, Lavender-Oatmeal Bar Soap, Magnify Your Purpose, Mirah Shave Oil, Oola Balance, Oola Field, Oola Finance, Oola Friends, Oola Grow, Reconnect, Relaxation Massage Oil, Rose Ointment, Sandalwood Moisture Cream, Sensation, Sensation Bath & Shower Gel, Sensation Hand & Body Lotion, Sensation Massage Oil, Shutran Aftershave Lotion, Shutran Bar Soap, Shutran Shave Cream, T-Away, T.R. Care, Valor II, White Angelica, Wolfberry Eye Cream |
| **Cumin** | *Cuminum cyminum* | Detoxzyme, ImmuPower, ParaFree, ParaGize, Protec |
| **Cypress** | *Cupressus sempervirens* | Aroma Life, Aroma Siez, Breathe Again Roll-On, Cel-Lite Magic Massage Oil, Cypress, Oola Fitness, R.C., Release, SARA, SniffleEase |
| **Dalmatia Bay Laurel** | *Laurus nobilis* | Dalmatia Bay Laurel |
| **Dalmatia Juniper** | *Juniperus oxycedrus* | Dalmatia Juniper |
| **Dalmatia Sage** | *Salvia officinalis* | Dalmatia Sage |
| **Davana** | *Artemisia pallens* | Acceptance, ART Creme Masque, ART L'Brianté Lip Gloss (Red), ART Sheerlumé Brightening Cream, Australian Blue, Awaken, Build Your Dream, Dream Catcher, Highest Potential, Lavender Bath & Shower Gel, Lavender Hand & Body Lotion, Mirah Shave Oil, Peace & Calming II, R.C., Release, SARA, Shutran, Shutran Aftershave Lotion, Shutran Bar Soap, Shutran Shave Cream, T-Away, T.R. Care, Trauma Life, Valor II |
| **Dill**<br><br>**Dill Vitality** | *Anethum graveolens* | Dill, Dill Vitality |
| **Dorado Azul** | *Hyptis suaveolens* | Cool Azul, Cool Azul Pain Relief Cream, Cool Azul Sports Gel, Common Sense, Deep Relief, Deep Relief Roll-On, Dorado Azul, Gary's Equine Essentials Massage Oil, ImmuPower, Infect Away, ParaFree, SniffleEase |
| **Douglas Fir** | *Pseudotsuga menziesii* | Regenolone Moisturizing Cream |
| **Elemi** | *Canarium luzonicum* | Cool Azul, Cool Azul Pain Relief Cream, Cool Azul Sports Gel, Elemi, Gary's Equine Essentials Massage Oil, Ortho Sport Massage Oil, Owie |
| **Eucalyptus Blue** | *Eucalyptus bicostata* | Breathe Again Roll-On, Eucalyptus Blue, SniffleEase |

578 | **Appendix B** | Single Oil Data

Single Oil Data | **Appendix B**

| Single Oil Name | Botanical Name | Products Containing Single Oil |
|---|---|---|
| **Eucalyptus Citriodora** | *Eucalyptus citriodora* | R.C. |
| **Eucalyptus Globulus** | *Eucalyptus globulus* | Breathe Again Roll-On, Eucalyptus Globulus, Ortho Ease Massage Oil, Ortho Sport Massage Oil, R.C., SniffleEase, Thieves Dentarome Ultra Toothpaste |
| **Eucalyptus Radiata** | *Eucalyptus radiata* | AromaGuard Mountain Mint Deodorant, Breathe Again Roll-On, Gary's Equine Essentials Shampoo, Eucalyptus Radiata, Inner Defense, KidScents Slique Toothpaste, Ortho Ease Massage Oil, Raven, R.C., SniffleEase, Thieves, Thieves AromaBright Toothpaste, Thieves Automatic Dishwashing Powder, Thieves Cleansing Soap, Thieves Cough Drops, Thieves Dental Floss, Thieves Dentarome Plus Toothpaste, Thieves Dentarome Ultra Toothpaste, Thieves Dish Soap, Thieves Foaming Hand Soap, Thieves Fruit & Veggie Soak, Thieves Fruit & Veggie Spray, Thieves Fresh Essence Plus Mouthwash, Thieves Household Cleaner, Thieves Hard Lozenges, Thieves Laundry Soap, Thieves Mints, Thieves Spray, Thieves Waterless Hand Purifier, Thieves Vitality, Thieves Wipes |
| **Eucalyptus Staigeriana** | *E. staigeriana* | Breathe Again Roll-On |
| **Fennel**<br><br>**Fennel Vitality** | *Foeniculum vulgare* | Allerzyme, AromaEase, Cortistop, Detoxzyme, Digest & Cleanse, DiGize, DiGize Vitality, Dragon Time, Dragon Time Bath & Shower Gel, Dragon Time Massage Oil, Essentialzyme, Essentialzymes-4, Estro, FemiGen, Fennel, Fennel Vitality, ICP, JuvaFlex, JuvaPower, JuvaSpice, K&B, Master Formula, Mister, MindWise, ParaFree, ParaGize, Prenolone Plus Body Cream, Prostate Health, SclarEssence, Slique CitraSlim, Thieves Fruit & Veggie Soak, TummyGize |
| **Frankincense**<br><br><br><br><br><br>**Frankincense Vitality** | *Boswellia carterii* | 3 Wise Men, Abundance, Acceptance, AromaSleep, ART Chocolate Masque, ART Gentle Cleanser, ART Intensive Moisturizer, ART Light Moisturizer, ART Refreshing Toner, ART Sheerlumé Brightening Cream, Awaken, Believe, Boswellia Wrinkle Cream, Brain Power, Build Your Dream, ClaraDerm Spray, Common Sense, Cortistop, Divine Release, Egyptian Gold, Exodus II, Forgiveness, Frankincense, Frankincense Vitality, Freedom, GeneYus, Gratitude, Harmony, Highest Potential, Humility, ImmuPower, Inner Harmony, Inspiration, Into the Future, KidScents Tender Tush, Live Your Passion, Longevity, Longevity Softgels, Mendwell, Oola Balance, Oola Faith, Oola Family, Oola Field, Oola Finance, Oola Friends, Oola Grow, Progessence Plus, Protec, Reconnect, SleepyIze, T-Away, The Gift, Transformation, T.R. Care, Trauma Life, Valor, Valor II, Valor Moisturizing Soap, Valor Roll-On, Wolfberry Eye Cream |
| **Frereana Frankincense** | *Boswellia frereana* | Slique Gum |
| **Galbanum** | *Ferula galbaniflua* | |

Seventh Edition | **Essential Oils Desk Reference** | 579

| Single Oil Name | Botanical Name | Products Containing Single Oil |
|---|---|---|
| Geranium | *Pelargonium graveolens* | Acceptance, Amoressence, Animal Scents Ointment, Animal Scents Shampoo, AromaGuard Meadow Mist Deodorant, AromaSleep, ART Chocolate Masque, ART Creme Masque, ART Renewal Serum, ART Sheerlumé Brightening Cream, Australian Blue, Awaken, Believe, Boswellia Wrinkle Cream, Build Your Dream, Clarity, Copaiba Vanilla Moisturizing Conditioner, Copaiba Vanilla Moisturizing Shampoo, Divine Release, Dragon Time Bath & Shower Gel, EndoFlex, EndoFlex Vitality, Envision, Evening Peace Bath & Shower Gel, Forgiveness, Gary's Equine Essentials Shampoo, Gary's Equine Essentials Tail & Mane Sheen, Gathering, Genesis Hand & Body Lotion, GeneYus, Gentle Baby, Geranium, Gratitude, Harmony, Highest Potential, Humility, Inner Harmony, Inspiration, Joy, JuvaFlex, JuvaTone, K&B, KidScents Bath Gel, KidScents Lotion, KidScents Tender Tush, L'Brianté Lip Gloss (Red), Lady Sclareol, Lavender-Oatmeal Bar Soap, Magnify Your Purpose, Melaleuca-Geranium Moisturizing Soap, Mendwell, Oola Balance, Oola Faith, Oola Family, Oola Field, Oola Finance, Oola Friends, Oola Grow, Prenolone Plus Body Cream, Prostate Health, Reconnect, Relaxation Massage Oil, Release, Sandalwood Moisture Cream, SARA, Sensation, Sensation Bath & Shower Gel, Sensation Hand & Body Lotion, Sensation Massage Oil, SleepyIze, T-Away, T.R. Care, Trauma Life, Valor II, White Angelica, Wolfberry Eye Cream |
| German Chamomile (Matricaria) German Chamomile Vitality | *Chamomilla recutita (Syn. Matricaria recutita)* | Acceptance, Australian Blue, Awaken, Build Your Dream, Comfor-Tone, Cool Azul, Cool Azul Pain Relief Cream, Cool Azul Sports Gel, Dream Catcher, EndoFlex, EndoFlex Vitality, Gary's Equine Essentials Massage Oil, German Chamomile, German Chamomile Vitality, Highest Potential, JuvaTone, OmegaGize[3], Peace & Calming II, Release, SARA, Surrender, T-Away, T.R. Care, Valor, Valor II |
| Ginger Ginger Vitality | *Zingiber officinale* | Abundance, Allerzyme, AromaEase, ComforTone, Digest & Cleanse, DiGize, DiGize Vitality, Ecuadorian Dark Chocolessence (Tangerine and Ginger), EndoGize, Essentialzymes-4, Ginger, Ginger Vitality, ICP, Live with Passion, Oola Field, ParaFree, ParaGize, Magnify Your Purpose, Master Formula, Thieves Fruit & Veggie Soak, TummyGize |
| Goldenrod | *Solidago canadensis* | Common Sense, Goldenrod |
| Grapefruit Grapefruit Vitality | *Citrus paradisi* | Acceptance, Australian Blue, Awaken, Build Your Dream, Cel-Lite Magic Massage Oil, Citrus Fresh, Citrus Fresh Vitality, Divine Release, Dream Catcher, GLF, Grapefruit, Grapefruit Lip Balm, Grapefruit Vitality, Highest Potential, KidScents Slique Toothpaste, Moisturizing Lip Balm Collection, Oola Fun, Oola Grow, Release, SARA, Slique Essence, Super C, T.R. Care, Ultra Young |
| Helichrysum | *Helichrysum italicum* | Aroma Life, Awaken, Brain Power, ClaraDerm Spray, Deep Relief, Deep Relief Roll-On, Divine Release, Forgiveness, GLF, Helichrysum, JuvaCleanse, JuvaFlex, LavaDerm Cooling Mist, Live with Passion, M-Grain, Owie, PanAway, T-Away, T.R. Care, Trauma Life |

Single Oil Data | **Appendix B**

| Single Oil Name | Botanical Name | Products Containing Single Oil |
|---|---|---|
| Hinoki | *Chamaecyparis obtusa* | ART Intensive Moisturizer, Divine Release, Gary's Equine Essentials Tail & Mane Sheen, Hinoki, Lady Sclareol, Light the Fire, Mendwell, Mirah Shave Oil, Oola Faith, Owie, Shutran, Shutran Aftershave Lotion, Shutran Bar Soap, Shutran Shave Cream |
| Hong Kuai | *Chamaecyparis formosensis* | Build Your Dream, Hong Kuai |
| Hyssop | *Hyssopus officinalis* | Awaken, Egyptian Gold, Exodus II, GLF, Harmony, Hyssop, ImmuPower, Mendwell, Oola Balance, Oola Faith, Oola Friends, Reconnect, Relieve It, T-Away, T.R. Care, White Angelica |
| Idaho Balsam Fir (Balsam Canada) | *Abies balsamea* | Animal Scents Ointment, ART L'Brianté Lip Gloss (Neutral), Believe, Build Your Dream, Deep Relief, Deep Relief Roll-On, Egyptian Gold, En-R-Gee, Gratitude, Idaho Balsam Fir, Oola Balance, Oola Faith, Oola Field, Oola Finance, Oola Fitness, Owie, Regenolone Cream, Sacred Mountain, Sacred Mountain Moisturizing Soap, Slique CitraSlim, The Gift |
| Idaho Blue Spruce | *Picea pungens* | Amoressence, ART L'Brianté Lip Gloss (Red), Believe, Build Your Dream, Evergreen Essence, Freedom, GeneYus, Idaho Blue Spruce, Inner Harmony, Into the Future, InTouch, Lady Sclareol, Live Your Passion, Mirah Shave Oil, Oola Balance, Oola Field, Oola Fitness, Oola Grow, Reconnect, Shutran, Shutran Aftershave Lotion, Shutran Bar Soap, Shutran Shave Cream, Transformation, Valor II |
| Idaho Ponderosa Pine | *Pinus ponderosa* | Evergreen Essence |
| Idaho Tansy | *Tanacetum vulgare* | Bite Buster, RepelAroma |
| Ishpingo | *Ocotea quixos* | |
| Jade Lemon | *Citrus limon Eureka var. formosensis* | Jade Lemon, Jade Lemon Vitality |
| Jade Lemon Vitality | | |
| Jasmine | *Jasminum officinale* | Acceptance, Amoressence, ART Cream Masque, ART L'Brianté Lip Gloss (Red), ART Renewal Serum, ART Sheerlumé Brightening Cream, Australian Blue, Awaken, Build Your Dream, Clarity, Dragon Time, Dragon Time Bath & Shower Gel, Dragon Time Massage Oil, Dream Catcher, Evening Peace Bath & Shower Gel, Forgiveness, Genesis Hand & Body Lotion, Gentle Baby, Harmony, Highest Potential, Inner Child, Into the Future, Jasmine, Joy, Lady Sclareol, Lavender Conditioner, Lavender Shampoo, Live with Passion, Mirah Shave Oil, Oola Balance, Oola Faith, Oola Family, Oola Finance, Oola Friends, Oola Fun, Oola Grow, Release, SARA, Sensation, Sensation Bath & Shower Gel, Sensation Hand & Body Lotion, Sensation Massage Oil, The Gift, T.R. Care, T-Away |

Seventh Edition | **Essential Oils Desk Reference** | 581

**Essential Oils Desk Reference** | Seventh Edition

| Single Oil Name | Botanical Name | Products Containing Single Oil |
|---|---|---|
| Juniper | *Juniperus osteosperma* | 3 Wise Men, Allerzyme, Awaken, Build Your Dream, Cel-Lite Magic Massage Oil, DiGize, DiGize Vitality, Dream Catcher, En-R-Gee, Grounding, Hope, Into the Future, Juniper, K&B, Morning Start Bath & Shower Gel, Morning Start Moisturizing Soap, Oola Faith, Oola Grow, Ortho Ease Massage Oil, ParaFree, ParaGize, Thieves Fruit & Veggie Soak |
| Laurus Nobilis (Bay Laurel) <br><br> Laurus Nobilis Vitality | *Laurus nobilis* | Breathe Again Roll-On, Laurus Nobilis, Laurus Nobilis Vitality, ParaFree |
| Lavandin | *Lavandula intermedia* | Animal Scents Shampoo, Gary's Equine Essentials Shampoo, PuriClean, Purification, Release, Thieves Fruit & Veggie Soak |
| Lavender <br><br><br><br> Lavender Vitality | *Lavandula angustifolia* | AromaGuard Meadow Mist Deodorant, Aroma Siez, AromaSleep, ART Beauty Masque, ART Gentle Cleanser, ART Refreshing Toner, Awaken, Brain Power, Build Your Dream, ClaraDerm, Cool Azul, Cool Azul Pain Relief Cream, Cool Azul Sports Gel, Copaiba Vanilla Moisturizing Conditioner, Copaiba Vanilla Moisturizing Shampoo, Dragon Time, Dragon Time Bath & Shower Gel, Dragon Time Massage Oil, Egyptian Gold, Envision, Essential Beauty Serum (Dry Skin), Estro, Forgiveness, Freedom, Gary's Equine Essentials Massage Oil, Gary's Equine Essentials Tail & Mane Sheen, Gathering, Gentle Baby, Harmony, Highest Potential, Inner Harmony, KidScents Tender Tush, LavaDerm Cooling Mist, Lavender, Lavender Bath & Shower Gel, Lavender Conditioner, Lavender Foaming Hand Soap, Lavender Hand & Body Lotion, Lavender Lip Balm, Lavender Mint Daily Conditioner, Lavender Mint Daily Shampoo, Lavender-Oatmeal Bar Soap, Lavender Conditioner, Lavender Shampoo, Lavender Vitality, Mendwell, M-Grain, Mirah Shave Oil, Mister, Motivation, Oola Balance, Oola Family, Oola Finance, Oola Friends, Oola Grow, Orange Blossom Facial Wash, Prostate Health, PuriClean, R.C., Reconnect, Relaxation Massage Oil, R.C., RutaVaLa, RutaVaLa Roll-On, Sandalwood Moisture Cream, SARA, Shutran Aftershave Lotion, Shutran Bar Soap, Shutran Shave Cream, SleepEssence, SleepyIze, SniffleEase, Stress Away, Stress Away Roll-On, Surrender, T-Away, T.R. Care, Tranquil Roll-On, Trauma Life, Wolfberry Eye Cream |
| Ledum | *Rhododendrum groenlandicum* | Divine Release, GLF, JuvaCleanse, Ledum |

**582** | **Appendix B** | Single Oil Data

Single Oil Data | **Appendix B**

| Single Oil Name | Botanical Name | Products Containing Single Oil |
|---|---|---|
| **Lemon**<br><br><br><br><br><br><br><br>**Lemon Vitality** | *Citrus limon* | Acceptance, AlkaLime, Allerzyme, Animal Scents Shampoo, AromaGuard Meadow Mist Deodorant, AromaGuard Mountain Mint Deodorant, ART Gentle Cleanser, ART Refreshing Toner, Australian Blue, Awaken, Build Your Dream, Citrus Fresh, Citrus Fresh Vitality, Clarity, Digest & Cleanse, Deep Relief, Deep Relief Roll-On, Dragon Time Bath & Shower Gel, Dream Catcher, Evening Peace Bath & Shower Gel, Forgiveness, Gary's Equine Essentials Shampoo, Gary's Equine Essentials Tail & Mane Sheen, Gary's True Grit NingXia Berry Syrup, Genesis Hand & Body Lotion, Gentle Baby, Harmony, Highest Potential, Inner Defense, Joy, JuvaTone, KidScents Shampoo, KidScents Slique Toothpaste, Lavender Bath & Shower Gel, Lavender Foaming Hand Soap, Lavender Hand & Body Lotion, Lavender Conditioner, Lavender Shampoo, Lemon, Lemon-Sandalwood Cleansing Soap, Lemon Vitality, MegaCal, MindWise, Mineral Essence, Mirah Shave Oil, MultiGreens, NingXia Red, Oola Balance, Oola Faith, Oola Family, Oola Finance, Oola Friends, Oola Fun, Oola Grow, Orange Blossom Facial Wash, Raven, Release, SARA, Shutran, Shutran Aftershave Lotion, Shutran Bar Soap, Shutran Shave Cream, Slique Essence, Super C, Surrender, T-Away, T.R. Care, Thieves, Thieves AromaBright Toothpaste, Thieves Automatic Dishwashing Powder, Thieves Cleansing Soap, Thieves Cough Drops, Thieves Dental Floss, Thieves Dentarome Plus Toothpaste, Thieves Dentarome Ultra Toothpaste, Thieves Dish Soap, Thieves Foaming Hand Soap, Thieves Fresh Essence Plus Mouthwash, Thieves Fruit & Veggie Soak, Thieves Fruit & Veggie Spray, Thieves Household Cleaner, Thieves Hard Lozenges, Thieves Laundry Soap, Thieves Mints, Thieves Spray, Thieves Vitality, Thieves Waterless Hand Purifier, Thieves Wipes, Transformation |
| **Lemon Myrtle** | *Backhousia citriodora* | Slique CitraSlim |
| **Lemongrass**<br><br><br>**Lemongrass Vitality** | *Cymbopogon flexuosus* | Allerzyme, DiGize, DiGize Vitality, En-R-Gee, Essentialzymes-4, ICP, Inner Child, Inner Defense, Lemongrass, Lemongrass Vitality, Morning Start Bath & Shower Gel, Morning Start Moisturizing Soap, MultiGreens, Oola Family, Oola Friends, Ortho Ease Massage Oil, Ortho Sport Massage Oil, ParaFree, ParaGize, PuriClean, Purification, Super C, Super Cal, Thieves Fruit & Veggie Soak |
| **Lime**<br><br><br>**Lime Vitality** | *Citrus latifolia (Syn. C. aurantifolia)* | AlkaLime, ART Beauty Masque, ART L'Brianté Lips Gloss (Pink), Common Sense, Copaiba Vanilla Moisturizing Conditioner, Copaiba Vanilla Moisturizing Shampoo, Lime, Lime Vitality, Live Your Passion, NingXia Zyng, MindWise, Stress Away, Stress Away Roll-On, Thieves Fruit & Veggie Spray |
| **Mandarin** | *Citrus reticulata* | ART L'Brianté Lip Gloss (Pink), Citrus Fresh, Citrus Fresh Vitality |
| **Manuka** | *Leptospermum scoparium* | Manuka |
| **Marjoram**<br><br>**Marjoram Vitality** | *Origanum majorana* | Aroma Life, Aroma Siez, Dragon Time, Dragon Time Bath & Shower Gel, Gratitude, Marjoram, Marjoram Vitality, M-Grain, Oola Fitness, Ortho Ease Massage Oil, R.C., RepelAroma, SniffleEase, SuperCal |

Seventh Edition | **Essential Oils Desk Reference** | **583**

**Essential Oils Desk Reference** | Seventh Edition

| Single Oil Name | Botanical Name | Products Containing Single Oil |
|---|---|---|
| **Mastrante** | *Lippia alba* | Light the Fire, Mastrante |
| **Melaleuca Ericifolia** | *Melaleuca ericifolia* | Melaleuca-Geranium Moisturizing Soap |
| **Melaleuca Quinquenervia (Niaouli)** | *Melaleuca viridiflora* | AromaGuard Meadow Mist Deodorant, Cool Azul, Cool Azul Pain Relief Cream, Cool Azul Sports Gel, Gary's Equine Essentials Massage Oil, Melaleuca Quinquenervia, Melrose |
| **Melissa** | *Melissa officinalis* | ART Gentle Cleanser, ART Refreshing Toner, Awaken, Brain Power, Build Your Dream, Divine Release, Forgiveness, GeneYus, Hope, Humility, Inner Harmony, InTouch, Live with Passion, Melissa, MultiGreens, Oola Finance, Reconnect, White Angelica |
| **Micromeria** | *Micromeria fruticosa* | |
| **Mountain Savory** | *Satureja montana* | ImmuPower, Mountain Savory, Mountain Savory Vitality, PuriClean, Surrender |
| **Mountain Savory Vitality** | | |
| **Myrrh** | *Commiphora myrrha* | 3 Wise Men, Abundance, Animal Scents Ointment, Boswellia Wrinkle Cream, ClaraDerm, Egyptian Gold, EndoGize, Essential Beauty Serum (Dry Skin), Exodus II, GeneYus, Gratitude, Hope, Humility, Infect Away, Inner Harmony, Lavender Bath & Shower Gel, Lavender Foaming Hand Soap, Lavender Hand & Body Lotion, Mendwell, Myrrh, Oola Balance, Oola Faith, Oola Finance, Protec, Reconnect, Rose Ointment, Sandalwood Moisture Cream, The Gift, Thyromin, White Angelica |
| **Myrtle** | *Myrtus communis* | Breathe Again Roll-On, EndoFlex, EndoFlex Vitality, Inspiration, JuvaTone, Mister, Myrtle, Oola Fun, Prostate Health, PuriClean, Purification, R.C., SniffleEase, Super Cal, Thieves Fruit & Veggie Soak, Thyromin |
| **Neroli (Bitter Orange)** | *Citrus aurantium amara* | Acceptance, Awaken, Humility, Inner Child, Live with Passion, Oola Family, Oola Field, Oola Finance, Oola Friends, Oola Grow, Present Time |
| **Niaouli** (See Melaleuca Quinquenervia) | *Melaleuca viridiflora* | |
| **Northern Lights Black Spruce** | *Picea mariana* | Animal Scents Shampoo, Egyptian Gold, Exodus II, Gary's Equine Essentials Shampoo, Gary's Equine Essentials Tail & Mane Sheen, Gathering, Gratitude, Highest Potential, Humility, LavaDerm Cooling Mist, Live Your Passion, Northern Lights Black Spruce, Oola Balance, Oola Finance, Oola Grow, Reconnect, Shutran Aftershave Lotion, Shutran Bar Soap, Shutran Shave Cream, The Gift, T.R. Care, Valor II |
| **Nutmeg** | *Myristica fragrans* | Ecuadorian Dark Chocolessence (Cinnamon Bark, Nutmeg, and Clove), EndoFlex, EndoFlex Vitality, En-R-Gee, Light the Fire, Live Your Passion, Magnify Your Purpose, NingXia Nitro, Nutmeg, Nutmeg Vitality, Oola Field, Oola Fitness, Oola Fun, ParaFree, Super B |
| **Nutmeg Vitality** | | |

584 | **Appendix B** | Single Oil Data

Single Oil Data | **Appendix B**

| Single Oil Name | Botanical Name | Products Containing Single Oil |
|---|---|---|
| **Ocotea** | *Ocotea quixos* | Acceptance, Amoressence, ART Beauty Masque, ART Creme Masque, ART L'Brianté (Neutral, Red), Australian Blue, Awaken, Build Your Dream, ComforTone, Common Sense, Dream Catcher, EndoGize, Highest Potential, Infect Away, KidScents Slique Toothpaste, Light the Fire, Mirah Shave Oil, Ocotea, Oola Balance, Oola Family, Oola Finance, Oola Friends, Oola Grow, ParaFree, Release, SARA, Shutran, Shutran Aftershave Lotion, Shutran Bar Soap, Shutran Shave Cream, Slique CitraSlim, Slique Essence, Slique Tea, Stress Away, Stress Away Roll-On, T.R. Care, Thieves AromaBright Toothpaste, Transformation, Ultra Young |
| **Orange**<br><br>**Orange Vitality** | *Citrus sinensis* | Abundance, Awaken, Balance Complete, Christmas Spirit, Cinnamint Lip Balm, Citrus Fresh, Citrus Fresh Vitality, Envision, Gary's True Grit NingXia Berry Syrup, Harmony, ImmuPro, Inner Child, Inner Harmony, Into the Future, Lady Sclareol, Live Your Passion, Longevity, Longevity Softgels, NingXia Red, Oola Balance, Oola Grow, Oola Finance, Orange, Orange Vitality, Peace & Calming, Peace & Calming II, Pure Protein Complete (Vanilla), Pure Protein Complete (Chocolate), SARA, Slique Bars, Slique Bars–Chocolate-Coated, Super C, Super C Chewable, T-Away, Thieves Foaming Hand Soap, T.R. Care |
| **Oregano**<br><br>**Oregano Vitality** | *Origanum vulgare (Syn. O. majorana)* | Cool Azul, ImmuPower, Inner Defense, Oregano, Oregano Vitality, Ortho Sport Massage Oil, Regenolone Moisturizing Cream |
| **Palmarosa** | *Cymbopogon martini* | Animal Scents Ointment, Awaken, Clarity, Dragon Time Bath & Shower Gel, Evening Peace Bath & Shower Gel, Forgiveness, Genesis Hand & Body Lotion, Gentle Baby, Harmony, Joy, Oola Balance, Oola Faith, Oola Family, Oola Finance, Oola Friends, Palmarosa, Rose Ointment, T-Away, T.R. Care |
| **Palo Santo** | *Bursera graveolens* | Bite Buster, Freedom, GeneYus, Infect Away, Oola Faith, Oola Friends, Palo Santo, PuriClean, Reconnect, RepelAroma, SniffleEase, Transformation |
| **Patchouli** | *Pogostemon cablin* | Abundance, Allerzyme, Animal Scents Ointment, ART L'Brianté Lip Gloss (Pink), DiGize, DiGize Vitality, Infect Away, Live with Passion, Magnify Your Purpose, Orange Blossom Facial Wash, ParaFree, ParaGize, Patchouli, Peace & Calming, Peace & Calming II, PuriClean, Rose Ointment, T-Away, Thieves Fruit & Veggie Soak, T.R. Care |

Seventh Edition | **Essential Oils Desk Reference** | **585**

**Essential Oils Desk Reference** | Seventh Edition

| Single Oil Name | Botanical Name | Products Containing Single Oil |
|---|---|---|
| Peppermint<br><br><br><br><br><br><br><br>Peppermint Vitality | *Mentha piperita* | Allerzyme, Aroma Ease, Aroma Siez, AromaGuard Mountain Mint Deodorant, Breathe Again Roll-On, Cinnamint Lip Balm, Clarity, ComforTone, Cool Azul, Cool Azul Pain Relief Cream, Cool Azul Sports Gel, Cortistop, Deep Relief, Deep Relief Roll-On, Digest & Cleanse, DiGize, DiGize Vitality, Essentialzyme, Freedom, Gary's Equine Essentials Massage Oil, Lavender Mint Daily Conditioner, Lavender Mint Daily Shampoo, Live Your Passion, M-Grain, Mightyzyme, MindWise, Mineral Essence, Mister, Morning Start Bath & Shower Gel, Morning Start Moisturizing Soap, NingXia Nitro, Oola Finance, Oola Fitness, Ortho Ease Massage Oil, Ortho Sport Massage Oil, PanAway, ParaFree, ParaGize, Peppermint, Peppermint-Cedarwood Moisturizing Soap, Peppermint Vitality, Progessence Plus, Prostate Health, R.C., Raven, Regenolone Moisturizing Cream, Relaxation Massage Oil, Relieve It, Satin Facial Scrub–Mint, SclarEssence, Slique Gum, SniffleEase, Thieves AromaBright Toothpaste, Thieves Automatic Dishwashing Powder, Thieves Dental Floss, Thieves Dentarome Plus Toothpaste, Thieves Dentarome Ultra Toothpaste, Thieves Fresh Essence Plus Mouthwash, Thieves Fruit & Veggie Soak, Thieves Hard Lozenges, Thieves Mints, Thieves Waterless Hand Purifier, Thyromin, Transformation, TummyGize, Vanillamint Lip Balm |
| Petitgrain | *Citrus aurantium amara (Syn. C. sinensis)* | Petitgrain |
| Pine | *Pinus sylvestris* | Evergreen Essence, Grounding, Oola Family, Pine, R.C., SniffleEase |
| Plectranthus Oregano | *Plectranthus amboinicus* | Cool Azul, Cool Azul Pain Relief Cream, Cool Azul Sports Gel, Gary's Equine Essentials Massage Oil, Infect Away |
| Ravintsara | *Cinnamomum camphora* | ImmuPower, Raven, Ravintsara, SniffleEase |
| Roman Chamomile | *Anthemis nobilis (Syn. Chamaemelum nobile)* | Amoressence, AromaSleep, ART Creme Masque, ART L'Brianté Lip Gloss (Red), Awaken, ClaraDerm, Clarity, Divine Release, Dragon Time Bath & Shower Gel, Evening Peace Bath & Shower Gel, Forgiveness, Genesis Hand & Body Lotion, Gentle Baby, Harmony, Inner Harmony, Joy, JuvaFlex, K&B, KidScents Tender Tush, M-Grain, Motivation, Oola Balance, Oola Faith, Oola Family, Oola Finance, Oola Friends, Oola Grow, Rehemogen, Satin Facial Scrub–Mint, SleepyIze, Surrender, T-Away, T.R. Care, Tranquil Roll-On, Wolfberry Eye Cream |
| Rose | *Rosa damascena* | Acceptance, Australian Blue, Awaken, Build Your Dream, Divine Release, Dream Catcher, Egyptian Gold, Envision, Forgiveness, Gathering, GeneYus, Gentle Baby, Harmony, Highest Potential, Humility, Inner Harmony, Joy, Mirah Shave Oil, Oola Balance, Oola Faith, Oola Finance, Oola Friends, Oola Grow, Reconnect, Release, Rose, Rose Ointment, SARA, T-Away, T.R. Care, Trauma Life, White Angelica |

| Single Oil Name | Botanical Name | Products Containing Single Oil |
|---|---|---|
| Rosemary<br><br>Rosemary Vitality | *Rosmarinus officinalis* | AromaGuard Meadow Mist Deodorant, AromaGuard Mountain Mint Deodorant, Clarity, ComforTone, En-R-Gee, Essentialzymes-4, Gary's Equine Essentials Shampoo, ICP, Inner Defense, JuvaFlex, JuvaTone, KidScents Slique Toothpaste, Melrose, Morning Start Bath & Shower Gel, Morning Start Moisturizing Soap, MultiGreens, Oola Finance, Orange Blossom Facial Wash, ParaGize, PuriClean, Purification, Rehemogen, Rosemary, Rosemary Vitality, Sandalwood Moisture Cream, Satin Facial Scrub–Mint, Shutran Bar Soap, Thieves, Thieves AromaBright Toothpaste, Thieves Automatic Dishwashing Powder, Thieves Cleansing Soap, Thieves Cough Drops, Thieves Dental Floss, Thieves Dentarome Plus Toothpaste, Thieves Dentarome Ultra Toothpaste, Thieves Dish Soap, Thieves Foaming Hand Soap, Thieves Fresh Essence Plus Mouthwash, Thieves Fruit & Veggie Soak, Thieves Fruit & Veggie Spray, Thieves Hard Lozenges, Thieves Household Cleaner, Thieves Laundry Soap, Thieves Mints, Thieves Spray, Thieves Waterless Hand Purifier, Thieves Wipes |
| Rosewood | *Aniba rosaeodora* | Valor, Valor Moisturizing Soap, Valor Roll-On |
| Royal Hawaiian Sandalwood | *Santalum paniculatum* | 3 Wise Men, Acceptance, ART Chocolate Masque, ART Gentle Cleanser, ART L'Brianté Lip Gloss (Neutral), ART Intensive Moisturizer, ART Light Moisturizer, ART Refreshing Toner, ART Sheerlumé Brightening Cream, Awaken, Boswellia Wrinkle Cream, Brain Power, Build Your Dream, Divine Release, Dream Catcher, Essential Beauty Serum (Dry Skin), Evening Peace Bath & Shower Gel, Forgiveness, Gary's Equine Essentials Tail & Mane Sheen, Gathering, GeneYus, Harmony, Highest Potential, Inner Child, Inner Harmony, Inspiration, InTouch, KidScents Tender Tush, Lady Sclareol, Lemon-Sandalwood Cleansing Soap, Live with Passion, Live Your Passion, Magnify Your Purpose, Mirah Shave Oil, Oola Balance, Oola Family, Oola Finance, Oola Friends, Oola Grow, Reconnect, Release, Royal Hawaiian Sandalwood, Sandalwood Moisture Cream, T-Away, Gary's Equine Essentials Tail & Mane Sheen, T.R. Care, Transformation, Trauma Life, White Angelica |
| Ruta | *Ruta graveolens* | AromaSleep, Common Sense, Freedom, RutaVaLa, RutaVaLa Roll-On, SleepEssence, SleepyIze, T-Away, T.R. Care |
| Sacred Frankincense | *Boswellia sacra* | ART Sheerlumé Brightening Cream, Build Your Dream, Freedom, GeneYus, Inner Harmony, Oola Balance, Oola Faith, Progessence Plus, Reconnect, Sacred Frankincense, SleepyIze, The Gift, Transformation |
| Sage<br><br>Sage Vitality | *Salvia officinalis* | Cool Azul, Cool Azul Pain Relief Cream, Cool Azul Sports Gel, Dragon Time Bath & Shower Gel, Dragon Time Massage Oil, EndoFlex, EndoFlex Vitality, Envision, Gary's Equine Essentials Massage Oil, FemiGen, K&B, Magnify Your Purpose, Mister, Oola Faith, Prenolone Plus Body Cream, Protec, Sage |
| Spanish Sage (Sage Lavender) | *Salvia lavandulifolia* | Awaken, Harmony, Lady Sclareol, Oola Balance, Oola Friends, SclarEssence, T-Away, T.R. Care |

**Essential Oils Desk Reference** | Seventh Edition

| Single Oil Name | Botanical Name | Products Containing Single Oil |
|---|---|---|
| Spearmint<br><br>Spearmint Vitality | *Mentha spicata* | Acceptance, Animal Scents Dental Pet Chews, AromaEase, ART L'Brianté Lip Gloss (Neutral, Pink, Red), ART Sheerlumé Brightening Cream, Australian Blue, Awaken, Build Your Dream, Cinnamint Lip Balm, Citrus Fresh, Citrus Fresh Vitality, Dream Catcher, EndoFlex, EndoFlex Vitality, GLF, Highest Potential, KidScents Slique Toothpaste, Lady Sclareol, Lavender Mint Daily Conditioner, Lavender Mint Daily Shampoo, NingXia Nitro, OmegaGize$^3$, Oola Fun, Oola Grow, ParaGize, Red Shot, Relaxation Massage Oil, Slique CitraSlim, Slique Essence, Slique Gum, Spearmint, Spearmint Vitality, Thieves AromaBright Toothpaste, Thieves Fresh Essence Plus Mouthwash, Thyromin, T.R. Care, TummyGize, Ultra Young |
| Spikenard | *Nardostachys jatamansi* | |
| Tangerine<br><br>Tangerine Vitality | *Citrus reticulata* | Acceptance, AromaSleep, ART L'Brianté Lip Gloss (Neutral, Pink, Red), Australian Blue, Awaken, Build Your Dream, Citrus Fresh, Citrus Fresh Vitality, ComforTone, Dragon Time Bath & Shower Gel, Dream Catcher, Ecuadorian Dark Chocolessence (Tangerine and Ginger), Highest Potential, Inner Child, Inner Harmony, Joy, KidScents Shampoo, KidScents Slique Toothpaste, NingXia Red, Oola Family, Oola Friends, Oola Fun, Oola Grow, Peace & Calming, Peace & Calming II, Red Shot, Relaxation Massage Oil, Release, SARA, SleepEssence, SleepyIze, Slique Essence, Super C, Tangerine, Tangerine Vitality, T-Away, T.R. Care, TummyGize, Ultra Young |
| Tarragon<br><br>Tarragon Vitality | *Artemisia dracunculus* | Allerzyme, ComforTone, DiGize, DiGize Vitality, Essentialzyme, Essentialzymes-4, ICP, ParaFree, ParaGize, Tarragon, Tarragon Vitality, Thieves Fruit & Veggie Soak |
| Tea Tree | *Melaleuca alternifolia* | Animal Scents Ointment, AromaGuard Meadow Mist Deodorant, ClaraDerm, Melaleuca-Geranium Moisturizing Soap, Melrose, Owie, ParaFree, PuriClean, Purification, Rehemogen, Rose Ointment, Shutran Shave Cream, Tea Tree, Thieves Fruit & Veggie Soak |
| Thyme<br><br>Thyme Vitality | *Thymus vulgaris* | Inner Defense, Longevity, Longevity Softgels, Ortho Ease Massage Oil, Ortho Sport Massage Oil, ParaFree, Rehemogen, Thieves Dentarome Ultra Toothpaste, Thyme, Thyme Vitality |
| Tsuga | *Tsuga canadensis* | Tsuga |
| Valerian | *Valeriana officinalis* | AromaSleep, Freedom, RutaVaLa, RutaVaLa Roll-On, SleepEssence, SleepyIze, T-Away, T.R. Care, Trauma Life, Valerian |
| Vanilla | *Vanilla planifolia* | ART Beauty Masque, ART Creme Masque, Copaiba Vanilla Moisturizing Conditioner, Copaiba Vanilla Moisturizing Shampoo, Gary's True Grit Einkorn Granola, NingXia Nitro, Slique Bars, Slique Bars–Chocolate-Coated, Slique Tea, Stress Away, Stress Away Roll-On |

588 | Appendix B | Single Oil Data

Single Oil Data | **Appendix B**

| Single Oil Name | Botanical Name | Products Containing Single Oil |
|---|---|---|
| **Vetiver** | *Vetiveria zizanoides (Syn. V. zizanioides)* | Amoressence, Animal Scents Shampoo, ART Creme Masque, ART L'Brianté Lip Gloss (Neutral, Pink, Red), ART Sheerlumé Brightening Cream, Cool Azul, Cool Azul Pain Relief Cream, Cool Azul Sports Gel, Deep Relief, Deep Relief Roll-On, Egyptian Gold, Gary's Equine Essentials Shampoo, Gary's Equine Essentials Massage Oil, Freedom, Humility, InTouch, Inspiration, Lady Sclareol, Melaleuca-Geranium Moisturizing Soap, Ortho Ease Massage Oil, Oola Balance, Oola Finance, Oola Grow, Ortho Sport Massage Oil, ParaFree, Peace & Calming II, Reconnect, SleepEssence, Thieves Fresh Essence Plus Mouthwash, T.R. Care, Valor II, Vetiver |
| **Western Red Cedar** | *Thuja plicata* | Evergreen Essence, KidScents Lotion |
| **White Fir** | *Abies concolor* | AromaGuard Mountain Mint Deodorant, ART L'Brianté Lip Gloss (Neutral), Australian Blue, Evergreen Essence, Grounding, Highest Potential, Into the Future, Oola Grow, T.R. Care |
| **White Lotus** | *Nymphaea lotus* | Build Your Dream, Into the Future, Oola Grow, SARA |
| **Wintergreen** | *Gaultheria procumbens* | Cool Azul, Cool Azul Sports Gel, Cool Azul Pain Relief Cream, Deep Relief, Deep Relief Roll-On, Gary's Equine Essentials Massage Oil, Ortho Ease Massage Oil, Ortho Sport Massage Oil, PanAway, Raven, Regenolone Moisturizing Cream, Super Cal, Thieves Dentarome Plus Toothpaste, Thieves Dentarome Ultra Toothpaste, Wintergreen |
| **Xiang Mao** | *Cymbopogon citratus* | Oola Family, Oola Friends, Xiang Mao |
| **Yarrow** | *Achillea millefolium* | Dragon Time, Dragon Time Massage Oil, Mister, Prenolone Plus Body Cream |
| **Ylang Ylang (Also Amazonian/ Ecuadorian Ylang Ylang)** | *Cananga odorata (Cananga odorata Equitoriana)* | Acceptance, Animal Scents Ointment, Aroma Life, AromaGuard Meadow Mist Deodorant, Aroma Life, ART Creme Masque, ART L'Brianté Lip Gloss (Red, Neutral), ART Intensive Moisturizer, ART Light Moisturizer, ART Renewal Serum, Australian Blue, Awaken, Believe, Boswellia Wrinkle Cream, Build Your Dream, Clarity, Common Sense, Dragon Time Bath & Shower Gel, Dragon Time Massage Oil, Dream Catcher, Evening Peace Bath & Shower Gel, FemiGen, Forgiveness, Gathering, Genesis Hand & Body Lotion, GeneYus, Gentle Baby, Gratitude, Grounding, Harmony, Highest Potential, Humility, Inner Child, Inner Harmony, Inspiration, Into the Future, Joy, KidScents Lotion, KidScents Tender Tush, Lady Sclareol, Lavender-Oatmeal Bar Soap, Live Your Passion, Magnify Your Purpose, Mirah Shave Oil, Motivation, Oola Balance, Oola Faith, Oola Field, Oola Finance, Oola Friends, Oola Grow, Peace & Calming, Peace & Calming II, Prenolone Plus Body Cream, Present Time, Reconnect, Relaxation Massage Oil, Release, Rose Ointment, Sacred Mountain, Sacred Mountain Moisturizing Soap, Sandalwood Moisture Cream, SARA, Sensation, Sensation Bath & Shower Gel, Sensation Hand & Body Lotion, Sensation Massage Oil, Shutran, Shutran Aftershave Lotion, Shutran Bar Soap, Shutran Shave Cream, T-Away, T.R. Care, Valor II, White Angelica, Wolfberry Eye Cream, Ylang Ylang |
| **Yuzu** | *Citrus junos* | NingXia Red |

Seventh Edition | **Essential Oils Desk Reference** | 589

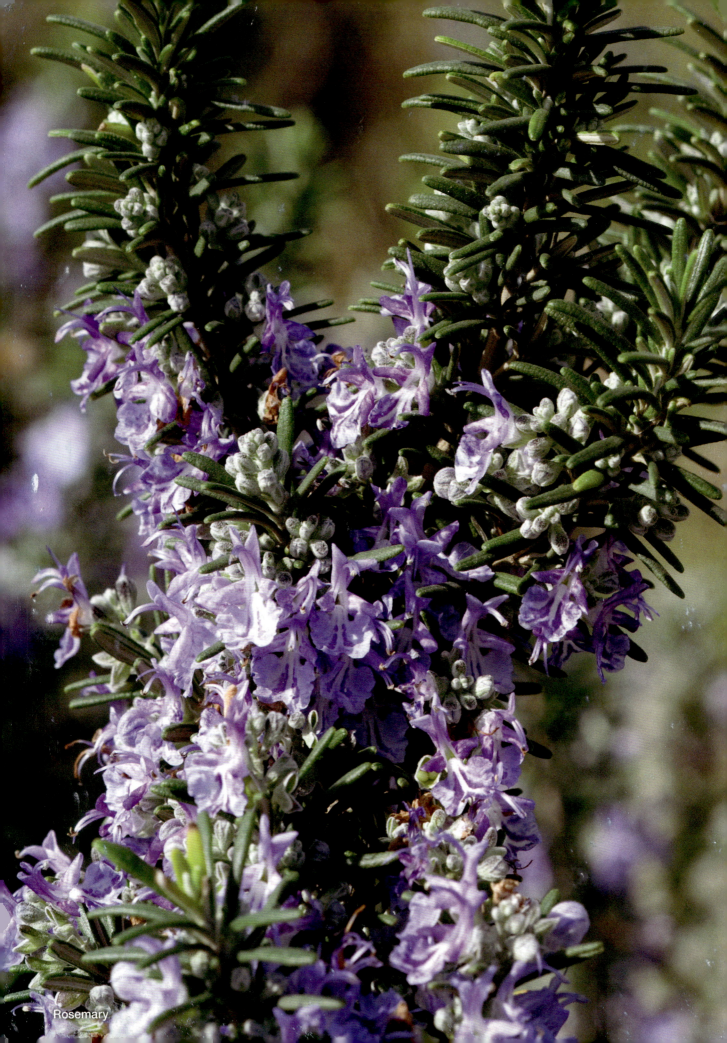
Rosemary

# Appendix C
## Essential Oil Blends Data

| Blend Name | Ingredients |
|---|---|
| 3 Wise Men | sweet almond oil, Royal Hawaiian Sandalwood, Juniper, Frankincense, Black Spruce, Myrrh |
| Abundance | Orange, Frankincense, Patchouli, Clove, Ginger, Myrrh, Cinnamon Bark, Black Spruce |
| Acceptance | sweet almond oil, Coriander, Geranium, Bergamot, Frankincense, Royal Hawaiian Sandalwood, Bitter Orange (Neroli), Grapefruit, Tangerine, Spearmint, Lemon, Blue Cypress, Davana, Kaffir Lime, Ocotea, Jasmine, Matricaria (German Chamomile) |
| Amoressence | Vetiver, Idaho Blue Spruce, Jasmine, Davana, Ocotea, Ylang Ylang, Roman Chamomile, Vanilla, Geranium |
| Aroma Ease | Peppermint, Spearmint, Ginger, Cardamom, Fennel |
| Aroma Life | sesame seed oil, Cypress, Marjoram, Ylang Ylang, Helichrysum |
| Aroma Siez | Basil, Marjoram, Lavender, Peppermint, Cypress |
| AromaSleep | Lavender, Geranium, Roman Chamomile, Bergamot, Tangerine, Sacred Frankincense, Valerian, Ruta |
| Australian Blue | Blue Cypress, Ylang Ylang, Cedarwood, White Fir, Geranium, Grapefruit, Tangerine, Spearmint, Davana, Kaffir Lime, Lemon, Ocotea, Jasmine, Matricaria (German Chamomile), Blue Tansy, Rose |
| Awaken | Joy, Forgiveness, Present Time, Dream Catcher, Harmony |
| Believe | Balsam Canada (Idaho Balsam Fir), Coriander, Bergamot, Frankincense, Idaho Blue Spruce, Ylang Ylang, Geranium |
| Bite Buster | caprylic/capric glycerides, Idaho Tansy, Citronella, Palo Santo |
| Brain Power | Royal Hawaiian Sandalwood, Cedarwood, Frankincense, Melissa, Blue Cypress, Lavender, Helichrysum |
| Breathe Again Roll-On | caprylic/capric triglyceride, Eucalyptus Staigeriana, Eucalyptus Globulus, Laurus Nobilis (Bay Laurel), Rose Hip Seed Oil, Peppermint, Eucalyptus Radiata, Copaiba, Myrtle, Blue Cypress, Eucalyptus Blue |
| Build Your Dream | Lavender, Sacred Frankincense, Melissa, Blue Cypress, Hong Kuai, Idaho Blue Spruce, Ylang Ylang, Dream Catcher, Believe, Blue Lotus |
| Christmas Spirit | Orange, Cinnamon Bark, Black Spruce |
| Citrus Fresh | Orange, Tangerine, Grapefruit, Lemon, Mandarin, Spearmint |
| Citrus Fresh Vitality | Orange, Tangerine, Grapefruit, Lemon, Mandarin, Spearmint |
| Clarity | Basil, Cardamom, Rosemary, Peppermint, Coriander, Geranium, Bergamot, Lemon, Ylang Ylang, Jasmine, Roman Chamomile, Palmarosa |
| Common Sense | Frankincense, Ylang Ylang, Ocotea, Goldenrod, Ruta, Dorado Azul, Lime |

**Essential Oils Desk Reference** | Seventh Edition

| Blend Name | Ingredients |
|---|---|
| Cool Azul | Wintergreen, Peppermint, Sage, Copaiba, Oregano, Niaouli, Plectranthus Oregano, Lavender, Blue Cypress, Elemi, Vetiver, Caraway, Dorado Azul, Matricaria (German Chamomile) |
| Deep Relief Roll-On | Peppermint, caprylic/capric triglyceride, Lemon, Balsam Canada (Idaho Balsam Fir), Clove, Copaiba, coconut oil, Wintergreen, Helichrysum, Vetiver, Dorado Azul |
| DiGize | Tarragon, Ginger, Peppermint, Juniper, Fennel, Lemongrass, Anise, Patchouli |
| DiGize Vitality | Tarragon, Ginger, Peppermint, Juniper, Fennel, Lemongrass, Anise, Patchouli |
| Divine Release | Royal Hawaiian Sandalwood, Roman Chamomile, Frankincense, Melissa, Geranium, Grapefruit, Blue Cypress, Hinoki, Helichrysum, Bergamot, Rose, Ledum, Angelica |
| Dragon Time | Fennel, Clary Sage, Marjoram, Lavender, Yarrow, Jasmine |
| Dream Catcher | Royal Hawaiian Sandalwood, Tangerine, Ylang Ylang, Black Pepper, Bergamot, Anise, Juniper, Geranium, Blue Cypress, Davana, Citrus Hystrix, Jasmine, Matricaria (German Chamomile), Blue Tansy, Rose, Grapefruit, Spearmint |
| Egyptian Gold | Frankincense, Balsam Canada (Idaho Balsam Fir), Lavender, Myrrh, Hyssop, Northern Lights Black Spruce, Cedarwood, Vetiver, Rose, Cinnamon Bark |
| En-R-Gee | Rosemary, Juniper, Lemongrass, Nutmeg, Balsam Canada (Idaho Balsam Fir), Clove, Black Pepper |
| EndoFlex | Spearmint, sesame seed oil, Sage, Geranium, Myrtle, Matricaria (German Chamomile), Nutmeg |
| EndoFlex Vitality | Spearmint, sesame seed oil, Sage, Geranium, Myrtle, Matricaria (German Chamomile), Nutmeg |
| Envision | Black Spruce, Geranium, Orange, Lavender, Sage, Rose |
| Evergreen Essence | Idaho Blue Spruce, Ponderosa Pine, Scotch Pine, Red Fir, Western Red Cedar, White Fir, Black Pine, Pinyon Pine, Lodgepole Pine |
| Exodus II | olive oil, Myrrh, Cassia, Cinnamon Bark, Calamus, Northern Lights Black Spruce, Hyssop, Vetiver, Frankincense |
| Forgiveness | sesame seed oil, Melissa, Geranium, Frankincense, Royal Hawaiian Sandalwood, Coriander, Angelica, Lavender, Bergamot, Lemon, Ylang Ylang, Jasmine, Helichrysum, Roman Chamomile, Palmarosa, Rose |
| Freedom | Copaiba, Sacred Frankincense, Idaho Blue Spruce, Vetiver, Lavender, Peppermint, Palo Santo, Valerian, Ruta |
| Gathering | Lavender, Northern Lights Black Spruce, Geranium, Royal Hawaiian Sandalwood, Ylang Ylang, Vetiver, Cinnamon Bark, Rose |
| GeneYus | fractionated coconut oil, Sacred Frankincense, Blue Cypress, Cedarwood, Idaho Blue Spruce, Palo Santo, Melissa, Northern Lights Black Spruce, almond oil, Bergamot, Myrrh, Vetiver, Geranium, Royal Hawaiian Sandalwood, Ylang Ylang, Hyssop, Coriander, Rose |
| Gentle Baby | Coriander, Geranium, Palmarosa, Lavender, Ylang Ylang, Roman Chamomile, Bergamot (furocoumarin-free), Lemon, Jasmine, Rose |
| GLF | Grapefruit, Ledum, Helichrysum, Celery Seed, Hyssop, Spearmint |
| GLF Vitality | Grapefruit, Ledum, Helichrysum, Celery Seed, Hyssop, Spearmint |
| Gratitude | Balsam Canada (Idaho Balsam Fir), Frankincense, Coriander, Myrrh, Ylang Ylang, Bergamot (furocoumarin-free), Northern Lights Black Spruce, Vetiver, Geranium |

592 | Appendix C | Oil Blends Data

Oil Blends Data | **Appendix C**

| Blend Name | Ingredients |
|---|---|
| **Grounding** | White Fir, Black Spruce, Ylang Ylang, Pine, Cedarwood, Angelica, Juniper |
| **Harmony** | Royal Hawaiian Sandalwood, Lavender, Ylang Ylang, Frankincense, Orange, Angelica, Geranium, Hyssop, Spanish Sage, Black Spruce, Coriander, Bergamot, Lemon, Jasmine, Roman Chamomile, Palmarosa, Rose |
| **Highest Potential** | Blue Cypress, Ylang Ylang, Jasmine, Cedarwood, Geranium, Lavender, Northern Lights Black Spruce, Frankincense, Royal Hawaiian Sandalwood, White Fir, Vetiver, Cinnamon Bark, Davana, Citrus Hystrix, Rose, German Chamomile, Blue Tansy, Grapefruit, Tangerine, Spearmint, Lemon, Ocotea |
| **Hope** | sweet almond oil, Melissa, Juniper, Myrrh, Black Spruce |
| **Humility** | caprylic/capric triglyceride, Coriander, Ylang Ylang, Bergamot (furocoumarin-free), Geranium, Melissa, Frankincense, Myrrh, Northern Lights Black Spruce, Vetiver, Bitter Orange (Neroli), Rose |
| **ImmuPower** | Hyssop, Mountain Savory, Cistus, Camphor (Ravintsara), Frankincense, Oregano, Clove, Cumin, Dorado Azul |
| **Inner Child** | Orange, Tangerine, Ylang Ylang, Royal Hawaiian Sandalwood, Jasmine, Lemongrass, Black Spruce, Bitter Orange (Neroli) |
| **Inner Harmony** | Geranium, Lavender, Royal Hawaiian Sandalwood, Ylang Ylang, Idaho Blue Spruce, Sacred Frankincense, Roman Chamomile, Tangerine, Orange, Northern Lights Black Spruce, Myrrh, Rose, Angelica, Vetiver, Melissa |
| **Inspiration** | Cedarwood, Black Spruce, Myrtle, Coriander, Royal Hawaiian Sandalwood, Frankincense, Bergamot (furocoumarin-free), Vetiver, Ylang Ylang, Geranium |
| **Into the Future** | sweet almond oil, Clary Sage, Ylang Ylang, White Fir, Idaho Blue Spruce, Jasmine, Juniper, Frankincense, Orange, Cedarwood, White Lotus |
| **InTouch** | caprylic/capric triglyceride, Vetiver, Melissa, Royal Hawaiian Sandalwood, Cedarwood, Idaho Blue Spruce |
| **Joy** | Bergamot, Ylang Ylang, Geranium, Lemon, Coriander, Tangerine, Jasmine, Roman Chamomile, Palmarosa, Rose |
| **JuvaCleanse** | Helichrysum, Ledum, Celery Seed |
| **JuvaCleanse Vitality** | Helichrysum, Ledum, Celery Seed |
| **JuvaFlex** | sesame seed oil, Fennel, Geranium, Rosemary, Roman Chamomile, Blue Tansy, Helichrysum |
| **JuvaFlex Vitality** | sesame seed oil, Fennel, Geranium, Rosemary, Roman Chamomile, Blue Tansy, Helichrysum |
| **Lady Sclareol** | Geranium, Coriander, Vetiver, Orange, Clary Sage, Bergamot, Ylang Ylang, Royal Hawaiian Sandalwood, Spanish Sage, Jasmine, Idaho Blue Spruce, Spearmint, Hinoki |
| **Light the Fire** | Nutmeg, Cassia, Mastrante, Ocotea, Canadian Fleabane, Lemon, Hinoki, Black Pepper, Northern Lights Black Spruce |
| **Live with Passion** | Royal Hawaiian Sandalwood, Clary Sage, Ginger, Jasmine, Angelica, Patchouli, Cedarwood, Helichrysum, Melissa, Bitter Orange (Neroli) |
| **Live Your Passion** | Orange, Royal Hawaiian Sandalwood, Nutmeg, Lime, Idaho Blue Spruce, Northern Lights Black Spruce, Ylang Ylang, Frankincense, Peppermint |
| **Longevity** | Thyme, Orange, Clove, Frankincense |
| **Longevity Vitality** | Thyme, Orange, Clove, Frankincense |
| **M-Grain** | Basil, Marjoram, Lavender, Roman Chamomile, Peppermint, Helichrysum |

Seventh Edition | **Essential Oils Desk Reference** | 593

**Essential Oils Desk Reference** | Seventh Edition

| Blend Name | Ingredients |
|---|---|
| **Magnify Your Purpose** | Royal Hawaiian Sandalwood, Sage, Coriander, Patchouli, Nutmeg, Bergamot, Cinnamon Bark, Ginger, Ylang Ylang, Geranium |
| **Melrose** | Rosemary, Tea Tree, Clove, Niaouli |
| **Mister** | sesame seed oil, Sage, Fennel, Lavender, Myrtle, Yarrow, Peppermint |
| **Motivation** | Roman Chamomile, Black Spruce, Ylang Ylang, Lavender |
| **Oola Balance** | fractionated coconut oil, Lavender, Ylang Ylang, Frankincense, Ocotea, Idaho Blue Spruce, Royal Hawaiian Sandalwood, Balsam Canada (Idaho Balsam Fir), Sacred Frankincense, Jasmine, Northern Lights Black Spruce, Orange, Angelica, Geranium, Hyssop, Spanish Sage, Myrrh, Vetiver, Cistus, Coriander, Bergamot, Lemon, Roman Chamomile, Palmarosa, Rose |
| **Oola Faith** | caprylic/capric triglyceride, Sacred Frankincense, Balsam Canada (Idaho Balsam Fir), Myrrh, Juniper, Hyssop, Cedarwood, Black Sage, Hinoki, Rose, Geranium, Palo Santo, Coriander, Bergamot, Lemon, Ylang Ylang, Jasmine, Roman Chamomile, Palmarosa |
| **Oola Family** | caprylic/capric triglyceride, Ylang Ylang, Lavender, Orange, Geranium, Cardamom, Tangerine, Frankincense, Cedarwood, Coriander, Pine, Royal Hawaiian Sandalwood, Lemongrass, Bergamot, Xiang Mao, Lemon, Black Spruce, Lime, Roman Chamomile, Palmarosa |
| **Oola Field** | caprylic/capric triglyceride, Cardamom, Frankincense, Ylang Ylang, sweet almond oil, Nutmeg, Ginger, Bitter Orange (Neroli), Balsam Canada (Idaho Balsam Fir), Coriander, Black Spruce, Bergamot, Idaho Blue Spruce, Geranium |
| **Oola Finance** | fractionated coconut oil, Frankincense, Orange, Ocotea, Balsam Canada (Idaho Balsam Fir), Royal Hawaiian Sandalwood, Basil, Geranium, Lavender, Cardamom, Coriander, Ylang Ylang, Northern Lights Black Spruce, Rosemary, Citronella (nardus), Citronella (winterianus), Bergamot (furocoumarin-free), Vetiver, Peppermint, Melissa, Myrrh, Cinnamon Bark, Lemon, Jasmine, Roman Chamomile, Palmarosa, Bitter Orange (Neroli), Rose |
| **Oola Fitness** | caprylic/capric triglyceride, Cypress, Copaiba, Basil, Cistus, Marjoram, Peppermint, Clary Sage, Idaho Blue Spruce, Balsam Canada (Idaho Balsam Fir), Nutmeg, Black Pepper |
| **Oola Friends** | caprylic/capric triglyceride, Lavender, Frankincense, Blue Cypress, Orange, Royal Hawaiian Sandalwood, Palo Santo, Xiang Mao, Ylang Ylang, Mandarin, Angelica, Geranium, Hyssop, Spanish Sage, Black Spruce, Jasmine, Lemongrass, Bitter Orange (Neroli), Coriander, Bergamot, Lemon, Roman Chamomile, Palmarosa, Rose |
| **Oola Fun** | caprylic/capric triglyceride, Spearmint, Cedarwood, Myrtle, Lemon, Grapefruit, Tangerine, Jasmine, Nutmeg |
| **Oola Grow** | fractionated coconut oil, White Fir, Blue Cypress, Ylang Ylang, Roman Chamomile, almond oil, Northern Lights Black Spruce, Coriander, Geranium, Jasmine, Cedarwood, Lavender, Frankincense, Bergamot (furocoumarin-free), Clary Sage, Royal Hawaiian Sandalwood, Grapefruit, Tangerine, Spearmint, Vetiver, Lemon, Neroli, Idaho Blue Spruce, Ocotea, Juniper, Orange, Cinnamon Bark, Citrus Hystrix, Rose, White Lotus |
| **Owie** | caprylic/capric glycerides, Balsam Canada (Idaho Balsam Fir), Tea Tree, Helichrysum, Elemi, Cistus, Hinoki, Clove |
| **PanAway** | Wintergreen, Helichrysum, Clove, Peppermint |
| **Peace & Calming** | Tangerine, Orange, Ylang Ylang, Patchouli, Blue Tansy |
| **Peace & Calming II** | Tangerine, Orange, Ylang Ylang, Patchouli, Northern Lights Black Spruce, Matricaria (German Chamomile), Vetiver, Cistus, Bergamot, Cassia, Davana |

Oil Blends Data | **Appendix C**

| Blend Name | Ingredients |
|---|---|
| Present Time | sweet almond oil, Bitter Orange (Neroli), Black Spruce, Ylang Ylang |
| Purification | Citronella, Rosemary, Lemongrass, Tea Tree, Lavandin, Myrtle |
| Raven | Camphor (Ravintsara), Lemon, Wintergreen, Peppermint, Eucalyptus Radiata |
| R.C. | Eucalyptus Globulus, Myrtle, Marjoram, Pine, Eucalyptus Radiata, Eucalyptus Citriodora, Lavender, Cypress, Black Spruce, Peppermint |
| Reconnect | fractionated coconut oil, Sacred Frankincense, Lavender, Blue Cypress, Cedarwood, Melissa, Idaho Blue Spruce, Palo Santo, Northern Lights Black Spruce, almond oil, Bergamot, Myrrh, Vetiver, Geranium, Royal Hawaiian Sandalwood, Ylang Ylang, Hyssop, Coriander, Rose |
| Red Shot | Tangerine, Mandarin, Lime, Grapefruit, Cassia, Spearmint |
| Release | Ylang Ylang, olive oil, Lavandin, Geranium, Royal Hawaiian Sandalwood, Grapefruit, Tangerine, Spearmint, Lemon, Blue Cypress, Davana, Kaffir Lime, Ocotea, Jasmine, Matricaria (German Chamomile), Blue Tansy, Rose |
| Relieve It | Black Spruce, Black Pepper, Hyssop, Peppermint |
| RutaVaLa | Lavender, Valerian, Ruta |
| RutaVaLa Roll-On | caprylic/capric triglyceride, Lavender, Valerian, Ruta |
| Sacred Mountain | Black Spruce, Ylang Ylang, Balsam Canada (Idaho Balsam Fir), Cedarwood |
| SARA | sweet almond oil, Ylang Ylang, Geranium, Lavender, Orange, Cedarwood, Blue Cypress, Davana, Citrus Hystrix, Jasmine, Rose, Matricaria (German Chamomile), Blue Tansy, Grapefruit, Tangerine, Spearmint, Lemon, Ocotea, White Lotus |
| SclarEssence | Clary Sage, Peppermint, Spanish Sage, Fennel |
| SclarEssence Vitality | Clary Sage, Peppermint, Spanish Sage, Fennel |
| Sensation | Coriander, Ylang Ylang, Bergamot (furocoumarin-free), Jasmine, Geranium |
| Shutran | Idaho Blue Spruce, Ylang Ylang, Ocotea, Hinoki, Davana, Cedarwood, Lavender, Coriander, Lemon, Northern Lights Black Spruce |
| SleepyIze | caprylic/capric glycerides, Lavender, Geranium, Roman Chamomile, Tangerine, Bergamot, Sacred Frankincense, Valerian, Ruta |
| Slique Essence | Grapefruit, Tangerine, Spearmint, Lemon, Ocotea, Stevia Extract |
| SniffleEase | caprylic/capric glycerides, Eucalyptus Blue, Palo Santo, Lavender, Dorado Azul, Ravintsara, Myrtle, Eucalyptus Globulus, Marjoram, Pine, Eucalyptus Citriodora, Cypress, Eucalyptus Radiata, Black Spruce, Peppermint |
| Stress Away | Copaiba, Lime, Cedarwood, Vanilla, Ocotea, Lavender |
| Stress Away Roll-On | Copaiba, Lime, Cedarwood, Vanilla, Ocotea, Lavender |
| Surrender | Lavender, Lemon, Black Spruce, Roman Chamomile, Angelica, Mountain Savory |
| The Gift | Balsam Canada (Idaho Balsam Fir), Sacred Frankincense, Jasmine, Northern Lights Black Spruce, Myrrh, Vetiver, Cistus |
| Thieves | Clove, Lemon, Cinnamon Bark, Eucalyptus Radiata, Rosemary |
| Thieves Vitality | Clove, Lemon, Cinnamon Bark, Eucalyptus Radiata, Rosemary |

| Blend Name | Ingredients |
|---|---|
| **T.R. Care** | Roman Chamomile, Tangerine, Lavender, Bergamot, Royal Hawaiian Sandalwood, Ylang Ylang, Frankincense, Valerian, Blue Cypress, Orange, Geranium, Northern Lights Black Spruce, Davana, Ruta, Jasmine, Angelica, Cedarwood, Helichrysum, Hyssop, Spanish Sage, Patchouli, Citrus Hystrix, White Fir, Blue Tansy, Vetiver, Coriander, Bergamot (furocoumarin-free), Rose, Lemon, Cinnamon Bark, Palmarosa, Matricaria (German Chamomile), Grapefruit, Spearmint, Ocotea |
| **Tranquil Roll-On** | Lavender, Cedarwood, caprylic/capric triglyceride, Roman Chamomile, coconut oil |
| **Transformation** | Lemon, Peppermint, Royal Hawaiian Sandalwood, Clary Sage, Sacred Frankincense, Idaho Blue Spruce, Cardamom, Ocotea, Palo Santo |
| **Trauma Life** | Royal Hawaiian Sandalwood, Frankincense, Valerian, Black Spruce, Davana, Lavender, Geranium, Helichrysum, Citrus Hystrix, Rose |
| **TummyGize** | caprylic/capric glycerides, Spearmint, Peppermint, Tangerine, Fennel, Anise, Ginger, Cardamom |
| **Valor** | caprylic/capric triglyceride, Black Spruce, Rosewood, Blue Tansy, Frankincense |
| **Valor II** | caprylic/capric triglyceride, Ylang Ylang, Coriander, Bergamot, Northern Lights Black Spruce, Matricaria (German Chamomile), Idaho Blue Spruce, Frankincense, Vetiver, Cistus, Cassia, Davana, Geranium |
| **Valor Roll-On** | caprylic/capric triglyceride, Black Spruce, Rosewood, Frankincense, Blue Tansy |
| **White Angelica** | sweet almond oil, Bergamot, Myrrh, Geranium, Royal Hawaiian Sandalwood, Ylang Ylang, Coriander, Black Spruce, Melissa, Hyssop, Rose |
| **White Light** | White Fir, White Cedar, White Spruce, White Pine |

# Appendix D
## Flash Points for Essential Oils

## Single Oils

| | | | | |
|---|---|---|---|---|
| Angelica | 111°F | | Fennel/Fennel Vitality | 168°F |
| Anise | >200°F | | Frankincense/Frankincense Vitality | 102°F |
| Basil/Basil Vitality | 177°F | | Geranium | 181°F |
| Bergamot/Bergamot Vitality | 149°F | | German Chamomile/G. Chamomile Vitality | >200°F |
| Black Pepper/Black Pepper Vitality | 112°F | | Ginger/Ginger Vitality | 168°F |
| Black Spruce | 102°F | | Goldenrod | 118°F |
| Blue Cypress | >200°F | | Grapefruit/Grapefruit Vitality | 133°F |
| Blue Tansy | 137°F | | Helichrysum | 150°F |
| Calamus | 194°F | | Hinoki | 110.9°F |
| Canadian Fleabane (Conyza) | 118°F | | Hong Kuai | 291°F |
| Cardamom/Cardamom Vitality | 154°F | | Hyssop | 158°F |
| Carrot Seed/Carrot Seed Vitality | 144°F | | Idaho Balsam Fir | 118°F |
| Cassia | 152°F | | Idaho Blue Spruce | 111°F |
| Cedarwood | >200°F | | Idaho Tansy | 168°F |
| Celery Seed/Celery Seed Vitality | 123.1°F | | Jade Lemon/Jade Lemon Vitality | 127.3°F |
| Cinnamon Bark/Cinnamon Bark Vitality | 179°F | | Jasmine | >200°F |
| Cistus | 114°F | | Juniper | 104°F |
| Citronella | 147°F | | Laurus Nobilis/Laurus Nobilis Vitality | 142°F |
| Clary Sage | 190°F | | Lavandin | 168°F |
| Clove/Clove Vitality | >200°F | | Lavender/Lavender Vitality | 157°F |
| Coriander/Coriander Vitality | 153°F | | Ledum | 147°F |
| Cumin | 142°F | | Lemon/Lemon Vitality | 109°F |
| Cypress | 103°F | | Lemon Myrtle | 256.8°F |
| Davana | >200°F | | Lemongrass/Lemongrass Vitality | 181°F |
| Dill/Dill Vitality | 150°F | | Lime/Lime Vitality | 109°F |
| Dorado Azul | 121.5°F | | Mandarin | 113°F |
| Elemi | 114°F | | Manuka | 208.4°F |
| Eucalyptus Blue | 114.8°F | | Marjoram/Marjoram Vitality | 149°F |
| Eucalyptus Citriodora | 176°F | | Mastrante | >252°F |
| Eucalyptus Globulus | 114°F | | Melaleuca Ericifolia | 127°F |
| Eucalyptus Radiata | 130°F | | Melaleuca Quinquenervia (Niaouli) | 168°F |

**Essential Oils Desk Reference** | Seventh Edition

| | | | | |
|---|---|---|---|---|
| Melissa | 189°F | | Rosemary/Rosemary Vitality | 116°F |
| Micromeria | >293°F | | Royal Hawaiian Sandalwood | >284 |
| Mountain Savory/Mountain Savory Vitality | 170°F | | Ruta | 159.3°F |
| Myrrh | >200°F | | Sacred Frankincense | 101.9°F |
| Myrtle | 100°F | | Sage/Sage Vitality | 146°F |
| Neroli | 143.1°F | | Spanish Sage | 108°F |
| Northern Lights Black Spruce | 102°F | | Spearmint/Spearmint Vitality | 149°F |
| Nutmeg/Nutmeg Vitality | 110°F | | Tangerine/Tangerine Vitality | 115°F |
| Ocotea | 138.7°F | | Tarragon/Tarragon Vitality | 148°F |
| Orange/Orange Vitality | 142°F | | Tea Tree | 157°F |
| Oregano/Oregano Vitality | 168°F | | Thyme/Thyme Vitality | 162°F |
| Palmarosa | 199°F | | Tsuga | 103°F |
| Palo Santo | 140.1°F | | Valerian | 112°F |
| Patchouli | >200°F | | Vetiver | >200°F |
| Peppermint/Peppermint Vitality | 172°F | | White Fir | 107°F |
| Petitgrain | 150°F | | Wintergreen | 191°F |
| Pine | 103°F | | Xiang Mao | 188.7°F |
| Ravintsara | 124°F | | Yarrow | 172°F |
| Roman Chamomile | 150°F | | Ylang Ylang | >200°F |
| Rose | 156°F | | Yuzu | 114.2°F |

# Blends

| | | | | |
|---|---|---|---|---|
| Abundance | 144°F | | Divine Release | 126.5°F |
| Acceptance | 166°F | | Dragon Time | 171°F |
| Amoressence | 116.1°F | | Dream Catcher | 142°F |
| Aroma Ease | 155.6°F | | Egyptian Gold | 125.1°F |
| Aroma Life | 142°F | | En-R-Gee | 121°F |
| Aroma Siez | 157°F | | EndoFlex/EndoFlex Vitality | 149°F |
| AromaSleep | 141°F | | Envision | 122°F |
| Australian Blue | 150°F | | Exodus II | 165°F |
| Awaken | 164°F | | Forgiveness | 172°F |
| Believe | 129°F | | Freedom | 130.2°F |
| Brain Power | 152°F | | Gathering | 142°F |
| Breathe Again Roll-On | 135.2°F | | Gentle Baby | 170°F |
| Build Your Dream | 134°F | | GLF/GLF Vitality | 134°F |
| Christmas Spirit | 125°F | | Gratitude | 115°F |
| Citrus Fresh/Citrus Fresh Vitality | 125°F | | Grounding | 134°F |
| Clarity | 156°F | | Harmony | 144°F |
| Common Sense | 100.4 °F | | Highest Potential | 155°F |
| Deep Relief Roll-On | 133.4 °F | | Hope | 142°F |
| DiGize/DiGize Vitality | 163°F | | Humility | 194°F |

Flash Points for Essential Oils | **Appendix D**

| | | | | |
|---|---|---|---|---|
| ImmuPower | **132°F** | Peace & Calming | **128°F** |
| Inner Child | **131°F** | Present Time | **142°F** |
| Inner Harmony | **128.3°F** | Purification | **132°F** |
| Inspiration | **153°F** | Raven | **127°F** |
| Into The Future | **152°F** | R.C. | **119°F** |
| InTouch | **168°F** | Reconnect | **125.9°F** |
| Joy | **146°F** | Red Shot | **132.6°F** |
| JuvaCleanse/JuvaCleanse Vitality | **135°F** | Release | **209°F** |
| JuvaFlex/JuvaFlex Vitality | **165°F** | Relieve It | **123°F** |
| Lady Sclareol | **150.8°F** | RutaVaLa Roll-On | **159.3°F** |
| Light the Fire | **126.6°F** | Sacred Mountain | **124°F** |
| Live with Passion | **160.7°F** | SARA | **185°F** |
| Live Your Passion | **126.9°F** | SclarEssence/SclarEssence Vitality | **169°F** |
| Longevity/Longevity Vitality | **137°F** | Sensation | **181°F** |
| M-Grain | **159°F** | Shutran | **125°F** |
| Magnify Your Purpose | **163°F** | Slique Essence | **134.6°F** |
| Melrose | **137°F** | Stress Away | **73.4°F** |
| Mister | **155°F** | Stress Away Roll-On | **74.5°F** |
| Motivation | **131°F** | Surrender | **131°F** |
| Oola Balance | **168.9°F** | The Gift | **109.3°F** |
| Oola Faith | **133.8°F** | Thieves/Thieves Vitality | **144°F** |
| Oola Family | **159.2°F** | T.R. Care | **130.6°F** |
| Oola Field | **148.6°F** | Tranquil Roll-On | **158.4 °F** |
| Oola Finance | **139.1°F** | Transformation | **125.1 °F** |
| Oola Fitness | **148.1°F** | Trauma Life | **133°F** |
| Oola Friends | **160.7°F** | Valor | **143°F** |
| Oola Fun | **149.9°F** | Valor Roll-On | **117.2 °F** |
| PanAway | **187°F** | White Angelica | **180°F** |

Seventh Edition | **Essential Oils Desk Reference** | 599

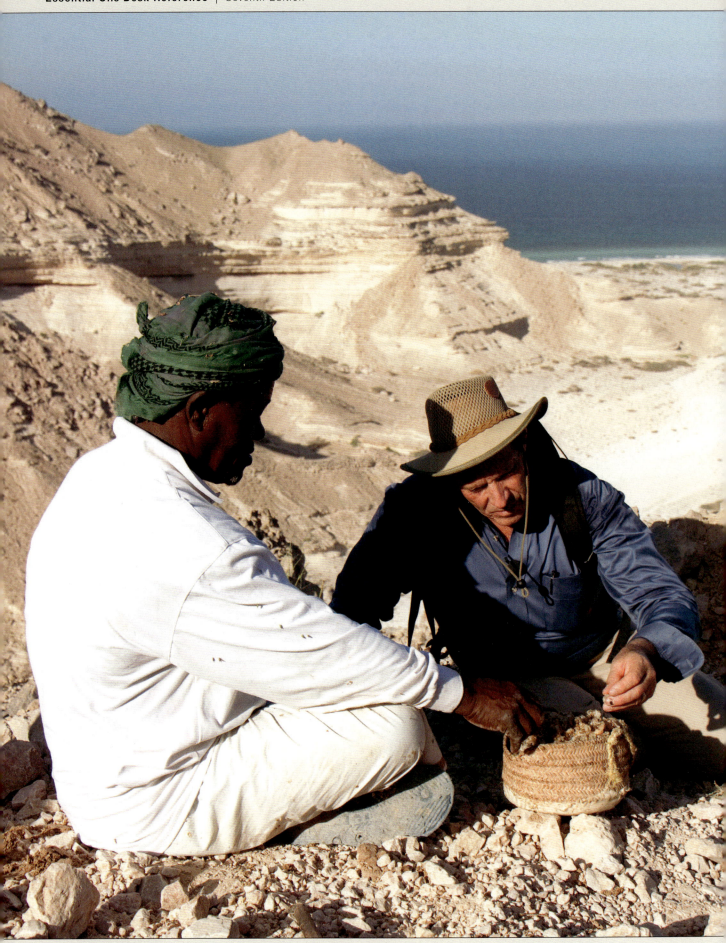

# Appendix E
## Product Usage for Body Systems

**Product Type Key:**

**S** Essential Oil Single  **L** Lotions/Creams/Massage Oils
**B** Essential Oil Blend  **G** Bath and Shower Gels/Soaps
**D** Dietary Supplement  **A** Antiseptic/Sanitizing
**P** Personal Care/Hair and Skin  **O** Oral Care

| Product | Product Type | Nervous System | Cardiovascular System | Respiratory System | Digestive / Elimination | Immune / Anti-infectious | Glandular / Hormonal | Emotional Balance | Muscle and Bone | Antiaging | Oral Hygiene | Skin and Hair |
|---|---|---|---|---|---|---|---|---|---|---|---|---|
| 3 Wise Men | B | | | | | | | ■ | | | | |
| Abundance | B | | | | | ■ | | ■ | | | | |
| Acceptance | B | ■ | | | | | | ■ | | | | |
| AgilEase | D | | | | | ■ | | | ■ | | | |
| AlkaLime | D | | | | ■ | ■ | | | | | | |
| Allerzyme | D | | | | ■ | | | | | | | |
| Amazonian Ylang Ylang | S | | ■ | | | | ■ | ■ | | | | |
| Amoressence | B | | | | | | | ■ | | | | |
| Angelica | S | ■ | | | | | | ■ | | | | |
| Animal Scents Dental Pet Chews (for animals) | O | | | | | | | | | | ■ | |
| Animal Scents Ointment (for animals) | L | | | | | | | | | | | ■ |
| Animal Scents Shampoo (for animals) | G | | | | | | | | | | | ■ |
| Anise | S | | | | ■ | | | | | ■ | | |
| AromaEase | B | | | | | | | | | | | |
| AromaGuard Meadow Mist Deodorant | P | | | | | | | | | | | ■ |
| AromaGuard Mountain Mint Deodorant | P | | | | | | | | | | | ■ |
| Aroma Life | B | | ■ | | | | | ■ | | | | |
| Aroma Siez | B | ■ | | | | | | | ■ | | | |
| AromaSleep | B | ■ | | | | | | ■ | | | | |
| ART Beauty Masque | P | | | | | | | | | | | ■ |
| ART Creme Masque | P | | | | | | | | | | | ■ |
| ART Gentle Cleanser | P | | | | | | | | | | | ■ |
| ART Intensive Moisturizer | P | | | | | | | | | | | ■ |
| ART L'Brianté (all colors and scents) | P | | | | | | | | | | | ■ |
| ART Light Moisturizer | P | | | | | | | | | | | ■ |
| ART Refreshing Toner | P | | | | | | | | | | | ■ |
| ART Renewal Serum | P | | | | | | | | | | | ■ |

# Product

**Product Type Key:**

- **S** Essential Oil Single
- **B** Essential Oil Blend
- **D** Dietary Supplement
- **P** Personal Care/Hair and Skin
- **L** Lotions/Creams/Massage Oils
- **G** Bath and Shower Gels/Soaps
- **A** Antiseptic/Sanitizing
- **O** Oral Care

| Product | Product Type | Nervous System | Cardiovascular System | Respiratory System | Digestive / Elimination | Immune / Anti-infectious | Glandular / Hormonal | Emotional Balance | Muscle and Bone | Antiaging | Oral Hygiene | Skin and Hair |
|---|---|---|---|---|---|---|---|---|---|---|---|---|
| ART Sheerlumé Brightening Cream | P | | | | | | | | | | | ■ |
| Australian Blue | B | | | | | | | ■ | | | | |
| Awaken | B | | | | | | ■ | ■ | | | | |
| Balance Complete | D | ■ | ■ | | ■ | ■ | | | | ■ | | |
| Basil | S | | | | ■ | | | | | | | |
| Basil Vitality | D | | | | ■ | | | | | | | |
| Bath & Shower Gel Base | G | | | | | | | | | | | ■ |
| Believe | B | | | | | | | ■ | | | | |
| Bergamot | S | | | | | | | ■ | | | | |
| Bergamot Vitality | D | | | | ■ | | | ■ | | | | ■ |
| Biblical Sweet Myrrh | S | ■ | | | | ■ | ■ | ■ | | | ■ | |
| Bite Buster | B | ■ | | | | | | | | | | |
| Black Pepper | S | ■ | | | ■ | | | | | | | |
| Black Pepper Vitality | D | ■ | | | ■ | | | | | | | |
| Black Spruce | S | | | ■ | | ■ | | ■ | | | | |
| Blue Agave | D | | | | ■ | ■ | | | | | | |
| Blue Cypress | S | | | | | ■ | | | | | | |
| Blue Tansy | S | ■ | | | | ■ | ■ | | | | | |
| Boswellia Wrinkle Cream | L | | | | | | | | | ■ | | ■ |
| Brain Power | B | ■ | | | | | | ■ | | | | |
| Breathe Again Roll-On | B | | | ■ | | | | | | | | |
| Build Your Dream | B | | | | | | | ■ | | | | |
| Canadian Fleabane (Conyza) | S | | | | | ■ | ■ | | | | | |
| Cardamom | S | | | | ■ | ■ | ■ | | | | | |
| Cardamom Vitality | D | | | | ■ | ■ | ■ | | | | | |
| Carrot Seed | S | | | | ■ | ■ | | | | | | |
| Carrot Seed Vitality | D | | | | ■ | ■ | | | | | | |
| Cassia | S | | | | | ■ | | | | | | |
| Cedarwood | S | ■ | | | | | | ■ | | | | ■ |
| Celery Seed | S | | | | ■ | ■ | | | | | | |
| Celery Seed Vitality | D | | | | ■ | ■ | | | | | | |
| Cel-Lite Magic Massage Oil | L | | | | | | | ■ | | | | ■ |
| Christmas Spirit | B | ■ | | | | | | ■ | | | | |
| Cinnamint Lip Balm | P | | | | | | | | | | | ■ |
| Cinnamon Bark | S | | | | | ■ | ■ | | | | ■ | |
| Cinnamon Bark Vitality | D | | | | | ■ | ■ | | | ■ | | |

## Body Systems Chart | Appendix E

**Product Type Key:**

**S** Essential Oil Single    **L** Lotions/Creams/Massage Oils
**B** Essential Oil Blend    **G** Bath and Shower Gels/Soaps
**D** Dietary Supplement    **A** Antiseptic/Sanitizing
**P** Personal Care/Hair and Skin    **O** Oral Care

| Product | Product Type | Nervous System | Cardiovascular System | Respiratory System | Digestive / Elimination | Immune / Anti-infectious | Glandular / Hormonal | Emotional Balance | Muscle and Bone | Antiaging | Oral Hygiene | Skin and Hair |
|---|---|---|---|---|---|---|---|---|---|---|---|---|
| Cistus | S | | | | | ■ | | | | ■ | | |
| Citronella | S | | | | ■ | | | | ■ | | | ■ |
| Citrus Fresh | B | | | ■ | ■ | | | ■ | | | | |
| Citrus Fresh Vitality | D | | | | ■ | ■ | | ■ | | | | |
| ClaraDerm | P | | | | | | | | | | | ■ |
| Clarity | B | ■ | | | | | | ■ | | | | |
| Clary Sage | S | | | | | ■ | ■ | | | | | |
| Clove | S | | ■ | ■ | ■ | ■ | | | | ■ | ■ | |
| Clove Vitality | D | | ■ | ■ | ■ | ■ | | | | ■ | ■ | |
| ComforTone | D | | | | ■ | | | ■ | | | | |
| Common Sense | B | ■ | | | | | | ■ | | | | |
| Cool Azul | B | | | | | | | | ■ | | | |
| Cool Azul Pain Relief Cream | L | | | | | | | | ■ | | | |
| Cool Azul Sports Gel | L | | | | | | | | ■ | | | |
| Copaiba | S | | | | ■ | | | | ■ | ■ | | |
| Copaiba Vanilla Moisturizing Conditioner | P | | | | | | | | | | | ■ |
| Copaiba Vanilla Moisturizing Shampoo | P | | | | | | | | | | | ■ |
| Copaiba Vitality | D | | | | ■ | | | ■ | ■ | ■ | | |
| Coriander | S | | | | ■ | | ■ | ■ | | | | |
| Coriander Vitality | D | | | | ■ | | ■ | ■ | | | | ■ |
| CortiStop | D | | | | | | ■ | | | | | |
| Cumin | S | | | | ■ | ■ | ■ | | | | | |
| Cypress | S | | ■ | | | | ■ | ■ | | | | |
| Dalmatia Bay Laurel | S | | | | | ■ | | | | ■ | | ■ |
| Dalmatia Juniper | S | | | | ■ | | | | | | | ■ |
| Dalmatia Sage | S | ■ | | | | | | | | | | ■ |
| Deep Relief Roll-On | B | | | | | | | | ■ | | | |
| Detoxzyme | D | | | | ■ | | ■ | | | | | |
| Digest & Cleanse | D | ■ | | | ■ | | ■ | | | | | |
| DiGize | B | | | | ■ | | | | | | | |
| DiGize Vitality | D | | | | ■ | | | | | | | |
| Dill | S | | | | ■ | ■ | | | | | | |
| Dill Vitality | D | | | | ■ | ■ | | | | | | |
| Divine Release | B | ■ | | | | | | ■ | | | | |
| Dorado Azul | S | | | ■ | | ■ | ■ | | ■ | | | |
| Douglas Fir | S | | | ■ | | ■ | | | ■ | | | |

| Product | Product Type | Nervous System | Cardiovascular System | Respiratory System | Digestive / Elimination | Immune / Anti-infectious | Glandular / Hormonal | Emotional Balance | Muscle and Bone | Antiaging | Oral Hygiene | Skin and Hair |
|---|---|---|---|---|---|---|---|---|---|---|---|---|
| Dragon Time | B | | | | | | ■ | ■ | | | | |
| Dragon Time Bath & Shower Gel | G | | | | | | | | | | | ■ |
| Dragon Time Massage Oil | L | | | | | | | ■ | | | | ■ |
| Dream Catcher | B | | | | | | | ■ | | | | |
| Ecuadorian Dark Chocolessence | D | | | | ■ | | | | | ■ | | |
| Egyptian Gold | B | ■ | | ■ | | ■ | | ■ | | | | |
| Elemi | S | | | | | ■ | | | ■ | | | ■ |
| EndoFlex | B | | | | ■ | | ■ | | | | | |
| EndoFlex Vitality | D | | | | ■ | | ■ | | | | | |
| EndoGize | B | | | | | | ■ | | | | | |
| En-R-Gee | B | ■ | | | | | | ■ | | | | |
| Envision | B | | | | | | | ■ | | | | |
| Essential Beauty Serum (Dry Skin) | P | | | | | | | | | | | ■ |
| Essentialzyme | D | | | | ■ | | | | | | | |
| Essentialzymes-4 | D | | | | ■ | | | | | | | |
| Estro | D | | | | | | ■ | ■ | | | | |
| Eucalyptus Blue | S | | | ■ | | ■ | | ■ | | | | |
| Eucalyptus Citriodora | S | | | ■ | | ■ | | | | | | |
| Eucalyptus Dives | S | | | ■ | | ■ | | | | | | |
| Eucalyptus Globulus | S | | | ■ | | ■ | | | | | | |
| Eucalyptus Polybractea | S | | | ■ | | ■ | | | | | | |
| Eucalyptus Radiata | S | | | ■ | | ■ | | | | | | ■ |
| Evening Peace Bath & Shower Gel | G | | | | | | | | | | | ■ |
| Evergreen Essence | B | ■ | | | | | | ■ | | | | |
| Exodus II | B | ■ | | | | ■ | | | | | | |
| FemiGen | D | | | | | | ■ | ■ | | | | |
| Fennel | S | | | | ■ | ■ | ■ | | | | | |
| Fennel Vitality | D | | | | ■ | ■ | ■ | | | | | |
| Forgiveness | B | | | | | | | ■ | | | | |
| Frankincense | S | ■ | | | | ■ | | ■ | | ■ | | ■ |
| Frankincense Vitality | D | ■ | | | | ■ | | ■ | | ■ | | ■ |
| Freedom | B | ■ | | | | | | ■ | | | | |
| Frereana Frankincense | S | | | | | ■ | | ■ | | | | |
| Gary's Equine Essentials (for animals) | P | | | | | | | | | | | ■ |
| Gary's True Grit Chocolate-Coated Wolfberry Crisp Bars | D | | | | ■ | | | | | | | |
| Gary's True Grit Einkorn Flour | D | | | | ■ | | | | | | | |

**Product Type Key:**

**S** Essential Oil Single  **L** Lotions/Creams/Massage Oils
**B** Essential Oil Blend  **G** Bath and Shower Gels/Soaps
**D** Dietary Supplement  **A** Antiseptic/Sanitizing
**P** Personal Care/Hair and Skin  **O** Oral Care

# Product

| Product | Product Type | Nervous System | Cardiovascular System | Respiratory System | Digestive / Elimination | Immune / Anti-infectious | Glandular / Hormonal | Emotional Balance | Muscle and Bone | Antiaging | Oral Hygiene | Skin and Hair |
|---|---|---|---|---|---|---|---|---|---|---|---|---|
| Gary's True Grit Einkorn Granola | D | | | | ■ | | | | | | | |
| Gary's True Grit Einkorn Pancake and Waffle Mix | D | | | | ■ | | | | | | | |
| Gary's True Grit Einkorn Rotini Pasta | D | | | | ■ | | | | | | | |
| Gary's True Grit Einkorn Spaghetti | D | | | | ■ | | | | | | | |
| Gary's True Grit Gluten-Free Pancake and Waffle Mix | D | | | | ■ | | | | | | | |
| Gary's True Grit NingXia Berry Syrup | D | | | | ■ | | | | | | | |
| Gathering | B | | | | | | | ■ | | | | |
| Genesis Hand & Body Lotion | L | | | | | | | | | | | ■ |
| GeneYus | B | ■ | | | | | | ■ | | | | |
| Gentle Baby | B | | | | | | | ■ | | | | ■ |
| Geranium | S | | | | ■ | ■ | | ■ | | | | ■ |
| German Chamomile | S | ■ | | | ■ | | | ■ | | | | ■ |
| German Chamomile Vitality | D | ■ | | | ■ | | | ■ | | | | |
| Ginger | S | ■ | | | ■ | | | | | | | |
| Ginger Vitality | D | ■ | | | ■ | | | | | | | |
| GLF | B | | | | ■ | ■ | | | | | | |
| Goldenrod | S | | ■ | | | | ■ | | | | | |
| Grapefruit | S | | ■ | ■ | | | ■ | ■ | | ■ | | |
| Grapefruit Lip Balm | P | | | | | | | | | | ■ | |
| Grapefruit Vitality | D | | ■ | ■ | | | ■ | | | ■ | | |
| Gratitude | B | | | | | | | ■ | | | | |
| Grounding | B | | | | | | | ■ | | | | |
| Harmony | B | | | | | | | ■ | | | | |
| Helichrysum | S | | ■ | | | ■ | | | | | | ■ |
| Highest Potential | B | | | | | | | ■ | | | | |
| Hinoki | S | ■ | | | | ■ | | ■ | | ■ | | ■ |
| Hong Kuai | S | | | ■ | | | | ■ | | | | ■ |
| Hope | B | | | | | | | ■ | | | | |
| Humility | B | | | | | | | ■ | | | | |
| Hyssop | S | ■ | ■ | ■ | | ■ | | | | | | |
| ICP | D | | | | ■ | | | | | | | |
| Idaho Balsam Fir | S | ■ | | | | ■ | ■ | ■ | | | | |
| Idaho Blue Spruce | S | | | ■ | | ■ | | ■ | ■ | | | |
| Idaho Tansy | S | | | ■ | | ■ | | | | | | |
| ImmuPower | B | | | | | ■ | | | ■ | | | |
| ImmuPro | D | | | | | ■ | | | | ■ | | |

**Essential Oils Desk Reference** | Seventh Edition

## Product Type Key:
**S** Essential Oil Single
**B** Essential Oil Blend
**D** Dietary Supplement
**P** Personal Care/Hair and Skin
**L** Lotions/Creams/Massage Oils
**G** Bath and Shower Gels/Soaps
**A** Antiseptic/Sanitizing
**O** Oral Care

## Product

| Product | Product Type | Nervous System | Cardiovascular System | Respiratory System | Digestive / Elimination | Immune / Anti-infectious | Glandular / Hormonal | Emotional Balance | Muscle and Bone | Antiaging | Oral Hygiene | Skin and Hair |
|---|---|---|---|---|---|---|---|---|---|---|---|---|
| Infect Away (for animals) | A | | | | | ■ | | | | | | ■ |
| Inner Child | B | | | | | | | ■ | | | | |
| Inner Defense | D | | | ■ | | ■ | | | | | | |
| Inner Harmony | B | | | | | | | ■ | | | | |
| Inspiration | B | | | | | | | ■ | | | | |
| InTouch | B | | | | | | | ■ | | | | |
| Into the Future | B | | | | | | | ■ | | | | |
| Jade Lemon | S | | | ■ | ■ | ■ | | | | ■ | | |
| Jade Lemon Vitality | D | | | ■ | ■ | ■ | | | | ■ | | |
| Jasmine | S | | | | | | ■ | ■ | | | | |
| Joy | B | | | | | | | ■ | | | | |
| Juniper | S | | | | ■ | | | ■ | | | | |
| JuvaCleanse | B | | | | ■ | | | | | ■ | | |
| JuvaCleanse Vitality | D | | | | ■ | | | | | ■ | | |
| JuvaFlex | B | | | | ■ | | | ■ | | | | |
| JuvaFlex Vitality | D | | | | ■ | | | ■ | | | | |
| JuvaPower | D | | | | ■ | | ■ | | | ■ | | |
| JuvaSpice | D | | | | ■ | | | | | | | |
| JuvaTone | D | | | | ■ | | ■ | | | | | |
| K&B | D | | | | ■ | | | | | | | |
| KidScents Bath Gel | G | | | | | | | | | | | ■ |
| KidScents Lotion | L | | | | | | | | | | | ■ |
| KidScents MightyVites | D | ■ | ■ | ■ | ■ | ■ | ■ | | ■ | | | |
| KidScents MightyZyme | D | | | | ■ | | | | | | | |
| KidScents Shampoo | P | | | | | | | | | | | ■ |
| KidScents Slique Toothpaste | O | | | | | | | | | | ■ | |
| KidScents Tender Tush | L | | | | | | | | | | | ■ |
| Lady Sclareol | B | | | | | | ■ | ■ | | | | |
| Laurus Nobilis (Bay Laurel) | S | | | ■ | ■ | ■ | | | | | ■ | |
| LavaDerm Cooling Mist | P | | | | | | | ■ | | | | |
| Lavender | S | ■ | ■ | | | ■ | | ■ | | | | ■ |
| Lavender Bath & Shower Gel | G | | | | | | | | | | | ■ |
| Lavender Conditioner | P | | | | | | | | | | | ■ |
| Lavender Foaming Hand Soap | G | | | | | | | | | | | ■ |
| Lavender Hand & Body Lotion | L | | | | | | | | | | | ■ |
| Lavender Lip Balm | P | | | | | | | | | | ■ | |

**Product Type Key:**

**S** Essential Oil Single  **L** Lotions/Creams/Massage Oils
**B** Essential Oil Blend  **G** Bath and Shower Gels/Soaps
**D** Dietary Supplement  **A** Antiseptic/Sanitizing
**P** Personal Care/Hair and Skin  **O** Oral Care

# Product

| Product | Product Type | Nervous System | Cardiovascular System | Respiratory System | Digestive / Elimination | Immune / Anti-infectious | Glandular / Hormonal | Emotional Balance | Muscle and Bone | Antiaging | Oral Hygiene | Skin and Hair |
|---|---|---|---|---|---|---|---|---|---|---|---|---|
| Lavender Mint Daily Conditioner | P | | | | | | | | | | | ■ |
| Lavender Mint Daily Shampoo | P | | | | | | | | | | | ■ |
| Lavender-Oatmeal Bar Soap | G | | | | | | | | | | | ■ |
| Lavender Shampoo | P | | | | | | | | | | | ■ |
| Lavender Vitality | D | ■ | ■ | | | ■ | | ■ | | | | |
| Ledum | S | | | | | ■ | ■ | | | ■ | | |
| Lemon | S | | | ■ | ■ | ■ | | ■ | | ■ | | |
| Lemongrass | S | | | | ■ | ■ | | ■ | | | | |
| Lemongrass Vitality | D | | | | ■ | ■ | | ■ | | | | |
| Lemon Myrtle | S | | | ■ | | ■ | | | | | | |
| Lemon-Sandalwood Cleansing Soap | G | | | | | | | | | | | ■ |
| Lemon Vitality | D | | | ■ | ■ | ■ | | ■ | | | | |
| Life 9 | D | | | | ■ | | | | | ■ | | |
| Light the Fire | B | | | | | | | ■ | | | | |
| Lime | S | | | ■ | ■ | ■ | | | | ■ | ■ | |
| Lime Vitality | D | | | ■ | ■ | ■ | | | | ■ | ■ | |
| Live with Passion | B | | | | | | | ■ | | | | |
| Live Your Passion | B | | | | | | | ■ | | | | |
| Longevity | B | | ■ | | ■ | | | | | ■ | | |
| Longevity Softgels | D | | ■ | | ■ | | | | | ■ | | |
| Longevity Vitality | D | | ■ | | ■ | | | | | | | |
| Magnify Your Purpose | B | ■ | | | | | | ■ | | | | |
| Mandarin | S | | | | ■ | | | | | ■ | | ■ |
| Manuka | S | | | ■ | | ■ | | | ■ | | | ■ |
| Marjoram | S | | ■ | | ■ | | | | ■ | | | ■ |
| Marjoram Vitality | D | | ■ | | ■ | | | | ■ | | | ■ |
| Master Formula | D | ■ | ■ | ■ | ■ | ■ | | | ■ | ■ | | |
| Mastrante | S | ■ | ■ | ■ | | ■ | | ■ | | | | |
| MegaCal | D | | ■ | | | | | | ■ | | | |
| Melaleuca Cajuput | S | | | ■ | ■ | ■ | | | ■ | | ■ | ■ |
| Melaleuca Ericifolia | S | | | ■ | | ■ | | | | | | ■ |
| Melaleuca-Geranium Moisturizing Soap | G | | | | | | | | | | | ■ |
| Melaleuca Quinquenervia (Niaouli) | S | | | ■ | ■ | | | | ■ | | | |
| Melissa | S | | | | | ■ | ■ | ■ | | ■ | | ■ |
| Melrose | B | | | ■ | | | | | | | | ■ |
| Mendwell (for animals) | P | | | | | | | | | | | ■ |

**Product Type Key:**

**S** Essential Oil Single  **L** Lotions/Creams/Massage Oils
**B** Essential Oil Blend  **G** Bath and Shower Gels/Soaps
**D** Dietary Supplement  **A** Antiseptic/Sanitizing
**P** Personal Care/Hair and Skin  **O** Oral Care

# Product

| Product | Product Type | Nervous System | Cardiovascular System | Respiratory System | Digestive / Elimination | Immune / Anti-infectious | Glandular / Hormonal | Emotional Balance | Muscle and Bone | Antiaging | Oral Hygiene | Skin and Hair |
|---|---|---|---|---|---|---|---|---|---|---|---|---|
| Micromeria | S | | | | ■ | | | ■ | | ■ | | |
| M-Grain | B | ■ | | | | | | | | ■ | | |
| MindWise | D | ■ | ■ | | | | | | | | | |
| Mineral Essence | D | ■ | ■ | | | | ■ | ■ | ■ | ■ | | |
| Mirah Shave Oil | P | | | | | | | | | | | ■ |
| Mister | B | | | | | | ■ | | | | | |
| Morning Start Bath & Shower Gel | G | | | | | | | | | | | ■ |
| Morning Start Moisturizing Soap | G | | | | | | | | | | | ■ |
| Motivation | B | ■ | | | | | | ■ | | | | |
| Mountain Savory | S | | | | | ■ | | | | ■ | | |
| MultiGreens | D | ■ | ■ | | ■ | ■ | | | ■ | | | |
| Myrrh | S | ■ | | | | ■ | ■ | | | | | ■ |
| Myrtle | S | | | ■ | ■ | ■ | ■ | | ■ | | | |
| Neroli | S | | | | ■ | ■ | | ■ | | | | ■ |
| Niaouli (see also Melaleuca Quinquenervia) | S | | | | ■ | | | | ■ | | | |
| Ningxia Dried Wolfberries (Organic) | D | ■ | ■ | | | ■ | ■ | | | ■ | | |
| NingXia Nitro | D | ■ | ■ | | | ■ | ■ | | | ■ | | |
| NingXia Red | D | ■ | ■ | | | ■ | ■ | | | ■ | | |
| NingXia Zyng | D | ■ | ■ | | | ■ | ■ | | | ■ | | |
| Northern Lights Black Spruce | S | | | ■ | | ■ | | ■ | | | | |
| Nutmeg | S | ■ | | | ■ | ■ | ■ | | | | | |
| Nutmeg Vitality | D | ■ | | | ■ | ■ | ■ | | | | | |
| Ocotea | S | | | | ■ | ■ | | | | ■ | | |
| OmegaGize[3] | D | ■ | ■ | | | ■ | ■ | | ■ | ■ | | ■ |
| Oola Balance | B | | | | | | | ■ | | | | |
| Oola Faith | B | | | | | | | ■ | | | | |
| Oola Family | B | | | | | | | ■ | | | | |
| Oola Field | B | | | | | | | ■ | | | | |
| Oola Finance | B | | | | | | | ■ | | | | |
| Oola Fitness | B | | | | | | | ■ | | | | |
| Oola Friends | B | | | | | | | ■ | | | | |
| Oola Fun | B | | | | | | | ■ | | | | |
| Oola Grow | B | | | | | | | ■ | | | | |
| Orange | S | | | | ■ | ■ | | ■ | | ■ | | ■ |
| Orange Blossom Facial Wash | P | | | | | | | | | | | ■ |
| Orange Vitality | D | | | | ■ | ■ | | ■ | | ■ | | ■ |

## Product Type Key:

**S** Essential Oil Single    **L** Lotions/Creams/Massage Oils
**B** Essential Oil Blend    **G** Bath and Shower Gels/Soaps
**D** Dietary Supplement    **A** Antiseptic/Sanitizing
**P** Personal Care/Hair and Skin    **O** Oral Care

| Product | Product Type | Nervous System | Cardiovascular System | Respiratory System | Digestive / Elimination | Immune / Anti-infectious | Glandular / Hormonal | Emotional Balance | Muscle and Bone | Antiaging | Oral Hygiene | Skin and Hair |
|---|---|---|---|---|---|---|---|---|---|---|---|---|
| Oregano | S | | | ■ | ■ | ■ | | ■ | ■ | ■ | | |
| Oregano Vitality | D | | | ■ | ■ | ■ | | ■ | ■ | ■ | | |
| Ortho Ease Massage Oil | L | | | | | | | | ■ | | | ■ |
| Ortho Sport Massage Oil | L | | | | | | | | ■ | | | ■ |
| Owie | B | | | | | | | | | | | ■ |
| Palmarosa | S | | ■ | | | ■ | | ■ | | | | ■ |
| Palo Santo | S | ■ | | | | ■ | | ■ | | ■ | | |
| PanAway | B | ■ | | | | | | | ■ | | | |
| ParaFree | D | | | | ■ | ■ | | | | | | |
| ParaGize (for animals) | D | | | | ■ | | | | | | | |
| Patchouli | S | | | | | ■ | | | | ■ | | ■ |
| PD 80/20 | D | | | ■ | | ■ | ■ | ■ | | | | |
| Peace & Calming | B | ■ | | | | | | ■ | | | | |
| Peace & Calming II | B | ■ | | | | | | ■ | | | | |
| Peppermint | S | ■ | | ■ | ■ | ■ | | | ■ | | ■ | ■ |
| Peppermint-Cedarwood Moisturizing Soap | G | | | | | | | | | | | ■ |
| Peppermint Vitality | D | ■ | | ■ | ■ | ■ | | | ■ | | ■ | ■ |
| Petitgrain | S | | | | | | ■ | ■ | | ■ | | |
| Pine | S | | | ■ | | ■ | | ■ | | | | |
| Plectranthus Oregano | S | | | ■ | ■ | ■ | | | ■ | ■ | | |
| PowerGize | D | ■ | | | | | | | ■ | | | |
| Prenolone Plus Body Cream | L | ■ | | | | | ■ | ■ | ■ | | | |
| Present Time | B | | | | | | | ■ | | | | |
| Progessence Plus | P | | | | | | ■ | | | | | |
| Prostate Health | D | | | | | | ■ | | | | | |
| Protec | B | | | | | | ■ | | | | | |
| Pure Protein Complete | D | | | | | | | | ■ | ■ | | |
| PuriClean (for animals) | A | | | | | ■ | | | | | | ■ |
| Purification | B | | | | | ■ | | | | | | ■ |
| Raven | B | | | ■ | | ■ | | | | | | |
| Ravintsara | S | | | ■ | | ■ | | | | | ■ | |
| R.C. | B | | | ■ | | ■ | | | | | | |
| Reconnect | B | | | | | | | ■ | | | | |
| Red Shot | B | | | | ■ | | | | | | | |
| Regenolone Moisturizing Cream | L | ■ | | | | | ■ | | ■ | | | ■ |
| Rehemogen | D | | ■ | | ■ | | | | | | | |

# Product

**Product Type Key:**

**S** Essential Oil Single    **L** Lotions/Creams/Massage Oils
**B** Essential Oil Blend    **G** Bath and Shower Gels/Soaps
**D** Dietary Supplement    **A** Antiseptic/Sanitizing
**P** Personal Care/Hair and Skin    **O** Oral Care

| Product | Product Type | Nervous System | Cardiovascular System | Respiratory System | Digestive / Elimination | Immune / Anti-infectious | Glandular / Hormonal | Emotional Balance | Muscle and Bone | Antiaging | Oral Hygiene | Skin and Hair |
|---|---|---|---|---|---|---|---|---|---|---|---|---|
| Relaxation Massage Oil | L | | | | | | | ■ | | | | ■ |
| Release | B | | | | | | ■ | ■ | | | | |
| Relieve It | B | | | | | | | | ■ | | | |
| RepelAroma (for animals) | B | | | | | | | | | | | ■ |
| Roman Chamomile | S | ■ | | | ■ | ■ | | ■ | | | | ■ |
| Roman Chamomile Vitality | D | ■ | | | ■ | ■ | | ■ | | | | ■ |
| Rose | S | | | | | | | ■ | | ■ | | ■ |
| Rosemary (CT cineol) | S | | ■ | | ■ | | ■ | | ■ | | | |
| Rosemary Vitality | D | | ■ | | ■ | | ■ | | ■ | | | |
| Rose Ointment | P | | | | | | | | | | | ■ |
| Royal Hawaiian Sandalwood | S | ■ | | | | ■ | | ■ | ■ | | | ■ |
| Royal Hawaiian Sandalwood Soaps | G | | | | | | | | | | | ■ |
| RutaVaLa | B | ■ | | | | | | ■ | | | | |
| RutaVaLa Roll-On | B | ■ | | | | | | ■ | | | | |
| Sacred Frankincense | S | | | | | ■ | | ■ | ■ | | | ■ |
| Sacred Mountain | B | | | | | | | ■ | | | | |
| Sacred Mountain Moisturizing Soap | G | | | | | | | | | | | ■ |
| Sage | S | | | | ■ | ■ | ■ | ■ | | | | |
| Sage Vitality | D | | | | ■ | ■ | ■ | ■ | | | | |
| Sandalwood Moisture Cream | P | | | | | | | | | | | ■ |
| SARA | B | | | | | | | ■ | | | | |
| Satin Facial Scrub, Mint | P | | | | | | | | | | | ■ |
| SclarEssence | B | | | | | | ■ | ■ | | | | |
| Sensation | B | | | | | | | ■ | | | | ■ |
| Sensation Bath & Shower Gel | G | | | | | | | | | | | ■ |
| Sensation Hand & Body Lotion | L | | | | | | | | | | | ■ |
| Sensation Massage Oil | L | | | | | | | ■ | | | | ■ |
| Shutran | B | | | | | | | ■ | | | | |
| Shutran Aftershave Lotion | P | | | | | | | | | | | ■ |
| Shutran Bar Soap | P | | | | | | | | | | | ■ |
| Shutran Shave Cream | P | | | | | | | | | | | ■ |
| SleepEssence | D | | | | | | | ■ | | | | |
| SleepyIze | B | | | | | | | ■ | | | | |
| Slique Bars | D | | | | ■ | | | | | | | |
| Slique Bars - Chocolate-Coated | D | | | | ■ | | | | | | | |
| Slique CitraSlim | D | | | | ■ | | | | | | | |

## Product Type Key:

**S** Essential Oil Single
**B** Essential Oil Blend
**D** Dietary Supplement
**P** Personal Care/Hair and Skin

**L** Lotions/Creams/Massage Oils
**G** Bath and Shower Gels/Soaps
**A** Antiseptic/Sanitizing
**O** Oral Care

## Product

| Product | Product Type | Nervous System | Cardiovascular System | Respiratory System | Digestive / Elimination | Immune / Anti-infectious | Glandular / Hormonal | Emotional Balance | Muscle and Bone | Antiaging | Oral Hygiene | Skin and Hair |
|---|---|---|---|---|---|---|---|---|---|---|---|---|
| Slique Essence | B | | | | ■ | | | | | | | |
| Slique Gum | O | | | | ■ | | | | | | ■ | |
| Slique Shake | D | | | | ■ | | | | | | | |
| Slique Tea | D | | | | ■ | | | | | | | |
| SniffleEase | B | | | ■ | | | | | | | | |
| Spanish Sage | S | ■ | ■ | ■ | ■ | ■ | ■ | ■ | ■ | ■ | | ■ |
| Spearmint | S | | | | ■ | ■ | | ■ | | | | |
| Spearmint Vitality | D | | | | ■ | ■ | | ■ | | | | |
| Stevia Extract | D | | | | ■ | ■ | ■ | | | | | |
| Stress Away (and Roll-On) | B | | | | | | | ■ | | | | |
| Sulfurzyme (Capsules and Powder) | D | ■ | | | | ■ | | | ■ | ■ | | ■ |
| Super B | D | ■ | ■ | | | | | ■ | | | | |
| Super C (and Chewable) | D | | | | ■ | ■ | | | | ■ | | |
| Super Cal | D | ■ | ■ | | | | | ■ | ■ | | | |
| Surrender | B | ■ | | | | | | ■ | | | | |
| Tangerine | S | | | | ■ | ■ | | ■ | | ■ | | ■ |
| Tangerine Vitality | D | | | | ■ | ■ | | ■ | | ■ | | ■ |
| Tarragon | S | ■ | | | ■ | | | | | | | |
| Tarragon Vitality | D | ■ | | | ■ | | | | | | | |
| T-Away (for animals) | B | | | | | | | ■ | | | | ■ |
| Tea Tree | S | | | ■ | | ■ | | | ■ | | ■ | ■ |
| The Gift | B | ■ | | | | ■ | ■ | ■ | | | | |
| Thieves | B | | | | | ■ | | | | ■ | ■ | |
| Thieves AromaBright Toothpaste | O | | | | | ■ | | | | | ■ | |
| Thieves Automatic Dishwasher Powder | A | | | | | ■ | | | | | | |
| Thieves Cleansing Soap | A | | | | | ■ | | | | | | ■ |
| Thieves Cough Drops | D | | | ■ | | ■ | | | | ■ | | |
| Thieves Dental Floss | O | | | | | | | | | | ■ | |
| Thieves Dentarome Plus Toothpaste | O | | | | | | | | | | ■ | |
| Thieves Dentarome Ultra Toothpaste | O | | | | | | | | | | ■ | |
| Thieves Dish Soap | A | | | | | ■ | | | | | | |
| Thieves Foaming Hand Soap | A | | | | | ■ | | | | | | ■ |
| Thieves Fresh Essence Plus Mouthwash | O | | | | | ■ | | | | | ■ | |
| Thieves Fruit & Veggie Soak (and Spray) | A | | | | | ■ | | | | | | |
| Thieves Hard Lozenges | O | | | ■ | | ■ | | | | | ■ | |
| Thieves Household Cleaner | A | | | | | ■ | | | | | | |

**Product Type Key:**
- **S** Essential Oil Single
- **B** Essential Oil Blend
- **D** Dietary Supplement
- **P** Personal Care/Hair and Skin
- **L** Lotions/Creams/Massage Oils
- **G** Bath and Shower Gels/Soaps
- **A** Antiseptic/Sanitizing
- **O** Oral Care

# Product

| Product | Product Type | Nervous System | Cardiovascular System | Respiratory System | Digestive / Elimination | Immune / Anti-infectious | Glandular / Hormonal | Emotional Balance | Muscle and Bone | Antiaging | Oral Hygiene | Skin and Hair |
|---|---|---|---|---|---|---|---|---|---|---|---|---|
| Thieves Laundry Soap | A | | | | | ■ | | | | | | |
| Thieves Mints | O | | | | | ■ | | | | | ■ | |
| Thieves Spray | A | | | | | ■ | | | | | ■ | ■ |
| Thieves Vitality | D | | | | | ■ | | | | ■ | ■ | |
| Thieves Waterless Hand Purifier | A | | | | | ■ | | | | | | ■ |
| Thieves Wipes | A | | | | | ■ | | | | | | |
| Thyme | S | | | | ■ | ■ | | | ■ | ■ | | |
| Thyme Vitality | D | | | | ■ | ■ | | | ■ | ■ | | |
| Thyromin | D | | | | | | ■ | | | | | |
| T.R. Care | B | ■ | | | | | | ■ | | | | |
| Tranquil Roll-On | B | ■ | | | | | | ■ | | | | |
| Transformation | B | ■ | | | | | | ■ | | | | |
| Trauma Life | B | ■ | | | | | | ■ | | | | |
| Tsuga | S | | ■ | ■ | | | | | | | | |
| TummyGize | B | | | | ■ | | | | | | | |
| Ultra Young | D | | | | | | ■ | | | ■ | | |
| V-6 Vegetable Oil Complex | L | | | | | | | | ■ | | | ■ |
| Valerian | S | ■ | | | | | | ■ | | | | |
| Valerian Vitality | D | ■ | | | | | | ■ | | | | |
| Valor | B | ■ | | | | | | ■ | | | | |
| Valor II | B | ■ | | | | | | ■ | | | | |
| Valor Moisturizing Soap | P | | | | | | | | | | | ■ |
| Valor Roll-On | B | ■ | | | | | | ■ | ■ | | | ■ |
| Vetiver | S | ■ | | | | ■ | | ■ | | | | ■ |
| Western Red Cedar | S | | | | | ■ | | | | | | ■ |
| White Angelica | B | | | | | | | ■ | | | | |
| White Fir | S | | | | | | | ■ | ■ | ■ | | |
| White Light | B | | | | | | | ■ | | | | |
| White Lotus | S | | | | ■ | ■ | | ■ | | ■ | | |
| Wintergreen | S | | | | | | | | ■ | | | |
| Wolfberry Eye Cream | L | | | | | | | | | ■ | | ■ |
| Xiang Mao | S | | | | | ■ | | ■ | | | | ■ |
| Yacon Syrup | D | | | | ■ | | | | | | | |
| Yarrow | S | | | | | | ■ | ■ | | | | |
| Ylang Ylang | S | | ■ | | | | ■ | ■ | | | | |
| Yuzu | S | ■ | | | | ■ | ■ | ■ | | | | |

# Index

3 Wise Men: 143, **144**, 151, **311**, 314, 333, 373, 412, 414, 415, 430, 437, 468, 469, 480, 497, 511, 525, 536, 542, 548, 554, 565, 576, 579, 582, 584, 587, 591, 601

Abscesses: 124, **544**

Absentmindedness: **429**

Absolutes: 18, **41**

Abundance: 8, 12, 50, 89, 91, 100, **143**, 144, 145, 157, 171, 175, 281, 312-316, 373, 412, 415, 492, 493, 576, 577, 579, 580, 584, 585, 591, 598, 601

Abuse: 130, 161, 164, 311, **312**, **415**, 430, 537, 565

Acceptance: 144, **145**, 271, 313-316, 373, 412, 415, 417-419, 434, 447, 511, 521, 522, 538, 539, 575-581, 583-589, 591, 598, 601

Acidosis: **415**, 450

Acne: 31, 32, 76, 78-80, 87, 93, 94, 103-106, 108, 109, 115, 119, 120, 125, 126, 128, 130, 133, 134, 137, 243, 382, 417, 510, **545**, 547, 554, 567

Acquired Immune Deficiency Syndrome: 418

Acupressure: 5, **54**, **282**

Acupuncture: 5, **53**, 54, **285**, 407

ADD: 357, **424**, 489, 522

Addictions: 154, **416**, 419, 467, 554

Addison's Disease: **416**

ADHD: 76, 85, 125, 137, **424**

Adrenal Gland Disorders: **416**

Adulterated Oils: v, **25**, 123

Adulteration: v, 4, **24**, 32, 33, 35, 47, 48

Aftershave Lotion: 235, 576, 578, 581-585, 589, 610

Agave: 4, 49, 155, 171, 204, 326, 331, 335, 338, 341, **393-394**, 397, 410, 416, 425, 426, 485, 507, 540, 561, 602

Age-Related Macular Degeneration: 196, 206, 363, **472**

AgilEase: **169**, 267, 409, 412, 423, 424, 427, 428, 433, 449, 454, 455, 476, 483, 495, 512-514, 517, 520-523, 529, 536, 556-559, 566, 601

Aging: iv, 33, 73, 137, 146, 155, 173, 175, 178, 181, 183, 185, 198-201, 204, 206, 208, 210, 212, 237, 320, 331, 347, 349, 354, **361-364**, 389, 395, 398, 405, 406,

473, 552, 553, 567

Agitation: 70, 73, 97, **312**, 375, **418**

Agrichemicals: **22**

AIDS: 11, 130, 179, 184, 211, 225, 249, 346, 349, 354, 389, **418**, 421, 452, 506, 518

Alcoholism: **419**, 518

Alcohols: **17-20**, 41, 47

Aldehydes: **17-19**, 35, 47, 140, 310, 326

AlkaLime: **169**, 322, 334, 388, 412, 415, 416, 420, 425-428, 431, 437, 448, 452, 453, 456, 460-464, 476, 479, 482, 483, 488, 491, 495, 515, 526, 551, 583, 601

Alkalinity: iii, 169, **321**, 322, 419

Alkalosis: **419**

Alkanes: **17-18**, 237-239

Allergic Rhinitis: **420**

Allergies: 49, **51**, 88, 112, 146, 169, 276, 320, 321, 332, 345, 348, 349, 351, 355, 382, **419**, 420, 427, 478, 484, 489, 501, 523, 524, 545, 549-551, 561, 564

Allerzyme: 168, **169**, 325, 327, 332, 335, 344, 346, 351, 387, 412, 413, 415, 419, 420, 427, 450, 459, 463, 471, 484, 485, 511-513, 520, 575, 579, 580, 582, 583, 585, 586, 588, 601

Alopecia Areata: 76, 126, **484**, 567

ALS: 516, **519**, 520

Aluminum: 22, 44, 51, 52, 219, 220, 358, 429, **487**

Aluminum Toxicity: 219, **487**

Alzheimer's: 32, 77, 82, 84, 96, 126, 130-134, 210, 220, 357, 393, **429**, 487, 523

Amazonian Ylang Ylang: 43, 67, **68**, 237, 415, 422, 434, 441, 443, 444, 446, 457, 511, 519, 520, 531, 571, 573, 589, 601

Amber Waves of Grain: **175-176**

AMD: **472-473**

Amino Acids: 174, 180, 184-186, 191, 193-196, 201, 203, 222, **327-354**, 378, 379, 382, 388, 397

Amoressence: **144**, 225, 412, 415, 418, 419, 469, 531, 565, 580, 581, 585, 586, 589, 591, 598, 601

Amygdala: 26, 27, 292, **309**, 374, 406, 467, 470, 525, 565

Analgesic: 19, 69, 71, 73, 78, 80, 82, 85, 88, 90, 93, 99, 101, 104, 111, 114-116, 124,

127, 129, 135, 139, 206, 244, **420**

Anemia: 220, **438**, 482, 506, 536

Aneurysm: **438**, 446

Angelica: 20, 43, 49, 50, 57, **67-69**, 144, 148, 150, 152, 153, 155-157, 162, 164, 206, 237, 239, 266, 293, 295, 297, 298, 303, 308, 311-316, 333, 373, 411, 412, 414, 415, 418, 419, 422, 433, 434, 464, 469, 525, 531, 532, 553, 554, 571, 573, 575, 576, 578, 580, 581, 584, 586, 587, 589, 592-597, 599, 601, 612

Anger: 27, 68, 83, 84, 94, 125, 141, 148, 152, 154, 160, 164, 282, 309, 311, **312**, 332, 433, 519, 558, 566

Angina: 103, 395, **438**

Animal Scents Dental Pet Chews: **265**, 588, 601

Animal Scents Essential Oil Blends: iii, **266**

Animal Scents Ointment: 264, **265**, 267, 268, 270-272, 575, 576, 578, 580, 581, 584, 585, 588, 589, 601

Animal Scents Shampoo: **265**, 268, 577, 580, 582-584, 589, 601

Animals: iii, 29, 32, 75, 78, 197, 199, 200, 207, 210, 242, **257-278**, 321, 353, 363-365, 383, 462, 601, 604, 606, 607, 609-611

Animal Treatment: iii, **267**

Anise: 19, 20, 43, 50, 67, **69**, 148, 149, 164, 169, 171-174, 177-179, 183, 185, 186, 214, 217, 250, 253, 265, 266, 330-332, 342, 350, 351, 498, 572, 573, 575, 592, 596, 597, 601

Anorexia Nervosa: **467**

Anthrax: **420**, 421

Anti-infectious: 8, **22**, 83, 85, 153, 163, 248, 601

Anti-inflammatory: v, 4, 19, 20, 22, 32, 40, 69, 71-73, 75, 77-83, 85-87, 89-95, 97-99, 104-109, 111-126, 128, 129, 131, 133, 134, 137-142, 145, 147, 148, 156, 160, 170, 171, 184, 186, 196, 225, 229, 242, 243, 267, 273, 278, 291, **307**, 324, **370-371**, 398, 412, **422**, 436, 444, 445, 454, 475, 490, 512, 532, 546

Antiaging: 73, 80, 89, 118, 134, 200, 205, 241, **389-390**, 601

Antibacterial: v, 3, 8, 9, 20, 29, 30, 69, 70, 73, 75-78, 84, 85, 88-90, 93, 97-99, 102-106, 108-114, 118-121, 124-129, 131-133, 162, 163, 178, 222, 227, 228, 231, 232, 234, 244, 245, 247, 248, 251-253, 291, 292, 304, 322, 324, 337, 385, **412**, 489, 505, 535, 544, 550

Antibiotic Reactions: **421**

Antibiotics: 9, 11, **29**, 30, 69, 95, 115, 181, 275, 322, 336, **421**, 478, 480, 482, 523

Anticancer: 31, 81, 87, 88, 93, 98, 105, 107, 110, 115, 123, 126, 128, 129, 132, 142, 163, 196, 198, 200, 208, 215, 261, **433-434**, 567

Anticoagulant: 68, 69, 75, 77, 79, 80, 95, 97, 99, 101, 103, 116, 118, 139

Antidepressant: 19, 70, 79, 91, 96, 97, 102, 111, 118, 120, 126, 371

Antifungal: 9, 19, 20, 32, 71, 73-75, 77-80, 82, 83, 85, 87-89, 93, 95, 97, 98, 100, 101, 103, 104, 106-111, 113, 115-121, 123, 126, 127, 129, 131, 133, 134, 138, 140, 162, 178, 243, 244, 247, 322-324, **477**, **480**, **550**, 567

Antimicrobial: 8, 17, 19, 30-33, 69-71, 73-75, 78-84, 86-91, 94, 97-103, 105-107, 110, 111, 114, 115, 118, 120, 124, 128, 133-135, 137, 138, 140, 150, 229, 231, 247, 290-292, 304, 322, 323, 377, 381, **398**, **421**, **423**, **452**, **489**, **501**, **503**, **535**

Antioxidant: iv, 31, 33, 68-72, 74-87, 90, 91, 93-99, 101, 103-105, 109-111, 114, 117, 118, 120, 123, 124, 126, 127, 129-132, 134, 138, 139, 142, 155, 170, 175, 179-181, 184, 188, 189, 192, 195, 198-201, 203, 206, 209, 213, 226, 236, 242, 243, 331, 334, 336, 337, 354, 361-365, 378, 385, 388, 389, 397, 398, 406, **413**, 429, **436**, **472**, 473, 500, 533-535, **544**

Antiseptic: 4, 9, 17, 18, 20, 29, 31, 72, 74, 81, 83, 86, 87, 89, 90, 93, 96, 98, 101, 103-105, 107, 116, 123, 130, 131, 133, 135, 137, 153, 156, 159, 163, 227-229, 240, 243, 244, 247, 248, 253, 254, 276, 307, 323, 354, **422**, **491**, **492**, 546, 550, 601-612

Antispasmodic: 20, 68, 69, 72-74, 78, 79, 83, 85, 87, 90, 93, 97, 108, 111, 115, 116, 122, 125, 131-134, 136, 137, 139, 141, 156

Antitumoral: 69, 79, 80, 83, 87, 90, 91, 93, 94, 96, 99, 101, 104, 105, 112, 114, 118, 120-122, 124, 126, 128, 129, 132, 138, 365

Antiviral: v, 8, 9, 18, 20, 29, 69, 71, 72, 75, 77, 78, 80, 83, 85, 88, 89, 97, 98, 101, 102, 108, 109, 111-114, 118-121, 124, 127, 128, 130, 133, 134, 146, 159, 163, 178, 248, 290, 291, 304, 324, **412**, **418**, **452**, **489**, 505, **539**, 567

Anxiety: 5, 27, 32, 68, 70, 78, 79, 81, 82, 94, 96, 102, 104, 106-109, 112, 115-118, 122, 123, 125-127, 130, 132, 136, 137, 140-

142, 147, 151, 158, 163, 208, 209, 212, 268, 307, 310, **312**, 357, 419, 460, 474, 487, 510, 532, 563, 564

Apathy: **312**

Apnea: **422**, 555

Appetite, Loss of: 103, 320, 417, 443, 452, 456, 464, **468**, 498, 499

Application: **279-304**, **410-411**

Argumentative: **313**

Aroma Ease: 144, **145**, 333, 576, 586, 591, 598

Aroma Life: 144, **145**, 373, 413, 438-447, 469, 488, 506, 548, 578, 580, 583, 589, 591, 598, 601

Aroma Siez: 144, **145**, 273, 276, 293, 295, 296, 298, 302, 373, 409, 412, 420, 423, 424, 427, 428, 447, 449, 454, 455, 487, 488, 490, 495, 511-514, 516-518, 520-522, 529, 531, 533, 536, 548-550, 555-559, 575, 578, 582, 583, 586, 591, 598, 601

Aroma Sleep: 144, **145**

AromaBright Toothpaste: **229**, 412, 422, 485, 525-528, 543, 544, 577, 579, 583, 585-588, 611

AromaGuard Meadow Mist Deodorant: **220**, 575, 577, 578, 580, 582-584, 587-589, 601

AromaGuard Mountain Mint Deodorant: **220**, 577, 579, 583, 586, 587, 589, 601

Aromatherapist: 109, **258**

Aromatherapy: v, 3-5, 9, 25, 27, 29, 32, 36, 68, 71, 72, 95, 102, 106, 122, 142, 217, 221, **259**, 290, 567

ART Beauty Masque: **237**, 414, 576, 578, 582, 583, 585, 588, 601

ART Chocolate Masque: **237**, 579, 580, 587

ART Creme Masque: **237**, 414, 578, 580, 585, 586, 588, 589, 601

ART Gentle Cleanser: **238**, 414, 545, 547, 554, 579, 582-584, 587, 601

ART Intensive Moisturizer: **238**, 576, 579, 581, 587, 589, 601

ART L'Brianté: **224**, **225**, 578, 581, 583, 585-589, 601

ART L'Brianté – Neutral/Winter Scent: **224**

ART L'Brianté – Pink/Summer Scent: **224**

ART L'Brianté – Red/Amoressence Scent: **225**

ART Light Moisturizer: 55, **238**, 414, 551, 554, 579, 587, 589, 601

ART Refreshing Toner: **238**, 414, 545, 547, 552, 554, 579, 582-584, 587, 601

ART Renewal Serum: 55, 237, **239**, 414, 575, 578, 580, 581, 589, 601

ART Sheerlumé Brightening Cream: 55, **239**, 414, 554, 576, 577, 579-581, 587-589, 602

Arteriosclerosis: 75, 76, 94, 97, 101, 104, 106, 118, 139, 361, **439**, 478, 482, 525

Arthritis: 69, 71, 72, 76, 78, 80-82, 89, 90,

92, 94, 95, 99-101, 103, 110, 112, 116, 118, 120, 121, 123-125, 129, 130, 137, 139, 158, 170, 190, 196, 204, 214, 235, 261, 264, **267**, 382, 383, 416, 417, **422**, 423, 428, 433, 452, 476, 495, 517, 528, 563

Aspartame: **392-393**

Asthma: 32, 86, 130, 142, **269**, 283, 355, 382, 417, 420, **501**, 524

Athletes Foot: 109, **477**, 545

Attention Deficit Disorder: 357, **424**, 489, 522

Australia: **11**, 37, 72, 90, 107, 109, 111, 112, 130, 134, 545

Australian Blue: 144, **146**, 312-316, 412, 450, 452, 532, 533, 536, 541, 546, 549, 576-578, 580, 581, 583, 585, 586, 588, 589, 591, 598, 602

Autism: **425**, 449

Automatic Dishwasher Powder: **251**, 421, 422, 611

Awaken: vii, 144, **146**, 149, 157, 165, 244, 313, 315, 331, 373, 392, 413, 451, 466, 474, 515, 520-522, 575-589, 591, 598, 602

Babies: 151, 168, 208, 317, **332**, 344, 345, 352, 378, 391, 494, 549

Backache: 235, **556**

Back Injuries and Pain: **556**

Bacteria: 3, 5, 11, 29-32, 56, 78, 79, 82, 87, 89, 100, 109, 118, 122, 124, 127, 131, 140, 150, 178, 181, 196, 208, 226-228, 230, 232, 234, 251, 253, 254, 267, 272, 291, 292, 317, 319, 321-323, 327, 331, 333, 335, 336, 348, 357, 360, 377, 379, 383, 393, 395, 397, 398, **421**, **422**, 426, **452**, 453, 460-462, 464, 479, 482, **489**, 496, **501-503**, **525**, 526, 535, 539, 545, 561, 563, 565, 566

Bad Breath: 228, 320, 327, **485**, 525, 543

Balance Complete Vanilla Cream Meal Replacement: **169**, **201**

Balancing Body Energy: **297**

Baldness/Hair Loss: **484**

Balm of Gilead: **571**, **573**

Balsam Canada: **99**, 146, 148, 149, 151, 156-158, 160, 163, 170, 571, 573, 581, 591, 592, 594, 595

Balsam Copaiba: **81**, 235, 270, 571, 573, 577, 578

Baser, K. Hüsnü Can: **10**

Basil: 4, 17, 18, 20, 31, 32, 43, 49, 50, 54, 67, **69**, 70, 145, 147, 156, 157, 182, 189, 255, 258, 261, 263, 276, 292, 293, 295, 296, 298, 300, 304, 313, 316, 326, 330, 339, 340, 342, 373, 407, 412, 428, 430, 431, 433, 455, 462, 463, 465-467, 470, 474, 478, 483, 486, 488, 494, 504-506, 510, 512-514, 517, 520-522, 530, 532, 536, 542, 551, 556-559, 572, 573, 575, 591, 593, 594, 597, 602

# Index

Basil Vitality: **70**, 255, 412, 428, 430, 431, 433, 455, 462, 463, 465, 474, 483, 488, 504, 510, 520-522, 530, 556, 557, 559, 572, 573, 575, 597, 602

Bath: ii, 51, **55**, 138, 155, 205, 217, 218, 225, 242, **247**, 276, 388, 411, 448, 449, 452, 464, 477, 479, 485, 491, 494, 495, 505, 508, 544, 547, 554, 560, 575-589, 601-612

Bath & Shower Gel Base: **217**, 485, 602

Bay Laurel: 17, 43, 67, 84, **103**, 147, 185, 414, 452, 477, 479, 493, 502, 507, 541, 544, 545, 549, 572, 573, 578, 582, 591, 603, 606

Beauty Masque: **237**, 414, 576, 578, 582, 583, 585, 588, 601

Becker, Robert O.: **373**, 378

Bedbug Bites: **492**

Bedbugs: **426**

Bee Stings: **491**

Belaiche, Paul: **9**, 10

Believe: vi, 26, 50, 109, 144, **146-147**, 150, 221, 273, 275, 291, 312-316, 321, 357, 361, 366, 405, 406, 412, 425, 433, 434, 451, 456, 467, 505, 521, 559, 575, 578-581, 589, 591, 598, 602

Bell's Palsy: **516**

Benign Prostate Hyperplasia (BPH): 211, 214, **532**

Bereavement: **310**, **565**

Bergamot: 19, 20, 31, 43, 49, 50, 57, 67, **70**, 71, 89, 145-159, 161, 164, 165, 213-215, 217-220, 223, 226, 239-241, 243, 247, 248, 250, 252, 253, 265, 266, 311, 312, 314-316, 330, 332, 412, 417, 419, 430, 457, 458, 460, 487, 510, 511, 525, 564, 571, 573, 575, 591-597, 602

Bergamot Vitality: **70**, 412, 417, 419, 430, 457, 458, 460, 487, 510, 511, 525, 564, 571, 573, 575, 597, 602

Bible: **8**, 98, 175, 308

Biblical References: **12-15**

Biblical Sweet Myrrh: 43, 67, **71**, 571, 573, 575, 602

Binge Eating Disorder: **468**

Birds: 13, 14, 257, **259**, 268, 275, 347

Birthing: 151, **267**

Bite Buster: 144, **146**, **250**, 491-494, 577, 581, 585, 591, 602

Bites: 3, 17, 69, 81, 90, 108, 129, 159, 225, 419, 426, **491-493**, 555

Black Pepper: 18, 20, 43, 67, **71**, 72, 115, 149, 155, 157, 160, 169, 173, 184, 203, 212, 313, 363, 412, 420, 429, 433, 442, 453, 474, 484, 496, 513, 515, 519, 535, 537, 552, 566, 572, 573, 575, 592-595, 597, 602

Black Pepper Vitality: **71**, 412, 429, 433, 442, 453, 474, 484, 519, 535, 566, 572, 573, 575, 597, 602

Black Spruce: 43, 45, 67, **72**, 116, 143, 145, 147, 149-153, 155-165, 169, 224, 235, 236, 240, 244, 250, 265, 266, 270, 312-316, 333, 412, 418, 420, 422-424, 427, 428, 444, 452, 465, 471, 489, 493, 501, 502, 504, 505, 507, 511, 513, 529, 531, 539, 541, 544, 550, 560, 561, 565, 572-576, 584, 591-598, 602, 608

Black Widow Spider Bite: **492**

Bladder/Urinary Tract Infection (Cystitis): **426**

Blanc, Bernard H: **379**

Bleeding: 93, 105, **267**, 271, 320, **439**, 456, 482, 488, 508, 509, 524-526, 536, 539, 549

Bleeding Gums: **525**, 536

Blends: ii, iv, 5, 30, 32, 50, 52, 53, 56, 57, 59, 85, **143-166**, 184, 215, 226, 234, 236, 247, 250, 253, 255, 259, 266, 268, 293, 298, 310, 312-316, 322, 325, 326, 328, 330, 332-334, 336, 373, 374, 381, 384, 386, 388, 406, 407, 410-433, 437-566, 569, **591-596**, 598

Blisters: 450, 477, 526, 539, 540, **545-547**, 549, 551

BLM Capsules: **170**, 171

BLM Powder: **170**, 171

Bloating/Swelling: **427**, **463**

Blocked Tear Ducts: **472**

Blood Circulation Poor: **439**

Blood Cleanse: **326**

Blood Clots (Embolism, Hematoma, Thrombus): **440**

Blood Detoxification: **440**

Blood Platelets: **441**

Blood Platelets (Low): **441**

Blood Pressure High (Hypertension): 117, 361, **441**

Blue Agave: 49, 155, **171**, 204, 326, 331, 335, 338, 341, **393**, 397, 410, 416, 425, 426, 485, 507, 540, 561, 602

Blue Cypress: 18, 43, 67, **72**, 145-149, 151, 152, 157-161, 164, 204, 219, 235, 239, 250, 270, 437, 450, 452, 453, 477, 479, 501, 511, 512, 531, 533, 535, 539, 541, 542, 549, 571, 573, 576, 591-597, 602

Blue Spruce, Idaho: 43, 67, **99**, 100, 145-147, 150, 151, 153-159, 161, 164, 165, 185, 215, 224, 225, 235, 236, 244, 250, 312-316, 412-414, 432, 433, 436, 437, 439, 442, 447, 454, 465, 469, 470, 472, 474, 476-478, 480, 483, 489-491, 495, 496, 507, 510, 511, 513, 518, 519, 529, 537, 556-559, 564, 565, 572, 573, 581, 591-597, 605

Blue Tansy: 43, 67, **73**, 146, 149, 152, 154, 158, 160, 161, 164, 165, 179, 217, 244, 266, 331, 464, 560, 572, 573, 576, 591-597, 602

Body Systems: **601-612**

Boils: 544, **546**

Bone Chips: **269**

Bone Pain: 170, **428**, **529**

Bone Problems: **427**

Bones: 4, **170**, 171, 182, 267, 278, 308, 321, 347, 353, 354, 357, 365, 366, 405, 406, 412, 422, **427-428**, 430, 455, 476, 517, **529**, 566

Bones, Ligaments, and Muscles: **170**

Boredom: **313**

Boswellia Wrinkle Cream: 55, **204**, **239**, 414, 523, 536, 545, 547, 548, 551, 552, 554, 579, 580, 584, 587, 589, 602

Botanical Names: **571-574**

BPH: 211, 214, **532**, 533

Brain: iv, 4, 26, 27, 32, 33, 51, 71, 76, 77, 84, 91, 102, 105, 106, 114, 121, 124, 126, 128, 136, 137, 142, 144, 146, 147, 149, 154-156, 175, 180-182, 184, 185, 194, 195, 207, 209-211, 215, 236, 249, 283, 288, 289, 303, 307-309, 311, 313-316, 322, 326, 329, 333, 353, 355, 357, 358, **362-364**, 371, 373, 374, 381, 388, 389, 393, 398, 406, 413, 415, 417, 418, 420, 424, 425, **429-432**, 434, 438, 440, 445, 446, 448, 449, 451, 453, 457, 465, 467, 470, 474, 476, 486, 494, 504, 515, 516, 518-523, 525, 536, 553, 555, 564, 565, 567, 576, 579, 580, 582, 584, 587, 591, 598, 602

Brain Disorders and Problems: **429**

Brain Function: iv, 84, 181, 194, 207, 249, 353, **363**

Brain Power: 144, **146**, 147, 313-316, 373, 381, 413, 415, 417, 420, 424, 425, 429-432, 434, 446, 453, 465, 467, 470, 474, 486, 515, 519, 520, 522, 523, 553, 564, 565, 576, 579, 580, 582, 584, 587, 591, 598, 602

Brain Stem Pump: **303**

Brazil: 37, 73, 81, 82, 90, 111, 127, 132, 136, 328,

Breast Cancer: 33, 81, 95, 110, 112, 118, 123, 128, 129, 206, 208, 209, 211, 215, 370, 398, **433-437**, 508, 567

Breastfeeding: **432**

Breathe Again Roll-On: 144, **147**, 326, 412, 422, 452, 471, 486, 489, 491, 501-504, 511, 523, 536, 542-544, 560, 561, 576, 578, 579, 582, 584, 586, 591, 598, 602

Brigham Young University: **33**, **128**, 436

Broken Bones: 278, **427**

Bronchitis: 32, 33, 81, 86, 111, 159, **501**, 502

Brown Recluse Spider Bite: **492**

Bruised Ankle: **269**

Bruised Muscles: 441, **512**

Bruising: 267, 269, 320, **441**, 490, 512

Brushing Teeth: **227**

Build Your Dream: 144, **147**, 312-314, 316, 458, 469, 525, 537, 538, 542, 565, 575-589, 591, 598, 602

Building Blocks of Health: iii, 305, **343-360**

Seventh Edition | **Essential Oils Desk Reference** | 615

Bulimia: 467, **468**

Bunions: **477**

Burns: 9, 17, 25, 55, 90, 104, 122, 156, 240, 354, 381, 387, 482, 542, **545-547**

Bursitis: 190, 204, 382, 383, **433**, 477, 517

Cairo University: **10**, 82, 377, 418

Calamus: 8, 13-15, 43, 67, **73**, 150, 571, 573, 576, 592, 597

Calluses: **478**

Canada: vii, **11**, 37, **45**, 72, 73, 96, 99, 100, 105, 116, 123, 135, 138, 146, 148, 149, 151, 156-158, 160, 163, 170, 176, 219, 290, 381, 386, 396, 493, 498, 552, 571, 573, 581, 591, 592, 594, 595

Canadian Fleabane: 43, 46, 67, **73**, 155, 171, 173, 192, 212, 417, 425, 429, 449, 470, 484, 509, 515, 518, 571, 573, 576, 593, 597, 602

Cancer: 32, 33, 69, 75, 77, 81, 83, 86, 89-91, 93, 95, 98, 105, 108, 110, 112-114, 117, 118, 121, 123, 124, 126-129, 133, 175, 178, 194, 196-198, 200, 201, 206, 208-211, 213-215, 219, 223, 226, 227, 259, **268**, **269**, 275, 321, 323, 326, 327, 346, 351, 354, 357-359, 365-367, 369, 370, 372, 373, 377, 383, 386, 388, 395, 398, **433-437**, 448, 456, 474, 475, 478, 495, 508, 526, 532, 533, 540, 550, 554, 567

Candida Albicans (Candidiasis): **479**

Candidiasis: **478-480**, 550

Canker Sores: **448**, 526

Carbohydrate: 81, 168, 187, 193, 335, **344-350**, 391

Carboxylic Acids: **19**

Cardamom: 43, 50, 67, **74**, 145, 147, 157, 164, 182, 186, 212, 215, 250, 314, 316, 424, 429-431, 465, 474, 487, 500, 519, 523, 542, 571, 573, 576, 591, 594, 596, 597, 602

Cardamom Vitality: **74**, 424, 429-431, 465, 487, 500, 519, 523, 571, 573, 576, 597, 602

Cardiovascular Conditions and Problems: **438**

Carpal Tunnel Syndrome: 94, 214, 516, **517**

Carrot Seed: 43, 50, 67, **74**, 75, 240, 265, 330, 412, 453, 462, 481, 488, 498-500, 526, 571, 573, 576, 597, 602

Carrot Seed Vitality: **75**, 412, 453, 462, 481, 488, 498-500, 526, 571, 573, 576, 597, 602

Cartilage Injury on Knee, Elbow, Etc.: **454**

Casabianca, Hervé: **10**, 23, 47, 369

Cassia: 8, 15, 17, 19, 20, 43, 50, 67, **75**, 121, 150, 155, 158, 160, 165, 173, 185, 188, 189, 202, 212, 228, 342, 361, 422, 563, 566, 571, 573, 576, 592-597, 602

Cataracts: 75, 80, 175, 196, **473**

Cats: **257-261**, 263, 264, 348, 349

Cattle: 258, **264**

Cedarwood: v, 4, 12, 18, 43, 50, 67, **76**, 78,

146, 149, 151-155, 157-164, 214, 219, 223-225, 235-238, 244, 247, 250, 312-314, 316, 322, 422, 424, 425, 429, 432, 457, 458, 461, 464, 470, 483-485, 489, 494, 518, 522, 523, 545, 547, 560, 561, 563-565, 571, 573, 576, 591-597, 602

Cel-Lite Magic Massage Oil: **225**, 412, 448, 449, 475, 506, 525, 552, 575-578, 580, 582, 602

Celery Seed: 20, 43, 50, 67, **76**, 77, 151, 154, 321, 328, 331, 499, 500, 571, 573, 576, 592, 593, 597, 602

Celery Seed Vitality: **76,** 499, 500, 571, 573, 576, 597, 602

Cellulite: 96, 225, **448**, 449

Cerebral Palsy: 425, **449**, 559

Cervical Cancer: 435, **437**, 540

Chakras: 68-83, 85-142, 149, 152, **308**, 311, 333, 415

Chao, Sue: **30**, 204, 237, 292, 377

Chapped, Cracked, or Dry Skin: **547**

Charley Horse: 401, **513**

Chemical Sensitivities: **51**, **564**

Chemical Sensitivity Reaction: **449**

Chemical Structure: vi, **36**, 136, 345

Chemistry of Essential Oils: 3, **17-27**, 150

Chemotypes: **20**

Chernobyl: **336**, **384-388**

Chicken Pox (Herpes Zoster): **450**

Chigger and Tick Bites: **492**

Children: ii, 12, 49, 52-54, 59, 67, 76, 88, 100, 107, 108, 118, 120, 125, 126, 136, 137, 139, 144, 146, 150, 151, 153, 154, 158-162, 164, 167, 168, 172, 173, 177, 180, 181, 183, 184, 190, 191, 201, 207-209, 213, 219, 231, 234, 235, **247-251**, 255, 263, 276, 292, 293, 309, 311, 321, 324, **332-335**, 337, 338, 344, 345, 349, 351, 352, 354, 357, 360, 365-367, 380, 381, 385-388, 391, 398, 405-407, 410, 411, 420, 424, 425, 450, 459, 462, 494, 496, 504, 520, 524, 528, 529, 534, 535, 543, 548, 554

China: 8, **9**, **11**, 29, 32, 75, 80, 88, 89, 95, 101, 118, 131, 138, 139, 142, **193-200**, 212, 354, 369, 389, 395, 396, 458, 497, 500

Chlorine: **357-360**, 392, 405

Chocolate-Coated Wolfberry Crisp Bars: **176**, 192, **201**, 204, 458, 467, 468, 474, 525, 604

Chocolessence, Ecuadorian Dark: **172**, 173, 341, 458, 577, 580, 584, 588, 604

Cholecystitis: **481**

Cholera: 71, 357, **450**

Cholesterol: 79, 104, 140, 172, 195, 196, 206, 207, 209, 210, 317, 318, 320, 323, 342, 354, 358, 363, 379, 395, 397, 435, 440, **442-445**, 481, 567

Cholesterol, High: 79, 320, **442**, 443, 445

Christmas Spirit: 50, 144, **147**, 312-316,

373, 450, 468, 469, 520, 543, 576, 577, 585, 591, 598, 602

Chronic Fatigue Syndrome: 357, 393, **451**, 564

Chronic Pain: 71, 393, 426, **529**, 530, 557

Cinnamint Lip Balm: 205, **224**, 475, 547, 577, 585, 586, 588, 602

Cinnamon Bark: 21, 43, 50, 67, **77**, 145, 147, 149, 150, 152, 156-158, 163, 164, 170, 173, 178, 183, 186, 188, 191, 202, 203, 205, 222, 224, 226, 227, 229, 231, 232, 234, 244, 245, 248, 251-255, 268, 270, 386, 412, 413, 421, 422, 441, 453, 458, 480, 485, 498, 503, 525, 541, 548, 554, 562, 564, 566, 571, 573, 576, 577, 584, 591-597, 602

Cinnamon Bark Vitality: **77**, 173, 255, 412, 413, 421, 441, 453, 458, 480, 485, 503, 525, 541, 554, 562, 564, 566, 571, 573, 576, 577, 597, 602

Circular Hand Massage: 296, **302**

Cistus: 37, 43, 50, 67, **78**, 126, 153, 156-158, 163, 165, 248, 250, 266, 267, 312-316, 334, 407, 412, 418, 426, 438-440, 442, 445-447, 475, 481, 482, 488, 490, 497, 508, 509, 524, 535, 536, 548, 549, 571, 573, 574, 577, 593-597, 603

Citronella: 43, 50, 67, **78**, 79, 101, 146, 157, 159, 250, 253, 265, 266, 270, 421, 491, 492, 494, 524, 552, 571, 573, 577, 591, 594, 595, 597, 603

Citrus Fresh: 50, 144, **147**, 255, 259, 313, 314, 316, 335-337, 373, 384, 385, 413, 426, 427, 437, 441, 447, 450, 451, 463, 465, 468, 481, 483, 485, 496, 498, 500, 506, 514, 520, 524, 534-536, 548, 565, 580, 583, 585, 588, 591, 598, 603

Citrus Fresh Vitality: **147,** 255, 413, 427, 437, 441, 450, 451, 463, 465, 468, 481, 483, 496, 498, 500, 506, 514, 520, 536, 565, 580, 583, 585, 588, 591, 598, 603

Citrus Hystrix: 43, 67, **79**, 149, 152, 158, 161, 164, 266, 571, 573, 577, 592-596

ClaraDerm: **239**, 414, 477, 479, 481, 531, 549-551, 579, 580, 582, 584, 586, 588, 603

Clarity: 56, 106, 126, 144, 146, **147**, 150, 151, 157, 208, 215, 295, 313, 314, 316, 324, 334, 351, 373, 381, 413, 417, 422, 424, 425, 429-432, 446, 465, 474, 475, 486, 515, 519, 520, 523, 542, 564, 565, 575, 576, 578, 580, 581, 583, 585-587, 589, 591, 598, 603

Clary Sage: 19, 21, 38, 43, 50, 67, **79**, 80, 148, 153, 155, 157, 158, 161, 164, 171, 173, 174, 205, 212-215, 217, 222, 223, 225, 278, 312, 315, 412, 427, 435, 457, 458, 470, 483, 484, 507-511, 531-533, 537, 538, 554, 572, 573, 577, 592-597, 603

Cleaning: v, 56, 57, 101, 105, 107, 230, 240,

**616** | Index

253, 254, 267, 354, 545

Cleanse: 12, 14, 19, 52, 93, 105, 120, 135, 151, 156, 170, 172, 185, 187, 205, 217, 225, 238, 242, 244, 265, **320**, **323-332**, 350, 355, 387, 389, 406, 407, 412, 413, 415-417, 419, 421, 423, 430, 432, 434, 438, 441, 442, 445, 447, 448, 451, 453, 456, 459-462, 464, 469, 471, 474-477, 479, 482, 485, 488, 491, 495-497, 499, 500, 502-504, 506-508, 510, 512, 515, 525, 530, 533, 542, 544, 545, 550, 551, 553, 555, 564, 575, 579, 580, 583, 586, 603

Cleansing: iii, 18, 19, 52, 76, 96, 134, 151, 154, 167, 171, 172, 177-179, 183, 185, 187, 205, 217, 218, 222, 231, 234, 238-241, 243, 244, 247, 252, 266, 267, 270, 305, **317-342**, 351, 376, 386, 406, 407, 412, 415, 416, 420-422, 431, 432, 434, 436, 441, 447, 480, 483, 484, 486-488, 500, 530, 545, 553, 577, 579, 583, 587, 607, 611

Clogged Pores: **547**

Clove: iv, v, 17, 19, 31, 32, 37, 40, 43, 50, 67, **80**, 81, 136, 145, 148, 149, 153, 155, 156, 158, 163, 169-171, 173, 178, 179, 181, 182, 185, 186, 191, 214, 219, 220, 222, 223, 226-229, 231, 232, 234, 239, 244, 245, 248, 250-255, 258, 268-270, 316, 322, 332, 334, 340, 359, **361-365**, 377, 386, 398, 407, 412, 413, 417, 418, 420-422, 424, 426, 436-448, 450-453, 458, 460-462, 465, 471-473, 476, 477, 480, 485-487, 489, 490, 493, 502-507, 512, 518-520, 525-529, 535, 544, 546, 548, 550, 553-555, 562, 563, 565-567, 571-573, 577, 584, 591-595, 597, 603

Clove Vitality: **80**, 173, 255, 412, 413, 417, 421, 422, 424, 426, 436-448, 450-453, 458, 460-462, 465, 471-473, 476, 480, 485-487, 489, 490, 502, 503, 505, 507, 519, 520, 525-529, 535, 554, 562, 563, 565, 566, 572, 573, 577, 595, 597, 603

Cold Packs: **54**, 455, 512, 516, 519, 522

Colds: 86, 99, 105, 112, 124, 130, 147, 159, **268,** 320, 333, 372, **452**, 489-491, 560

Cold Sores (Herpes Simplex Type 1): **451**

Colic: 90, 267, **268**, **269**, 278

Colitis: 118, 135, 169, 321, **452**, 453, 456, 461, 478, 495

Colon Cleanse: **326-329**, 499, 530, 555

Colorado: 258, 291, **304**, 429

Coma: **453**

ComforTone: 167, **171**, 177, 179, 326, 329-332, 335, 387, 388, 406, 407, 412, 413, 416, 419, 420, 423, 427, 434, 442, 450-453, 455, 456, 459-463, 468, 470, 471, 476, 480-483, 485-488, 499, 500, 503, 508, 530, 539, 544, 545, 550-555, 557, 562, 565, 575, 580, 585-588, 603

Common Sense: 49, 144, **147**, 261, 264,

281, 313-316, 333, 350, 381, 409, 413, 415, 417, 419, 422, 425, 429-431, 433, 434, 446, 458, 465, 468, 470, 474, 515, 520, 523, 532, 560, 564, 578-580, 583, 585, 587, 589, 591, 598, 603

Compress: **54**, 148, 154, 156, 158-161, 278, 332, 411, 416, 418, 419, 424, 427, 431, 433, 439-442, 445, 453-461, 463, 464, 466, 469, 475-478, 481, 482, 486, 489-491, 495-500, 502-504, 506, 508-512, 514-518, 529, 531, 541, 543, 544, 549, 551, 552, 556-558, 560-564

Concentration: 10, 56, 70, 71, 104, 122, 126, 136, 146, 156, 171, 194, 200, 220, 257, 261, **313**, 320, 329, 355, 357, 358, 363, 393, **430**, 431

Concentration, Impaired: **430**

Confusion: 122, 141, 153, 179, 258, **313**, 413, **430**, 474, 510, 523

Congestive Cough: **560**

Congestive Heart Failure: **443**

Conjunctivitis/Pink Eye: **473**

Connective Tissue Damage: **454**

Constipation (Impacted Bowel): **459**

Constituents: v, **4**, **17-35**, **36-47**, 65, 68-80, 82-143, 145, 197, 198, 212, 228, 234, 361, 364, 371, 457, 497, 525

Convulsions: **431**

Cooking: iv, 22, 41, 42, 44, 83, 105, 107, 123, 130, 142, 184, 192, 203, 254, **255**, 322, 335, 339, 340, **342**, 343, 345, 352, 377, 378, 380, 387, 397

Cool Azul: 144, **148**, **235**, 268, 269, 409, 412, 420, 422-424, 427, 428, 433, 442, 447, 449, 454, 455, 457, 476-478, 483, 490, 495, 496, 506, 508, 511-514, 516-518, 520, 521, 526, 528, 529, 556-560, 566, 576, 578, 580, 582, 584-587, 589, 592, 603

Cool Azul Pain Relief Cream: **235**, 268, 269, 409, 412, 420, 422-424, 427, 428, 433, 442, 447, 449, 454, 455, 457, 476-478, 483, 490, 496, 506, 508, 511-514, 516-518, 520, 521, 529, 556-560, 566, 576, 578, 580, 582, 584, 586, 587, 589, 603

Cool Azul Sports Gel: **235**, 268, 269, 409, 412, 420, 422-424, 427, 428, 433, 442, 449, 454, 455, 457, 476-478, 483, 490, 496, 506, 512-514, 516-518, 521, 529, 556-560, 566, 576, 578, 580, 582, 584, 586, 587, 589, 603

Copaiba: 43, 50, 67, **81**, 82, 147, 148, 150, 157, 162, 169, **204**, 214, **221**, 223, 235, 237, 261, 267, 270, 313-316, 412, 413, 420, 424, 427, 428, 431-433, 436, 444, 445, 450, 453-456, 463, 464, 475, 476, 478, 482, 483, 485, 486, 490-492, 502, 512, 513, 518, 529, 555-560, 571, 573, 577, 578, 580, 582, 583, 588, 591, 592, 594, 595, 603

Copaiba Vanilla Moisturizing Conditioner:

**204**, **221**, 483, 485, 578, 580, 582, 583, 588, 603

Copaiba Vanilla Moisturizing Shampoo: **204**, **221**, 483, 485, 578, 580, 582, 583, 588, 603

Copaiba Vitality: **81**, 412, 413, 431-433, 444, 445, 450, 453-456, 463, 464, 475, 476, 486, 490, 502, 529, 556-558, 560, 571, 573, 577, 578, 603

Coriander: 19, 43, 50, 67, **82**, 145-147, 150-158, 161, 164, 165, 215, 217-220, 224, 226, 235, 236, 239-241, 243, 244, 247, 248, 265, 266, 340, 412, 458, 459, 564, 571, 573, 578, 591-597, 603

Coriander Vitality: **82**, 412, 458, 459, 564, 571, 573, 578, 597, 603

Corns and Calluses: **478**

Cortisol: **211**

CortiStop: **171**, 211, **212**, 413, 417, 470, 560, 576, 577, 579, 586, 603

Cosmetics: v, 8, 51, 52, 130, 142, 236, 251, 317, 381, 390, 406, 407, 434, 449, 545

Coughs, Congestive and Dry: **560**

Coumarins: **20**, 69

Cramps: **513**

Cramps, Stomach: **460**

Creme Masque: **237**, 414, 578, 580, 585, 586, 588, 589, 601

Croatia: **11**, 37, 45, **46-47**, 84, 97, 103, 130, 136

Crohn's Disease: 327, 452, **456**, 461

Cumin: 19, 32, 43, 50, 67, **83**, 153, 172, 173, 185, 214, 223, 265, 266, 328, 332, 351, 418, 453, 462, 463, 481, 497, 530, 571, 573, 578, 593, 597, 603

Cushing's Syndrome: **417**, 470

Cuts, Scrapes, and Wounds: **548**

Cypress: 18, 41, 43, 67, 72, **83**, 84, 145-149, 151, 152, 157-162, 164, 204, 219, 225, 235, 239, 245, 250, 258, 261, 263, 270, 271, 276, 293, 295, 296, 298, 301, 304, 313-315, 407, 418, 427, 428, 437-443, 445-450, 452, 453, 463, 469, 472-474, 477-479, 482-484, 488, 494, 501, 505, 506, 508-512, 514, 516, 517, 519, 521, 522, 524, 529, 531, 533, 535, 536, 539, 541, 542, 547-549, 552, 553, 557-562, 565, 571, 573, 576, 578, 591-597, 602, 603

Cystitis: 81, 135, 383, **426**

Cysts: 435, **457**, 508

Daily Maintenance: iii, 185, 326, 327, **334-335**

Dalmatia Bay Laurel: 67, **84**, 414, 452, 477, 479, 493, 502, 507, 541, 544, 545, 549, 572, 573, 578, 603

Dalmatia Juniper: 67, **84**, 312-315, 412, 422, 483, 484, 572, 573, 578, 603

Dalmatia Sage: 67, **84**, 315, 412, 414, 415, 422, 519, 541, 572, 573, 578, 603

Dandruff: 109, 130, **484**, 485, 501

Davana: 43, 67, **84**, 85, 145, 146, 149, 152, 158, 160, 161, 164, 165, 205, 218, 224, 225, 235-237, 239, 244, 266, 571, 573, 578, 591-597

Day-Dreaming: **313**

Deep Relief Roll-On: 144, **148**, 409, 412, 420, 423, 424, 427, 428, 433, 439, 442, 449, 454, 455, 476-478, 486, 490, 491, 495, 508, 510-514, 516-518, 529, 536, 553, 555-559, 566, 577, 578, 580, 581, 583, 586, 589, 592, 598, 603

Dental Visits: **526**

Dentarome Plus Toothpaste: **229**, 412, 422, 485, 525-528, 543, 544, 577, 579, 583, 586, 587, 589, 611

Dentarome Ultra Toothpaste: **229**, 412, 422, 485, 526-528, 543, 544, 577, 579, 583, 586-589, 611

Deodorants: ii, 51, 52, **219**, 251, 487

Depression: 27, 70, 91, 96, 102, 105, 106, 108, 112, 115, 116, 118, 122, 125, 130, 132, 133, 136, 137, 141, 152, 154, 158, 163, 208, 211-213, 242, 282, 283, 307, 309-311, **313**, 332, 357, 374-376, 396, 405, 406, 417, 419, **457**, 458, 487, 494, 510, 522, 525, 542, 563, 564

Dermatitis: 51, 93, 109, 121, 125, 225, 242, 382, 388, 419, 489, 498, **549**, **551**

Despair: 130, **313**, 332

Despondency: **314**

Detoxzyme: 168, **172**, 269, 325, 327, 331, 332, 335, 336, 344, 346, 351, 387, 406, 407, 409, 412, 413, 416, 419-421, 423-425, 427, 428, 431, 434, 437-439, 441, 442, 445, 450-453, 455-457, 459-463, 467, 469, 471, 476, 477, 479, 480, 482, 485-488, 491, 495, 497-501, 504-506, 508, 511, 512, 515, 516, 525, 527, 530, 536, 545, 550, 551, 553, 555, 563-565, 575, 578, 579, 603

DeVita, Sabina: **381**

DHEA: 171, 173, 185, 205, 207, 209, **210-213**, 223, 474, 507

Diabetes: 75, 80, 82-86, 90, 114, 124, 125, 175, 193, 206, 208, 267, 318-321, 342, 391, 392, 395-398, 440, **458**, 474, 478, 482, 503, 517, 518, 563

Diaper Rash: 151, 248, **549**

Diarrhea: 93, 135, 169, 171, 177, 183, 187, 272, 321, 325, 330, 346, 348, 351, 419-421, 450, 452, 456, **459-461**, 463, 476, 478, 495, 530, 567

Diet: iii, 69, 73, 108, 118, 142, 170, 171, 174, 177-181, 185, 188, 189, 194, 196, 198, 200, 201, 206, 208, 210, 236, 265, 275, 293, 305, **317-342**, 345-347, 352, 353, 365, 375, 385, 388-393, 395, 396, 405, 406, 416, 419, 424, 425, 428, 430, 431, 434, 461, 478, 480, 490, 495, 496, 498, 500, 513, 514, 534-536, 545, 553

Diffusing: i, 5, 6, **56-57**, **259**, 261, 263, 264, 276, 386, 410, 453, 457, 489, 504, 525, 535

Digest & Cleanse: **172**, 330, 332, 387, 406, 407, 412, 413, 415-417, 419, 421, 430, 438, 442, 445, 448, 451, 453, 456, 459-462, 464, 469, 471, 475-477, 479, 482, 485, 488, 491, 495-497, 500, 502-504, 506, 507, 512, 515, 525, 530, 542, 544, 545, 550, 551, 553, 564, 575, 579, 580, 583, 586, 603

Digestive problems: 71, 76, 83-85, 90, 93, 106, 108, 118, 119, 121, 128, 131, 132, 140, 148, 211, 345, **459**, 476

DiGize: 50, 144, **148**, 253, 261, 268, 269, 271, 272, 330-332, 334, 335, 387, 388, 406, 407, 412, 413, 415-417, 419-421, 426, 427, 434, 437, 438, 440, 445, 447, 451, 453, 456, 459-465, 468, 469, 471, 476, 479, 481, 482, 485, 487, 488, 491, 494-496, 501, 506, 511, 514-516, 530, 532, 533, 543, 550, 575, 579, 580, 582, 583, 585, 586, 588, 592, 598, 603

DiGize Vitality: **148**, 261, 268, 269, 271, 272, 406, 412, 413, 415-417, 419-421, 426, 427, 434, 437, 438, 440, 445, 447, 451, 453, 456, 459-465, 468, 469, 471, 476, 479, 481, 482, 485, 487, 488, 491, 495, 496, 506, 511, 514-516, 530, 533, 543, 575, 579, 580, 582, 583, 585, 586, 588, 592, 598, 603

Dill: 24, 43, 50, 67, **85**, 86, 178, 179, 265, 316, 339, 350, 412, 414, 437, 458, 564, 571, 573, 578, 597, 603

Dill Vitality: **86**, 412, 414, 437, 458, 564, 571, 573, 578, 597, 603

Diphtheria: **464**

Disappointment: **314**

Disc Deterioration: **557**

Discouragement: **314**

Dish Soap: **252**, 421, 422, 575, 577, 579, 583, 587, 611

Dishwasher Powder: **251**, 421, 422, 611

Disinfectant: 117, 358, **422**, 527

Distemper: **269**

Distillation: i, vii, 3-5, 7-10, 17, 18, 22, 35-37, **40-47**, 65, 70, 72, 95, 101, 109, 125, 136, 141

Diverticulosis/Diverticulitis: 452, 456, **461**

Divine Release: 144, **148**, **311**, 316, 332, 333, 412, 414, 415, 425, 434, 458, 467-469, 487, 575, 576, 579-582, 584, 586, 587, 592, 598, 603

Dizziness: 179, 278, 355, **465**, 493, 516, 521, 542, 564

Dogs: 110, 202, 257, 258, **263-264**

Dorado Azul: viii, 43, 67, **86**, 88, 147, 148, 153, 159, 162, 185, 235, 250, 266, 270, 315, 316, 412, 413, 417, 420, 422-424, 430, 433, 439, 442, 444, 445, 447, 454, 465, 474, 475, 485, 486, 489-492, 494, 495, 501-505, 511, 513, 514, 524, 528,

529, 539, 540, 542, 543, 548, 554, 556, 557, 559, 562, 563, 571-573, 578, 591-593, 595, 597, 603

Douglas Fir: 67, **87**, 214, 224, 572, 573, 578, 603

Dragon Time: 144, **148**, **215**, **217**, 225, 313, 315, 373, 411, 413, 457, 458, 509-511, 538, 547, 575-583, 585-589, 592, 598, 604

Dragon Time Bath & Shower Gel: **217**, 575-583, 585-589, 604

Dragon Time Massage Oil: **225**, 413, 577, 579, 581, 582, 587, 589, 604

Dream Catcher: 144, 146, 147, **149**, 151, 313, 314, 373, 413, 434, 464, 494, 532, 553, 575-578, 580-583, 585-589, 591, 592, 598, 604

Dry, Cracked Nipples: **432**

Dry Nose: **523**

Dysentery: 357, **461**

Dysfunction, Sexual (Men): **537**

Dysfunction, Sexual (Women): **537**

Earache: 70, **465**

Ear Chart: **282-283**

Ear Infection: 31, **466**

Ear problems: **465**

Eating Disorders: **467**

Eating Habits: 335, **467**

Ecclesiastes: **8**

Ecuador: vii, **10**, **11**, **23**, 37, 68, 86-88, 101, 111, 117, 120, 124, 128, 137, 141, 266, 369, 389, 397, 571, 573

Ecuadorian Dark Chocolessence: **172**, 173, 341, 458, 577, 580, 584, 588, 604

Eczema/Dermatitis: 93, 125, 382, **549**, 551

Edema (Swelling): **469**

Edfu: **5**, **7**

Effleurage: **290**

Egypt: **6-7**, 20, 25, 83, 85, 94, 110, 138, 139

Egyptian: v, 5, 74, 75, 82, 90, 91, 93, 114, 134, 144, **149**, 307, 313-315, 348, 361, 398, 412, 464, 576, 577, 579, 581, 582, 584, 586, 589, 592, 598, 604

Egyptian Gold: 144, **149**, 313-315, 412, 464, 576, 577, 579, 581, 582, 584, 586, 589, 592, 598, 604

Einkorn: 166, 173, **175-177**, 192, 201, 341, 350, 588, 604, 605

Einkorn Flour: **176**, 177, 604

Einkorn Grain: 173, **175-177**

Einkorn Grain Products: **175**

Einkorn Granola: **176**, 201, 588, 605

Einkorn Pancake and Waffle Mix: **176**, 605

Einkorn Rotini Pasta: 176, **177**, 605

Einkorn Spaghetti: 176, **177**, 605

Einkorn Grain (Wheat): **175-177**

Elemi: 19, 43, 50, 67, **87**, 148, 158, 226, 235, 250, 270, 420, 428, 433, 447, 455, 495, 513, 514, 529, 536, 541, 542, 553, 557, 571, 573, 578, 592, 594, 597, 604

Embalming: v, 5, 6, 72, 76, 87, 134

# Index

Embolism: **440**

Emotional: iii, vii, 3, 19, 26, 27, 69, 72, 83, 85, 98-100, 112, 116, 123, 131, 137, 138, 143, 149, 150, 152, 153, 158, 160, 161, 164, 178, 215, 225, 266, 282, 285, 290, 292, 293, 297, 303, 305, 307-316, 322, 326, 361, 374, 378, 405, 406, 412, 420, 425, 433, 434, 450, 451, 457, **467-469**, 471, 487, 519, 522, 525, 536-538, 542, 545, 553, 558, 564-566, 601

Emotional Challenges: iii, **312**

Emotional Ear Chart: **282**

Emotional Health: 143, 178, 215, **309-310**, 405

Emotional Release: 282, 292, **310-312**

Emotional Trauma: 27, 83, 137, 164, 292, **309-310**, **469**, 542, 565

Endocrine System: 155, 173, 185, 212, 215, 308, 332, 337, 385, **470**, 534

EndoFlex: 50, 144, **149**, 335-337, 373, 384, 385, 387, 412, 413, 415, 417-419, 421, 426, 438, 440, 448, 459, 469-471, 474-476, 504, 509-511, 520, 532-534, 538, 564, 565, 580, 584, 587, 588, 592, 598, 604

EndoFlex Vitality: **149**, 412, 413, 415, 417-419, 421, 426, 438, 440, 448, 459, 469-471, 474-476, 504, 509-511, 520, 532, 533, 538, 564, 565, 580, 584, 587, 588, 592, 598, 604

En-R-Gee: 144, **149**, 313-316, 373, 413, 417, 431, 440, 473, 474, 506, 513, 537, 538, 575, 577, 581-584, 587, 592, 598, 604

EndoGize: **173**, **212**, 406, 407, 413, 415, 417, 418, 423, 424, 428, 430, 432, 451, 457, 458, 469, 474-476, 484, 507-511, 516, 537, 538, 576, 577, 580, 584, 585, 604

Endometriosis: **508**

Endorphins: **56**

EndoShield: **336-337**, **384-385**, 534, 535

Energy Centers: 146, 152, 157, 161, 296, **308**, 310, 311, 333

Environmental Pollution: 336, 337, 385, 405, 406, **534**, 553

Environmental Protection Kits: iii, iv, **336-337**, **384-385**, **534**

Envision: 144, 145, **149**, 312-315, 373, 413, 415, 434, 474, 565, 576, 580, 582, 585-587, 592, 598, 604

Enzyme Cleanse: **327**

Enzyme Quick Reference Guide: ii, iii, 168, **344**, 409

Enzyme Ramping: **327**

Enzymes: iii, 35, 37, 92, 168, 169, **172-174**, 180, 199, 201, 207-210, 229, 249, 253, 264, 319, **323-331**, 337, 338, **343-355**, 364, 365, 367, 371, 377, 378, 385, 389, 391, 395, 398, 405, 406, 409, 416, 425, 428, 434-436, 447, 459, 462, 463, 476,

481, 500, 513, 529, 530, 534

Epilepsy: 93, 130, 209, 215, 393, **470**

Epstein-Barr Virus: 451, **471**, 474

Essential Beauty Serum: **204**, **219**, 414, 432, 547, 576, 577, 582, 584, 587, 604

Essential Oil Chemistry: **17-22**

Essential Oil Testimonials About Animals: iii, **275**

Essential Oils for Cooking: **255**

Essential Oils Skin Rejuvenation: **552**

Essentialzyme: 168, **173**, 208, 271, 325, 327, 331, 334-336, 344, 346, 350, 351, 387, 406, 407, 409, 412, 413, 415, 416, 418-421, 423-425, 427-429, 434-439, 441, 442, 446-451, 453, 455-457, 459-465, 467-476, 479-484, 486-488, 491, 495, 497-506, 508, 511-516, 519-522, 527, 530, 535-537, 539, 541, 544, 545, 550-559, 562, 564-566, 575, 577, 579, 586, 588, 604

Essentialzymes-4: 168, **174**, 208, 271, 327, 331, 332, 334-336, 344, 346, 350, 351, 387, 406, 407, 412, 413, 415, 416, 418-421, 423-425, 427-429, 434, 437-439, 441, 442, 446-453, 455, 456, 459-465, 467-476, 479-484, 486-488, 491, 495, 498-505, 508, 511-516, 519, 521, 522, 527, 530, 535-537, 544, 545, 550-557, 564-566, 575, 579, 580, 583, 587, 588, 604

Esters: **19**, 20, 35, 197, 238, 310, 337, 385, 534

Estro: **174**, 423, 428, 457, 458, 508, 538, 577, 579, 582, 604

Ethers: **19**

Eucalyptus Blue: 43, 67, **87**, 88, 147, 159, 162, 250, 334, 412, 413, 420, 426, 431, 452, 454, 465, 474, 475, 484-487, 489-492, 501-505, 513, 514, 519, 520, 528, 535, 542-544, 548, 551, 555, 560-562, 571, 573, 578, 591, 595, 597, 604

Eucalyptus Citriodora: 21, 43, 67, **88-90**, 159, 162, 250, 571, 573, 579, 595, 597, 604

Eucalyptus Globulus: 21, 30, 32, 43, 50, 56, 67, 88, **89**, 123, 147, 159, 162, 225-227, 250, 254, 268, 315, 422-425, 429, 450, 486, 490-492, 501-505, 511, 524-526, 543, 548, 552, 560-562, 571, 573, 579, 591, 595, 597, 604

Eucalyptus Radiata: 21, 43, 57, 67, **89**, 90, 147, 159, 162, 163, 178, 191, 220, 222, 225, 227, 229, 231, 232, 234, 244, 245, 248, 250-254, 268, 292, 304, 412, 422, 452, 455, 465, 473, 477, 486, 489-492, 494, 501-503, 519, 526, 527, 542-545, 548, 560-562, 571, 573, 579, 591, 595, 597, 604

Eucalyptus Staigeriana: 43, 67, **90**, 147, 571, 573, 579, 591

Europe: vii, 8, **29**, **44**, 69, 71, 76, 77, 85, 87,

90, 94, 104, 110, 125, 128-130, 133, 134, 141, 149, 167, 174, 209, 225, 396

Evening Peace Bath & Shower Gel: **217**, 547, 575-578, 580, 581, 583, 585-587, 589, 604

Evergreen Essence: 144, **150**, 412, 414, 425, 434, 451, 458, 467-469, 479, 487, 542, 565, 581, 586, 589, 592, 604

Excessive Bleeding: **508**, 509

Excessive Sexual Desire: **539**

Exodus II: 52, 144, **150**, 153, 267, 268, 272, 333, 334, 373, 386, 387, 406, 407, 413, 417, 418, 421, 437, 452, 461, 465, 466, 471, 473, 479, 480, 482, 489, 491-493, 502, 503, 505, 511, 524, 526, 527, 530, 535, 536, 539, 541-544, 552, 555, 560-563, 566, 576, 577, 579, 581, 584, 592, 598, 604

Exotic Pets: 257, **259**

Expressed Oils: **41**

Eye Cream: **205**, **241**, 554, 575, 578-580, 582, 586, 589, 612

Eye Disorders: **471**

Facial Scrub: **241**, 545, 547, 586, 587, 610

Facial Wash: **205**, **240**, 547, 582, 583, 585, 587, 608

Fainting: 79, 367, 446, **474**, 498, 542

Fan Strokes: **300**

Farag, Radwan: **10**, 362, 377, 418

Fasting: 77, 206, **324-325**, 389, 390, 434, 435, 447, 530

Fat: 7, 8, 77, 95, 104, 175, 182, 188, 194, 206-208, 210, 211, 225, 241, 317-321, 325-327, 330, **344-350**, 351, **355**, 358, 363, 378, 392, 393, 398, 448, 449, 481, 501, 506, 525

Fatigue: 27, 69, 71, 99, 116, 122, 123, 126, 130, 131, 134, 145, 169, 171, 179, 191, 211, 320, 321, 348, 357, 382, 393, 417, 419, 421, 422, 431, 443, 450-452, 471, **474**, 478, 487, 490, 498, 499, 510, 516, 530, 541, 543, 555, 564, 565

FDA: 30, 32, 35, 50, 51, 219, 292, **319**, **355**, 367, **380**, 383, 392, 393, 396, 409

Fear: 27, 153, 156, 282, 309, **314**, 325, 405, 406, 433, 519

Feather Spray: **259**, 275

Feather Strokes: **299**

FemiGen: **174**, **213**, 413, 428, 457, 458, 508, 509, 538, 577, 579, 587, 589, 604

Fennel: 18-20, 43, 50, 67, **90**, 91, 145, 148, 154, 156, 161, 164, 169, 171-174, 177-179, 182, 183, 185, 186, 189, 202, 212-215, 217, 223, 225, 250, 253, 265, 266, 315, 326, 328, 330-332, 339, 342, 350, 351, 406, 407, 412, 413, 415-417, 419, 420, 427, 429, 435, 448, 453, 456, 458, 459, 461-463, 468-470, 482, 495, 497, 506-509, 511, 513, 519, 525, 530-532, 538, 543, 544, 564, 572, 573, 579, 591-597, 604

Fennel Vitality: **90**, 412, 413, 415-417, 419, 420, 427, 429, 448, 453, 456, 458, 459, 461-463, 468-470, 482, 495, 506-509, 511, 519, 525, 530, 531, 538, 543, 544, 564, 572, 573, 579, 597, 604

Fever: 84, 111, 195, 293, 420, 461, **475**, 476, 482, 490, 493, 499, 505-507, 517, 526, 530, 531, 535, 541, 543, 548, 562, 566

Fibrillation: **443**

Fibroids: **475**, 508

Fibromyalgia: 327, 382, 416, 417, **476**, 528

Finger Straddle: 296, **301**

First Aid: 267, **548**

First-aid Spray: **245**, **548**

First-Degree Burns: **546**

Fish: 168, 178, 184, 185, 220, **259**, 276, 328, 335, 340, 344, 350, 353, 354, 388

Flash Points: **597-599**

Flatulence: 330, 346, **462**, 464

Fleas: 123, **268**

Flu: 11, 86, 130, **268**, 304, 333, 354, 382, 429, 452, 490, 502

Fluoride: iv, 227-229, 231, 358, **365-367**, 398, 405

Foaming Hand Soaps: **245**

Food Allergies: **420**

Food Poisoning: **476**

Foot Conditions and Problems: **477**, 479

Forgetfulness: **314**, 320

Forgiveness: 144, 146, 148, **150**, 151, 152, **311**, 313, 315, 316, 373, 412, 415, 418, 419, 433, 434, 468, 469, 519, 520, 531, 565, 575, 578-584, 586, 587, 589, 591, 592, 598, 604

FOS: 170, 186, 190, 192, 323, **395-397**, 458, 462, 479

Fractures: 153, **269**, 367, 398

France: vii, 9, **10**, **11**, **23**, 25, 27, 37, 41, 43, **47**, 68, 70, 75, 79, 83, 98, 104, 105, 110, 112, 114, 119, 125, 127, 130, 134, 228, 291, 369

Franchomme, Pierre: **9**, **17**, 337, 385, 534

Frankincense: iv, v, 4, 5, 8, 13-16, 18, 21, 24, 31-33, 41, 43, 50, 56, 57, 67, 71, 87, **91-93**, 108, 115, 120, 128, 129, 143, 145-153, 155-159, 161, 163-165, 169, 171, 181, 189, 202, 204, 205, 212, 214, 215, 223, 234, 236-241, 243, 244, 248, 250, 259, 261, 266, 268, 269, 275, **307**, 308, 310, 312-316, 330, 332-334, 361, **368-373**, 381, 386-388, 398, 412-415, 417-420, 422-425, 427-434, 436-438, 447, 449, 450, 452-455, 457, 458, 461, 464, 465, 468-478, 481-485, 487, 489-493, 496-498, 501, 503, 504, 506, 507, 514, 516, 518-521, 523-526, 528, 529, 531, 533, 535-538, 542, 544, 546, 548-550, 552-555, 557, 560-562, 565, 566, 571, 573, 574, 579, 587, 591-598, 604, 610

Frankincense Vitality: **91**, 261, 412-415, 417-420, 422-425, 428-434, 436-438, 447, 449, 450, 452-454, 457, 458, 461, 464, 465, 468-476, 481, 483, 484, 487, 489, 490, 497, 498, 501, 503, 506, 507, 514, 516, 519-521, 523, 525, 526, 528, 529, 531, 533, 535, 537, 538, 555, 560-562, 571, 573, 579, 597, 604

Freedom: 36, 144, **150**, 175, 266, 310-316, 332, 379, 412, 414, 415, 434, 458, 467-469, 487, 537, 542, 565, 578, 579, 581, 582, 585-589, 592, 598, 604

Frequency: iv, 27, 52, 72, 93, 116, 143, 150, 152, 165, 169, 209, 211, 220, 257-259, 285, 311, 332, 333, 358, **372-377**, 381, 383

Frereana Frankincense: 43, 67, **92**, 189, 371, 398, 571, 573, 579, 604

Friedmann, Terry: **76**, **137**, 236, 291, 424, 444, 471

Frigidity (Women): **538**

Fructose: 133, 170, 171, 176, 180, 186, 213, 249, 328, 346, **391-397**

Fruit & Veggie Soak: **253**, 421, 422, 575, 577, 579, 580, 582-588, 611

Fruit & Veggie Spray: **253**, 577, 579, 583, 587

Frustration: 152, **314**, 332, 376, 418, 474

FTIF Spectroscopy: **47**

Fujimoto, Edward: **378**

Fungal Infections: 71, 72, 75, 88, 93, 98, 109, 110, 114, 116, 119, 121, 127, 133, 243, 259, **478**, 479, 484, 485, 564

Fungal Skin Infections: **550**

Furanoids: **20**

Galbanum: 8, 67, **93**, 373, 572, 573, 579

Gallbladder Infection (Cholecystitis): **481**

Gallstones: 209, 320, 330, 351, **481**, 567

Ganglion Cysts: **457**

Gangrene: 9, **482**, 518

Gary's Equine Essentials: iii, **270**, 576-584, 586, 587, 589, 604

Gary's Equine Essentials Massage Oil: **270**, 576, 578, 580, 582, 584, 586, 587, 589

Gary's Equine Essentials Shampoo: **270**, 577, 579, 580, 582-584, 587, 589

Gary's Tail & Mane Sheen: **270**, 583

Gary's True Grit: 173, **175-177**, 192, 201, 204, 583, 585, 588, 604, 605

Gary's True Grit Chocolate-Coated Wolfberry Crisp Bars: **176**, 192, **201**, 204, 604

Gary's True Grit Einkorn Flour: **176**, 604

Gary's True Grit Einkorn Grain Products: **175**

Gary's True Grit Einkorn Granola: **176**, **201**, 588, 605

Gary's True Grit Einkorn Pancake and Waffle Mix: **176**, 605

Gary's True Grit Einkorn Rotini Pasta: 176, **177**, 605

Gary's True Grit Einkorn Spaghetti: 176, **177**, 605

Gary's True Grit NingXia Berry Syrup: **177**, **201**, 583, 585, 605

Gas: 4, 9, 10, 18, 19, 23-27, 33, 41, 42, 47, 48, 91, 104, 108, 129, 148, 169, 172, 177, 180, 249, 320, 330, 335, 346, 348, 351, 352, 396, 398, 412, 449, 457, 459, 460, **462**, 463, 471, 482, 495, 530

Gas (Flatulence): **462**

Gas Chromatography: 4, 10, **23-25**, 27, 33, 47, 48, 91, 108, 129, 398

Gastritis: 327, 464, **482**

Gathering: 144, **150**, 312-316, 333, 373, 412, 413, 430, 434, 464, 489, 519, 520, 525, 532, 539, 565, 577, 580, 582, 584, 586, 587, 589, 592, 598, 605

Gattefossé, René-Maurice: **9-10**

Genesis Hand & Body Lotion: **218**, 414, 545, 547, 575, 578, 580, 581, 583, 585, 586, 589, 605

GeneYus: 144, **151**, **250**, 312-316, 413, 415-417, 424, 425, 429-432, 446, 453, 465, 470, 474, 486, 515, 519, 520, 523, 575, 576, 578-581, 584-587, 589, 592, 605

Genital Human Papillomavirus (HPV): **540**

Genital Warts/Blisters (Herpes Simplex Type 2): **540**

Gentle Baby: 144, **151**, 267, 268, 313, 314, 373, 412, 414, 515, 531, 532, 536, 546, 547, 549, 551, 553, 554, 575, 578, 580-583, 585, 586, 589, 592, 598, 605

Geranium: 19, 30, 43, 50, 67, **93**, 94, 145-161, 164, 165, 179, 186, 204, 205, 213-215, 217-221, 223, 225, 226, 236, 237, 239-241, 243, 247, 248, 250, 265-268, 270, 292, 312-316, 330, 331, 337, 385, 431, 439-442, 445, 447, 450, 457, 466, 467, 469, 475, 479, 480, 483, 486, 487, 489, 494, 496-498, 500, 506, 507, 509, 510, 512, 518, 520, 521, 524, 530, 531, 534, 538, 541, 545, 547-549, 552-554, 572, 573, 580, 591-597, 605

German Chamomile: d, 19, 21, 40, 43, 46, 50, 67, **94**, 145, 146, 148, 149, 152, 158, 160, 161, 164, 165, 171, 179, 185, 235, 240, 242, 266, 270, 331, 373, 412, 414, 417, 420, 422, 423, 429, 438-440, 442, 444-446, 453, 455, 456, 464, 469, 475, 476, 478, 481, 486, 489-492, 495, 497, 499, 500, 502, 507, 508, 512, 513, 528, 531, 533, 541, 545, 546, 548-551, 556, 557, 564, 571-574, 580, 591-597, 605

German Chamomile Vitality: **94**, 414, 417, 420, 423, 429, 438-440, 442, 444-446, 453, 456, 464, 469, 475, 476, 486, 490, 499, 500, 502, 507, 508, 528, 533, 551, 557, 564, 572, 573, 580, 605

Germany: 20, **31**, 119, 195, 196, 232, 434, 485

Giardia: 360, **462**, 476

Gift, The: iv, 30, 57, 144, 145, 151, **163**, 310, 312, 314-316, 332-334, 368, 381, 388, 398, 412, 413, 415, 419, 421, 425,

Index

432, 434, 453, 458, 464, 469, 470, 483, 485, 486, 489, 492, 493, 513, 524, 525, 531, 537, 538, 548, 555, 560, 565, 577, 579, 581, 584, 587, 595, 599, 611

Ginger: 17, 18, 43, 50, 67, **95**, 145, 148, 155-157, 164, 169, 171-174, 177-179, 182, 185, 186, 212, 250, 253, 265, 266, 313, 314, 326, 330, 331, 340, 350, 412, 419, 427, 429, 456, 459, 460, 462, 463, 467, 468, 476, 513-516, 519, 530, 537, 552, 572, 573, 580, 588, 591-594, 596, 597, 605

Ginger Vitality: **95**, 173, 412, 419, 427, 429, 456, 459, 460, 462, 463, 467, 468, 476, 515, 516, 519, 530, 572, 573, 580, 597, 605

Gingivitis and Periodontitis: 229, **526**

Glands: 41, 71, 114, 146, 150, 200, 207, 209-211, 287, 308, 333, 337, 385, **416-418**, **470**, **496**, 506, 511, 534

GLF: 144, **151**, 325, 328, 334, 388, 389, 406, 412, 413, 416, 419, 421, 425, 427, 434, 437, 440, 441, 447, 453, 481, 483, 487, 496, 499-501, 514, 515, 522, 524, 536, 554, 576, 580-582, 588, 592, 598, 605

GLF Vitality: **151**, 406, 412, 413, 416, 419, 421, 425, 427, 434, 437, 440, 441, 447, 453, 481, 483, 487, 496, 499, 500, 514, 515, 522, 536, 554, 576, 588, 592, 598

Glycemic Index: 171, **197-198**, **203**, 335, 393, 395-397

Goldenrod: 43, 46, 50, 67, **95**, 147, 185, 438, 440, 443, 445, 446, 518, 537, 554, 560, 563, 572, 573, 580, 591, 597, 605

Gonorrhea and Syphilis: **541**

Good Eating Habits: **335**

Gout: 120, 382, **482**, 483

Grade B Maple Syrup: 324, 325, **396**

Grain: 41, 173, **175-177**, 230, 254, 269, 271, 273, 342, 348, 354, 436

Grapefruit: 18, 20, 31, 41, 43, 49, 50, 56, 57, 67, **96**, 97, 145-149, 151, 152, 158, 160-162, 164, 182, 186, 188-192, 205, 224, 225, 231, 247, 248, 313, 325, 326, 328, 334, 350, 412, 413, 429, 433, 437, 440, 446, 448, 449, 463, 469, 471, 475, 481, 496, 499, 500, 505, 506, 525, 547, 571, 573, 580, 591-597, 605

Grapefruit Juice Recipe: **326**

Grapefruit Lip Balm: 205, **224**, 475, 547, 580, 605

Grapefruit Vitality: **96**, 412, 413, 429, 437, 440, 446, 448, 463, 469, 471, 481, 496, 505, 525, 571, 573, 580, 592, 597, 605

GRAS: i, **50**, 81, 292, 397, 406

Gratitude: 50, 144, **151**, 312, 314, 315, 412, 434, 575, 578-581, 583, 584, 589, 592, 598, 605

Graves' Disease: **563-564**

Grief: 154, **315**

Grounding: 72, 83, 87, 99, 111, 116, 123, 128, 136, 137, 144, **152**, 160, **311**, 313, 315, 316, 326, 333, 373, 381, 412, 417, 433, 465, 469, 489, 531, 575, 576, 582, 586, 589, 593, 598, 605

Guilt: 282, **315**, 558, 566

Hahn, Scott: **307**

Hair and Scalp Problems: **483**

Hair Care: ii, 51, 146, 208, 221, **483**, 485, 601-612

Hair Loss: 76, 104, 126, 130, 141, **484**, 507

Halitosis (Bad Breath): **485**, 525

Háloa Áina Royal Hawaiian Sandalwood: **243**

Háloa Áina Royal Hawaiian Sandalwood Soap Collection: **243**

Hand Purifier: ii, **222**, 253, 421, 422, 577, 579, 583, 586, 587, 612

Hardening of the Arteries: 358, **439**

Harmony: 126, 140, 144, 146, **152**, 153, 165, 171, 239, 281, **310**, 312-316, 332, 333, 373, 375, 376, 381, 412, 414-417, 420, 425, 429, 430, 432, 434, 458, 464, 465, 467-470, 487, 494, 516, 519, 532, 537, 539, 542, 545, 554, 555, 560, 565, 575, 576, 578-589, 591, 593, 598, 599, 605, 606

Hashimoto's Disease: **564**

Hawaii: **11**, 128, **243**, 378

Hay Fever (Allergic Rhinitis): **420**

Headache: 32, 79, 94, 121, 195, 257, 325, 450, **485-487**, 490, 493, 505, 531, 543, 564, 566, 567

Health Issues: 304, **358**

Healthy Snacks: **341**

Hearing Impairment: **466**

Heart Attack (Myocardial Infarction): **443**

Heartburn: 148, 322, 330, 346, 348, 415, **463**, 464

Heart Health: 443, **444**

Heart Stimulant: **444**

Heart Vita Flex: 439, 441, **443-445**, 447, 470

Heavy Metals: 48, 179, 317, **324-328**, 357, 389, **487**

Heavy Metals Cleanse: **327**

Hebrew University: **307**, 371

Helichrysum: 5, 19, 37, 43, 46, 47, 50, 67, **97**, 145, 146, 148, 150, 151, 154-156, 158, 164, 240, 250, 266-268, 270, 271, 313, 316, 321, 328, 331, 373, 409, 412-414, 418-420, 423, 424, 427-429, 431, 438-449, 453, 455, 465-467, 469, 475, 478, 481, 483, 486-488, 490, 497-499, 508, 509, 512-514, 516-519, 521, 522, 524-529, 531, 536, 545, 546, 548, 549, 551-553, 555-559, 566, 572, 573, 580, 591-594, 596, 597, 605

Hematoma: **440**

Hemorrhagic Strokes: **446**

Hemorrhaging: **439**, 447

Hemorrhoids: **488**

Hepatitis: 73, 76, 80, 93-95, 102, 105, 114, 116, 124, 126, 131, 134, 139, 154, 196, 283, 318-321, 377, 498, **499**

Herb Farming: **37**

Herbicides: 22, 37, 44, 207, **317**, 348, 358, 448, **449**

Herniated Disc/Disc Deterioration: **557**

Herpes Simplex Type 1: **451**

Herpes Simplex Type 2: **539**, 540

Herpes Zoster: 72, 121, 128, **450**, **541**

Hertel, Hans Ulrich: **379**

HFCS: **391**, 392

Hiccups: **488**

Hide Injuries: **270**

Hieroglyphics: **5**, 348, 361

Highest Potential: 144, 146, **152**, 271, 312-314, 316, 333, 414, 524, 531, 532, 554, 565, 576-589, 593, 598, 605

High-Fructose Corn Syrup: **391-392**, 396, 398

Highland Flats Tree Farm: **44-45**

Hildegard of Bingen: **8**, 69, 80, 85, 90, 110, 114, 116, 118, 126, 134

Hinoki: 43, 67, **97**, 148, 155, 157, 158, 161, 215, 224, 235, 236, 238, 244, 250, 266, 270, 312-316, 412-414, 418, 477-480, 489, 490, 571, 573, 581, 592-595, 597, 605

Hippocampus: 27, 95, **309**, 406, 470

Hirsch, Alan: **27**, 121, 525

Hives: **489**, 493, 498

Hobble Injury: **269**

Home: **251-256**

Hong Kuai: 43, 67, **98**, 147, 571, 573, 581, 591, 597, 605

Hoof Infections: **270**

Hope: 93, 144, 146, **152**, 163, 282, **311**, 316, 352, 373, 412, 413, 415, 433, 434, 449, 453, 458, 469, 474, 487, 519, 520, 540, 554, 565, 576, 582, 584, 593, 598, 605

Hormonal Edema: **509**

Hormone Balancing: ii, **223**

Hormones: ii, viii, 27, 59, 71, 112, 114, 161, 173, 174, **207-215**, 225, 318, 348, 351, 354, 361, 367, 390, 416, 417, 430, 435, 436, 470, 474, 507, 508, 510, 519, 538, 560, 563, 565

Horses: iii, 13-15, 241, 242, 257, 258, **264**, **269**, 272, 273, 304, 348, 435, 513

HPV: **540**

Human Rights: **379**

Humidifier: **57**, 88, 90, 115

Humility: 144, **152**, 157, 313-316, 373, 412, 415, 418, 441, 464, 552-554, 560, 575, 578-580, 584, 586, 589, 593, 598, 605

Huntington's Chorea: **520**

Hunza: **389**, 390

Hyperactivity: 5, 76, 97, 136, 137, 242, **489**

Hypertension: 32, 73, 83, 95, 97, 101, 106, 112, 115-118, 120, 126, 133, 139, 141, 162, 206, 320, 355, 361, **441**, 530

Seventh Edition | **Essential Oils Desk Reference** | 621

**Essential Oils Desk Reference** | Seventh Edition

Hyperthyroid: **563**
Hypoglycemia: 206, 450, 471, 485, **564**
Hypothyroid: 115, **564**
Hyssop: 8, 12, 14, 15, 19, 43, 50, 67, **98**, 99, 149-153, 156, 157, 159, 160, 164, 165, 250, 266, 388, 437, 452, 471, 481, 490, 505, 512, 532, 535, 560, 572, 573, 581, 592-597, 605
Hysterectomy: **509**
Iceland: **31**, 498
ICP: **177**, 208, 272, 325, 330, 332, 335, 387, 388, 406, 407, 409, 412, 413, 416, 419, 420, 423, 427, 441, 442, 450, 451, 453, 455, 456, 459-465, 469-471, 476, 480-483, 485-488, 491, 495, 497, 499-503, 506, 508, 530, 533, 539, 545, 550-555, 557, 562, 564, 565, 575, 579, 580, 583, 587, 588, 605
Idaho: vii, **11**, 19, 39, **43-45**, 49, 50, 57, 67, 87, 94, **99-101**, 105, 112, 138, 145-151, 153-161, 163-165, 170, 171, 185, 188, 215, 224, 225, 235, 236, 244, 250, 265-270, 273, 311-316, 326, 330, 332-334, 373, 381, 412-415, 417, 418, 422-428, 432, 433, 436, 437, 439, 440, 442, 447, 449, 453, 454, 463, 465, 468-470, 472, 474-478, 480, 481, 483, 489-496, 502, 503, 507, 510, 511, 513, 514, 518, 519, 528, 529, 532, 533, 535, 537, 538, 542-544, 546, 547, 549, 551, 555-560, 564, 565, 571-573, 581, 591-597, 605
Idaho Balsam Fir: 43, 50, 57, 67, **99**, 146, 148, 149, 151, 156-158, 160, 163, 170, 171, 188, 224, 244, 250, 265, 267, 269, 270, **311**, 316, 326, 330, 332, 333, 381, 412, 415, 417, 418, 422-425, 427, 428, 433, 436, 437, 439, 440, 449, 453, 454, 468, 469, 474-476, 481, 491, 493, 495, 496, 502, 503, 513, 514, 528, 529, 532, 533, 535, 538, 542-544, 546, 547, 549, 555-557, 559, 560, 565, 571, 573, 581, 591, 592, 594, 595, 597, 605
Idaho Blue Spruce: 43, 67, **99**, 100, 145-147, 150, 151, 153-159, 161, 164, 165, 185, 215, 224, 225, 235, 236, 244, 250, 312-316, 412-414, 432, 433, 436, 437, 439, 442, 447, 454, 465, 469, 470, 472, 474, 476-478, 480, 483, 489-491, 495, 496, 507, 510, 511, 513, 518, 519, 529, 537, 556-559, 564, 565, 572, 573, 581, 591-597, 605
Idaho Ponderosa Pine: 43, 67, **100**, 312-315, 423, 424, 572, 573, 581
Idaho Tansy: 19, 43, 45, 49, 67, **101**, 146, 224, 250, 266-268, 273, 316, 332, 334, 373, 426, 463, 470, 491, 492, 494, 551, 572, 573, 581, 591, 597, 605
Immune System: 17, 78, 79, 132, 163, 170, 175, 178, 181, 185, 190, 201, 204, 210, 211, 259, 284, 291, 292, 308, 309, 311, 320, 333, 334, 337, 343, 346, 354, 378-

380, 383, 385, 387-389, 393, 395, 397, **406**, **420**, 423, 448, **450**, **451**, 456, 479, 480, 489, 503, 507, 512, 521, 534, 553, 554, 560
ImmuPower: 144, **153**, 268, 333, 334, 373, 381, 412, 413, 421, 422, 432, 437, 451, 452, 456, 461, 465, 466, 471, 475, 476, 479, 482, 489, 491, 503, 506, 507, 526-528, 530, 531, 535, 540, 541, 552, 561-563, 577-579, 581, 584-586, 593, 599, 605
ImmuPro: **178**, **201**, **213**, 268, 333, 387, 406, 407, 409, 412, 414, 417, 418, 421-424, 426, 432, 437, 441, 448, 450-452, 460, 462, 465, 466, 471, 473, 475, 479, 482, 486, 487, 489, 490, 495, 499-501, 503, 504, 506-508, 511, 512, 523, 526-528, 530, 531, 533, 535, 538-544, 553-555, 560-563, 566, 585, 605
Impacted Bowel: **459**
Impotence (Men): **537**
Imprinting on New Foals: **271**
Indigestion (Bloating): **463**
Infect Away: **266**, 268, 272, 578, 584-586, 606
Infected Breast: **432**
Infection (Bacterial and Viral): **489**
Infectious Parotitis: **511**
Infertility (Men): **537**
Infertility (Women): **538**
Inflammation: 25, 32, 79, 88, 91, 93, 95, 98, 99, 106, 118, 120, 125, 128, 139, 142, 148, 156, 158, 169, 170, 176, 185, 186, 194, 196, 200, 214, 227, 229, 242, 267-269, 275, 291, 292, 317, 321, 324, 327, 371, 377, 382, 392, 398, 420, 422, 423, 426, 433, 435, 436, 439, 444, 445, 452, 454-456, 465, 473, 481, 489, **490**, 495, 496, 501, 502, 511, 512, 516, 517, 519, 521, 522, 524, 529, 531-533, 535, 542-546, 548, 556, 558, 559, 561, 562, 566
Inflammation Due to Infection: **512**
Inflammation Due to Injury: **512**
Inflammation of Veins: **445**
Influenza: 11, 112, 128, 134, 159, **490**, 491
Inhalation: 4, 27, 31, 32, 49, 57, **58**, 71, 76, 98, 102, 105, 106, 116, 123, 134, 142, 162, 281, 359, 374, 388, 406, 424
Inner Child: 144, **153**, **311**, 315, 326, 333, 373, 412, 415, 433, 450, 464, 469, 472, 509, 547, 576, 581, 583-585, 587-589, 593, 599, 606
Inner Defense: **178**, 332-334, 336, 387, 412, 413, 417, 418, 420-422, 426, 431, 432, 440, 448, 450-453, 460-462, 464-466, 471, 476, 480-482, 489, 491, 492, 497, 502-505, 507, 511, 526-528, 530, 531, 535, 540-544, 553, 560-563, 566, 577, 579, 583, 585, 587, 588, 606
Inner Harmony: 144, **153**, 312-316, 332, 333, 412, 415, 425, 434, 458, 464, 467-

469, 487, 537, 542, 565, 575, 579-582, 584-589, 593, 599, 606
Insect: 3, 17, 69, 78, 79, 81, 88-90, 101, 108, 120, 129, 146, 154, 225, 250, **259**, 266, 268, 419, 426, 491-494, 506
Insect Bites and Stings: **491**
Insect Repellent: 78, 88, 89, 101, 120, 268, **493**, 494
Insomnia: 17, 70, 79, 94, 104, 108, 112, 115, 118, 122, 125, 131, 132, 136, 137, 158, 164, 457, **494**, 495, 554, 563
Inspiration: 144, **153**, 157, 314-316, 333, 373, 412, 427, 453, 480, 483, 501, 552, 575, 576, 578-580, 584, 587, 589, 593, 599, 606
Intestinal Fiber Cleanse: **330**
Intestinal Worms: **530**
Into the Future: 144, 145, **153**, 312, 314, 316, 373, 412, 413, 576, 577, 579, 581, 582, 585, 589, 593, 599, 606
InTouch: 144, **154**, 312-316, 333, 412, 414-416, 418, 419, 424, 425, 429-432, 434, 451, 458, 467-469, 487, 537, 542, 565, 576, 581, 584, 587, 589, 593, 599, 606
Iran: **31**, 69, 78, 84, 102, 104, 106, 112, 119, 126
Irregular Periods: 148, **509**
Irritability: 125, 132, 169, 179, 242, **315**, 321, 325, 417, 419, 450, 471, 474, 478, 510, 555, 564
Irritable Bowel Syndrome: 122, 169, 209, 320, 452, 461, **463**, **495**, 567
Ishpingo: 43, 67, **101**, 117, 572, 573, 581
Israel: **7**, **11**, 12, 13, 113, 368
Itching: 109, 120, 225, 239, 244, 320, 419, 426, 451, 488, 489, 491, 492, 498, 539, **550**
Jade Lemon: 43, 50, 67, **101**, 102, 252, 253, 312-316, 412-415, 419, 421, 426, 430, 438, 440, 441, 445, 447, 448, 450, 451, 457, 458, 460, 462-464, 467, 469, 473, 474, 481-483, 485, 487, 488, 496, 498, 500, 506, 511, 515, 536, 561, 565, 571, 573, 581, 597, 606
Jade Lemon Vitality: **102**, 412-415, 419, 421, 426, 430, 438, 440, 441, 445, 447, 448, 450, 451, 457, 458, 460, 462-464, 467, 469, 473, 474, 481-483, 485, 487, 488, 496, 498, 500, 506, 511, 515, 536, 561, 565, 571, 573, 581, 597, 606
Japan: **11**, 97, 98, 292, 317, 370, 396, 545
Jasmine: 7, 18, 19, 41, 43, 50, 67, **102**, 108, 145-158, 160, 161, 163, 164, 215, 217-219, 222, 225, 226, 235, 237, 239, 266, 312, 313, 315, 316, 414, 457, 487, 509, 536-538, 572, 573, 581, 591-597, 606
Jaundice: 139, 320, 481, 498, **499**, 530
Jealousy: 14, 309, **315**
Jitteriness: **264**, **271**
Joint Stiffness or Pain: **495**
Joy: 27, 50, 57, 110, 116, 144-147, **154**,

**622** | Index

**Index**

163, **215**, 271, 281, **311**, 316, 333, 370, 373, 412-415, 433, 434, 445, 451, 458, 519, 520, 524, 525, 531, 532, 536, 538, 539, 552, 565, 575, 578, 580, 581, 583, 585, 586, 588, 589, 591, 593, 599, 606

Juniper: 5, 18, 19, 21, 43, 50, 67, 84, **103**, 143, 148, 149, 152, 153, 157, 158, 169, 179, 185, 218, 225, 244, 253, 265, 266, 271, 312-315, 330, 350, 373, 412, 413, 422, 426, 427, 445, 446, 448, 449, 466, 467, 469, 471, 474, 481, 483, 484, 495-498, 513, 514, 518-521, 572, 573, 578, 582, 591-594, 597, 603, 606

JuvaCleanse: 50, 144, **154**, 321, 325, 328, 329, 331, 332, 334, 388, 406, 412, 415, 416, 419-421, 434, 438, 440, 441, 443, 446, 447, 453, 459, 462, 463, 481-484, 487, 499, 500, 511, 515, 524, 525, 530, 549-551, 554, 576, 580, 582, 593, 599, 606

JuvaCleanse Vitality: **154**, 406, 412, 415, 416, 419-421, 434, 438, 440, 441, 443, 446, 447, 453, 459, 462, 463, 481-484, 487, 499, 500, 511, 515, 525, 530, 551, 554, 593, 599, 606

JuvaFlex: 50, 144, **154**, 325, 326, 328, 330, 331, 334, 373, 406, 412, 413, 416, 434, 438, 443, 460, 462, 481, 488, 495, 496, 499, 500, 530, 550, 551, 576, 579, 580, 586, 587, 593, 599, 606

JuvaFlex Vitality: **154**, 406, 412, 413, 416, 434, 438, 443, 460, 462, 481, 488, 495, 496, 499, 500, 530, 551, 593, 599, 606

JuvaPower: **178**, 179, 208, 322, 325, 330, 331, 335, 387, 388, 407, 412, 413, 415-417, 420, 423, 427, 429, 434, 438, 439, 441, 442, 445, 447, 450-453, 455, 459, 461-465, 469-471, 473, 480, 481, 483, 487, 488, 491, 495, 497, 499-502, 506-508, 511, 513, 515, 522, 523, 525, 530, 533, 545, 550-556, 564, 565, 575, 579, 606

JuvaSpice: **179**, 322, 331, 335, 338-341, 387, 412, 413, 417, 420, 427, 429, 438, 439, 441, 442, 447, 450, 451, 453, 455, 459, 465, 470, 481, 499, 500, 502, 506, 511, 513, 522, 523, 533, 550-552, 554-556, 564, 565, 575, 579, 606

JuvaTone: **179**, 327, 331, 332, 334, 406, 412, 413, 416, 418-420, 423, 434, 441-443, 450, 451, 455, 471, 481, 483, 488, 499, 500, 508, 544, 550, 551, 554, 555, 565, 576, 580, 583, 584, 587, 606

K&B: **179**, 271, 426, 496-498, 500, 577, 579, 580, 582, 586, 587, 606

Ketones: **19**, 20, 47, 85

Kidney Disorders: 81, **496**

Kidney Failure: **271**, **496**, 497

Kidney Inflammation/Infection (Nephritis): **496**

Kidney Stones: 330, **497**

KidScents: ii, **180**, 201, 227, 231, **247-250**, 332, 387, 406, 407, 412, 413, 432, 485, 488, 489, 501, 525-528, 536, 543, 547, 550, 551, 553, 575-580, 582, 583, 585-589, 606

KidScents Bath Gel: **247**, 576, 580, 606

KidScents Body Care for Children: ii, **247**

KidScents Lotion: **247**, 547, 575, 576, 578, 580, 589, 606

KidScents MightyVites: **180**, **201**, **249**, 387, 406, 407, 413, 606

KidScents MightyZyme: **180**, **249**, 332, 406, 407, 412, 413, 501, 550, 606

KidScents Oil Collection: ii, **250**

KidScents Shampoo: **247**, 583, 588, 606

KidScents Slique Toothpaste: 227, **231**, **247**, 248, 485, 525-528, 543, 577, 579, 580, 583, 585, 587, 588, 606

KidScents Tender Tush: **248**, 432, 488, 489, 536, 550, 551, 553, 575, 577-580, 582, 586, 587, 589, 606

Kitty Litter: **261**, 386

Kitty Raindrop: 258, **261**, 263

Kopp, William: **380**

Korea: **396**

Lack of Libido/Desire (Women): **538**

Lack of Libido (Men): **537**

Lactones: **20**

Lady Sclareol: 144, **155**, **215**, 315, 412, 508-511, 538, 575, 577, 578, 580, 581, 585, 587-589, 593, 599, 606

Lakota Indians: **72**, 116, 290

Lapraz, Jean-Claude: **9-10**, 290

Laryngitis: 130, **561**

Laundry: **253**, 254, 421, 422, 575, 577, 579, 583, 587, 612

Laundry Soap: **253**, 421, 422, 575, 577, 579, 583, 587, 612

Laurus Nobilis (Bay Laurel): **103**, 412, 414, 452, 477, 479, 493, 502, 507, 541, 544, 545, 549, 572, 573, 578, 582, 591, 597, 606

Laurus Nobilis Vitality (Bay Laurel): **103**, 412, 414, 502, 507, 572, 573, 582, 597, 606

LavaDerm Cooling Mist: 55, **240**, 387, 413, 450, 455, 457, 545-551, 580, 582, 584, 606

Lavandin: 18, 20, 21, 23, 25, 43, 50, 53, 67, **104**, 105, 159, 160, 253, 265, 266, 270, 422, 552, 572, 573, 582, 595, 597

Lavender: vi, 4, **9**, **10**, **17-21**, **23-25**, 27, 31, 32, 34, 35, 37, 41-43, 50, 53, 56, 57, 67, **104**, 105, 108, 130, 145-153, 156-164, 174, 186, 188, 202, 204, 205, 214-222, 224-226, 235-241, 243-245, 248, 250, 254, 255, 259, 266-268, 270, 275, 278, 310, 312-316, 326, 333, 373, 387, 412-414, 418-420, 422, 424, 425, 431-434, 438-451, 454-457, 460, 464-467, 469, 470, 472, 473, 475, 477-480, 482-487,

489-495, 498, 501, 502, 504, 505, 507, 508, 510-516, 518, 519, 522, 523, 525, 526, 528, 531, 536, 539-541, 544-556, 560, 562, 564, 566, 572-574, 577, 578, 581-584, 586-588, 591-597, 606, 607

Lavender Bath & Shower Gel: **205**, **217**, 578, 582-584, 606

Lavender Conditioner: **222**, 483, 485, 577, 581-583, 586, 588, 606

Lavender Foaming Hand Soap: **245**, 582-584, 606

Lavender Hand & Body Lotion: **205**, **218**, 414, 578, 582-584, 606

Lavender Lip Balm: 205, **224**, 475, 547, 582, 606

Lavender Mint Invigorating Conditioner: **205**, **221**

Lavender Mint Invigorating Shampoo: **205**, **221**

Lavender-Oatmeal Bar Soap: **243**, 575, 578, 580, 582, 589, 607

Lavender Shampoo: 205, 221, **222**, 483, 485, 577, 581-583, 607

Lavender Vitality: **105**, 255, 412-414, 418-420, 422, 424, 425, 431-434, 438, 439, 441-448, 450, 451, 454, 455, 457, 460, 464, 465, 469, 470, 472, 473, 475, 479, 480, 483, 484, 486, 487, 490, 494, 495, 501, 502, 504, 505, 507, 508, 510, 511, 515, 516, 519, 522, 525, 526, 528, 536, 539, 540, 551, 555, 560, 562, 564, 572, 573, 582, 597, 607

Laxative for Foals: **271**

Layering: 52, **54**, 541

Ledoux, Joseph: **309**

Ledum: 43, 46, 67, **105**, 106, 148, 151, 154, 268, 321, 325, 328, 330-332, 388, 412, 416, 419, 436, 448, 481, 499, 500, 560, 565, 572, 573, 582, 592, 593, 597, 607

Lee, Lita: **378**

Lemon: v, 17, 18, 20, 21, 30, 31, 41, 43, 49, 50, 52, 56, 57, 67, 90, 101, 102, **105-108**, 111, 112, 136, 140, 145-148, 150-152, 154-164, 169, 172, 177-179, 182-184, 186, 188-191, 201-203, 205, 215, 217, 218, 220, 222, 224, 227, 229, 231, 232, 234-236, 238, 240, 243-245, 247, 248, 251-255, 259, 265, 266, 270, 312-316, 324, 325, 329-331, 334, 337, 338, 342, 352, 359, 361, 373, 385, 388, 409, 412-415, 419, 421, 426, 430-432, 434, 438, 440, 441, 445, 447, 448, 450-452, 457, 458, 460, 462-464, 467, 469, 472-474, 477, 479, 481-483, 485, 487, 488, 492, 494, 496-498, 500, 503, 506, 507, 511, 514, 515, 523, 531, 534, 536, 547-549, 551, 555, 560-562, 565, 567, 571, 573, 581, 583, 591-597, 606, 607

Lemon-Sandalwood Cleansing Soap: **243**, 583, 607

Lemon Myrtle: 30, 43, 67, **107**, 108, 158,

Seventh Edition | **Essential Oils Desk Reference** | 623

188, 313, 314, 479, 571, 573, 583, 594, 597, 607

Lemon Vitality: 102, **106**, 255, 409, 412-415, 419, 421, 426, 430-432, 438, 440, 441, 445, 447, 448, 450-452, 457, 458, 460, 462-464, 467, 469, 472-474, 481-483, 485, 487, 488, 496, 498, 500, 503, 506, 507, 511, 514, 515, 531, 536, 560-562, 565, 571, 573, 581, 583, 597, 606, 607

Lemonade Diet: **324**

Lemongrass: 4, 19, 21, 30, 31, 43, 50, 56, 67, 97, 106, **107**, 119, 140, 148, 149, 153, 157, 159, 169, 174, 177, 178, 183, 185, 188, 190, 191, 218, 225, 226, 244, 251, 253, 265-268, 292, 330, 334, 342, 350, 388, 407, 412, 419, 421, 427, 428, 431, 435, 442, 448, 450, 453-455, 458, 464, 473, 474, 477, 479, 489, 493-495, 497, 505, 512-514, 517, 538, 548, 550, 554, 564-566, 571, 573, 583, 592-595, 597, 607

Lemongrass Vitality: **107**, 412, 419, 421, 427, 431, 442, 448, 450, 453-455, 458, 464, 473, 474, 479, 489, 497, 505, 538, 564, 565, 571, 573, 583, 597, 607

Letting Go: iii, **310-311**

Leukemia: 76, 79, 84, 116, 130, 393, **437**, 451, 525

Lewis, Roger: **154**, 321, 499

Lice: 31, 80, 123, 265, **498**, 552

Life 9: 178, **181**, 209, 322, 323, 331, 334, 336, 387, 406, 407, 412, 417, 419-421, 429, 445, 447-450, 453, 455, 456, 458-460, 462-464, 469-471, 475, 476, 479-482, 485, 487, 489, 491, 495, 497, 499, 500, 502, 503, 505-507, 511-513, 515, 522, 527, 530, 531, 535-537, 539-541, 544, 545, 550-557, 560, 562, 564-566, 607

Ligament Sprain or Tear: **455**

Ligaments: 4, 106, 140, 145, 148, 170, 225, 268, **454**, 559

Light the Fire: 144, **155**, 312-314, 316, 412, 434, 458, 537, 538, 576, 581, 584, 585, 593, 599, 607

Limbic System: 4, **26-27**, 71, 114, 309, 311, 322, 333, 374, 406, 415, 424, 467, 470

Lime: 18, 20, 41, 43, 50, 57, 67, 79, **108**, 145-147, 155, 157, 160, 162, 169, 182-184, 191, 203, 204, 221, 224, 237, 253, 312-316, 388, 412-414, 419, 421, 426, 430, 438, 450, 451, 457, 458, 460, 462-464, 467, 469, 474, 481-483, 485, 487, 488, 500, 506, 511, 515, 536, 561, 565, 571, 573, 583, 591, 593-595, 597, 607

Lime Vitality: **108**, 412-414, 419, 421, 426, 430, 438, 450, 451, 457, 458, 460, 462-464, 467, 469, 474, 481-483, 485, 487, 488, 500, 506, 511, 515, 536, 561, 565, 571, 573, 583, 597, 607

Limonene: **20**, **31**, 68, 70-73, 76, 78, 82-84, 86-91, 96, 98-103, 105, 106, 108, 109, 111, 112, 115-118, 120, 123, 127, 129-136, 140, 142, 292, 433, 481

Lin, HK: **31**, **32**, 398

Linalool: 4, **17-20**, 22, 68, 82, 124, 127, 142, 186, 292

Linalyl Acetate: **17**, **19-21**, 24, 25, 70, 74, 79, 104, 105, 116, 122, 130, 141

Lip Balm: **205**, **224**, 475, 547, 577, 580, 582, 585, 586, 588, 602, 605, 606

Lip Balm, Cinnamint: **205**, **224**, 475, 547, 577, 585, 586, 588, 602

Lip Balm, Grapefruit: **205**, **224**, 475, 547, 580, 605

Lip Balm, Lavender: **205**, **224**, 475, 547, 582, 606

Lip Gloss: ii, **224-225**, 578, 580, 581, 583, 585-589

Lipase: 169, 170, 172, 174, 177, 180, 186-188, 249, 253, **343**, **346**, **349**, **351**

Lipid: **24**, 32, 94-96, 98, 102, 106, 162, 198, 200, 204, 219, 247, 318, 319, 398, **544**, **547**

Liposomes: **232**, 233

Live with Passion: 144, **155**, 312-314, 316, 373, 412, 434, 458, 537, 538, 575-577, 580, 581, 584, 585, 587, 593, 599, 607

Live Your Passion: 144, **155**, 312-314, 316, 412, 434, 458, 537, 538, 579, 581, 583-587, 589, 593, 599, 607

Liver: iii, 20, 70, 73, 74, 76, 77, 82, 83, 85, 86, 88, 93-97, 99, 103, 105, 115-118, 121, 124-126, 130, 132, 139, 149, 151, 154, 160, 171, 172, 178, 179, 181, 193, 196, 197, 203, 208, 210, 211, 219, 220, 236, 242, 257, 269, 283, 287, 289, 304, 308, 311, **317-327**, 329-332, 342, 343, 346, 348, 351, 354, 355, 362-365, 377, 389, 392, 395-398, 406, 407, 415, 416, 418-420, 423, 434-436, 438, 441, 442, 452, 460, 471, 474-476, 478, 481-483, 485, 488, 489, 494, **498-501**, 505, 506, 508, 510, 544, 549, 550, 553, 555

Liver Diseases and Disorders: **317-327**, **498**

Liver Health: iii, 83, **318**, 331, 396

Liver Spots (Solar Lentigines): **501**

Livestock: 29, **264**

Longevity: iv, 27, 30, 50, 110, 130, 144, **155**, 181, 269, 305, 324, 334-337, 352, 357, **361-398**, 412, 413, 418, 421, 423, 424, 431, 432, 439, 440, 442-447, 452, 453, 455, 462, 471-475, 481, 484, 488, 489, 497, 500, 502-504, 506, 507, 512, 518, 520, 526, 532-536, 546, 554, 556, 561, 562, 577, 579, 585, 588, 593, 599, 607

Longevity Softgels: 155, **181**, 269, 334-337, 384, 385, 387, 413, 418, 423, 424, 431, 432, 439, 440, 442, 444, 445, 447, 452, 453, 455, 462, 471, 472, 474, 475, 481, 488, 489, 500, 502-504, 506, 507, 512,

518, 520, 526, 532-536, 546, 554, 556, 561, 562, 577, 579, 585, 588, 607

Longevity Vitality: **155**, 412, 421, 439, 440, 442-446, 462, 471-473, 484, 497, 535, 593, 599, 607

Loss of Smell: **523**, 543

Lotion: **205**, **218**, **219**, **235**, **247**, 414, 450, 545-547, 552, 554, 575, 576, 578, 580-586, 589, 605, 606, 610

Lou Gehrig's Disease: 516, **519**

Lumbago (Lower back pain): 72, 99, 113, 116, 121, 283, **557**

Lung Cancer: 436, **437**, 567

Lung Infections and Problems: **501**

Lupus: 382, 416, 417, **504-506**

Lyme Disease: 423, 493, **505**, 535

Lymphatic Massage: 4, **506**

Lymphatic Pump: iii, 279, **284**, 303, 411, 447

Lymphatic System: 108, 380, **505**, 506

Magnify Your Purpose: 144, 145, **155**, 312-316, 373, 466, 532, 575, 577, 578, 580, 584, 585, 587, 589, 594, 599, 607

Maintenance Protocol: **335**

Malaria: 71, 89, 357, 493, **506**, 517

Malaysia: **11**, 79, 81

Male Hormone Imbalance: 470, **507**, 563

Mandarin: 19, 20, 41, 43, 50, 67, **108**, 109, 132, 142, 147, 157, 160, 188, 224, 329, 339, 445, 467, 481, 485, 554, 571, 573, 583, 591, 594, 595, 597, 607

Manuka: 43, 67, **109-110**, 572, 573, 583, 597, 607

Maple Syrup: 155, 324, 325, 331, 335, 341, **396-397**, 410, 416, 425, 426, 448, 540, 561

Marjoram: 4, 21, 43, 50, 54, 67, **110**, 145, 148, 156, 157, 159, 162, 191, 215, 217, 225, 250, 258, 261, 263, 273, 276, 278, 292, 293, 295, 296, 298, 302, 304, 312, 315, 412, 418, 420, 428, 433, 438, 441-443, 445, 446, 454, 455, 464, 469, 486, 496, 506, 512-514, 517, 519, 521, 522, 539, 556-560, 566, 572, 573, 583, 591-595, 597, 607

Marjoram Vitality: **110**, 412, 418, 420, 428, 433, 438, 441-443, 445, 446, 454, 455, 464, 469, 519, 521, 522, 539, 556, 557, 559, 560, 572, 573, 583, 597, 607

Mass Spectrometry: 4, 10, **23-25**, 48, 92, 108, 115, 197, 378, 398

Mass Spectroscopy: 4, **24**

Massage: 4, 49, **51-54**, 84, 105, 123, 143, 148, 151, 154, 158, 160, 163, 213, 215, 223, 225, 226, 235, 238, 240, 241, 245, 264, 265, 267, 269-271, 273, 278, 281, 285, 290, 292, 293, 295, 296, 301, 302, 311, 332, 333, 407, 409, 411-414, 418, 420, 422-425, 427, 428, 430-433, 438-450, 452-455, 461, 464-487, 490, 496-498, 500-518, 520-525, 528-533, 535-

541, 543-545, 548, 552-554, 556-560, 565, 566, 575-589, 601-612

Massage Oils: 49, 51, **53**, 84, 154, 158, 225, 226, 269, 411, 454, 501, 521, 601-612

Master Cleanse: **324-326**, 331, 332

Master Formula: **181**, 182, **201**, 331, 406, 407, 412-415, 419, 424, 428, 429, 432, 437-439, 443, 445, 446, 452, 454, 459, 465, 469-472, 484, 489, 499, 500, 504, 505, 514, 520, 523, 524, 529, 532, 533, 535, 536, 553, 554, 556-560, 576, 577, 579, 580, 607

Mastitis: **432**

Mastrante: 67, **111**, 155, 313-315, 479, 480, 486, 487, 504, 560, 572, 574, 583, 584, 593, 597, 607

Matricaria: d, 21, 89, **94**, 145, 146, 148, 149, 158, 160, 161, 164, 165, 235, 247, 270, 571-574, 580, 591, 592, 594-596

MCT (Mixed Connective Tissue Disease): **506**

Measles: 425, **507**, 508

Meat: 8, 12, 14, 15, 32, 168, 188, 242, 255, 331, 342, **344**-354, 388, 419, 434, 463, 500, 532

MegaCal: **182**, 322, 334, 406, 407, 409, 412-418, 423, 424, 427-430, 433, 439, 441-444, 446, 453-455, 459, 460, 464, 465, 467-469, 482, 486-489, 495, 506, 512-521, 523, 527-529, 536, 538, 541, 546, 553-560, 564-566, 583, 607

Mein, Carolyn L: **312**

Melaleuca-Geranium Moisturizing Soap: **243**, 545, 547, 580, 584, 588, 589, 607

Melaleuca Alternifolia: 32, 56, 57, 67, 111, **133**, 134, 381, 550, 572, 574, 588

Melaleuca Ericifolia: 43, 67, **111**, 112, 243, 336, 477, 479, 572, 574, 584, 597, 607

Melaleuca Quinquenervia: 43, 67, **112**, 148, 156, 220, 235, 270, 453, 465, 477, 479, 506, 535, 545-547, 549, 550, 572, 574, 584, 597, 607, 608

Melanoma: 128, 137, 141, 369, 436, **437**

Melatonin: 76, 116, 128, 146, 178, 188, 201, **209-211**, 213, 215, 333, 494, 554

Melissa: 4, 19, 30, 37, 43, 47, 50, 67, **112**, 113, 146-148, 150-155, 157, 159, 165, 183, 212, 238, 239, 250, 268, 313-316, 330, 332, 334, 342, 373, 388, 413, 415, 418, 425, 426, 429, 432, 435, 448, 450, 451, 453, 457, 458, 474, 477, 479, 480, 489, 503, 505, 511, 523, 531, 536, 539-542, 548, 549, 551, 560, 572, 574, 584, 591-596, 598, 607

Melrose: 56, 57, 144, **156**, 267-273, 334-337, 373, 381, 384-388, 412, 413, 421, 422, 426-428, 437, 448, 450-455, 461, 462, 464-466, 473, 475, 477-480, 482-486, 488-494, 497, 502-505, 507, 508, 524, 525, 534, 535, 539-541, 543-553, 555, 560-563, 565, 566, 577, 584, 587,

588, 594, 599, 607

Memory Impaired: 126, **431**

Mendwell: **266**, 268, 272, 579-582, 584, 607

Menopause: 174, 208, 211-215, 475, 508, **510**, 517, 525

Menstrual and Female Hormone Conditions: 427, 457, 470, 475, 485, **508**, 563

Menstrual Cramps: 174, **510**

Mental: iii, 11, 31, 56, 69, 80, 104, 105, 121-123, 126, 129, 130, 146, 147, 152, 158, 161, 162, 164, 179, 183, 185, 199, 203, 208, 211, 212, 215, 225, 305, 307-316, 325, 334, 349, 354, 357, 361, 378, 382, 391, 405, 413, 415, **431**, 432, **474**, 487, 493, 520

Mental Fatigue: 69, 122, 126, 130, 211, **431**, **474**

Methyl Chavicol: 4, 20, 69, 90, 133

Mexico: **11**, 108, 111, 171, 175, 206, 384, 388, 389, 398

M-Grain: 50, 144, **156**, 373, 412, 429-431, 450, 465, 475, 484, 486, 487, 513, 515, 523, 575, 580, 582, 583, 586, 593, 599, 608

Microbes: iv, **29**, 227-229, 292, 323, 342, 346, 374, **377**, 423

Micromeria: 43, 67, **113**, 572, 574, 584, 598, 608

Microwave: iv, 345, **377-381**, 383

Microwave Cooking: iv, 345, **377-380**

Microwave Ovens: **377-380**

MightyVites: **180**, **201**, 249, 332, 337, 385, 387, 406, 407, 413, 534, 606

MightyZyme: 168, **180**, 208, 249, 325, 327, 332, 344-346, 351, 352, 387, 406, 407, 412, 413, 459, 501, 550, 586, 606

Migraine (Vascular-type Headache): **486**

MindWise: **182**, 413, 415-417, 424, 425, 429-432, 438-441, 443, 444, 446, 447, 465, 467, 470, 472, 495, 515-523, 536, 553, 554, 556, 560, 564, 565, 575, 579, 583, 586, 608

Mineral Essence: **183**, 256, 268, 322, 331, 334, 355, 387, 406, 407, 409, 412-417, 419-421, 424, 427-431, 438, 440-444, 446, 449, 454, 455, 457-459, 462-465, 467, 468, 473, 474, 479, 482, 484-487, 489, 497, 502, 506, 511-524, 527-529, 533, **535-539**, 541, 545, 547, 550-559, 563, 564, 566, 577, 583, 586, 608

Minerals: iii, 37, 169, 172, 174, 178, 180-184, 187, 189-196, 201, 203, 214, 223, 229, 240, 249, 320, 322-325, 327, 331, 333, 334, 337, 343, **350-355**, 358, 359, 377, 380, 382, 383, 385, 387, 389, 391, 395-397, 405, 406, 409, 416, 423, 424, 428, 446, 478, 513, 518, 534

Mirah Shave Oil: **235**, 576, 578, 581-583, 585-587, 589, 608

Mister: 144, **156**, **215**, 315, 316, 373, 484, 507, 511, 532, 533, 537, 538, 579, 582,

584, 586, 587, 589, 594, 599, 608

Mites: 267, **268**, 420, 501, 552

Mixed Connective Tissue Disease: **504**, **506**

Moisture Cream: 55, **205**, **240**, 414, 547, 548, 551, 554, 575, 578, 580, 582, 584, 587, 589, 610

Moisturizing Bar Soaps: **242**, 547

Moles: **550**, 551

Mononucleosis: **471**

Monoterpenes: **18**

Mood Swings: 148, 169, 179, 210, 211, 213, **315**, 321, 450, 471, 478, 510, 564

Morning Sickness: **515**

Morning Start Bath & Shower Gel: **218**, 547, 582, 583, 586, 587, 608

Morning Start Moisturizing Soap: **244**, 582, 583, 586, 587, 608

Mosquito Bites: **493**

Motion Sickness: **516**

Motivation: 30, 124, 144, 145, 150, 155, **156**, 164, 312-315, 317, 373, 405, 406, 412, 413, 419, 434, 450, 467, 471, 474, 515, 564, 576, 582, 586, 589, 594, 599, 608

Mountain Savory: 17, 30, 43, 50, 52, 67, **113**, 114, 153, 162, 266, 267, 269, 272, 273, 304, 334, 377, 386, 407, 413, 422-424, 426, 427, 432, 438, 440, 451, 452, 457, 460, 462, 465, 466, 471, 477, 479-482, 489, 490, 502, 503, 525, 526, 530, 531, 535, 541, 548, 552, 555, 562, 563, 566, 572, 574, 584, 593, 595, 598, 608

Mountain Savory Vitality: **114**, 413, 422-424, 426, 432, 438, 440, 451, 452, 457, 460, 462, 465, 471, 479, 480, 489, 490, 502, 503, 525, 526, 530, 531, 535, 541, 555, 562, 563, 566, 572, 574, 584, 598

Moussaieff, Arieh: **307**, 368, 371

Mouth Rinse: 228, **232**

Mouth Ulcers: 448, **526**

Mouthwash: 31, 134, 137, 227, 229, **232-234**, 365, 412, 422, 448, 465, 466, 477, 479-481, 498, 502-504, 526-529, 542-544, 560-563, 577, 579, 583, 586-589, 611

MS: 516, **521-522**

MSM: iv, 170, 171, 186, 190, 204, 205, 213, 214, 218, 219, 222, 223, 236, 240, 241, 247, 249, 333, **382-383**, 423, 441, 456, 476, 504, 528, 564

Mucus: 122, 229, 232, 320, 322, 324, 501, 504, **511**, 543

Mucus (Excess): **511**

Mugwort: 43, **67**

MultiGreens: 167, **183**, 331, 334, 387, 388, 406, 407, 413-417, 420, 422, 424, 429, 431, 432, 437, 438, 441, 442, 447, 449, 451, 454-456, 458, 459, 464, 465, 471, 472, 474-476, 479, 482, 483, 487-489, 495, 497, 499-501, 503-507, 511-516, 518, 520, 521, 523, 529, 530, 536-538,

**Essential Oils Desk Reference** | Seventh Edition

545, 551, 556, 560-562, 564, 565, 583, 584, 587, 608

Multiple Sclerosis (MS): **521-522**

Mumps: 425, **511**

Muscles: 4, 88, 89, 106, 109, 123, 140, 145, 148, 170, 182, 212, 217, 225, 273, 278, 284, 290, 292, 293, 296, 304, 308, 353, 405, 406, 409, 411, 412, 417, 431, 433, 441, 449, 455, 459, 476, 487, 490, 501, 504, **512-514**, 519, 531, 536, 542, 556

Muscle Spasms, Cramps, and Charley Horses: **513**

Muscle Weakness: **513**, 514, 517, 521, 542

Muscular Dystrophy: **514**

Myocardial Infarction: **443**

Myrrh: v, 4-6, 8, 13-15, 18-21, 41, 43, 50, 67, 71, 87, **114**, 115, 143, 145, 149-153, 156, 157, 159, 163, 165, 173, 192, 204, 205, 212, 214, 218, 219, 223, 236, 239, 240, 245, 250, 265-268, 272, 307, 312-315, 322, 332, 334, 361, 373, 414, 418, 424-429, 432, 436, 439, 449, 455-457, 462, 464, 466, 473, 475, 477-482, 486, 488-490, 492, 493, 496, 497, 499, 502-505, 511, 512, 514, 517, 522, 523, 525-527, 531-533, 536, 537, 539, 543-549, 551-553, 560-565, 571, 573-575, 584, 591-596, 598, 602, 608

Myrtle: 12, 13, 15, 30, 31, 43, 50, 67, 107, 108, **115**, 147, 149, 153, 156, 158, 159, 162, 179, 186, 188, 191, 192, 212, 214, 215, 250, 253, 266, 268, 313, 314, 334, 337, 381, 385, 414, 437, 464, 470, 479, 501, 503, 505, 524, 533, 534, 565, 571-574, 583, 584, 591-595, 597, 598, 607, 608

Nails: 8, 295, 308, 334, 353, 382, 383, **514-515**

Narcolepsy: **515**, 563

Nasopharyngitis: **542**, 543

Natural Soaps: **241**

Nature-identical: **35**, 390

Nausea: 51, 79, 95, 102, 106, 120-122, 131, 133, 145, 172, 320, 325, 327, 346, 407, 409, 417, 419, 434, 435, 452, 463, 476, 486, 493, 497-499, **515**, 516, 530

Neck Pain and Stiffness: **557**

Nephritis: **496**

Neroli: 8, 43, 50, 67, **115**, 116, 145, 152, 153, 155, 157-159, 511, 531, 547, 554, 571, 574, 575, 584, 591, 593-595, 598, 608

Nerve Disorders: **516**, 519

Nervous Anxiety: **268**

Nervous System: v, 19, 71, 78, 85, 107, 113, 119, 135, 136, 149, 181, 209, 225, 242, 285, 287, 290, 307, 308, 310, 329, 357, 371, 378, 382, 398, 418, 420, 492, **518**, 519, 521, 538, 541, 560, 601

Nervous System, Parasympathetic: 71, **518**

Nervous System Autonomic: 85, 308, **518**

Nervous System Connection Points: **287**

Neuralgia: 516, **517**, 557

Neuritis: 516, **517**

Neuro Auricular Technique: iii, 279, **282**

Neurologic Diseases: **519**

Neuropathy: 116, 516, **518**, 567

Neurotoxin: iv, **220**, 365

New Testament: **8**, 131, 151, 308

Niaouli: 43, **112**, 148, 156, 212, 220, 235, 270, 337, 385, 453, 465, 506, 534, 545, 546, 550, 572, 574, 584, 592, 594, 597, 607, 608

NingXia Berry Syrup: **177**, **201**, 583, 585, 605

Ningxia Hui Autonomous Region: **193**

NingXia Nitro: **183**, **203**, 429, 430, 432, 451, 458, 474, 475, 575, 584, 586, 588, 608

NingXia Red: ii, 155, 160, 182, **184**, 202, **203**, 264, 275, 331, 332, 334-338, 345, 355, 385, 387, 388, 406, 407, 409, 410, 412, 413, 415-418, 421, 424, 425, 429-432, 434, 437-440, 442, 444, 446, 447, 449, 451, 456, 458, 463, 465, 467, 468, 470, 472-475, 485-487, 489, 503, 510, 512, 514, 519-521, 523, 524, 534-536, 541, 553, 554, 556, 559, 564, 566, 583, 585, 588, 589, 608

Ningxia Wolfberries (Organic Dried): ii, 184, 185, **199**, 201, **203**, 341, 345, 429, 430, 432, 438-441, 443, 459, 472, 473, 475, 486, 489, 514, 520, 523, 535, 545, 554, 564, 608

Ningxia Wolfberry: **193-206**

NingXia Zyng: **184**, **203**, 406, 407, 412, 413, 429, 430, 432, 451, 458, 474, 475, 583, 608

Nipples: **432**

Northern Lights Black Spruce: 43, 67, **116**, 149-153, 155-159, 161, 163-165, 169, 224, 235, 236, 240, 244, 250, 265, 270, 312-316, 333, 412, 418, 420, 422-424, 427, 428, 444, 452, 465, 471, 489, 493, 501, 502, 504, 505, 507, 511, 513, 529, 531, 539, 541, 544, 550, 560, 561, 565, 572, 574, 584, 592-596, 598, 608

Northern Lights Farm: **45**

Nose and Sinus Problems: **523**

Nosebleeds: **524**

Nutmeg: 19, 40, 43, 50, 67, **116**, 117, 149, 155-158, 173, 184-187, 190, 203, 255, 314, 315, 332, 363, 413, 417, 418, 422-424, 427, 429, 437, 440, 444-446, 456, 460-463, 468, 471, 474-476, 490, 495, 498, 501, 504-506, 512, 513, 515, 517, 518, 525, 530, 532, 537, 538, 550, 554, 557, 558, 567, 572, 574, 577, 584, 592-594, 598, 608

Nutmeg Vitality: **117**, 173, 255, 413, 417, 423, 424, 427, 429, 437, 440, 444-446, 456, 460-463, 468, 471, 474-476, 490,

495, 504, 505, 515, 525, 530, 538, 554, 572, 574, 584, 598, 608

NutraSweet®: **393**

Nutrition: ii, 133, **167**, **170**, 175, 180, 187-189, 193-195, 197, 203, 206, 337, 338, 345, 358, 385, 392, 398, 405, 534

Nutritional Support: ii, 201, **167-192**, 397

Oberg, Craig J.: **30**

Obesity: 31, 71, 77, 90, 96, 97, 105, 106, 108, 121, 131, 132, 175, 208, 210, 211, 318-320, 349, 391, 392, 397, 398, 405, 406, 417, **525**

Obsessiveness: **315**

Ocotea: 43, 67, 101, **117**, 145-147, 152, 155-158, 160-162, 164, 171, 185, 188, 189, 192, 202, 215, 224, 225, 229, 231, 235-237, 244, 248, 266, 267, 269, 312-316, 334, 342, 412, 413, 418, 420, 441, 444, 458, 459, 461, 465, 471, 477, 485, 489, 492, 494, 495, 506, 515, 520, 526, 537, 542, 562, 563, 565, 572-574, 581, 584, 585, 591, 593-596, 598, 608

Oil Pulling: **227**

Ointment: 8, 15, 100, 151, 156, **240**, 248, 264, **265**, 267, 268, 270-272, 414, 432, 451, 452, 488, 489, 523, 536, 539, 545-551, 553, 554, 575, 576, 578, 580, 581, 584-586, 588, 589, 601, 610

Old Testament: **93**, 308

Olive Oil: 3, **7**, 8, 49-51, 83, 84, 143, 150, 160, 180, 185, 214, 218, 222, 223, 225, 226, 235, 236, 239, 240, 243, 244, 249, 264, 269, 329, 338, 339, 466, 502, 503, 533, 546, 592, 595

Oman: **11**

OmegaGize³: **184**, 185, 333, 406, 407, 413, 415-417, 423, 424, 427, 429, 430, 439-444, 446, 448, 449, 456, 459, 464, 467, 472, 473, 476, 489, 495, 502, 506, 508, 516-518, 520-523, 525, 526, 530, 535, 536, 545, 546, 551, 554, 556-558, 560-562, 564, 566

Onycha: 19, 43, **50**, 572, 574

Oola: 144, **156-158**, 165, 312-316, 415, 429-432, 458, 469, 474, 525, 565, 575-589, 594, 599, 608

Oola Balance: 144, **156**, 312-316, 429-432, 458, 469, 474, 525, 565, 575, 577-587, 589, 594, 599, 608

Oola Faith: 144, **157**, 312-316, 415, 429-432, 458, 469, 474, 565, 575, 576, 579-587, 589, 594, 599, 608

Oola Family: 144, **157**, 312-316, 415, 429-432, 458, 469, 474, 565, 575, 576, 579-589, 594, 599, 608

Oola Field: 144, **157**, 313-316, 415, 429-432, 458, 469, 474, 565, 575, 576, 578-581, 584, 589, 594, 599, 608

Oola Finance: 144, **157**, 312-316, 415, 429-432, 458, 469, 474, 565, 575-587, 589, 594, 599, 608

626 | Index

# Index

Oola Fitness: 144, **157**, 313-316, 415, 429-432, 458, 469, 474, 565, 575, 577, 578, 581, 583, 584, 586, 594, 599, 608

Oola Friends: 144, **157**, 312-316, 415, 429-432, 458, 469, 474, 565, 575, 576, 578-589, 594, 599, 608

Oola Fun: 144, **158**, 312-316, 415, 429-432, 458, 469, 474, 565, 576, 580, 581, 583, 584, 588, 594, 599, 608

Oola Grow: 144, **158**, 312-314, 316, 415, 429-432, 458, 469, 474, 565, 575-589, 594, 608

Optical Rotation: **47**

ORAC: 69-80, 82-84, 86-91, 93-100, 102, 103, 105-110, 112, 114, 115, 117-119, 121, 122, 124-128, 130-133, 135-139, 141, 142, 181, **198-200**, 389

Oral Care, Teeth and Gums: 485, **525**

Oral Health Care: ii, **226-229**, 231, 440

Oral Hygiene: **226-229**, 232, 525, 601

Oral Infection Control: **527**

Orange: 18, 20, 21, 25, 31, 32, 41, 43, 49, 50, 52, 56, 67, 96, 115, 116, **118**, 145, 147, 149, 152, 153, 155-159, 161, 164, 170, 177, 178, 180-182, 184, 186-188, 190, 191, 199, 201-203, 205, 212, 213, 215, 222, 224, 236, 239, 240, 245, 249, 251, 252, 255, 259, 266, 276, 308, 312-316, 325, 329, 334, 337, 338, 341, 342, 350, 353, 359, 385, 412-414, 416, 419, 433, 434, 438, 446, 448, 449, 451, 468, 478, 480, 481, 487, 494, 495, 498, 500, 505, 506, 530, 534, 536, 547, 554, 565, 571, 574, 575, 582-585, 587, 591-596, 598, 608

Orange Blossom Facial Wash: **205**, **240**, 547, 582, 583, 585, 587, 608

Orange Vitality: **118**, 255, 412-414, 416, 419, 438, 446, 448, 451, 468, 480, 481, 487, 494, 495, 498, 500, 505, 530, 536, 565, 574, 585, 591, 598, 608

Oregano: 25, 43, 50, 52, 65, 67, 103, **118**, 119, 123, 124, 148, 153, 178, 182, 214, 224, 226, 228, 235, 255, 258, 261, 263, 266, 269, 270, 272, 273, 276, 292, 293, 295, 296, 298, 299, 304, 334, 340, 377, 386, 407, 412, 413, 418, 421-424, 426, 433, 451-453, 457, 460-462, 465, 471, 475, 476, 478-482, 489, 490, 492-494, 502-505, 526, 527, 529-532, 535, 541, 544, 546, 548, 550-552, 559, 561-563, 566, 572, 574, 585, 586, 592, 593, 598, 609

Oregano Vitality: **119**, 255, 272, 412, 413, 418, 421-424, 426, 433, 451-453, 457, 460-462, 465, 471, 475, 476, 480, 481, 489, 490, 502-505, 526, 527, 529-532, 535, 541, 559, 561-563, 566, 572, 574, 585, 598, 609

Ortho Ease Massage Oil: **225**, 295, 412, 420, 423, 424, 427, 428, 433, 442, 447, 449, 450, 454, 455, 477-480, 483, 490, 496, 501, 506, 512-514, 516-518, 521, 529, 556-560, 566, 579, 582, 583, 586, 588, 589, 609

Ortho Sport Massage Oil: **225**, 267, 409, 412, 420, 423, 424, 427, 428, 433, 442, 449, 454, 455, 477, 478, 480, 483, 490, 496, 512-514, 517, 518, 521, 529, 556-560, 566, 578, 579, 583, 585, 586, 588, 589, 609

OSHA: 380

Osteoarthritis: 95, 129, 382, **422**, 423, 495

Osteoporosis: 129, 207, 208, 211, 213, 353, 417, **428**, 510

Ovarian and Uterine Cysts: **457**, 508

Owie: 144, **158**, **250**, 414, 432, 442, 493, 545, 547-551, 577, 578, 580, 581, 588, 594, 609

Oxides: **19**, 225, 243

Oxygen: 17, 24, 56, 65, 71, 84, 99, 104, 150, 198, 199, 242, 285, **309**, 323, **337**, 342, **343**, 350, 353-355, 385, 389, 423, 431, 432, 438, 443, 474, 501, **534**, 567

Pain: ii, v, 5, 10, 11, 25, 31, 71, 73, 76, 78, 80, 81, 86, 87, 91, 97, 99, 100, 102, 109, 110, 112, 116, 121, 138, 139, 143, 148, 156, 158, 160, 170, 171, 179, 180, 187, 191, 211, 214, 234, **235**, 242, 244, 249, 267, **268**, 271, 276-278, 283, 285, 291, 293, 304, 309, 330, 348, 382-384, 387, 393, 409, 412, 420, 422-428, 432, 433, 438, 442, 445-447, 449, 451, 454-457, 459, 463-466, 469, 476-478, 481-483, 485, 486, 488, 490, 492, 493, 495-498, 500, 505, 506, 508, 510-514, 516-522, **528-530**, 532, 541, 543, 548, 556-560, 566, 567, 576, 578, 580, 582, 584, 586, 587, 589, 603

Pain Relief: ii, 81, 99, 109, **235**, 268, 269, 304, 409, 412, 420, 422-424, 427, 428, 433, 442, 447, 449, 454, 455, 457, 469, 476-478, 483, 490, 496, 506, 508, 511-514, 516-518, 520, 521, **529**, 556-560, 566, 576, 578, 580, 582, 584, 586, 587, 589, 603

Pain Relief Cream: **235**, 268, 269, 409, 412, 420, 422-424, 427, 428, 433, 442, 447, 449, 454, 455, 457, 476-478, 483, 490, 496, 506, 508, 511-514, 516-518, 520, 521, 529, 556-560, 566, 576, 578, 580, 582, 584, 586, 587, 589, 603

Pakistan: **7**, 175, 389

Palm: 13, 53, 58, 176, 180, 182, 189, 203, 214, 221-223, 236, 242-244, 249, 254, 263, 265, 271, 284, 288, 289, 296-298, **302**, 333, 410, 444

Palm Slide: 296, **302**

Palmarosa: 43, 50, 67, **119**, 147, 150-152, 154, 156, 157, 164, 215, 217, 218, 240, 265, 266, 312-316, 479, 487, 547, 552, 554, 571, 574, 585, 591-594, 596, 598,

609

Palo Santo: 43, 67, **120**, 146, 147, 150, 151, 153, 157, 159, 162, 164, 215, 250, 266-268, 273, 312-316, 334, 381, 386, 412, 413, 420, 423, 424, 426-428, 431, 433, 434, 436, 437, 444, 454, 455, 463, 465, 471, 480, 484, 489-492, 494, 495, 498, 501-503, 512-514, 516, 520, 528, 529, 531, 533, 535, 540, 543, 549, 551, 552, 556, 561, 565, 571, 574, 585, 591, 592, 594-596, 598, 609

PanAway: 52, 144, **158**, 267, 268, 277, 278, 373, 409, 411-413, 420, 422-424, 427, 428, 432, 433, 440, 442, 444, 449, 450, 454-456, 465, 476-478, 481, 486-488, 490-492, 495, 502, 504-506, 508, 510-514, 516-518, 521, 525-529, 549, 556-559, 566, 577, 580, 586, 589, 594, 599, 609

Pancreatitis: 173, 481, **529**, 530

Panic: **315**

ParaFree: **185**, 268, 326, **332**, 406, 412, 459, 462, 530, 575, 577-580, 582-586, 588, 589, 609

ParaGize: **266**, 268, 272, 575, 578-580, 582, 583, 585-588, 609

Parasites: 70, 78, 80, 84, 90, 98, 106, 112, 123, 132, 140, 259, 266, **268**, 269, 317, 319, 324-327, **332**, 346, 357, 459, 484, **530**, 539, 552

Parasympathetic Nervous System: 71, **518**

Parkinson's Disease: 89, 516, **522**, 523

Patchouli: 3, 18, 43, 50, 67, **120**, 121, 132, 136, 145, 148, 155, 156, 158, 164, 169, 185, 224, 240, 253, 265, 266, 315, 350, 388, 412, 413, 419, 425, 429, 432, 437, 448, 449, 455, 456, 461, 462, 464, 469, 477, 478, 482, 483, 487, 494, 515, 516, 519, 544, 545, 549-553, 555, 565, 572, 574, 585, 591-594, 596, 598, 609

PD 80/20: **185**, **213**, 413, 417, 427, 429, 450, 454, 455, 457, 469, 475, 484, 495, 508-511, 517, 518, 520, 522, 532, 538, 541, 609

Peace & Calming: 144, **158**, 264, 267, 268, 271, 277, 281, 312-316, 326, 333, 373, 412, 414-418, 424, 425, 433, 434, 439, 441, 443-447, 458, 464, 469, 470, 487, 489, 494, 509, 512, 513, 516-519, 522, 528, 531, 536, 539, 548, 554, 555, 560, 565, 575-578, 580, 585, 588, 589, 594, 599, 609

Peace & Calming II: 144, **158**, 271, 312-316, 326, 333, 412, 414-418, 424, 425, 433, 434, 439, 441, 443-447, 458, 464, 469, 470, 487, 489, 494, 509, 512, 513, 516-519, 522, 528, 531, 536, 539, 548, 554, 555, 560, 565, 575-578, 580, 585, 588, 589, 594, 609

Pénoël, Daniel: **9-10**, 17, 20, 115, 290, 337, 385, 386, 524, 534, 539, 543

Peppermint: 4, 19, 20, 27, 31, 32, 43, 49, 50, 54, 57, 67, 68, **121**, 122, 131, 142, 145, 147, 148, 150, 155-162, 164, 169, 171-173, 178, 179, 181, 183-186, 189, 191, 192, 202, 203, 205, 212, 214, 215, 218, 220-227, 229, 231, 232, 234, 235, 238, 239, 241, 242, 244, 249, 250, 253-255, 258, 259, 261, 263, 265, 266, 268-270, 276, 292, 293, 295, 296, 298, 303, 312-315, 330, 341, 342, 350, 351, 359, 373, 377, 386, 406, 407, 412, 413, 415, 416, 418-421, 423-425, 427-433, 442, 444, 447, 449, 451-457, 459-469, 474, 475, 477-480, 482-495, 498, 499, 502-504, 506, 509, 511-526, 528-533, 535, 536, 541-544, 548, 550-552, 554, 556-562, 565-567, 572, 574, 586, 591-596, 598, 609

Peppermint-Cedarwood Moisturizing Soap: **244**, 576, 586, 609

Peppermint Vitality: **122**, 255, 268, 412, 413, 415, 416, 418-421, 423-425, 427-433, 442, 444, 447, 449, 451-457, 459-465, 468, 469, 474, 475, 479, 480, 482-488, 490, 495, 499, 502-504, 509, 511, 515, 516, 519-523, 525, 526, 529-531, 533, 535, 544, 554, 556, 557, 559-562, 565, 566, 572, 574, 586, 598, 609

Periodontitis: 228, 229, **526**

Perry, Bruce D: **309**

Personal Care: **217-246**

Pert, Candace: **309**

Petitgrain: 20, 43, 50, 67, **122**, 571, 574, 586, 598, 609

pH Balance: 169, 247, **321-323**, **326-327**, 388, 421, 547, 551

Phenols: 11, **17**, 119, 258, 348, 362, 421, 492

Phlebitis (Inflammation of Veins): **445**

Physical Ear Chart: **283**

Physical Fatigue: **474**

Physical Relief: **292**

Pigs: 32, 258, **264**, 349

Pine: 5, 12, 13, 18, 19, 25, 43, 50, 57, 67, 100, **123**, 146, 150, 152, 157, 159, 162, 165, 250, 267, 268, 292, 312-315, 412, 423, 424, 427, 428, 474, 475, 495, 502, 511, 513, 514, 516, 529, 537, 572-574, 581, 586, 592-596, 598, 609

Pink Eye: **473**

Plant Parts: **43**

Plaque: 30-32, 140, 227, **228-234**, **445**, 511, 525

Plectranthus Oregano: 43, 67, **123**, 124, 148, 235, 258, 261, 263, 266, 269, 270, 272, 273, 293, 295, 296, 298, 299, 304, 418, 421, 422, 426, 433, 451-453, 457, 460-462, 465, 471, 475, 476, 478-482, 489, 490, 493, 502-505, 526, 527, 529-532, 535, 541, 544, 548, 550, 552, 559, 561-563, 566, 572, 574, 586, 592, 609

Pleurisy: **502**

PMS: 17, 68, 79, 90, 93, 102, 104, 110, 130, 131, 133, 141, 148, 155, 174, 213, 214, 460, **510**

Pneumonia: 30, 121, 124, 134, 159, 333, **502**, 503

Pointer Technique: **557**

Poison Oak/Poison Ivy/Poison Sumac: **551**

Polio: 5, **531**

Polyps Nasal: **524**

Postpartum Depression: **458**

PowerGize: **185**, 412, 420, 423, 424, 427, 428, 447, 449, 454, 455, 487, 490, 495, 511-514, 516-518, 520-523, 529, 531, 533, 536, 537, 550, 556-559, 609

Power Meal: **185-187**, 267, 269, 271, 275, 406, 407, 409, 412, 413, 416, 418, 419, 421, 424, 425, 429, 442, 446, 448-450, 455, 467, 472, 474, 475, 490, 505, 511, 513-515, 520-523, 525, 527, 535, 536, 553, 556, 557, 559

Pregnancy: 102, 106, 151, 171, 185, 208, 211, 330, 458, 515, 517, **531**, 532, 537, 553, 555, 558

Pregnenolone: 171, **185**, **205**, **207-215**, 223, 435, 474, 507, 508, 510, 518, 528, 567

Premenstrual Syndrome (PMS): **510**

Prenolone: **205**, **213**, **223**, 413, 414, 428, 445, 455, 457, 458, 486, 495, 507-511, 517, 518, 520, 525, 532, 533, 537, 538, 545, 560, 575, 577, 579, 580, 587, 589, 609

Prenolone + Body Cream: **205**, **213**, **223**

Present Time: 144, 146, **159**, **311**, 315, 355, 373, 381, 412, 415, 422, 434, 469, 542, 576, 584, 589, 591, 595, 599, 609

Progessence Plus: **214**, **223**, 406, 407, 413, 414, 427, 428, 445, 451, 454, 457, 458, 486, 495, 508-511, 521, 525, 538, 545, 575-579, 586, 587, 609

Prostate Cancer: 209, 211, 214, 435, **437**

Prostate Health: **186**, **214**, 223, 413, 484, 507, 532, 533, 537, 579, 580, 582, 584, 586, 609

Prostate Problems: 115, 141, 212, **532**, 537

Prostatitis: **533**

Protec: **214**, **223**, 413, 437, 457, 507, 532, 533, 537, 578, 579, 584, 587, 609

Protecting Your Home: iii, **251**

Protein: 168-170, 175, 176, 185-187, 189, **193**, 194, 201, 203-205, 211, 213, 214, 221-223, 240, 241, 264, 267, 269, 272, 317, 319, 320, 325, 328, 334, 335, 338, 341, 342, **344-351**, 354, 361, 363, 377, 378, 380, 382, 383, 406, 407, 413, 416, 418, 419, 424, 425, 438, 444, 446, 449, 459, 474, 483, 506, 511, 513, 514, 525, 528, 536, 585, 609

Psalms: **8**, **13-15**

Psoriasis: 74, 81, 93, 97, 104, 115, 121, 127,

242, 348, **551**

Puncture Wounds: **272**

Pure Protein Complete: **186**, 187, 267, 269, 325, 334, 338, 406, 407, 413, 416, 418, 419, 424, 425, 438, 446, 449, 459, 474, 483, 506, 511, 513, 525, 536, 585, 609

PuriClean: **266**, 268, 272, 577, 582-585, 587, 588, 609

Purification: v, 50, 56, 57, 89, 99, 106, 107, 144, **159**, 198, 207, 253, 259, 267, 268, 271, 276, 324, 334, 359, 360, 373, 386, 388, 412, 413, 421, 422, 426-428, 438, 439, 451-453, 455, 457, 462, 465-467, 473, 477, 479, 480, 482, 483, 485, 486, 488-494, 497, 498, 502, 503, 511, 524, 539, 544-553, 555, 561, 565, 577, 582-584, 587, 588, 595, 599, 609

Purity: iii, **22**, 24, 25, 35-37, 44, 47, 48, 65, 134, 167, 355, 357, 368, 396

Pyorrhea: **527**

QuadShield: **336-337**, **384-385**, 534, 535

Quality Control: **47-48**

Quick Usage Guide: **412-414**

Radiation: iv, 141, 156, 200, 209, 317, 336, 337, 357, 376-378, 380, 381, **383-389**, 398, 405, 406, 434, 436, **533**, 534, 546

Radiation Exposure Damage: **533**

Raindrop Technique: iii, 4, 99, 119, 145, 149-151, 153, 154, 159, 164, 165, 258, 261, 263, 264, 267, 269, 272, 273, 279, 285, **290-293**, 295-297, 303, 304, 407, 411, 418, 425, 427, 430, 449, 452-454, 456, 471-473, 476, 489-491, 499, 500, 502, 504-506, 512, 519-523, 530, 531, 535, 536, 540, 541, 544, 556, 557, 559, 561-563

Raindrop Technique for Horses: iii, **273**

Raven: 57, 144, **159**, 268, 269, 373, 386, 411-413, 420-422, 452, 465, 471, 475, 477, 479, 486, 489, 491, 501-504, 511, 523, 524, 542-544, 560-562, 579, 583, 586, 589, 595, 599, 609

Ravintsara: 43, 67, **124**, 153, 159, 162, 250, 304, 334, 373, 413, 421, 422, 451, 452, 465, 471, 479, 489-491, 499, 501-503, 507, 508, 511-513, 531, 539-544, 560, 561, 563, 566, 571, 574, 586, 593, 595, 598, 609

R.C.: 30, 144, 147, **159**, 267-269, 304, 373, 412, 413, 420, 422, 426, 452, 453, 465, 471, 474, 479, 486, 489, 491, 493, 501-504, 511, 523, 524, 527, 536, 542-544, 548, 551, 560-562, 576, 578, 579, 582-584, 586, 595, 599, 609

Recipes: ii, iii, 5, 8, 74, 75, 90, 91, 114, 134, 171, 176, 177, 192, 202, 255, 325, 326, 331, **338**, 342, 397, 514

Recipes—Delicious and Nutritious: iii, **338**

Reconnect: 144, 152, 153, **159**, 311-316, 332, 333, 412, 414-416, 418, 419, 424, 425, 429-432, 434, 451, 458, 467-469,

487, 537, 542, 565, 575, 576, 578-582, 584-587, 589, 595, 599, 609

Red Shot: **160**, 576, 588, 595, 599, 609

Refractive Index: **47**

Regenolone Moisturizing Cream: **205**, **214**, **223**, 413, 414, 454, 455, 496, 506, 510, 513, 517, 518, 521, 529, 550, 556-558, 578, 585, 586, 589, 609

Rehemogen: **187**, 326, 327, 334, 423, 424, 438, 441, 444, 446, 508, 565, 586-588, 609

Relaxation Massage Oil: **226**, 414, 424, 501, 512, 513, 575, 578, 580, 582, 586, 588, 589, 610

Release: v, 8, 19, 41, 56, 68, 93, 94, 98, 102, 106, 125, 128, 144-146, 148, 150, 157, **160**, 161, 164, 172-174, 186, 195, 203, 206, 211, 225, 232, 233, 268, 282, 292, 296, 303, 304, 309, **311**, 316, 326, 332, 333, 343, 359, 373, 412, 414, 415, 418-420, 425, 433, 434, 445, 458, 467-470, 487, 488, 500, 529, 563, 565, 575-589, 592, 595, 598, 599, 603, 610

Relieve It: 50, 52, 144, **160**, 268, 373, 411, 412, 420, 423, 424, 427, 428, 433, 440, 442, 444, 449, 454, 455, 476-478, 486, 490, 495, 506, 508, 510-514, 516-518, 525, 529, 549, 553, 556-559, 566, 575, 576, 581, 586, 595, 599, 610

RepelAroma: **266**, 268, 577, 581, 583, 585, 610

Research: i, vii, 1, 3, 4, 11, 23, 24, **29-34**, 47, 56, 68-143, 154, 163, 175, 181, 185, 190, 197, 206-211, 214, 221, 226-228, 281, 282, 290, 291, 304, 307, 309, 321, 323, 337, 348, 349, 354, 355, 361-363, 365-372, 374, 375, 377-382, 384, 385, 388, 389, 392, 396-398, 406, 425, 430, 434-436, 456, 499, 525, 534, 536, 545, 559, 567

Resentment: **316**

Restless Legs Syndrome: **522**

Restlessness: 125, 135, 154, 163, 164, **316**, 563

Retention: 23, 47, **58**, 74, 83, 90, 96, 103, 105, 106, 108, 110, 118, 120, 132, 133, 140, 210, 214, 233, 320, 354, 382, 407, 411, 427, 431, 457, 461, 481, 504, 517, 530-533, 537, 540, 541

Rheumatic Fever: **535**, 562

Rheumatoid Arthritis: 103, 112, 129, 422, **423**, 495, 517

Rhinitis: 73, 109, 420, 523, **543**

Ringing in the Ears: **467**

Ringworm and Skin Candida: **479**

Robertson, John: **368**, 369

Rocky Mountain Spotted Fever: **505**, 535

Roman Chamomile: 19, 21, 43, 50, 65-67, 85, **125**, 145, 147, 148, 150-154, 156-158, 161-164, 179, 187, 205, 213-215, 217, 218, 223, 225, 236, 237, 239-241,

247, 248, 250, 266-268, 312-316, 326, 331, 412-414, 418-420, 432, 442, 453, 457, 464, 465, 483, 486, 487, 489, 490, 494, 495, 507, 509, 510, 517, 518, 522, 525, 528, 545-547, 549, 551, 553, 554, 560, 571, 574, 586, 591-596, 598, 610

Romans: **6**, 110, 129, 130

Rose: 3, 8, 15, 17-19, 43, 47, 50, 67, 78, **125**, 126, 146-154, 156-161, 164, 165, 191, 215, 218, 219, 227, 235, 236, 239, 240, 247, 250, 265, 266, 307, 309, 311-316, 329, 332, 373, 414, 431, 432, 434, 451, 452, 464, 467, 469, 488, 489, 511, 516, 519, 523, 531, 536, 538, 539, 545-555, 560, 565, 571, 572, 574-576, 578, 584-586, 588, 589, 591-596, 598, 610

Rose of Sharon: **78**, 126, 571, 574

Rose Ointment: 151, 156, **240**, 414, 432, 451, 452, 488, 489, 523, 536, 539, 545-551, 553, 554, 575, 576, 578, 584-586, 588, 589, 610

Rosemary: 8, 19, 20, 31, 32, 43, 49, 50, 67, 103, **126**, 127, 130, 147, 149, 154, 156, 157, 159, 163, 171, 174, 177-179, 183, 187, 191, 205, 218, 220-222, 227, 229, 231, 232, 234, 240-245, 248, 251-255, 265, 266, 268, 270, 272, 292, 313-316, 323, 326, 330, 331, 334, 342, 350, 351, 361, 362, 388, 407, 413, 414, 418, 422-424, 426, 428-432, 438, 440-446, 448, 449, 451-453, 455, 457, 460, 461, 470, 471, 474, 477, 479-487, 489, 491-494, 496-498, 500, 501, 503-507, 510, 511, 513-517, 519-521, 523-525, 530, 532, 533, 535, 539, 542-544, 548, 550-552, 558, 572, 574, 587, 590-595, 598, 610

Rosemary Vitality: **127**, 255, 413, 414, 422-424, 426, 428-432, 438, 440-444, 446, 448, 451-453, 455, 457, 460, 461, 471, 474, 479-481, 483-486, 489, 497, 500, 501, 503-507, 510, 511, 519-521, 523, 525, 530, 533, 535, 539, 543, 544, 572, 574, 587, 598, 610

Rosewood: 18, 43, 67, **127**, 164, 165, 214, 244, 431, 551, 571, 574, 587, 596

Royal Hawaiian Sandalwood: 67, **128**, 130, 143, 145, 146, 148-160, 164, 165, 204, 215, 217, 219, 224, 235, 237-240, **243**, 248, 250, 266, 270, 381, 414, 415, 418, 422, 424, 425, 429, 432, 437, 446, 448, 450, 451, 453, 455, 456, 458, 463-465, 470, 471, 474, 477, 478, 483, 484, 501, 516, 519-522, 531, 535, 536, 539-541, 545, 547, 549, 551-555, 560, 565, 566, 572, 574, 587, 591-596, 598, 610

Royal Hawaiian Sandalwood Soap: **243**

Russia: **82**

Ruta: 20, 43, 49, 67, **128**, 145, 147, 150, 160, 161, 164, 188, 250, 266, 310, 572, 574, 587, 591, 592, 595, 596, 598

RutaVaLa: 57, 144, **160**, 312, 313, 315, 316,

326, 333, 411, 412, 414, 415, 418, 422, 429-432, 434, 439, 445, 458, 464, 468, 470, 475, 486, 487, 489, 494, 516-522, 528, 532, 536, 548, 554, 555, 560, 565, 582, 587, 588, 595, 599, 610

RutaVaLa Roll-On: 144, **160**, 312, 313, 315, 316, 326, 414, 418, 422, 429-432, 434, 439, 445, 458, 464, 468, 470, 475, 486, 487, 489, 494, 516-522, 528, 536, 548, 554, 555, 560, 565, 582, 587, 588, 595, 599, 610

Sacred Frankincense: 32, 43, 57, 67, 128, 129, 145, 147, 150, 151, 153, 156, 157, 159, 161, 163, 164, 189, 214, 215, 223, 239, 250, 269, 307, 308, **310**, 312-316, 333, 334, 370, 371, 381, 386, 388, 412-415, 417-420, 422-425, 427-434, 437, 438, 447, 449, 450, 452-455, 457, 458, 461, 464, 465, 468·478, 481-485, 487, 489-493, 497, 498, 501, 503, 504, 506, 507, 514, 516, 518-521, 523-526, 528, 529, 531, 533, 535-538, 542, 544, 548-550, 552-555, 557, 560-562, 565, 571, 574, 587, 591-596, 598, 610

Sacred Mountain: 50, 57, 144, 151, **160**, 244, 271, 312-316, 332, 373, 412, 414, 422, 428, 433, 445, 452, 469, 472, 487, 489, 501, 503, 513, 525, 529, 531, 555, 565, 576, 581, 589, 595, 599, 610

Sacred Mountain Moisturizing Soap: **244**, 576, 581, 589, 610

Saddle Sores: **272**

Safe Use: **49-51**

Sage: 19, 21, 31, 32, 38, 43, 49, 50, 67, 79, 80, 84, 103, **129-131**, 148, 149, 152, 153, 155-158, 161, 164, 171, 173, 174, 179, 205, 212-215, 217, 222, 223, 225, 235, 266, 270, 278, 312, 315, 362, 412, 414, 415, 418, 422, 427, 435, 437, 457, 458, 463, 470, 471, 474, 483, 484, 506-511, 517, 519, 531-533, 537-539, 541, 554, 560, 572-574, 577, 578, 587, 592-598, 603, 610, 611

Sage Vitality: **130**, 412, 414, 415, 418, 427, 437, 457, 458, 463, 470, 471, 474, 483, 506-511, 519, 532, 533, 537, 538, 554, 560, 587, 598, 610

Sagging Skin: **552**

Sandalwood: v, 3, 4, 7, 18, 31, 33, 43, 50, 55, 67, 84, 93, 108, 128, **130**, 143, 145, 146, 148-160, 164, 165, 204, 205, 215, 217-219, 224, 235-241, 243, 248, 250, 266, 268, 270, 312, 313, 322, 332, 373, 381, 414, 415, 418, 422, 424, 425, 429, 432, 437, 446, 448, 450, 451, 453, 455, 456, 458, 463-465, 470, 471, 474, 477, 478, 483, 484, 501, 516, 519-522, 531, 535, 536, 539-541, 545, 547-549, 551-555, 560, 565-567, 572, 574, 575, 578, 580, 582, 584, 587, 589, 591-596, 598, 610

Sandalwood Moisture Cream: 55, **205**, **240**,

414, 547, 548, 551, 554, 575, 578, 580, 582, 584, 587, 589, 610

SARA: 144, **161**, **311**, 313, 315, 333, 373, 412, 415, 433, 576-578, 580-583, 585, 586, 588, 589, 595, 599, 610

Satin Facial Scrub Mint: **241**, 545, 547, 586, 587, 610

Saunas: **149**

Scabies: **552**

Scalp Problems: **483**

Scar Tissue: 93, 94, 97, 151, 240, 318, 382, **536**

Scarring: 104, 126, 140, 151, 275, 499, 546, 548, **549**

Schizophrenia: **523**

Schreuder, Marc: **368**, 370

Sciatica: 72, 99, 116, 139, 214, 283, 288, 289, 291, 304, **558**

SclarEssence: 144, **161**, **215**, 412, 413, 428, 455, 457, 458, 507-511, 537, 538, 577, 579, 586, 587, 595, 599, 610

SclarEssence Vitality: **161**, 412, 413, 428, 457, 458, 507-511, 537, 538, 595, 599

Scleroderma: 382, **455**, 456

Scoliosis: 5, 99, 113, 121, 291, 304, **559**

Scorpion Sting: **493**

Scours: 177, **272**

Screw Worm: **272**

Scurvy: 99, 105, **536**

Second-Degree Burns: **547**

Seed to Seal: i, **36**, 46-48, 370

Seizures: 393, 431, 449, **536**

Sensation: 26, 49, 54, 121, 144, 148, **161**, 190, **218**, **219**, 225, **226**, 239, 373, 411, 412, 414, 424, 454, 501, 522, 524, 538, 547, 553, 554, 558, 575, 577, 578, 580, 581, 589, 595, 599, 610

Sensation Bath & Shower Gel: **218**, 547, 575, 578, 580, 581, 589, 610

Sensation Hand & Body Lotion: **219**, 414, 575, 578, 580, 581, 589, 610

Sensation Massage Oil: **226**, 414, 424, 454, 501, 575, 577, 578, 580, 581, 589, 610

Sesquiterpenes: **18**

Sexual Dysfunction: **536**, 537

Sexually Transmitted Diseases: **539**, 540

Shampoo: 51, 55, **204**, **205**, **221**, 222, **247**, **265**, 268, **270**, 411, 483-485, 498, 553, 577-584, 586-589, 601, 603, 606, 607

Shave Cream: **236**, 576, 578, 581-585, 588, 589, 610

Shave Oil: **235**, 576, 578, 581-583, 585-587, 589, 608

Shaving: ii, 197, **235**, 273

Sheerlumé Brightening Cream: 55, **239**, 414, 554, 576, 577, 579-581, 587-589, 602

Shingles (Herpes Zoster): **541**

Shiny Coats: **268**

Shock: **316**, 355, 398, 433, 450, 474, **542**, 546, 547, 558

Shower: ii, **55**, 155, 205, 217, 218, 259, 359,

360, 411, 485, 498, 521, 547, 554, 575-589, 601-612

Shutran: 144, **161**, 163, **224**, 235, 236, 244, 312-316, 470, 474, 507, 522, 537, 545, 547, 576, 578, 581-585, 587-589, 595, 599, 610

Shutran Aftershave Lotion: **235**, 576, 578, 581-585, 589, 610

Shutran Bar Soap: **244**, 545, 547, 576, 578, 581-585, 587, 589, 610

Shutran Shave Cream: **236**, 576, 578, 581-585, 588, 589, 610

Singapore: **11**

Single Oils: ii, 50, 52, 53, 59, **65-142**, 143, 255, 293, 330, 374, 381, 386, 406, 407, 411, 445, 446, 451, 466, 478, 488, 498, 527, 540, 548, 558, 566, **575-589**, 597

Sinus: 72, 74, 80, 87, 89, 99, 106, 107, 112, 115, 116, 123, 133, 140, 147, 159, 227, **268**, 288, 289, 377, 452, 486, 487, 489, 523, 542, **543**

Sinus Congestion: **543**

Sinus Headache: **486**, 487

Sinus Infections: 87, 89, 99, 112, 115, 123, 452, 486, **542**, 543

Sinusitis / Rhinitis: **543**

Skin Cancer: 81, 196, **268**, **437**, 550

Skin Candida: **479**

Skin Care: ii, v, 20, 52, 87, 105, 108, 137, 217, 218, 220, 236, 238, **414**, 487, 547, 549, 550, 554

Skin Disorders and Problems: **544**

Skin Ulcers: **553**

Skin Warming: **291**

Sleep Disorders: **554**

SleepEssence: **188**, 418, 422, 476, 487, 495, 523, 528, 553-555, 582, 587-589, 610

SleepyIze: 144, **161**, **250**, 312-316, 415, 416, 418, 424, 425, 429-432, 451, 458, 469, 487, 575, 579, 580, 582, 586-588, 595, 610

Slique Bars: **188**, **203**, 341, 412, 413, 416, 442, 446, 448, 449, 458, 467, 468, 472, 474, 475, 525, 535, 577, 585, 588, 610

Slique Bars—Chocolate-Coated: **188**, **203**, 341, 458, 467, 468, 474, 525, 577, 585, 588, 610

Slique Bars—Tropical Berry Crunch: **188**, **203**

Slique CitraSlim: **188**, 412, 413, 416, 442, 446, 448, 449, 468, 472, 474, 475, 490, 525, 535, 576, 579, 581, 583, 585, 588, 610

Slique Essence: 144, **162**, 189, 231, 247, 255, 441, 442, 459, 468, 482, 485, 525-528, 580, 583, 585, 588, 595, 599, 611

Slique Gum: **189**, **234**, 468, 485, 525-528, 579, 586, 588, 611

Slique Shake: **189**, **203**, 331, 334, 335, 341, 406, 407, 409, 412, 413, 416, 418, 419, 421, 424, 425, 429, 442, 446, 448-450,

455, 467, 472, 474, 475, 490, 505, 511, 513-515, 520-523, 525, 527, 535, 536, 553, 556, 557, 559, 611

Slique Tea: 162, **189**, 416, 441, 442, 459, 463, 468, 585, 588, 611

Slique Toothpaste: 227, **231**, 247, 248, 485, 525-528, 543, 577, 579, 580, 583, 585, 587, 588, 606

Smoking Cessation: **554**

Snacks: **341**, 391, 397

Snake Bites: 3, **555**

SniffleEase: 144, **162**, **250**, 576, 578, 579, 582-586, 595

Snoring: **555**

Soaps: ii, v, 29, 30, 52, 107, 130, **241-245**, 251, 252, 347, 381, 407, 434, 545, 547, 549, 601-612

Solar Lentigines: **501**

Solvent Extraction: **4-5**, 25

Sore Feet: **478**

Sore Muscles: 88, 89, 145, **513**, 514

Sore Throat: 81, 191, 195, 234, 409, 476, 490, 531, **561**, 562

Sorrow: **163**, 315

Spa Foot Scrub: **245**

Spanish Sage: 21, 43, 67, **130**, 131, 152, 155-157, 161, 164, 215, 266, 572, 574, 587, 593-596, 598, 611

Spastic Colon Syndrome: **463**

Spearmint: 24, 43, 50, 67, **131**, 145-147, 149, 151, 152, 155, 158, 160-162, 164, 184, 185, 189, 192, 203, 205, 215, 221, 222, 224-226, 229, 231, 234, 239, 248, 250, 255, 265, 266, 313, 326, 337, 342, 385, 412, 413, 417, 421, 431, 448, 453, 462, 463, 465, 468, 469, 474, 479, 480, 482, 485, 486, 488, 494, 503, 515, 516, 534, 536, 565, 572, 574, 588, 591-596, 598, 611

Spearmint Vitality: **131**, 255, 412, 413, 417, 421, 431, 448, 453, 462, 463, 465, 468, 469, 474, 482, 485, 486, 503, 515, 516, 536, 565, 572, 574, 588, 592, 598, 611

Species: i, iii, **19-21**, 23, 31, 36, 37, 46, 71, 73, 76, 78, 82, 84, 88-90, 92, 96-102, 104, 117, 121, 123, 130, 131, 135, 138, 140, 142, 175, 184, 196, 243, 257-259, 266, 307, 337, 368-371, 385, 398, 423, 493, 506, 534, 567

Specific Gravity: **47**

Spider Veins: **447**

Spikenard: 8, 13-15, 67, **131**, 132, 387, 572, 574, 588

Spina Bifida: **555**

Spinal Tissue Pull: 296, **300**

Spine Injuries and Pain: **556**

Spiritual: iii, vii, 3, 5, 68, 71, 91, 93, 103, 114, 120, 129, 138, 141, 143, 150, 158, 160, 163, 165, 297, 305, **307-316**, 361, 371, 374, **376**, 405, 412

Splenda: 358, **392-393**

Sports Gel: **235**, 268, 269, 409, 412, 420, 422-424, 427, 428, 433, 442, 449, 454, 455, 457, 476-478, 483, 490, 496, 506, 512-514, 516-518, 521, 529, 556-560, 566, 576, 578, 580, 582, 584, 586, 587, 589, 603

Sprain: 455, 517, **559**

Stanford University: **378**

Stanley Burroughs: **285**, 324

Steam Distillation: 3, 7, 17, 36, **40-44**, 72, 101, 109

Stenosing Tenosynovitis: **566**

Stevia: 162, 169, 178, 183, 184, 187, 189-192, 203, 229, **231**, 234, 248, **396-397**, 458, 595, 611

Stings: **491**

Stomachache: 352, **464**

Stomach Cramps: **460**

Stomach Ulcers: 81, **464**

Storage: **49**, **65**, 207, 210, 319, 349, 388

Strangles: **272**

Strength-building Protocol: **334**

Strep Throat: 535, **562**

Stress: 4, 17, 19, 26, 27, 32, 69, 71, 73, 79, 85, 88, 93, 94, 98, 105, 109, 110, 112, 116, 119, 120, 123, 125, 127, 128, 132, 136-138, 141, 142, 144, 145, 151, 152, 158, 162-164, 171-173, 181, 188, 190, 198-200, 211, 213, 215, 217, 225, 226, 237, 269, 273, 276, 285, 292, 310, 312, **316**, 319, 321, 322, 325, 326, 333, 347, 361, 389, **414**, 418, 422, 430, 439, 445, 446, 448, 450, 457, 460, 464, 467-469, 476, 482, 485-487, 489, 495, 499-501, 503, 510, 517, 519, 522, 528, 532, 535-537, 545, 548, 554, 555, 557, **560**, 564, 576, 578, 582, 583, 585, 588, 595, 599, 611

Stress Away: 144, **162**, 217, 237, 312, 316, 326, 333, 414, 418, 422, 439, 445, 446, 467, 469, 476, 486, 487, 489, 495, 522, 528, 535, 536, 548, 554, 555, 557, 576, 578, 582, 583, 585, 588, 595, 599, 611

Stress Away Roll-On: 144, **162**, 316, 326, 414, 418, 422, 439, 445, 446, 467, 469, 476, 486, 487, 489, 495, 522, 528, 535, 536, 548, 554, 555, 557, 576, 578, 582, 583, 585, 588, 595, 599

Stretch Marks: 104, 108, 114, 115, 151, 248, 531, **553**

Strokes: 239, 261, 263, 273, 296, 299-301, 440, **446**, 447

Sucralose: **392-393**

Sugar: 85, 117, 119, 130, 171, 173, 176, 177, 180, 181, 188, 189, 191, 192, 194, 196-198, 201, 203, 204, 211, 222, 227, 229, 231, 234, 236, 318, 320, 321, 323, 325, 328-331, 335, 345-347, 350, 358, **391-393**, 395-397, 416, 420, 431, 435, 458, 462, 478, 480, 481, 485, 501, 510, 536, 545, 551, 564, 565

Suhail, Mahmoud: **32**, **368**, **370**

Sulfurzyme Capsules and Powder: **190**, **204**, 611

Sunburn: **546**

Super B: **190**, 326, 333, 334, 406, 407, 413, 414, 417-419, 422, 425, 427, 430, 432, 438, 441, 447, 449, 451, 454, 455, 458, 464, 470, 474, 475, 483, 489, 511, 512, 514, 516-523, 529, 530, 536-538, 553-556, 558-560, 584, 611

Super C: **190**, 191, 268, 332, 334-337, 384, 385, 387, 406, 407, 413, 421, 429, 437, 440, 442, 451, 452, 454, 455, 457, 464, 465, 469, 471, 472, 475, 476, 479, 482, 486, 487, 489, 490, 497, 502-504, 506-508, 511, 516-522, 525, 526, 529, 530, 534-536, 539, 542-544, 552, 553, 559-563, 565, 566, 580, 583, 585, 588, 611

Super C Chewable: **191**, 334, 335, 337, 385, 387, 413, 421, 429, 437, 440, 442, 451, 452, 454, 455, 465, 469, 471, 472, 475, 476, 479, 482, 486, 487, 489, 490, 497, 502-504, 506-508, 511, 517-522, 526, 529, 530, 534-536, 539, 542-544, 552, 553, 560-563, 565, 566, 585

SuperCal: **191**, 583, 584, 589, 611

Surrender: 144, **162**, 271, 312-316, 373, 412, 415, 418, 453, 466, 539, 554, 575, 576, 580, 582-584, 586, 595, 599, 611

Sweeteners: iv, 184, 189, 203, 234, 324, 329, 331, 335, **391-393**, 396, 397, 416, 425

Swelling: 54, 99, 158, 270-272, 419, 422, 423, **427**, 432, 445, 454, 455, 457, 465, 469, 482, 493, 496, 498, 511, 512, 517, 530, 532, 533, 558, 561

Switzerland: **10**, 379

Swollen Sheath: **272**

Sympathetic Nervous System: 78, **519**

Synthetic: ii, v, vii, 4, 20, **22-25**, **35**, 36, 44, 48, 51, 52, 65, 102, 105, 146, 174, 179, 205, 207, 208, 211, 217, 221, 229, 231, 232, 235, 236, 242, 247, 251, 258, 259, 265, 291, 335, 345, 357, 378, 381, 390-392, 396, 397, 407, 421, 425, 435, 508, 532, 554

Syphilis: 81, 541

T-Away: **266**, 268, 271, 575-583, 585-589, 611

Tachycardia: **446**

Tail & Mane Sheen: 268, **270**, 580-584, 587

Taiwan: **11**, **37**, 98, 101, 102, 140, 189, 200, 396

Tangerine: 18, 20, 41, 43, 49, 50, 67, **132**, 145-147, 149, 152-154, 157, 158, 160-162, 164, 171, 173, 180, 182, 184, 189-192, 202, 215, 217, 224-226, 231, 247-250, 255, 266, 313-315, 326, 329, 334, 412, 427, 431, 433, 445, 447, 448, 461, 465, 467, 469, 481, 487, 505, 509, 536, 552, 565, 571, 574, 580, 588, 591-596, 598, 611

Tangerine Vitality: **132**, 173, 255, 412, 427, 431, 445, 447, 448, 461, 465, 467, 469, 481, 487, 505, 509, 536, 565, 571, 574, 588, 598, 611

Tarragon: 19, 43, 50, 67, **133**, 148, 169, 171, 173, 174, 177, 185, 253, 265, 266, 330, 331, 350, 412, 415, 416, 419, 427, 437, 453, 459, 461, 463, 482, 488, 495, 510, 530, 532, 557, 558, 571, 574, 588, 592, 598, 611

Tarragon Vitality: **133**, 412, 415, 416, 419, 427, 437, 453, 459, 461, 463, 482, 488, 495, 510, 530, 571, 574, 588, 592, 598, 611

Tea Tree: 30-32, 43, 50, 56, 57, 109, 111, **133**, 134, 156, 158, 159, 185, 187, 220, 236, 240, 243, 245, 250, 253, 254, 265, 266, 268, 272, 273, 332, 334, 336, 381, 412, 413, 418, 422-424, 426, 432, 437, 441, 450-453, 457, 465, 471, 477, 479-481, 483-487, 489-494, 498, 502, 504, 507, 508, 511, 517, 524, 526, 528, 530, 531, 535, 539-546, 548, 550, 551, 554, 555, 560, 561, 563, 566, 567, 572, 574, 588, 594, 595, 598, 611

Techniques for Different Animal Species: iii, **259**

Techniques for Essential Oil Application: iii, 279, **281-296**, 298-304

Teeth Grinding: **528**

Teething: **528**

Temple of Edfu: **5**

Tender Tush: **248**, 432, 488, 489, 531, 536, 547-551, 553, 575, 577-580, 582, 586, 587, 589, 606

Tendonitis: 190, 204, 382, 383, 454, **455**, 517, 566

Tendons: 268, 278, 433, 454, **455**, 457, 476, 517, 566

Tension (Stress) Headache: **487**

Terpenes: 11, **17-19**, 25, 92, 100, 304, 362

Testimonials About Animals: iii, **275**

Testing: **47-48**

Testing Your pH: **323**

Texas: **31**, 111, 309

Texas Southern University: **31**

The Gift: 57, 144, 145, 151, **163**, 312, 314-316, 332-334, 381, 388, 412, 413, 415, 419, 421, 425, 432, 434, 453, 458, 464, 469, 470, 483, 485, 486, 489, 492, 493, 513, 524, 525, 531, 537, 538, 548, 555, 560, 565, 577, 579, 581, 584, 587, 595, 599, 611

Therapeutic: v, vii, 3, 4, 10, 11, 18, 20, 22, 23, 25, 29, 33, **35-37**, 40-44, 47, 49, 56, 57, 65, 102, 125, 163, 218, 225, 233, 242, 257, 290, 292, 310, 381, 383, 406, 411, 435, 527, 551, 567

Therapeutic-Grade: i, v, vii, 1, 4, 22, 23, **35-48**, 126, 129, 143, 165, 167, 179, 183, 189, 191, 214, 220-223, 225, 227, 229,

236, 238, 242, 243, 253, 257, 281, 282, 292, 323, 409, 556

Thieves: iii, 11, 50, 52, 56, 57, 80, 126, 144, 153, 159, **163**, 178, 191, 202, 222, 227, 229, 231, 232, 234, 244, 245, 247, 251-255, 267, 268, 270-272, 276, 333, 334, 373, 386, 388, 406, 407, 409, 412, 413, 416, 418, 420-422, 426, 437, 440, 448, 450-453, 455, 457, 459-462, 464-466, 471, 475-477, 479-483, 485-487, 489, 491-494, 497, 498, 502-505, 507, 508, 511, 525-531, 535, 536, 539-544, 546, 548-555, 560-563, 565, 566, 575, 577, 579, 580, 582-589, 595, 599, 611, 612

Thieves AromaBright Toothpaste: **229**, 412, 422, 485, 525-528, 543, 544, 577, 579, 583, 585-588, 611

Thieves Automatic Dishwasher Powder: **251**, 421, 422, 611

Thieves Cleansing Soap: **244**, 421, 422, 577, 579, 583, 587, 611

Thieves Cough Drops: **191**, **234**, 412, 422, 452, 465, 476, 485, 491, 502-504, 531, 560-563, 577, 579, 583, 587, 611

Thieves Dental Floss: **231**, 485, 526, 527, 577, 579, 583, 586, 587, 611

Thieves Dentarome Plus Toothpaste: **229**, 412, 422, 485, 525-528, 543, 544, 577, 579, 583, 586, 587, 589, 611

Thieves Dentarome Ultra Toothpaste: **229**, 412, 422, 485, 526-528, 543, 544, 577, 579, 583, 586-589, 611

Thieves Dish Soap: **252**, 421, 422, 575, 577, 579, 583, 587, 611

Thieves Foaming Hand Soap: **245**, **252**, 421, 422, 577, 579, 583, 585, 587, 611

Thieves Fresh Essence Plus Mouthwash: 227, **232-234**, 412, 422, 465, 466, 477, 479-481, 498, 502-504, 526-529, 542-544, 561, 577, 579, 583, 586-589, 611

Thieves Fruit & Veggie Soak: **253**, 421, 422, 575, 577, 579, 580, 582-588, 611

Thieves Fruit & Veggie Spray: **253**, 577, 579, 583, 587

Thieves Hard Lozenges: **191**, **234**, 412, 422, 452, 465, 476, 480, 485, 491, 502-504, 526, 527, 531, 543, 544, 560-563, 577, 579, 583, 586, 587, 611

Thieves Household Cleaner: 57, **253**, 272, 276, 421, 422, 494, 577, 579, 583, 587, 611

Thieves Laundry Soap: **253**, 421, 422, 575, 577, 579, 583, 587, 612

Thieves Mints: **191**, **234**, 476, 485, 491, 504, 526, 527, 531, 543, 544, 560-563, 577, 579, 583, 586, 587, 612

Thieves Spray: **253**, 255, 412, 421, 422, 448, 450-452, 457, 465, 466, 475, 477, 479, 480, 485, 502-504, 507, 526-528, 539-544, 548, 549, 551, 555, 560-563, 577, 579, 583, 587, 612

Thieves Vitality: 62, **163**, 272, 409, 412, 413, 416, 418, 421, 422, 426, 437, 448, 450-453, 459-462, 464, 465, 471, 476, 479-481, 483, 485, 487, 489, 491, 497, 502-505, 507, 508, 511, 525-528, 530, 535, 536, 539-541, 543, 544, 554, 560-563, 565, 566, 577, 579, 583, 588, 595, 599, 612

Thieves Waterless Hand Purifier: **222**, **253**, 421, 422, 577, 579, 583, 586, 587, 612

Thieves Wipes: **254**, 421, 422, 577, 579, 583, 587, 612

Third-Degree Burns: **547**

Three Mile Island: **336**, **384**

Throat: 6, 49, 68, 69, 80, 81, 99, 112, 115, 123, 124, 126, 137, 146, 147, 149, 151, 159, 191, 195, 234, 272, 303, 308, 332, 333, 345, 377, 378, 409, 442-446, 448, 452, 465, 466, 474, 476, 479, 480, 488-490, 493, 499, 500, 512, 531, 535, 541, 542, 544, **560-563**

Throat Infections and Problems: **560**

Thrombotic Strokes: **446**

Thrombus: **440**, 445

Thrush: **480**, 526

Thyme: 17, 20, 22, 31, 33, 43, 50, 52, 67, 103, **134**, 135, 155, 173, 178, 181, 185, 187, 225-228, 232, 255, 258, 261, 263, 272, 273, 276, 292, 293, 295, 296, 298, 300, 304, 312-315, 322, 332, 334, 342, 361-364, 377, 398, 407, 412, 413, 421, 422, 426-428, 432, 437, 438, 441, 445, 448, 451-453, 457, 461, 462, 465, 466, 471, 474, 476, 477, 479, 480, 482, 484, 489-494, 497, 498, 502-507, 511, 512, 518, 521, 524-527, 531-533, 535, 541-544, 546, 548, 550, 552, 555, 558, 559, 561-563, 566, 572, 574, 588, 593, 598, 612

Thyme Vitality: **135**, 255, 272, 412, 413, 421, 422, 426-428, 432, 437, 438, 441, 445, 448, 451-453, 457, 461, 462, 465, 471, 474, 476, 479, 480, 484, 489, 490, 497, 502-507, 511, 521, 525-527, 531-533, 535, 541, 544, 555, 559, 561-563, 566, 572, 574, 588, 593, 598, 612

Thyroid Problems: 115, 470, 494, 515, **563**

Thyromin: **191**, 192, 333, 335-337, 384, 385, 387, 406, 407, 413, 414, 417, 422, 428, 430-432, 448, 449, 451, 455, 458, 469-471, 475, 476, 484, 505, 509, 511, 515, 523, 525, 534, 537, 538, 554, 564, 565, 584, 586, 588, 612

Ticks: 265, 267, **268**, **492**

Tinnitus (Ringing in the Ears): **467**

Tisserand, Robert B.: **9**

To Disinfect: 126, 243, 270, 271, **548**

To Promote Healing: 264, 290, 292, **549**

To Reduce Bleeding: 267, **549**

To Reduce Scarring: **549**

Tonsillitis: 81, 109, **563**

Toothache and Teething Pain: **528**

Tooth Enamel: 227, **230**, 232, 366

Toothpaste: 51, **227-231**, 247, 248, 365, 366, 412, 422, 485, 525-528, 543, 544, 577, 579, 580, 583, 585-589, 606, 611

Topical Application: i, 4, 5, **53-55**, 209, 213, 407

Toxemia: **565**

Toxic Liver: iii, **320**, 435, **500**

Tranquil Roll-On: 144, **163**, 312, 314-316, 326, 414, 415, 418, 431, 432, 464, 469, 486, 487, 489, 495, 516, 520, 522, 528, 548, 554, 555, 560, 576, 582, 586, 596, 599, 612

Transformation: 128, 144, **163-164**, **215**, 312, 313, 315, 316, 333, 412, 434, 458, 484, 510, 511, 537, 555, 576, 577, 579, 581, 583, 585-587, 596, 599, 612

Trauma: 27, 68, 79, 83, 137, 144, 160, 161, 163, **164**, 194, 267, **268**, 271, 292, 309-312, 314-316, 332, 333, 373, 388, 406, 412, 414, 415, 433, 439, 453, 458, 464, 469, 474, 487, 494, 495, 514, 517, 536, 537, 542, 548, 553, 554, 560, 565, 576-580, 582, 586-588, 596, 599, 612

Trauma, Emotional: 27, 83, 137, **164**, 292, 309, 310, 469, 542, **565**

Trauma Life: 144, **164**, 267, 268, 271, 312, 314-316, 373, 412, 414, 415, 433, 439, 453, 458, 464, 469, 474, 487, 495, 536, 542, 548, 554, 560, 565, 576-580, 582, 586-588, 596, 599, 612

T.R. Care: 144, **164**, 312-316, 332, 333, 414, 415, 433, 439, 453, 458, 464, 469, 474, 487, 495, 536, 542, 548, 554, 560, 565, 575-589, 596, 599, 612

Trigger Finger (Stenosing Tenosynovitis): **566**

Truman, Karol K: **312**

Tsuga: 43, 50, 67, **135**, 313-315, 412, 437, 533, 572, 574, 588, 598, 612

Tuberculosis: 11, 30, 70, 81, 118, 121, 139, 159, 291, 304, 395, **503**

TummyGize: 144, **164**, **250**, 412, 413, 415, 417, 419-421, 426, 427, 434, 437, 438, 445, 447, 451, 453, 456, 459-464, 468, 471, 476, 482, 485, 488, 491, 495, 496, 511, 515, 516, 575, 576, 579, 580, 586, 588, 596, 612

Tumors: 209, 215, **268**, 275, 317, 434, **437**, 475, 518, 523

Typhoid Fever: 517, **566**

Ulcerative Colitis: 452, **453**, 456

Ultra Young: **192**, 413, 417, 422, 451, 469, 470, 474, 489, 509, 516-518, 535, 537, 553, 564, 565, 576, 580, 585, 588, 612

Umbilical Cords of Newborn Foals: **272**

United Kingdom: **11**, 363

University of Delaware: **31**

University of Minnesota: **378**

University of Nevada Las Vegas: **33**

University of Oklahoma: **31**, 369

Urinary Tract Infection: 90, 123, 133, **426**, 497

Usage: c, iv, v, vii, **49**, 65, 101, 117, 231, 233, 255, 304, 374, 380, 381, 386, 396, 399, 400, 402, 404-569, 601

USDA: **35**, 206, 389, 391, 392

Utah: vii, **10**, **11**, 18, 19, **23**, **44**, 47, 70, 79, 94, 98, 103, 105, 112, 125, 128, 131, 138, 154, 214, 227, 253, 254, 292, 321, 348, 398, 436, 499

Uterine Cancer: **437**

Uterine Cysts: **457**, 508

V-6 Vegetable Oil Complex: 49-54, 65, 67-80, 82-90, 92, 93, 95, 96, 98-101, 103, 105-113, 115-120, 122-124, 126, 128, 130-135, 138, 139, 141, 143-145, 147-156, 158-161, 163-165, 215, **226**, 258, 261, 263, 264, 268-270, 276, 291, 295, 332, 387, 406, 407, 409-411, 420, 423, 424, 428, 432, 438, 442, 450, 452, 453, 469, 473, 479, 481, 484, 497, 504, 514, 516, 526, 530, 532, 541, 542, 544, 545, 547, 552, 554, 612

Vaginal Yeast Infection: **480**, 481

Valerian: 19, 43, 50, 67, **135**, 136, 145, 150, 160, 161, 164, 188, 250, 266-268, 271, 315, 316, 326, 414, 418, 423, 424, 437, 443, 444, 453, 455, 464, 469, 486, 487, 489, 494, 495, 510, 518, 519, 522, 523, 528, 532, 539, 549, 554, 555, 557, 560, 572, 574, 588, 591, 592, 595, 596, 598, 612

Valnet, Jean: **9-10**, 25, 89, 93, 121, 227, 290, 406, 421

Valor: 144, 145, 151, **164**, 165, 244, 261, 263, 264, 268, 271, 273, 276, 293, 295-297, 303, 304, **310**, 312-316, 326, 332, 333, 373, 381, 411, 412, 414, 415, 419, 420, 422, 425, 429-434, 439, 440, 444, 445, 453, 458, 464, 467, 469, 470, 474, 475, 487, 494, 501, 504, 506, 516, 518, 519, 521-523, 525, 531, 532, 535-538, 542, 545, 546, 549, 553, 555, 556, 559, 560, 565, 575-581, 584, 587, 589, 596, 599, 612

Valor II: **165**, 261, 264, 293, 295-297, 303, 304, **310**, 312-316, 326, 333, 411, 412, 414, 415, 419, 420, 422, 425, 429-434, 439, 440, 444, 445, 453, 458, 464, 467, 469, 470, 474, 475, 487, 494, 501, 504, 506, 516, 518, 519, 521-523, 525, 531, 535-538, 542, 545, 546, 549, 553, 555, 556, 559, 560, 565, 575-581, 584, 589, 596, 612

Valor Moisturizing Soap: **244**, 576, 579, 587, 612

Valor Roll-On: 144, **165**, 312-316, 415, 419, 420, 422, 425, 429-432, 439, 440, 444, 445, 453, 458, 464, 467, 469, 470, 474, 475, 487, 494, 504, 506, 516, 518, 519, 521-523, 525, 531, 536-538, 542, 546,

556, 559, 560, 565, 576, 579, 587, 596, 599, 612

Vanilla: 67, **136**, 137, 145, 162, 169, 170, 176, 177, 183, 184, 187-189, 201, 203, 204, 221, 225, 237, 239, 341, 483, 485, 525, 572, 574, 578, 580, 582, 583, 585, 588, 591, 595, 603

Vaporizer: **57**

Varicose Veins: 97, 106, 121, 140, 141, **447**

Vascular Cleansing: 431, 432, **447**

Vegetarian: 169, 180, 185, 188, 195

Vertebrae: 145, **287**, 293, 300, 304, 431, 511, 555, 557, 559

Veterinary Medicine: iii, **257-258**, 436

Vetiver: 3, 4, 18, 19, 43, 50, 67, **137**, 145, 148-159, 163-165, 185, 188, 215, 224-226, 234, 235, 237, 239, 243, 250, 265, 267, 270, 315, 332, 414, 418, 423-425, 427-429, 431, 432, 453, 455, 469, 473, 477, 478, 482, 485, 489-491, 496, 510, 512-514, 516-519, 523, 528-530, 532, 545, 546, 549-553, 557, 558, 572, 574, 589, 591-596, 598, 612

Viaud, Henri: **10**

Viral Colitis: **453**

Vita Flex: iii, 4, 5, 53, 54, 68-83, 85-142, 146-150, 152-156, 158, 159, 161, 164, 165, 215, 263, 273, 279, 282, **285**, 286, 290, 295, 296, 298, 299, 301, 332, 407, 411, 415, 418, 420, 430, 432, 439-441, 443-448, 452, 453, 457, 459-461, 463, 464, 466-475, 479-482, 496-506, 510, 511, 523, 524, 529, 531-533, 537-544, 556-558, 561-563, 565

Vita Flex Foot Chart: **286**

Vita Flex Thumb Roll: **296**, 301

Vital Life Juice Recipe: **326**, 331

Vitality: iv, 11, **50**, 70, 71, 74-77, 80, 82, 86, 90, 91, 94-96, 102, 103, 105-108, 110, 114, 117-119, 122, 127, 130-133, 135, 143, 146, 147, 149, 151, 154, 155, 161, 163, 164, 170, 173, 178, 181, 183, 189, 201, 226, 255, 261, 268, 269, 271, 272, 281, 282, 285, 305, 317, 326, 334, 347, 355, **361-398**, 406, 409, 410, 412-434, 436-465, 467-476, 479-491, 494-511, 514-516, 519-523, 525-533, 535-541, 543, 544, 551, 554-566, 571-588, 591-593, 595, 597-599, 602-612

Vitassage: **281**

Vitex: **43**, **67**

Vitiligo: 93, **553**, 563

Warm Packs: **406**, 407

Water: iii, 4, 7, 8, 12, 14, 15, 25, 30, 37, 38, 40-44, 46, 47, 49-55, 57, 58, 74, 75, 81, 86, 102, 105, 106, 112, 120, 125, 129, 133, 139, 143, 155, 159, 162, 167, 169-172, 174, 177-179, 181-192, 194, 200, 204, 207, 213-215, 217-223, 225, 227, 229, 231-241, 243-245, 247, 248, 251-255, 259, 264, 265, 268-270, 272, 275,

276, 278, 293, 295, 303, 308, 317, 320, 323-328, 330, 331, 333-335, 338, 339, 341, 342, 345, 349-353, **355-360**, 362, 365-367, 374, 375, 377, 378, 383, 384, 386-388, 390, 398, 405-407, 409-411, 415-421, 423-427, 429-433, 438-454, 456, 458-466, 468-491, 493-512, 514-516, 519-531, 533, 535, 538-545, 547, 548, 552, 555, 556, 558-567

Water Distillers: **359**

Water Filtration: **359**

Waterless Hand Purifier: **222**, **253**, 421, 422, 577, 579, 583, 586, 587, 612

Weber State University: **11**, **163**, **227**, **229**, 253, 254, 292, 377

West Nile Virus: **493**

Western Red Cedar: 39, 43, 67, **137**, 138, 150, 247, 313-315, 414, 431, 437, 555, 565, 572, 574, 589, 592, 612

White Angelica: 50, 57, 144, **165**, 293, 295, 297, 298, 303, 308, **311**, 312, 314-316, 333, 373, 411, 412, 414, 415, 418, 419, 422, 433, 434, 464, 469, 525, 531, 532, 553, 554, 575, 576, 578, 580, 581, 584, 586, 587, 589, 596, 599, 612

White Fir: 43, 46, 67, **138**, 146, 150, 152, 153, 158, 164, 165, 220, 224, 571, 574, 589, 591-594, 596, 598, 612

White Light: 144, **165**, 312-316, 412, 414, 415, 418, 419, 422, 433, 434, 464, 469, 525, 531, 553, 596, 612

White Lotus: 43, 67, **138**, 139, 153, 158, 161, 572, 574, 589, 593-595, 612

Whooping Cough: **269**, **504**

Wintergreen: 4, 5, 19, 43, 50, 67, **139**, 148, 158, 159, 169-171, 191, 205, 214, 223-227, 229, 232, 235, 258, 261, 263, 267-270, 276, 293, 295, 296, 298, 301, 304, 412, 420, 422-424, 427, 428, 431, 433, 436, 438, 440, 444-446, 450, 452-456, 460, 463, 466, 469, 476-478, 485, 486, 490, 491, 495, 496, 502, 504, 506, 511-514, 517, 525-527, 529, 531-533, 548, 556-562, 564, 572, 574, 589, 592, 594, 595, 598, 612

Wipes: 219, **254**, 421, 422, 577, 579, 583, 587, 612

Wolfberry: ii, 59, 170, 176-178, 180, 182-184, 186, 189, 190, **192-206**, 213, 214, 218, 219, 221-224, 236, 237, 239-241, 243, 244, 249, 333, 334, 341, 351, 355, 383, 389, 397, 429, 434, 458, 467, 468, 472, 474, 497, 500, 525, 554, 575, 578-580, 582, 586, 589, 604, 612

Wolfberry Crisp: **176**, 192, 201, **204**, 341, 458, 467, 468, 474, 525, 604

Wolfberry Crisp Bars, Chocolate-Coated: 176, **192**, 201, **204**, 458, 467, 468, 474, 525, 604

Wolfberry Eye Cream: **205**, **241**, 554, 575, 578-580, 582, 586, 589, 612

World War II: **9**, 377, 379, 550

Worms: 74, 77, 78, 80, 90, 98, 121, 266, **268**, 461, **530**

Wounds: **268, 271-272**

Wrinkles: 74, 87, 93, 102, 105, 114, 115, 118, 120, 126, 128, 137, 151, 204, 212, 239, 383, 552, **553**

Xiang Mao: 43, 67, **140**, 157, 571, 574, 589, 594, 598, 612

Yacon: 51, 155, **192**, 324, 326, 331, 335, 338, 341, **397**, 410, 416, 425, 426, 458, 459, 507, 536, 540, 561, 612

Yarrow: 43, 46, 50, 67, **140**, 141, 148, 156, 213, 215, 223, 225, 315, 506, 507, 512, 513, 518, 532, 533, 536, 538, 571, 574, 589, 592, 594, 598, 612

Yeast: 31, 35, 48, 87, 100, 122, 169, 172, 178, 180, 181, 249, 321-323, 327, 348, 354, 377, 395, 404, **421**, **478**, **480**, 481, 485, **550**, 564, 565, 633

Yemen: **6**, 71, 369

Ylang Ylang: 17, 43, 50, 57, 67, 68, 136, **141**, 142, 145-147, 149-161, 164, 165, 174, 204, 205, 213, 215, 217-220, 223-226, 235-241, 243, 244, 247, 248, 250, 265, 266, 311-316, 412, 414, 415, 422, 434, 441, 443-446, 457, 483, 511, 519, 520, 531, 537, 538, 552, 555, 571, 573, 574, 589, 591-596, 598, 601, 612

Young: v, vii, 6, 7, **9-12**, 14, 15, **18-20**, 22-24, 27, 30, **32**, 33, 35-37, 40, 42, **44-48**, 68, 71, 86, 87, 92, 100, 128, 129, 136, 140, 145, 147, 151, 154, 167, 172, 183, 188-190, 192, 199, 200, 203, 206-208, 214, 215, 219, 221, 225, 235, 238, 239, 247, 248, 250, 258, 263, 265, 275, 278, 281, 282, 290, 292, 304, 307, 318, 321, 323, 324, 326, 328, 331, 333, 338, 342, 348-350, 363, 365-372, 377, 380, 386, 389, 398, 406, 409, 413, 417, 422, 436, 451, 469, 470, 474, 475, 489, 499, 509, 516-518, 535, 537, 553, 564, 565, 576, 580, 585, 588, 612

Young, D. Gary: vii, 6, 7, **9-11**, 30, **32**, 36, 44, 47, 86, 92, 128, 147, 167, 172, 183, 188, 203, 207, 214, 215, 281, 282, 290, 292, 304, 318, 326, 331, 338, 342, 348, 368, 369, 377, 386, 389

Young, Gary: vii, 6, 7, **9-11**, 30, **32**, 36, 37, 44, 47, 68, 86, 92, 128, 147, 167, 172, 183, 188, 203, 207, 214, 215, 281, 282, 290, 292, 304, 318, 326, 331, 338, 342, 348, 368-371, 377, 386, 389

Young Living: v, **10-11**, **18-20**, 22-24, 35-37, 40, 42, 44-48, 68, 71, 87, 100, 128, 129, 136, 145, 147, 167, 172, 189, 190, 199, 221, 235, 238, 239, 258, 265, 275, 278, 281, 333, 342, 350, 368-372, 377, 406, 409

Young Living Essential Oils: **10-11**, 22, 23, 36, **44**, 100, 136, 147, 172, 190, 199, 258, 275, 281, 368-370, 377

Yuzu: 43, 67, **142**, 184, 412, 414, 571, 574, 589, 598, 612